Gray's
Anatomy Review

Gray's Anatomy Review

THIRD EDITION

Marios Loukas, MD, PhD

Professor, Department of Anatomical Sciences
Dean of Basic Sciences; Dean of Research
St. George's University School of Medicine
Grenada, West Indies

R. Shane Tubbs, MS, PA-C, PhD

Professor
Departments of Neurosurgery, Neurology and Structural
and Cellular Biology
Tulane University School of Medicine, New Orleans,
Louisiana, United States
Department of Neurosurgery and Ochsner Neuroscience Institute, Ochsner Health System, New Orleans,
Louisiana, United States
Department of Anatomical Sciences
St. George's University
Grenada, West Indies

Peter H. Abrahams, MBBS, FRCS(ED), FRCR, DO(Hon), FHEA, FRSA

Peter Abrahams MBBS FRCS(ED) FRCR DO(Hon)
FHEA FRSA
Prof. "Emeritus" of Clinical Anatomy, Warwick Medical
School,
National Teaching fellow & Life Fellow, Girton College,
Cambridge
Visiting Prof. LKC School of Medicine NTU Singapore
Consultant Brunel Médical School

Stephen W. Carmichael, PhD, DSc

Professor Emeritus of Anatomy and Orthopedic Surgery
Mayo Clinic
Rochester, Minnesota, United States

Thomas Gest, PhD

Professor of Anatomy
University of Houston
College of Medicine
Houston, Texas, United States

For additional online content visit StudentConsult.com

ELSEVIER

London   New York   Oxford   Philadelphia   St Louis   Sydney   2022

First edition 2010
Second edition 2016

Notices

Practitioners and researchers must always rely on their own experience and knowledge in evaluating and using any information, methods, compounds or experiments described herein. Because of rapid advances in the medical sciences, in particular, independent verification of diagnoses and drug dosages should be made. To the fullest extent of the law, no responsibility is assumed by Elsevier, authors, editors or contributors for any injury and/or damage to persons or property as a matter of products liability, negligence or otherwise, or from any use or operation of any methods, products, instructions, or ideas contained in the material herein.

ISBN: 978-0-323-63916-3

Content Strategist: Jeremy Bowes
Content Development Specialist: Kim Benson
Project Manager: Andrew Riley
Design: Amy Buxton
Illustration Manager: Deanna Sorenson
Marketing Manager: Kathleen Patton

Printed in India

Last digit is the print number: 9 8 7 6 5 4 3

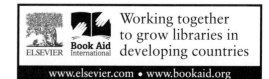

To my father Christos that gave me the foundations, love, empathy and care to become a physician, and more importantly the inspiration and continuous thirst to create knowledge and share it with the rest of the world. Love you Dad, I am thinking of you every day.

ML

To Ruth Jones. You are the best.

RST

To "Lucy in the Sky with Diamonds," and all the descendants of "Papi and Lulu"

PA

Susan Lee Stoddard, Allen St. P. Carmichael, and Magnolia Quinn Carmichael

SWC

To my family, for all of their support, and to my students, for all of their inspiration

TG

Preface

Rote memorization of anatomic facts has been the cardinal feature of exhaustive, and exhausting courses in human anatomy for many generations of students in medicine, dentistry, and other allied health science programs. Often, little distinction was made between the wheat and the chaff, and little attention was given to the practical, clinical application of the information. *Gray's Anatomy Review* was designed for use by students who wish to test their knowledge of clinical anatomy. The questions, answers, and explanations in this book are intended to serve multiple purposes for students in various programs.

1. This review provides a thought-provoking source for study by students in preparation for examinations in various programs of gross anatomy around the globe.
2. To avoid pointless memorization by the student, all the questions are framed within clinical vignettes that guide the student toward practical applications of the textual material.
3. The multiple-choice, single-best-answer format of the questions is designed to facilitate student review in preparation for the United States Medical Licensing Examination (USMLE) and similar qualifying examinations.
4. The explanations of the answers emphasize the critical importance of understanding normal and dysfunctional human anatomy.
5. Student understanding is further enhanced by critical examination of alternative, incorrect answers that students might be tempted to choose.

6. Finally, the review provides a succinct distillation of the plethora of facts in clinical anatomy, assisting the student's learning and understanding of important concepts in the practice of medicine, irrespective of the student's career choice. The majority of the questions in this review book are correlated with the following textbooks:
   - *Gray's Anatomy for Students*, ed 4, by Richard L. Drake, A. Wayne Vogl, and Adam W. M. Mitchell
   - *Netter Atlas of Human Anatomy*, ed 7, by Frank Netter
   - *Abrahams' and McMinn's Clinical Atlas of Human Anatomy*, ed 8, by Peter H. Abrahams, Jonathan D. Spratt, Marios Loukas, and Albert N. Van Schoor

Each answer is referenced to pages in Gray's *(GAS)*, Netter's *(N)* and Abrahams' and McMinn's *(ABR/McM)*.

For the embryology chapter we have correlated the clinical vignettes with *Before We Are Born: Essentials of Embryology and Birth Defects*, ed 9, by Keith L Moore, TVN Persaud, and Mark G. Torchia.

We have incorporated or adapted many drawings, full-color illustrations, and radiological images in an attempt to accelerate the learning process and to enhance understanding of both the anatomy and the clinical applications. The primary sources on which we have drawn for illustrative material are from *Abrahams'and McMinn's ed 8, "Clinical Atlas of Human Anatomy."*

Acknowledgments

A clinical review book is the work not only of the authors but also of numerous scientific and clinical friends and colleagues who have been so generous with their knowledge and given significant feedback and help. This book would not have been possible were it not for the contributions of the colleagues and friends listed below.

A very special group of medical students, members of the Student Clinical Research Society at the Department of Anatomical Sciences at St. George's University, helped enormously with the completion of this project through their comments and criticism of each chapter as part of the advisory board of this book.

Advisory Board (for the First and Second editions)

Nkosi Alvarez *(Neck)*
Meha Bhargava *(Pelvis and Perineum)*
Liann Chin Casey *(Lower Limb)*
Rana Chakrabarti *(Upper Limb)*
Ramya Chitters *(Embryology)*
Monica Dandapani *(Abdomen)*
Piyumika De Silva *(Upper Limb)*
Uta Guo *(Embryology)*
Rich Hajjar *(Abdomen)*
Roland Howard *(Lower Limb)*
Lijo C. Illipparambi *(Upper Limb)*
Theofannis Kollias *(Upper Limb)*
Jun Lee *(Back)*
Olivia Lu *(Lower Limb)*
Prateek Mathur *(Head)*
Spiro Mavromatis *(Neck)*
Lewis Musoke *(Lower Limb)*
Anastasiya Nelyubina *(Pelvis and Perineum)*
Georgia Paul *(Pelvis and Perineum)*
Tony Sadek *(Thorax)*
Shanojan Thiyagalingam *(Back)*
David Thornton *(Abdomen)*
Randy Tigue *(Head)*
Ryan Uyan *(Thorax)*
Lindsey Van Brunt *(Head and Neck)*
Danielle Van Patten *(Head and Neck)*

Advisory Board for the Third edition

Yusuf Alimi, MD
Cassandra Ang, MD

Tanya Cabrito, MD
Mark Carrasco, MD
Stacey Charles, MD
Vincent Courant, MD
Seif Eid, MD
Sasha Lake, MD
Sang Lee, MD
Gaurav Mandal, MD
Anniesha Noel, MD
Rabjot Rai, MD
Asad Rizvi, MD
Melissa Roberts, MD
Wallisa Roberts, MD., MBA
Sonja Salandy, MD
Tiwadayo Sam-Odusina, MD
Krishna Thakore, MD
Edidiong Udoyen, MD

The following faculty from the Department of Anatomical Sciences at St. George's University have also been very helpful with their comments and criticism as part of the advisory board:

Chrystal Antoine-Frank, MD
Emanuel Baidoo, MD
Kathleen Bubb, MD
Danny Burns, MD, PhD
James Coey, MBBS
Maira Du Plessis, MSc
Deon Forrester, MD
Iketchi Gbenimacho, MD
Rachael George, MD
Robert Hage, MD, PhD
Geobrina Hargrove, MD
Robert Jordan, PhD
Theofanis Kollias, MD
Ahmed Mahgoud, MD
Ewarld Marshall, MD, MSc
Michael Montalbano, MD
Olufemi Obadina, MBBS
Vid Persaud, MD, PhD
Madonna Petula Phillip, MD
Kazzara Raeburn, MD, MSc
Ramesh Rao, MD
Vish Rao, PhD
Deepak Sharma, MD
Feimatta Sowa, MD

Kristna Thompson, MD
Alena Wade, MD

Dr. Anthony D'Antoni, PhD, Professor, at Physician Assistant Program, Wagner College, One Campus Road, Staten Island, NY, has always been a great friend and colleague. His continuous support, comments, criticism, and enthusiasm have contributed enormously to the completion of this project.

Dr. Kitt Shaffer, MD, Ph.D. Professor of Radiology and Vice Chair of Department of Radiology at Boston University, for her comments and criticism, and invaluable expertise contributed toward this project.

We are especially thankful to Ms. Madelene Hyde, at Elsevier, for her invaluable insights, advice, and encouragement.

The authors would also like to thank Jeremy Bowes Kim Benson and Andrew Riley, our commissioning and developmental editors, and all the team at Elsevier for guiding us through the preparation of this book.

The authors thank the following individuals and their institutions for kindly supplying various clinical, operative, endoscopic, and imaging photographs:

Dr. Ray Armstrong, Rheumatologist, Southampton General Hospital, Southampton, and Arthritis Research Campaign

Professor Paul Boulos, Surgeon, Institute of Surgical Studies, University College London Medical School, London

Professor Norman Browse, Emeritus Professor of Surgery, and Hodder Arnold Publishers, for permission to use illustrations from *Symptoms and Signs of Surgical Disease,* 4th edition, 2005.

Mr. John Craven, formerly Consultant Surgeon, York District Hospital, York

Mr. John Craven, formerly Consultant Surgeon, York District Hospital, York

Professor Michael Hobsley, formerly Head of the Department of Surgical Studies, The Middlesex Hospital Medical School, London

Mr. Ralph Hutchings, photographer for Imagingbody.com

Mr. Umraz Khan, Plastic Surgeon, Charing Cross Hospital, London

Professor John Lumley, formerly Director, Vascular Surgery Unit, St. Bartholomew's and Great Ormond Street Hospitals, University of London

Dr. J. Spratt, Consultant Radiologist and Clinical Director of Radiology City Hospitals, Sunderland

Dr. William Torreggiani, Radiologist, The Adelaide and Meath Hospital, Tallaght, Dublin

Miss Gilli Vafidis, Ophthalmologist, formerly at Central Middlesex Hospital, London

Professor Jamie Weir, Emeritus Professor of Clinical Radiology, Grampian University Hospitals Trust, Aberdeen, Scotland, and editor of Weir and Abrahams *Imaging Atlas of Human Anatomy*, ed 5, Elsevier.

Contents

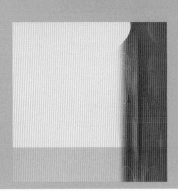

1

Back

Introduction

1. A 35-year-old man is admitted to the emergency department 30 minutes after being involved in a motor vehicle collision. Physical examination shows a damaged serratus anterior muscle. Which of the following nerves would be most likely to be injured along with injury to the serratus anterior muscle?
   A. Long thoracic
   B. Axillary
   C. Accessory
   D. Dorsal scapular
   E. Thoracodorsal

Explanation

A. The long thoracic is the only nerve that innervates the serratus anterior.
B. The axillary nerve innervates the deltoid and teres minor.
C. The accessory nerve innervates the sternocleidomastoid and trapezius.
D. The dorsal scapular nerve supplies the rhomboid muscles and the lower portion of the levator scapulae.
E. The thoracodorsal nerve innervates the latissimus dorsi.

2. A 35-year-old man is admitted to the emergency department 30 minutes after being involved in a motor vehicle collision. Physical examination shows a damaged serratus anterior muscle. Which of the following functions does the serratus anterior serve?
   A. Adducts scapula
   B. Depresses ribs
   C. Protraction and rotation of scapula
   D. Elevation of scapula
   E. Adducts, extends, and medially rotates arm

Explanation

A. The trapezius and rhomboid major and minor retract the scapula.
B. The serratus posterior inferior depresses the lower ribs.
C. The serratus anterior protracts and rotates the scapula upward.

D. The levator scapulae elevates the superior angle of the scapula, while trapezius elevates its lateral angle or the acromion.
E. The latissimus dorsi adducts, extends, and medially rotates the arm.

3. A 35-year-old man is admitted to the emergency department 30 minutes after being involved in a motor vehicle collision. Physical examination shows a damaged serratus anterior muscle. Which of the following functions will the patient most likely be unable to perform?
   A. Retraction of the scapula
   B. Elevation of the scapula
   C. Depression of the scapula
   D. Protraction of the scapula
   E. Downward rotation of the scapula

Explanation

Different muscles contribute to the movement of the scapula such as the serratus anterior, trapezius, levator scapulae, rhomboids, and pectoralis minor.
A. Retraction of the scapula is carried out by the rhomboids and trapezius.
B. Elevation of the scapula is carried out mainly by the trapezius and levator scapulae muscles.
C. Depression of the scapula is performed primarily by the lower fibers of the trapezius.
D. The serratus anterior muscle pulls the scapula forward (protraction) on the thoracic wall.
E. Upward rotation of the scapula is accomplished by the trapezius and serratus anterior together, while downward rotation of the scapula is performed by the rhomboid muscles and levator scapulae.

4. A 35-year-old man is admitted to the emergency department 30 minutes after being involved in a motor vehicle collision. Physical examination shows injury to the chest wall in the axillary region and winged scapula. Which of the following muscles is most likely injured?
   A. Levator scapulae
   B. Serratus anterior

C. Trapezius
D. Rhomboid major and minor
E. Serratus posterior superior

Explanation

A. The levator scapulae elevates the scapula.
B. The serratus anterior muscle pulls the scapula forward (protraction) and counterbalances the pull of the trapezius to keep the costal surface of the scapula closely opposed to the thoracic wall, preventing winging of the scapula.
C. Atrophy of the trapezius muscle may lead to scapular winging, but its nerve, the accessory, travels through the posterior triangle of the neck.
D. The rhomboid major and minor elevate and retract the scapula and their atrophy may lead to slight scapular winging, but their nerve, the dorsal scapular, travels through the neck.
E. The serratus posterior superior elevates the 2nd through 5th ribs.

Second Order Question

5. A 35-year-old man is admitted to the emergency department 30 minutes after being involved in a motor vehicle collision. Physical examination shows injury to the chest wall in the axillary region and winged scapula. Which of the following nerves is most likely injured?
A. Long thoracic
B. Axillary
C. Accessory
D. Dorsal scapular
E. Thoracodorsal

Explanation

A. The long thoracic nerve innervates the serratus anterior muscle, which protracts and upwardly rotates the scapula. Patients with injury to this nerve will have their scapulae protrude on their back like a wing.
B. The axillary nerve supplies the deltoid and teres minor muscles. The deltoid abducts, flexes, and extends the arm while the teres minor laterally rotates the arm.
C. The accessory nerve is responsible for supplying the trapezius and sternocleidomastoid muscles, and it travels through the posterior cervical triangle, not the axilla. The trapezius elevates and upwardly rotates the scapula while the sternocleidomastoid flexes and pulls the chin upward to the opposite side. The balance of pull between trapezius and serratus anterior prevents scapular winging.
D. The dorsal scapular nerve travels through the root of the neck to supply the rhomboid major and minor muscles which are responsible for retraction of the scapula and help to prevent scapular winging.
E. The thoracodorsal nerve supplies the latissimus dorsi muscle, which adducts, medially rotates, and extends the arm.

Third Order Question

6. A 35-year-old man is admitted to the emergency department 30 minutes after being involved in a motor vehicle collision.

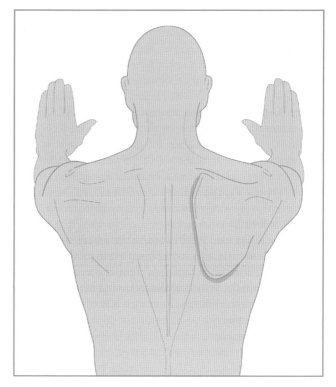

• **Fig. 1.1**

Physical examination shows the findings in Fig. 1.1. Which of the following nerves is most likely injured?
A. Long thoracic
B. Axillary
C. Accessory
D. Dorsal scapular
E. Thoracodorsal

Explanation

A. The long thoracic nerve innervates the serratus anterior muscle, which protracts the scapula, holds the scapula close to the thoracic wall preventing it from "winging," and abducts and upwardly rotates the scapula. Patients with injury to this nerve will have their scapula protruding on their back like a wing.
B. The axillary nerve supplies the deltoid and teres minor muscles. The deltoid abducts, flexes, and extends and the teres minor laterally rotates the arm.
C. The accessory nerve is responsible for supplying the trapezius and sternocleidomastoid muscles. The trapezius elevates and upwardly rotates the scapula while the sternocleidomastoid flexes and pulls the chin upward to the opposite side. While atrophy of the trapezius may result in scapular winging, lesion of the long thoracic nerve is more commonly the cause of winged scapula.
D. The dorsal scapular nerve supplies the rhomboid major and minor muscles and are responsible for retraction of the scapula. Atrophy of the rhomboid muscles may result in slight scapular winging.
E. The thoracodorsal nerve supplies the latissimus dorsi muscle, which adducts, medially rotates, and extends the arm.

Fourth Order Question

7. A 35-year-old man is admitted to the emergency department 30 minutes after being involved in a motor vehicle collision. Physical examination shows the findings in Fig. 1.1. Which of the following functions will the patient most likely be unable to perform during physical examination?
   A. Lateral rotation of the arm
   B. Abduction of the arm from 0 to 15 degrees
   C. Flexion of the arm
   D. Extension of the arm
   E. Abduction of the arm above 90 degrees

Explanation

A. Performed by the infraspinatus, teres minor, and posterior fibers of deltoid muscle.

B. Performed by the supraspinatus muscle.
C. Performed by the anterior deltoid fibers, pectoralis major, biceps brachii and coracobrachialis muscles.
D. Performed by the posterior deltoid fibers, latissimus dorsi, and teres major muscles.
E. In this image, the patient has a winged scapula. This usually occurs as a result of damage to the long thoracic nerve, which innervates the serratus anterior muscle. The functions of this muscle are protraction of the scapula and superior rotation of the glenoid fossa. Elevating the arm further than 90 degrees requires upward rotation of the scapula (superior rotation of the glenoid fossa) that is normally done by the serratus anterior and trapezius, working together.

Main Questions

Questions 1–25

1. A 55-year-old man is brought to the emergency department because of a 5-day history of severe cough, night sweats, and hemoptysis. A chest x-ray shows tuberculosis of the right lung, with extension into the thoracic vertebral bodies of T6 and T7, producing a "gibbus deformity." Which of the following conditions is most likely to be confirmed by radiologic examination?
   A. Hyperlordosis
   B. Hyperkyphosis
   C. Scoliosis
   D. Spina bifida
   E. Osteoarthritis

2. A 68-year-old man is brought to the hospital due to severe back pain. The patient says the pain began insidiously 4 months ago. He has no history of recent trauma or strenuous activities. Physical examination shows muscular strength of 5/5 and sensory findings within normal limits. An x-ray of the spine shows severe osteoporosis of the vertebral column, with compression fractures to vertebrae L4 and L5. Which of the following parts of the vertebrae are most likely fractured in this patient?
   A. Spinous process
   B. Vertebral bodies
   C. Transverse process
   D. Superior articular processes
   E. Intervertebral disc

3. A 45-year-old man is brought to the hospital because of 2-week history of severe pain in the back and lower limb. Physical examination shows slight bilateral loss of sensation of the skin over the lower limbs. An x-ray of the spine shows spinal canal stenosis in the lumbar region. Which of the following conditions is most likely to be confirmed by a magnetic resonance imaging (MRI) examination?

A. Hypertrophy of supraspinous ligament
B. Hypertrophy of interspinous ligament
C. Hypertrophy of ligamentum flavum
D. Hypertrophy of anterior longitudinal ligament
E. Hypertrophy of nuchal ligament

4. A 35-year-old man is brought to the emergency department after being involved in a motor vehicle collision. Physical examination shows the scapula retracted laterally on the affected side. An x-ray of the neck shows an injury to the dorsal surface of the neck and a fracture of the medial border of the right scapula. Which of the following nerves is most likely injured on that side?
   A. Axillary
   B. Long thoracic
   C. Dorsal scapular
   D. Greater occipital
   E. Suprascapular

5. A 64-year-old man is brought to the emergency department because of a 4-day history of painful rash and skin eruptions that are localized entirely on one side of his body, closely following the dermatome level of the spinal nerve C7. The patient was diagnosed with a herpes zoster viral infection known as "shingles." In which of the following structures has the virus most likely proliferated to cause the patient's current condition?
   A. The sympathetic trunk
   B. The dorsal root ganglion of the C7 spinal nerve
   C. The lateral horn of the C7 spinal cord segment
   D. The posterior cutaneous branch of the dorsal ramus of C7
   E. The ventral horn of the C7 spinal cord segment

6. A 45-year-old woman comes to the physician because she has experienced moderate pain for 2 years over her left lower back. The pain radiates to her left lower limb and has become a nuisance more recently. She says that after lifting a case of soft drinks, the pain suddenly became intense. An MRI of the lumbar region

shows an intervertebral disc herniation between vertebral levels L4 and L5. Which of the following nerves is most likely affected by the disc herniation?

A. L1
B. L2
C. L3
D. L4
E. L5

7. A 3-year-old boy is brought by his mother to the emergency department with severe headache, high fever, lethargy, malaise, and confusion. He has a history of multiple middle ear infections. His temperature is 40.1°C (104.2°F). A diagnosis of bacterial meningitis is suspected. Further evaluation with a lumbar puncture and laboratory analysis of the cerebrospinal fluid confirms the diagnosis. Which of the following vertebral levels is the most appropriate location for the lumbar puncture?

A. T12–L1
B. L1–L2
C. L2–L3
D. L4–L5
E. L5–S1

8. A 3-year-old boy is brought by his mother to the emergency department with severe headache, high fever, lethargy, malaise, and confusion. He has a history of multiple middle ear infections. His temperature is 40.1°C (104.2°F). A diagnosis of bacterial meningitis is suspected. Further evaluation with a lumbar puncture and laboratory analysis of the cerebrospinal fluid confirms the diagnosis. Which of the following external landmarks is the most reliable to determine the position of the L4 vertebral spine?

A. The inferior angles of the scapulae
B. The highest points of the iliac crests
C. The lowest pair of ribs bilaterally
D. The sacral hiatus
E. The posterior inferior iliac spines

9. A 39-year-old man is brought to the emergency department with severe neck pain after a whiplash injury, sustained when his car was struck from behind. He was placed in a cervical collar and anesthetic injection (Lidocaine) was administered. Imaging studies show trauma to the ligament lying on the anterior surface of the cervical vertebral bodies. Which of the following ligament is most likely disrupted?

A. Anterior longitudinal ligament
B. Ligamentum flavum
C. Nuchal ligament
D. Posterior longitudinal ligament
E. Transverse cervical ligament

10. A 65-year-old man is brought to the emergency department because of severe back pain and the weakness in lower limb motions, especially pointing his left toes. Physical examination shows weakness in standing on tiptoes on his left leg. Right lower limb shows

no motor strength deficits. The patient has numbness on the lateral side of the left limb and foot. Sensation is intact on the right. An MRI of his spine shows compression of nerve elements at the intervertebral foramen between vertebrae L5 and S1. Which of the following structures is most likely responsible for this space-occupying lesion?

A. Annulus fibrosus
B. Nucleus pulposus
C. Posterior longitudinal ligament
D. Anterior longitudinal ligament
E. Ligamentum flavum

11. A 27-year-old man is brought to the emergency department after being involved in a motor vehicle collision. His vital signs are within normal limits. Physical examination shows weakness during medial rotation, extension, and adduction of the humerus. His radial pulses are symmetrical and normal. Which of the following nerves is most likely injured?

A. Thoracodorsal
B. Axillary
C. Dorsal scapular
D. Accessory
E. Radial

12. A 39-year-old woman comes to the physician because of 2-month history of inability to reach the top of her head to brush her hair with her right hand. Two months ago, she had a mastectomy procedure with axillary lymph node dissection of her right breast. Physical examination shows winging of her right scapula and a normal left scapula. Which of the following nerves is most likely damaged during surgery?

A. Axillary
B. Accessory
C. Long thoracic
D. Dorsal scapular
E. Thoracodorsal

13. A 19-year-old man is brought to the emergency department after dislocating his shoulder when he was hit by the top of a helmet during an offensive play by the opposing team while playing football. Following treatment of the dislocation, he cannot initiate abduction of his arm. An MRI of the affected shoulder shows a torn muscle. Which of the following muscles is most likely damaged by the injury?

A. Coracobrachialis
B. Long head of the triceps brachii
C. Pectoralis minor
D. Supraspinatus
E. Teres major

14. A 1-year-old girl is brought to the physician by her mother for a routine examination. The mother says she did not always take her prenatal vitamins as she was advised to. Physical examination shows a dimpling of the skin in the midline of the lumbar region

with a tuft of hair growing over the dimple. Which of the following is the most likely diagnosis?

A. Meningomyelocele
B. Meningocele
C. Spina bifida occulta
D. Spina bifida cystica
E. Rachischisis

15. A 26-year-old woman comes to the physician because of an itch on her back that appears to be caused by an insect bite. Five days ago, she returned from a vacation in Latin America where she hiked in a rainforest. Which of the following nerve fibers carry the sensation of a mosquito bite on the back, just lateral to the spinous process of the T4 vertebra?

A. Somatic afferent
B. Somatic efferent
C. Visceral afferent
D. Visceral efferent
E. Somatic efferent and visceral afferent

16. A 15-year-old girl is brought to the emergency department because of 3-day history of progressive fever, headache, and lethargy. The patient's parents are against vaccinations and say their daughter is not up to date on all vaccinations. She has no history of major illnesses and is not taking any known medications. Her temperature is 40.3°C (104.5°F), blood pressure is 101/64 mm Hg, pulse is 110/min, and respirations are 25/min. A diagnosis of meningitis is suspected. To obtain a sample of cerebrospinal fluid by spinal tap in the lumbar region, the tip of the needle must be placed in which of the following locations?

A. In the epidural space
B. Between anterior and posterior longitudinal ligaments
C. Superficial to the ligamentum flavum
D. Between arachnoid mater and dura mater
E. In the subarachnoid space

17. A 59-year-old man comes to the physician because of severe back pain after lifting heavy luggage. The patient describes the pain in his neck as an electric-like shooting pain. He has no loss of motor function or sensation. Physical examination shows no neurologic abnormalities or injury to the spinal cord. An MRI of the cervical spine shows a herniated disc. Which of the following ligaments is in an anatomic position to protect the spinal cord from direct compression in this patient?

A. Supraspinous
B. Posterior longitudinal
C. Anterior longitudinal
D. Ligamentum flavum
E. Nuchal ligament

18. A 15-year-old girl is brought to the emergency department because of 3-day history of progressive fever, headache, and lethargy. The patient's parents are against vaccinations and say their daughter is not up to date on all vaccinations. She has no history of

major illnesses and is not taking any known medications. Her temperature is 40.3°C (104.5°F), blood pressure is 101/64 mm Hg, pulse is 110/min, and respirations are 25/min. A diagnosis of meningitis is suspected and a lumbar puncture is ordered. In lumbar puncture, the needle is often inserted between the spinous processes of the L4 and L5 vertebrae to ensure that the spinal cord is not injured. This level is safe because in the adult the spinal cord usually terminates at the disc between which of the following vertebral levels?

A. T11 and T12
B. T12 and L1
C. L1 and L2
D. L2 and L3
E. L3 and L4

19. A 45-year-old woman comes to the physician because of a 6-year history of discoloration of her fingers and toes in low temperatures due to chronic vasospasm. She was diagnosed with scleroderma and Raynaud disease at the age of 39. Relief from the symptoms in the hands would require surgical division of which of the following neural elements?

A. Lower cervical and upper thoracic sympathetic fibers
B. Lower cervical and upper thoracic ventral roots
C. Lower cervical and upper thoracic dorsal roots
D. Lower cervical and upper thoracic spinal nerves
E. Bilateral accessory nerves

20. A 69-year-old woman comes to the physician because of neck pain that has been progressively getting worse for the past few weeks. Her temperature is 37°C (98.6°F), blood pressure is 126/84 mm Hg, pulse is 92/min, and respirations are 21/min. An MRI of the spine shows osteophytes in the intervertebral foramen between vertebrae C2 and C3. Which of the following muscles will most likely be affected by this condition?

A. Rhomboid major
B. Serratus anterior
C. Supraspinatus
D. Diaphragm
E. Latissimus dorsi

21. A 42-year-old woman comes to the physician with lower back pain that has been progressively getting worse for the past 2 months. Her pain is worse when walking down hill and is alleviated when she bends over. Physical examination shows normal reflexes and sensation bilaterally in the upper and lower limbs. An MRI shows stenosis of the lumbar vertebral canal. A laminectomy of two vertebrae is performed. Which of the following ligaments will most likely also be removed?

A. Anterior longitudinal
B. Denticulate
C. Ligamentum flavum
D. Nuchal
E. Cruciform

22. A 28-year-old primigravida woman at 40 weeks' gestation is admitted to the hospital for delivery. Her vital signs are within normal limits. A tocometer and fetal heart rate monitor are placed on her abdomen. In the final stages of labor, a caudal anesthetic is administered via the sacral hiatus. Into which of the following spaces in the sacral canal is the anesthetic most likely placed?
    A. Vertebral canal
    B. Vertebral venous plexus
    C. Epidural space
    D. Subarachnoid space
    E. Subdural space

23. A 12-year-old boy was brought to the emergency department by his parents because of high fever and severe stiffness in his back. His initial temperature is 38.8°C (101.8°F), respirations are 19/min, pulse is 94/min, and blood pressure is 141/91 mm Hg. A diagnosis of meningitis is suspected, and a lumbar puncture is ordered. Microscopic examination of the cerebrospinal fluid shows hematopoietic cells. Which of the following ligaments is most likely penetrated by the needle?
    A. Supraspinous
    B. Denticulate
    C. Anterior longitudinal
    D. Posterior longitudinal
    E. Nuchal

24. A 25-year-old man is admitted to the hospital 30 minutes after being involved in a motor vehicle collision. Physical examination shows a sluggish response to stimuli. Neurologic examination shows no other abnormalities. An MRI shows damage to the tip of the transverse process of the third cervical vertebra, with a significantly large pulsating hematoma. Which of the following arteries is most likely damaged?
    A. Anterior spinal
    B. Vertebral
    C. Ascending cervical
    D. Deep cervical
    E. Posterior spinal

25. A 79-year-old man comes to the physician because of 3-month history of increasingly painful ambulation. Physical examination shows an abnormally increased posterior convexity to the thoracic curvature resulting from osteoporosis. Which of the following is the most likely condition of this patient's spine?
    A. Scoliosis
    B. Hyperkyphosis
    C. Spinal stenosis
    D. Lordosis
    E. Herniated disc

Questions 26–50

26. A 42-year-old woman is brought to the emergency department because of an injury sustained after sliding into second base headfirst during her company's softball game 2 hours ago. She has severe pain and stiffness in her neck. Her vital signs are within normal limits. Physical examination shows drooping of her right shoulder and difficulty in elevating that shoulder. An x-ray of the spine shows no fractures and an MRI shows soft tissue damage. Which of the following nerves is most likely damaged in this patient?
    A. Thoracodorsal
    B. Accessory
    C. Dorsal scapular
    D. Greater occipital
    E. Axillary

27. A 53-year-old man is admitted to the hospital 50 minutes after being involved in a motor vehicle collision. Physical examination shows sluggish response to stimuli. An x-ray of the lower limb shows a left femoral fracture and a cervical open-mouth x-ray shows compression of the spinal cord by the odontoid process. An MRI of the pelvis shows urethral injury and hematoma. Which of the following ligaments is most likely torn?
    A. Anterior longitudinal ligament
    B. Transverse ligament of the atlas
    C. Ligamentum flavum
    D. Supraspinous ligament
    E. Nuchal ligament

28. An 18-year-old woman is brought to the emergency department after being injured in a rollover motor vehicle. Physical examination shows multiple maxillofacial lacerations and considerable weakness in her ability to flex her neck, associated with injury to CN XI. Which of the following muscles is most likely affected?
    A. Iliocostalis thoracis
    B. Sternocleidomastoid
    C. Rhomboid major
    D. Rhomboid minor
    E. Teres major

29. A 23-year-old man was killed in a high-speed motor vehicle collision after racing his friend on a local highway. When the medical examiner arrives at the scene, it is determined that the most likely cause of death was a spinal cord injury. Upon confirmation by autopsy, the medical examiner officially reports that the patient's cause of death was a fracture of the pedicles of the axis (C2). Rupture of which of the following ligaments would be most likely implicated in this fatal injury?
    A. Ligamentum flavum
    B. Nuchal ligament
    C. Cruciform ligament
    D. Posterior longitudinal ligament
    E. Supraspinous ligament

30. A 65-year-old man is injured when a vehicle traveling at a high rate of speed hits his car from behind. He is brought to the emergency department where he is stabilized, and an x-ray of the spine shows that two

of his articular processes are now locked together, a condition known as "jumped facets." Surgical repair is scheduled the same day. In which of the following regions of the spine has this injury most likely occurred?

A. Cervical
B. Thoracic
C. Lumbar
D. Lumbosacral
E. Sacral

31. A 47-year-old woman is brought to the emergency department after being involved in a motor vehicle collision 40 minutes ago. She has severe headache and back pain. Her blood pressure is 99/78 mm Hg, pulse is 122/min, and respirations are 32/min. An MRI of the spine shows a large hematoma from bleeding from the internal vertebral venous plexus (of Batson). In which of the following space is the blood most likely accumulating?

A. Subarachnoid space
B. Subdural space
C. Central canal
D. Epidural space
E. Lumbar cistern

32. A 32-year-old man is brought to the emergency department because of 3-hour history of severe pain radiating to the posterior aspect of his right thigh and leg. He has been an elite athlete and he was lifting heavy weights during an intense training session when the pain appeared. His vitals are within normal limits. Physical exam shows no motor weakness or sensory loss in his lower limbs. Reflexes are fully intact bilaterally in upper and lower limbs. MRI of the lumbar spine shows a ruptured L4–L5 intervertebral disc. Which of the following nerves is most likely affected?

A. L3
B. L4
C. L2
D. L5
E. S1

33. A 24-year-old is brought to the emergency department because of a lower back strain after a severe fall while skiing. The patient was not wearing a helmet and lost consciousness for an unknown amount of time. Physical examination shows pain when the patient is laterally bending the trunk. An MRI of the lower thoracic spine shows injury to the muscles responsible for extending and laterally bending the trunk. Which of the following arteries provide blood supply to these muscles?

A. Subscapular
B. Thoracodorsal
C. Anterior intercostal
D. Suprascapular
E. Posterior intercostal

34. A 22-year-old man is brought to the emergency department unconscious following a head-to-head collision with another player while playing football. An x-ray of the head and neck shows slight dislocation of the atlantoaxial joint. Physical examination shows decreased range of motion at that joint. He has no loss of sensation or motor strength in his upper or lower limbs. Which of the following movements of the head would most likely be severely affected?

A. Rotation
B. Flexion
C. Abduction
D. Extension
E. Adduction

35. A 42-year-old man is brought to the emergency department because of 2-hour history of having been struck in the back with an unknown object during an aggravated robbery. An MRI of the spine shows ruptures of the internal vertebral venous plexus (of Batson) leading to a hematoma causing compression of the spinal cord. When aspiration of the excess blood is performed, the needle should stop just before puncturing which of the following structures?

A. Spinal cord
B. Pia mater
C. Arachnoid mater
D. Dura mater
E. Ligamentum flavum

36. A 65-year-old man is brought to the emergency department after being hit by a car in a busy intersection. The patient's current medications include warfarin, metoprolol, metformin, and aspirin (325mg mg). His pulse is 112/min, respirations are 24/min and shallow, and blood pressure is 112/72 mm Hg. An MRI shows dislocation of the fourth thoracic vertebra. Which of the following costal structures is most likely to be involved in the injury?

A. Head of the fourth rib
B. Neck of the fourth rib
C. Head of the third rib
D. Tubercle of the third rib
E. Head of the fifth rib

37. A 20-year-old hiker is brought to the emergency department 45 minutes after he sustained a deep puncture wound to his back during a fall. Physical examination shows a lesion between the trapezius and latissimus dorsi muscles on the right lateral side of his back. Physical examination shows weak adduction and medial rotation of his arm. Which of the following muscles is most likely injured?

A. Teres minor
B. Triceps brachii
C. Supraspinatus
D. Infraspinatus
E. Teres major

38. A 22-year-old man is brought to the emergency department after he was thrown through a plate glass wall in a fight 2 hours ago. An x-ray of the thorax shows that the lateral border of his right scapula is

shattered. Physical examination shows difficulty rotating his arm laterally. He has no loss of sensation in his right upper limb. Which of the following muscles is most likely injured?

A. Teres major
B. Infraspinatus
C. Latissimus dorsi
D. Trapezius
E. Supraspinatus

39. A 20-year-old woman comes to the emergency department with a 6-day history of headache, photophobia, and stiffness of her back. She recently moved into a dormitory on campus where she lives with one other roommate, who has not been sick. She is not up to date on her vaccinations. Physical examination shows positive signs for meningitis and a lumbar puncture is performed to determine if a pathogen is in the cerebrospinal fluid. What is the last structure the needle will penetrate before reaching the lumbar cistern?

A. Arachnoid mater
B. Dura mater
C. Pia mater
D. Ligamentum flavum
E. Posterior longitudinal ligament

40. A 19-year-old man is brought to the emergency department with high fever, severe headache, nausea, and stiff neck that have persisted for 3 days. Physical examination shows there is a purpuric rash on his trunk and extremities. A diagnosis of meningitis is suspected and a sample of cerebrospinal fluid using a lumbar puncture is obtained. From which of the following spaces was the cerebrospinal fluid collected?

A. Epidural
B. Subdural
C. Subarachnoid
D. Pretracheal
E. Central canal of the spinal cord

41. A 38-year-old man is admitted to the emergency department after sustaining injuries from a motor vehicle collision. Physical examination shows several lacerations and ecchymosis over his back. Pain from lacerations or irritations of the skin of the back is conveyed to the central nervous system (CNS) by which of the following?

A. Dorsal rami
B. Communicating rami
C. Ventral rami
D. Ventral roots
E. Intercostal nerves

42. A 66-year-old woman comes to the physician because she had been diagnosed recently with a tumor on her spine. She has started to retain urine and is experiencing rectal incontinence. Ultrasound of the bladder shows no physical obstructions in the bladder. Both of her symptoms are signs of conus medullaris syndrome. At which of the following vertebral levels is the tumor most likely located?

A. L3–L4
B. L3
C. L4
D. T12–L2
E. T11

43. Examination of a 3-day-old male shows protrusion of his spinal cord and meninges from a defect in the lower back. Which of the following best describes this congenital anomaly?

A. Avulsion of meninges
B. Meningitis
C. Spina bifida occulta
D. Spina bifida with myelomeningocele
E. Spina bifida with meningocele

44. A 32-year-old woman comes to the physician because of 2-week history of pain in the coccygeal area after giving birth. To determine whether the coccyx is involved, a local anesthetic is first injected in the region of the coccyx and then dynamic MRI studies are performed. Physical examination shows pain with palpation to the region of the coccyx. The local anesthetic is used to interrupt which of the following nerve pathways?

A. Visceral afferent
B. Somatic efferent
C. Somatic afferent
D. Sympathetic preganglionic
E. Parasympathetic preganglionic

45. A 65-year-old man comes to the physician for a routine examination. He is 1.8 m (5 ft, 11 in) and 78 kg (172 lb). He has a history of exercise-induced asthma and uses an albuterol inhaler as needed. His vital signs are within normal limits for his age. He is tested for ease and flexibility of the movements of his lumbar region. Which of the following movements is most characteristic of the intervertebral joints in the lumbar region?

A. Circumduction
B. Lateral flexion
C. Abduction
D. Adduction
E. Inversion

46. A 72-year-old man with a history of cancer of the prostate gland is brought to the emergency department with loss of consciousness and seizures. Physical examination shows loss of vibration and proprioception on his left side below the umbilical line. A computed tomography (CT) scan of the brain shows metastatic tumors and a CT scan of the pelvis shows a primary tumor. Which of the following best explains the metastasis to the brain?

A. The internal venous plexus contains the longest veins in the body.
B. The internal venous plexus has valves that ensure one-way movement of blood.
C. The internal venous plexus is located in the subarachnoid space.

D. The internal venous plexus is, in general, valveless.

E. The internal venous plexus is located in the subdural space.

47. A 26-year-old man is brought to the emergency department after he slipped and fell from a ladder onto the pavement below while painting his house. Physical examination shows no abnormalities. An x-ray of the scapula shows that the portion of his left scapula that forms the tip, the highest point of the shoulder has been fractured. Which of the following bony parts is most likely fractured?
A. Coracoid process
B. Superior angle of the scapula
C. Glenoid
D. Spine of the scapula
E. Acromion

48. A 43-year-old man who is a construction worker is brought to the emergency department after a fall from a two-story building. Physical examination shows loss of all sensation in his lower limbs. An MRI of the cervical spine shows a crushed spinal cord at C6 vertebral level. Which of the following muscles will most likely be paralyzed?
A. Sternocleidomastoid
B. Trapezius
C. Diaphragm
D. Latissimus dorsi
E. Deltoid

49. A 36-year-old woman, at 14 weeks' gestation comes to the physician for a prenatal visit. She has had one previous pregnancy resulting in full term delivery. Today, her vital signs are within normal limits. Physical examination shows a uterus consistent in size with a 14-week gestation. She has no bleeding or vaginal discharge. A maternal serum sample with high alpha-fetoprotein is indicative of a possible neural tube defect. Fetal ultrasonography shows a fetus with myelomeningocele protruding from the back of the child. Which of the following is the most likely diagnosis of this congenital anomaly?
A. Cranium bifida
B. Spina bifida occulta
C. Spina bifida cystica
D. Hemothorax
E. Caudal regression syndrome

50. A 7-year-old girl is brought to the physician by her parents because of a soft lump above the buttocks. Physical examination shows the lump is located just superior to the iliac crest unilaterally on the left side. The protrusion is deep to the skin and pliable to the touch. Which of the following is the most likely diagnosis?
A. Tumor of the external abdominal oblique muscle
B. Herniation at the lumbar triangle (of Petit)
C. Indirect inguinal hernia
D. Direct inguinal hernia
E. Femoral hernia

Questions 51–75

51. A 74-year-old woman comes to the physician because of a 1-year history of back pain. Her temperature is 37.1°C (98.8°F), pulse is 74/min, respirations are 15/min, and blood pressure is 138/74 mm Hg. Physical examination shows no neurologic abnormalities. An MRI of the spine shows that the intervertebral discs have been decreased in size because of age, resulting in mild spinal stenosis and disc herniation. At which locations are the spinal nerves most likely to be compressed?
A. Between the denticulate ligaments
B. As they pass through the vertebral foramen
C. Between the superior and inferior articular facets
D. Between the inferior and superior vertebral notches
E. Between the superior and inferior intercostovertebral joints

52. A 37-year-old pregnant woman, gravida 1, para 0, at 39 weeks' gestation, comes to the hospital with regular uterine contractions at 12-minute intervals that have been steadily increasing in strength. Physical examination shows a cervix dilated to 4 cm and 50% effaced. She is given a caudal epidural block to alleviate pain during vaginal delivery. Which of the following landmarks is most commonly used for the caudal epidural block?
A. Anterior sacral foramina
B. Posterior sacral foramina
C. Cornua of the sacral hiatus
D. Intervertebral foramina
E. Median sacral crest

53. A 38-year-old woman comes to the physician because of a 3-month history of persistent back pain and headaches. She has not had any fever, chills, or weight loss. She has no history of major medical illness. Physical examination shows areas of localized tenderness in the cervical spine. A CT scan shows breast cancer with metastasis to the brain and cervical spine. An MRI of the cervical spine confirms localized metastasis to the certain parts of the cervical spine. Metastasis is most likely located in which of the following locations?
A. Odontoid process
B. Transverse process
C. Lateral mass
D. Pedicle
E. Spinous process

54. A 22-year-old man is brought into the emergency department following a brawl in a tavern. He has severe pain radiating across his back and down his left upper limb. He supports his left upper limb with his right hand, holding it close to his body. Any attempt to move the left upper limb greatly increases the pain. An x-ray of the scapula shows an unusual sagittal fracture through the spine of the left scapula. The fracture extends superiorly toward the superior scapular

notch. Which of the following nerves is most likely affected?

A. Suprascapular

B. Thoracodorsal

C. Axillary

D. Subscapular

E. Suprascapular and thoracodorsal

55. A 5-year-old boy is brought to the emergency department because of 2-day history of pain in the upper back and a "stiff" neck. His mother says he has lost some of his hearing and is concerned with these constellations of symptoms. Physical examination shows the boy has a low posterior hairline and a short-webbed neck. An x-ray of the cervical spine shows abnormal fusion of the C5 and C6 vertebrae and a high-riding scapula. Which of the following is the most likely diagnosis?

A. Lordosis

B. Kyphosis

C. Scoliosis

D. Spina bifida

E. Klippel-Feil syndrome

56. A 53-year-old man comes to physician because of 3-month history of progressive back pain. His pain is radiating down his legs and he can walk for about 6 minutes before the pain becomes unbearable. Physical examination shows normal patellar tendon reflexes, pedal pulses are present, and there is difficulty in heel-walking. An MRI examination shows anterior dislocation of the body of the L5 vertebra upon the sacrum. Which of the following is the most likely diagnosis?

A. Spondylolysis

B. Spondylolisthesis

C. Herniation of intervertebral disc

D. Lordosis

E. Scoliosis

57. A 1-year-old boy is brought to the physician by his mother because of his bilateral arm weakness, difficulty swallowing milk, and stridor. Physical exam shows the boy is barely able to lift his arms off the exam table. He is diagnosed with a congenital malformation. An MRI of the brain and spinal cord shows the cerebellum and medulla oblongata are protruding inferiorly through the foramen magnum into the vertebral canal. Which of the following is the most likely diagnosis?

A. Meningocele

B. Klippel-Feil syndrome

C. Chiari II malformation

D. Hydrocephalus

E. Tethered cord syndrome

58. A 62-year-old woman is admitted to the hospital because a 5-month history of back pain has gotten progressively worse. She feels relieved when she bends forward and worse when she walks for a few minutes. Physical examination shows she has 5/5 motor strength bilaterally in the lower extremities. There is

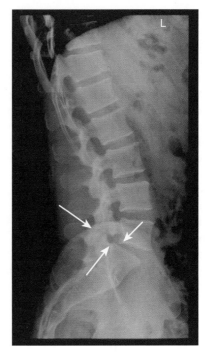

• Fig. 1.2

a slight sensation deficit on the left medial aspect of the thigh. An x-ray of the spine shows the L4 vertebral body has slipped anteriorly, with fracture of the zygapophysial joint (Fig. 1.2). Which of the following is the most likely diagnosis?

A. Spondylolysis and spondylolisthesis

B. Spondylolisthesis

C. Crush vertebral fracture

D. Intervertebral disc herniation

E. Klippel-Feil syndrome

59. A 40-year-old woman is brought to the emergency department after being injured in a motor vehicle collision in which her neck was hyperextended when her vehicle was struck from behind. An x-ray of her cervical spine shows a fracture of the odontoid process (dens). Which of the following structures is also most likely injured?

A. Anterior arch of the atlas

B. Posterior tubercle of the atlas

C. Atlantooccipital joint

D. Inferior articular process of the axis

E. Anterior tubercle of the atlas

60. A 34-year-old woman is admitted to the emergency department after a motor vehicle collision. She rear-ended a stopped vehicle at a low rate of speed. Physical examination shows she has paraspinal tenderness in the cervical and thoracic region. She has significantly limited range of motion in all axes and she is unable to perform a task when she is asked to turn her head to the left. Neurologic examination is within normal limits in the upper and lower extremities. An MRI of the spine shows a whiplash injury in addition to

hyperextension of her cervical spine. Which of the following ligaments is most likely injured?
- **A.** Ligamentum flavum
- **B.** Anterior longitudinal ligament
- **C.** Posterior longitudinal ligament
- **D.** Annulus fibrosus
- **E.** Interspinous ligament

61. A 23-year-old woman is admitted to the emergency department 50 minutes after jumping from a 50-foot high waterfall. Physical examination shows a number of lacerations and ecchymosis over her back and upper extremities with 3/5 motor strength in her lower extremities and 5/5 motor strength in her upper extremities. Sensory and reflex examinations are within normal limits in the upper and lower extremities. MRI of the spine shows a lateral shift of the spinal cord to the left. Which of the following structures has most likely been torn to cause the deviation?
- **A.** Posterior longitudinal ligament
- **B.** Tentorium cerebelli
- **C.** Denticulate ligaments
- **D.** Ligamentum flavum
- **E.** Nuchal ligament

62. A 6-year-old boy is brought to the hospital by his parents because of a 2-day history of coughing and dyspnea. The patient says he feels like there is glass in his lungs. Physical examination shows abnormal lung sounds on auscultation heard most clearly during inhalation with the scapulae protracted. Which of the following form the borders of a triangular space where one should place the stethoscope to best hear the lung sounds?
- **A.** Latissimus dorsi, trapezius, medial border of scapula
- **B.** Deltoid, levator scapulae, trapezius
- **C.** Latissimus dorsi, external abdominal oblique, iliac crest
- **D.** Quadratus lumborum, internal abdominal oblique, inferior border of the twelfth rib
- **E.** Rectus abdominis, inguinal ligament, inferior epigastric vessels

63. A 45-year-old man comes to the physician because of a 2-week severe shoulder pain and lateral arm paresthesia. The pain has been bothering him for years and is exacerbated when he plays basketball. He played basketball for many years in his college years. Physical examination shows weakened shoulder movements with normal sensation in the upper extremities. Axial T1-weighted MRI shows signs of quadrangular space syndrome, causing weakened shoulder movements. Which of the following nerves is most likely affected?
- **A.** Suprascapular
- **B.** Subscapular
- **C.** Axillary
- **D.** Radial
- **E.** Ulnar

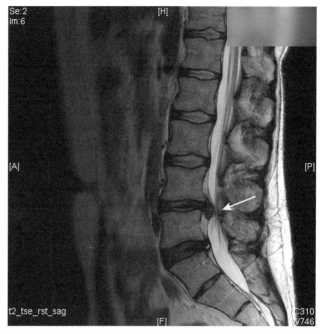

• Fig. 1.3

64. A 29-year-old woman who is an elite athlete was lifting heavy weights during an intense training session when she felt severe pain radiate suddenly to the lateral aspect of her right thigh and leg. She was brought to the hospital where an MRI of her spine was performed (Fig. 1.3). Which of the following nerves was most probably affected?
- **A.** L3
- **B.** L4
- **C.** L2
- **D.** L5
- **E.** S1

65. A 58-year-old man in the intensive care unit exhibits little voluntary control of urinary or fecal activity following repair of an abdominal aortic aneurysm in the days prior. Physical examination shows widespread paralysis of his lower limbs. These functions were essentially normal prior to admission to the hospital. The most likely cause of this patient's current condition is which of the following?
- **A.** Injury to the left vertebral artery
- **B.** Injury of the great radicular artery (of Adamkiewicz)
- **C.** Ligation of the posterior spinal artery
- **D.** Transection of the conus medullaris of the spinal cord
- **E.** Division of the thoracic sympathetic trunk

66. A 23-year-old woman is brought to the emergency department because of a 2-day history of severe back pain. She had polio when she was 8 years of age and was diagnosed with a muscular dystrophy. Physical examination shows no neurological deficits. CT of her spine shows a clinical condition affecting her vertebral

column. Which of the following is most likely present in this patient?

A. Hyperlordosis
B. Hyperkyphosis
C. Scoliosis
D. Spina bifida
E. Osteoarthritis

67. A 26-year-old man comes to the physician because of pain, weakness, numbness, and tingling in his upper limb for the past 2 months. Physical examination shows no abnormalities. MRI of the spine shows a cervical disc herniation compressing the nerve roots and a portion of the spinal cord. An anterior cervical discectomy and fusion (ACDF) surgery is performed. The intervertebral disc is examined upon removal and the annulus fibrosus and nucleus pulposus are severely damaged posterolaterally. What type of cartilage most likely gives the tensile strength of the intervertebral disc?

A. Hyaline
B. Elastic
C. Fibrous
D. Epiphysial
E. Elastic and fibrous

68. A 23-year-old man comes to the physician because of a 3-month history of pain, weakness, numbness, and tingling in his upper limb. MRI of the spine shows a cervical disc herniation compressing the nerve roots and a portion of the spinal cord. An ACDF surgery is performed. The intervertebral disc is examined and the annulus and nucleus polposus are severely damaged. What is the embryologic origin of the annulus fibrosus and nucleus pulposus, respectively?

A. Notochord and neural crest cells
B. Neural crest cells and ectoderm
C. Sclerotome and myotome
D. Mesenchymal cells from sclerotome and neural crest cells
E. Mesenchymal cells from sclerotome and notochord

69. A 55-year-old woman comes to physician because of 1-week history of noticeable changes at her face. She had a middle ear infection for the past month that has been producing drainage and two transient ischemic attacks in the last year. Physical examination shows right-sided miosis, partial ptosis of her eyelid, anhidrosis of the right side of her face and redness in her conjunctiva. Three days, after her visit, she suddenly develops a stroke. Despite appropriate care, she dies. At autopsy examination of which of the following structures would show the cell bodies of neurons affected by the physical examination findings?

A. Anterior gray horn of the spinal cord
B. Lateral gray horn of the spinal cord
C. Posterior gray horn of the spinal cord
D. Spinal ganglia
E. Lateral column of spinal cord white matter

70. A 62-year-old man is brought to the emergency department after a severe motor vehicle collision resulting in a whiplash injury. Physical examination shows no neurological deficits. An MRI of the head and neck shows several hairline vertebral fractures in the cervical region impinging upon the dorsal rami of the same levels. Two months after the injury the patient recovers well, but there is still some weakness in the function of a muscle. Which of the following muscles is most likely affected?

A. Rhomboid major
B. Levator scapulae
C. Rhomboid minor
D. Semispinalis capitis
E. Latissimus dorsi

71. A 22-year-old man is brought to the emergency department because of a 1-month history of progressive weakness with extending and rotating his head. He has headaches and some muscle weakness to the upper muscles of his back for the last 6 months. Physical examination shows decreased motor strength in left and right rotation of the head with no neurological deficits. An MRI of the head and neck shows a large tumor compressing the suboccipital and greater occipital nerves. Which of the following muscles will most likely still be functioning normally?

A. Rectus capitis posterior major and minor
B. Semispinalis capitis
C. Splenius capitis
D. Obliquus capitis superior
E. Obliquus capitis inferior

72. A 36-year-old woman is brought to the emergency department because of a severe episode of major depressive disorder. She has been hospitalized several times in the past 8 years. Despite therapy, her condition worsens, and she hangs herself. Autopsy shows a cervical vertebra fracture as a result of hanging. The mechanism of injury resulting in death is forcible hyperextension resulting in a fracture of which of the following structures?

A. Odontoid process
B. Transverse process
C. Lateral mass
D. Pedicle (pars articularis)
E. Spinous process

73. A 72-year-old woman comes to the physician after falling in her bathroom 2 days ago. Her vital signs are within normal limits. An x-ray series of her vertebral column shows a wedge fracture at the fourth thoracic vertebra and thin cortical bone showing signs of osteoporotic changes. What will be the most likely type of abnormal spinal curvature in such a patient?

A. Hyperkyphosis
B. Scoliosis
C. Hyperlordosis
D. Normal
E. Primary

74. A 65-year-old woman comes to the physician because of a 3-day history of a group of painful blisters over

her back in the distribution of the T9 dermatome. She noticed that a few days prior to the eruption of the blisters she experienced an intense burning sensation over her skin. Physical examination shows a maculopapular rash in a dermatomal distribution. A diagnosis of herpes zoster (shingles) is made. Where are the neural cell bodies located that are responsible for the pain sensation?

A. Dorsal horn
B. Lateral horn
C. Dorsal root ganglia
D. Sympathetic trunk ganglia
E. White rami communicantes

75. A 53-year-old man was is admitted to the hospital 30 minutes after being involved in a motor vehicle collision resulting in the dens crushing the spinal cord. An x-ray of the head and neck shows an atlantodental interval of 7.3 mm and on open-mouth odontoid x-ray shows lateral mass displacement of 8 mm. Which of the following is most likely torn for the dens to compress the spinal cord?

A. Anterior and posterior longitudinal ligaments
B. Transverse ligament of the atlas
C. Interspinous ligament
D. Supraspinous ligament
E. Nuchal ligament

Questions 76–100

76. A 16-year-old girl is brought the physician for a routine physical examination prior to the beginning of her school year. She has no history of major medical illnesses and receives no medication. Her vital signs are within normal limits. Physical examination shows one shoulder is higher than the other. When she asked to bend forward at the waist to touch her toes a posterior bulging of the ribs on the right side is shown. Which of the following is the most likely diagnosis?

A. Kyphosis
B. Spondylosis
C. Lordosis
D. Spondylolisthesis
E. Scoliosis

77. A 30-year-old woman is admitted to the hospital because of a 3-month history of thoracic back pain and persistent cough. She says that the cough is getting progressively worse. Laboratory studies show a positive Mantoux (PPD: purified protein derivative) skin test after 48 hours. An x-ray of the chest shows signs of tuberculosis in the lungs and dissemination in the thoracic vertebrae. Which of the following will most likely be a long-term effect in the thoracic spine if this condition left untreated?

A. Spondylolysis
B. Spondylolisthesis
C. Herniation of intervertebral disc
D. Vertebral collapse
E. Wedge fracture

78. A 70-year-old man with prostate cancer is brought to the emergency department because of a 4-hour history of sharp shooting pains radiating from his neck into the upper limb. His vital signs are within normal limits. Physical examination shows no neurological abnormalities. An MRI of his spine shows a small metastatic mass in the cervical region extending into the left intervertebral foramen between C6 and C7. The intervertebral discs appear normal. Which neural structure is most likely being compressed by the metastatic mass to account for the pain?

A. C8 spinal nerve
B. Dorsal horn of C6 spinal cord segment
C. C6 spinal nerve
D. Dorsal horn of C7 spinal nerve
E. C7 spinal nerve

79. A 3-day-old girl is brought to the physician by her mother because of a 2-day history of poor feeding, irritability, and lethargy. Her mother says she developed a fever that is unresponsive to over-the-counter medication. Her temperature is 40.0°C (104.0°F), blood pressure is 100/60 mm Hg, pulse is 94, and respirations are 38/min. Meningitis is suspected and a lumbar puncture is performed. The puncture must be performed below the termination of the spinal cord which usually ends at which vertebral level in a patient of this age?

A. L1
B. S1
C. L3
D. S3
E. L5

80. A 26-year-old man comes to the office because of a 3-day history of an itchy, red rash on his back. Three days ago, he returned from an expedition safari in Okavango Delta in Botswana., during which he was bit by many insects while outside. Shortly after arriving back to the United States, he noticed the area where he was bitten has become infected and purulent material was draining. A surgical procedure to debride the abscess involving the erector spinae muscle at vertebral level T8 is performed. The nerve branch supplying the skin and the underlying muscle are severed from the abscess. In which of the following structures are the cell bodies of this nerve branch located?

A. Ventral horn and dorsal horn
B. Ventral horn, dorsal horn, and lateral horn
C. Ventral horn, dorsal root ganglion, and lateral horn
D. Ventral horn, dorsal root ganglion, and sympathetic paravertebral ganglion
E. Ventral horn, dorsal horn, and dorsal root ganglion

81. A 28-year-old man is brought to the emergency department after being involved in a motor vehicle collision resulting in hyperextension of his neck. Physical examination shows midline tenderness over the cervical vertebrae. He was placed in a cervical

collar. The next day his neck was stiff and painful. Which of the following structures is most likely damaged resulting in pain?

A. Anterior longitudinal ligament
B. Posterior longitudinal ligament
C. Ligamentum flavum
D. Intervertebral disc
E. Supraspinous ligament

82. A 38-year-old man comes to the physician because of chronic lower back pain with radiating pain to the heel. The pain is so debilitating that he now has trouble ambulating. An MRI of the lower back shows severe narrowing of an intervertebral foramen, which causes compression of the exiting nerve root. A surgical procedure is performed, and during the procedure the intervertebral foramen is accessed using a lateral approach. The superior margin (roof) of the intervertebral foramen is decompressed from the exiting nerve root. Which of the following vertebral bony features is most likely removed?

A. Superior articular process
B. Lamina
C. Inferior articular process
D. Pedicle
E. Spinous process

83. A 35-year-old man is brought to the emergency department because of a 45-minute history of injury of his neck when he was playing football. An MRI shows an acute posterolateral herniation of the most superiorly located intervertebral disc which is located within the corresponding intervertebral foramen and compressing the exiting nerve. Which of the following nerves in most likely injured?

A. C1
B. C2
C. C3
D. C4
E. C5

84. A 14-year-old girl is brought to the emergency room after she flipped her bicycle off a curb, fell, and landed on her face 45 minutes ago. Although she was wearing a helmet, she landed in such a way that her neck was forced into hyperextension. Physical examination shows no neurological deficits but there is neck rigidity. Which of the following ligaments of the cervical spine is most likely stretched to the greatest degree during her injury?

A. Posterior longitudinal
B. Nuchal
C. Ligamentum flavum
D. Supraspinous
E. Anterior longitudinal

85. In preparation for a lumbar puncture, the iliac crests are palpated, and a line is drawn across the patient's back with a skin marker to connect the highest points of the left and right crests. The needle is inserted above the point at which the subarachnoid space terminates inferiorly. Which of the following most likely represents the level at which the subarachnoid space ends inferiorly?

A. Three spinous processes superior to the horizontal line
B. Two spinous processes inferior to the horizontal line
C. Three spinous processes inferior to the horizontal line
D. Two spinous processes superior to the horizontal line
E. The spinous process bisected by the horizontal line

86. A 68-year-old man is brought to the emergency department with acute mid-back pain that began a few hours ago. Physical examination shows decreased sensation of the skin bilaterally over the lower limbs. Motor strength is assessed at 5/5 in all four limbs. MRI of the thoracic spine shows a large tumor arising from the anterior median fissure of the spinal cord at the level of the T3 vertebra. The artery compressed by the tumor is most likely formed superiorly by direct branches from which of the following arteries?

A. Ascending cervical
B. Segmental medullary
C. Vertebral
D. Segmental spinal
E. Posterior spinal

87. A 12-year-old girl is brought to the emergency department by her parents for mid-back pain that has been ongoing for weeks and is progressively getting worse. Her vital signs are within normal limits. Physical examination shows no neurological abnormalities. An x-ray of the spine shows a hemivertebra of the lower thoracic spine. Which additional finding would most likely be present on the x-ray?

A. Osteoporosis
B. Scoliosis
C. Hyperlordosis
D. Spondylolisthesis
E. Sacralization

88. A 35-year-old man is brought to the emergency department because of a 45-minute history of injury at his neck when he was playing football. MRI shows severe narrowing of the C7–T1 intervertebral foramen on the left. Which of the following nerves is most likely compressed?

A. C6
B. C7
C. C8
D. T1
E. T2

89. A 15-month-old girl is brought to the physician by her mother because of a curvature in her low back. The mother says that this curvature was not present previously and that she noticed it when the girl started standing and walking. She has received all scheduled childhood immunizations. She attends

a day-care center and has no siblings. Her vitals are within normal limits. Physical examination shows a slight curvature of the spine. The mother is reassured that the spinal curvature was normal. Which curvature did the mother most likely observe?

A. Thoracic kyphosis
B. Cervical lordosis
C. Lumbar lordosis
D. Cervical kyphosis
E. Thoracic lordosis

90. A 24-year-old man comes to the physician for a routine physical examination. Physical examination shows a large hypertrophied muscle of his back. This muscle inserts onto the floor of the intertubercular sulcus of the humerus. Which of the following structures is most likely the vertebral origin of the hypertrophied muscle?

A. Spinous processes of T7–L5
B. Spinous processes of C7–T12
C. Transverse processes of C1–C4
D. Spinous processes of T2–T5
E. Spinous processes of C7 and T1

91. A 34-year-old woman, gravida 2, para 1, at 13 weeks' gestation, comes to the office for a prenatal visit. She says that her job involves exposure to known teratogens and dangerous chemicals. She has no vaginal bleeding or cramping pains. Today, her vital signs are within normal limits. Physical examination shows a uterus consistent with a 13-week gestation. A drug that preferentially destroys sclerotomes during embryogenesis would most likely result in underdevelopment of which of the following structures?

A. Nucleus pulposus of intervertebral discs
B. Vertebral bodies
C. Dorsal root ganglia
D. Spinal cord
E. Sympathetic ganglia

92. A 24-year-old man is brought to the emergency department after a penetrating injury to his upper back while working at his construction site 30 minutes ago. Physical examination shows no neurological or musculoskeletal abnormalities. Which of the following muscles is most likely located immediately deep to the semispinalis muscles, passes from a lateral point of origin in a superomedial direction to attach to spinous processes, and crosses between two and four vertebrae?

A. Multifidus
B. Rotatores
C. Longissimus
D. Iliocostalis
E. Spinalis

93. A 32-year-old construction worker is brought to the emergency department after he fell from a scaffold. He has severe lower back pain. Physical examination shows normal neurological examination and no motor deficits. An x-ray of the lumbar spine shows

bilateral pars interarticularis fractures of the L5 vertebra. Which of the following radiographic views would most likely show these fractures?

A. Anteroposterior
B. Lateral
C. Posteroanterior
D. Oblique
E. Anteroposterior open mouth

94. A 45-year-old man comes to the physician because of a small growth that he noticed slowly growing in the posterior cervical region for the last week. MRI of the cervical spine shows a small 1-cm tumor that is located within a muscle on the lateral border of the right suboccipital triangle. This muscle inserts on which of the following bony features?

A. Transverse process of atlas
B. Lateral portion of the inferior nuchal line of the occipital bone
C. Occipital bone between the superior and inferior nuchal lines
D. Medial portion of the inferior nuchal line of the occipital bone
E. Posterior tubercle of atlas

95. A 68-year-old woman comes to the physician because of lower back pain that has been bothering her for the last 2 weeks. An x-ray of the lumbar spine in the anteroposterior view shows marked bilateral enlargement of the transverse processes of a single vertebra. The length and width of both transverse processes of this single vertebra are enlarged and the inferior aspects of these bony features appear to be articulating with the bone immediately below it, so much so that the single vertebra appears to have morphologic characteristics similar to the bone immediately below it. The single vertebra identified on x-ray is most likely which of the following?

A. L1 vertebra
B. L4 vertebra
C. S2 vertebra
D. S1 vertebra
E. L5 vertebra

96. A 45-year-old man was brought to the emergency department 45 minutes after being injured in a motor vehicle collision. An x-ray of the upper cervical spine shows a type III dens fracture demonstrated by a horizontal radiolucent line on the superior half of the posterior aspect of the C2 vertebral body. Which of the following ligaments most likely has direct attachment to the bony area where the fracture was located?

A. Apical ligament
B. Superior longitudinal band of cruciform ligament
C. Transverse ligament of atlas
D. Inferior longitudinal band of cruciform ligament
E. Ligamentum flavum

97. A 65-year-old man comes to the physician because of a history of 1-year back pain that has been progressively getting worse. Physical examination shows

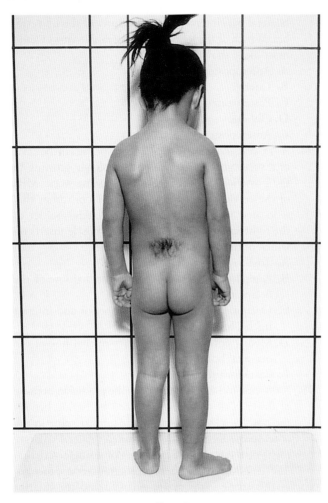

• Fig. 1.4

normal reflexes, reduced sensation of the skin over the abdomen, and no detectable motor deficits. A laminectomy of the T8 to T9 vertebrae is performed because the posterior roots were compressed at that level due to a space-occupying lesion. Which of the following arteries is most likely being directly compressed by the lesion?

A. Radicular
B. Segmental spinal
C. Segmental medullary
D. Anterior spinal
E. Posterior spinal

98. An 8-year-old girl was brought to the physician for a routine examination. Her vital signs are within normal limits. Physical examination shows a well-groomed resting child in no physical distress. The figure associated with this question is a photograph of the child (Fig. 1.4). Which of the following best describes the embryologic basis for this child's condition?

A. Underdevelopment of the secondary ossification center in the vertebral arch
B. Underdevelopment of the primary ossification center in the spinous process

C. Underdevelopment of the primary ossification center in the vertebral body
D. Underdevelopment of the secondary ossification center in the vertebral body
E. Underdevelopment of the primary ossification center in the vertebral arch

99. A 54-year-old man comes to the physician for neck pain that has been getting worse for the last year. The pain was initially only when he turned his head to the left, but now is elicited when he turns left or right. Over-the-counter anti-inflammatory medications no longer alleviate the pain. Physical examination shows decreased cervical range of motion in all axes. MRI of the cervical spine shows a large osteophyte emanating from the posterolateral area of the vertebral body of the vertebra immediately above the C3 spinal nerve and severely compressing it. The osteophyte is most likely emanating from which of the following vertebrae?

A. C2
B. C3
C. C4
D. C5
E. C1

100. A 38-year-old woman, gravida 4, para 3, abortus 1, at 40 weeks' gestation, is brought to the hospital after she began having sustained contractions every 10 minutes and getting stronger and in shorter intervals. She is confirmed to be in labor and has been so for 14 hours. She has agreed to have an epidural anesthetic injection for pain control. Which of the following structures is most likely to be the last penetrated by the needle before it reaches the epidural space?

A. Supraspinous ligament
B. Interspinous ligament
C. Anterior longitudinal ligament
D. Posterior longitudinal ligament
E. Ligamentum flavum

Questions 101–123

101. A 48-year-old man comes to the physician because of a 1-week history of vertigo, nausea, and emesis. Physical examination shows complete hearing loss on the left with hemianesthesia on the left side of the face. MRI of the brain shows a tumor at the opening of the internal acoustic meatus. He undergoes a craniotomy whereby a midline incision through the nuchal ligament that began 1-cm inferior to the external occipital protuberance and ended at the level of the C2 vertebra is performed. A self-retaining retractor is placed into the incision to forcibly separate the tissues. During recovery, the patient experiences severe occipital pain and the diagnosis of postsurgical occipital neuralgia is made. Which of the following nerves was most likely directly stretched by the retractors during the surgery and resulted in this patient's post-surgical pain?

A. Third occipital
B. Suboccipital
C. Greater occipital
D. Lesser occipital
E. Accessory

102. A 7-year-old boy is brought to the physician for lower back pain over the course of 2 weeks. His vital signs are within normal limits. Physical examination shows no neurological deficits. MRI of the spine shows a mass in his spinal cord. He undergoes surgery to remove a tumor from his spinal cord. During surgery of the spinal cord, which of the following structures is used as a landmark to identify anterior rootlets from posterior rootlets?
    A. Denticulate ligament
    B. Filum terminale internum
    C. Conus medullaris
    D. Posterior longitudinal ligament
    E. Ligamentum flavum

103. A 45-year-old man is brought the emergency department 45 minutes after he was involved in a motor vehicle collision. MRI of the head and neck shows a complete tear of the right alar ligament. None of the other ligaments of the upper cervical spine was torn. Physical examination would show which of the following cervical spine movements to be most likely increased as a result of the tear?
    A. Flexion
    B. Extension
    C. Lateral flexion
    D. Rotation
    E. Abduction

104. A 25-year-old man comes to the physician because of a 2-week history of difficulty moving his right shoulder. Physical examination shows the muscles of the left upper back and shoulder were notably larger than the right side. There was a notable decrease of muscle power on his right-sided upper back and shoulder muscles when he was asked to pull the shoulder blades toward the middle of his back against resistance. Nerve conduction examination confirms neurapraxia of the nerves supplying the rhomboid major and minor muscles. In which of the following functions will he most likely also demonstrate weakness?
    A. Abduction of the right arm above the horizontal level and protraction of the scapula
    B. Medial rotation and adduction of the right arm
    C. Extensions, adduction, and medial rotation of the right arm
    D. Elevation of the scapula and inferior rotation of the right shoulder
    E. Abduction of the right arm from 0 to 15 degrees

105. A 38-year-old woman comes to the physician because of a 6-month history of a hard mass in the left breast. She has a history of carcinoma of the left breast and had a lumpectomy 2 years previously. Ultrasonography of the axilla shows a 3- × 4-cm hard mass in the upper outer quadrant extending into the axillary tail (of Spence) of the breast. A radical mastectomy is performed successfully, and the tumor is removed. Three weeks postoperatively, the patient experiences difficulty raising her left arm above her head. Which of the following additional findings is most likely to be found during physical examination?
    A. Weak protraction of both scapulae
    B. Protrusion of the medial border of the left scapula when the hands are pushed against a wall
    C. Weak abduction of the left upper limb in the 15–90-degree range
    D. Weak retraction of the scapula
    E. Weak adduction of the humerus

106. A 2-month-old girl is brought to the emergency department because of a fever and rash that began 2 days prior. He has been irritable and feeding poorly the last 24 hours. His temperature is 39.6°C (103.2°F), pulse is 152/min, and respirations are 54/min. Physical examination shows a slightly bulging anterior fontanelle. A lumbar puncture is performed to confirm the diagnosis. The needle is inserted into the lumbar cistern (dural sac). At which vertebral level will the conus medullaris typically be found in this patient?
    A. L3
    B. L4
    C. L5
    D. S1
    E. S2

107. A 3-day-old girl is brought to the physician because of a large lump on her back. She has been feeding well and has not been irritable. Physical examination shows a large cystic mass of approximately 15 × 10 cm in the sacrococcygeal region. The mass was removed, and histopathological studies identified tissue from all three embryological germ layers. Which of the following embryonic tissues is most likely responsible for this condition?
    A. Remnants of the primitive streak
    B. Chorionic villi
    C. Neural folds
    D. Intraembryonic coelom
    E. Neural crest

108. A 53-year-old man is brought to the emergency department with severe back pain that began suddenly earlier in the day. MRI examination of the lumbar spine shows fracture of the pars interarticularis and normal alignment of the body of the L5 vertebra upon the sacrum. What is the most likely diagnosis?
    A. Spondylolysis
    B. Spondylolisthesis
    C. Herniation of intervertebral disc
    D. Lordosis
    E. Scoliosis

109. A 22-year-old pregnant woman at 40 weeks' gestation comes to the hospital for delivery. Her cervix is 60%

effaced and dilated 5 cm. She undergoes epidural anesthesia in anticipation of labor. After delivery, she developed back pain and right lower extremity weakness. An MRI of her spine shows a hematoma in the epidural space resulting in compression of the nerve that exits at the level of L2–L3. Which of the following vessels is most likely responsible for the hematoma?

A. Internal vertebral plexus
B. Great radicular artery (of Adamkiewicz)
C. Anterior spinal artery
D. Posterior spinal artery
E. External vertebral plexus

110. A 71-year-old man is brought to the emergency department 30 minutes after he was involved in a motor vehicle collision. He was idling at a stoplight in his vintage car without headrests and was struck from behind by a truck. Physical examination shows severe hyperextension neck injury due to the crash. A T2-weighted MRI shows a rupture of the anterior annulus fibrosus of the C4–C5 intervertebral disc and a prevertebral hematoma which compromised his airway and required intubation. Which of the following ligaments is most likely disrupted in this injury?

A. Anterior longitudinal
B. Posterior longitudinal
C. Ligamentum flavum
D. Interspinous
E. Intertransverse

111. A 28-year-old primigravida woman at 40 weeks' gestation is admitted to the hospital for delivery. Her vital signs are within normal limits. A tocometer and fetal heart rate monitor are placed on her abdomen. In the final stages of labor, an epidural anesthetic is administered immediately lateral to the spinous processes of L3 and L4 vertebrae. During this procedure, what would be the last ligament perforated by the needle to access the epidural space?

A. Ligamentum flavum
B. Anterior longitudinal
C. Posterior longitudinal
D. Interspinous
E. Intertransverse

112. A 38-year-old man is brought to the physician because of a 5-day history of lower back pain during the past 5 days. Physical examination shows tenderness of the spine over the L5 vertebra with an obvious "step-off" defect at that level. There was some weakness of the limbs. MRI of the lumbar spine shows an anterior displacement of the L5 vertebral body and narrowing of the vertebral canal. This pathology will most likely be associated with which of the following?

A. Compression of the spinal cord and bilateral lower limb weakness
B. Compression of the spinal cord and unilateral lower limb weakness

C. Compression of the spinal nerve roots and L5 with unilateral lower limb weakness
D. Compression of the cauda equina and bilateral lower limb weakness
E. Compression of the cauda equina and low back pain only

113. A 62-year-old man comes to the physician for a routine examination. Physical examination shows noticeable pulsations on palpation of the lower abdomen. Ultrasonography of the abdomen shows a large abdominal aortic aneurysm. The patient is operated on and during the repair his aorta is temporarily clamped. Which of the following arterial anastomoses will most likely prevent ischemia of the spinal cord if the blood pressure drops dangerously low?

A. Segmental arteries from the vertebral, intercostals, superficial epigastric, lumbar, and median sacral arteries
B. Segmental arteries from the vertebral, posterior intercostal, lumbar, and lateral sacral arteries
C. Anterior and posterior spinal arteries
D. Great radicular artery (of Adamkiewicz)
E. Segmental arteries from the vertebral and intercostal arteries

114. A 22-year-old woman comes to the physician because of pain in her index finger over the last week that has gotten worse. She has no recent trauma or insect bites. Physical examination shows a left index finger with a pale blue well-circumscribed mass at the distal interphalangeal joint. A diagnosis of chondroma is suspected. An x-ray and an MRI of the finger localized the tumor and surgical excision were recommended. Which of the following structures is most likely sharing the same embryologic origin with the tumor?

A. Dorsal root ganglia
B. Sympathetic ganglia
C. Nucleus pulposus
D. Apical ligament
E. Calvaria

115. A 40-year-old woman is brought to the emergency department after she survived a motor vehicle collision in which her neck was hyperextended when her vehicle was struck from behind. She is brought in on a backboard and has a cervical collar secured around her neck. Physical examination shows she is breathing spontaneously. Her vitals are within normal limits with the exception of a heart rate of 109/min. An x-ray of her cervical spine is shown (Fig. 1.5). Which of the following was also most likely injured?

A. Anterior arch of the atlas
B. Posterior tubercle of the atlas
C. Atlantooccipital joint
D. Inferior articular process of the axis
E. Anterior tubercle of the atlas

116. A 32-year-old man is brought to the emergency department because of severe pain radiating to the lateral aspect of his right thigh and leg when he was

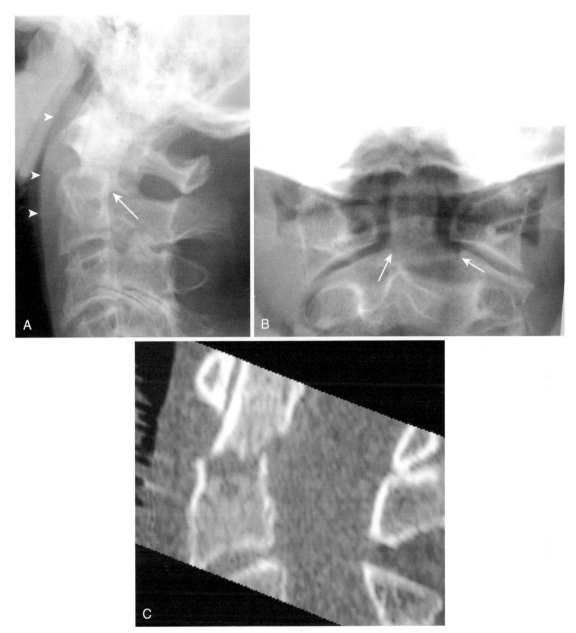

• **Fig. 1.5**

lifting heavy weights during an intense training session. Physical examination shows no saddle anesthesia, loss in sensation, or muscle weakness in his lower extremities. MRI of the lumbar spine (see Fig. 1.3) shows a ruptured intervertebral disc. Which of the following nerves is most likely affected?

A. L2
B. L3
C. L4
D. L5
E. S1

117. A 16-year-old boy is brought to the emergency department by his parents because of an injury sustained from diving head-first into shallow water. He has a severe bruise on the top of his head and intense neck pain but has no noticeable cutaneous sensory loss. A CT of his neck shows fractures bilaterally to the atlas, with the fracture lines located immediately posterior to the superior articular surfaces of the atlas. What artery and nerve would be at greatest risk of injury with this fracture?

A. Anterior spinal; hypoglossal
B. Posterior spinal; C1
C. Posterior spinal; C2
D. Vertebral; C1
E. Vertebral; C2

118. A 25-year-old man is admitted to the hospital 30 minutes after being involved in a motor vehicle collision while driving in a vintage car, which was equipped with lap-seat belts rather than shoulder belts as in modern cars. His car hit a tree head-on, and although he was wearing his lap-belt, he sustained injuries. The

patient is conscious and has intense back pain. A CT of his thoracolumbar region shows a Chance fracture of the 12th thoracic vertebra. The anterior portion of the vertebral body, a piece of the spinous process, and the neural arch immediately posterior to the vertebral body are fractured. What portion of the neural arch has most likely been injured?

A. Lamina
B. Pedicle
C. Spinous process
D. Superior articular process
E. Transverse process

119. A 70-year-old man is brought to the emergency department because of an injury he sustained while digging a foundation for a patio. He felt a pop followed by intense pain in his upper back or lower neck posteriorly as he was digging and then was unable to move. A CT of his lower neck shows an avulsion fracture of the tip of the spinous process of C7. Which of the following ligaments is most likely injured?

A. Denticulate ligament
B. Interspinous ligament
C. Ligamentum flavum
D. Nuchal ligament
E. Posterior longitudinal ligament

120. A 42-year-old woman is brought to the emergency department because of an 8-hour history of severe back pain, urinary and fecal incontinence, and is passing flatus that she cannot control. She has been lifting weights professionally for the past 20 years. Physical examination shows retained urine within the urinary bladder, poor rectal tone, perineal skin numbness, weakness in muscles of the lower limb, and an absent calcaneal tendon reflex bilaterally. Which of the following is the most likely diagnosis?

A. Cauda equina syndrome
B. Obturator hernia
C. Piriformis syndrome
D. Pudendal nerve palsy
E. Sciatica

121. A 67-year-old man has been diagnosed with ankylosing spondylitis for the past 30 years, and lately he has noticed difficulty in breathing. A CT scan of his thorax shows his rib cage is becoming more rigid as a result of the progression of the disease. There are also early signs of a straightening of his spine. If this straightening occurs primarily in his lumbar region, what curvature will be reduced?

A. Kyphosis
B. Lordosis
C. Primary
D. Scoliosis
E. Tertiary

122. A 13-year-old girl is brought to the emergency department because of suspected meningitis. A lumbar puncture is performed to obtain a sample of cerebrospinal fluid for culture. As the needle is introduced through the tissues of the back, a first pop is felt, and then a second pop. The second pop indicates that the needle is introduced into the subarachnoid space. The first pop is the result of the needle passing through a highly elastic tissue. Which of the following structures is most likely the elastic tissue?

A. Dura mater
B. Interspinous ligament
C. Ligamentum flavum
D. Posterior longitudinal ligament
E. Supraspinous ligament

123. A 12-year-old boy is diagnosed with osteopetrosis, which is the result of a failure of osteoclasts to perform normal bone resorption. The patient has developed very dense bone, but also brittle bone because the bone fails to remodel in response to functional stresses as in normal bone (Wolff's Law) One year ago, the lateral portions of two adjacent vertebral bodies fractured and the bodies collapsed laterally. What type of curvature did this produce in the spine?

A. Kyphosis
B. Lordosis
C. Primary
D. Scoliosis
E. Secondary

Answers

Answers 1–25

1. **B.** Hyperkyphosis is characterized by a "hunchback" due to an abnormal increase in concave anterior curvature of the thoracic region of the vertebral column.
   A. Hyperlordosis, or "swayback," is an increase in lumbar curvature of the spine. Lordosis can be physiologic, such as seen in a pregnant woman.
   C. Scoliosis is a lateral curvature of the spine with rotation of the vertebrae.
   D. Spina bifida is a neural tube defect characterized by failure of closure of the vertebral arch.

   E. Osteoarthritis is a degenerative disorder that affects the articular cartilage of joints and is not specifically related to the thoracic region of the spine.
   GAS 75; N 162; ABR/McM 87

2. **B.** A crush fracture is characterized by compression of the entire vertebral body. The wedge fracture is similar in that it affects the vertebral bodies, but it involves small fractures around the perimeter of the vertebral body. Both of these fractures cause reductions in overall height.
   A, C, D. Fracture of the spinous, transverse, or superior articular surfaces can be due to

an oblique, transverse, or comminuted fracture.

    E. Intervertebral discs are associated with disc herniation, not compression fractures.
GAS 78; N 164, 168; ABR/McM 92, 113

3. **C.** The ligamentum flavum connects the laminae of two adjacent vertebrae and forms the posterior wall of the vertebral canal. It is the only answer choice that is in direct contact with the vertebral foramen. Therefore hypertrophy of only the ligamentum flavum would present as spinal canal stenosis.

    A, B. The supraspinous and interspinous ligaments connect spinous processes.

    D. The anterior longitudinal ligament connects the anterior portion of the vertebral bodies and intervertebral discs.

    E. The nuchal ligament is a posterior extension of the supraspinous ligament above the level of C7.
GAS 81–83; N 29; ABR/McM 103

4. **C.** The dorsal scapular nerve (from the ventral ramus of C5) is responsible for innervating rhomboids major and minor and usually the lower portion of the levator scapulae. The rhomboids, assisted by the trapezius, are responsible for retraction of the scapula. Therefore, if this nerve is damaged, individuals present with a laterally displaced scapula. In this case, the levator scapulae remains functional due to additional innervation provided by C3–C4 spinal nerves. Injury to any of these other nerves would not present with a laterally retracted scapula.

    A. The axillary nerve innervates the deltoid and teres minor muscles. The deltoid muscle abducts the humerus primarily, and the teres minor laterally rotates the humerus.

    B. The long thoracic nerve innervates the serratus anterior, which functions to protract and upwardly rotate the scapula.

    D. The greater occipital nerve is mainly sensory but also contributes to the innervation of the semispinalis capitis. In addition, the greater occipital nerve can be involved in occipital neuralgia.

    E. The suprascapular nerve innervates the supraspinatus and infraspinatus muscles. The supraspinatus abducts the humerus, and the infraspinatus muscle laterally rotates the humerus.
GAS 91–92, 101; N 468; ABR/McM 100

5. **B.** Herpes zoster is a viral disease that remains latent in the dorsal root ganglia of spinal nerves and when the virus becomes active presents as a painful skin lesion. It is associated only with sensory nerve fibers and has no motor involvement. The only answer choice that is solely responsible for sensory innervation is the dorsal root ganglion.

    A. Sympathetic preganglionic fibers are visceral efferent fibers and do not contain sensory information.

    C. The lateral or intermediolateral horns found in T1–L2 are responsible for sympathetic outflow as well as at levels S2–S4 for parasympathetic outflow.

    D. Herpes zoster virus does not reside in the dorsal ramus, although its cutaneous sensory branches will transmit the virus to the back skin. The dorsal rami innervate a small section of skin and native muscles of the back.

    E. The ventral horn, or the anterior horn, contains motor neurons for controlling skeletal muscles.
GAS 61, 112; N 171; ABR/McM 98

6. **E.** Disc herniation in the lumbar region between L4 and L5 affects the L5 spinal nerve roots. Even though the L4 spinal nerve root lies directly between the L4 and L5 vertebrae, it exits from the spinal canal through the intervertebral foramen superior to the intervertebral disc, whereas the L5 spinal nerve root lies directly posterior to the disc and is in greatest jeopardy in a posterolateral disc herniation.

    A. The L1 spinal nerve exits between L1 and L2 vertebrae.

    B. The L2 spinal nerve exits between L2 and L3 vertebrae.

    C. The L3 spinal nerve exits between L3 and L4 vertebrae.

    D. The L4 spinal nerve exits between L4 and L5 vertebrae.
GAS 80; N 170, 165; ABR/McM 101–102

7. **D.** A lumbar puncture is performed by taking a sample of cerebrospinal fluid from the lumbar cistern (the subarachnoid space below the spinal cord) between vertebrae L4 and L5 or sometimes between L3 and L4. It is done in this region because the spinal cord typically ends at the level of L1–L2 and the dural sac ends at the level of S2. Therefore, it is the safest place to do the procedure because it lies between these areas and the risk of injuring the spinal cord is minimized. (Remember in children the cord ends slightly more caudally.)

    A. The spinal cord typically ends at the level of L1–L2 and the dural sac ends at the level of S2.

    B. The spinal cord typically ends at the level of L1–L2 and the dural sac ends at the level of S2.

    C. The spinal cord typically ends at the level of L1–L2 and the dural sac ends at the level of S2.

    E. This would be too low as the spinal cord typically ends at the level of L1–L2 and the dural sac ends at the level of S2.
GAS 107, 119; N 170; ABR/McM 103

8. **B.** The highest points of the iliac crests are used as a landmark for locating the position of the spine of L4 for a lumbar puncture; it is identified and traced medially toward the vertebral column (Tuffier line).

    A. The inferior angles of the scapulae lie at vertebral level T7.

    C. The lowest ribs lead one to T12.

    D. The sacral hiatus is located lower at the distal portion of the sacrum.

    E. The posterior inferior iliac spines lie below S2.
GAS 109, 117–118; N 161; ABR/McM 103

9. A. The anterior longitudinal ligament lies anterior to the vertebral bodies along the vertebral column.
   B. The ligamentum flavum connects the laminae of two adjacent vertebrae.
   C. The nuchal ligament is a posterior continuation of the supraspinous ligament above C7, which connects spinous processes.
   D. The posterior longitudinal ligament lies on the posterior surface of the vertebral bodies.
   E. The transverse cervical (cardinal) ligament is associated with the uterus and not the spinal column (GAS Figs. 2.35 and 2.38).
      GAS 81; N 29, 193; ABR/McM 98, 102

10. B. Compression of nerves at the intervertebral foramen indicates a disc herniation. A disc herniation is characterized by protrusion of the nucleus pulposus through a torn annulus fibrosus posterolaterally into the spinal canal or intervertebral foramen. In general, the posterior longitudinal ligament may be affected by the herniation but is not responsible for the compression of the spinal nerve roots.
    A. A herniated disc is a rupture of the annulus fibrosus of the intervertebral disc, commonly causing a posterolateral displacement of the nucleus pulposus into the vertebral canal.
    C. The posterior longitudinal ligament is the only ligament spanning the posterior aspect of the vertebral bodies. The posterior longitudinal ligament traverses the length of the vertebral canal.
    D. The anterior longitudinal ligament traverses the length of the vertebral canal.
    E. The ligamentum flavum connect the laminae of adjacent vertebrae.
       GAS 80; N 28, 164, 168; ABR/McM 103

11. A. The thoracodorsal nerve innervates the latissimus dorsi, one of major muscles that extends, adducts, and medially rotates the humerus. Whereas the axillary nerve innervates the deltoid muscle which can medially rotate the humerus, it does not extend or adduct the humerus. The medial and lateral pectoral nerves and the lower subscapular nerve supply the other medial rotators of the humerus.
    B. The axillary nerve supplies the deltoid muscle which can rotate the humerus in either direction but is primarily known as the abductor of the humerus.
    C. The dorsal scapular nerve supplies the rhomboids and levator scapulae muscles which elevate and retract the scapula.
    D. The accessory nerve innervates the trapezius which retracts, elevates, and depresses the scapula.
    E. The radial nerve is responsible for the innervation of the muscles and skin over the posterior aspect of the arm and forearm. These muscles are nearly all extensors of the elbow, wrist, and digits.
       GAS 91, 101; N 414; ABR/McM 144, 146

12. C. The long thoracic nerve innervates the serratus anterior, which is responsible for elevation and protraction of the scapula beyond the horizontal level while maintaining its position against the thoracic wall. Along with the thoracodorsal nerve, the long thoracic nerve runs superficially along the thoracic wall and is subject to injury during a mastectomy procedure. Aside from the long thoracic and thoracodorsal nerves, the remaining nerves do not course along the lateral thoracic wall.
    A. The axillary nerve supplies the deltoid and teres minor muscles.
    B. The accessory nerve innervates the trapezius and sternocleidomastoid muscles.
    D. The dorsal scapular nerve is responsible for innervation of the rhomboids and sometimes, the levator scapulae.
    E. The thoracodorsal nerve innervates the latissimus dorsi.
       GAS 726; N 189; ABR/McM 144–149

13. D. The rotator cuff muscles are common sites of damage during shoulder injuries. These muscles include the supraspinatus, infraspinatus, teres minor, and subscapularis (SITS). Initiation of abduction of the humerus (the first 15 degrees) is performed by the supraspinatus, followed by the deltoid from 15 to 90 degrees. Above the horizontal, the scapula is upwardly rotated by the trapezius and serratus anterior muscles, causing the glenoid fossa to turn superiorly and allowing the humerus to move above 90 degrees.
    A. The coracobrachialis is responsible for adduction and flexion of the arm.
    B. The triceps brachii is responsible for extension of the arm and forearm.
    C. The pectoralis minor is responsible for medial rotation and adduction of the humerus. This muscle is therefore not involved in abduction at the glenohumeral joint.
    E. Teres major is responsible for medial rotation and adduction of the humerus. This muscle is therefore not involved in abduction at the glenohumeral joint.
       GAS 711–712, 717; N 180, 409, 412–413; ABR/McM 138

14. C. Spina bifida is a developmental condition resulting from incomplete fusion of the vertebral arches within the lumbar region. Spina bifida occulta commonly presents asymptomatically with midline, lumbar, cutaneous stigmata such as a tuft of hair, and a small skin dimple.
    A. Spina bifida with myelomeningocele is characterized by protrusion of both the meninges and CNS tissues and is often associated with neurologic deficits.
    B. Meningocele is the protrusion of the meninges through the skull or the spinal column, most commonly due to a developmental defect, forming a cyst or a sac filled with cerebrospinal fluid.

D. Spina bifida cystica presents with protrusion of the meninges through the unfused vertebral arches.

E. Rachischisis, also known as spina bifida cystica with myeloschisis, results from a failure of neural folds to fuse and is characterized by protrusion of the spinal cord or spinal nerves and meninges.
GAS 72; N 164; ABR/McM 93

15. **A.** Somatic afferents are responsible for conveying pain, pressure, touch, temperature, and proprioception to the CNS. Afferent fibers carry only sensory stimuli.

B. Somatic efferent fibers convey motor information.

C. Visceral afferents generally carry information regarding the physiologic changes of the internal viscera.

D. Visceral efferents deliver autonomic motor function to three types of tissue: smooth muscle, cardiac muscle, and glandular epithelium. Visceral innervation is associated with the autonomic nervous system, whereas visceral efferents deliver autonomic motor function to three types of tissue: smooth muscle, cardiac muscle, and glandular epithelium.

E. Somatic efferent fibers convey motor information and visceral afferent transmit physiologic changes of the internal viscera.
GAS 31–33; N 6

16. **E.** cerebrospinal fluid is found within the subarachnoid space and is continuous with the ventricles of the brain (cerebrospinal fluid flows from the ventricles into the subarachnoid space).

A. The epidural space, positioned between the dura mater and periosteum of the vertebrae, contains fat and the internal vertebral venous plexus (of Batson).

B. The anterior and posterior longitudinal ligaments traverse the length of the vertebral bodies.

C. The ligamentum flavum connects the laminae of two adjacent vertebrae.

D. The subdural space, between the arachnoid mater and dura mater, exists only as a potential space and does not contain cerebrospinal fluid.
GAS 107, 109, 119; N 170; ABR/McM: 103

17. **B.** The posterior longitudinal ligament is the only ligament spanning the posterior aspect of the vertebral bodies and intervertebral discs. With intervertebral disc herniation, the nucleus pulposus of the intervertebral disc usually protrudes posterolaterally.

A. The supraspinatus connects the spinous processes of adjacent vertebrae.

C. The anterior longitudinal ligament traverses the anterior side of the vertebral bodies and thus would not protect the spinal cord from direct compression.

D. The ligamentum flavum ligaments connect the laminae of adjacent vertebrae.

E. The nuchal ligament is a posterior continuation of the supraspinous ligaments near the C7 vertebrae and runs to the external occipital protuberance.
GAS 81–82; N 30; ABR/McM 98

18. **C.** This is the location of the conus medullaris, a tapered conical projection of the terminal spinal cord at its inferior termination. Although the conus medullaris usually rests at the level of L1 and L2 in the adult, the cauda equina and filum terminale internum extend below beyond the conus medullaris.

A. The spinal cord is present at the levels of T11 and T12.

B. The spinal cord is present at the levels of T11 and T12.

D. The conus medullaris is often situated at L3 in newborns.

E. The conus medullaris is often situated at L3 in newborns.
GAS 101; N 165, 169–170; ABR/McM 101

19. **A.** The sympathetic division of the autonomic nervous system is primarily responsible for vasoconstriction. Division of selected sympathetic trunk ganglia, however, would decrease the sympathetic outflow to the upper limbs.

B. Separation of ventral roots would lead to loss of motor activity.

C. Separation of dorsal roots would lead to loss of sensation.

D. Surgical division of spinal nerves would have unwanted consequences, but such are not related to the increased arterial constriction and the painful ischemia in the digits.

E. Surgical division of the accessory nerves would denervate the sternocleidomastoid and trapezius muscles.
GAS 36–37; N 175; ABR/McM 100–101

20. **D.** The diaphragm is innervated by the phrenic nerve, which arises from C3 to C5.

A. Rhomboid major is innervated by a branch of the ventral ramus of C5 which contributes to the brachial plexus.

B. Serratus anterior is innervated by branches of the ventral rami of C5, 6, and 7 which contribute to the brachial plexus.

C. Supraspinatus is innervated by branches of the ventral rami of C5 and C6 from the brachial plexus.

E. Latissimus dorsi is innervated by branches of the ventral rami of C7 and C8 from the brachial plexus.
GAS 161–162; N 196

21. **C.** The ligamentum flavum is one of the two ligaments found in the vertebral canal and is adherent to the anterior aspect of the vertebral arches and often greatly thickened in spinal pathology. It is thus simultaneously removed upon excision of the lamina.

A. The anterior longitudinal ligament runs along the anterior-most aspect of the vertebral column from C1 to the sacrum and would therefore be unaffected by a laminectomy.

B. Denticulate ligaments are lateral extensions from the pia mater to the dura mater through the arachnoid mater from the foramen magnum to T12.

D. The nuchal ligament is a posterior longitudinal extension continuing from the supraspinous ligament at the level of C7 to the external occipital protuberance (inion).

E. The cruciform ligament is an incorrect answer because it is located anterior to the spinal cord, and thus would not be involved in laminectomy. *GAS 81–83; N 29; ABR/McM 103*

22. **C.** The spinal epidural space is found superficial to the dura mater. It is a fat-filled space extending from C1 to the sacrum.

A. The vertebral canal is the longitudinal canal that extends through the vertebrae, containing the meninges, spinal cord, and associated ligaments. This answer choice does not describe a specific space.

B. The internal vertebral venous plexus is the mostly valveless network of veins extending longitudinally along the vertebral canal. This answer choice does not describe a specific space.

D. The subarachnoid space is a true space containing cerebrospinal fluid It is found within the CNS and extends to the level of S2.

E. The subdural space is a potential space between the dura and the arachnoid mater. Normally, these two layers are fused due to the pressure of cerebrospinal fluid in the subarachnoid space. *GAS 57, 104; N 166; ABR/McM 101*

23. **A.** The supraspinous ligament connects the spinous processes of the vertebrae. The needle, if directed in the midline, will penetrate this structure and the interspinous ligament at this level connecting the adjacent spinous processes.

B. The denticulate ligaments are not correct because they terminate at T12 and are located laterally.

C. The anterior longitudinal ligament extends along the most anterior aspect of the vertebral bodies and can be reached only ventrally.

D. Lumbar puncture is generally performed at the level of L4 or L5. The posterior longitudinal ligament is present at the correct vertebral level but will be punctured only if the procedure is performed incorrectly as in this case, where hematopoietic cells were aspirated from the vertebral body anterior to the ligament.

E. The nuchal ligament extends cranially from the supraspinous ligament in the lower cervical region to the skull. *GAS 81–83; N 29, 165, 167; ABR/McM 102, 103*

24. **B.** The vertebral arteries run through the transverse foramina of cervical vertebrae C6 through C1 and are therefore most closely associated with injury to transverse processes.

A. The anterior spinal artery is located anteriorly along the spinal cord and is not directly associated with the vertebrae.

C. The ascending cervical artery is usually a very small branch of the inferior thyroid artery from the thyrocervical trunk of the subclavian artery, running on the anterior aspect of the vertebrae.

D. The deep cervical artery arises from the costocervical trunk and is also a very small artery that courses along the posterior aspect of the cervical vertebrae to supply deep neck muscles.

E. The posterior spinal arteries are adherent to the posterior aspect of the spinal cord. *GAS 102; N 29, 176; ABR/McM 98–99, 111*

25. **B.** Hyperkyphosis is an increased primary curvature of the spinal column (posterior convexity). This curvature is associated with thoracic and sacral regions and is most likely this patient's clinical condition.

A. Scoliosis is defined as a lateral deviation of the spinal column to either side.

C. Spinal stenosis is a narrowing of the vertebral canal and is not directly associated with a displacement of the spinal column.

D. Hyperlordosis is an increased secondary curvature (concave posteriorly) affecting the cervical and lumbar regions.

E. A herniated disc is a rupture of the annulus fibrosus of the intervertebral disc, commonly causing a posterolateral displacement of the nucleus pulposus into the vertebral canal. *GAS 75; N 162; ABR/McM 87*

Answers 26–50

26. **B.** The accessory nerve is the eleventh cranial nerve (CN XI) and innervates both the trapezius and sternocleidomastoid muscles. The loss of CN XI results in drooping of the shoulder due to paralysis of the trapezius, whose superior fibers represent the only muscle to raise the point of the shoulder. In addition to the clinical findings of the MRI, one can test the innervation of this nerve by asking the patient to shrug his or her shoulders against resistance (testing the trapezius), as well as turning his or her head against resistance (testing the sternocleidomastoid).

A. The thoracodorsal nerve innervates the latissimus dorsi, which has no direct action on the shoulder girdle.

C. The dorsal scapular nerve innervates the rhomboid muscles and usually the levator scapulae muscle.

D. The greater occipital nerve is primarily a sensory nerve innervating the posterior aspect of the scalp.

E. The axillary nerve is a branch of the brachial plexus and innervates the deltoid and teres minor muscles. It is not involved in shoulder elevation. *GAS 89, 101; N 138, 140, 183; ABR/McM 100*

27. B. The transverse ligament of the atlas anchors the dens anteriorly laterally to prevent posterior displacement of the dens. This ligament has been torn in this injury.
   A. The anterior longitudinal ligament runs on the anterior aspect of the vertebrae and is not affected.
   C. The ligamentum flavum is found on the posterior aspect of the vertebral canal and does not contact the anteriorly placed dens.
   D. The supraspinous ligament is located along the spinous processes of the vertebrae.
   E. The nuchal ligament is a longitudinal extension of the supraspinous ligament above the level of C7.
   GAS 68, 69; N 30; ABR/McM 98

28. B. The sternocleidomastoid muscle is innervated by CN XI and functions in contralateral rotation (unilateral contraction) and flexion (bilateral contraction) of the neck.
   A. The iliocostalis thoracis muscle is found in the deep back and functions to maintain posture. It is not associated with neck flexion.
   C. Rhomboid major is innervated by the dorsal scapular nerve and serves to adduct the scapulae.
   D. Rhomboid minor is innervated by the dorsal scapular nerve and serves to adduct the scapulae.
   E. Teres major is innervated by the lower subscapular nerve and serves to medially rotate and adduct the humerus.
   GAS 89, 91, 101, 122; N 171; ABR/McM 39, 138

29. C. The cruciform (also called the transverse ligament of the atlas) ligament is a stabilizing ligament found at the skull base and C1/C2. It attaches to the pedicles and helps stabilize the dens. Rupture of this ligament often severs the spinal cord and therefore can be fatal.
   A. The pedicles are bony structures connecting the vertebral arches to the vertebral body. The ligamentum flavum runs on the posterior aspect of the vertebral canal and is more closely associated with the laminae than to the pedicles of the vertebrae.
   B. The nuchal ligament is a longitudinal extension of the supraspinous ligament from C7 to the occiput, both running on the most posterior aspect of the vertebrae along the spinous processes.
   D. The posterior longitudinal ligament extends the length of the anterior aspect of the vertebral canal and is medial to the pedicles.
   E. The supraspinous ligament is located along the spinous processes of the vertebrae from C7 inferiorly.
   GAS 68; N 30; ABR/McM 98

30. A. Spondylolysis is the anterior displacement of one or more vertebrae. Due to more horizontally oriented articular facets, the cervical vertebrae are less tightly locked than other vertebrae. This can lead to dislocations with locking of the displaced articular processes a condition known as "jumped facets."

   B. It is much less common in the thoracic vertebrae due to the stabilizing factor of the ribs.
   C. Lumbar vertebrae are somewhat susceptible to this problem because of the pressures at lower levels of the spine and the sagittal angles of the articular facets.
   D. It is not seen in the sacral vertebrae because they are fused together.
   E. It is not seen in the sacral vertebrae because they are fused together.
   GAS 83–84; N 167; ABR/McM 91, 113

31. D. The internal vertebral plexus (of Batson) surrounds the dura mater in the epidural space; hence the bleeding would cause the hematoma in this space.
   A. The subarachnoid space, containing the cerebrospinal fluid is located between pia and arachnoid mater. A subarachnoid hemorrhage would most likely result from a ruptured intracerebral aneurysm.
   B. A subdural hematoma would result most likely from a venous bleed from a torn cerebral vein as it enters the superior sagittal sinus within the skull.
   C. The central canal is located within the gray matter of the spinal cord.
   E. The lumbar cistern is an enlargement of the subarachnoid space between the conus medullaris of the spinal cord and the caudal end of the subarachnoid space.
   GAS 104; N 175; ABR/McM 102

32. D. In the lumbar region spinal nerves exit the vertebral column below their named vertebrae. In an L4, L5 intervertebral disc herniation, the L5 spinal nerve would be affected as it descends between L4 and L5 vertebrae to exit below the L5 level.
   A. L2, L3, and L4 spinal nerves have already exited above the level of herniation.
   B. L2, L3, and L4 spinal nerves have already exited above the level of herniation.
   C. L2, L3, and L4 spinal nerves have already exited above the level of herniation.
   E. S1 will exit below the L4, L5 intervertebral disc herniation.
   GAS 80, 111; N 164, 170

33. E. Posterior intercostal arteries supply the deep back muscles in the thoracic region, which are responsible for extending and laterally bending the trunk. The other muscles listed are not responsible for extension and lateral flexion of the trunk.
   A. The subscapular artery supplies the subscapularis muscle.
   B. The thoracodorsal artery supplies the latissimus dorsi.
   C. The anterior intercostal supplies the upper nine intercostal spaces.
   D. The suprascapular artery supplies the supraspinatus and infraspinatus muscles.
   GAS 102–103; N 168, 197

34. A. The atlantoaxial joint is a synovial joint responsible for rotation of the head, not flexion, abduction, extension, or adduction.
B. The atlantooccipital joint is primarily involved in flexion and extension of the head on the neck.
C. Lateral flexion of the head is not affected by atlantoaxial joint dislocation.
D. The atlantooccipital joint is primarily involved in flexion and extension of the head on the neck.
E. Adduction (lateral reduction) of the head is not affected by atlantoaxial joint dislocation.
GAS 69; N 22, 26, 28–29; ABR/McM 112

35. D. The internal vertebral plexus (of Batson) lies external to the dura mater in the epidural space. To aspirate excess blood, the physician must pass the needle through the ligamentum flavum to reach the epidural space where the blood would accumulate.
A. The spinal cord is located within the dural sac.
B. The pia mater is located on the surface of the spinal cord, which lies within the dural sac.
C. The arachnoid mater is located within the dural sac.
D. The ligamentum flavum is located within the dural sac deep to the epidural space.
GAS 104; N 175; ABR/McM 102

36. E. The T4 thoracic vertebra articulates with the head of the fifth rib. The head of the rib has two facets. The rib articulates with the superior facet on the body of its own vertebra (the fourth rib articulates with the superior facet T4 vertebra) and with the inferior facet on the body of the vertebra above (the fourth rib articulates with the inferior facet of T3 vertebra). Taking the T4 vertebra into consideration, the superior facet of this vertebra articulates with the head of the fourth rib and the inferior facet articulates with the head of the fifth rib.
A. The fourth rib has two points of articulation (the rib head forms a joint with the vertebral body and the rib tubercle forms a costotransverse joint) on the T4 vertebra, so when the latter is injured, the vertebra and rib move as a unit, whereas the fifth rib has only one articulation with T4.
B. The neck of the fourth rib will likely not be injured.
C. The head of the third rib will likely not be injured.
D. The tubercle of the third rib will likely not be injured.
GAS 126–127; N 192; ABR/McM 102

37. E. The teres major is responsible for adduction and medial rotation of the humerus.
A. The teres minor is responsible for lateral rotation of the humerus.
B. The triceps brachii is responsible for extension of the elbow.
C. The supraspinatus is responsible for the first 15 degrees of abduction of the humerus.
D. The infraspinatus is a lateral rotator of the humerus.
GAS 717; N 180, 413; ABR/McM 105–107

38. B. The infraspinatus is responsible for lateral rotation of the humerus (along with the teres minor, not a choice here).
A. The teres major is responsible for adduction and medial rotation of the humerus.
C. The latissimus dorsi is responsible for adduction, extension, and medial rotation of the humerus.
D. The trapezius is an elevator of the scapula and rotates the scapula during abduction of the humerus above the horizontal plane.
E. The supraspinatus is responsible for the first 15 degrees of abduction.
GAS 717; N 413, 422; ABR/McM 104–106

39. A. When a lumbar puncture is performed, the needle must penetrate the ligamentum flavum, the dura mater, and finally the arachnoid mater to reach the subarachnoid space where the cerebrospinal fluid is located. The lumbar cistern is a continuation of the subarachnoid space below the conus medullaris.
B. The internal vertebral plexus (of Batson) lies external to the dura mater in the epidural space.
C. The pia mater is adherent to the spinal cord.
D. The ligamentum flavum is located deep to the epidural space.
E. The posterior longitudinal ligament is attached to the posterior aspect of the vertebral bodies.
GAS 109, 117–119; N 174; ABR/McM 103

40. C. The subarachnoid space, containing the cerebrospinal fluid is located between the pia and the arachnoid mater. cerebrospinal fluid circulates within the subarachnoid space and can be aspirated only from this location.
A. The epidural space does not contain cerebrospinal fluid. The epidural space contains the epidural fat and the internal vertebral venous plexus (Batson veins) and is the site to inject an anesthetic for epidural anesthesia.
B. The subdural space does not contain cerebrospinal fluid. The subdural space is only a potential space between the dura and arachnoid mater.
D. The pretracheal space does not contain cerebrospinal fluid.
E. Although the central canal, contained within the substance of the spinal cord, does contain cerebrospinal fluid extraction of cerebrospinal fluid from this space would result in spinal cord injury.
GAS 109; N 120; ABR/McM 101

41. A. General somatic afferent fibers are conveyed from the skin of the back via the dorsal rami.

B. Communicating rami contain general visceral efferent (sympathetic) fibers and general visceral afferent fibers of the autonomic nervous system.

C. Ventral rami convey mixed sensory and motor nerves to/from all other parts of the trunk and limbs excluding the back.

D. The ventral roots contain only efferent (motor) fibers.

E. Intercostal nerves are the ventral rami of T1–T11. The ventral ramus of T12 is the subcostal nerve. *GAS 31–33; ABR/McM 99*

42. D. The conus medullaris is usually located at the L1–L2 vertebral level; therefore any choice that contains this region is the correct answer.

A. L3–L4 is a common location to perform lumbar puncture, but it is caudal to the apex of the conus medullaris.

B. L3 is caudal to the conus medullaris.

C. L4 is caudal to the conus medullaris.

E. T11 is superior to the conus medullaris. *GAS 101; N 169, 170; ABR/McM 101*

43. D. Because the meninges and spinal cord are included in the protrusion, the patient's condition is a classic presentation of spina bifida with myelomeningocele.

A. Avulsion of the meninges would not involve protrusion of the spinal cord.

B. Meningitis is an inflammation of the meninges caused by bacteria, viral, or numerous other irritants (e.g., blood). It does not cause deformation of the vertebrae or result in protrusion of spinal cord contents.

C. Spina bifida occulta is a normally asymptomatic condition in which the vertebral laminae fail to fuse completely during embryologic development. A tuft of hair is commonly seen growing over the affected region (usually midline lumbar in position).

E. If the protrusion contains only meninges but no CNS tissue, it is known as spina bifida with meningocele. *GAS 72; N 164; ABR/McM 93*

44. C. Somatic afferent fibers convey localized pain, typically from the body wall and limbs.

A. Visceral afferents convey autonomic nervous system sensory information. Pain from these fibers will present as dull and diffuse.

B. Somatic efferent fibers convey motor innervation to skeletal muscle.

D. Sympathetic preganglionic fibers are visceral efferent fibers and do not contain sensory information.

E. Parasympathetic preganglionic fibers are also visceral efferents and do not contain sensory information. *GAS 31–33; N 6*

45. B. In addition to lateral flexion, the lumbar vertebrae allow for flexion, extension, and rotation.

A. Circumduction is limited due to the orientation of the articular facets.

C. Abduction is limited due to the orientation of the articular facets.

D. Adduction is limited due to the orientation of the articular facets.

E. Inversion is limited due to the orientation of the articular facets. *GAS 62–69; N 162; ABR/McM 87*

46. D. The internal vertebral venous (Batson) venous plexus, in general, is a valveless network of veins located in the epidural space of the vertebral canal. The lack of valves can provide a route for the metastasis of cancer (e.g., from the prostate or breast to the brain) because the flow of blood is bidirectional due to local pressures.

A. The length of the internal vertebral venous (Batson) plexus is irrelevant to the question.

B. This is incorrect because the internal vertebral venous (Batson) plexus, in general, does not have valves or one-way movement of blood.

C. The internal vertebral venous (Batson) plexus is located within the epidural space, not the subarachnoid.

E. The internal vertebral venous (Batson) plexus is located within the epidural, not the subdural space. *GAS 104; N 175; ABR/McM 102*

47. E. The acromion (the highest point of the shoulder) is the part of the scapula that forms the "point" of the shoulder.

A. The coracoid process is located more inferomedially.

B. The superior (or medial) angle of the scapula is located near the midline of the back.

C. The glenoid fossa of the scapula articulates with the head of the humerus to form the glenohumeral joint.

D. The spine of the scapula is located posteriorly and separates supraspinous and infraspinous fossae. *GAS 702–711; N 36, 192, 409*

48. D. All of the spinal nerves from C6 and below will be affected, so the thoracodorsal nerve (C7–C8) which innervates latissimus will be lost.

A. The trapezius and sternocleidomastoid muscles will be intact because they are innervated by the accessory nerve.

B. The trapezius and sternocleidomastoid muscles will be intact because they are innervated by the accessory nerve.

C. The diaphragm will work properly as its motor nerve supply is derived from the phrenic nerve (C3–C5).

E. The deltoid will not be affected because its nerve motor supply is from the axillary nerve derived from C5 and C6. *GAS 91, 101; N 414*

49. C. Spina bifida cystica refers to spina bifida with a meningocele or myelomeningocele and is the correct answer.

 A. Cranium bifida could present with meningocele in the skull, but it would not be located in the lower back.

 B. Spina bifida occulta is a defect in the formation of the vertebral arches and does not usually present with meningocele.

 D. Hemothorax refers to blood accumulation in the pleural space surrounding the lungs.

 E. Caudal regression syndrome presents with loss or deformation of the lower part of the spine, spinal cord, and the lower limbs and is not related to a meningocele or myelomeningocele, in general.
 GAS 72; N 164; ABR/McM 93

50. B. The lumbar triangle (of Petit) is bordered medially by the latissimus dorsi, laterally by the external abdominal oblique, and inferiorly by the iliac crest. The floor of Petit triangle is formed by the internal abdominal oblique, and this is a possible site of herniation.

 A. This is not the best answer because this lump is described as soft and pliable, which would not likely indicate a tumor, as tumors tend to be hard masses.

 C. An indirect inguinal hernia is located in the inguinal canal of the anterior abdominal wall.

 D. A direct inguinal hernia is located in the inguinal (Hesselbach) triangle of the anterior abdominal wall.

 E. A femoral hernia occurs below the inguinal ligament.
 GAS 87–88; N 161, 180; ABR/McM 105

Answers 51–75

51. D. This question tests anatomic knowledge relating to typical vertebra and the spinal cord. Intervertebral disc herniations occur when the nucleus pulposus of the intervertebral disc protrudes through the annulus fibrosus into the intervertebral foramen or vertebral canal. The most common protrusion is posterolaterally, where the annulus fibrosus is not reinforced by the posterior longitudinal ligament. The inferior and superior vertebral notches frame the intervertebral foramen, so this is the most likely location of compression.

 A. The denticulate ligaments are lateral extensions of pia mater that anchor to the dura mater, and help maintain the spinal cord in position within the subarachnoid space.

 B. The vertebral foramen is the canal through which the spinal cord passes; while this may also be a place of compression, it is not the most likely site of herniation.

 C. Articular facets are the locations where the articular processes of the vertebrae articulate with each other.

 E. Intercostovertebral joints are locations where vertebral bodies articulate with ribs.
 GAS 101–103, 111–112; N 28, 164; ABR/McM 103

52. C. Caudal anesthesia is used to block the sacral spinal nerves that carry sensation from the perineum. This procedure is commonly used by anesthesiologists to relieve pain during labor and childbirth. Administration of local anesthetic to the epidural space is via the sacral hiatus, which opens between the sacral cornua.

 A. The anterior sacral foramina are located on the pelvic surface of the sacrum and are not palpable from a dorsal approach.

 B. The posterior sacral foramina are the openings through which dorsal rami of sacral nerves exit and are not palpable landmarks.

 D. The intervertebral foramina are the openings through which spinal nerves exit in cervical, thoracic, and lumbar regions.

 E. The median sacral crest is cranial to the injection site.
 GAS 109–113; N 166; ABR/McM 95

53. D. Patients with persistent headache or back pain with areas of localized tenderness in women who recently had breast cancer suggests metastasis to either brain or cervical spine. The typical place of metastasis in the cervical spine is the vertebral pedicles.

 A. The typical place of metastasis in the cervical spine is the vertebral pedicles.

 B. The typical place of metastasis in the cervical spine is the vertebral pedicles.

 C. The typical place of metastasis in the cervical spine is the vertebral pedicles.

 E. The typical place of metastasis in the cervical spine is the vertebral pedicles.
 GAS 55, 60, 66; N 27, 164; ABR/McM 89

54. A. The suprascapular nerve passes through the superior scapular notch, deep to the superior transverse scapular ligament. This nerve is most likely affected in a fracture of the scapula as described in the question.

 B. The thoracodorsal nerve runs behind the axillary artery and lies superficial to the subscapularis muscle and would therefore be protected.

 C. The axillary nerve passes posteriorly through the quadrangular space, which is distal to the superior scapular notch.

 D. The subscapular nerve originates from the posterior cord of the brachial plexus, which is distal to the site of fracture.

 E. The suprascapular nerve is correct, but not in combination with the thoracodorsal nerve, which runs behind the axillary artery and lies superficial to the subscapularis muscle and would therefore be protected.
 GAS 717–718; N417, 468

55. E. Klippel-Feil syndrome is a congenital defect in which there is a reduction, or extensive fusion of one or more cervical vertebrae. It often manifests as a short, stiff neck with limited motion.
- **A.** Hyperlordosis is an abnormal increase in lumbar curvature.
- **B.** Hyperkyphosis ("hunchback") is an abnormal increase in thoracic curvature.
- **C.** Scoliosis is a lateral curvature of the spine.
- **D.** Spina bifida can present with deformities in the lumbar region.
  GAS 76; N BP19

56. A. Spondylolysis is a condition in which the region between the superior and inferior articular facets (on the posterior arch of the L5 vertebra) is damaged or missing, which is not the case in this example.
- **B.** Spondylolisthesis is an anterior vertebral displacement created by an irregularity in the anterior margin of the vertebral column such that L5 and the overlying L4 (and sometimes L3) protrude forward rather than being restrained by S1.
- **C.** Herniation is a protrusion of the nucleus pulposus through the annulus fibrosus, and this is not associated with vertebral dislocation.
- **D.** Hyperlordosis is an abnormal increase in lumbar curvature.
- **E.** Scoliosis is an abnormal lateral curvature of the spine.
  GAS 83–84; N 167; ABR/McM 91, 113

57. C. Chiari II malformation includes herniation of the brainstem and cerebellum vermis below the foramen magnum.
- **A.** Meningocele is a small defect in the cranium in which only the meninges herniate.
- **B.** Klippel-Feil syndrome results from an abnormal number of cervical vertebral bodies.
- **D.** Hydrocephalus results from obstruction of its flow, or interference with cerebrospinal fluid absorption.
- **E.** Tethered cord syndrome is a congenital anomaly often caused by a defective closure of the neural tube. This syndrome is often characterized by a low-lying conus medullaris and a thickened filum terminale internum.
  N 117

58. A. Spondylolisthesis is an anterior displacement created by an irregularity in the anterior margin of the vertebral column such that L5 and the overlying L4 (and sometimes L3) protrude forward. There is a fracture at the zygapophyseal joint including the area of the pars interarticularis. This condition is known as spondylolysis. Additionally, anterior displacement of the vertebrae is known as spondylolisthesis. Therefore, in this patient, a spondylolysis has led to a spondylolisthesis.

- **B.** Spondylolysis is a condition in which the region between the superior and inferior articular facets (on the posterior arch of the L5 vertebra) is damaged or missing, which is not the case in this example.
- **C.** Compression vertebral fracture is a collapse of vertebral bodies as a result of trauma.
- **D.** Intervertebral disc herniations occur when the nucleus pulposus protrudes through the annulus fibrosus into the intervertebral foramen or vertebral canal. The most common protrusion is posterolaterally, where the annulus fibrosus is not reinforced by the posterior longitudinal ligament.
- **E.** Klippel-Feil syndrome results from an abnormal number of cervical vertebral bodies.
  GAS 83–84; N 167; ABR/McM 91, 113

59. A. The odontoid process, or the dens, projects superiorly from the body of the axis and articulates with the anterior arch of the atlas.
- **B.** The posterior tubercle of the atlas is a bony eminence on the outer surface of the posterior arch of the atlas.
- **C.** The atlantooccipital joint is primarily involved in flexion and extension of the head on the neck.
- **D.** The inferior articular facet is where the axis articulates with the C3 vertebra (*GAS* Fig. 2.21).

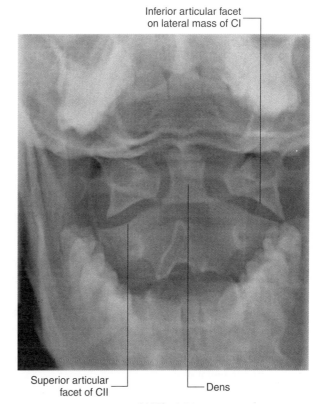

Inferior articular facet on lateral mass of CI

Superior articular facet of CII

Dens

• **GAS Fig. 2.21**

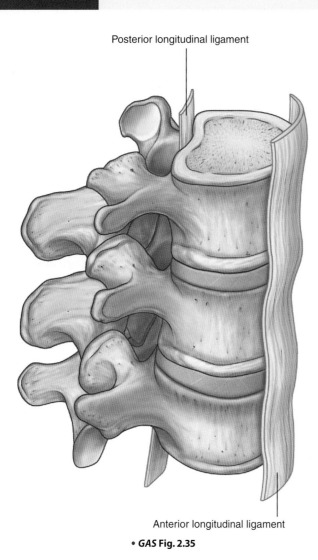

Posterior longitudinal ligament

Anterior longitudinal ligament

• *GAS* Fig. 2.35

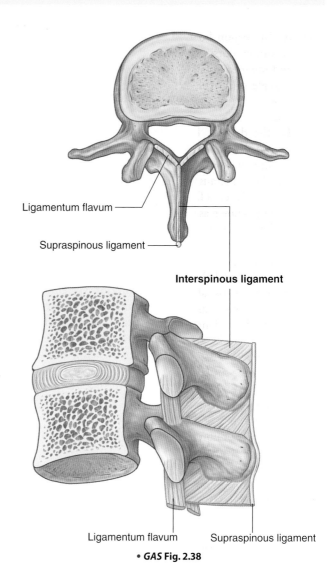

Ligamentum flavum

Supraspinous ligament

Interspinous ligament

Ligamentum flavum   Supraspinous ligament

• *GAS* Fig. 2.38

E. The anterior tubercle of the atlas is a bony eminence on the outer surface of the anterior arch of the atlas.
GAS 69; N BP34; ABR/McM 89, 112

60. B. The anterior longitudinal ligament is a strong fibrous band that covers and connects the anterolateral aspect of the vertebral bodies and intervertebral discs; it maintains stability and prevents hyperextension. It can be torn by cervical hyperextension.
A. The ligamentum flavum helps maintain upright posture by connecting the laminae of two adjacent vertebrae.
C. The posterior longitudinal ligament runs within the vertebral canal supporting the posterior aspect of the vertebral bodies and prevents hyperflexion.
D. The annulus fibrosus is the outer fibrous part of an intervertebral disc.
E. The interspinous ligament connects adjacent spinous processes.
GAS 81; N 193; ABR/McM 98, 102

61. C. The denticulate ligaments are lateral extensions of pia mater that attach to the dura mater between the dorsal and ventral roots of the spinal nerves. These ligaments are thought to function in keeping the spinal cord stabilized.
A. The posterior longitudinal ligament supports the posterior aspect of the vertebral bodies within the vertebral canal.
B. The tentorium cerebelli is a layer of dura mater that supports the occipital lobes of the cerebral hemispheres and covers the cerebellum.
D. The ligamentum flavum helps maintain upright posture by connecting the laminae of two adjacent vertebrae.
E. The nuchal ligament is a posterior extension of the supraspinous ligaments extending from the C7 vertebra to the external occipital protuberance.
GAS 106–107; N 174–175; ABR/McM 98, 100, 111

62. A. The region bounded by the upper border of the latissimus dorsi, the lateral border of the trapezius, and the medial border of the scapula is known as the triangle of auscultation. Lung sounds can be heard most clearly from this location because minimal tissue intervenes between the skin of the back and the lungs.

B. The deltoid, levator scapulae, and trapezius do not form the borders of the so-called "triangle of auscultation."

C. The latissimus dorsi, external abdominal oblique, and iliac crest form the border of the lumbar triangle (also known as the inferior lumbar triangle of Petit).

D. The quadratus lumborum, internal abdominal oblique, and inferior border of the twelfth rib form the border of the superior lumbar triangle (of Grynfeltt).

E. The rectus abdominis, inguinal ligament, and inferior epigastric vessels form the border of the inguinal triangle (of Hesselbach).

GAS 87, 90; N 161, 257; ABR/McM 105–106

63. C. The weakness in shoulder movement results from denervation of the teres minor and deltoid by the axillary nerve, which passes through the quadrangular space. Quadrangular space syndrome occurs when there is hypertrophy of the muscles that border the quadrangular space or fibrosis of portions of the muscles that are in contact with the nerve. Numbness of the skin over the deltoid muscle may result if the superior lateral brachial cutaneous branch of the axillary nerve is affected.

A. The suprascapular nerve innervates the supraspinatus and infraspinatus muscles. The supraspinatus abducts the humerus, and the infraspinatus muscle laterally rotates the humerus.

B. Teres major is innervated by the lower subscapular nerve and serves to medially rotate and adduct the humerus.

D. The radial nerve is responsible for the innervation of the muscles and skin on the posterior aspect of the arm and forearm.

E. Ulnar nerve damage would manifest with hand movement abnormalities.

GAS 718; N 414

64. D. In this MRI a posterolateral herniation between L4 and L5 exists. In the lumbar region, spinal nerves exit the vertebral column below their named vertebrae. In an L4–L5 intervertebral disc herniation, the L5 spinal nerve would be affected as it descends between L4 and L5 vertebrae to exit below the L5 level.

A. Compression of nerve L3 would produce numbness on the anterior thigh.

B. Compression of nerve L4 would produce numbness over the knee.

C. Compression of nerve L2 would produce numbness of the upper anterior thigh.

E. Compression of nerve S1 would produce numbness on the lateral ankle and foot.

GAS 80; N 165; ABR/McM 101–102

65. B. The great radicular artery (of Adamkiewicz) is important for blood supply to anterior and posterior spinal arteries. The location of this artery should be noted during surgery because damage to it can result in dire consequences, including paraplegia (loss of all sensation and voluntary movement inferior and at the level of the injury).

A. Injury to the left vertebral artery would not be likely due its superior location to the surgical site.

C. Ligation of the posterior spinal artery would not occur because of its protected location inside the vertebral canal.

D. Transection of the conus medullaris of the spinal cord would not occur as this structure is located at L1, L2 levels and is, again, protected inside the vertebral canal.

E. Division of the thoracic sympathetic trunk would not be likely as the symptoms described include limb paralysis, which would not be a consequence of sympathetic disruption (*GAS* Fig. 2.55A).

GAS 102–103; N 176

66. C. Scoliosis can be a secondary condition in such disorders as muscular dystrophy and polio in which abnormal muscle action does not keep the normal alignment of the vertebral column and results in a lateral curvature.

A. Hyperlordosis is increased secondary curvature of the lumbar region. It can be caused by stress on the lower back and is quite common during late pregnancy.

B. Hyperkyphosis is increased primary curvature of the thoracic regions and produces a hunchback deformity. It can be secondary to tuberculosis, producing a "gibbus deformity," which results in angulated kyphosis at the lesion site.

D. Spina bifida is a congenital defect and would not present as a result of muscular dystrophy or polio.

E. Osteoarthritis most commonly presents with age from normal "wear and tear." It is highly unlikely in a 23-year-old woman.

GAS 74; N 162; ABR/McM 87

67. C. The intervertebral disc consists of an outer annulus fibrosus and inner nucleus pulposus. The tensile strength comes from the annulus fibrosus, which limits rotation between vertebrae.

A. Hyaline cartilage is found on articular surfaces in synovial joints and epiphysial plates.

B. Elastic cartilage is found in, for example, the epiglottis.

D. The epiphysial plate is a type of hyaline cartilage.

E. Elastic fibers are found in the epiglottis.

GAS 79; N 164, 168; ABR/McM 103

68. E. Notochord remnant forms the gelatinous nucleus pulposus and the surrounding mesenchyme which is derived from the adjacent sclerotome forms the concentric rings of the annulus fibrosus.

A. Nucleus pulposus is a remnant of the notochord, and there is no direct involvement of neural crest cells in its development.

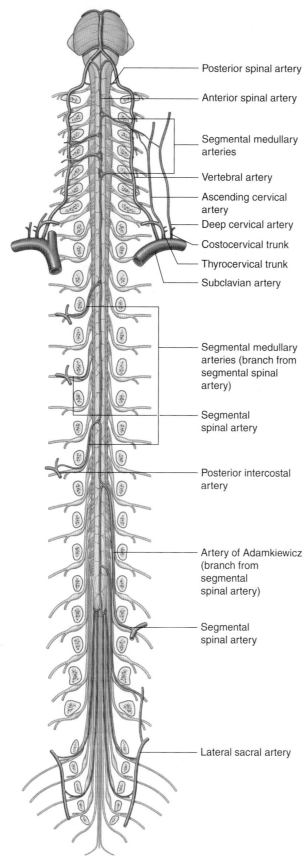

Posterior spinal artery

Anterior spinal artery

Segmental medullary arteries

Vertebral artery

Ascending cervical artery

Deep cervical artery

Costocervical trunk

Thyrocervical trunk

Subclavian artery

Segmental medullary arteries (branch from segmental spinal artery)

Segmental spinal artery

Posterior intercostal artery

Artery of Adamkiewicz (branch from segmental spinal artery)

Segmental spinal artery

Lateral sacral artery

• *GAS* **Fig. 2.55A**

B. There is no direct neural crest or ectoderm involvement in development of either.

C. The sclerotome is involved in development of the annulus fibrosus, but there is no sclerotome or myotome involvement in the development of the nucleus pulposus.

D. While the sclerotome is involved in the development of the annulus fibrosus, there is no neural crest cell involvement in the development of the nucleus pulposus.
GAS 79; N 164, 168; ABR/McM 103

69. B. Horner syndrome is characterized by, among other things, constricted pupils, sunken eyes, partially drooping eyelid (blepharoptosis), and dryness of the skin on the face. It is caused by problems in sympathetic autonomic pathways such as damage to the lateral horn. Horner syndrome is a result of disruption to the sympathetic supply of the head whose presynaptic cell bodies are located in the lateral gray horn of the spinal cord in the upper thoracic region.

A. The anterior gray horn has cell bodies for somatic efferent fibers.

C. Cells in the posterior gray horn receive the signals from sensory fibers whose cell bodies are located in the spinal ganglia.

D. There are no sympathetic nerve cell bodies located in the spinal ganglia.

E. There are no sympathetic nerve cell bodies located in the white matter of the spinal cord.
N 172; ABR/McM 100

70. D. Semispinalis capitis is the only muscle among the choices that is supplied by dorsal rami of cervical nerves. All of the other muscles are supplied by the ventral rami.

A. The rhomboid major is innervated by the dorsal scapular nerve, a branch of the ventral ramus of C5.

B. The levator scapulae is often innervated by branches of C3 and C4, as well as from branches of the dorsal scapular nerve.

C. The rhomboid minor is innervated by the dorsal scapular nerve, a branch of the ventral ramus of C5.

E. The latissimus dorsi is innervated by the thoracodorsal nerve, which contains fibers from the ventral rami of C7 and C8.
GAS 95; N 184; ABR/McM 110

71. C. The splenius capitis is supplied by the dorsal rami of C3 and C4.

A. Rectus capitis posterior major and minor muscles are innervated by branches of the suboccipital nerve.

B. The greater occipital nerve supplies the semispinalis capitis.

D. The obliquus capitis muscles are innervated by branches of the suboccipital nerve which also supplies the rectus capitis posterior major and minor.

E. The obliquus capitis muscles are innervated by branches of the suboccipital nerve which also supplies the rectus capitis posterior major and minor. *GAS 95, 100; N Table 3.2–3.3; ABR/McM 109*

72. D. With the type of injury described, the most likely fracture is of the pars interarticularis (pedicle) of the C2 vertebrae. This is also known as a "hangman's" fracture. In a hanging, the pedicles of C2 are fractured and the cruciform ligament is torn which results in the upper spinomedullary junction being crushed by the odontoid process, killing the person.

A. The odontoid process is typically not fractured in such cases.

B. There is no transverse process involvement.

C. The C1 vertebra is not necessarily involved so there may be no lateral mass involvement.

E. There is no spinous process involvement. *GAS 84, 105; N 26 (Table 2.1); ABR/McM 113*

73. A. The thoracic vertebrae contribute to the primary curvature, convex posteriorly. Wedge fracture here from osteoporosis, infection, or trauma leads to hyperkyphosis.

B. Scoliosis is an abnormal lateral curvature of the vertebrae, which also involves rotation of the vertebrae on one another.

C. Hyperlordosis occurs when the secondary curvature, concave posteriorly, is accentuated in the lumbar region.

D. This would not lead to normal spinal curvature.

E. This would not lead to a primary spinal curvature. *GAS 75; N 162; ABR/McM 87*

74. C. Somatic afferent fibers convey localized pain, typically from the body wall and limbs, and the cell bodies are found in the dorsal root ganglia.

A. The dorsal horn is found at all spinal cord levels and is comprised of sensory nuclei that receive and process incoming somatosensory information.

B. The lateral horn comprises presynaptic autonomic neurons, not sensory neurons.

C. The sympathetic trunk ganglia deliver the sympathetic innervation to the body.

D. White rami communicantes carry preganglionic sympathetic fibers and are called *white* because the fibers contain more myelin. *GAS 35, 112; N 171; ABR/McM 98*

75. B. The transverse ligament of the atlas anchors the dens anteriorly laterally to prevent posterior displacement of the dens, which has been torn in this injury.

A. The anterior longitudinal ligament runs on the anterior aspect of the vertebral bodies and is not affected.

C. The interspinous ligaments attach adjacent spinous processes to each other from C2 to the sacrum. It restricts the degree of separation of the spinous processes during flexion.

D. The supraspinous ligament is located along the tips of spinous processes of vertebrae.

E. The nuchal ligament is a longitudinal extension of the supraspinous ligaments above the level of C7. *GAS 68-69; N 30; ABR/McM 98*

Answers 76–100

76. E. Scoliosis is defined as a lateral deviation of the spinal column to either side and is often associated with a "rib-hump" as seen on examination when bending forward to touch the toes.

A. Hyperkyphosis is an increased primary curvature (convex posteriorly) of the spinal column. This curvature is associated with thoracic and sacral regions and is not likely this patient's clinical condition.

B. Spondylosis is the general term meaning degeneration of the spinal column for any number of reasons.

C. Hyperlordosis is the increased secondary curvature (concave posteriorly) affecting the cervical and lumbar regions.

D. Spondylolisthesis is an anterior displacement of a portion of the vertebra consequent to a fracture of the pars interarticularis (spondylolysis). *GAS 74; N 162; ABR/McM 87*

77. D. This is a typical case of Pott disease, which is disseminated tuberculosis in the spine. This eventually leads to destruction of the thoracic vertebral bodies and intervertebral discs and collapse of the vertebrae.

A. Spondylolysis is a fracture of the neural arch. Tuberculosis of the vertebral column typically affects the vertebral bodies.

B. Spondylolisthesis is an anterior displacement of one or more vertebrae, often following fracture of the neural arch or spondylolysis. Tuberculosis of the vertebral column typically affects the vertebral bodies.

C. Herniation of intervertebral discs is not usually a consequence of tuberculosis infection.

E. Wedge fractures are typically the result of hyperflexion and crushing of the anterior portion of vertebral bodies, often related to osteoporosis. *GAS 73, 77; N 162*

78. E. In the cervical region, spinal nerves exit the vertebral column above their named vertebrae.

A. From the thoracic region and below, the spinal nerves exit the vertebral column below their named vertebrae, but in the cervical region, spinal nerves exit above their named vertebrae.

B. The dorsal horn of the spinal cord would not be affected by a mass at the intervertebral foramen.

C. From the thoracic region and below, the spinal nerves exit the vertebral column below their named vertebrae, but in the cervical region, spinal nerves exit above their named vertebrae.

D. The dorsal horn of the spinal cord would not be affected by a mass at the intervertebral foramen. *GAS 111–112; N 170*

79. C. Lumbar puncture is generally performed at the level of L4–L5. The spinal cord ends at the level of L1–L2 in adults and often at the level of L2–L3 in newborns.
  A. The spinal cord typically ends at the level of L1–L2 in adults but may extend to L3 in the newborn.
  B. The spinal cord typically ends at the level of L1–L2 in adults but may extend to L3 in the newborn.
  D. The dural sac usually ends at the level of S2, so the spinal cord must end higher.
  E. The spinal cord typically ends at the level of L1–L2 in adults but may extend to L3 in the newborn.
  GAS 109; N 170

80. D. The erector spinae muscle is supplied by the dorsal rami, which carry motor, sensory, and autonomic fibers. The cell bodies of the motor part are found in the anterior horn, while the cell bodies of the sensory fibers are found in the dorsal root ganglia. The cell bodies of the sympathetic fibers are found in the paravertebral ganglia.
  A. This answer does not account for the cell bodies of the sympathetic fibers, which are found in the paravertebral ganglia.
  B. This answer does not account for the cell bodies of the sympathetic fibers, which are found in the paravertebral ganglia. The lateral horns found in T1–L2 are responsible for sympathetic outflow while levels S2–S4 are responsible for parasympathetic outflow in the pelvis.
  C. The lateral horns found in T1–L2 are responsible for sympathetic outflow while levels S2–S4 are responsible for parasympathetic outflow in the pelvis.
  E. This answer does not account for the cell bodies of the sympathetic fibers, which are found in the paravertebral ganglia.
  GAS 95–97; N 174

81. A. The anterior longitudinal ligament is a strong fibrous band that covers and connects the anterolateral aspect of the vertebral bodies and intervertebral discs; it maintains stability and prevents hyperextension. It can be torn by cervical hyperextension.
  B. The posterior longitudinal ligament runs within the vertebral canal supporting the posterior aspect of the vertebral bodies and prevents hyperflexion.
  C. The ligamentum flavum helps maintain upright posture by connecting the laminae of two adjacent vertebrae.
  D. The annulus fibrosus is the outer fibrous part of an intervertebral disc.
  E. The interspinous ligament connects adjacent spinous processes.
  GAS 81–84; N 167–168; ABR/McM 98

82. D. The boundaries of an intervertebral foramen (clockwise) include the following: the superior margin (roof) is formed by the inferior vertebral notch of the pedicle of a vertebra, the anterior margin by the intervertebral disc between the vertebral bodies of the adjacent vertebrae, the inferior margin (floor) by the superior vertebral notch of the pedicle of the vertebra below, and the posterior margin by the zygapophysial (facet) joint of the adjacent articular processes. Each pedicle contains superior and inferior vertebral notches.
  A. The superior articular process articulates with the inferior articular process of adjacent vertebrae. Articular processes project from the laminae of vertebrae.
  B. The laminae are flat sheets of bone that extend from the pedicles to join in the midline to form the roof of the vertebral arch.
  C. The inferior articular process articulates with the superior articular process of adjacent vertebrae. Articular processes project from the laminae of vertebrae.
  E. The spinous process projects from the midline union of two laminae and is the site for ligament and muscle attachment.
  GAS 62–70; N 163–164; ABR/McM 102

83. C. The most superiorly positioned intervertebral disc is between the C2 and C3 vertebrae. In the cervical region the spinal nerves exit superior to their corresponding vertebrae and take a somewhat horizontal path. The C3 nerve therefore exits between the C2 and C3 intervertebral foramen and would be affected by a posterolateral disc herniation at this level.
  A. The C1 nerve exists between the C1 vertebra and the occipital bone of the cranium and would not be affected.
  B. The C2 nerve passes superior to the second vertebra and would not be affected by a herniated disc between C2 and C3.
  D. C4 exits superior to its corresponding vertebra which is below the level of the herniated disc and will therefore not be affected.
  E. C5 exits superior to its corresponding vertebra which is below the level of the herniated disc and will therefore not be affected.
  GAS 69; N 170; ABR/McM 99–100

84. E. Ligaments serve to restrict movement. The anterior longitudinal ligament courses downward on the anterior surface of the vertebral bodies attaching to the intervertebral discs along its way. It stretches from the base of the skull inferiorly to the anterior surface of the sacrum. The anterior longitudinal ligament is the most anteriorly positioned ligament of the vertebral column and limits its extension.

A. The posterior longitudinal ligament travels on the posterior surface of the vertebral bodies attaching to the intervertebral discs along the way. This ligament serves to prevent excessive flexion of the vertebral column and extends from C2 to the sacrum.

B. The nuchal ligament limits excessive flexion of the cervical spine and serves as an attachment for muscles.

C. The ligamentum flava attach the internal surfaces of adjacent laminae to each other and prevent them from pulling apart during flexion.

D. The supraspinous ligament attaches the tips of the spinous processes to each other from C7 to the sacrum. Superiorly the ligament broadens sagittally, becoming more distinct and triangular and is termed the nuchal ligament.
GAS 81–82; N 167–168; ABR/McM 98

85. C. A horizontal line that connects the highest points of the iliac crests typically bisects the spinous process of the L4 vertebra or L4–L5 interspace (Tuffier line). The lumbar cistern, which represents the subarachnoid space, terminates at the level corresponding to the S2 spinous process. Three spinous processes inferiorly from the drawn line between the iliac crests would correspond to S2 spinous processes.

A. Three spinous processes above the drawn line would be at the vertebral level L1, which would correspond to the approximate location where the spinal cord ends and therefore the pia mater.

B. Two spinous processes would not be low enough.

D. Two spinous processes above the drawn line would be at the vertebral level L2, which would correspond to the approximate location where the spinal cord ends and therefore the pia mater.

E. The marked line intersects with the spinous process of the L4 vertebra. The dural sac ends at the S2 level.
GAS 101; N 170; ABR/McM 101

86. C. The anterior spinal artery lies in the anterior median fissure and would likely be compressed by the tumor. This artery is formed superiorly by the union of two anterior spinal branches that directly arise from the vertebral arteries.

A. The ascending cervical artery is not found within the vertebral canal and does not often contribute to the blood supply of the spinal cord.

B. The segmental spinal arteries follow the spinal nerves and provide the segmental medullary vessels which run along the dorsal and ventral roots to supply the lateral aspect of the spinal cord.

D. The segmental spinal arteries follow the spinal nerves and provide the segmental medullary vessels which run along the dorsal and ventral roots to supply the lateral aspect of the spinal cord.

E. There are two posterior spinal arteries; each is located in the posterolateral sulcus on the posterior aspect and have only small branches to the direct area.
GAS 102–103; N 176; ABR/McM 98

87. B. Hemivertebra is a condition where part of one or more vertebrae does not develop completely. This causes an abnormal lateral bending of the spinal column known as scoliosis, which may also include rotational deformities.

A. Osteoporosis is a condition where bones become gradually less dense and may result in fractures even in minor traumas.

C. Hyperlordosis is characterized by an increase in the convex anterior curvature of the lumbar or cervical spines. It is a result of an increase in thickness anterior, or a decrease in thickness posterior, on the vertebral bodies.

D. Spondylolisthesis is an anterior displacement of a portion of the vertebra consequent to a fracture of the pars interarticularis (spondylolysis).

E. Sacralization is when the fifth lumbar vertebra fuses to the sacrum.
GAS 73–77; N 162; ABR/McM 87

88. C. There are seven (7) cervical vertebrae and eight (8) cervical spinal nerves. Nerves C1–C7 exit superior to their corresponding vertebrae, whereas nerve C8 exits inferiorly to the C7 vertebra.

A. Nerves C1–C7 exit superior to their corresponding vertebrae.

B. Nerves C1–C7 exit superior to their corresponding vertebrae.

D. The nerves of the thoracic and subsequent regions all exit inferior to their corresponding vertebrae.

E. The nerves of the thoracic and subsequent regions all exit inferior to their corresponding vertebrae.
GAS 111; N 170

89. C. When a child is born, only one curvature is present in the vertebral column, the primary curvature, which is concave anteriorly and termed kyphosis. During postnatal development two additional curvatures form, secondary curvatures, which are convex anteriorly and termed lordosis. The first forms in response to the child lifting its head and is in the cervical spine; the second forms once the child is sitting and completes once the child starts to walk.

A. Thoracic kyphosis is the normal curvature with which we are born.

B. Cervical lordosis develops when the baby begins to hold its neck up.

D. Cervical kyphosis would be considered abnormal curvatures in a child of this age.

E. Thoracic lordosis would be considered abnormal curvatures in a child of this age.
GAS 54; N 162; ABR/McM 87

90. A. The hypertrophied muscle is the latissimus dorsi, which is attached to the spinous processes of vertebrae T7–L5 and the iliac crest and then attaches to the floor of the intertubercular sulcus.

B. None of the other options describes attachments sites for muscles attaching to the upper limb.

C. None of the other options describes attachments sites for muscles attaching to the upper limb.

D. None of the other options describes attachments sites for muscles attaching to the upper limb.

E. None of the other options describes attachments sites for muscles attaching to the upper limb.
GAS 86–92; N 180 (Table 3.2); ABR/McM 105–107

91. B. Sclerotomes are the derivatives of somites that develop into connective tissues like bone and cartilage and, if eliminated, will result in underdevelopment of the vertebral column.

A. The nucleus pulposus is a remnant of the notochord. It becomes encased within the annulus fibrosis, which develops from the sclerotome.

C. The dorsal root ganglia are formed by neural crest cells that migrate during development.

D. The neural tube is the precursor for the spinal cord.

E. The sympathetic ganglia develop from neural crest cells, as do all peripheral ganglia.
GAS 65

92. A. Multifidus is a deep back muscle, which attaches from transverse processes superomedially to spinous processes and usually crosses four to six segments.

B. The rotatores muscles typically attach between spinous processes or laminae of vertebrae and transverse processes of vertebra one or two segments below.

C. Longissimus is not deep to semispinalis but is superficial.

D. Iliocostalis is not deep to semispinalis but is superficial.

E. Spinalis is not deep to semispinalis but is superficial.
GAS 97–98; N 182; ABR/McM 107

93. D. The oblique radiographic view is ideal to show the pars interarticularis. In this projection a "Scottie dog" can be seen; the neck of the dog is the pars interarticularis, where the fracture may be seen.

A. In the anteroposterior view, the vertebral bodies make it difficult to see the pars interarticularis.

B. In the lateral view, the pedicles are superimposed on the pars interarticularis and so it cannot be easily seen.

C. In the posteroanterior view, the vertebral bodies make it difficult to see the pars interarticularis.

E. The anteroposterior open mouth is a radiographic view of the upper cervical region.
GAS 84; N 26; ABR/McM 113

94. A. The muscle that inserts on the transverse process of the atlas is the obliquus capitis inferior which forms the inferior border of the suboccipital triangle.

B. The rectus capitis posterior major inserts on the lateral portion of the inferior nuchal line and the rectus capitis posterior minor inserts on the medial portion of the inferior nuchal line of the occipital bone. These muscles form the medial border of the triangle.

C. The muscle that forms the lateral border of the suboccipital triangle is the obliquus capitis superior. This muscle originates from the transverse process of the atlas and inserts onto the occipital bone between the superior and inferior nuchal lines.

D. The rectus capitis posterior minor arises from the posterior tubercle of the atlas and inserts on the inferior nuchal line medially.

E. The rectus capitis posterior minor originates from the posterior tubercle of the atlas.
GAS 99–100; N 184; ABR/McM 109–110

95. E. Sacralization is a process where the L5 vertebra completely or incompletely fuses with the sacrum. This takes place in about 5% of the population. This vertebra adapts the characteristics of the sacrum with an increase in the length and width of both transverse processes. In other people the S1 is more or less separated from the sacrum and is partly or completely fused with L5 vertebra. This process is called lumbarization. Typically, when the L5 vertebra is sacralized, the L5–S1 levels are strong; however this puts pressure on the level above at L4–L5 which eventually degenerates, often producing painful symptoms.

A. The L1 vertebrae is not involved in sacralization.

B. The L4 vertebrae is not involved in sacralization.

C. The S2 vertebrae is not involved in sacralization.

D. The S1 vertebrae is not involved in sacralization.
GAS 76; N 166; ABR/McM 93, 95

96. D. The inferior longitudinal band of the cruciform ligament runs inferiorly from the transverse ligament of the atlas and attaches to the posterosuperior aspect of the vertebral body of the axis (C2).

A. The apical ligament runs from the tip of the dens to the anterior margin of the foramen magnum.

B. The superior longitudinal band of the cruciform ligament runs superiorly to attach onto the occiput.

C. The transverse ligament of the atlas spans the distance between the medial aspects of the lateral masses, holding the dens in place.

E. The ligamentum flavum is located in the vertebral canal and connects the laminae of adjacent vertebrae.
GAS 68–70; N 30; ABR/McM 98

97. A. The radicular arteries are branches of the segmental spinal arteries. They occur at every vertebral level and follow and provide blood supply to the anterior and posterior roots. A space-occupying lesion that compresses the posterior roots will also compress the arteries that supply them.

B. The segmental spinal arteries are feeder arteries that reinforce the blood supply to the spinal cord and arise from the vertebral and deep cervical arteries in the neck, the posterior intercostals in the thorax, the lumbar arteries in the abdomen, and the lateral sacral arteries in the pelvis.

C. The segmental medullary arteries are also branches of the segmental spinal arteries that anastomose directly with the anterior and posterior spinal arteries.

D. The anterior spinal artery arises from the vertebral artery and supplies the spinal cord directly.

E. The posterior spinal artery arises from the vertebral artery and supplies the spinal cord directly.
GAS 102–104; N 176–177; ABR/McM 98

98. E. The patient in the figure above has spina bifida occulta. This is a developmental condition resulting from incomplete ossification and failure of fusion of the vertebral arches. Three primary ossification centers should be present in the fetus by the eighth week: one in the centrum (to form the vertebral body) and one in each half of the vertebral arch. Five secondary ossification centers develop in the vertebrae after puberty: one at the tip of the spinous processes, the tips of the transverse processes, and on the inferior and superior rims of the vertebral body.

A. There are no secondary ossification centers in the vertebral arch, only two bilateral primary ossification centers.

B. There is no primary ossification center in the spinous processes, only secondary ossification centers.

C. Although the vertebral bodies possess primary centers of ossification, this child exhibits spina bifida occulta, which is not related to vertebral body development.

D. Vertebral bodies possess primary, not secondary, centers of ossification.
GAS 72; N 164; ABR/McM 93

99. A. In the cervical region, the spinal nerve exits in the intervertebral foramen above the correspondingly named vertebrae. Therefore the C3 spinal nerve exits above the C3 vertebrae and lies directly below the C2 vertebrae.

B. In the cervical region, the spinal nerve exits in the intervertebral foramen above the correspondingly named vertebrae. Therefore the C3 spinal nerve exits above the C3 vertebrae and lies directly below the C2 vertebrae.

C. In the cervical region, the spinal nerve exits in the intervertebral foramen above the correspondingly named vertebrae. Therefore the C3 spinal nerve exits above the C3 vertebrae and lies directly below the C2 vertebrae.

D. In the cervical region, the spinal nerve exits in the intervertebral foramen above the correspondingly named vertebrae. Therefore the C3 spinal nerve exits above the C3 vertebrae and lies directly below the C2 vertebrae.

E. In the cervical region, the spinal nerve exits in the intervertebral foramen above the correspondingly named vertebrae. Therefore the C3 spinal nerve exits above the C3 vertebrae and lies directly below the C2 vertebrae.
A. GAS 112; N 170; ABR/McM 89

100. E. The ligamentum flavum lies within the vertebral canal on the anterior aspect of the vertebral arches connecting the lamina of adjacent vertebrae. Puncturing this ligament allows the needle to enter into the epidural/extradural space for the injection of the anesthetic.

A. The supraspinous ligament connects and passes along the tips of the vertebral spinous processes. This ligament does not lie within the vertebral canal.

B. The interspinous ligament lies between adjacent spinous processes. This ligament does not lie within the vertebral canal.

C. The anterior longitudinal ligament connects the anterior aspect of the vertebral bodies. This ligament does not lie within the vertebral canal.

D. Although the posterior longitudinal ligament lies within the spinal canal, it lies anterior to the spinal cord and dural sac and it will not be punctured during the procedure.
GAS 81–83; N 168; ABR/McM 103

Answers 101–123

101. A. The third occipital nerve is the medial branch of the dorsal ramus of C3. It pierces the trapezius muscle medially in the neck below the external occipital protuberance and supplies the skin of this region.

B. The suboccipital nerve lies within and supplies the muscles of the suboccipital triangle.

C. The greater occipital nerve lies lateral to the midline and is less likely to be affected in this patient.

D. The lesser occipital nerves lie behind the ear and are less likely to be affected in this patient.

E. The accessory nerve supplies the trapezius and sternocleidomastoid muscles and has no cutaneous supply in the neck (*GAS* Fig. 2.52).
GAS 87; N 184; ABR/McM 108

102. A. The denticulate ligament is an extension of pia mater running longitudinally on either side of the spinal cord, connecting it to the dura mater. Medially, the denticulate ligament lies between the origin of the anterior and posterior rootlets serving as a landmark to differentiate between them.

B. The filum terminale internum is an extension of the pia mater that connects the conus medullaris to the end of the spinal dural sac.

C. The conus medullaris is the terminal end of the spinal cord.

D. The posterior longitudinal ligament lies posterior to the vertebral bodies.

E. The ligamentum flavum connects the lamina of adjacent vertebrae.
GAS 106–107; N 174; ABR/McM 100

103. D. The alar ligament connects the dens to the medial surface of the occipital condyles. It limits excessive rotation of the atlantoaxial joints.

A. Flexion of the upper cervical spine occurs at the atlantooccipital joints and the zygapophesial joints. These are not limited by the alar ligaments (*GAS* Fig. 2.20B).

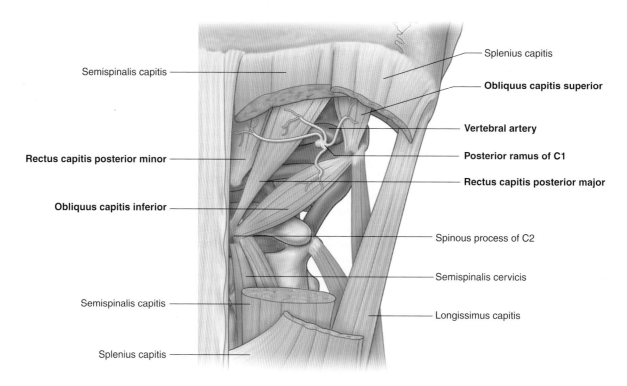

Semispinalis capitis

Splenius capitis

Obliquus capitis superior

Vertebral artery

Posterior ramus of C1

Rectus capitis posterior major

Rectus capitis posterior minor

Obliquus capitis inferior

Spinous process of C2

Semispinalis cervicis

Semispinalis capitis

Longissimus capitis

Splenius capitis

• *GAS* Fig. 2.52

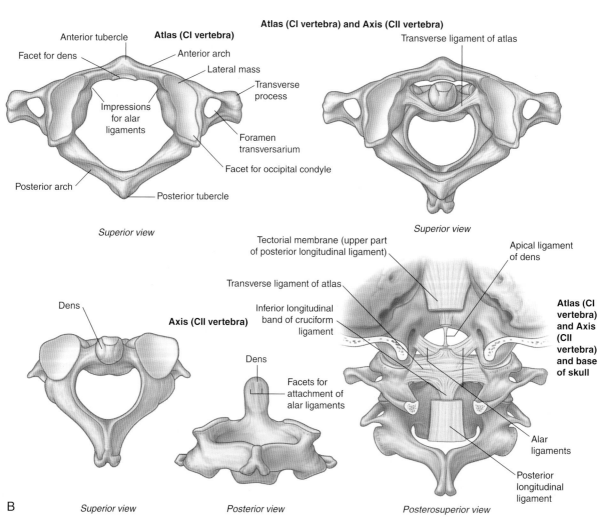

Atlas (CI vertebra) and Axis (CII vertebra)

Anterior tubercle

Atlas (CI vertebra)

Facet for dens

Anterior arch

Lateral mass

Impressions for alar ligaments

Transverse process

Foramen transversarium

Facet for occipital condyle

Posterior arch

Posterior tubercle

Transverse ligament of atlas

Superior view

Superior view

Dens

Axis (CII vertebra)

Tectorial membrane (upper part of posterior longitudinal ligament)

Apical ligament of dens

Transverse ligament of atlas

Inferior longitudinal band of cruciform ligament

Dens

Facets for attachment of alar ligaments

Atlas (CI vertebra) and Axis (CII vertebra) and base of skull

Alar ligaments

Posterior longitudinal ligament

B   *Superior view*   *Posterior view*   *Posterosuperior view*

• *GAS* Fig. 2.20B

B. Extension of the upper cervical spine occurs at the atlantooccipital joints and the zygapophysial joints.

C. Lateral flexion is a combination movement at the uncovertebral joints (of Luschka). Lateral flexion is not limited by the alar ligament (*GAS* Fig. 2.20B).

E. Abduction is a combination movement at the uncovertebral joints (of Luschka). It is not limited by the alar ligaments (*GAS* Fig. 2.20B).
GAS 68–69; N 23; ABR/McM 85

104. D. The rhomboid major and minor are supplied by the dorsal scapular nerve which sometimes also supplies the lower portion of levator scapulae. The function of levator scapulae is elevation and inferior rotation of the scapula.

A. Abduction of the arm above 90 degrees and protraction of the scapula are possible due to the combined actions of serratus anterior and trapezius, which are supplied by the long thoracic and accessory nerves, respectively.

B. Medial rotation and adduction of the arm is performed mainly by the pectoralis major and latissimus dorsi, which also extends the arm. These are supplied by the medial and lateral pectoral nerves and thoracodorsal nerve, respectively.

C. Medial rotation and adduction of the arm is performed mainly by the pectoralis major and latissimus dorsi, which also extends the arm.

E. Abduction of the arm through 15 degrees is produced by the supraspinatus, which is supplied by the suprascapular nerve.
GAS 90–92; N 468; ABR/McM 106

105. B. During surgery the long thoracic nerve was damaged which supplies the serratus anterior muscle. During abduction of the arm, serratus anterior elevates and laterally rotates the scapulae to allow for full abduction, such as when the hand is lifted above the head. If the nerve supply to this muscle is damaged this will not be achieved when the patient pushes her hands against the wall, resulting in what is called a "winged scapula."

A. The serratus anterior is responsible for protracting the scapula and therefore holding it against the thoracic wall when working together with trapezius.

C. Initiation of abduction of the humerus (the first 15 degrees) is performed by the supraspinatus, followed by the deltoid from 15 to 90 degrees.

D. Retraction of the scapula is mainly accomplished by rhomboid major, minor, and the trapezius.

E. Adduction is accomplished by the pectoralis major, latissimus dorsi, teres major, and the subscapularis.
GAS (Upper Limb Chapter); N 417; ABR/McM 106

106. A. During development, the spinal cord fills the vertebral canal entirely. Due to differential growth of the vertebral column and the spinal cord, the cord ends at L3 in an infant. It gradually changes its position to the level of the L1–L2 intervertebral disc, which is the adult level.

B. L4 is caudal to the conus medullaris in adults.

C. L5 is caudal to the conus medullaris in adults.

D. S1 is caudal to the conus medullaris in adults.

E. S2 is the level at which the dural sac normally terminates.
GAS 101; N 169–170; ABR/McM 101

107. A. The primitive streak is the epiblast structure responsible for the development of the mesoderm and endoderm, resulting in the trilaminar disc which contains all three germ layers.

B. Chorionic villi do not contribute to the formation of the embryo itself but the membranes of the embryo and therefore does not contain cells that would give rise to the germ layers.

C. Neural folds are formed from ectoderm and gives rise to neural crest cells.

D. The intraembryonic coelom forms the embryonic cavities and is therefore a space.

E. Neural folds are formed from ectoderm and gives rise to neural crest cells.
N 153

108. A. A fracture of the pars interarticularis without displacement of the vertebrae is termed spondylolysis.

B. Spondylolisthesis is when the anterior portion of the vertebra is displaced after fracture of the pars interarticularis.

C. A herniated disc is when the nucleus pulposus protrudes through the annulus fibrosus.

D. Lordosis is the normal curvature of the cervical and lumbar spine.

E. Scoliosis is an abnormal lateral curvature of the spine which usually also has a degree of rotation of the vertebrae.
GAS 83–84; N 164; ABR/McM 113

109. A. An epidural anesthetic procedure is performed in the epidural space which contains fat and the internal vertebral (Batson) plexus. A hematoma in this region would cause compression on the spinal nerves and possibly the spinal cord resulting in severe pain and deficits.

B. The great anterior medullary artery or great radicular artery (of Adamkiewicz) is the largest of the spinal segmental arteries and is usually located at around T12, much higher than L2–L3.

C. The anterior spinal artery is located in the anterior median fissure of the spinal cord, and is not located in the epidural space.

D. The posterior spinal arteries are located in the posterolateral fissures of the spinal cord, and are not located in the epidural space.

E. The external vertebral plexus is located external to the vertebral column and a hematoma of this plexus will not produce the symptoms of this patient. *GAS 102–104; N 178*

110. **A.** Ligaments serve to restrict movement. The anterior longitudinal ligament courses downward on the anterior surface of the vertebral bodies attaching to the intervertebral discs along its way. It stretches from the base of the skull inferiorly to the anterior surface of the sacrum. The anterior longitudinal ligament is the most anteriorly positioned ligament of the vertebral column and limits its extension.
   B. The posterior longitudinal ligament travels on the posterior surface of the vertebral bodies attaching to the intervertebral discs along the way. This ligament serves to prevent excessive flexion of the vertebral column and extends from C2 to the sacrum.
   C. Ligamentum flavum attaches the internal surfaces of adjacent laminae to each other and prevents them from pulling apart during flexion.
   D. The interspinous ligaments attach adjacent spinous processes to each other from C2 to the sacrum; it restricts the degree of separation of the spinous processes during flexion.
   E. The intertransverse ligaments connect adjacent transverse processes and prevent excessive rotation. *GAS 81; N 167–168; ABR/McM 102*

111. **A.** The order of structures pierced during an epidural procedure is skin, subcutaneous tissue, muscle, supraspinous ligament, interspinous ligament, and ligamentum flavum (although there is often a midline gap in the ligamentum flavum).
   B. The anterior longitudinal ligament is anterior to the vertebral bodies and cannot be reached by this approach.
   C. The posterior longitudinal ligament is posterior to the vertebral bodies and can also not be reached by this procedure.
   D. The interspinous ligaments attach adjacent spinous processes to each other from C2 to the sacrum; it restricts the degree of separation of the spinous processes during flexion.
   E. The intertransverse ligaments are too lateral and may not be perforated by this technique. *GAS 81–83; N 168; ABR/McM 103*

112. **D.** The spinal cord ends at the level between the L1–L2 intervertebral disc but the spinal nerves continue as the caudal equina below this level. As a result, narrowing of the canal at the level of L5 will impact on all of the nerves below this level resulting in bilateral lower limb weakness.
   A. The lesion described is at the L5 level, below the end of the spinal cord.
   B. The lesion described is at the L5 level, below the end of the spinal cord.

C. Narrowing of the canal at the level of L5 will impact on all of the nerves resulting in bilateral lower limb weakness, not unilateral weakness.
   E. Narrowing of the canal at the level of L5 will impact on all of the nerves resulting in bilateral lower limb weakness, not only back pain. *GAS 108–111, 121; N 170; ABR/McM 101*

113. **A.** Segmental arteries at all levels of the vertebral column send anastomotic branches to resupply the anterior and posterior spinal arteries, but these do not include the superficial epigastric or median sacral artery.
   B. The anterior and posterior spinal arteries do not provide sufficient blood supply to the spinal cord below cervical levels and will receive additional supply segmentally along its course from the multiple sources listed. The largest of these vessels is usually termed the artery of Adamkiewicz and arises at the lower thoracic or upper lumbar region.
   C. The anterior and posterior spinal arteries do not provide sufficient blood supply to the spinal cord below cervical levels and receive additional supply segmentally along their course from multiple sources.
   D. While the great radicular artery (of Adamkiewicz) is an important anastomotic channel for the lowest portion of the spinal cord, it is not the only vessel to provide collateral circulation to the cord.
   E. Anastomotic supply to the spinal cord is provided by segmental vessels along the entire length of the vertebral column, not simply in the neck and chest regions. *GAS 102–104; N 176–177*

114. **D.** A chondroma is typically a benign tumor of cartilaginous origin, which is encapsulated. It has the same origin from mesoderm as the apical ligament of the atlas which is considered as a rudimentary intervertebral fibrocartilage derived from the sclerotome.
   A. Dorsal root ganglia develop from neural crest cells.
   B. Sympathetic paravertebral ganglia arise from neural crest cells.
   C. Nucleus pulposus is derived from the mesodermal cells of the notochord.
   E. The bones of the cranial vault develop from cranial unsegmented paraxial mesoderm and neural crest cells. *GAS 101–104*

115. **A.** The odontoid process, or dens, projects superiorly from the body of the axis and articulates with the anterior arch of the atlas.
   B. The posterior tubercle of the atlas is a bony eminence on its posterior arch.
   C. The atlantooccipital joint is primarily involved in flexion and extension of the head on the neck.

D. The inferior articular facet is where the axis joins to the C3 vertebra.

E. The anterior tubercle of the atlas is a bony eminence on its anterior arch.

A, Lateral x-ray shows that this patient has only mild prevertebral swelling, which is centered at the odontoid (see *arrowheads* in Fig. 1.5, p. 19). The odontoid is displaced posteriorly relative to the C2 body *(arrow)* and is angled posteriorly. These findings indicate a fracture. **B,** The fracture is extremely subtle on the open-mouth odontoid x-ray *(arrows)*. **C,** Sagittal CT reconstruction shows the fracture.
GAS 66–71; N BP34–BP35

116. D. The herniated disc is between vertebrae L4 and L5. In the lumbar region spinal nerves exit below their corresponding vertebrae, in which case the L4 nerve would pass superior to the herniation. As the L5 nerve crosses the intervertebral disc to exit below the fifth lumbar vertebra it will be compressed by the herniation.

A. Compression of nerves L2, L3, L4, and S1 would produce symptoms different to those seen in this patient.

B. Compression of nerves L2, L3, L4, and S1 would produce symptoms different to those seen in this patient.

C. Compression of nerves L2, L3, L4, and S1 would produce symptoms different to those seen in this patient.

E. Compression of nerves L2, L3, L4, and S1 would produce symptoms different to those seen in this patient.
GAS 80; N 165; ABR/McM 99

117. D. The vertebral artery lies on the superior surface of the atlas as it passes posterior to its superior articular facet. The C1 spinal nerve lies beneath it, against the atlas. Both of these structures may be injured in this type of fracture. This is a typical Jefferson fracture in which the anterior and posterior arches of C1 are fractured.

A. The anterior spinal artery is located within the dural sac and would not be damaged in this sort of fracture. The hypoglossal nerve runs anterolaterally above the occipital condyles and would usually not be injured in an atlas fracture.

B. The paired posterior spinal arteries lie on the spinal cord within the dural sac and would not be injured in a fracture of the atlas.

C. The paired posterior spinal arteries lie on the spinal cord within the dural sac and would not be injured in a fracture of the atlas.

E. The C2 spinal nerve lies between C1 and C2 and is less likely to be injured than C1, which lies on the atlas.
GAS 69, 102–104; N 176–177

118. B. The pedicle is the part of the neural arch that connects to the vertebral body, and it is the part injured in a Chance fracture.

A. The lamina is the posterior portion of the neural arch and does not contact the vertebral body directly.

C. The spinous process projects posteriorly from the neural arch, where the paired laminae meet in the midline.

D. The articular processes project superiorly and inferiorly from the laminae and do not attach to the vertebral bodies.

E. The transverse processes project laterally from the union of the pedicle and lamina on each side, and do not attach to the vertebral bodies.
GAS 66–67; N 163; ABR/McM 90

119. D. The nuchal ligament is a posterior extension elaboration of the supraspinous ligament. It attaches along the tips of all of the cervical vertebrae. An avulsion fracture of the tip of the spinous process of C7 is often referred to as a Clay Shoveler's fracture.

A. The denticulate ligament is a lateral extension of pia and lies within the dural sac.

B. The interspinous ligaments connect adjacent spinous processes, not their tips.

C. The ligamentum flavum connects adjacent laminae of vertebrae.

E. The posterior longitudinal ligament lies anterior to the dural sac and posterior to the vertebral bodies and intervertebral discs.
GAS 81–81; N 29; ABR/McM 108–109

120. A. Cauda equina syndrome involved wide-ranging functional deficits because it involves compression of the nerves of the cauda equina by a mass such as a herniated intervertebral disc, or a tumor. It typically involves compression of spinal roots L2 and below. It presents with unilateral radicular pain, absent knee and ankle reflex, and loss or reduced urinary bladder and anal sphincter control. The treatment involves emergent surgery and steroids.

B. An obturator hernia may cause weakness in the medial thigh muscles due to compression of the obturator nerve, but it would not affect structures in the perineum.

C. Piriformis syndrome is compression of the common fibular nerve in instances where part of this neve passes through the piriformis muscle. It would not affect perineal structures.

D. While pudendal neve palsy might explain the perineal structures affected, there would not be lower limb involvement in this type of nerve injury.

E. Sciatica is a term used loosely for pain along the path of the sciatic nerve and not in the perineum.
GAS 121

121. B. Lordosis is a normal secondary curvature, concave posteriorly, that is acquired as the person begins to crawl and then walk. Ankylosing spondylitis may reverse this curvature in the lumbar region and even produce lumbar kyphosis. Ankylosing spondylitis is a type of arthritis that affects the spine. Typical symptoms of the disease include pain and stiffness. The vertebrae eventually fuse together, resulting in a rigid spine or bamboo spine. Furthermore, progression of the ankylosing spondylitis into costovertebral and costosternal joints can cause restrictive lung disease because of inability of the chest wall to expand.
  - **A.** Kyphosis is a convex posterior curvature that is the primary curvature in the thoracic and sacral regions.
  - **C.** The primary curvature of the vertebral column is concave anteriorly. As the infant begins to crawl, a cervical lordosis, a secondary curvature, develops, and then as walking begins, a lumbar lordosis is acquired.
  - **D.** Scoliosis is an abnormal lateral bending and torsion of the spine.
  - **E.** There is no tertiary curvature in the spine.
    GAS 75; N 162; ABR/McM 87

122. C. The ligamentum flavum is highly elastic and is the cause of the first of two pops as a needle is introduced into the subarachnoid space.
  - **A.** The dura mater, with the arachnoid mater lying against its inner surface, produces the second pop felt in a lumbar puncture, because it is like puncturing a water balloon, because it and the arachnoid are filled with cerebrospinal fluid.
  - **B.** The interspinous ligament is not highly elastic and is fairly continuous with the more superficial supraspinous ligament.
  - **D.** The posterior longitudinal ligament lies anterior to the dural sac, and posterior to the vertebral bodies and intervertebral discs.
  - **E.** The supraspinous ligament lies along the tips of the vertebral spinous processes, and is not highly elastic. A needle passing through it would simply enter the interspinous ligament beneath it.
    GAS 81–83; N 168; ABR/McM 103

123. Osteopetrosis is characterized by failure of normal bone resorption due to defective osteoclasts function. The defective osteoclasts are due to a mutation in the gene for carbonic anhydrase II that impairs their ability to generate acidic environment and as a result, defects the bone resorption. This produces thick and dense bones because of overgrowth of cortical bones that fill the bone marrow spaces and creates susceptibility to fractures. Once cranial foramina are involved patients exhibit cranial nerve compression and palsies. X-rays show diffuse symmetric sclerosis known also as bone-in-bone or "stone bone." Laboratory studies show pancytopenia and extramedullary hematopoiesis.
  - **D.** Scoliosis is a lateral curvature of the spine that may result from a congenital condition or trauma to the spine.
  - **A.** Kyphosis is a primary, posteriorly convex curvature that is found in the thoracic and sacral regions of the adult spine.
  - **B.** Lordosis is a secondary, concave posterior curvature that is acquired in the cervical region when an infant begins to crawl, and in the lumbar region when the child begins to walk.
  - **C.** The primary curvature of the spine is convex posteriorly.
  - **E.** The spine acquires secondary curvatures in the cervical and lumbar regions as the infant begins to crawl and later to walk.
    GAS 74

2

Thorax

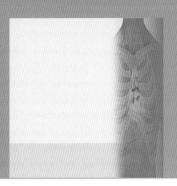

Questions

Questions 1–25

1. A 31-year-old woman delivers a full-term boy via normal spontaneous vaginal delivery without complications during birth. Two hours after delivery the boy is admitted to the neonatal intensive care unit because of cyanosis. The pregnancy was complicated with type 2 diabetes mellitus. An echocardiogram shows transposition of the great arteries. Which structure is primarily responsible for the division of the truncus arteriosus into the great arteries?
   A. Septum secundum
   B. Septum primum
   C. Bulbar septum
   D. Aorticopulmonary septum
   E. Endocardial cushions

2. A 32-year-old woman, gravida 1, para 0, aborta 0, at 30 weeks' gestation, comes to the office for a prenatal visit. Today, her vital signs are within normal limits. Physical examination shows a uterus consistent in size with a 30-week gestation. Fetal ultrasonography shows a fetus with enlarged, echogenic lungs, an inverted diaphragm, and fetal ascites with no other abnormalities. Which of the following conditions is most consistent with these findings?
   A. Laryngeal atresia
   B. Tracheal atresia
   C. Polyhydramnios
   D. Lung hypoplasia
   E. Oligohydramnios

3. A 2-year-old African American child is brought to the physician for a routine examination. Previous visits showed no abnormalities and the mother had a normal spontaneous vaginal delivery with no complications during the pregnancy. Physical examination shows a cardiac murmur. The child has no other associated medical conditions. Which of the following congenital cardiac anomalies occurs most commonly?
   A. Membranous ventricular septal defect
   B. Tetralogy of Fallot
   C. Muscular ventricular septal defect
   D. Ostium secundum defect
   E. Ostium primum defect

4. A 27-year-old woman gives birth to a full-term girl. Physical examination of the girl 2 days after birth shows central cyanosis, tachypnea, and a loud, single S2 sound on auscultation of the heart. An echocardiogram shows transposition of the great arteries. Which of the following structures must remain patent for the girl to survive until surgical correction of the malformation is performed?
   A. Ductus arteriosus
   B. Umbilical arteries
   C. Umbilical vein
   D. Coarctation of the aorta
   E. Pulmonary artery stenosis

5. A 29-year-old woman delivers a newborn girl via vaginal delivery with no complications during birth. At 6 months old, the girl is brought to the emergency department by her mother because her skin appeared to have a slight bluish discoloration while feeding. Physical examination shows a harsh systolic murmur at the left upper sternal border. An echocardiogram shows pulmonary artery stenosis, an overriding aorta, a ventricular septal defect and hypertrophy of the right ventricle. An x-ray of the chest shows a boot-shaped heart. Which condition is most likely responsible for the development of this clinical picture?
   A. Tetralogy of Fallot
   B. Atrial septal defect
   C. Transposition of the great vessels
   D. Pulmonary atresia
   E. ventricular septal defect

6. A 6-day-old girl is brought to the emergency department by her mother because of a sudden episode of turning blue. The mother says the girl's lips turned blue while breastfeeding. An echocardiogram shows pulmonary artery stenosis, overriding of the aorta, ventricular septal defect and hypertrophy of the right ventricle. Which of the following embryologic mechanisms is most likely responsible for the development of this cluster of anomalies?
   A. Superior malalignment of the subpulmonary infundibulum
   B. Defect in the aorticopulmonary septum
   C. Endocardial cushion defect
   D. Total anomalous pulmonary venous connections
   E. Atrioventricular (AV) canal malformation

7. A 5-year-old boy is brought to the emergency department by his mother because of severe shortness of breath when playing soccer with friends. The mother says that the child is easily fatigued during physical activities. He has no prior hospitalizations or history of major illness. Physical examination shows a loud systolic murmur and a wide, fixed split of the S_2 sound. An x-ray of the chest shows an enlarged right heart. What is the most likely diagnosis?
   A. ventricular septal defect
   B. Atrial septal defect
   C. Tetralogy of Fallot
   D. Transposition of the great arteries
   E. Aortic stenosis

8. A 3-month-old boy is brought to the physician by his mother for routine examination. The child was born at full term via spontaneous vaginal delivery. Physical examination shows epicanthic folds, macroglossia, a flat profile, depressed nasal bridge, and a single palmar crease. Cardiac examination shows a murmur. Chromosomal analysis confirms the diagnosis of Down syndrome. What other cardiac finding is most likely to occur in this condition?
   A. Tetralogy of Fallot
   B. Transposition of the great arteries
   C. Atrial septal and ventricular septal defects
   D. Truncus arteriosus
   E. Coarctation of the aorta

9. A 3-month-old boy is brought to the physician by his mother for a routine examination. Physical examination shows narrow palpebral fissures, elongated facial features, micrognathia, and low-set ears. Laboratory studies show hypocalcemia and an echocardiogram shows severe congenital cardiac malformations. The boy is diagnosed with a deletion at the 22q11 chromosome. Which of the following malformations will most likely be associated with this condition?
   A. Tetralogy of Fallot and truncus arteriosus
   B. Transposition of the great arteries
   C. Atrial septal and ventricular septal defects
   D. Coarctation of the aorta
   E. Aortic atresia

10. A 28-year-old woman, gravida 2, para 1, aborta 0, at 32 weeks' gestation, is brought to the emergency department because of dizziness for several days. Her vital signs are within normal limits. Laboratory studies show elevated serum glucose concentrations confirming the diagnosis of gestational diabetes. Which of the following fetal cardiac malformations is most likely associated with the mother's condition?
    A. Tetralogy of Fallot
    B. Transposition of the great arteries
    C. Atrial septal and ventricular septal defects
    D. Truncus arteriosus
    E. Coarctation of the aorta

11. A 2-year-old boy is brought to emergency department by his mother because of shortness of breath. Physical examination shows tachypnea, nasal flaring, abdominal retractions during breathing. Cardiac examination shows a continuous machinery-like murmur. A cardiac catheterization is performed and shows the contrast medium to be visible immediately in the left pulmonary artery when released into the arch of the aorta. What is the most likely explanation for this finding?
    A. Atrial septal defect
    B. Mitral stenosis
    C. Patent ductus arteriosus
    D. Patent ductus venosus
    E. ventricular septal defect

12. A 3-year-old boy is brought to the physician by his mother for a routine examination. Cardiac examination shows a loud systolic murmur and a wide, fixed, split S2 sound. An x-ray of the chest shows an enlarged right heart and the patient is diagnosed with an atrial septal defect. This condition usually results from incomplete closure of which of the following structures?
    A. Foramen ovale
    B. Ligamentum arteriosum
    C. Ductus arteriosus
    D. Sinus venarum
    E. Coronary sinus

13. A 2-hour premature boy, born at 24 weeks gestation, is brought to the emergency department because of progressive difficulty in breathing. The boy was born to a 17-year-old mother via cesarean delivery. Physical examination of the boy shows tachypnea, nasal flaring, and grunting. The boy is diagnosed with respiratory distress syndrome. Which of the following cell type is responsible for synthesizing surfactant in this syndrome?
    A. Alveolar capillary endothelial
    B. Bronchial mucous
    C. Bronchial respiratory epithelium
    D. Type I alveolar
    E. Type II alveolar

14. An infant is admitted to the intensive care unit 1 hour after delivery because of respiratory distress. An x-ray of the chest shows a hypoplastic left lung and gastric contents in the left hemithorax. Physical examination shows the left hemidiaphragm ascending into the thorax during inspiration, while the right hemidiaphragm contracts normally. Which of the following is the most likely cause of this condition?
    A. Absence of a pleuropericardial fold
    B. Absence of musculature in one half of the diaphragm
    C. Failure of migration of diaphragm
    D. Failure of the septum transversum to develop
    E. Absence of a pleuroperitoneal fold

15. A 35-year-old man is brought to the emergency department because of a severe nosebleed and a worsening headache over the weekend. Physical examination shows a more developed upper body, cold lower extremities, absent femoral pulses, and a loud midsystolic murmur on his anterior chest wall and back. Which of the following embryologic structure(s) is most likely affected to produce these symptoms?
    A. Bulbus cordis
    B. Ductus arteriosus
    C. Third, fourth, and sixth pharyngeal arches
    D. Right and left horns of sinus venosus
    E. Right cardinal vein

16. A 5-day-old boy is brought to the emergency department by his mother because of excessive drooling and choking during feeding. The mother says the newborn became cyanotic when swallowing milk. An x-ray of the chest shows a nasogastric tube coiling in the thorax with air bubbles in the stomach. Which of the following structures failed to develop in this patient?
    A. Esophagus
    B. Trachea
    C. Tongue
    D. Tracheoesophageal septum
    E. Pharynx

17. A 5-day-old boy is brought to the emergency department by his mother because of excessive drooling and choking during feeding. The mother says the newborn became cyanotic when swallowing milk. An x-ray of the chest shows a nasogastric tube coiling in the thorax with air bubbles in the stomach. A tracheoesophageal fistula (TEF) is suspected. Which of the following conditions is most likely to be associated with this condition?
    A. Oligohydramnios
    B. Rubella
    C. Polyhydramnios
    D. Thalidomide exposure
    E. Toxoplasmosis

18. A 2-day-old girl is brought to the emergency department by her parents 1 hour after they noted a bluish discoloration of her chest and abdomen and severe shortness of breath. The pregnancy was uncomplicated, and the girl was born at full term via spontaneous vaginal delivery. Physical examination shows tachypnea, nasal flaring, abdominal retractions during breathing, and a continuous machine-like heart murmur. Which of the following infections will most likely lead to this congenital anomaly?
    A. Toxoplasmosis
    B. Rubella
    C. Cytomegalovirus
    D. Varicella virus
    E. Treponema pallidum

19. A 5-year-old boy is brought to the physician by his mother because of frequent episodes of fatigability and shortness of breath. Cardiac examination shows a loud systolic murmur and a wide, fixed, split S_2 sound. An ultrasound examination shows an atrial septal defect located at the opening of the superior vena cava. Which of the following types of atrial septal defects are characteristic for this description?
    A. Ostium secundum
    B. Ostium primum
    C. AV canal
    D. Common atrium
    E. Sinus venosus

20. A 1-hour-old newborn with ectopia cordis is brought to the emergency department. His birth weight was 3500 kg (7 lb, 11oz), and Apgar scores were 5 and 4 at 1 and 5 minutes, respectively. Physical examination shows multiple cardiac abnormalities. Despite appropriate care, the newborn dies 3 days later from cardiac failure and hypoxemia. Which of the following embryologic events is most likely responsible for the development of such conditions?
    A. Faulty development of the sternum and pericardium, secondary to incomplete fusion of the lateral folds
    B. Interruption of third pharyngeal arch development
    C. Interruption of fourth pharyngeal arch development
    D. Interruption of fifth pharyngeal arch development
    E. Faulty development of sinus venosus

21. A 2-day-old boy is brought to the neonatal intensive care unit because of cyanosis and tachypnea. The pregnancy course was uncomplicated, and the boy was born via spontaneous vaginal delivery at full term. Physical examination shows nasal flaring, grunting, and retractions with breathing. An echocardiogram and magnetic resonance imaging (MRI) show totally anomalous pulmonary connections. Which of the following embryologic events is responsible for this malformation?
    A. Abnormal septation of the sinus venosus
    B. Abnormal development of the septum secundum
    C. Abnormal development of the left sinus horn
    D. Abnormal development of the coronary sinus
    E. Abnormal development of common cardinal vein

22. A 3-day-old newborn girl is brought to the emergency department by her mother because of difficulty with breathing. Physical examination shows nasal flaring and abdominal retractions upon inspiration. A computed tomography (CT) scan of her chest and abdomen shows absence of the central tendon of the diaphragm. Which of the following structures failed to develop normally?
    A. Pleuroperitoneal folds
    B. Pleuropericardial folds
    C. Septum transversum
    D. Cervical myotomes
    E. Dorsal mesentery of the esophagus

23. A 30-year-old man comes to the physician because of easy fatigability. Physical examination shows the

brachial arterial pressure is markedly increased, the femoral artery pressure is decreased, and the femoral pulses are delayed. He is diagnosed with a blockage of arterial flow in the proximal part of the thoracic aorta. Which of the following structures failed to develop normally?

A. Second aortic aorta
B. Third aortic arch
C. Fourth aortic arch
D. Fifth aortic arch
E. Ductus venosus

24. A 1-year-old boy is brought to the physician by his mother because of severe shortness of breath. Physical examination shows a continuous machine-like murmur in the second intercostal space in the left upper sternal border. An ECG shows arrhythmias and right ventricular hypertrophy. An angiogram shows a patent ductus arteriosus. Which of the following embryologic arterial structures does the ductus arteriosus originate from?

A. Left sixth aortic arch
B. Right sixth aortic arch
C. Left fifth aortic arch
D. Right fourth aortic arch
E. Left fourth aortic arch

25. A 4-year-old girl is brought to the emergency department by her father because of a high fever. Her temperature is 39.4°C (102.9°F). The remaining vital signs are within normal limits. Cardiac examination shows a loud, harsh murmur heard on auscultation. An x-ray of the chest shows prominent pulmonary arteries. Echocardiography shows all the valves to be normal. Blood culture shows Staphylococcus aureus and antibiotic therapy is initiated. Which of the following congenital malformations most likely explains these findings?

A. Atrial septal defect
B. Tetralogy of Fallot
C. Coarctation of the aorta
D. Patent ductus arteriosus
E. Aortic atresia

Questions 26–50

26. A 3-day-old full-term boy is brought into the neonatal intensive care unit because of an episode of severe cyanosis where the boy's face and extremities turned blue. The boy was given supplemental oxygen, which did not improve his symptoms. Echocardiographic examination shows a right-to-left shunt. Which of the following conditions will most likely produce this type of shunt?

A. Interatrial septal defect
B. Interventricular septal defect
C. Patent ductus arteriosus
D. Corrected transposition of the great arteries
E. Common truncus arteriosus

27. A 2-day-old boy is brought into the neonatal intensive care unit because of dyspnea and cyanosis. Physical examination shows nasal flaring and retractions. An x-ray of the chest shows a left hypoplastic lung and herniation of the abdominal intestines into the left thoracic cavity. Which of the following embryological structures most likely failed to develop properly?

A. Septum transversum
B. Pleuroperitoneal membrane
C. Tracheoesophageal septum
D. Laryngotracheal groove
E. Foregut

28. A 3-month-old girl is brought to the physician by her mother because of difficulty breathing during feeding and excessive fatigue. Physical examination shows a holosystolic murmur. An echocardiogram shows a ventricular septal defect at the area of the subpulmonary infundibulum. Which of the following structures must be avoided carefully by the surgeon when the sutures are placed at the site of the defect?

A. Right bundle branch
B. Right coronary artery
C. Tricuspid valve
D. Left interventricular (anterior descending) artery
E. Aortic valve

29. A 5-day-old boy is brought to the physician because of difficulty with feeding. Physical examination shows anal atresia and radial aplasia. An x-ray of the spine shows vertebral abnormalities and an echocardiogram shows cardiac abnormalities. A diagnosis of incomplete division of the foregut into respiratory and digestive portions is made. Which of the following conditions of the gastrointestinal tract is associated with this syndrome?

A. Esophageal atresia
B. Esophageal achalasia
C. Pyloric stenosis
D. Congenital diaphragmatic hernia
E. Esophageal fistula

30. A 2-year-old boy is brought unconscious to the emergency department after a motor vehicle collision. His blood pressure is 62/30 mm Hg, pulse is 105/min, and oxygen saturation is 88%. Physical examination shows multiple lacerations on the chest wall. An emergency tracheostomy is performed. Which of the following structures is most commonly at high risk of injury during this procedure?

A. Left brachiocephalic vein
B. Left common carotid artery
C. Vagus nerve
D. Phrenic nerve
E. Thoracic duct

31. A 45-year-old woman is brought to the emergency department because of difficulty breathing. Her vital signs are within normal limits. Physical examination shows clear breath sounds bilaterally. An x-ray of the chest shows a tumor invading the lung surface anterior to the hilum. Which nerve is most likely compressed by the tumor to result in dyspnea?

A. Phrenic
B. Vagus
C. Intercostal
D. Recurrent laryngeal
E. Cardiopulmonary

32. A 62-year-old man comes to the physician because of 3-month history of progressive voice softening. Vital signs are within normal limits. Physical examination shows clear lung sounds bilaterally and no murmurs are heard. A CT scan of the chest shows a growth located within the aortic arch adjacent to the left pulmonary artery. Which neural structure is most likely being compressed to cause the changes in the patient's voice?
A. Left phrenic nerve
B. Esophageal plexus
C. Left recurrent laryngeal nerve
D. Left vagus nerve
E. Left sympathetic trunk

33. A 39-year-old woman comes to the physician because of a 2-month history of being unable to reach a pantry shelf just above her head due to pain. Two months ago, she underwent a mastectomy procedure. Physical examination shows weakness of shoulder abduction beyond 90 degrees in her right arm. Which nerve was most likely damaged during surgery to result in the patient's condition?
A. Axillary
B. Spinal accessory
C. Long thoracic
D. Radial
E. Thoracodorsal

34. A 41-year-old woman is brought to the emergency department because of severe, sharp, but poorly localized pain on the chest wall. Physical examination shows decreased breath sounds, dullness to percussion, and decreased tactile fremitus in the right lower lung fields. An x-ray of the chest shows right pleural effusion. What is the location of the neuronal cell bodies responsible for the nerve fibers that carry this pain to the central nervous system?
A. Dorsal root ganglia
B. Sympathetic trunk ganglia
C. Dorsal horn of the spinal cord
D. Lateral horn of the spinal cord
E. Ventral horn of the spinal cord

35. A 23-year-old man is brought to the emergency department after being involved in a motor vehicle collision. His pulse is 115/min, blood pressure is 120/78 mm Hg, and respirations are 25/min. Physical examination shows bruising of the chest. What is the location of the preganglionic neuronal cell bodies involved in increasing the heart rate?
A. Deep cardiac plexus
B. Dorsal motor nucleus of vagus
C. Lateral horn T5–T9
D. Lateral horn T1–T4
E. Inferior cervical ganglia

36. A 55-year-old man is brought to the emergency department because of severe, substernal, pressure-like chest pain that radiates to his left arm. His pulse is 110/min, respirations are 30/min, and blood pressure is 90/70 mm Hg. An ECG shows ST-elevations and laboratory studies show elevated troponins confirming a myocardial infarction. Which of the following nerves carry the pain fibers from the heart to the central nervous system?
A. Vagus
B. Greater thoracic splanchnic
C. Least thoracic splanchnic
D. Thoracic visceral (cardiopulmonary)
E. T5–T9 ventral rami

37. A 17-year-old girl is brought to the emergency department by her boyfriend because of 2-hour history of severe dyspnea. Her pulse is 110/min, respirations are 35/min, and blood pressure is 120/80 mm Hg. Physical examination shows diffuse expiratory wheezing on lung auscultation. A diagnosis of acute asthma attack is made. Which of the following nerves is responsible for the innervation of the bronchial smooth muscle cells?
A. Greater thoracic splanchnic
B. Phrenic
C. Vagus
D. Intercostal
E. Lesser thoracic splanchnic

38. A 42-year-old woman is brought to the emergency department by her husband because of 2-month history of hoarseness. Vital signs are within normal limits. Physical examination shows normal lung sounds bilaterally. A CT scan of the chest shows a mass at the aorticopulmonary window. Which of the following nerves is most likely compressed?
A. Vagus
B. Phrenic
C. Left recurrent laryngeal
D. Right recurrent laryngeal
E. Greater thoracic splanchnic

39. A 42-year-old woman comes to the physician because of 10-day history of dysesthesia in the inner aspect of the arm and axilla. She had a total mastectomy including excision of the axillary tail (of Spence) after being diagnosed with carcinoma of the breast two weeks ago. Vital signs are within normal limits. Which of the following nerves was most likely injured during the procedure?
A. Ulnar
B. Long thoracic
C. Intercostobrachial
D. Lateral cutaneous nerve of T4
E. Axillary nerve

40. A 39-year-old man is brought to the emergency department because of 3-day history of progressively sharp retrosternal pain that radiates to the left

shoulder. The pain is relieved by leaning forward and worse with inspiration. Vital signs are within normal limits. Physical examination shows a pericardial friction rub. Which of the following nerves is responsible for the radiating pain to the shoulder?

A. Intercostobrachial
B. Phrenic
C. Long thoracic
D. Greater thoracic splanchnic
E. Thoracic visceral (cardiopulmonary)

41. A 72-year-old man is brought to the emergency department because of 30-min history of sharp, substernal pressure-like chest pain. The pain radiates to his left arm. Physical examination shows a diaphoretic man with dyspnea. An ECG shows myocardial infarction of the posterior wall of the left ventricle. Laboratory studies show elevated cardiac troponins. Which of the following nerves is responsible for the radiation of pain to the arm during myocardial infarction?

A. Phrenic
B. Vagus
C. Intercostobrachial
D. Greater thoracic splanchnic
E. Suprascapular

42. A 43-year-old man comes to the physician because of 1-week history of numbness and anhidrosis in the left axilla. He fell over a barbed wire fence last week and sustained several deep lacerations along the left midaxillary line. Physical examination shows loss of sensation in the left axilla and several healing wounds. Which structures were most likely damaged to result in these signs?

A. Dorsal roots
B. Ventral roots
C. Cutaneous branches of dorsal rami
D. Cutaneous branches of ventral rami
E. Rami communicantes

43. A 62-year-old patient is brought to the emergency department because of a sudden-onset, tearing chest pain radiating to the back. He has a history of hypertension and smokes a pack a day. His blood pressure is 150/100 mm Hg, pulse is 100/min, and respirations are 22/min. A CT scan examination of the chest shows an aortic aneurysm. An urgent placement of an endovascular stent-graft is performed. Which of the following nerves are most likely responsible for the tearing sensation radiating to his back?

A. Somatic afferents
B. Thoracic visceral afferents
C. Sympathetic postganglionics
D. Sympathetic preganglionics
E. Parasympathetic afferents

44. A 22-year-old woman comes to the physician because of 2-month history of loss of sensation bilaterally in the nipples and areolae following elective breast enhancement. Physical examination shows reduction of sensation of the skin from the areolae laterally to the midaxillary lines. There is no erythema and incisions are dry and healing. Which of the following nerves were most likely subject to iatrogenic injury?

A. Anterior cutaneous branches of second and third intercostal nerves
B. Anterior and lateral cutaneous branches of the fourth intercostal nerves
C. Lateral pectoral nerves
D. Lateral cutaneous branches of the ventral ramus of the second thoracic spinal nerves (intercostobrachial nerves)
E. Lateral cutaneous branches of the second and third intercostal nerves

45. A 32-year-old woman is brought to the emergency department because of 5-hour history of severe dyspnea and anxiety. For the past 2 months she has been on a liquid diet because of dysphagia and has lost 15 kg (33 lb). Over the past several weeks, she has had bloody sputum during attacks of coughing and hoarseness. Fluoroscopy and a barium swallow show a 4-cm mass in the trachea compressing the thoracic esophagus. Which of the following nerves is most likely to be affected?

A. Right recurrent laryngeal nerve
B. Left vagus nerve, posterior to the hilum of the lung
C. Left recurrent laryngeal nerve
D. Greater thoracic splanchnic nerve
E. Phrenic nerve

46. A 35-year-old man comes to the physician because of a 4-month history of progressive difficulty with swallowing solid food. Vital signs are within normal limits. Physical examination shows a diastolic murmur at the apex of the heart. A CT scan of the chest shows a dilated left atrium. Which structure is most likely being compressed by the expansion of the left atrium to result in the patient's symptoms?

A. Esophagus
B. Root of the lung
C. Trachea
D. Superior vena cava
E. Inferior vena cava

47. A 69-year-old woman is admitted to the hospital because of laryngeal cancer. Physical examination shows a thin-appearing woman with a hoarse voice. A CT scan examination of the chest and abdomen shows multiple masses in the lungs and liver. For nutritional needs a nasogastric tube is inserted. What is the last site at which resistance would be expected as the tube passes from the nose to the stomach?

A. Pharyngoesophageal junction
B. Level of the superior thoracic aperture
C. Posterior to the aortic arch
D. Posterior to the left main bronchus
E. Esophageal hiatus of the diaphragm

48. A 59-year-old man is brought to the emergency department because of shortness of breath. Physical examination shows crackles at the lung bases, increased jugular venous distention, an S3 gallop, and pitting edema. A slight rhythmic pulsation on the chest wall at the left fifth intercostal space in the midclavicular line can be seen. What part of the heart is responsible for this pulsation?
A. Right atrium
B. Left atrium
C. Aortic arch
D. Apex of the heart
E. Mitral valve

49. A 42-year-old man is brought to the emergency department after a head-on motor vehicle collision. He was an unrestrained driver and sustained blunt trauma to his sternum from the steering wheel. Physical examination shows extensive ecchymoses on the anterior chest wall. What part of the heart would be most likely to be injured by the impact?
A. Right ventricle
B. Apex of left ventricle
C. Left ventricle
D. Right atrium
E. Anterior margin of the left atrium

50. A 54-year-old woman is brought to the emergency department because she feels her heart beating. She experiences shortness of breath with exertion, orthopnea, and an intermittent cough. Vital signs are within normal limits. Physical examination shows a murmur with a mid-systolic click and echocardiographic studies shows severe mitral valve prolapse. Auscultation of this valve is best performed at which of the following locations?
A. Left fifth intercostal space, just below the nipple
B. Right lower part of the body of the sternum
C. Right second intercostal space near the lateral border of the sternum
D. Directly over the middle of the manubrium
E. Left second intercostal space near the lateral border of the sternum

Questions 51–75

51. A 48-year-old man is brought to the emergency department by his wife because of 5-day history of chest pain. The pain is worse with exertion and improves with rest. His pulse is 98/min, blood pressure is 130/80 mm Hg, and respirations are 25/min. Coronary angiography shows nearly total blockage of the circumflex artery near its origin from the left coronary artery. When this artery is exposed to perform a bypass procedure, what accompanying vein must be protected from injury?
A. Middle cardiac
B. Great cardiac
C. Small cardiac
D. Anterior cardiac
E. Posterior vein of the left ventricle

52. A 55-year-old man was brought to the emergency department 5-days ago with chest pain. Cardiac catheterization showed the vessel that supplies much of the left ventricle and the right and left bundle branches of the cardiac conduction system to be blocked. The patient is scheduled to undergo a coronary bypass operation. Which artery is the surgeon most concerned with?
A. Right marginal
B. Anterior interventricular
C. Circumflex
D. Artery to the sinuatrial (SA) node
E. Posterior (inferior) interventricular

53. A 58-year-old man is brought to the emergency department with severe chest pain that is worse with exertion. Upon cardiac catheterization, it is found that he has a significant occlusion in his right coronary artery, distal to the right sinus of the aortic valve. His collateral cardiac circulation is minimal. Assuming the patient is right coronary dominant, which of the following arteries would be most likely to still have normal blood flow?
A. Right (acute) marginal artery
B. AV nodal artery
C. Inferior (posterior) interventricular artery
D. Sinuatrial nodal artery
E. Anterior interventricular artery

54. A 55-year-old man is brought to the emergency department with severe chest pain. Coronary angiography shows the left coronary artery to be 70%–80% occluded at three points proximal to its bifurcation into the circumflex and left anterior descending (LAD) arteries. Having a left dominant coronary circulation and no surgical intervention, what is the most likely explanation for a poor prognosis of recovery for this patient?
A. All the branches of the coronary artery are end arteries, precluding the chance that anastomotic connections will occur.
B. It is probable that the anterior and posterior papillary muscles of the tricuspid valve have been damaged.
C. The blood supply of the sinuatrial node is inadequate.
D. The development of effective collateral circulation between anterior and inferior (posterior) interventricular arteries will not be possible.
E. The blood supply of the AV node will be inadequate.

55. A 35-year-old woman is brought to the physician for a routine examination. Vital signs are within normal limits. Physical examination shows a prominent S1 heart sound located in the left fifth intercostal space along the left mid-clavicular line. This location best corresponds to the location for auscultation of which of the following valves?

A. Mitral valve
B. Aortic
C. Pulmonary
D. Aortic and pulmonary
E. Tricuspid

56. A 72-year-old man is brought to the emergency department because of severe chest pain with radiation to the jaw. His pulse is 105/min, blood pressure is 90/60 mm Hg, and respirations are 30/min. Physical examination shows a diaphoretic man in severe discomfort. An ECG shows severe myocardial infarction of the lower part of the muscular interventricular septum. The function of which of the following valves will be most severely affected?
    A. Pulmonary
    B. Aortic
    C. Tricuspid
    D. Mitral
    E. Eustachian

57. A 35-year-old woman is brought to the emergency department because of shortness of breath. Her pulse is 95 beats/min, respirations are 21 breaths/min, and blood pressure is 120/80 mm Hg. Physical examination shows wide splitting in her S_2 heart sound. An ECG shows a right bundle branch block. Which of the following valves is most likely defective?
    A. Mitral valve
    B. Pulmonary
    C. Aortic and mitral
    D. Tricuspid
    E. Tricuspid and aortic

58. A 3-month-old girl born full term via spontaneous vaginal delivery is diagnosed with a membranous ventricular septal defect and undergoes a cardiac repair. The septal defect is patched inferior to the noncoronary cusp of the aorta. Two days postoperatively, the girl develops severe arrhythmias affecting both ventricles. Which part of the conduction tissue was most likely injured during the procedure?
    A. Right bundle branch
    B. Left bundle branch
    C. AV bundle (of His)
    D. Posterior internodal pathway
    E. AV node

59. A 62-year-old man is brought to the emergency department because of severe chest pain. ECG and echocardiography show a myocardial infarction and pulmonary valve regurgitation. Emergency coronary angiography is performed and shows that the artery supplying the upper portion of the anterior right ventricular free wall is occluded. Which of the following arteries is most likely to be occluded?
    A. Circumflex
    B. Anterior interventricular artery
    C. Inferior (posterior) interventricular artery
    D. Artery of the conus
    E. Right marginal branch of the right coronary artery

60. A 3-month-old boy dies unexpectedly in his sleep. An autopsy was performed and tissue samples were taken from the heart of the boy. It was found that a portion of the conduction tissue that penetrates the right fibrous trigone had become necrotic. The cause of death was probably a fatal arrhythmia. Which of the following parts of the conduction tissue was most likely interrupted?
    A. Right bundle branch
    B. The bundle of Bachmann
    C. The left bundle branch
    D. The AV bundle of His
    E. The posterior internodal pathway

61. A 42-year-old woman is brought to the emergency department after a motor vehicle collision. She sustained blunt trauma to her sternum by the steering wheel during the crash. Her blood pressure is 75/55 mm Hg, pulse is 105/min, and respirations are 22 minutes. Physical examination shows muffled heart sounds and jugular vein distention. Ultrasound examination shows a cardiac tamponade. Which of the following cardiac structures will most likely be injured?
    A. Right ventricle
    B. Obtuse margin of the left ventricle
    C. Right atrium
    D. Left atrium
    E. Apex of the left ventricle

62. A 69-year-old man is brought to the emergency department because of severe substernal, "crushing" chest pain. Physical examination shows a diaphoretic man with crackles in the lung bases. An ECG shows hypokinetic ventricular septal muscle, myocardial infarction in the anterior two-thirds of the interventricular septum and left anterior ventricular wall. A left bundle branch block is also noted on ECG. Which of the following arteries is most likely occluded?
    A. Circumflex
    B. Proximal right coronary
    C. Proximal left coronary
    D. Proximal anterior interventricular artery
    E. Inferior (posterior) interventricular artery

63. A 49-year-old woman is brought to the emergency department because of severe, crushing, retrosternal pain for the last hour. An ECG shows that she is suffering from an acute myocardial infarction in the posterior aspect of her left ventricle and posteromedial papillary muscle. A coronary angiogram is performed, and the patient is found to have left dominant coronary circulation. Which of the following arteries is the most likely to be occluded?
    A. Artery of the conus
    B. Right coronary artery
    C. Circumflex
    D. Right marginal
    E. Diagonal

64. A 75-year-old man comes to the physician because of mild shortness of breath and an inability to walk due to swollen legs. Vital signs are within normal limits. Echocardiogram shows a large, mobile structure in

the right atrium near the opening of the inferior vena cava identified as a normal component of the heart. Which of the following structures would most likely resemble a thrombus in this location?
A. Tricuspid valve
B. Eustachian valve
C. Thebesian valve
D. Septum primum
E. Fossa ovalis

65. A 4-year-old boy with a small muscular interventricular septal defect is taken to the operating room for surgical repair. To access the right side of the interventricular septum, a wide incision is first made in the anterior surface of the right atrium. Instruments are then inserted through the tricuspid valve to correct the ventricular septal defect. Which of the following structures is the most crucial to protect during the opening of the right atrium?
A. Crista terminalis
B. Pectinate muscles
C. Tricuspid valve
D. Eustachian valve
E. Coronary sinus

66. A 52-year-old patient is brought to the emergency department because of severe chest pain. His blood pressure is 90/60 mm Hg, pulse is 100/min, and respirations are 22/min. Physical examination shows muffled heart sounds and jugular vein distention. ECG shows ST segment elevations and labs show elevated troponins confirming a myocardial infarction. Cardiac tamponade is suspected and an emergency pericardiocentesis is performed. At which of the following locations should the needle be inserted to relieve the tamponade?
A. Right seventh intercostal space in the midaxillary line
B. Left fifth intercostal space at the sternal border
C. Right third intercostal space, 1 inch lateral to the sternum
D. Left sixth intercostal space in the midclavicular line
E. Triangle of auscultation

67. A 55-year-old man is brought to the emergency department after a motor vehicle collision. His blood pressure is 70/55 mm Hg and pulse is 98/min and irregular. Ultrasound examination shows internal abdominal bleeding and the patient is taken to the operating room. The descending thoracic aorta is clamped to minimize blood loss and to preserve cerebral blood flow. The fibrous pericardium is elevated with forceps and punctured. A midline, longitudinal incision of the pericardium would be made to prevent injury to which of the following structures?
A. Auricular appendage of the left atrium
B. Coronary sinus
C. Anterior interventricular artery
D. Left phrenic nerve
E. Left sympathetic trunk

68. A 45-year-old man is brought to the emergency department because of acute onset chest pain. ECG shows ST elevation confirming a myocardial infarction. Cardiac catheterization shows severe blockage of the left coronary artery and the anterior interventricular artery. The patient is taken for a coronary bypass surgery. The surgeon can place her fingers in the transverse pericardial sinus allowing easy placement of a vascular clamp. Which of the following vessels are clamped?
A. Right and left pulmonary veins
B. Superior and inferior vena cava
C. Right and left coronary arteries
D. Pulmonary trunk and ascending aorta
E. Pulmonary trunk and superior vena cava

69. A 48-year-old man is brought to the emergency department because of substernal chest pain. ECG shows a myocardial infarction. Coronary arteriography shows nearly total blockage of the inferior (posterior) interventricular artery. The patient is scheduled to have a coronary arterial bypass. When exposing this artery to perform the bypass procedure, which accompanying vessel is most susceptible to injury?
A. Middle cardiac vein
B. Great cardiac vein
C. Small cardiac vein
D. Anterior cardiac vein
E. Coronary sinus

70. A 54-year-old man is brought to the emergency department because of severe chest pain. ECG shows ST segment elevations and labs show elevated troponins confirming a myocardial infarction. If the inferior (posterior) interventricular branch arises from the right coronary artery, which part of the myocardium will have reduced blood supply if the circumflex branch of the left coronary artery becomes occluded?
A. Anterior part of the interventricular septum
B. Diaphragmatic surface of the right ventricle
C. Infundibulum
D. Lateral wall of the left ventricle
E. Posterior part of the interventricular septum

71. A 70-year-old woman is brought to the emergency department because of severe chest pain. The symptoms began a few hours ago. She describes the pain as crushing with radiation down the left arm. An ECG shows a new myocardial infarction with a ventricular arrhythmia. Coronary angiography shows that the right coronary artery is blocked just distal to the origin of the right marginal artery in a right coronary dominant circulation. Which of the following structures would most likely be affected after such a blockade?
A. Right atrium
B. Sinuatrial node
C. AV node
D. Lateral wall of the left ventricle
E. Anterior interventricular septum

72. A 43-year-old woman comes to the physician because of shortness of breath and fatigue. Vital signs are within normal limits. Physical examination shows a mid-diastolic rumble with an abnormally loud S1 and opening snap sound heard after S2. An echocardiogram shows a mitral valve stenosis. Which of the following heart valves are responsible for the production of the first heart sound?
A. Aortic and mitral
B. Aortic and tricuspid
C. Tricuspid and mitral
D. Mitral and pulmonary
E. Tricuspid and pulmonary

73. A 75-year-old woman is brought to the emergency department because of substernal, pressure-like chest pain radiating to the left arm. ECG shows a myocardial infarction and a right bundle branch block. Physical examination shows a loud second heart sound. Which of the following heart valves are responsible for the production of the second heart sound?
A. Aortic and pulmonary
B. Aortic and tricuspid
C. Tricuspid and mitral
D. Mitral and pulmonary
E. Tricuspid and pulmonary

74. A 3-month-old girl is brought to the emergency department because her mother found her unresponsive in her crib. Ten days ago, the girl had a cardiac malformation corrected. Despite the doctor's effort, the girl dies shortly after arrival. An autopsy is performed and shows a significant portion of the conduction tissue to be necrotic. The area of the necrotic tissue was located inferior to the central fibrous body, membranous septum, and septal leaflet of the tricuspid valve. Further examination showed infarction of the surrounding tissue. The rest of the heart was unremarkable. Which of the following arteries was most likely occluded?
A. Artery of the conus
B. Sinuatrial nodal artery
C. Atrioventricular nodal artery
D. First septal perforator of the anterior interventricular artery

75. A 75-year-old man is brought to the emergency department because of chest pain, shortness of breath, and an episode of fainting. Physical examination shows a systolic crescendo-decrescendo murmur best heard at the right second intercostal space and which radiates to the carotids. Echocardiogram shows the aortic valve area to be 0.7 cm² confirming aortic valve stenosis. Patient undergoes an aortic valve replacement. As the surgeon explores the oblique pericardial sinus, which of the following is not directly palpable with the tips of the fingers?
A. Inferior vena cava
B. Superior vena cava

C. Posterior wall of the left atrium
D. Inferior right pulmonary vein
E. Right atrium

Questions 76–100

76. A 42-year-old man is brought to the emergency department after a stab wound to his chest during a violent domestic dispute. His blood pressure is 70/55 mm Hg, pulse is 115/min, and respirations are 35/min. Physical examination shows cool and clammy extremities. Echocardiogram shows fluid in the pericardial space. Which of the following will most likely be found during physical examination?
A. There will be a visible or palpable decrease in the dimensions of the external jugular and internal jugular vein
B. There will be gradual enlargement of the ventricles in diastole
C. The difference between systolic and diastolic arterial pressures will increase significantly
D. There will be diminished heart sounds
E. The pulses in the internal carotid arteries will become increasingly distinct, as detected behind the angles of the mandible

77. A 15-year-old boy is brought to the hospital by his parents for a previously scheduled surgical repair of a congenital cardiac anomaly. Pre-operative angiography shows that the boy has a right dominant coronary arterial system. During the procedure, the physician accidentally injured a vessel that usually supplies part of the conduction system. This results in intermittent periods of AV block and severe arrhythmia. The injured artery was most likely a direct branch of which of the following arteries?
A. Distal anterior interventricular artery
B. Circumflex artery
C. Left coronary artery
D. Marginal artery
E. Right coronary artery

78. A 42-year-old woman is brought to the emergency department because of shortness of breath. Physical examination shows a holosystolic murmur best heard at the left fifth intercostal space at the midclavicular line with radiation to the left axilla. Echocardiogram shows severe mitral valve regurgitation. Which of the following structures prevents regurgitation of the mitral valve cusps into the left atrium during systole?
A. Crista terminalis
B. Crista supraventricularis
C. Pectinate muscles
D. Chordae tendineae
E. Trabeculae carneae

79. A 58-year-old woman is brought to the emergency department because of fainting. ECG shows a third-degree heart block and she is scheduled for a pacemaker placement. The electrical conducting leads of the pacemaker must be passed into the heart. Which of the following is the correct order of structures for passage of the leads into the right ventricle?

A. Right brachiocephalic vein, superior vena cava, mitral valve, right ventricle

B. Superior vena cava, right atrium, mitral valve, right ventricle

C. Superior vena cava, right atrium, tricuspid valve, right ventricle

D. Right brachiocephalic vein, superior vena cava, right atrium, tricuspid valve, right ventricle

E. Right brachiocephalic vein, superior vena cava, right atrium, mitral valve, right ventricle

80. A 68-year-old man is brought to the emergency department because of difficulty swallowing food. His pulse is 85/min, respirations are 22/min, and blood pressure is 126/78 mm Hg. A barium swallow shows esophageal constriction secondary to compression. Echocardiogram shows significant cardiac hypertrophy. Which of the following is the most likely cause of the patient's dysphagia?

A. Mitral valve stenosis

B. Pulmonary valve stenosis

C. Regurgitation of the aorta

D. Occlusion of the anterior interventricular artery

E. Occlusion of the inferior (posterior) interventricular artery

81. A 35-year-old woman is brought to the emergency department because of palpitations, lightheadedness, and weakness. Her pulse is 120/min and irregular, blood pressure is 130/80 mm Hg, and respirations are 25/min. ECG examination shows absent P-waves confirming atrial fibrillation. Where is the mass of specialized conducting tissue that initiates the cardiac cycle located?

A. At the junction of the coronary sinus and the right atrium

B. At the junction of the inferior vena cava and the right atrium

C. At the junction of the superior vena cava and the right atrium

D. Between the left and right atria

E. In the interventricular septum

82. A 45-year-old woman comes to the physician because of bilateral lower extremity swelling. Physical examination shows a holosystolic murmur best heard at the left lower sternal border. Echocardiogram shows an enlarged right atrium and an incompetent tricuspid valve. Into which of the following areas would the regurgitation of blood flow in this cardiac abnormality?

A. Pulmonary trunk

B. Left atrium

C. Ascending aorta

D. Right atrium

E. Left ventricle

83. A 34-year-old man is brought to the emergency department because of a sharp, localized pain over the anterior thoracic wall, cough, and shortness of breath. Physical examination shows decreased breath sounds, dullness to percussion, and decreased tactile fremitus in the right lower lung fields. An x-ray of the chest shows blunting of the right costophrenic angle confirming right sided pleural effusion. Through which intercostal space along the midaxillary line is it most appropriate to insert a chest tube to drain the effusion fluid?

A. Fourth

B. Sixth

C. Eighth

D. Tenth

E. Twelfth

84. A 51-year-old man is brought to the emergency department because of chest pain and severe shortness of breath. His blood pressure is 86/52 mm Hg, and pulse is 115/min. Physical examination shows absent breath sounds on the right side and distended jugular veins. An x-ray of the chest shows a tension pneumothorax. Adequate local anesthesia of the chest wall prior to insertion of a chest tube is necessary for pain control. Which of the following is the deepest layer that must be infiltrated with the local anesthetic to achieve adequate anesthesia?

A. Endothoracic fascia

B. Intercostal muscles

C. Costal parietal pleura

D. Subcutaneous fat

E. Visceral pleura

85. A 5-year-old boy is brought to the emergency department by his mother for difficulty breathing and coughing which started half an hour ago. The boy was seen earlier playing with his small toy cars. Physical examination shows decreased breath sounds. A foreign body aspiration is suspected. Where in the tracheobronchial tree is the most common site for a foreign object to lodge?

A. The right primary bronchus

B. The left primary bronchus

C. The carina of the trachea

D. The beginning of the trachea

E. The left tertiary bronchus

86. A 3-year-old child is brought to the emergency department by his father because of a sudden onset shortness of breath. Physical examination shows diffuse wheezing and intercostal retractions. The boy is suspected of having a severe asthma attack. The patient is placed on oxygen and given bronchodilators. Which of the following is the most important factor in increasing the intrathoracic capacity in inspiration?

A. "Pump handle movement" of the ribs—thereby increasing anterior-posterior dimensions of the thorax

B. "Bucket handle movement" of the ribs—increasing the transverse diameter of the thorax

C. Straightening of the forward curvature of the thoracic spine, thereby increasing the vertical dimensions of the thoracic cavity

D. Descent of the diaphragm, with protrusion of the abdominal wall, thereby increasing vertical dimensions of the thoracic cavity

E. Orientation and flexibility of the ribs in the baby, thus allowing expansion in all directions

87. A 54-year-old woman is brought to the emergency department because of a stab wound she sustained after a bar fight. Her blood pressure is 90/60 mm Hg, pulse is 105/min, and respirations are 25/min. Physical examination shows a laceration in the right fourth costal cartilage with associated decreased breath sounds. Which of the following pulmonary structures is present at this site?
    A. The horizontal fissure of the left lung
    B. The horizontal fissure of the right lung
    C. The oblique fissure of the left lung
    D. The apex of the right lung
    E. The root of the left lung

88. A 55-year-old woman comes to the physician because of a painful lump in her right breast and a bloody discharge from her right nipple. Physical examination shows unilateral inversion of the nipple with an orange-peel appearance of the skin *(peau d'orange)* in the vicinity of the areola. Mammogram shows a tumor in the right upper quadrant of the breast. Which of the following best explains the inversion of her nipple?
    A. Retention of the fetal and infantile state of the nipple
    B. Intraductal cancerous tumor
    C. Retraction of the suspensory ligaments of the breast by cancer
    D. Obstruction of the cutaneous lymphatics, with edema of the skin
    E. Inflammation of the epithelial lining of the nipple and underlying hypodermis

89. A 58-year-old woman is brought to the emergency department because of severe shortness of breath. Her blood pressure is 120/80 mm Hg, pulse is 76/min, and respirations are 35/min. Bronchoscopy shows that the carina is distorted and widened. Enlargement of which group of lymph nodes is most likely responsible for altering the carina?
    A. Pulmonary
    B. Bronchopulmonary
    C. Inferior tracheobronchial
    D. Superior tracheobronchial
    E. Paratracheal

90. A 72-year-old man with Parkinson disease is brought to the emergency department from a nursing home because of difficulty with breathing. An hour ago, he was found aspirating his lunch. Bronchoscopic examination shows partially digested food blocking the origin of the right superior lobar bronchus. Which of the following groups of bronchopulmonary segments will be affected by this obstruction?
    A. Superior, medial, lateral, medial basal
    B. Apical, anterior, posterior
    C. Posterior, anterior, superior, lateral
    D. Apical, lateral, medial, lateral basal
    E. Anterior, superior, medial, lateral

91. A 35-year-old woman comes to the physician because of a mass in her right breast. Physical examination shows a firm and fixed mass in her right breast, with swollen lymph nodes in the ipsilateral axilla. A mammogram and biopsy confirm carcinoma of the breast. Which group of axillary lymph nodes is the first to receive lymph drainage and most likely to contain metastasized tumor cells?
    A. Lateral
    B. Central
    C. Apical
    D. Anterior (pectoral)
    E. Posterior (subscapular)

92. An 18-year-old man is brought to the emergency department because of nosebleed, fatigue, and a headache that has worsened over several days. Physical examination shows that brachial artery pressure is markedly increased, femoral pressure is decreased, and the femoral pulses are delayed. The patient shows no external signs of inflammation. Which of the following is the most likely diagnosis?
    A. Coarctation of the aorta
    B. Cor pulmonale
    C. Dissecting aneurysm of the right common iliac artery
    D. Obstruction of the superior vena cava
    E. Pulmonary embolism

93. A 22-year-old man is brought to the emergency department because of nosebleed, fatigue, and a headache that has worsened over several days. Physical examination shows that brachial artery pressure is markedly increased, femoral pressure is decreased, and the femoral pulses are delayed. The patient shows no external signs of inflammation. Which of the following conditions will most likely be observed on an x-ray of the chest?
    A. Flail chest
    B. Pneumothorax
    C. Hydrothorax
    D. Notching of the ribs
    E. Mediastinal shift

94. A 56-year-old woman presents to the physician with pain and weakness in the right shoulder. Two weeks ago, the patient underwent a radical mastectomy with extensive axillary dissection after being diagnosed with carcinoma of the right breast. Physical examination shows winging of the scapula when she pushes against the wall. Injury to which of the following nerves would result in this condition?

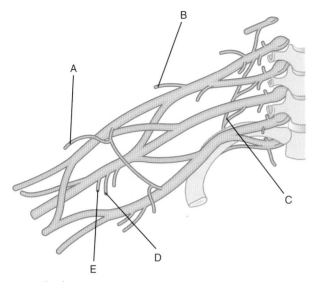

A. A
B. B
C. C
D. D
E. E

95. A 22-year-old woman is brought to the emergency department after sustaining a chest injury upon impact with the steering wheel during a motor vehicle collision. Physical examination shows profuse swelling, erythema, and deformation of the chest wall. An x-ray shows an uncommon fracture of the sternum at the manubriosternal joint. Which of the following ribs would most likely also be involved in such an injury?
A. First
B. Second
C. Third
D. Fourth
E. Fifth

96. A 47-year-old man is brought to the emergency department because of difficulty swallowing. Physical examination shows swelling of the lower extremities. A barium swallow shows esophageal dilation with severe inflammation due to constriction at the esophageal hiatus from a large lipoma. What is the most likely cause of the severe edema of the lower limbs?
A. Thoracic aorta constriction
B. Thoracic duct blockage
C. Superior vena cava occlusion
D. Aortic aneurysm
E. Femoral artery disease

97. A 49-year-old man comes to the physician to undergo coronary artery bypass. He has a history of hypertension and diabetes. During the procedure, the left internal thoracic artery is used as the coronary artery bypass graft. The anterior intercostal arteries in the third to sixth intercostal spaces are ligated. Which of the following arteries will most likely provide collateral supply to these intercostal spaces?

A. Musculophrenic
B. Superior epigastric
C. Posterior intercostal
D. Lateral thoracic
E. Thoracodorsal

98. A 10-year-old boy is brought to the physician because of retrosternal discomfort. There is no family history of cancer. Physical examination shows normal development and no gross deformities of the neck. A CT scan shows a midline tumor of the thymus. Which of the following veins would most likely be compressed by the tumor?
A. Right internal jugular
B. Left internal jugular
C. Right brachiocephalic
D. Left brachiocephalic
E. Right subclavian

99. A 25-year-old man is brought to the emergency department after sustaining a gunshot wound in the neck. His temperature is 37°C (98.6°F), pulse is 120/min, and blood pressure is 85/45 mm Hg. Physical examination shows a bullet wound in the neck just above the middle of the right clavicle and first rib. An x-ray of the chest shows collapse of the right lung and a tension pneumothorax. Which of the following structures was most likely injured to result in the tension pneumothorax?
A. Costal pleura
B. Cupula
C. Right mainstem bronchus
D. Right upper lobe bronchus
E. Mediastinal parietal pleura

100. A 51-year-old woman is brought to the emergency department because of chest pain. She has a history of brain tumor and severe oropharyngeal dysphagia. She received chemotherapy two days ago and has had intractable episodes of vomiting. Physical examination of the chest shows dullness to percussion over the right lung field. Crackles are heard on auscultation. An x-ray of the chest shows pneumonia of the right lower lobe. Which of the following is the most likely explanation of pneumonia affecting the right lower lung lobe?
A. Pulmonary vascular resistance is higher in the right lung than the left lung
B. The right main bronchus is straighter than the left main bronchus
C. The right main bronchus is narrower than the main bronchus
D. The right main bronchus is longer than the left main bronchus
E. The right lower lung lobe has poorer venous drainage than the other lobes

Questions 101–125

101. A 41-year-old man is brought to the emergency department with complaints of shortness of breath, dizziness, and sharp chest pain. Patient has a long

history of smoking and hypertension. His temperature is 37°C (96.8°F), pulse is 120/min, respirations are 24/min, and blood pressure is 100/65 mm Hg. The large arrow in the x-ray of the chest indicates the region of pathology (Fig. 2.1). What is this structure?

A. Superior vena cava
B. Right ventricle
C. Left ventricle
D. Arch of the aorta
E. Pulmonary artery

102. A 42-year-old woman comes to the physician because she has a painful lump in her right breast and a bloody discharge from her right nipple. Physical examination shows unilateral inversion of the right nipple and a hard, woody texture of the skin over a mass of tissue in the right upper quadrant of the breast. Which of the following conditions is most likely characterized by these findings?

A. Peau d'orange
B. Cancer en cuirasse
C. Intraductal cancerous tumor
D. Obstruction of the lymphatics draining the skin of the breast, with edema of the skin
E. Inflammation of the epithelial lining of the nipple and underlying hypodermis

103. A 25-year-old woman is brought to the emergency department after being involved in a motor vehicle collision. Her temperature is 37°C (98.6°F), pulse is 110/min, and blood pressure is 115/85 mm Hg. An x-ray of the chest shows four broken ribs of the left

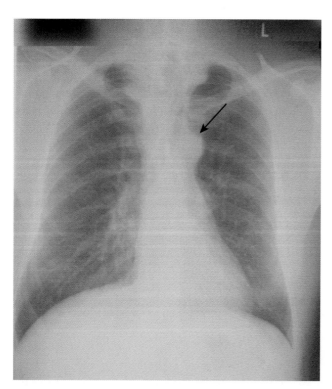

• **Fig. 2.1**

thoracic wall. Which of the following will be most likely observed during physical examination?

A. During deep inspiration, the flail segment moves in the opposite direction of the chest wall
B. During deep inspiration, the flail segment moves in the same direction as the chest wall
C. "Pump handle movements" of the ribs will not be affected by the rib fractures
D. The descent of the diaphragm will be affected on the side of the broken ribs
E. The descent of the diaphragm will be affected on the side of the broken ribs and also on the opposite side

104. A 33-year-old man is brought to the emergency department with severe traumatic injuries after being involved in a motor vehicle collision. His temperature is 37°C (98.6°F), pulse is 115/min, and blood pressure is 89/39 mm Hg. A central venous line is placed for fluid resuscitation. Which of the following injuries is most likely to occur if a subclavian central venous line procedure is incorrectly performed?

A. Penetration of the subclavian artery
B. Injury of the phrenic nerve
C. Penetration of the superior vena cava
D. Penetration of the left common carotid artery
E. Impalement of the vagus nerve

105. A 50-year-old man is brought to the emergency department with painful swallowing. Patient has a long-standing history of smoking. A barium swallow shows an esophageal constriction at the level of the diaphragm. A CT scan and a biopsy further indicate the presence of an esophageal cancer in the distal third of the esophagus. Which of the following lymph nodes will most likely be affected first?

A. Posterior mediastinal and left gastric
B. Bronchopulmonary
C. Tracheobronchial
D. Inferior tracheobronchial
E. Superior tracheobronchial

106. A 42-year-old man is brought to the emergency department with retrosternal pain for 6 months. He has smoked 20 cigarettes daily for the past 20 years. Endoscopy and biopsy examinations of the trachea show a malignant growth at the right main bronchus. Which of the following lymph nodes will most likely be the first infiltrated by cancerous cells from the malignancy?

A. Inferior tracheobronchial
B. Paratracheal
C. Bronchomediastinal trunk
D. Bronchopulmonary
E. Thoracic duct

107. A 60-year-old man is brought to the emergency department with severe pain in his midsection. A CT scan shows a dissecting aneurysm of the descending thoracic aorta. During his hospital stay, the patient's aneurysm ruptured and he was transferred for surgery.

Postoperatively, the patient suffers from paraplegia. Which of the following arteries was most likely injured during the operation to result in the paralysis?

A. Right coronary artery
B. Left common carotid
C. Right subclavian
D. Great radicular (of Adamkiewicz)
E. Esophageal

108. A 47-year-old woman comes to the physician with pain in her neck. Physical examination shows an enlarged thyroid gland on the left side and displacement of the trachea. An x-ray of the chest shows a tracheal deviation to the right and a biopsy shows a benign tumor. Which of the following structures will most likely be compressed by the enlarged thyroid gland?

A. Left brachiocephalic vein
B. Left internal jugular vein
C. Left subclavian artery
D. Vagus nerve
E. Phrenic nerve

109. A 33-year-old man is brought to the emergency department after being involved in a motor vehicle collision. His temperature is 37°C (96.8°F), pulse is 80/min, and blood pressure is 119/89 mm Hg, and a central venous line is placed. Which of the following structures is used as a landmark to verify that the tip of the catheter of the central venous line is in the correct place?

A. Carina
B. Subclavian artery
C. Superior vena cava
D. Left atrium
E. Right atrium

110. A 42-year-old man comes to the physician for an abdominal pain. He is diagnosed with liver and pancreatic disease as a result of alcoholism. Physical examination shows an enlargement of his mammary glands, as a secondary result of his disease process. Which of the following clinical conditions will most likely describe this case?

A. Polythelia
B. Supernumerary breast
C. Polymastia
D. Gynecomastia
E. Amastia

111. A 21-year-old woman is brought to the emergency department with severe dyspnea after a fall from the uneven parallel bars during her gymnastic practice. An x-ray of the chest shows that her right lung is collapsed and the left lung is compressed by the great volume of air in her right pleural cavity. Physical examination does not show any signs of external injuries. Which of the following conditions will most likely describe this case?

A. Flail chest with paradoxical respiration
B. Emphysema

C. Hemothorax
D. Chylothorax
E. Tension pneumothorax

112. A 34-year-old man is brought to the emergency department after being found unconscious. His temperature is 37°C (96.8°F), pulse is 90/min, and blood pressure is 120/90 mm Hg. A central venous line is placed. A subsequent x-ray of the chest shows a chylothorax. Which of the following structures was most likely accidentally damaged during the placement of the central venous line?

A. Left external jugular vein
B. Site of origin of the left brachiocephalic vein
C. Right subclavian vein
D. Proximal part of right brachiocephalic vein
E. Right external jugular vein

113. A 28-year-old woman in the third trimester of pregnancy comes to the emergency department because of severe dizziness for several days. Physical examination shows that her blood pressure is normal when standing or sitting. When the patient is supine, her blood pressure drops to 90/50 mm Hg. Which of the following structures is most likely compressed?

A. inferior vena cava
B. superior vena cava
C. aorta
D. common carotid artery
E. internal jugular veins

114. A 17-year-old girl comes to the physician because of dyspnea and fever for 4 days. Physical examination shows rales and crackles at the level of the sixth intercostal space at the midaxillary line, and dull sounds are produced during percussion. An x-ray of the chest shows lobar pneumonia in one of the lobes of her right lung. Which of the following lobes is most likely to be involved by pneumonia?

A. Upper lobe of the right lung
B. Middle lobe of the right lung
C. Lower lobe of the right lung
D. Lower lobes of the right and left lungs
E. Upper lobes of the right and left lungs

115. A 35-year-old man is brought to the emergency department with severe chest pain, dyspnea, tachycardia, cough, and fever. An x-ray of the chest shows significant pericardial effusion. When pericardiocentesis is performed, the needle is inserted up from the infrasternal angle. The needle passes too deeply, piercing the visceral pericardium and entering the heart. Which of the following chambers would be the first to be penetrated by the needle?

A. Right ventricle
B. Left ventricle
C. Right atrium
D. Left atrium
E. The cardiac apex

116. A 45-year-old man is brought to the emergency department with severe chest pain radiating to his

left arm and left upper jaw. An ECG shows an acute myocardial infarction of the inferior ventricular wall. Which of the following spinal cord segments would most likely receive the sensations of pain in this case?

A. T1, T2, T3
B. T1, T2, T3, T4
C. T1, T2
D. T4, T5, T6
E. T5, T6, T7

117. A 55-year-old woman is brought to the emergency department with cough and severe dyspnea. An x-ray of the chest shows an emphysema. Physical examination shows "bucket handle\movements" during deep inspiration. Which of the following movements of the thoracic wall is characteristic for this type of breathing?

A. Increase of the transverse diameter of \ the thorax
B. Increase of the anteroposterior diameter of the thorax
C. Increase of the vertical dimension of the thorax
D. Decrease of the anteroposterior diameter of the thorax
E. Decrease of the transverse diameter of the thorax

118. A 15-year-old boy is brought to the emergency department with cough and severe dyspnea. Physical examination shows expiratory wheezes, and asthma was diagnosed. The expiratory wheezes are characteristic signs of bronchospasm of the smooth muscle of the bronchial airways. Which of the following nerves could be blocked to cause relaxation of the smooth muscle?

A. Phrenic
B. Intercostal
C. Vagus
D. T1–T4 sympathetic fibers
E. Recurrent laryngeal nerve

119. A 34-year-old man is brought to the emergency department with a sharp, localized pain over the thoracic wall. Physical examination shows dullness on percussion and an x-ray of the chest shows a pleural effusion. A chest tube is inserted to drain the effusion through an intercostal space. At which of the following locations is the chest tube most likely to be inserted?

A. Superior to the upper border of the rib
B. Inferior to the lower border of the rib
C. At the middle of the intercostal space
D. Between the internal and external intercostal muscles
E. Between the intercostal muscles and the internal intercostal membrane

120. A 42-year-old woman is brought to the emergency department after a fall from a balcony. The patient is in significant distress. Physical examination shows distant heart sounds, reduced systolic pressure, and engorged external jugular veins. Which condition is most likely characterized by these signs?

A. Hemothorax
B. Cardiac tamponade
C. Hemopneumothorax
D. Pneumothorax
E. Deep vein thrombosis

121. A 35-year-old woman is brought to the emergency department with a complaint of shortness of breath on exertion for 3 months. Vitals are within normal limits. Physical examination shows a wide splitting in S_2 heart sound. An x-ray of the chest showed normal findings. Which of the following valve(s) is/are responsible for production of the S_2 heart sound?

A. Mitral valve
B. Pulmonary and aortic
C. Aortic and mitral
D. Tricuspid
E. Tricuspid and aortic

122. A 35-year-old woman is brought to the emergency department with dyspnea for 2 months. Vitals are within normal limits. Physical examination shows a very loud S_1 heart sound. An x-ray of the chest showed normal findings. Which of the following valve(s) is/are responsible for production of the S_1 heart sound?

A. Mitral valve
B. Pulmonary and aortic
C. Aortic and mitral
D. Tricuspid
E. Tricuspid and mitral

123. A 57-year-old man is brought to the emergency department after he was struck by a truck while crossing a street. An x-ray of the chest shows a flail chest. Physical examination shows that the patient is experiencing severe pain during inspiration and expiration. Which of the following nerves is most likely responsible for the sensation of pain during respiration?

A. Phrenic
B. Vagus
C. Cardiopulmonary
D. Intercostal
E. Thoracic splanchnic

124. A 62-year-old woman is brought to the emergency department with severe dyspnea and pain over her left shoulder. Vitals are within normal limits. Physical examination shows no abnormalities. An x-ray of the chest shows an aneurysm of the aortic arch. Which of the following nerves is most likely affected by the aneurysm?

A. Phrenic
B. Vagus
C. Cardiopulmonary
D. Intercostal
E. Thoracic splanchnic

125. A 62-year-old woman is brought to the emergency department with severe chest pain that radiates to her left arm. An ECG shows an acute myocardial infarction. Coronary angiography is performed and a stent is placed at the proximal portion of the anterior

interventricular artery (LAD). Because of the irregular cardiac rhythm, a cardiac pacemaker is also placed in the heart. The function of which of the following structures is essentially replaced by the insertion of a pacemaker?

A. AV node
B. Sinuatrial node
C. Purkinje fibers
D. Bundle of His
E. Bundle of Kent

Questions 126–148

126. A 22-year-old man is brought to the emergency department with severe dyspnea. Physical examination shows that the patient is experiencing an acute asthma attack, and a bronchodilation drug is administered. Which of the following elements of the nervous system must be inhibited by the drug to achieve relaxation of the smooth muscle of the tracheobronchial tree?

A. Postganglionic sympathetic fibers
B. Preganglionic sympathetic fibers
C. Postganglionic parasympathetic fibers
D. Visceral afferent fibers
E. Somatic efferent fibers

127. A 3-day-old girl is brought to the emergency department because she was blue. The fact that the patient was cyanotic gives evidence of abnormalities within the heart. Blood tests show abnormally high levels of TGF-β factor *Nodal*. Which of the following conditions is most likely to be associated with these findings?

A. Dextrocardia
B. Ectopia cordis
C. Transposition of the great arteries
D. Unequal division of the truncus arteriosus
E. Coarctation of the aorta

128. A 35-year-old woman was brought to the emergency department for a drug overdose. The patient is unresponsive and an empty bottle of acetaminophen was found in her handbag. The patient required insertion of a nasogastric tube and administration of activated charcoal. What are the three sites in the esophagus where one should anticipate resistance due to compression on the organ?

A. At the aortic arch, the cricopharyngeal constriction, and the diaphragmatic constriction
B. The cardiac constriction, the cricoid cartilage constriction, and the thoracic duct
C. The pulmonary constriction, cricothyroid constriction, and the azygos vein arch
D. The cardiac constriction, the azygos vein arch, and the pulmonary trunk
E. The cricopharyngeal constriction, cricothyroid constriction, and thymus

129. A 69-year-old woman comes to the physician because of severe pain radiating across her back and chest.

Vitals are within normal limits. Physical examination shows a rash characteristic of herpes zoster infection passing from her upper left back and across her left nipple. Which of the following spinal nerve roots sheds the active virus?

A. Dorsal root of T3
B. Ventral root of T3
C. Dorsal root of T4
D. Ventral root of T4
E. Dorsal root of T5

130. A 3-year-old boy is brought to the emergency department after a fall from a tree. The patient complains of severe pain over the right side of his chest. Physical examination shows dullness on percussion in the lower lobes of lungs bilaterally. An x-ray of the chest shows a rib fracture at the midaxillary line, atelectasis, and hemothorax resulting from the accumulation of blood in his pleural space. What is the most likely source of bleeding to cause the hemothorax?

A. Left common carotid artery
B. Intercostal vessels
C. Pulmonary arteries
D. Pulmonary veins
E. Internal thoracic artery

131. A 45-year-old woman is brought to the emergency department with severe dyspnea for 4 months. The patient has smoked 1 pack of cigarettes a day for 30 years. Radiologic examination confirms the presence of a Pancoast tumor (Fig. 2.2). Physical examination shows that the patient has miosis of the pupil, partial ptosis of the eyelid, and anhidrosis of the face. Which of the following structures has most likely been injured?

A. Sympathetic trunk
B. Vagus nerve
C. Phrenic nerve
D. Arch of aorta
E. Cardiopulmonary plexus

132. A 35-year-old man is brought to the emergency department due to severe dysphagia. The patient lost 20 lb in last 6 months. Vitals are within normal limits. Physical examination shows no abnormalities. A CT scan (Fig. 2.3) shows carcinoma of the middle segment of the esophagus. Which of the following structures will most likely be affected if the carcinoma increases greatly in size?

A. Inferior vena cava
B. Left atrium
C. Pulmonary artery
D. Left ventricle
E. Vertebral body

133. A 62-year-old man is brought to the emergency department with a complaint of severe chest pain. ECG shows an acute myocardial infarction. After the patient is stabilized, angiography is performed and the ejection fraction of the left ventricle is reduced to 30% from 60% on previous echocardiogram 3

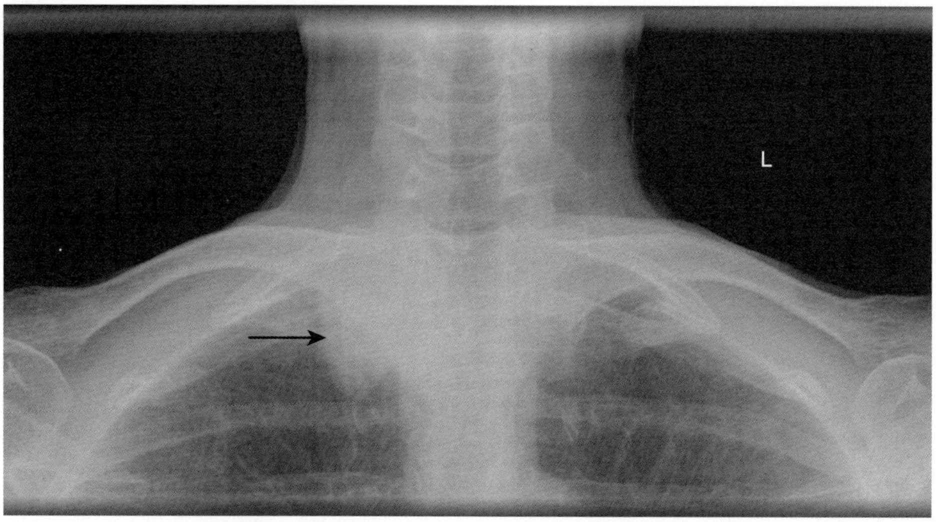

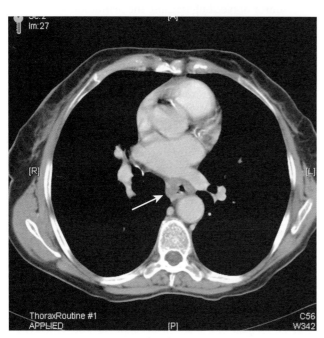

• Fig. 2.2

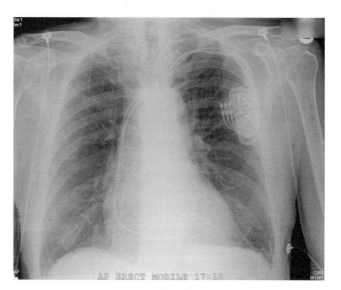

• Fig. 2.3

• Fig. 2.4

A. Esophagus
B. Pulmonary trunk
C. Superior vena cava
D. Trachea
E. Inferior vena cava

months ago. A cardiac pacemaker is placed to prevent fatal arrhythmias (Fig. 2.4). What is the location of the tip of the pacemaker?

A. Right atrium
B. Left atrium
C. Right ventricle
D. Left ventricle
E. Superior vena cava

134. A 68-year-old man comes to the physician for post-operative follow up after mitral valve replacement 8 weeks ago. The surgery went well without complications and the patient has been well since the surgery. The patient had a significant cardiac hypertrophy before the surgery (Fig. 2.5). Which of the following structures would be most likely compressed?

135. A 29-year-old man is brought to the emergency department after being involved in a motor vehicle collision. He has significant difficulty in breathing. His temperature is 37°C (96.8°F), pulse is 100/min, respirations are 25/min, and blood pressure is 120/90 mm Hg. Physical examination shows no signs of external injuries, but the dyspnea becomes progressively worse. An x-ray of the chest (Fig. 2.6) shows no fractured bones or mediastinal shift. Which of the following conditions would best describe this case?

A. Flail chest with paradoxical respiration
B. Emphysema
C. Hemothorax

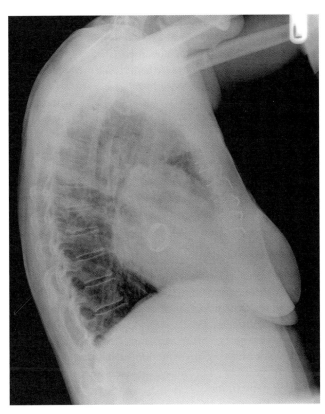

• **Fig. 2.5**

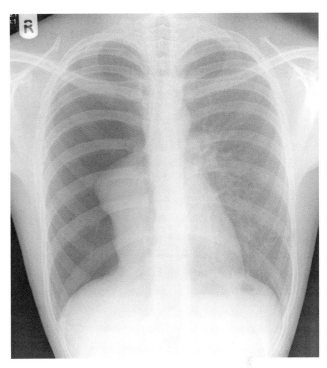

• **Fig. 2.6**

D. Spontaneous pneumothorax

E. Tension pneumothorax

136. A 56-year-old man is brought to the emergency department with dyspnea, cough, and high fever. Physical examination shows dullness on percussion, decreased intensity of breath sounds, and rhonchi. An x-ray of the chest shows lobar pneumonia (Fig. 2.7). Which of the following lobes of the lung is affected as shown in the image?

A. Right upper

B. Right middle

C. Right lower

D. Right upper, middle, and lower

E. Right upper and lower

137. A 62-year-old man is brought to the emergency department with severe chest pain after a fall while jogging. An ECG shows an acute myocardial infarction. After the patient is stabilized, angiography is performed and one of the major coronary arteries is found to be occluded (Fig. 2.8). Which of the following arteries is most obviously blocked by atherosclerotic plaque or clot?

A. Right coronary

B. Left anterior interventricular

C. Inferior (posterior) interventricular

D. Diagonal

E. Circumflex

138. A 47-year-old woman comes to the physician for an abnormal change in her right breast. The patient does not have a family history of cancer but has drunk a bottle of wine every day for 10 years. Physical examination shows *peau d'orange* characteristics in her right breast. This condition is primarily a result of which of the following occurrences?

A. Blockage of cutaneous lymphatic vessels

B. Shortening of the suspensory ligaments by cancer in the axillary tail of the breast

C. Contraction of the retinacula cutis of the areola and nipple

D. Invasion of the pectoralis major by metastatic cancer

E. Ipsilateral (same side) inversion of the nipple from cancer of the duct system of the breast

139. A 27-year-old man is brought to the emergency department after a small-caliber bullet wound to the chest in the region of the third intercostal space, several centimeters to the left of the sternum. His temperature is 37°C (96.8°F), pulse is 110/min, respirations are 26/min, and blood pressure is 100/70 mm Hg. The patient is admitted to the surgical floor and a preliminary notation of "Beck's triad" is entered on the patient's chart. Which of the following are features of this triad?

A. There was injury to the left pulmonary artery, left primary bronchus, and esophagus

B. The patient has bleeding into the pleural cavity, a collapsed lung, and mediastinal shift to the right side of the thorax

C. The patient has a small, quiet heart; decreased pulse pressure; and increased central venous pressure

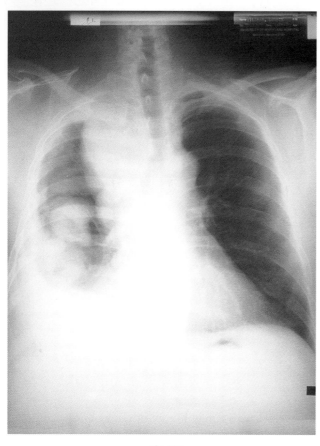

• Fig. 2.7

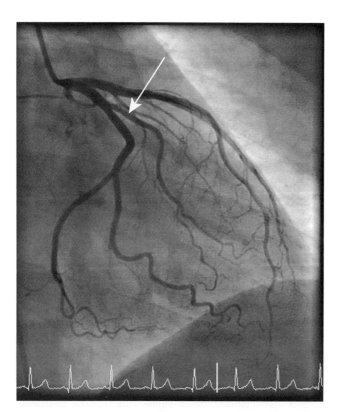

• Fig. 2.8

D. The young man is suffering from marked diastolic emptying, dyspnea, and dilation of the aortic arch

E. The left lung has collapsed, there is paradoxical respiration, and there is a mediastinal shift of the heart and trachea to the left

140. A 34-year-old man is brought to the emergency department for severe shortness of breath. The patient had been diagnosed earlier in the week with Guillain-Barré syndrome. His thoracic wall contracts and relaxes violently, but there is little movement of the abdominal wall. The degenerative disease has obviously affected the muscle that is most responsible for increasing the vertical dimensions of the thoracic cavity (and pleural cavities). Which of the following is the most likely cause of his disease?

A. Paralysis of his intercostal muscles and loss of the "bucket handle movement" of his ribs

B. Generalized intercostal nerve paralysis that resulted in loss of the "pump handle movement" of his ribs

C. Paralysis of his medial and lateral pectoral nerves, interrupting the function of his pectoralis major muscles, an important accessory muscle of respiration

D. Paralysis of his sternocleidomastoid muscles

E. Degeneration of the myelin of his phrenic nerves

141. A 34-year-old man is brought to the emergency department with shortness of breath. The patient has a history of Guillain-Barré syndrome. Two days after the patient's breathing had become assisted by mechanical ventilation, he began experiencing severe cardiac arrhythmia, with decreased cardiac contractions, resulting in reduced cardiac output. Which of the following most likely has caused an interruption of the contractile stimulus?

A. Left vagus nerve

B. Right phrenic nerve

C. Preganglionic sympathetic fibers in upper thoracic spinal nerves

D. Cardiac pain fibers carried by upper thoracic spinal nerves

E. Ventral horn neurons of spinal cord levels T1–T4

142. A 45-year-old man comes to the physician for a scheduled transesophageal echocardiography (TEE). During the procedure, an ultrasound transducer is placed through the nose or mouth to lie directly behind the heart. The closer a structure is to the transducer, the better the ultrasound image that can be obtained. Which heart valve can be best visualized by TEE?

A. Tricuspid

B. Pulmonary

C. Mitral

D. Aortic

E. Valve of the inferior vena cava

143. A 45-year-old man is brought to the emergency department because of continuous vomiting for the past 2 days. He has history of alcohol abuse and is severely dehydrated. The patient was placed on fluid replacement and he recovers well. An x-ray of the chest shows a mild pneumomediastinum. The presence of which of the following anatomic structures is a radiologic landmark for the diagnosis of pneumomediastinum?

A. Left superior intercostal vein
B. Vagus nerve
C. Superior vena cava
D. Pulmonary vein
E. Aortic arch

144. A newborn boy was born at 34 weeks of gestation and was found to have pneumonitis. A CT scan of the chest shows that the upper segment of the esophagus ends blindly and the presence of an abnormal communication between the trachea and the lower segment of esophagus. Which of the following clinical conditions is most commonly seen in association with this congenital anomaly?

A. Polyhydramnios
B. Oligodramnios
C. Anhydramnios
D. Hydatidiform mole
E. Choriocarcinomas

145. A 30-year-old man is brought to the emergency department because of a significant nosebleed and a headache that has worsened over several days. Physical examination shows markedly increased brachial artery pressure, decreased femoral pressure, and delayed femoral pulses. There were no external signs of inflammation. From which of the following embryological structures does this defect arise?

A. Fourth pharyngeal arch
B. Third pharyngeal arch
C. Left dorsal aorta
D. Left fifth pharyngeal arch
E. Sixth pharyngeal arch

146. A 3-day-old boy is brought to the emergency department for severe dyspnea and cyanosis. Physical examination shows a flat abdomen. An x-ray of the chest shows a left side pneumothorax and pockets of air in the left hemithorax. Which of the following conditions is the most likely diagnosis?

A. Congenital diaphragmatic hernia
B. Laryngeal atresia
C. Emphysema
D. Respiratory distress syndrome
E. Tracheoesophageal fistula

147. A 55-year-old man is brought to the emergency department with complaints of severe chest pain radiating to his left arm and increased sweating over his chest. ECG shows an acute myocardial infarction of the posterior wall of the left ventricle. Which nerve fibers are most likely responsible for the increased sweating?

A. Preganglionic parasympathetics
B. Postganglionic sympathetics in the cardiopulmonary nerve
C. Thoracic visceral afferents
D. Postganglionic sympathetic fibers from T1 to T4
E. Postganglionic sympathetic fibers from superior, middle, and inferior cervical ganglia

148. A 35-year-old woman comes to the physician after finding a small mass in her right breast when performing a self-examination while taking a shower. Mammogram shows mass about 1 cm in diameter slightly above, and lateral, to her right areola. She underwent lymph node biopsy and a specific dye was injected into the tissue around the tumor, which was taken up by the lymph vessels, draining the area. The vessels were traced to surgically expose the lymph nodes receiving the lymph from the tumor. Which nodes will most likely first receive lymph from the tumor?

A. Anterior axillary (pectoral)
B. Lateral axillary
C. Parasternal
D. Central axillary
E. Apical axillary (infraclavicular)

Questions 149–173

149. A 51-year-old woman comes to the physician complaining because of dyspnea on exertion for the past 2 months. She also has generalized fatigue. Vitals are within normal limits. Physical examination shows edema of the lower limbs and a systolic murmur was heard in the left second intercostal space. Which of the following valve abnormalities is she most likely suffering from?

A. Regurgitation through aortic valve
B. Regurgitation through pulmonary valve
C. Stenosis of aortic valve
D. Regurgitation through mitral valve
E. Stenosis of pulmonary valve

150. A 58-year-old man was brought to the emergency department because of shortness of breath and chest pain radiating to his left arm. A diagnosis of angina pectoris was made resulting from ischemia of the myocardium. Sublingual nitroglycerine relieved the condition by causing vasodilation and improving blood flow to the heart. Which of the following nerves referred the pain to the arm?

A. Vagus
B. Intercostals
C. Phrenic
D. Intercostobrachial
E. Cardiopulmonary

151. A 41-year-old woman comes to the physician for a lump in her right breast. Physical examination shows dimpling of skin of the breast over the mass. A CT scan of the breast shows a 3-cm mass at the right upper quadrant of her right breast with multiple calcifications. The dimpling of the breast is most likely caused by invasion of the tumor into which of the following structure(s)?

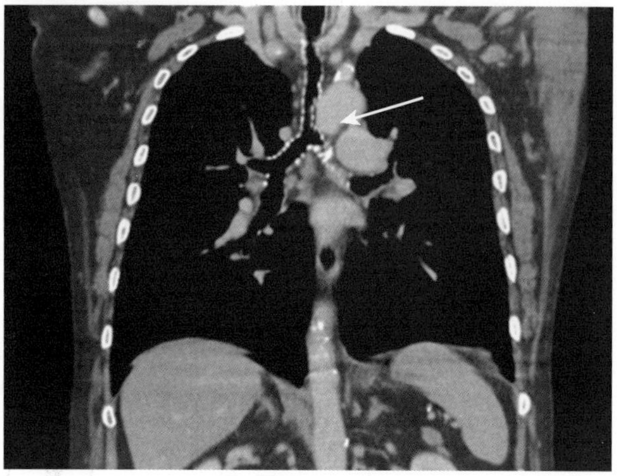

• Fig. 2.9

A. Lactiferous ducts
B. Mammary and apical lymph nodes
C. Suspensory ligaments
D. Clavipectoral fascia
E. Medial and lateral pectoral nerves

152. A 65-year-old woman is brought to the emergency department with severe chest pain radiating to her upper jaw and arms for 3 hours. ECG shows a myocardial infarction. Cardiac catheterization is performed and the portion of the heart immediately behind the sternum is found to be infarcted. Which artery is most likely occluded?
A. Circumflex
B. Anterior interventricular
C. Inferior (posterior) interventricular
D. Left marginal
E. Right coronary

153. A 42-year-old woman is brought to the emergency department with gradually worsening dysphagia for a month. She also has hoarseness. A CT scan (Fig. 2.9) of the thorax shows a small aortic aneurysm. Which of the following nerves will most likely be compressed if the aortic aneurysm continues to grow?
A. Vagus
B. Phrenic
C. Left recurrent laryngeal
D. Right recurrent laryngeal
E. Greater thoracic splanchnic

154. A 59-year-old man is brought to the emergency department with a chest pain. ECG showed severe inferior myocardial infarction. The patient was brought to the catheterization lab for an emergency catheterization of his coronary arteries. During passage of the catheter from his right radial artery it is noted that the patient has a right subclavian artery passing posteriorly to the esophagus and thus requires a longer catheter. Which of the following structures failed to regress in this condition?
A. Right dorsal aorta distal to the seventh intersegmental artery
B. Left dorsal aorta distal to the seventh intersegmental artery
C. Right dorsal aorta proximal to the seventh intersegmental artery
D. Fifth arch artery
E. Ventral part of the first arch artery

155. A 25-year-old man comes to the physician with severe headache, cold feet and legs, and pain in his legs when he runs a short distance. Physical examination shows that femoral pulses are much weaker than radial pulses. Three-dimensional CT scan angiography shows a coarctation of the aorta proximal to the left subclavian artery. The condition that creates these symptoms is a result of a failure of normal development of which structure?
A. Fourth pharyngeal arch
B. Third pharyngeal arch
C. Left dorsal aorta
D. Left fifth pharyngeal arch
E. Sixth pharyngeal arch

156. A newborn girl comes to the physician for cyanosis. The patient does not have any cardiac family history. She is diagnosed with tricuspid valve atresia. An ultrasonographic shows a widely patent foramen ovale, ventricular septal defect hypoplastic right ventricle, and hypertrophied left ventricle. The patient most likely reflects a developmental failure of which of the following structures?
A. Endocardial cushions
B. Foramen primum
C. Septum secundum
D. Truncus arteriosus
E. Bulbus cordis

157. A 35-year-old woman is brought to the emergency department with dyspnea and unintentional weight loss for 6 months. She smoked 2 packs of cigarettes a day for 20 years. Vitals are within normal limits. An x-ray of the chest shows a tumor invading the lung surface just anterior to the hilum. Which nerve is being compressed by the tumor?
A. Phrenic
B. Vagus
C. Intercostal
D. Recurrent laryngeal
E. Thoracic visceral

158. A 60-year-old woman comes to the physician for a routine follow up. She has a history of severe rheumatic heart disease. Her cardiac symptoms have been relatively stable since valve replacement surgery 2 years ago, but she has developed some new symptoms over the past few months. An x-ray of the chest shows sternotomy wires, prosthetic aortic and mitral valves, and a greatly enlarged left atrium. Which symptom would most likely develop as a direct result of her left atrial enlargement?
A. Nausea and vomiting
B. Pain and tenderness over thoracic vertebral spinous processes
C. Difficulty swallowing
D. Epigastric pain after eating fatty foods
E. Increased coughing

159. A 59-year-old man is brought to the emergency department with severe chest pain and sweating. He has a long history of hypertension and uncontrolled diabetes. Vitals are within normal limits. Physical examination shows a slight rhythmic pulsation on the chest wall at the left fifth intercostal space. An x-ray of the chest is within normal limits. What would be the cause of this pulsation?
    A. Right atrium
    B. Left atrium
    C. Aortic arch
    D. Apex of the heart
    E. Mitral valve

160. A 48-year-old man is brought to the emergency department with chronic angina for 6 months and it has gotten severely worse since yesterday. ECG shows an acute myocardial infarction. Coronary angiography shows nearly total blockage of the anterior interventricular artery just after it arises from the left coronary. In exposing this artery for a bypass procedure, which accompanying vein must be protected from injury?
    A. Middle cardiac
    B. Great cardiac
    C. Small cardiac
    D. Anterior cardiac
    E. Posterior vein of the left ventricle

161. A 25-year-old man is brought to the emergency department because of a 1-week history of fever and cough productive of purulent sputum. His temperature is 38.9°C (102°F), pulse is 110/min, respirations are 24/min, and blood pressure is 110/70 mm Hg. Crackles, decreased breath sounds, and decreased fremitus are present in the right lower lobe. An x-ray of the chest shows a pleural effusion over the lower third of the thorax on the right in the midclavicular line. A thoracocentesis is scheduled. Which intercostal space in the midclavicular line in this patient would be most appropriate for insertion of the needle during this procedure?
    A. Fifth
    B. Seventh
    C. Ninth
    D. Eighth
    E. Eleventh

162. A 70-year-old man is brought to the emergency department for abdominal pain. The patient has not been able to have bowel movements or flatus for 5 days. An x-ray of the abdomen showed a small bowel obstruction. When inserting a nasogastric tube by a surgical resident, which is the most distal site in, or in relation to, the esophagus that might offer resistance to the tube as it passes to the stomach?
    A. Posterior to the left atrium
    B. Level of the superior thoracic aperture
    C. Posterior to the aortic arch
    D. Posterior to the left main bronchus
    E. Esophageal hiatus of the diaphragm

163. A 55-year-old woman comes to the physician for chest pain and she is found to have an acute myocardial infarction. She has a history of morbid obesity, hypertension, and uncontrolled diabetes. She is scheduled for a coronary bypass operation. The artery of primary concern is the vessel that arises from the circumflex artery in a left dominant heart. Which artery is this?
    A. Right marginal
    B. Anterior interventricular
    C. Left marginal
    D. Sinuatrial nodal
    E. Inferior (posterior) interventricular

164. A 35-year-old woman is brought to emergency department with dyspnea for 3 months. The patient has a history of IV drug use and endocarditis. Vitals are within normal limits. Physical examination shows a systolic (S1) murmur, suggestive of regurgitation of the tricuspid valve. What is the best site to auscultate this valve?
    A. Fourth intercostal space at left border of sternum
    B. Fifth intercostal space at left midclavicular line
    C. Fifth intercostal space at right border of sternum
    D. Third intercostal space at right border of sternum
    E. Second intercostal space at right border of sternum

165. A 42-year-old woman is brought to the emergency department after a fall from the balcony of her apartment. Vitals are within normal limits. Physical examination shows absent heart sounds, reduced systolic pressure, and engorged jugular veins. The condition that was created can be alleviated with which of the following procedures?
    A. Chest tube insertion superior to the rib
    B. Central venous line
    C. Nasogastric tube
    D. Thoracocentesis
    E. Pericardiocentesis

166. A 55-year-old man comes to the physician with dizziness and was found to have bradycardia and reduced cardiac output. The patient has a history of hypertension and diastolic congestive heart failure. The last echocardiogram showed 60% ejection fraction. Which nerve fibers may have been damaged to cause these symptoms?
    A. Preganglionic parasympathetics from the vagus nerve in the cardiac plexus
    B. Somatic efferents in the phrenic nerve
    C. Visceral afferents in the thoracic visceral nerves
    D. Preganglionic sympathetics from T1 to T4 lateral horn
    E. T1–T4 ventral horn neurons

167. A 65-year-old woman underwent open lobectomy of the lung for an adenocarcinoma. During a dissection of the posterior mediastinum, a surgeon identifies a vessel that lies on the anterior surface of the vertebral bodies between the descending thoracic aorta on the left and the azygos vein on the right. This vessel would most likely contain which of the following?
    A. Lymph
    B. Deoxygenated blood
    C. Saliva
    D. Urine
    E. Oxygenated blood

168. A 10-year-old boy comes to the physician for a hard mass in his chest that existed for 2 months and was found to have a thymoma. CT scan of the chest shows a single but large tumor in a structure located in the most anterior part of the superior mediastinum immediately posterior to the manubrium. This structure is most likely derived from which of the following pharyngeal pouches?

A. First
B. Second
C. Third
D. Fourth
E. Fifth

169. A 25-year-old woman was brought to the emergency department after suffering a gunshot wound to the back. Her temperature is 38.9°C (102°F), pulse is 110/min, respirations are 24/min, and blood pressure is 90/70 mm Hg. The left thorax was notably larger than the right with decreased breath sounds on auscultation and hyperresonance to percussion of the left chest. A tracheal tug to the right side was noted. She was assessed as having a tension pneumothorax and the physician prepared to perform an emergency decompression of the left thorax. Between which layers will the needle have to be placed to relieve the pneumothorax?

A. Between the visceral and parietal layers of the pericardium
B. Between the serous and fibrous layers of the pericardium
C. Between the mediastinal pleura and fibrous pericardium
D. Between the parietal and visceral layers of the pleura
E. Between the endothoracic fascia and parietal pleura

170. A 38-year-old woman delivered a girl at 37 weeks by elective cesarean section. Ultrasound at 16 weeks' gestation showed that the fetal heart was located outside the chest cavity but the mother opted against termination of the pregnancy. Physical examination of the girl showed that he was pink without cardiopulmonary distress. Vital signs were within normal limits. A pulsatile mass of 5 × 6 cm was seen outside the skin in the midline of the thorax. An x-ray of the chest showed a "split" in the sternum. The girl was diagnosed with ectopia cordis. What was the most likely embryological cause of this defect?

A. Failed fusion of pleuropericardial folds at the midline
B. Failed fusion of the septum transversum with pleuropericardial folds
C. Failed fusion of lateral body wall folds in the midline
D. Failed fusion of pleuroperitoneal at the midline
E. Failed fusion of pericardial coelom and peritoneal coelom

171. A 42-year-old woman delivered a boy at term. Vital signs of the boy were normal. Although he moved all limbs equally, there was generalized decreased muscle tone. His face was broad and flat with oblique eye fissures, flattened nose bridge, and protruding tongue from a small jaw. Auscultation of the chest showed a systolic ejection murmur. Cardiac ultrasound showed a defect in the wall separating the right from the left atrium. The patient was diagnosed with trisomy 21 with an atrial septal defect. What is the most likely cause of the defect in this patient?

A. Failed fusion of septum primum with the AV septum
B. Failed fusion of septum primum with septum secundum
C. Excess resorption of the cranial part of the septum primum
D. Short septum secundum
E. Incomplete resorption of the sinus venosus into the right atrium

172. A 32-year-old woman delivers a girl by cesarean section. Physical examination shows a pansystolic murmur without cyanosis. Cardiac ultrasound showed a small jet of blood directly between left and right ventricles during systole, through a defect in the cranial part of the interventricular septum. Which of the following is most likely true concerning the cardiac defect discovered in this patient?

A. There is uneven partitioning of the bulbus cordis
B. It causes a right to left shunt of blood at birth
C. It is a cause of cyanosis at birth
D. The interventricular septum and endocardial cushions failed to fuse
E. The septum primum and septum secundum failed to fuse at birth

173. A 30-year-old woman delivered a 2.7-kg (6-lb) girl at term via spontaneous vaginal delivery. Physical examination of the girl showed an elevated respiratory rate and she was subsequently admitted to the neonatal intensive care unit. She developed a fever a day later with persistent tachypnea. An x-ray of the chest showed bilateral basal hazy opacification and a right-sided cardiac shadow. A whole-body CT scan shows a normal orientation of the other viscera. What is the most likely cause of this girl's cardiac condition?

A. Posterior and superior growth of the primordial atrium
B. Anterior and inferior growth of the primordial ventricle
C. Anterior and inferior growth of the bulbus cordis
D. Growth of primordial heart tube to the left
E. Growth of the primordial heart tube to the right

Questions 174–188

174. A 54-year-old man comes to the physician because of a 2-week history of progressively increased pain from acid reflux. He has a 20-year history of alcoholism and was diagnosed with Barrett esophagus 3 years ago. An esophageal surgery is performed and the distal part of the esophagus is excised. Postoperatively, he has gradually increased chest discomfort. His temperature is 37.5°C (99.5°F), pulse is 120/min, respirations are 24/min, and blood pressure is 120/80 mm Hg. An x-ray of the chest shows hazy opacity of the mediastinum. CT scan of the chest showed a collection of fluid in the posterior mediastinum. Which of the following structures is most likely damaged in this patient?

A. Thoracic duct
B. Esophagus
C. Descending aorta
D. Azygos vein
E. Bronchial lymphatics

175. A 4-day-old girl is brought to the emergency department because of dyspnea, tachycardia, tachypnea, and cyanosis. Physical examination shows a depressed caved in abdomen. An x-ray of the abdomen shows herniation of bowel into the left thoracic cavity and a hypoplastic left lung. Which embryologic structure most likely failed to develop and resulted in the herniation?

A. Septum transversum
B. Pleuroperitoneal membrane
C. Tracheoesophageal septum
D. Laryngotracheal groove
E. Ventral mesogastrium

176. A 30-year-old man is brought to the emergency department because he was stabbed in his right anterior chest wall with a sharp instrument in a domestic dispute. Physical examination shows a puncture wound in the third right intercostal space at the midclavicular line and distended neck veins. There is hyperresonance on percussion and absent breath sounds on right hemithorax. An x-ray of the chest shows a deviated trachea to the left and bilateral opacities which are consistent with acute respiratory distress. Which of the following is the most likely diagnosis?

A. Right tension pneumothorax
B. Right simple pneumothorax
C. Right simple pneumothorax and cardiac tamponade
D. Right tension pneumothorax and cardiac tamponade
E. Cardiac tamponade

177. A 35-year-old man is brought to the emergency department after being involved in a hit and run motor vehicle collision. Physical examination shows multiple skin lacerations but not any major bleeding. An x-ray of the chest shows broken ribs 5–7, but no evidence of punctured pleura. The lung field appears opacified. Several hours later the patient appears cyanotic. What is the most likely cause of the cyanosis?

A. Hemothorax
B. Flail chest
C. Paralysis of the diaphragm

D. Tension pneumothorax
E. Spontaneous pneumothorax

178. A 55-year-old man is brought to the emergency department because of chills followed by a dry cough, pleuritic chest pain and fever for the past 3 days. Physical examination shows a dullness on percussion in the lower lobe of the lung bilaterally. An x-ray of the chest shows blunted costophrenic angle. A lidocaine (a local anesthetic agent) is administered to reduce the pain to which of the following nerves?

A. Intercostal nerves
B. Phrenic nerve
C. Vagus nerve
D. Cardiopulmonary
E. Recurrent laryngeal nerve

179. A 3-week-old prematurely born boy is brought to the emergency department with respiratory distress. Physical examination shows a systolic murmur crossing the S_2 heart sound. The murmur is accompanied by a thrill, is best heard below the left clavicle, and radiates over the chest. An x-ray of the chest shows enlarged cardiac silhouette and increased pulmonary vascular markings. Echocardiography shows a congenital defect. A video-assisted thoracoscopic procedure is considered for correction of the underlying defect. Which of the following structures is most commonly at risk of injury during the procedure?

A. Left vagus nerve
B. Right vagus nerve
C. Left phrenic nerve
D. Right phrenic nerve
E. Left recurrent laryngeal nerve

180. A 27-year-old man is brought to the emergency department after being stabbed in the chest during a bar fight. He has a severe chest pain upon breathing. His temperature is 38.9°C (102°F), a pulse is 110/min, respirations are 25/min, and blood pressure is 80/50 mm Hg. Physical examination shows a jugular vein distention right-sided hyperresonance on percussion, and decreased breath sounds over the right lung. An x-ray of the chest shows decreased vascular markings on the right side and a tracheal deviation to the left. Which of the following is the most likely diagnosis?

A. Spontaneous pneumothorax
B. Tension pneumothorax
C. Cardiac tamponade
D. Lung contusion
E. Pneumonia

181. A 72-year-old man is brought to the emergency department because of a tight, burning substernal chest pain. The patient has a history of morbid obesity, diabetes, and hypertension. An ECG shows a myocardial infarction of the cardiac muscle forming the diaphragmatic surface of the heart. Which of the following coronary arteries is most likely occluded in this patient?

A. Anterior interventricular artery
B. Circumflex coronary artery
C. Left coronary artery
D. Right coronary artery
E. Right marginal branches

182. A 37-year-old woman delivered a 3.6-kg (8-lb) boy at term via spontaneous vaginal delivery. The newborn is transferred to the neonatal intensive care unit because he was cyanotic at birth. An x-ray of the chest shows that his right ventricle is enlarged, and his heart shows a characteristic boot shape. Which of the following embryological events most likely underlies this condition?
A. Abnormal neural crest cell migration
B. Endocardial cushion defect
C. Aortic arch constriction
D. Pulmonary hypertension
E. Abnormal primitive heart tube looping

183. A 70-year-old man is brought to the emergency department because of 2-day history of high fever, chills, and chest pain. Physical examination shows a holosystolic murmur that radiates toward the axilla. Two sets of blood cultures are positive for *Staphylococcus aureus*. A transesophageal echo is performed and the ultrasound transducer is placed in the mid-esophagus facing posteriorly. Which of the following structures will be immediately posterior to the transducer?
A. Left atrium
B. Pulmonary veins
C. Right atrium
D. Right ventricle
E. Aorta

184. A 52-year-old man is brought to the emergency department because of 2-day history of severe dysphagia and retrosternal "burning" pain. He has a history of alcoholism and liver disease. During upper endoscopy, the physician advances the endoscope until its tip reaches the esophageal hiatus of the diaphragm. Which of the following vertebral levels did the tip of the endoscope most likely end?
A. T7
B. T8
C. T10
D. T11
E. T12

185. A 55-year-old man is brought to the emergency department after the barb of a stingray's tail suddenly pierced his chest while he was snorkeling. The tip of the barb pierced the right ventricle and the man instinctively removed it in the water. When he was brought onto the boat, there were muffled heart sounds, reduced cardiac output, and engorged jugular veins. Which of the following is the most likely diagnosis?
A. Pneumothorax
B. Deep vein thrombosis
C. Cardiac tamponade

D. Pulmonary embolism
E. Hemothorax

186. A 38-year-old man comes to the physician for a routine examination. The physician auscultates the heart by placing a stethoscope on the anterior surface of the patient's chest between the left second and third costal cartilages. Which of the following heart valves is the physician most likely auscultating?
A. Pulmonary
B. Aortic
C. Mitral
D. Tricuspid
E. Bicuspid

187. A 70-year-old woman comes to the physician because of a 3-week history of cough. The patient is a nursing home resident and has a history of pneumonia, diabetes, and congestive heart failure. An x-ray of the chest shows a mass at the sternal angle (of Louis). Which of the following radiographic views would best demonstrate this landmark?
A. Anteroposterior
B. Posteroanterior
C. Lateral
D. Apical lordotic
E. Axial

188. A 50-year-old man was brought to the emergency department after being involved in a motor vehicle collision. Physical examination shows dullness on percussion and an x-ray of the chest shows a pleural effusion. A chest tube is placed to drain fluid. The following anatomic structures comprise the wall of the thorax.
1. Internal intercostal muscle
2. Skin
3. Innermost intercostal muscle
4. Parietal pleura
5. External intercostal muscle
6. Visceral pleura
Which of the following best represents the order of structures traversed by the chest tube during the procedure?
A. 4-6-5-1-3-2
B. 2-5-1-3-6-4
C. 2-3-1-5-6-4
D. 2-1-3-5-4-6
E. 2-5-1-3-4

189. A 14-year-old girl comes to the emergency department because of 4-hour history of severe difficulty breathing. Physical examination shows that she has a prolonged expiratory phase with a bronchospasm and the diagnosis of asthma was subsequently made. Which of the following nerves is responsible for the constriction of the bronchial smooth muscle cells?
A. Vagus
B. Phrenic
C. Greater thoracic splanchnic
D. Thoracic visceral
E. Intercostal

Answers

1. D. The aorticopulmonary septum functions to divide the truncus arteriosus and bulbus cordis into the ascending aorta and pulmonary trunk.
   A. The septum secundum forms an incomplete separation between the two atria.
   B. The septum primum divides the atrium into right and left halves.
   C. The bulbar septum is derived from the bulbus cordis and will give rise to the interventricular septum inferior to the aorticopulmonary septum eventually fusing with it.
   E. The endocardial cushions play a role in the division of the AV canal into right and left halves by causing the AV cushions to approach each other.
   GAS 208; N 216; ABR/McM196, 203

2. A. Laryngeal atresia (congenital high airway obstruction syndrome) is a rare obstruction of the upper fetal airway. Distal to the site of the atresia, the airways dilate, lungs enlarge and become echogenic, the diaphragm flattens or inverts, and fetal ascites and/or hydrops develop.
   B. Tracheal atresia is a rare obstruction of the trachea, commonly found with a TEF, probably resulting from the unequal division of foregut into esophagus and trachea.
   C. Polyhydramnios is an excess of amniotic fluid, often associated with esophageal atresia or TEF.
   D. Lung hypoplasia is reduced lung volume, often seen in infants with a congenital diaphragmatic hernia.
   E. Oligohydramnios, or a decrease in amniotic fluid, is associated with stunted lung development and pulmonary hypoplasia.
   GAS 175–182; N 237; ABR/McM 212, 213, 216

3. A. ventricular septal defects account for 25% of congenital heart defects. The most common of these are defects in the membranous portion of the interventricular septum (membranous ventricular septal defects).
   B. Tetralogy of Fallot makes up approximately 10% of congenital heart defects.
   C. Muscular ventricular septal defects occur less commonly than membranous ventricular septal defects.
   D. Ostium secundum defect is an atrial septal defect that makes up around 7% of congenital heart defects.
   E. Ostium primum defect is an atrial septal defect that is most commonly associated with Down syndrome (trisomy 12).
   GAS 208; N 216; ABR/McM 196, 203

4. A. A patent ductus arteriosus acts as a shunt between the aorta and pulmonary trunk, allowing oxygenated blood to reach the tissues. In transposition of the great arteries, oxygenated blood enters the pulmonary trunk from the left ventricle and goes to the lungs. In contrast, the aorta carries deoxygenated blood to the systemic circulation.
   B and C: Maintained patency of the umbilical vessels would not provide adequate oxygenated blood for survival.
   D. Coarctation of the aorta is a congenital narrowing of the aorta that will not deliver more oxygenated blood to the systemic circulation.
   E. Pulmonary artery stenosis will not enhance the delivery of oxygenated blood to the systemic circulation.
   GAS 208; N 233; ABR/McM 206

5. A. Tetralogy of Fallot is characterized by four cardiac defects: pulmonary stenosis, ventricular septal defect overriding aorta, and these in turn lead to right ventricular hypertrophy.
   B. An atrial septal defect is characterized by the communication between the two atria.
   C. In a case of transposition of the great vessels, the aorta arises from the right ventricle and the pulmonary trunk arises from the left ventricle.
   D. Pulmonary atresia involves failure of the pulmonary valve orifice to develop. It can occur alongside other congenital cardiac defects, but there is no typical pattern of presentation.
   E. A ventricular septal defect is characterized by communication between the two ventricles and may or may not occur alongside other cardiac defects.
   GAS 208; N 228; ABR/McM 200, 201

6. A. Superior malalignment of the subpulmonary infundibulum causes stenosis of the pulmonary trunk. This leads to the four symptoms mentioned and is known as *tetralogy of Fallot.*
   B. A defect in formation of the aorticopulmonary septum is characteristic of transposition of the great arteries.
   C. An endocardial cushion defect is associated with membranous ventricular septal defects.
   D. Total anomalous pulmonary venous connection is a congenital heart disorder that involves all four pulmonary veins making anomalous connections to the systemic venous circulation. It is fatal unless it is concurrent with an atrial septal defect patent foramen ovale, or patent ductus arteriosus.
   E. An AV canal defect can result in an atrial septal defect and/or a ventricular septal defect.
   GAS 197–198, 208; N 228; ABR/McM 200, 201

7. B. An atrial septal defect produces a widely fixed and split S2 murmur, systolic ejection murmur best heard at the left sternal border.
   A. A ventricular septal defect produces a pansystolic murmur at S2 along the lower left sternal border.
   C. Tetralogy of Fallot will not result in a characteristic murmur that occurs at S1 or S2.

D. Transposition of the great arteries may result in a mid-diastolic rumble and/or a loud, single S2.

E. Aortic stenosis most commonly produces a systolic, crescendo-decrescendo murmur.

GAS 202–203, 208; N 224, 225; ABR/McM 201

8. Down syndrome (more properly called "trisomy 21") is associated with cardiovascular abnormalities such as arrhythmias and endocardial cushion defects. It is also characterized by mental retardation, brachycephaly, flat nasal bridge, upward slant of the palpebral fissure, protruding tongue, simian crease, and clinodactyly of the fifth digit.

C. Down syndrome is associated with increased incidence of atrial septal defect and ventricular septal defect because it may result in endocardial cushion defects.

A. Tetralogy of Fallot is not associated with Down syndrome. It is most commonly associated with 22q11 syndrome.

B. Transposition of the great arteries is a cyanotic, congenital heart disorder that is not associated with Down syndrome.

D. Coarctation of the aorta is most commonly associated with Turner syndrome.

E. Aortic atresia is not associated with Down syndrome but may be associated with Marfan syndrome.

GAS 208; N 224, 225; ABR/McM 200

9. **A.** Tetralogy of Fallot and truncus arteriosus are associated with DiGeorge syndrome (22q11).

B. Transposition of the great arteries is associated with maternal diabetes.

C. Atrial septal defects and ventricular septal defects are present in individuals with Down syndrome.

D. Coarctation of the aorta is related to Turner syndrome.

E. Marfan syndrome is present in individuals with aortic atresia.

GAS 208; N 218; ABR/McM 200

10. **B.** Transposition of the great arteries is associated with maternal diabetes.

A. Tetralogy of Fallot is associated with DiGeorge syndrome (22q11 syndrome).

C. Atrial septal defects and ventricular septal defects are associated with Down syndrome.

D. Truncus arteriosus is associated with DiGeorge syndrome (22q11 syndrome).

E. Coarctation of the aorta is associated with Turner syndrome.

GAS 202–203, 208; N 218; ABR/McM 196, 203

11. **C.** The ductus arteriosus is an embryologic structure that acts as a communication between the pulmonary trunk and the aorta. If it remains patent, the injected contrast medium would flow from the aorta through this communication and into the pulmonary artery.

A. An atrial septal defect is a communication between the atria.

B. Mitral stenosis is a narrowing of the AV valve between the left atrium and left ventricle.

D. The ductus venosus transports blood from the left umbilical vein to the inferior vena cava, bypassing the liver.

E. A ventricular septal defect is a communication between the ventricles.

GAS 208; N 218; ABR/McM 207

12. **A.** An atrial septal defect is a communication between the right and left atria. In the formation of the partition between the two atria, the opening in the foramen secundum, also known as the foramen ovale, typically closes at birth. If it remains patent, an atrial septal defect will result.

B. The ligamentum arteriosum is the remnant of the ductus arteriosus and is closely related to the left recurrent laryngeal nerve and the aorta.

C. Patency of the ductus arteriosus is not associated with atrial septal defect formation but is necessary for survival in certain congenital heart conditions.

D. Sinus venarum is the posterior aspect of the right atrium and is not involved in atrial septal defect formation.

E. The coronary sinus is where the cardiac veins come together and drain into the right atrium. It is not involved in atrial septal defect formation.

GAS 208; N 224–225; ABR/McM 199

13. **E.** Type II alveolar cells are the only cells that produce surfactant.

A. Alveolar capillary endothelial cells contribute to the blood-air barrier, but do not produce surfactant.

B. Bronchial mucous cells (goblet cells) do not produce surfactant.

C. Bronchial respiratory epithelial cells act to moisten and protect the respiratory tract.

D. Type I alveolar cells are responsible for gas exchange and do not produce surfactant.

GAS 169–177; N 202; ABR/McM 212

14. **B.** An absence of musculature in one half of the diaphragm causes it to protrude into the thoracic cavity forming a pouch into which the abdominal viscera protrude.

A. Pleuropericardial folds are responsible for separating the pericardial cavity from the pleural cavity.

C. Typically, the diaphragm migrates to its position with the fibrous pericardium.

D. The septum transversum is the primordial central tendon of the diaphragm that separates the heart from the liver.

E. The pleuroperitoneal folds form the pleuroperitoneal membranes that separate the pleural cavity from the peritoneal cavity.

GAS 262; N191; ABR/McM 184

15. **C.** The anomalies present in this individual are all caused by a coarctation of the aorta. The portion of the aortic arch that is constricted arises from the third, fourth, and sixth pharyngeal arches.

A. The bulbus cordis becomes part of the ventricular system.

B. The ductus arteriosus becomes the ligamentum arteriosum.

D. Sinus venosus becomes part of the right atrium as the sinus venarum, and also contributes to the sinuatrial node and coronary sinus.

E. The right cardinal vein is not involved in this anomaly.

GAS 222; N 216; ABR/McM 207

16. D. The tracheoesophageal septum is a primordial structure that separates the trachea from the esophagus. If this structure fails to develop, a TEF will result, in which event the two structures will not separate completely. When the infant attempts to swallow milk, it spills into the esophageal pouch and is regurgitated. The child becomes cyanotic because an insufficient amount of oxygen reaches the lungs as a result of the malformed trachea.

A. Failure of esophageal formation would not result in a TEF but could result in esophageal atresia.

B. Failure of the trachea to form will not result in a TEF.

C. Improper formation of the tongue would not lead to a TEF.

E. Malformation of the pharynx should not be expected to specifically lead to fistula formation.

GAS 223; N 237; ABR/McM 209

17. C. Polyhydramnios is an excess of amniotic fluid, often associated with esophageal atresia or a TEF. This abnormality affects fetal ability to swallow the normal amount of amniotic fluid; therefore, excess fluid remains in the amniotic sac.

A. Oligohydramnios is the deficiency of amniotic fluid, and it may be associated with certain chromosomal abnormalities.

B. Congenital rubella infection may be associated with congenital heart defects such as pulmonary artery stenosis and patent ductus arteriosus.

D. Thalidomide exposure may cause characteristic birth defects, although TEF is not among them.

E. Congenital toxoplasmosis may cause adverse effects such as premature birth and low birth weight, but TEF is not associated with it.

GAS 335; N 238; ABR/McM 209

18. B. Congenital rubella infection is associated with congenital heart defects such as patent ductus arteriosus and pulmonary artery stenosis.

A. Congenital toxoplasmosis may cause adverse effects such as premature birth and low birth weight, but patent ductus arteriosus is not associated with it.

C. Congenital cytomegalovirus may cause premature birth and neurological sequelae, such as, mental retardation and sensorineural hearing loss. It is not associated with congenital heart defects such as patent ductus arteriosus.

D. Congenital varicella may cause low birth weight, premature birth, and neurological damage. It is not associated with patent ductus arteriosus.

E. Congenital syphilis with Treponema pallidum infection may cause a characteristic rash, saddle nose, and failure to thrive but is not specifically associated with patent ductus arteriosus.

GAS 208; N 218; ABR/McM 207

19. E. Sinus venosus ASDs occur close to the entry of the superior vena cava in the superior portion of the interatrial septum.

A. Ostium secundum ASDs are located near the fossa ovale and encompass both septum primum and septum secundum defects.

B. An ostium primum defect is a less common form of atrial septal defect and is associated with endocardial cushion defects because the septum primum fails to fuse with the endocardial cushions resulting in a patent foramen primum.

C. An AV canal defect is not a clinically significant type of atrial septal defect.

D. A common atrium is an uncommon type of atrial septal defect in which the interatrial septum is absent (Figs. 2.10 and 2.11).

GAS 196–198, 203; N 224, 225; ABR/McM 199

20. A. Ectopia cordis is a condition in which the heart is located abnormally, outside the thoracic cavity, commonly resulting from a failure of fusion of the lateral folds in forming the thoracic wall. This is incompatible with life because of the occurrence of infection, cardiac failure, and/or hypoxemia.

B. The third pharyngeal arch gives rise to the stylopharyngeus muscle, the hyoid bone, the thymus, and the common and internal carotid arteries.

C. The fourth pharyngeal arch gives rise to the cricothyroid muscle, thyroid and epiglottic cartilage, the subclavian artery, and the aortic arch.

D. The fifth pharyngeal arch derivatives are not clinically relevant.

E. Faulty development of the sinus venosus is related to ASDs that result from deficient absorption of the sinus venosus into the right atrium and/or unusual development of the septum secundum.

GAS 196–198; N 216; ABR/McM 184

21. A. The right horn of the sinus venosus has two divisions: One develops into the sinus venarum, the smooth interior aspect of the right atrial wall; the other half develops into the pulmonary veins. Abnormal septation of the sinus venosus can lead to inappropriate pulmonary connections.

B. Abnormal development of the septum secundum could result in an atrial septal defect.

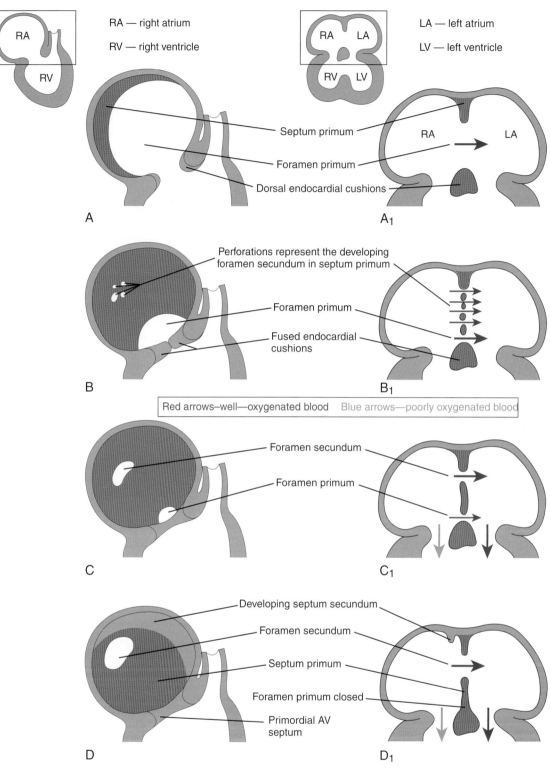

RA — right atrium

RV — right ventricle

LA — left atrium

LV — left ventricle

RA

LA

RV

LV

Septum primum

Foramen primum

Dorsal endocardial cushions

RA

LA

A

A₁

Perforations represent the developing
foramen secundum in septum primum

Foramen primum

Fused endocardial
cushions

B

B₁

Red arrows—well—oxygenated blood   Blue arrows—poorly oxygenated blood

Foramen secundum

Foramen primum

C

C₁

Developing septum secundum

Foramen secundum

Septum primum

Foramen primum closed

Primordial AV
septum

D

D₁

• **Fig. 2.10**

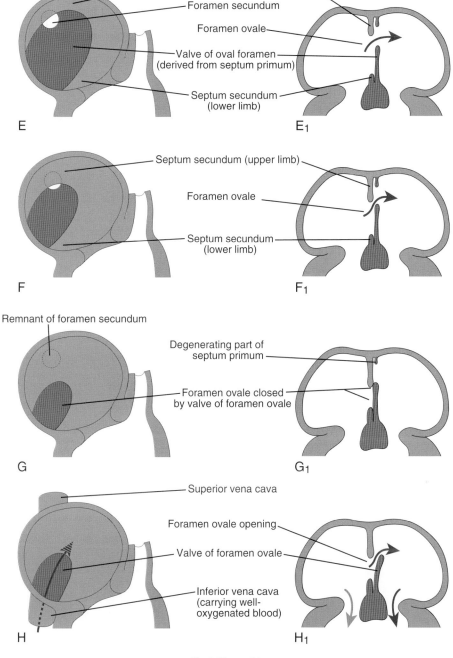

Fig. 2.10, cont'd

C. Abnormal development of the left sinus horn would present with abnormalities in the coronary sinus. The left sinus horn develops into the coronary sinus, and the right sinus horn is incorporated into the right atrial wall.

D. Abnormal development of the coronary sinus would potentially disrupt cardiac venous drainage but would not lead to totally anomalous pulmonary connections.

E. Abnormal development of the common cardinal vein would not lead to totally anomalous pulmonary connections.

GAS 196–198, 208; N 218; ABR/McM 203–205

22. C. The septum transversum is a thickened layer of mesoderm that gives origin to the central tendon of the diaphragm. It is situated between the thoracic cavity and the omphalomesenteric duct.

A. As the lungs grow into the pericardioperitoneal canal, they give rise to two folds: the pleuroperitoneal and pleuropericardial folds. The pleuroperitoneal folds are responsible for formation of the posterolateral aspect of the diaphragm.

B. The pleuropericardial folds develop into the fibrous pericardium and would not be involved with failure of the central tendon of the diaphragm to develop.

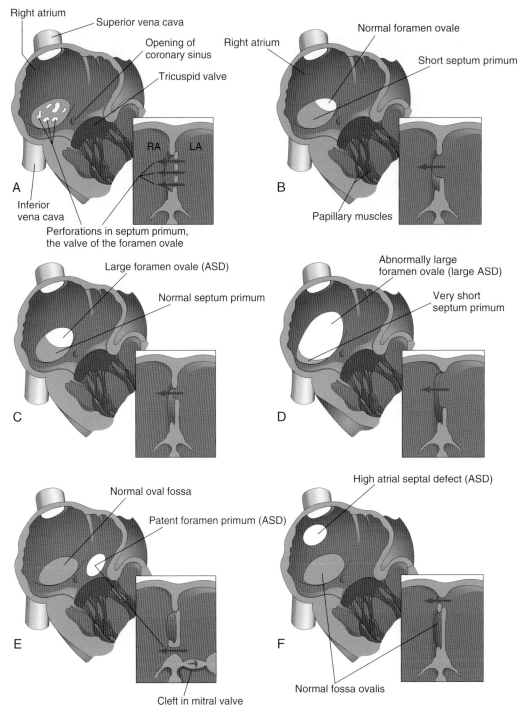

Right atrium
Superior vena cava
Opening of coronary sinus
Tricuspid valve
RA   LA
A
Inferior vena cava
Perforations in septum primum, the valve of the foramen ovale

Normal foramen ovale
Short septum primum
Right atrium
B
Papillary muscles

Large foramen ovale (ASD)
Normal septum primum
C

Abnormally large foramen ovale (large ASD)
Very short septum primum
D

Normal oval fossa
Patent foramen primum (ASD)
E
Cleft in mitral valve

High atrial septal defect (ASD)
F
Normal fossa ovalis

• **Fig. 2.11**

D. The cervical myotomes are responsible for the diaphragmatic musculature.

E. The crura provide origin of the dorsal mesentery of the esophagus, which is not involved in development of the central tendon of the diaphragm. *GAS 258, 208; N 201; ABR/McM 204–225*

23. C: The fourth aortic arch develops into the aortic arch on the left side and the brachiocephalic and subclavian arteries on the right side of the embryo. Improper development of the arch of the aorta will

cause increased pressure in the subclavian artery and, subsequently, the brachial artery. Similarly, decreased flow through the aorta will lead to decreased pressure in the femoral artery.

A. The second aortic arch, specifically the dorsal aspect, develops into aspects of the small stapedial artery.

B. The proximal part of the third aortic arch gives rise to the common carotid arteries, which supply the head.

D. The fifth aortic arch is said not to usually develop in human embryos. The proximal part of the sixth aortic arch develops into the left pulmonary artery.

E: The ductus venosus is a fetal cardiovascular structure that remains after development as the ligamentum venosum and would not cause this presentation.
GAS 217–220; N 211; ABR/McM 196, 205

24. **A.** The left sixth aortic arch is responsible for the development both of the pulmonary arteries and the ductus arteriosus. Without regression of the ductus arteriosus, a patent connection remains between aorta and the pulmonary trunk. The ductus arteriosus often reaches functional closure within 24 hours after birth, whereas anatomic closure and subsequent formation of the ligamentum arteriosum often occur by the twelfth postnatal week.
    B. The proximal part of the right sixth aortic arch becomes the proximal part of the right pulmonary artery.
    C. The fifth aortic arch does not contribute to any structures.
    D. The right fourth aortic arch forms the right subclavian artery.
    E. The left fourth aortic arch contributes to part of the aortic arch between the origin of the left carotid artery and the ductus arteriosus.
    GAS 208; N 218; ABR/McM 207

25. **D.** With a patent ductus arteriosus an abnormal connection persists between the aorta and the pulmonary trunk. Blood leaving the left ventricle of the heart and into the aorta is shunted back into the left pulmonary artery. This is responsible for the murmur heard during auscultation of the heart. The diversion of blood to the pulmonary arteries causes increased atrial pressure, leading to enlarged, and therefore noticeable, pulmonary arteries on the chest x-ray.
    A. Atrial septal defects are often characterized by a left-to-right shunt of blood, which often presents with dyspnea and abnormal heart sounds. A chest x-ray would not show prominent pulmonary arteries in such cases.
    B. The tetralogy of Fallot often presents with a right-to-left shunt of blood flow through the ventricles. It is also associated with pulmonary artery stenosis, right ventricular hypertrophy, interventricular septal defect, and an overriding aorta. This condition would not present with a murmur, however.
    C. Coarctation of the aorta results in aortic narrowing and may be associated with Turner syndrome.
    E. Aortic atresia results in narrowing of the aorta but would not lead to noticeable prominent pulmonary arteries on the x-ray. It may also be associated with other disorders such as hypoplastic left heart syndrome.
    GAS 208; N 218; ABR/McM 207

26. **E.** A common truncus arteriosus results from failure of separation of the pulmonary trunk and aorta. Without proper perfusion of the child by oxygenated blood, severe cyanosis will result.
    A. An atrial septal defect typically forms a left-to-right shunt due to pressure gradient between the left atrium and right atrium.
    B. A ventricular septal defect typically forms a left-to-right shunt due to pressure gradient between the left ventricle and right ventricle.
    C. Coarctation of the aorta is not associated with shunt formation.
    D. Transposition of the great arteries may cause a right-to-left shunt immediately after birth but this would not persist once corrected.
    GAS 208; N 218; ABR/McM 205, 207

27. **B.** The pleuroperitoneal membrane forms the posterolateral aspect of the diaphragm. A defect in this membrane would allow for communication between the upper left abdominal cavity and thoracic cavity and could result in a congenital diaphragmatic hernia.
    A. The septum transversum provides origin to the central tendon of the diaphragm but is not involved in herniation of the intestines.
    C. The tracheoesophageal septum is not associated with development of the diaphragm, and malformations of it would result in fistula formation.
    D. The laryngotracheal groove gives rise to the larynx and trachea and does not contribute to development of the diaphragm.
    E. The foregut refers to the gastrointestinal tract from the mouth to the proximal duodenum and is not associated with diaphragmatic development.
    GAS 258; N 191; ABR/McM 225

28. **A.** When closing a ventricular septal defect it is important not to suture over the right bundle branch because it carries the stimulating impulse from the AV node to the apex of the heart through the right AV bundle (of His). Following the course of the right bundle branch on the interventricular septum, the impulses travel along branches such as the septomarginal trabecula (moderator band) to end as Purkinje fibers innervating the papillary muscles and the ventricular walls, leading to ventricular contraction.
    B. The right coronary artery passes inferiorly and dorsally in the AV groove; therefore, it does not pass through the interventricular septum.
    C & E. The tricuspid and aortic valve is not directly associated with the interventricular septum.
    D. The anterior interventricular (LAD) coronary artery is superficial to the IV septum on the anterior surface of the heart.
    GAS 197–198, 208; N 224; ABR/McM 199, 200

29. **A.** Esophageal atresia is often the result of an incomplete division of the tracheoesophageal septum, thus causing an absence of, or blind ending of, the

esophagus. The findings in this patient correlate with the VACTERL syndrome. VACTERL includes vertebral anomalies, anal atresia, cardiac malformations, TEF, esophageal atresia, renal anomalies and radial aplasia, and limb anomalies.

B. Esophageal achalasia is a motility disorder of the esophagus that involves the smooth muscle lining the esophagus and the lower esophageal sphincter.

C. Pyloric stenosis is not seen in VACTERL syndrome. It is a congenital stenosis of the pyloric sphincter.

D. Congenital diaphragmatic hernia allows abdominal viscera to pass into the thoracic cavity and leads to both pulmonary hypoplasia and pulmonary hypertension.

E. The esophagus can form a fistulous connection with a number of structures that surround it.
GAS 175–177; N 237; ABR/McM 209

30. A. In a tracheotomy, an incision is made at the level of the sixth cervical vertebra, below the cricoid cartilage. The left brachiocephalic vein passes across the trachea immediately anterior to the brachiocephalic trunk. This vein is the most superficial structure and thus the most likely to be damaged.

B. The left common carotid artery is not situated near the midline incision of the tracheotomy.

C. The vagus nerve is not at risk during tracheotomy as it is not positioned midline.

D. The phrenic nerve is not at risk during tracheotomy, but it may be damaged iatrogenically by procedures such as a thymectomy.

E. The thoracic duct is located posterior and lateral to the esophagus and the trachea and is not likely to be damaged during a tracheotomy, other than the intentional opening made in it.
GAS 836–837, 1053, 1112; N 198; ABR/McM 207, 208

31. A. The phrenic nerve has a path between the anteromedial aspect of the lung and the mediastinum. Along the path of the nerve, it courses anterior to the root of the lung.

B. The vagus nerves run posterior to the roots of the lungs as they give off branches to the cardiac and pulmonary plexuses upon the trachea near the carina and on the lung roots.

C. The intercostal nerves would not be affected by a tumor located at the lung surface anterior to the hilum.

D. The recurrent laryngeal nerves arise from the vagus nerves before the vagus nerves pass behind the roots of the lungs.

E. The cardiopulmonary nerve would not be affected by a tumor located at the lung surface anterior to the hilum.
GAS 227; N 197; ABR/McM 219

32. C. The left recurrent laryngeal nerve passes beneath the ligamentum arteriosum and then loops superiorly toward the tracheoesophageal groove, medial to the arch of the aorta. It is the only nerve located near the described mass.

A. The left phrenic nerve passes anterior to the first part of the subclavian artery and posterior to the subclavian vein as it enters the thorax.

B. The esophageal plexus would not be affected by a growth within the aortic arch lying next to the left pulmonary artery.

D. The left vagus nerve enters the thorax between the left subclavian artery and the left common carotid artery. It gives rise to the left recurrent laryngeal nerve but would not directly be affected by this mass.

E. The left sympathetic trunk would not be affected by the mass described.
GAS 169–172, 225–230; N 190; ABR/McM 207

33. During mastectomy procedures, three nerves are most susceptible to ligation or laceration: the long thoracic nerve, intercostobrachial nerve, and thoracodorsal nerve.

C. In the event of injury to the long thoracic nerve, the patient complains of an inability to fully abduct the humerus above the horizontal. The serratus anterior (supplied by the long thoracic nerve) is necessary to elevate, rotate, and abduct the scapula, to facilitate abduction of the humerus above the shoulder.

A. Injury of the axillary nerve would cause loss of arm abduction from 15 to 90 degrees and weakness of shoulder movements due to paralysis of the deltoid and teres minor muscles.

B. Injury of the spinal accessory nerve would cause weakness of the trapezius muscle and poorly localized neck pain.

D. Radial nerve injury would produce characteristic symptoms depending on where the injury site is located but would not cause the symptoms described.

E. Because the patient does not indicate any loss of medial rotation or adduction of the humerus, ligation or injury of the thoracodorsal nerve can be eliminated.
GAS 183; N 194; ABR/McM 135

34. A. The dorsal root ganglia contain nerve cell bodies for general somatic afferent and general visceral afferent neuronal processes. Pain localized on the chest wall is transmitted back to the CNS via sensory fibers.

B. The sympathetic trunk ganglia will not carry sensory pain of the chest wall back to the CNS.

C. The dorsal horn of the spinal cord receives sensory input such as proprioception, light touch, and vibration.

D. The lateral horn of the spinal cord carries autonomic signals.

E. The ventral horn of the spinal cord carries motor signals to skeletal muscle.
GAS 137–138; N 197; ABR/McM 189

35. D. The lateral horns, or intermediolateral cell columns, contain the cell bodies of preganglionic neurons of the sympathetic system. Spinal cord segments T1–T4 are often associated with the upper limbs and thoracic organs.

A. The preganglionic cell bodies of the implicated neurons would not be found at the deep cardiac plexus.

B. The dorsal motor nucleus of the vagus nerve would not contain preganglionic cell bodies of the autonomic fibers involved in raising the heart rate.

C. The sympathetic neurons in spinal cord segments T5–T9 usually correlate with innervation of vascular smooth muscle, sweat glands, and arrector pili muscles of the chest and abdominal wall as well as organs in the abdominal cavity, specifically organs derived from the foregut.

E. The inferior cervical ganglion would not contain the preganglionic cell bodies of the fibers responsible for raising the heart rate but contains some of the postganglionic neurons that innervate the heart with sympathetics.
GAS 234–235; N 207; ABR/McM 100, 217

36. D. The thoracic visceral (or cardiopulmonary splanchnic) nerves are responsible for carrying the cardiac sympathetic efferent fibers from the sympathetic ganglia to the thoracic viscera, and afferent fibers for pain from these organs.

A: The vagus nerve is responsible for carrying parasympathetic fibers.

B & C: The greater, lesser, and least thoracic splanchnic nerves carry preganglionic sympathetic fibers (primarily) to the abdomen.

E: The sympathetic neurons in spinal cord segments T5–T9 usually correlate with innervation of vascular smooth muscle, sweat glands, and arrector pili muscles of the chest and abdominal wall as well as organs in the abdominal cavity, specifically organs derived from the foregut.
GAS 234–235; N 214; ABR/McM 205

37. C. The vagus nerve is the only nerve responsible for parasympathetic innervation of the lungs.

A. The greater thoracic splanchnic nerve carries sympathetic fibers to the abdomen and does not innervate the lungs.

B. The phrenic nerve is a somatic nerve that does not innervate the lungs or the heart.

D. The intercostal nerves are part of the somatic nervous system and do not innervate the bronchial smooth muscle.

E. The lesser thoracic splanchnic nerve carries preganglionic sympathetic fibers (primarily) to the abdomen and pain afferents from the abdomen. It does not innervate the lungs.
GAS 223–235; N 190; ABR/McM 205, 219

38. C. There is close proximity between the aorticopulmonary window and the left recurrent laryngeal nerve. A mass within or adjacent to this window is likely to compress the left recurrent laryngeal nerve, resulting in the hoarseness of the patient.

A. Though the vagus nerve is responsible for innervation of the larynx, it passes dorsal to the area of the aorticopulmonary window and is not likely to be compressed.

B. Compression of the phrenic nerve would not produce the hoarseness as described in this patient.

D. A mass at the aorticopulmonary window would not compress the right recurrent laryngeal nerve.

E. The greater and lesser thoracic splanchnic nerves arise inferior and posterior to the aorticopulmonary window and are thus unlikely to be compressed. The thoracic splanchnic nerves are not involved in the innervation of the larynx.
GAS 223–235; N 199; ABR/McM 207

39. C. The intercostobrachial nerve is responsible for innervation of the skin on the medial surface of the arm. Only the intercostobrachial nerve is responsible for sensory supply of the lateral aspect of the axilla.

A. The ulnar nerve is responsible for cutaneous sensation on the medial aspect of the hand.

B. The long thoracic nerve provides motor supply to the serratus anterior and is not involved in cutaneous innervation of the axillary region.

D. The lateral cutaneous branch of T4 innervates the dermatome corresponding to the nipple and areola and also supplies the medial aspect of the axilla.

E. The axillary nerve innervates the lateral aspect of the shoulder and provides sensory information over the shoulder joint and the "regimental badge" over parts of the deltoid muscle.
GAS 162, 734; N 195; ABR/McM 144

40. B. Pericarditis is an inflammation of the pericardium and often causes a pericardial friction rub, with the surface of the pericardium becoming gradually coarser. Because the phrenic nerve is solely responsible for innervation of the pericardium, it would transmit the pain fibers radiating from the pericardial friction rub.

A. The intercostobrachial nerve provides sensory innervation of the skin on the arm's medial surface. It would not carry pain fibers from this patient's condition.

C. The long thoracic nerve supplies the serratus anterior muscle. It would not carry pain fibers from a patient with pericarditis.

D. The greater thoracic splanchnic nerve is involved in abdominal innervation.

E. The thoracic visceral or cardiopulmonary nerves are postsynaptic sympathetic nerves that supply the heart and lungs but would not carry fibers associated with pericarditis.
GAS 189; N 215; ABR/McM 205, 207

41. C. The intercostobrachial nerve is the lateral cutaneous branch of the second intercostal nerve. It serves a cutaneous function both in the axilla and medial aspect of the arm.

A: The phrenic nerve arises from spinal nerves C3–C5 and innervates the diaphragm. This nerve has no branches that pass into the arm.

B. The vagus nerve is CN X and supplies autonomic function to the gut, up to the left colic flexure, and also provides some autonomic motor and sensory supply to organs in the head, neck, and thorax.

D. The greater thoracic splanchnic nerve originates in the thorax from the sympathetic trunk at the levels of T5–T9 and innervates abdominal structures.

E. The suprascapular nerve originates from the upper trunk of the brachial plexus and receives fibers primarily from C5 and C6. It innervates the supraspinatus and the infraspinatus muscles.
GAS 162, 225–235; N 195; ABR/McM 144

42. D. Ventral rami contain both sensory and motor fibers and also sympathetics to the body wall, supplying all areas of the body wall except for tissues of the back. In this case, both sensory fibers (numbness) and sympathetics (anhidrosis) are disrupted at the midaxillary line; therefore, cutaneous branches of ventral rami is the only correct choice.

A. The dorsal roots carry somatic and visceral sensory information from the periphery. Because only cutaneous sensation is lost the deficit cannot involve the dorsal roots.

B. The ventral roots of the spinal cord carry only somatic and visceral efferents. Because no motor functions are disrupted, this is not the correct answer.

C. The branches of dorsal rami provide cutaneous and muscle innervation to the back and thus have no relation to the midaxillary line.

E. The rami communicantes are components of the sympathetic nervous system and are not involved with general somatic afferent sensation.
GAS 58–59; N 197; ABR/McM 188

43. B. General visceral afferents, including the thoracic visceral afferents, are nerve fibers that carry sensation from organs, in this case pain from the abdominal aorta. These fibers get mixed with general somatic afferents in the dorsal roots. This is the phenomenon of "referred pain." The dorsal root ganglia (or their counterparts associated with sensory cranial nerves) contain the cell bodies associated with all sensory fibers from the body, including somatic and visceral sensation.

A. Somatic afferents are involved in sensation of pain, touch, and temperature from the body's surface. They would not be responsible for the pain of an aortic aneurysm.

C. The postganglionic sympathetic fibers are autonomic motor fibers and would not transmit pain associated with an aortic aneurysm.

D. Sympathetic preganglionics are autonomic motor fibers and would not transmit the pain of an aortic aneurysm.

E. Parasympathetic afferents would not transmit the signals from an aortic aneurysm.
GAS 58–59; N 214; ABR/McM 205

44. B. The anterior and lateral cutaneous branches of the fourth intercostal nerves provide the sensory and sympathetic supply to the areolae and nipples.

A. Anterior cutaneous branches of the second and third intercostal nerves innervate the skin above the nipples and areolae.

C. The lateral pectoral nerves provide motor innervation mainly to the pectoralis major muscle, not sensory supply.

D. Ventral primary rami of the second thoracic spinal nerves provide muscle innervation and sensory innervation above the nipples and areolae and sensory fibers for the medial side of the arm (GAS Fig. 3.9).

E. Lateral cutaneous branches of the second and third intercostal nerves would not supply the affected area.
GAS 132–140; N 197; ABR/McM 188

45. C. The left recurrent laryngeal nerve passes superiorly in the tracheoesophageal groove after looping around the aorta. The compression of this nerve and compression of the esophagus against the trachea would result in the presenting symptoms.

A. The right recurrent laryngeal nerve loops around the right subclavian artery before passing toward the larynx and therefore does not descend into the thorax.

B. The left vagus nerve courses posterior to the hilum of the lung, after it has already given off its left recurrent laryngeal branch at the level of the aortic arch; therefore, compression of this nerve would not result in the presenting symptoms.

D. The greater thoracic splanchnic nerve arises from sympathetic trunk ganglia at levels T5–T9 and therefore would not cause the presenting symptoms.

E. The phrenic nerve innervates the diaphragm; compression of this nerve would not result in the presenting symptoms.
GAS 223–226; N 199; ABR/McM 207

46. A. The patient's chief complaint is pain upon swallowing. With a dilated left atrium, the most probable structure being compressed is the esophagus. The esophagus descends into the abdomen immediately posterior to the left atrium below the level of the tracheal carina.

B. The root of the lung is the collection of structures that enter or leave the lung hilum, including the pulmonary arteries, veins, and primary bronchi. The lung root is not so intimately associated with the esophagus and would not be associated with pain during swallowing.

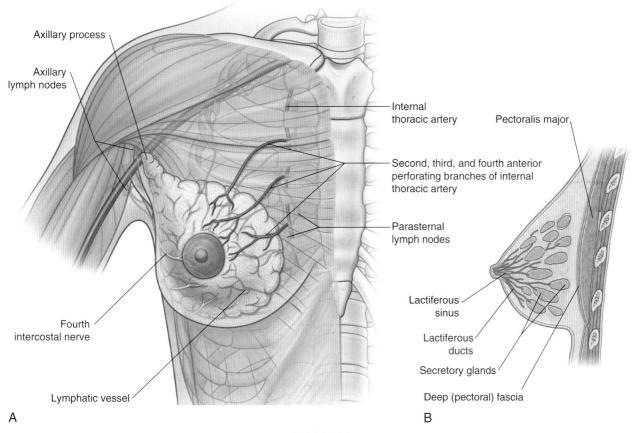

Axillary process

Axillary lymph nodes

Internal thoracic artery

Pectoralis major

Second, third, and fourth anterior perforating branches of internal thoracic artery

Parasternal lymph nodes

Fourth intercostal nerve

Lactiferous sinus

Lactiferous ducts

Secretory glands

Lymphatic vessel

Deep (pectoral) fascia

A

B

GAS Fig. 3.9

C. The trachea ends and bifurcates above the level of the left atrium and therefore would be unaffected by a dilated left atrium.

D. The superior vena cava is anterior in position and is not close in relation to the esophagus or the left atrium.

E. The inferior vena cava ascends from the abdomen to the right atrium and is not nearby the affected structures.

GAS 223–226; N 237; ABR/McM 205

47. E. The esophageal hiatus of the diaphragm is one of four openings associated with the diaphragm. It is located at the level of T10 and allows the esophagus to pass from the thoracic cavity into the abdominal cavity. It is the site of the most inferior of four esophageal constrictions.

A. The pharyngoesophageal junction is the site at which the pharynx ends and the esophagus begins in the neck, at the level of the sixth cervical vertebra. It is the first and the most superior of the esophageal constrictions.

B. There are no constrictions found at the level of the superior thoracic aperture; this is the opening for passage of the structures passing from the neck into the thorax.

C. The esophagus descends posterior to the arch of the aorta. It is at this level, where the trachea bifurcates anterior to the esophagus, that the second of the esophageal constrictions is found.

D. The third constriction occurs as the esophagus passes posteriorly to the left main bronchus.
GAS 128; N 199; ABR/McM 207

48. D. The apex of the heart is located in the left fifth intercostal space, about 3½ inches to the left of the sternum. When this area of the heart is palpated, any pulsations would be generated by throbbing of the apex of the heart against the thoracic wall.

A. The right atrium is located to the right of the sternum.

B. The left atrium is located on the posterior aspect of the heart, thus no direct palpation is realized.

C. The aortic arch would be located posterior to the manubrium of the sternum, above the second intercostal space.

E. Although the mitral valve is auscultated at the fifth left intercostal space along the mid-clavicular line, this would not be associated with palpation as the apex of the heart is.
GAS 190; N 216; ABR/McM 184

49. A. These components of the heart are readily viewed in a plain chest x-ray. It is important to understand the spatial arrangement of the heart as it rests in the thorax. The conus region of the right ventricle is located on the most anterior aspect of the heart, thus

it is the most anterior portion of the heart within the thorax.

B. The apex of the left ventricle is also located anteriorly, but it is located lateral to the sternum and occupies little area compared with the right ventricle.

C. The left ventricle is positioned on the left lateral side and slightly posterior position in the thorax.

D. The right atrium is located on the right lateral side of the heart.

E. The anterior margin of the left atrium is positioned posteriorly in the thorax.
GAS 190–195; N 235; ABR/McM 204

50. **A.** The left fifth intercostal space, just below the left nipple, is typically the best location to listen to the mitral valve. Although the mitral valve is located at the fourth intercostal space just to the left of the sternum, the sound is best realized "downstream" from the valve.

B. The right lower part of the body of the sternum is the location of the tricuspid valve.

C. The right second intercostal space near the lateral border of the sternum is the typical location of auscultation of the aortic valve.

D. It is difficult to hear valvular sounds through bone, so auscultating directly over the middle of the manubrium is not a good choice.

E. The left second intercostal space near the lateral border of the sternum is the site chosen typically for auscultation of the pulmonary valve (GAS Fig. 3.110).
GAS 208, 238; N 217; ABR/McM 184

Answers 51–75

51. **B.** The great cardiac vein takes a pathway initially beside the anterior interventricular artery (LAD) in its course, finally terminating in the coronary sinus when it is joined by the oblique vein (of Marshall) of the left atrium. This vein must be protected when performing bypass procedures.

A. The middle cardiac vein is located on the posterior aspect of the heart, and it also drains into the coronary sinus.

C. The small cardiac vein drains blood along the same path as the right marginal branch of the right coronary artery.

D. The anterior cardiac veins drain the blood from the right ventricle anteriorly and drain directly into the right atrium, and are not associated with the anterior interventricular artery.

E. The posterior (or inferior) vein of the left ventricle drains blood from mainly the left ventricle.
GAS 209; N 222; ABR/McM202, 203

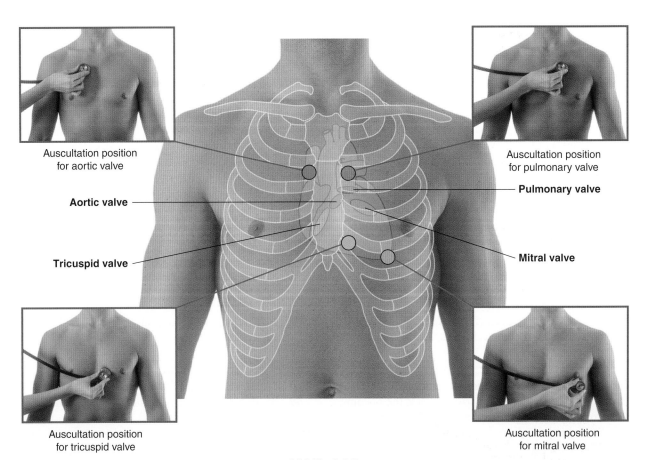

Auscultation position for aortic valve

Auscultation position for pulmonary valve

Aortic valve

Pulmonary valve

Tricuspid valve

Mitral valve

Auscultation position for tricuspid valve

Auscultation position for mitral valve

GAS Fig. 3.110

52. B. The anterior interventricular artery (left anterior interventricular artery, LAD) supplies the right and left ventricles and anterior two thirds of the IV septum.

    A. The right marginal artery supplies the right ventricle and apex of the heart; therefore, it does not supply the left ventricle.

    C. The left circumflex artery supplies the left atrium and left ventricle; it courses posteriorly in, or near to, the coronary sulcus and supplies the posterior portion of the left ventricle and left atrium.

    D. The artery to the sinuatrial node is (usually) a branch of the right coronary artery and does not supply the left ventricle.

    E. The inferior (posterior) interventricular (inferior interventricular or posterior descending) artery arises from the right coronary artery in about 85% of people (this is referred to as a right dominant pattern) and supplies the posterior aspect of both ventricles and the posterior third of the interventricular septum (GAS Fig. 3.78A).

GAS 203–207; N 222; ABR/McM 202, 203

53. E. The anterior interventricular artery (also called the left anterior descending, or LAD, nicknamed "the widow maker") arises from the left coronary artery. If there is occlusion in the right coronary artery, the anterior interventricular artery will still have normal blood flow.

    A. The right marginal artery branches from the right coronary artery; therefore, if there is occlusion of the right coronary artery, flow from the marginal artery will be compromised.

    B. The AV nodal artery is supplied by the coronary artery that crosses the crux of the heart posteriorly. If this artery arises from the right coronary, as it does in up to 85% of people, supply to the AV node might be reduced, depending upon collateral supply.

    C. The inferior (posterior) interventricular artery originates from the right coronary artery in about 85% of individuals, and this is known as a "right dominant pattern." It supplies the posterior aspect of both ventricles and the posterior third of the interventricular septum.

    D. The sinuatrial nodal artery is supplied by the right coronary artery in about 55% of the population

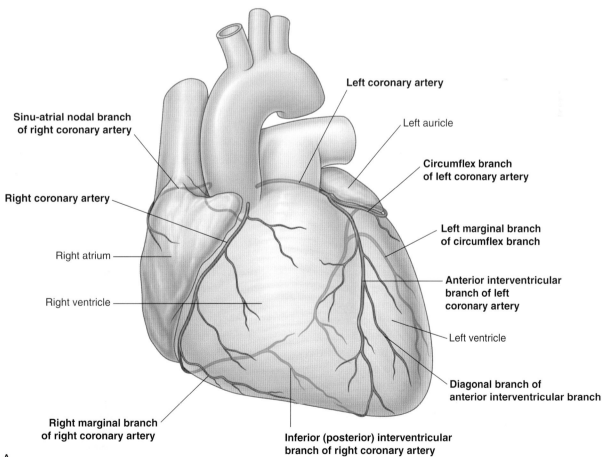

GAS Fig. 3.78A

(only 35% from the left); as the patient is right coronary dominant, it would be predicted that the sinuatrial nodal artery will not have normal blood flow.

GAS 203–207; N 222; ABR/McM 202, 203

54. D. Because the patient is left coronary artery dominant, if there is 70% to 80% occlusion of the left coronary, there will be deficiencies in flow both in the anterior interventricular and circumflex arteries. No possibility is available for collateral flow from the inferior (posterior) interventricular artery, as it would be derived from the left coronary, by way of the circumflex artery. If the patient does not undergo surgery to remove or bypass the occlusion, he will be unable to have any substantial type of collateral circulation between the two major branches of the left coronary.

A. The branches of the coronary arteries are not end arteries, and there are anastomoses between them.

B. The papillary muscles of the tricuspid valve would not be affected with left coronary artery occlusion.

C. The blood supply to the sinuatrial node would not be inadequate.

E. The blood supply of the region of the AV node might or might not be adequate, for it could still be supplied by a branch of the right coronary artery.

GAS 203–207; N 222; ABR/McM 202, 203

55. A. The mitral valve corresponds to the S_1 heart sound produced during systole.

B, C, and D: The aortic and pulmonary valves correspond to the S2 heart sound produced during diastole. The aortic valve also corresponds with the S2 sound, and therefore would be incorrect.

E. The tricuspid valve also corresponds with the S1 heart sound, best heard along the left lower sternal border.

GAS 207–209; N 225; ABR/McM 200, 201

56. C. The interventricular septum is intimately involved with the tricuspid valve on the right side, via the muscular connections of the septomarginal trabecula (moderator band) to the anterior papillary muscle. Therefore, if the electrical system of the heart is disrupted, as with a myocardial infarction in the upper portion of the muscular septum, the innervation of the interventricular septum will be compromised and the tricuspid valve will be directly affected.

A. The pulmonary valve is found between the right ventricle and pulmonary artery and is not directly attached to the interventricular septum.

B. The aortic valve is a semilunar valve that lies between the left ventricle and aorta. It is not involved directly with the interventricular septum.

D. The mitral valve is an AV valve found between the left atrium and left ventricle. It is not intimately associated with the interventricular septum.

E. The Eustachian valve, or the valve of the inferior cava, is found between the inferior vena cava and the right atrium. It is not associated with the interventricular septum.

GAS 211–213; N 224; ABR/McM 199, 201

57. B. The pulmonary valve is associated with the S_2 heart sound produced in diastole. A splitting in the S_2 sound indicates that the aortic and pulmonary valves are not closing simultaneously and would correlate with a possible defect in this valve.

A. The mitral valve is associated with the S1 heart sound, produced in systole; therefore, it cannot be defective if only the S2 sound is involved.

C. The aortic valve is associated with the S2 heart sound, but the mitral valve is not (as stated earlier); therefore, this answer cannot be correct.

D and E: The tricuspid valve is associated with the S1 heart sound and therefore is not associated with the occurrence of an abnormal S2 heart sound.

GAS 208; N 226; ABR/McM 201

58. C. The AV bundle (of His) is a collection of specialized cardiac muscle cells (Purkinje fibers) that carry electrical activity to the right and left bundle branches. Because both ventricles are affected, this is the logical site of injury, for this bundle leads to the bundle branches supplying both ventricles.

A. An injury to the right bundle branch would be limited to the right ventricle.

B. An injury to the left bundle branch would be limited to the left ventricle. Terminal Purkinje fibers transmit the electrical activity to the greater sections of the ventricles, yet dysfunction in the terminal part of the conduction system would affect only a small section of one ventricle, not both.

D. The posterior internodal pathway is in the roof of the right atrium and is not involved here.

E. The AV node is a group of specialized cardiac muscle cells that serve to decrease the rate of conduction to the ventricles and is located in the region deep in the septal wall of the right atrium.

GAS 211–213; N 229; ABR/McM 201

59. D. The artery of the conus is given off from the right coronary artery and courses around the conus arteriosus. The conus region is the superior part of the right ventricle that tapers into a cone (infundibulum) where the pulmonary valve leads into the pulmonary trunk. This conus artery supplies the upper portion of the anterior right ventricle and usually has a small anastomotic connection with the anterior interventricular (LAD) branch of the left coronary artery.

A. The circumflex artery supplies the left atrium and ventricle and does not supply the right ventricle except when the inferior (posterior) interventricular (posterior descending) artery arises from the circumflex, or in unusual cases in which the circumflex passes to the surface of the right ventricle.

B. The anterior interventricular artery supplies the right and left ventricles and the anterior two-thirds of the IV septum. It is given off by the left coronary artery and does not specifically supply the upper portion of the right ventricle.

C. The inferior (posterior) interventricular artery supplies the right and left ventricles and the posterior third of the IV septum. It does not supply the upper portion of the right ventricle.

E. The right marginal branch of the right coronary artery can supply both surface of the right ventricle but does not reach the upper portion of the right ventricle.

GAS 202–209; N 223, ABR/McM 202

60. **D.** The AV bundle of His is a strand of specialized cardiac muscle fibers (Purkinje fibers) that arises from the AV node and passes through the right fibrous trigone. The right fibrous trigone (central fibrous body) is a dense area of connective tissue that interconnects the mitral, tricuspid, and aortic valve rings.

A and C. After reaching the upper portion of the muscular interventricular septum, the AV bundle (of His) splits into right and left bundle branches. Damage to these structures would only affect the respective ventricles they are associated with.

B. The bundle of Bachmann is a collection of fibers running from the sinuatrial node to the left atrium and is the only collection of conducting fibers to innervate the left atrium.

E. The posterior internodal pathway, also known as Thorel's pathway, is the principal pathway of electrical activation between the sinuatrial node and AV node in humans.

GAS 211–213; N 227; ABR/McM 201

61. **A.** The sternocostal surface of the heart consists mostly of the right ventricle. Therefore, an anterior injury to the thorax would most likely first affect the right ventricle because it is adjacent to the deep surface of the sternum.

B. The obtuse margin of the left ventricle would not be directly affected as it is located posteriorly and laterally relative to the right ventricle.

C. If the question did not ask which part of the heart has been injured but which part of the heart will most likely be compressed by the cardiac tamponade, the correct answer would have been the right atrium. This is due to the fact that the right atrium has lower pressures than the other cardiac components.

D. The left atrium makes up the posterior aspect of the heart and would not be affected by direct trauma to the sternum.

E. The apex of the left ventricle would also not be directly affected by this injury.

GAS 190–195; N 235; ABR/McM 204, 208

62. **D.** The tissues affected in this case, the interventricular septum and anterior ventricular wall, are mostly supplied by the proximal portion of the anterior interventricular artery.

A. If the circumflex artery were blocked, the left atrium and left ventricle would be affected (in a right coronary dominant heart).

B. If the right coronary artery were occluded, again assuming right coronary dominance, it would affect the right atrium, the SA and AV nodes, part of the posterior left ventricle, and the posterior part of the interventricular septum.

C. If the left coronary artery were blocked, most of the left atrium and left ventricle, the anterior two-thirds of the interventricular septum, and the area of bifurcation of the AV bundle (of His) would be affected.

E. If the inferior (posterior) interventricular artery were occluded, it would affect the right and left ventricles and the posterior third of the interventricular septum. The circumflex and the anterior interventricular arteries are branches of the left coronary artery and the inferior (posterior) interventricular artery is most commonly a branch of the terminal segment of the right coronary artery.

GAS 203–209; N 222; ABR/McM 202

63. **C.** A "left coronary dominant" circulation means that the left coronary artery supplies the inferior (posterior) interventricular artery as a terminal branch of the circumflex. The posterior aspect of the heart is composed primarily of the left ventricle and is supplied by the inferior (posterior) interventricular branch.

A. The artery of the conus supplies the right ventricular free wall.

B. If the right coronary artery were occluded (in a right coronary dominant heart), it would affect the right atrium, right ventricle, the SA and AV nodes, the posterior part of the interventricular septum, and part of the posterior aspect of the left ventricle.

D. The right marginal artery supplies the inferior margin of the right ventricle.

E. The diagonal arteries arise most commonly from the anterior interventricular (left-anterior descending) artery but can also arise as branches of the left coronary or the circumflex.

GAS 203–209; N 222; ABR/McM 202

64. **B.** The valve of the inferior vena cava (Eustachian valve) is an embryologic remnant of the development of the heart and is not a functional valve. Typically, this valve regresses postnatally but rarely it persists and can cause obstruction to blood flow.

A. The tricuspid valve is located below the inferior vena cava between the right atrium and right ventricle.

C. The valve of the coronary sinus (Thebesian valve) is a semicircular fold at the orifice of the coronary sinus.

D. The septum primum is an embryologic structure that separates the single, primitive atrium into a right and left atrium.

E. The fossa ovalis is an embryonic remnant of the septum primum and septum secundum of the interatrial septum, located between the right and left atria.
GAS 196–197; N 224; ABR/McM 201

65. **A.** The crista terminalis is a muscular ridge that runs from the opening of the superior vena cava to the inferior vena cava. This ridge provides the path taken by the posterior internodal pathway (of Thorel) between the SA and AV nodes. The crista also provides the origin of the pectinate muscles of the right auricle.

B. The origin of the pectinate muscles associated with the right auricle is provided by the crista terminalis, thus the crista is a better answer choice.

C. The tricuspid valve is located below the inferior vena cava, between the right atrium and right ventricle.

D. The Eustachian valve or valve of the inferior vena cava is an embryologic remnant of the development of the heart.

E. The ostium of the coronary sinus is located between the right AV orifice and the inferior vena cava.
GAS 196–197; N 224; ABR/McM 201

66. **B.** During pericardiocentesis, the needle is inserted below the xiphoid process, or in the left fifth or sixth intercostal space at the sternal border.

A and D. The sixth and seventh intercostal spaces are locations that are not used clinically because of the increased likelihood of injury to the pleura or lungs.

C. The most effective way of draining the pericardium is by penetrating the thoracic wall at its lowest point anatomically, hence the third intercostal space would be too superior in position.

E. The triangle of auscultation is an area of the back where there is a lack of muscle layers. It is not the ideal location for performing pericardiocentesis.
GAS 185–189; N 216, 210; ABR/McM 196

67. **C.** The anterior interventricular (LAD) artery lies anteriorly and to the left and descends vertically to the left toward the apex. It can be more easily injured by a transverse incision of the pericardium, which would cross perpendicular to this artery.

A. The auricular appendage of the left atrium is located posteriorly; therefore, it would not be injured in an anterior longitudinal incision.

B. The coronary sinus is between the right AV orifice and the inferior vena cava and would not be affected.

D. The left phrenic nerve lies between the heart and the left lung, just anterior to the root of the lung, and is too deep to be injured in this incision.

E. The left sympathetic trunk is also too posterior to be injured.
GAS 185–189; N 222; ABR/McM 196

68. **D.** A finger passing through the transverse pericardial sinus passes directly behind the two great arteries exiting the heart, thus allowing the surgeon to easily place a vascular clamp upon the pulmonary trunk and ascending aorta.

A. The right and left pulmonary veins are not accessible through the transverse sinus.

B. The superior and inferior vena cavae cannot be accessed via the transverse sinus.

C. The right and left coronary arteries cannot be accessed through the transverse sinus.

E. Although the pulmonary trunk may be accessible, the superior vena cava will not be readily available via the transverse sinus.
GAS 185–189; N 219; ABR/McM 196

69. **A.** The middle cardiac veins run parallel with the inferior (posterior) interventricular (posterior descending) artery and drains directly into the coronary sinus.

B. The great cardiac vein is parallel to the anterior interventricular artery.

C. The small cardiac vein passes parallel with the right marginal artery.

D. The anterior cardiac veins are several small veins that drain directly into the right atrium.

E. The coronary sinus is a wide venous channel that runs from left to right in the posterior part of the coronary groove.
GAS 207-209; N 222; ABR/McM 198

70. **D.** The left coronary artery bifurcates into the anterior interventricular artery (LAD) and the circumflex branch. The circumflex branch gives off the left marginal branch, which supplies the lateral wall (obtuse margin) of the left ventricle.

A. The anterior part of the interventricular septum is supplied by the anterior interventricular artery (LAD).

B. The diaphragmatic surface of the right ventricle is supplied by the inferior (posterior) interventricular artery and the right marginal, a branch of the right coronary artery.

C. The infundibulum, also known as the conus arteriosus, is the outflow portion of the right ventricle.

E. The posterior part of the interventricular septum is supplied by the inferior (posterior) interventricular artery, in most cases a branch of the right coronary artery.
GAS 202–209; N 222; ABR/McM 198

71. **C.** The AV node is most commonly supplied by a branch of the right coronary artery. This branch arises at the crux of the heart (the point of junction of all four cardiac chambers posteriorly); this is the location of the occlusion.

A. The right atrium is supplied by the right coronary artery.

B. The right coronary artery also supplies the sinuatrial node.

D. The left marginal artery supplies the lateral wall of the left ventricle.

E. The anterior portion of the interventricular septum is supplied by the anterior interventricular artery.
GAS 211–214; N 229; ABR/McM 198

72. C. The first heart sound is caused by the closure of the tricuspid and mitral valves.
A and B; D and E. The second heart sound is caused by the closure of the aortic and pulmonary valves. Any answer choice including either the aortic and/or pulmonary valves would therefore be incorrect.
GAS 19, 240; N 222; ABR/McM 201

73. A. The second heart sound is caused by the closure of the aortic and pulmonary valves.
B, C, D, E: The first sound by the heart is caused by the closure of the tricuspid and mitral valves. Any answer choice including either the tricuspid and/or mitral valves would therefore be incorrect.
GAS 208, 240; N 222; ABR/McM 201

74. D. The first septal perforating branch of the anterior interventricular artery (LAD) is the first branch of the LAD that supplies the conducting tissue of the heart; it passes directly to the point of bifurcation of the common AV bundle (of His).
A. The artery of the conus is a small branch of the right coronary artery and supplies the conus arteriosus. It would not be implicated in the ischemic area.
B. The sinuatrial nodal artery would not be implicated in the ischemic area.
C. The AV nodal artery does not supply the area described in the pathology report.
GAS 202–206; N 224; ABR/McM 198

75. B. The superior vena cava empties into the right atrium on the superior aspect of the heart and is not directly palpable from the oblique sinus.
A. The inferior vena cava will be palpable as the oblique sinus provides access to it.
C. The oblique sinus provides access to the posterior wall of the left atrium.
D. The oblique sinus, which exists as a cul-de-sac, will also provide access to the inferior right pulmonary vein.
E. The right atrium can also be accessed via the oblique sinus.
GAS 184–188; N 212; ABR/McM 196

Answers 76–100

76. D. Cardiac tamponade is characterized by hypotension, tachycardia, muffled heart sounds, and jugular vein distention. Bleeding into the pericardial cavity would muffle the heart sounds because of the increased distance between the chest wall and the heart, leading to "distant" heart sounds. When the effusion is particularly severe, the heart may take on a "water bottle" appearance on an anterior-posterior x-ray.
A. There will be distension of the jugular veins, as opposed to decrease in the dimensions of the jugular veins.

B. Cardiac tamponade will not produce a gradual enlargement of the ventricles during diastole.
C. The difference between systolic and diastolic arterial pressures will not increase significantly during cardiac tamponade. There will be overall hypotension.
E. Pulses of the internal carotid artery will not become increasingly distinct.
GAS 184–189; N 223; ABR/McM 184

77. E. "Right coronary dominant circulation" refers simply to the fact that the right coronary artery provides origin for the inferior (posterior) interventricular (posterior descending) coronary artery. In such cases, it provides supply for the SA and AV nodes. It might be anticipated that right coronary blockage could result in dysfunction of the AV node, if collateral supply is poor or absent.
A. The distal anterior interventricular artery comes off the left coronary artery and would not be involved in this scenario.
B. The circumflex artery comes off the left coronary artery and also would not be involved.
C. The left coronary artery would not be implicated in this scenario.
D. The right marginal artery is a branch of the right coronary artery.
GAS 202–209; N 223; ABR/McM 198

78. D. The chordae tendineae are fibrous cords that connect papillary muscles to valve leaflets. The restraint provided by these cords on the valve leaflets, along with contraction of the papillary muscles, prevents the prolapse of the mitral valve cusps into the left atrium.
A. The crista terminalis is a ridge that runs from the opening of the inferior vena cava to the superior vena cava.
B. The crista supraventricularis is a muscular strip within the right ventricle that separates the conus arteriosus from the rest of the ventricle.
C. The pectinate muscles are parallel, linear muscles in the atrial wall that make up the atrial appendage.
E. Trabeculae carneae are irregular ridges of myocardium that are present within the ventricles.
GAS 195–200; N 225; ABR/McM 200

79. D. The correct path that leads to the right ventricle for the lead of the pacemaker is the brachiocephalic vein (could be right or left; pacemakers are more commonly placed on the left in which case it would be the left brachiocephalic vein), superior vena cava, right atrium, tricuspid valve, and right ventricle.
A. This answer is incorrect as it does not include the right atrium, which must be passed between the superior vena cava and tricuspid valve. It also lists the mitral valve, which is in the left heart.
B. This answer is incorrect because it does include the brachiocephalic vein, which is one of the first structures that must be entered. It also lists the mitral valve, which is on the left side of the heart.
C. This answer is incorrect as it does include the brachiocephalic vein, which is one of the first structures that must be entered.

E. This answer is incorrect because it includes the mitral valve, which is between the left atrium and left ventricle.
GAS 189–194; N 229; ABR/McM 205

80. **A.** Mitral stenosis leads to left atrial dilation, which can exert a compressive effect on the esophagus. Stenosis of the mitral valve (AV valve between left atrium and left ventricle) would lead to enlargement of the left atrium, which would in turn impinge upon the esophagus which lies directly posterior to the left atrium.

    B. The pulmonary valve is located between the outflow tract of the right ventricle and the pulmonary trunk. A stenosis of the pulmonary valve would have no effect upon the esophagus because of the anterior position of the pulmonary trunk in the thorax.

    C. The aortic valve is located between the left ventricle and the aorta. Regurgitation through any valve will ultimately decrease systemic blood flow.

    D and E. Anterior interventricular (LAD) and inferior (posterior) interventricular (posterior descending) arterial occlusions can cause a myocardial infarction, but not dysphagia. In the normal position of the heart the left atrium lies most posteriorly. An occlusion of a coronary artery will lead to ischemia and possibly myocardial infarction.
    GAS 202–209; N 228; ABR/McM 204

81. **C.** The sinuatrial node, the primary pacemaker of the heart, is a mass of specialized cardiac cells within the myocardium at the upper end of the crista terminalis, near the opening of the superior vena cava into the right atrium.

    A. The AV node is at the junction of the coronary sinus and the right atrium upon the right fibrous trigone (central fibrous body).

    B. The valve of the inferior vena cava (Eustachian) directs blood from the inferior vena cava through the right atrium toward the foramen ovale during fetal life, so that the umbilical venous blood carried by the IVC can reach the left atrium and ultimately the head as soon as possible.

    D. The interatrial septum is located between the left and right atria.

    E. The septomarginal trabecula (moderator band) arises from the muscular portion of the interventricular septum and passes to the base of the anterior papillary muscle in the right ventricle. The moderator band carries part of the right bundle branch of the conduction system just beneath its endocardial layer.
    GAS 211–213; N 229; ABR/McM 199

82. **D.** The tricuspid valve is the AV valve located between the right atrium and right ventricle. An incompetent valve would allow blood to regurgitate into the right atrium during systole and subsequently raise pressure in the venous system, increasing capillary pressure and causing edema.

    A. Regurgitation of blood into the pulmonary trunk would be a result of an incompetent pulmonary valve.

    B. Regurgitation of blood from the left ventricle back into the left atrium is a result of prolapse of the mitral valve.

    C. There is no direct anatomic relationship between the tricuspid valve and the ascending aorta.

    E. Blood would pool in the left ventricle in the event of aortic valve incompetence.
    GAS 196–198; N 228; ABR/McM 199

83. **C.** To avoid damaging the lungs, a chest tube should be placed below the level of the lungs, in the costodiaphragmatic recess. The point of entrance for the tube would be the eighth or ninth intercostal space. At the midclavicular line, the costodiaphragmatic recess is localized between intercostal spaces 6 and 8, at the midaxillary line between 8 and 10, and at the paravertebral line between ribs 10 and 12.

    A and B. The fourth and sixth rib spaces along the midaxillary line will be too high up to reach the costodiaphragmatic recess.

    D and E. The tenth and twelfth rib spaces may be too low to reach the costodiaphragmatic recess. Ideally the best position is between the eighth and tenth rib spaces along the midaxillary line.
    GAS 163–174, 241–242; N 221; ABR/McM 186

84. **C.** The costal parietal pleura is innervated by the intercostal nerves and is very sensitive to pain, in this case being somatic innervation. Therefore, the costal parietal pleura is the deepest layer that must be anesthetized to reduce pain during aspiration or chest tube placement.

    A. The endothoracic fascia must be penetrated prior to reaching the costal parietal pleura.

    B. The intercostal muscles must also be penetrated prior to reaching the costal parietal pleura.

    D. The subcutaneous fat is a relatively superficial layer that must be penetrated to reach the costal parietal pleura.

    E. The visceral pleura lies deep to the costal parietal pleura and does not need to be infiltrated to achieve adequate anesthesia.
    GAS 163–174; N 215; ABR/McM 191

85. **A.** The right main bronchus is the shorter, wider, and more vertical primary bronchus. Therefore, this is most often the location that foreign objects will likely be lodged.

    B. The left primary bronchus is not as vertical and therefore does not present the path of least resistance.

    C. The carina is a ridge separating the openings of left and right bronchi; the "fork in the road."

    D. The trachea is a tubular structure supported by incomplete cartilaginous rings, and the likelihood that an object will be lodged there is minimal.

    E. It is unlikely that a foreign object would descend so far as to obstruct a tertiary bronchus.
    GAS 163–179; N 208; ABR/McM 209

86. **D.** Contraction of the diaphragm (descent) pulls the dome inferiorly, increasing the vertical dimension of the thorax. This is the most important factor in inspiration for decreasing intrathoracic pressure, thereby increasing the internal pulmonary volume.

    A and B. The contraction of intercostal muscles is usually involved in forced inspiration, resulting in increases in the transverse and anteroposterior dimensions of the thoracic cavity.

C. Straightening of the spine's forward curvature would not have as significant of an impact on the vertical dimensions of the thoracic cavity.

E. Orientation and flexibility of the ribs to expand in all directions would not be specific to the movements needed to increase inspiratory capacity.

GAS 163–166; N 200; ABR/McM 225

87. B. The horizontal fissure of the right lung is a fissure separating the superior lobe from the middle lobe. It usually extends medially from the oblique fissure at the midaxillary line to the sternum, along the lower border of the fourth rib.

A. There is usually no horizontal fissure in the left lung.

C. The oblique fissure of the left lung would not be affected by stab wound to the right chest.

D. The apex of the right lung reaches to a level above the first rib and is therefore superior to the stab wound in the fourth costal cartilage.

E. The root of the left lung would not be affected by stab wound to the right thorax.

GAS 163–179; N 205; ABR/McM 186

88. C. The patient's symptoms are all indicative of inflammatory breast cancer. Common symptoms include inversion of the nipple and dimpling of the overlying skin, changes that are due to the retraction of the suspensory ligaments (of Cooper).

A. Retention of infantile and fetal state of the nipple would not cause pathologic inversion.

B. Intraductal cancerous tumors show symptoms including breast enlargement, breast lump, breast pain, and nipple discharge (GAS Fig. 3.16).

D. Obstruction of the cutaneous lymphatics would not cause inversion of the nipple and the changes seen in peau d'orange.

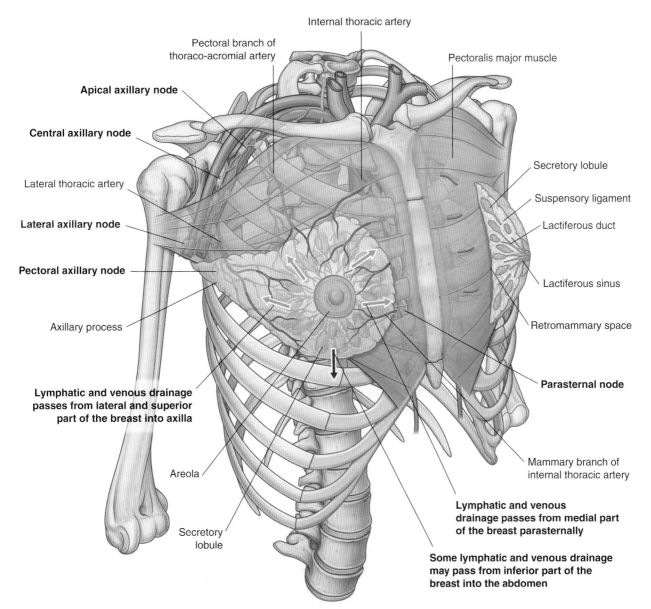

GAS Fig. 3.16

E. Inflammation of the nipple's epithelial lining would not produce the changes described here.
GAS 141–142; N 188; ABR/McM 185

89. C. The inferior tracheobronchial nodes are also known as the carinal nodes and are located inferior to the carina, the site of bifurcation of the trachea.
A. The pulmonary nodes lie within the lungs.
B. The bronchopulmonary (hilar) nodes lie at the hilum of the lungs.
D. The superior tracheobronchial nodes lie superior to the junction of the bronchi and the trachea.
E. The paratracheal nodes run beside the trachea.
GAS 141–142; N 212; ABR/McM 209

90. B. The superior lobar bronchus is one of the divisions of the right main bronchus. This bronchus branches into apical, anterior, and posterior tertiary or segmental bronchi.
A. The superior and medial basal segments arise from the right lower lobar bronchus, and the medial and lateral segments arise from the right middle lobar bronchus.
C. This answer choice includes segments from the right middle and right lower lobar bronchi.
D. The lateral segment arises from the right middle lobar branch and the lateral basal segment arises from the right lower lobar bronchus.
E. This answer choice includes segments from the right middle and right lower lobar bronchi.
GAS 169–179; N 209; ABR/McM 212

91. D. Lymphatic drainage of the breast is typically to the axillary nodes, more specifically to the anterior axillary (pectoral) nodes.
A. The lateral axillary node receives lymph from the upper limb, but not from the breast area.
B. The central axillary nodes receive lymph after it has passed through the anterior axillary (pectoral) nodes.
C. The apical axillary nodes receive lymph from the central axillary nodes, after it has passed through the anterior axillary (pectoral) nodes. The apical axillary nodes are located superior to the upper border of the pectoralis minor and inferior to the clavicle. From these nodes, lymph passes into the subclavian lymph trunk, although some breast lymph may enter supraclavicular nodes.
E. The posterior axillary (subscapular) nodes receive lymph from the posterior shoulder region and not from the breast area. This is the reason for the edema of the upper limb that occurs after a mastectomy, in which there may be a total removal of axillary lymph nodes.
GAS 141–142; N 191; ABR/McM 185

92. A. Increased arterial pressure in the upper limbs (as demonstrated in the brachial artery) and decreased pressure in the lower limbs (as demonstrated in the femoral artery) are common symptoms of coarctation of the aorta. Other symptoms include tortuous and enlarged blood vessels above the coarctation and an increased risk of cerebral hemorrhage. This condition of coarctation occurs when the aorta is abnormally constricted during development.
B. The patient does not complain of respiratory distress, so cor pulmonale would not be the most likely underlying condition.
C. Dissection of the right common iliac artery would not result in nosebleed or headache.
D. Obstruction of the superior vena cava would not account for decreased femoral pulse.
E. A pulmonary embolism will not present with these symptoms. Most commonly associated symptoms would be sudden onset shortness of breath and chest pain.
GAS 216; N 211; ABR/McM 207

93. D. The diagnosis for these symptoms is coarctation of the aorta. This condition occurs when the aorta is abnormally constricted. One of the cardinal radiographic signs is a characteristic rib notching. "Notching" of the ribs is due to the reversal of direction of blood flow through the anterior intercostal branches of the internal thoracic artery, as these usually small arteries carry collateral arterial blood flow through the posterior intercostal arteries and into the descending aorta inferior to the coarctation. Enlargement and vibration of the intercostal arteries against the rib results in erosion ("notching") of the costal grooves, which is visible on radiography.
A. Flail chest is seen when a segment of the ribs breaks and is detached from the rest of the thoracic wall. It is usually seen after traumatic injury.
B. Pneumothorax is an abnormal collection of air within the pleural space and would not be associated with coarctation of the aorta.
C. Hydrothorax refers to abnormal pooling of fluid within the pleural space and would not be associated with coarctation of the aorta.
E. Mediastinal shift is movement of thoracic contents in one half of the thorax toward the other side. It can be seen in conditions affecting the thoracic volume or pressure but is not associated with coarctation of the aorta.
GAS 216; N 197; ABR/McM 207

94. C. The long thoracic nerve arises from the C5, C6, and C7 ventral rami and innervates the serratus anterior muscle. Due to its location on the lateral chest wall, it may be injured in axillary dissection during radical mastectomy. Injury of this nerve will result in a characteristic winged scapula.
A. A is the lateral pectoral nerve, which innervates the pectoralis major muscle.
B. B is the suprascapular nerve, which innervates the supraspinatus and infraspinatus muscles.
D. D is the thoracodorsal nerve, which innervates latissimus dorsi.

E. E is the lower subscapular nerve that innervates the lower part of the subscapularis muscle and the teres major.

GAS 717, 727, 795; N 194; ABR/McM 144

95. B. The superior margin of the manubrium is characterized by the jugular notch. Laterally are the sternoclavicular joints and the articulations of the first ribs with the manubrium. The second pair of ribs articulates with the sternum at the sternal angle, the junction of the manubrium with the body of the sternum.

A. The first rib connects with the manubrium of the sternum below the sternoclavicular joint.

C, D, E. The third, fourth, and fifth ribs are too low to interact with the junction of the manubrium with the body of the sternum. They are not the most likely to be involved in direct traumatic injury to the sternal angle.

GAS 148–153; N 192; ABR/McM 183

96. B. The thoracic duct is important in lymph drainage of the entire body with the exception of the upper right quadrant. The thoracic duct ascends between the aorta and azygos vein behind the esophagus. Dilation of the esophagus here in the lower thorax from a large lipoma can compress the thoracic duct, leading to impairment of lymphatic drainage from below the blockage and resultant edema in the lower limbs.

A. Dilation of the esophagus would not compress the thoracic aorta to produce symptoms of lower limb swelling.

C. Superior vena cava occlusion is most often caused by mediastinal tumors and would not produce significant lower limb edema.

D. An aortic aneurysm is not associated with cancerous growths and would not cause lower limb edema.

E. Femoral artery disease would not produce lower limb edema.

GAS 231–232; N 242; ABR/McM 225, 226

97. C. The anterior intercostal arteries anastomose with the posterior intercostal arteries. Ligation of the anterior arteries would not affect the supply of the intercostal spaces because the posterior arteries would provide collateral arterial supply.

A. Branches of the musculophrenic artery provide anterior intercostal supply for the lower seventh, eighth, and ninth intercostal spaces.

B. The superior epigastric artery passes into the rectus sheath of the anterior abdominal wall.

D. The lateral thoracic artery arises from the second part of the axillary artery.

E. The thoracodorsal artery is a branch of the subscapular artery, a branch of the third part of the axillary artery.

GAS 157–158; N 205–206; ABR/McM 221

98. D. The thymus lies in the superior mediastinum and may extend into the anterior mediastinum. A midline tumor of this gland can compress the left brachiocephalic vein.

A and B. The internal jugular veins are located superior and lateral to the position of the thymus and would not be affected by this mass.

C. A midline tumor is more likely to cause compression of the left brachiocephalic vein, which crosses the midline, than the right brachiocephalic vein, which is not located in the midline.

E. The subclavian vein is distal or lateral to this location, and the thymus would not likely impinge upon it.

GAS 220–222; N 222; ABR/McM 228

99. B. The parietal pleura can be divided regionally into costal, diaphragmatic, mediastinal, and cervical portions, depending upon local topographic relations. Another name for the cervical pleura is the cupula. This forms the dome of the pleura, projecting into the neck above the first rib and corresponding to the area of injury.

A. The costal pleura lines the internal surfaces of the ribs and intercostal spaces.

C. The right mainstem bronchus is not located near the right clavicle or the first rib.

D. The right upper lobe bronchus is not located in the vicinity of the right clavicle nor the first rib.

E. The mediastinal parietal pleura lies between the lungs and the organs in the mediastinum.

GAS 166–169; N 222; ABR/McM 216

100. B. The right primary bronchus is shorter, wider, and more vertical than the left main bronchus. When a foreign body is aspirated, it is more likely to enter the right main bronchus (although in some cases the foreign body enters the left bronchus).

A. Pulmonary vascular resistance is not related to the question.

C. This is incorrect as the right main bronchus is wider, not narrower.

D. This is incorrect as the right main bronchus is shorter, not longer.

E. The right lower lung lobe does not have poorer venous drainage than the other lobes.

GAS 167–170; N 215; ABR/McM 221-222

Answers 101–125

101. D. The normal position of the heart as seen in a plain chest x-ray has the right border of the heart formed by the superior vena cava, right atrium, and inferior vena cava. The left border is formed by the aortic arch superiorly, left pulmonary artery, left auricle, left ventricle, and the apex of the heart inferolaterally. The area indicated by the arrow is just inferior to the clavicle (on the left side), and this marks the location of the arch of the aorta.

A. The superior vena cava would comprise the heart's upper right border and the arrow is pointing to a structure along the heart's left border.

B. The right ventricle would also comprise the heart's anterior surface and is not indicated by the arrow.

C. The left ventricle would lie more inferior to where the arrow is pointing.

E. The pulmonary artery would lie more inferior to the area pointed to by the arrow.

GAS 195–198; N 224; ABR/McM 208

102. **B.** All of the symptoms described in the question are indicative of breast cancer. The best choice of answers is cancer en cuirasse, a pathologic condition that presents as a hard, "wood like" texture.

A. Peau d'orange refers to the physical exam finding of abnormal texture of the skin that resembles an orange peel. This is caused by obstruction of lymphatic flow through invaded axillary lymph nodes.

C. Intraductal cancerous tumor is often a mild form of cancer detected by mammography.

D. This is a physical symptom and not an exam finding.

E. This is also a physical condition and not the best description of the symptoms depicted in the question.

GAS 143; N 197; ABR/McM 190–191

103. **A.** When multiple rib fractures produce a flail segment of the thoracic wall, paradoxical motion of the flail segment is commonly experienced upon deep inspiration; that is, the flail area is sucked in rather than expanding outward with inspiration, and the reverse movement occurs in expiration.

B. The flail segment will move in the opposite direction, not in the same direction, as the chest wall.

C. Because the ribs are fractured, they will not be able to facilitate the normal "pump handle" motion during inspiration.

D and E. The excursions of the diaphragm will not be affected on either side by the broken ribs, except as pain restricts the breathing effort of the patient.

GAS 154; N 201; ABR/McM 190–191

104. **A:** The subclavian artery lies directly posterior to the subclavian vein; therefore, it is the structure that would be most vulnerable to damage when placing a central venous line in the subclavian vein.

B. The phrenic nerve is medial to the site of line placement and will most likely not be damaged.

C. The superior vena cava lies medial and inferior to the site of placement and is too deep to be easily damaged.

D. The common carotid artery is also too medial to be damaged by the line.

E. The vagus nerve is medial to the site of line placement and is not likely to be damaged by this procedure.

GAS 221; N 204; ABR/McM 228

105. **A.** Lymph from the lower third of the esophagus drains into the posterior mediastinal and left gastric lymph nodes. The middle third of the esophagus drains into posterior and superior mediastinal lymph nodes. The upper third of the esophagus drains into the deep cervical nodes.

B. The bronchopulmonary nodes will not receive lymph from the esophagus.

C. The tracheobronchial nodes will also not receive lymphatic drainage from the esophagus.

D and E. The inferior and superior tracheobronchial nodes are not involved in drainage of the esophagus. They may be enlarged in pathology of the lungs.

GAS 183; N 219

106. **A.** Lymph from the right primary bronchus would drain first into the inferior tracheobronchial nodes.

B. The paratracheal nodes receive lymph from the superior tracheobronchial nodes.

C. The bronchomediastinal trunk is not a lymph node.

D. The bronchopulmonary nodes would not be the first site to receive lymphatic drainage from the right primary bronchus.

E. The thoracic duct receives lymph from the bronchomediastinal trunks, which in turn receive lymph from the paratracheal nodes.

GAS 183; N 219

107. **D.** The great radicular artery (of Adamkiewicz) is an important artery that provides oxygenated blood to the lower portion of the spinal cord, specifically the anterior cord where lower motor neurons are located, inferior to the vertebral level of origin of the artery (usually T12–L1), and provides collateral anastomoses with the anterior spinal artery. Care should be taken during surgery to prevent damage to this artery as this can lead to paraplegia and alteration of functions of pelvic organs.

A. Injury to the right coronary artery would not specifically lead to paraplegia but could disrupt cardiac function.

B. Injury to the left common carotid artery could be potentially fatal but is not specifically associated with paraplegia.

C. Injury to the right subclavian artery would not produce paraplegia.

E. Iatrogenic injury of the esophageal artery is also not likely to produce paraplegia as an associated symptom.

GAS 104–106; N 185

108. **B.** An enlarged thyroid gland will most likely compress the left internal jugular vein which lies immediately lateral to it in the neck.

A. The left brachiocephalic vein lies inferior to the thyroid gland and is not as likely to be affected by tracheal deviation.

C. The left subclavian artery will not be injured by tracheal deviation at the level of the thyroid.

D. The vagus nerve is not as likely to be affected by the scenario described here.

E. The phrenic nerve is also not the most likely structure to be affected.

GAS 173–177; N 199; ABR/McM 218

109. **A.** The carina is the only answer listed that can easily be seen in chest x-ray. The carina is at the level

of T4–T5 (plane associated with the sternal angle [of Louis]). This landmark is commonly used to guide the placement of a central venous line.

B. The subclavian artery is not the most ideal landmark to guide placement of a central venous line as it is not as easily seen on a chest x-ray.

C. The superior vena cava is not an ideal landmark to verify placement of a central line.

D and E. Cardiac structures such as the left and right atrium would not be ideal landmarks for central line placement as they may not be reliably seen on chest x-ray.
  GAS 173–179; N 216; ABR/McM 209

110. D: Gynecomastia is the abnormal growth of the mammary glands in men.

A. Polythelia refers to supernumerary, or extra, nipples.

B and C: Supernumerary breasts and polymastia refer to the same condition—an additional breast.

E. Amastia refers to the absence of breasts.
  GAS 135, 141–143; N 190; ABR/McM 185

111. E. A tension pneumothorax is caused by injury to the lung, leading to air in the pleural cavity. The site of the wound acts as a one-way valve, allowing air to enter the pleural cavity but not to leave the cavity. The lack of negative pressure in the pleural cavity causes the lung to collapse. The tension pneumothorax occurred during a violent fall; therefore, the clinical condition is not likely to be a spontaneous pneumothorax, in which case there is rupture of the pleura without the necessary occurrence of trauma.

A. Flail chest will not cause increased volume of air in the pleural cavity as it refers to the condition whereby multiple rib fractures produce a flail segment in the thoracic wall.

B. Emphysema is a respiratory condition that is not characterized by changes in the pleural cavity.

C. Hemothorax refers to blood within the thoracic cavity and is not associated with the signs seen here.

D. Chylothorax is seen after injury to the thoracic duct, with lymph entering the thoracic cavity.
  GAS 169; N 211; ABR/McM 212

112. B. Chylothorax is usually caused by injury to the thoracic duct. The thoracic duct enters the venous system at the junction of the left internal jugular vein and the left subclavian vein, where they form the left brachiocephalic vein. Penetrating injuries at the beginning of the left brachiocephalic vein commonly also disrupt the termination of the thoracic duct.

A. Injury to the left external jugular vein would not produce chylothorax.

C. Injury to the right subclavian vein would not result in chylothorax.

D. Injury to the proximal part of the right brachiocephalic vein is not as closely associated with the thoracic duct as the origin of the left brachiocephalic vein.

E. Injury to the right external jugular vein will not produce chylothorax.
  GAS 159; N 219; ABR/McM 228

113. A. The inferior vena cava may undergo compression by the growing fetus when the pregnant woman is in a supine position. In this case the compression leads to decreasing venous return when the woman is in in supine position. This condition is referred as Supine Hypotensive Syndrome.

B. There is no reason for compression of the superior vena cava to occur in this patient when she lies supine.

C. The patient's aorta may be compressed as she lies supine, but this would lead to elevated, not depressed, blood pressure in the upper limbs.

D. Compression of the common carotid artery will not produce the changes in blood pressure seen in this patient.

E. Compression of the internal jugular veins will not produce the changes in blood pressure described.
  GAS 134; N 274

114. C. Crackling noises in the lungs due to the buildup of fluid are referred to as rales. The fluid usually migrates to the inferior portion of the lung due to the effects of gravity. Auscultation over the sixth intercostal space at the midaxillary line would be associated with the lower lobe of the right lung. Remember that the oblique fissure runs from the level of T2 posteriorly to the sixth costal cartilage anteriorly. At the sixth intercostal space in the midaxillary line, one would be percussing below this fissure and therefore over the lower lobe.

A and B. Due to the effects of gravity, the fluid buildup heard as crackling is less likely to be built up in the upper lobe or the middle lobe of the right lung.

D and E. This question does not indicate any examination of the left lung.
  GAS 172–176; N 213–214; ABR/McM 223–224

115. A. Pericardiocentesis is usually performed through the infrasternal angle with the needle passing up through the diaphragm to the fibrous pericardium. The diaphragmatic surface of the heart is largely composed of the right ventricle and would therefore be entered if a needle is inserted too far.

B: The left ventricle would not be encountered when entering the heart through the diaphragmatic surface adjacent to the midline.

C: The right atrium would not be encountered during pericardiocentesis.

D: The left atrium lies on the heart's posterior surface and would not be encountered during pericardiocentesis.

E: The cardiac apex would not be encountered when approaching the heart via the diaphragmatic surface.
  GAS 190–194; N 223; ABR/McM 208

116. B. The pain experienced by the patient travels with the sympathetic innervation of the heart, derived from spinal nerve levels T1–T4. The pain fibers leave

the heart and the cardiac plexuses via the cardiopulmonary nerves. Subsequently, the pain fibers pass through the sympathetic trunk, enter the spinal nerve, and pass into the dorsal roots of the spinal nerves. The cell bodies of the pain fibers are located in the dorsal root ganglia of the spinal nerves from T1 to T4.

B. This answer is incorrect as it does not include the T4 spinal nerve.

C. This answer is incorrect as it does include the T3 and T4 spinal nerves.

D. Spinal nerves T5 and T6 are not involved in carrying this pain signal.

E. Spinal nerves T5, T6, and T7 will not be involved in carrying this pain signal (GAS Fig. 3.84). *GAS 138; 244–246; N 238*

117. A. The "bucket handle movement" of the ribs affects the transverse diameter of the thorax. Inspiration would act to increase the transverse diameter of the thorax.

B. The anteroposterior diameter of the thorax would be increased by the "pump handle movements" of the ribs and sternum.

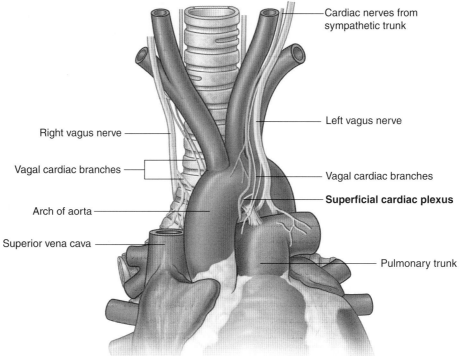

Cardiac nerves from sympathetic trunk

Left vagus nerve

Right vagus nerve

Vagal cardiac branches — Vagal cardiac branches

Superficial cardiac plexus

Arch of aorta

Superior vena cava

Pulmonary trunk

A

Cardiac nerves from sympathetic trunk

Right recurrent laryngeal nerve — Left recurrent laryngeal nerve

Right vagus nerve — Left vagus nerve

Vagal cardiac branches — Vagal cardiac branches

Deep cardiac plexus

B

GAS Fig. 3.84

C. The vertical dimensions of the thorax are increased by contraction and relaxation of the diaphragm.

D. The anteroposterior diameter of the thorax decreases during expiration due to "pump handle movements" of the ribs and sternum.

E. The transverse diameter of the thorax decreases during expiration due to the "bucket handle movement" of the ribs (GAS Fig. 3.35).
GAS 164–165; N 201

118. C. Bronchial constriction is induced by the parasympathetic innervation of the airways. This is supplied

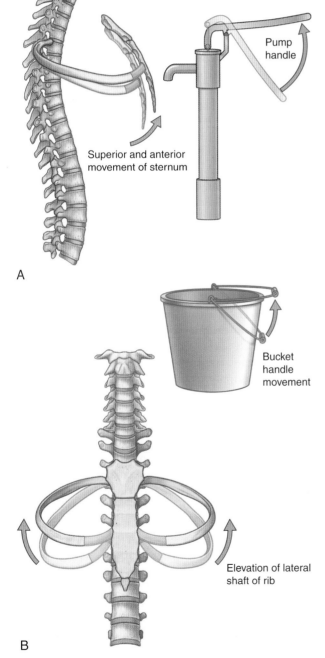

A

B

GAS Fig. 3.35

by the vagus nerves, which could be blocked to result in relaxation of the airways.

A. The phrenic nerve provides motor and sensory innervation to the diaphragm.

B. The intercostal nerves provide sensory and somatic motor innervation to their respective intercostal spaces.

D. Stimulation of sympathetic innervation results in bronchodilation.

E. The recurrent laryngeal nerve is a branch of the vagus and innervates parts of the larynx.
GAS 183; N 220

119. A. The location where one is least likely to damage important structures by making an incision or pushing a chest tube into the thorax is over the upper border of the rib.

B. At the inferior border of each rib, one will encounter intercostal vein, artery, and nerve, in that order (VAN structures), therefore this is not an ideal location for chest tube placement.

C. Entrance through the middle of the intercostal space does not eliminate the heightened possibility of piercing important structures.

D. Entering between the internal and external intercostal muscles will not permit entry to the pleural cavity.

E. Entering between the intercostal muscles and the internal intercostal membrane will not allow entry to the pleural cavity.
GAS 152–153; N 205; ABR/McM 232–233

120. B. Cardiac tamponade is a condition in which fluid accumulates in the pericardial cavity. It can result from pericardial effusion or from leakage of blood from the heart or proximal portions of the great vessels. The increased pressure within the pericardial sac leads to decreased cardiac filling during diastole and therefore reduced systolic blood pressure. Because of the reduced pumping capacity of the heart, there is increased pressure in the venous system, leading to the distension of the jugular venous system.

A. Hemothorax will not result in the symptoms described in the vignette.

C. Hemopneumothorax will not produce the reduced heart sounds, engorged jugular veins, and hypotension seen in this patient.

D. Pneumothorax will not produce the reduced heart sounds, engorged jugular veins, and hypotension seen in this patient.

E. Deep vein thrombosis often occurs in the lower limbs and increases the risk of pulmonary embolism.
GAS 190–194; N 223; ABR/McM 208

121. B. The S₂ heart sound refers to the second *(dub)* heart sound. This sound is produced by the closure of the aortic and pulmonary semilunar valves.

A. The closure of mitral/bicuspid and tricuspid valves produces the first S1 (lub) heart sound, therefore this answer is incorrect.

C. This is incorrect as it includes the mitral valve.

D. The tricuspid valve contributes to the first heart sound.

E. This answer is incorrect as it includes the tricuspid valve.

GAS 243; N 224; ABR/McM 190–191

122. **E.** The closure of the mitral/bicuspid and tricuspid valves produces the first S₁ (lub) heart sound, so this option is correct.

A. This is not correct as both the mitral and tricuspid valves produce the first heart sound.

B. Closure of the pulmonary and aortic valves produces the second heart sound, so this option is incorrect.

C. This answer is incorrect as it includes the aortic valve.

D. This is not correct as the mitral valve also contributes to the first heart sound.

GAS 243; N 224; ABR/McM 190–191

123. **D.** Flail chest is characterized by paradoxical breathing movements caused by multiple rib fractures. The sensory innervation provided to intercostal spaces and to the underlying parietal pleura is supplied via the corresponding intercostal nerves.

A. The phrenic nerve provides motor innervation to the diaphragm and sensory innervation to the diaphragmatic and mediastinal parietal pleura and pericardium.

B. The vagus nerves provide parasympathetic innervation to the thoracic viscera, and to the gastrointestinal tract as distal as the left colic flexure.

C. The cardiopulmonary nerves carry sympathetic innervation from T1 to T4 levels to the thoracic organs, and pain fibers from these organs.

E. Thoracic splanchnic nerves carry sympathetic innervation to the abdomen.

GAS 152–155; N 206; ABR/McM 200

124. **A.** An aneurysm of the aortic arch could impinge upon the phrenic nerve, causing referral of pain to the left shoulder. This referral occurs because the root levels of the phrenic nerve are C3–C5, nerve levels that are also distributed to the skin over the shoulder region.

B. Although the left vagus nerve lies against the aortic arch and may be affected by an aneurysm there, it does not transmit pain sensations except from certain organs in the abdomen and pelvis.

C. The thoracic visceral or cardiopulmonary nerves do not cause referred pain to the shoulder region, but they do carry pain fibers from thoracic organs.

D. The intercostal nerves carry sensory information from the intercostal spaces and parietal pleura, pain that would not be referred to the shoulder.

E. The thoracic splanchnics carry sympathetic innervation to the abdomen and sensory information from the abdominal organs supplied.

GAS 222; N 208; ABR/McM 202

125. **B.** The sinuatrial node functions as the primary intrinsic pacemaker of the heart, setting the cardiac rhythm. An artificial pacemaker assists in producing a normal rhythm when the sinuatrial node is not functioning normally.

A. The AV node receives the depolarization signals from the sinuatrial node. The signal is delayed within the AV node (providing the time for the atria to contract), and then travels throughout the cardiac muscle.

C. The Purkinje fibers are specialized conducting fibers that receive the signal via the bundle of His. They allow the ventricles to contract in a synchronized manner, but have no pacemaker function

D. The AV bundle (of His) sends the conduction signal from the AV node down to the Purkinje fibers, and is not involved in determining the rate of depolarization.

E. The bundle of Kent is an abnormal, accessory conduction pathway that is present in a small proportion of the population. It is associated with Wolff-Parkinson-White syndrome.

GAS 216–219; N 236; ABR/McM 211

Answers 126–148

126. **C.** Postganglionic parasympathetic fibers are involved in the constriction of smooth muscle in the tracheoesophageal tree. Therefore, inhibiting them will allow for relaxation of the tracheobronchial tree.

A and B. Sympathetic fibers cause dilation of this structure. Inhibiting either the preganglionic or the postganglionic sympathetic fibers will therefore cause further constriction of the tracheobronchial tree.

D. Visceral afferent fibers are sensory in modality, and therefore cannot modulate the dilation of smooth muscle as this is done via motor nerves.

E. Somatic efferent fibers are motor in function, but they supply skeletal muscle, not smooth muscle of the tracheobronchial tree.

GAS 183; N 221

127. **A.** Dextrocardia is a condition that results from a bending of the heart tube to the left instead of to the right. TGF-β factor Nodal plays a role in the looping of the heart during the embryonic period.

B. Ectopia cordis is an anomaly in which the heart is either partially or entirely located external to the thoracic cavity. It is not associated with Nodal.

C. Transposition of the great arteries is not associated with the Nodal factor.

D. An unequal division of the truncus arteriosus is also not associated with the Nodal factor.

E. Coarctation of the aorta is most often associated with Turner syndrome but is not associated with the Nodal factor.

GAS 208; N 233; ABR/McM 196

128. A. The esophagus typically has four constrictions. In the thorax the esophagus is compressed by (1) the arch of the aorta, (2) the left principal bronchus, and (3) the diaphragm. The cricopharyngeal constriction is in the neck. Answer A is correct as it includes these constrictions

  B. The heart, the thoracic duct, and the cricoid cartilage will not constrict the esophagus.

  C. The azygos vein arch will not constrict the esophagus.

  D. The heart and the azygos vein will not constrict the esophagus at any point along its length.

  E. The thymus and the cricothyroid muscle will not constrict the esophagus along its length.
  GAS 233–234; N 244

129. C. The dermatome that encompasses the nipple is supplied by spinal nerve T4. In this case the herpes zoster virus is harbored in the dorsal root ganglion of T4 and can be activated to cause the characteristic rash that is distributed along the dermatome including the nipple.

  A. The nipple and the surrounding area are supplied by the T4 dermatome, not the T3 dermatome.

  B. The nipple and the surrounding area are not supplied by the T3 dermatome.

  D. The virus is found in the dorsal root ganglion of T4, not the ventral root.

  E. The nipple and the surrounding area are not supplied by the T5 dermatome.
  GAS 138; N 180

130. B. Due to rib fracture, the intercostal vessels are damaged, parietal pleura is torn, and blood flows into the pleural space. The loss of negative pressure within the pleural cavity results in collapse of the lung.

  A. The left common carotid artery would not be affected by the injury described here.

  C and D. The pulmonary vessels are found within the parenchyma of the lungs and would not be injured due to an external injury such as that described.

  E. The internal thoracic artery is well protected by the sternum and is not the cause of this hemothorax.
  GAS 149–153; N 206; ABR/McM 200

131. A. Miosis, partial ptosis, and anhidrosis are a clinically important constellation of symptoms possibly indicating Horner syndrome. Horner syndrome is a lesion of the cervical sympathetic trunk and sympathetic trunk ganglia and is often a result of a Pancoast tumor, also known as a superior pulmonary sulcus tumor of the apex of the lung. The dilator pupillae, the superior tarsal muscle of the eyelid, and sweat glands are all under sympathetic nervous system control.

  B. The vagus nerve does carry parasympathetic fibers to muscles and glands of the trachea, bronchi, digestive tract, and heart but not to any structure in the head and neck (laryngeal supply, and Von Ebner glands in the tongue) other than mucous glands of the pharynx and larynx.

  C. The phrenic nerve does not carry autonomic fibers that would produce the symptoms described here. A lesion to the phrenic nerve would result in paralysis of the diaphragm.

  D. The aortic arch also would not produce the symptoms described in this patient.

  E. The thoracic visceral or cardiopulmonary nerves are splanchnic nerves that are postganglionic and sympathetic. They originate in cervical and upper thoracic ganglia and innervate thoracic organs. The cardiopulmonary plexus is the autonomic supply to the heart.
  GAS 140; N 204; ABR/McM 206

132. B. The esophagus lies posterior to the heart. Of the four chambers in the heart, the left atrium lies most posteriorly, just anterior to the esophagus when the heart is in its normal position in the mediastinum.

  A. The inferior vena cava runs on the right side within the thoracic cavity and empties its contents into the right atrium.

  C. The pulmonary arteries are too anterior to the esophagus to be affected by an esophageal tumor.

  D. The left ventricle is too anterior within the mediastinum to be affected by an esophageal tumor.

  E. The esophagus does lie against the vertebral bodies. A growing tumor would affect the esophagus first because it is a smooth muscle structure and therefore the path of least resistance, but this organ can be deviated relatively easily rather than compressed.
  GAS 228–229; N 223; ABR/McM 205

133. C. Artificial pacemakers are commonly used to treat patients who have weak or failing heart conduction systems. The electrode or "tip" of the pacemaker is threaded through the subclavian vein to the superior vena cava into the right atrium and then the right ventricle where it is used to stimulate the Purkinje fibers to result in ventricular contraction.

  A. The pacemaker passes through the right atrium to reach the right ventricle, but the right atrium is not the final location as it does not contain Purkinje fibers.

  B. The left atrium also contains no Purkinje fibers and would be relatively difficult to reach.

  D. The left ventricle is among the most difficult chambers to access, so the pacemaker will be inserted through the chambers of the right heart.

  E. The superior vena cava plays no role in cardiac pacing.
  GAS 211–212; N 236; ABR/McM 211

134. A. Cardiac hypertrophy is a compensatory mechanism of the myocardium in response to increasing demands on the heart due to ischemia, incompetent valves, or hypertension. The increased size of the heart muscle would most likely compress the esophagus, and due to the incompetent mitral valve, a backflow of blood into the left atrium can cause a left atrial dilation.

The left atrium lies just anterior to the esophagus in the mediastinum.

B. The pulmonary trunk is located superiorly and delivers blood to the lungs, so cardiac hypertrophy would not cause direct compression to this structure.

C. The superior vena cava delivers blood to the right atrium and would not be compressed in this scenario.

D. The heart lies inferior to the trachea and would not compress the trachea secondary to cardiac hypertrophy.

E. The inferior vena cava is also not likely to be compressed by this particular example of cardiac hypertrophy.
GAS 228–229; N 223; ABR/McM 205

135. E. Tension pneumothorax is a progressive accumulation of air in the pleural cavity that is trapped during inspiration. The resulting increase of pressure diminishes the negative pressure required to maintain an inflated lung, resulting in a collapsed lung as seen on the chest x-ray.

A. A flail chest is a result of ribs being broken in two or more locations, and no broken ribs are seen on this chest x-ray.

B. Emphysema is a chronic condition in which elastic tissues and alveoli in the lungs are destroyed, reducing the surface area for gas exchange. Emphysema may result in a secondary spontaneous pneumothorax.

C. A hemothorax is an accumulation of blood in the pleural space. On a chest x-ray it is identifiable by a meniscus of fluid.

D. Although spontaneous pneumothorax would present the same way on a chest x-ray the patient's history of trauma (car crash) indicates the patient does not have a spontaneous pneumothorax.
GAS 169; N 211; ABR/McM 218

136. D. As per the accompanying chest x-ray the right upper, middle, and lower lobes are affected. The right upper lobe extends from the apex of the lung (above the clavicle) to the fourth rib. The chest x-ray shows multiple opacities on the right side, eliminating the possibility of it being a left lung pneumonia. Opacity in the right middle lobe extends inferiorly to the sixth rib. In the present case the opacity is inferior to the sixth rib extending to the tenth rib in the midaxillary line affecting the lower lobe of the right lung.

A. This is incorrect as the opacity also occupies the right middle and lower lobes.

B. This is incorrect as the opacity also occupies the right upper and lower lobes.

C. This is incorrect as the opacity also occupies the right upper and middle lobes.

E. This is incorrect as the opacity also occupies the right middle lobe.
GAS 172–176; N 212–213; ABR/McM 223

137. D. In many people, the anterior interventricular branch of the left coronary artery gives rise to a diagonal branch that descends on the anterior surface of the heart. This branch is occluded.

A. The right coronary artery is not occluded in this angiogram. The right coronary artery arises from the right aortic sinus and runs in the coronary groove. It usually gives off a sinuatrial nodal branch; it then descends in the coronary groove and gives off a right marginal branch. At the crux of the heart, it gives off an AV nodal branch and a large inferior (posterior) interventricular branch (in the "right dominant" pattern).

B. The anterior interventricular artery is not occluded here. It comes off the left coronary artery, and is also known as the LAD artery. The LAD runs along the anterior interventricular groove to the apex of the heart.

C. The inferior (posterior) interventricular artery comes off the right coronary artery in the "right dominant" pattern at the crux of the heart.

E. The circumflex artery comes off of the left coronary artery and along with the anterior interventricular artery is one of the two branches of the left coronary artery. The left coronary artery arises from the left aortic sinus of the ascending aorta and passes between the left atrium and the pulmonary trunk.
GAS 207–211; N 229–230; ABR/McM 208–210

138. A. Blockage of cutaneous lymphatic vessels results in edema of the skin surrounding the hair follicles, leading to an appearance like an orange peel *(peau d'orange)*.

B. Shortening of the suspensory ligaments leads to dimpling of the overlying skin, not peau d'orange.

C. Contraction of retinacula cutis results in retraction and inversion of the nipple and/or areola.

D. Pectoralis major involvement has nothing to do with this condition but can result in fixing the tumor firmly to the chest wall.

E. Intraductal cancer of the breast will not directly lead to inversion of the nipple.
GAS 143; N 199–200; ABR/McM 196

139. C. The patient is suffering from cardiac tamponade, that is, filling of the pericardial cavity with fluid. The classic signs of this tamponade are referred to as "Beck's triad." This trio, by definition, includes a small heart from compression of the heart by the fluid-filled pericardial sac, and a quiet heart because the tamponade muffles the cardiac sounds; decreased pulse pressure resulting from the reduced difference between systolic and diastolic pressure because the tamponade restricts the ability of the heart to fill in diastole; and increased central venous pressure because venous blood cannot enter the compressed heart.

A. Beck's triad refers to cardiac signs and symptoms secondary to pericardial fluid accumulation.

B. A hemothorax is defined by bleeding into the pleural space, and the resultant physical findings. This would not be consistent with Beck's triad.

D. These changes are not characteristic of Beck's triad.

E. These symptoms describe a classic presentation of tension pneumothorax, which is not consistent with the findings seen in Beck's triad.

GAS 190–194; N 223; ABR/McM 208

140. **E.** Myelin degeneration of the phrenic nerves, as can occur in Guillain-Barré syndrome results in loss of phrenic nerve function and paralysis of the diaphragm. Diaphragmatic paralysis is predictable with lack of movement of the abdominal wall in respiratory efforts. **A and B.** The intercostal muscles are still functioning as the ribs are described as moving "violently" in this patient's presentation.

C. This patient's pectoral muscles are still functioning as his ribs are described as moving "violently" during respiration. The only disturbance seen here is in the diaphragm.

D. The sternocleidomastoid muscle is a neck muscle that acts as an accessory muscle of respiration by helping to raise the rib cage during breathing. In this presentation, the ribs are still moving so this muscle is not implicated.

GAS 164–165; N 208; ABR/McM 202

141. **C.** The loss of myelin from the preganglionic (normally myelinated) sympathetic fibers in T1–T4 results in interruption in their transmission of electrical stimulating impulses and, therefore, reduction of positive inotropic (force increasing) and chronotropic (rate increasing) stimulation of the heart.

A. Reduction of function of the vagus nerves would not result in slowing cardiac activity; just the opposite would occur.

B. Interruption of phrenic nerve activity has no effect on cardiac rate (as this nerve innervates the diaphragm).

D. Disturbing firing of the thinly myelinated pain fibers from the heart would have no influence on the cardiac rate.

E. The ventral horn neurons do not innervate the heart, but rather skeletal muscle; therefore, they would not be directly affected by the disease process affecting the heart.

GAS 164–165; N 208; ABR/McM 202

142. **C.** The mitral valve is best visualized by TEE because the transducer within the esophagus is directly posterior to the left atrium. The physical laws that apply to ultrasound imaging dictate that the closer the structure to the transducer, the better the ability to obtain a good image. This question asks which heart valve is most directly related to the posterior aspect of the left atrium, which is the mitral valve.

A. The tricuspid valve is found between the right atrium and right ventricle and as such is not the valve seen most clearly by the TEE.

B. The pulmonary valve transports blood to the lungs via the right ventricle and is not the valve that is best visualized by TEE.

D. Although the aortic valve is on the left side of the heart, it is not as clearly seen as the mitral valve as the left atrium is the posterior most chamber of the heart.

E. The Eustachian valve, or the valve of the inferior vena cava, is not the one that is best visualized by the TEE.

GAS 228–229; N 223; ABR/McM 205

143. **A.** Pneumomediastinum describes the presence of air in the mediastinum and may arise from a wide range of pathological conditions. Despite the well-described imaging of pneumomediastinum, it is sometimes difficult to differentiate from other conditions such as pneumopericardium and medial pneumothorax. The "aortic nipple" is the radiographic term used to describe the lateral nipple-like projection from the aortic knob, the left side of the aortic arch as seen on an PA/AP chest x-ray. The aortic nipple corresponds to the end-on appearance of the left superior intercostal vein coursing around the aortic knob and may be mistaken radiologically for lymphadenopathy or a neoplasm. In cases of pneumomediastinum, it takes on an "inverted aortic nipple" appearance and this helps differentiate it from similar conditions (*GAS* Fig. 3.89).

B. The presence of the vagus nerve is not a reliable indicator for diagnosis of pneumomediastinum.

C. The superior vena cava is not used as a diagnostic marker of pneumomediastinum.

D. The pulmonary vein is not used as a diagnostic marker for pneumomediastinum.

E. The aortic arch itself is not useful at differentiating a diagnosis of pneumomediastinum from similar conditions.

GAS 190–193; N 241–242; ABR/McM 219

144. **A.** A TEF is an abnormal communication between the trachea and esophagus. This is a congenital anomaly that results from incomplete fusion of the tracheoesophageal folds that separate the trachea from the esophagus embryologically. In most cases it is accompanied by esophageal atresia. Polyhydramnios is commonly associated with TEF and esophageal atresia, as the amniotic fluid is unable to pass into the stomach

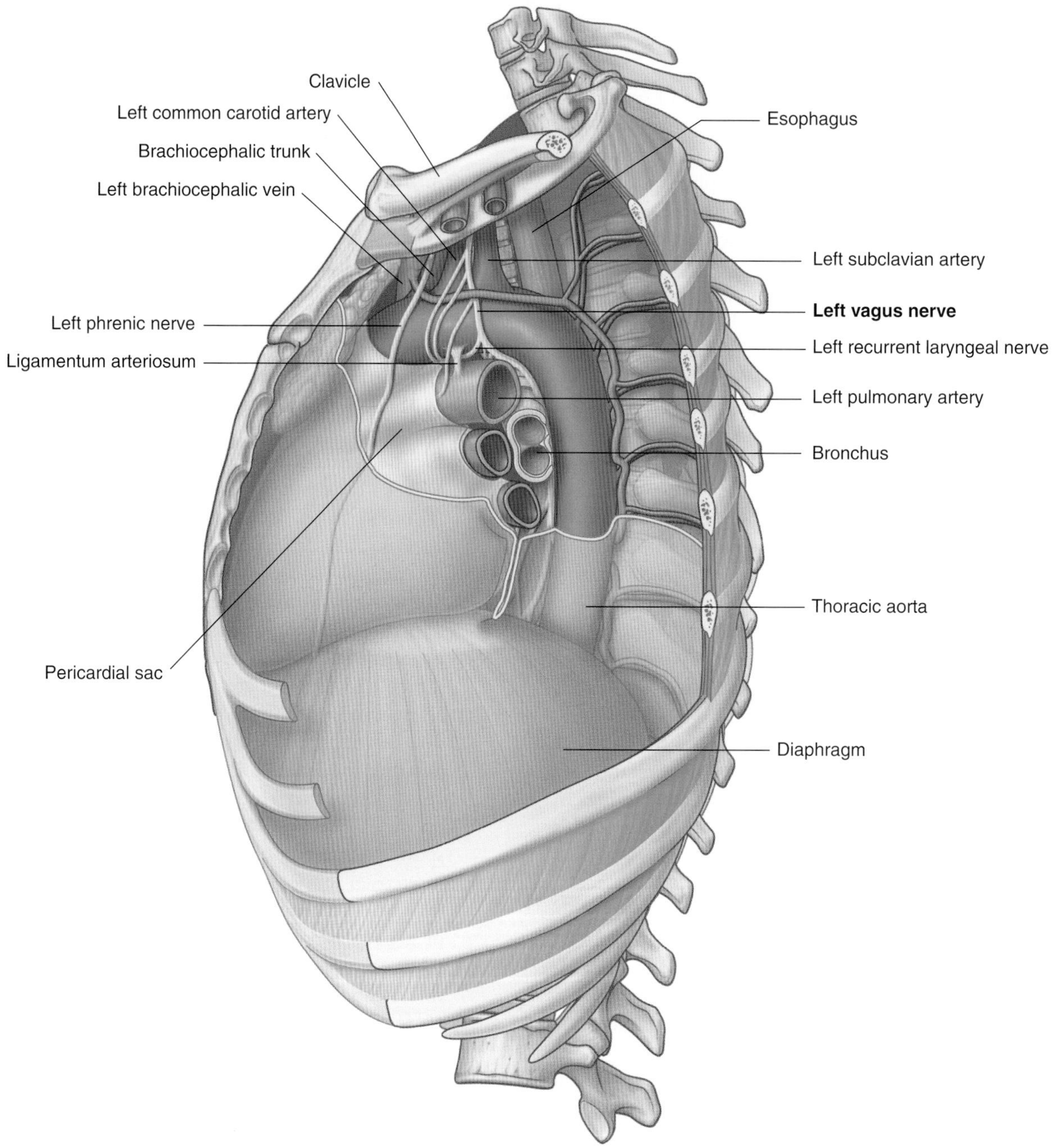

Clavicle

Left common carotid artery

Brachiocephalic trunk

Left brachiocephalic vein

Esophagus

Left subclavian artery

Left vagus nerve

Left phrenic nerve

Left recurrent laryngeal nerve

Ligamentum arteriosum

Left pulmonary artery

Bronchus

Thoracic aorta

Pericardial sac

Diaphragm

GAS Fig. 3.89

and intestines for absorption and collects in the amniotic sac.

B. Oligohydramnios refers to a deficiency of amniotic fluid and is associated with genitourinary anomalies, not with a TEF.

C. Anhydramnios refers to a complete absence of amniotic fluid and is also associated with genitourinary anomalies. It carries a poor prognosis.

D and E. Hydatidiform mole and choriocarcinomas are tumors of the placenta and are not usually associated with polyhydramnios.

GAS 223; N 237; ABR/McM 208

145. C. This is a typical description of a postductal coarctation. This type of coarctation is the most common type found in adults. It is associated with the typical symptoms of notching of the ribs, hypertension in the upper limb, and weak pulses in the lower limbs. During embryonic development, the left dorsal aorta gives rise to the descending thoracic aorta. Since this case is a postductal coarctation, the development of this area of the arch of the aorta is from the dorsal aorta.

A. Although the fourth pharyngeal arch contributes to the aortic arch, since this is a postductal coarctation, the left dorsal aorta is most likely the correct answer.

B. The third pharyngeal arch gives rise to the common carotid artery.

D. The fifth pharyngeal arch does not contribute to any structures in the developed adult.

E. The sixth pharyngeal arch contributes to the ductus arteriosus on the left and parts of the pulmonary trunk as well (Fig. 2.12).
GAS 227; N 240; ABR/McM 219

146. A. Congenital diaphragmatic hernia is a relatively common congenital anomaly. It is most often seen as a posterolateral defect in the diaphragm resulting from the defective formation or fusion of the pleuroperitoneal membranes with the other three embryological parts of the diaphragm. If this defect persists when the intestines return to the abdomen from the umbilical cord during the tenth week, some of the intestines and abdominal viscera may pass into the thorax. This compresses the developing lungs and results in

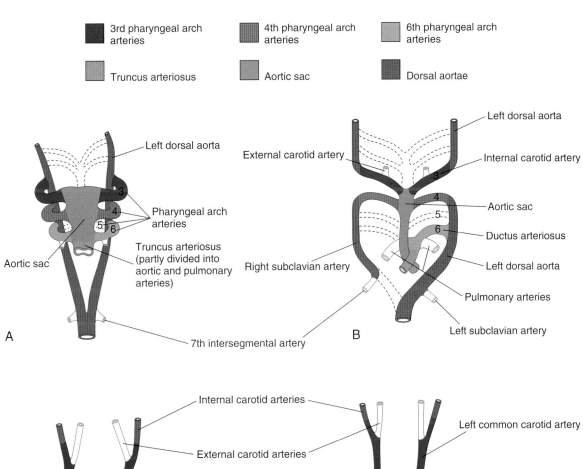

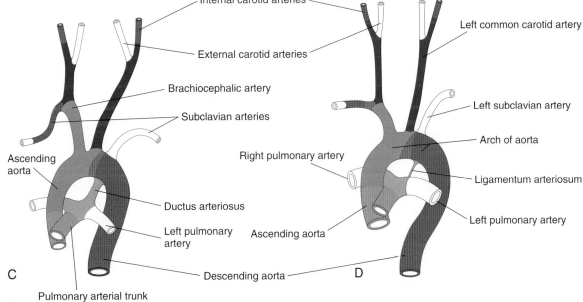

• **Fig. 2.12**

pulmonary hypoplasia. In cases of severe hypoplasia, some primordial alveoli may rupture, causing air to enter into the pleural cavity (pneumothorax). On physical exam, the patient has severe dyspnea and a flat "scaphoid" abdomen.

B. Laryngeal atresia is a rare anomaly that results in obstruction of the upper airways.

C. Emphysema is a condition usually seen in adults where the elasticity of the lung tissue is lost resulting in rupture of the alveoli and the development of large air pockets.

D. Respiratory distress syndrome is usually seen in premature infants due to a surfactant deficiency.

E. TEF is a congenital condition where there is an abnormal connection between the trachea and esophagus and is usually accompanied by esophageal atresia. Patients usually present with dyspnea and choking when attempting to feed.
GAS 372; N 222

147. D. The sympathetic system innervates the sweat glands located in the skin and subcutaneous tissue. The postganglionic cell bodies are located in the sympathetic trunk from T1 to T4, which corresponds to the chest wall. The postganglionic fibers leave the sympathetic trunk via the gray rami communicantes to enter the T1–T4 spinal nerves in order to get to their target.

A. There are no parasympathetic fibers in the body wall so this is incorrect.

B. Postganglionic sympathetics in the thoracic visceral (cardiopulmonary) nerves are responsible for increasing the heart rate.

C. Thoracic visceral afferents travel back to the spinal cord with sympathetic fibers but are responsible for the patient's complaint of severe chest pain.

E. Postganglionic sympathetic fibers from superior, middle, and inferior cervical ganglia are directed either to the head and neck or to the heart to increase the heart rate.
GAS 36–44, 214; N 231; ABR/McM 205

148. A. The lateral quadrants of the breast drain into the anterior axillary (pectoral), which is approximately 75% of the lymphatic drainage. The dye injected into the mass described will first drain to the anterior axillary (pectoral) nodes.

B. The lateral axillary nodes will not receive drainage from this mass.

C. The medial quadrants drain into the parasternal nodes with some drainage to the parasternal nodes of the opposite breast. This mass will not drain into these nodes.

D and E. The central and apical axillary nodes receive lymphatic from the anterior, lateral, and posterior axillary nodes. They will also not be among the first nodes to receive drainage from this mass.

GAS 142–143; N 199–200; ABR/McM 196

Answers 149–173

149. E. Pulmonary stenosis of the pulmonary valve results in a systolic murmur that can be auscultated at the left second intercostal space. During systole, blood is forcibly expelled from the ventricles and results in turbulent flow against a narrowed valve.

A. Regurgitation of the aortic valve will produce a diastolic murmur.

B. Regurgitation of the pulmonary valve will also produce a diastolic murmur.

C. Aortic stenosis also results in a systolic murmur but is auscultated at the right second intercostal space so this would not be correct.

D. Regurgitation through the mitral valve results in a systolic murmur that is auscultated at the left fifth intercostal space in the midclavicular line. Pulmonary and aortic valve regurgitation result in diastolic murmurs.
GAS 214, 243; N 233–234; ABR/McM 190–191

150. D. The intercostobrachial nerve is the lateral cutaneous branch of the second intercostal nerve and is responsible for the sensation to the medial side of the arm. Ischemia of the myocardium stimulates visceral afferents that travel back to the spinal cord with the sympathetics that innervate the heart. At the level of the spinal cord, this visceral stimulus is interpreted as coming from the body wall.

A. The vagus nerve is CN X and is a major supplier of autonomic function to the gut, up to the left colic flexure, and also provides some autonomic motor and sensory supply to organs in the head, neck, and thorax. It would not produce the referred pain phenomenon described here.

B. The intercostal nerves innervate the anterior and posterior chest wall, and would not produce the referred pain described

C. The phrenic nerve arises from spinal nerves C3–C5 and innervates the diaphragm. This nerve has no branches that pass into the arm.

E. The thoracic visceral or cardiopulmonary nerves are responsible for carrying the cardiac sympathetic efferent fibers from the sympathetic ganglia to the thoracic viscera and afferent fibers for pain from these organs (GAS Fig. 3.114C).
GAS 163; N 204, 408

151. C. The suspensory ligaments (of Cooper) are condensations of connective tissue that run from the investing fascia of the pectoralis major muscle to the dermis of the skin overlying the breast. They support and suspend the breast from the chest wall. Carcinoma of the breast produces tension on these ligaments and causes dimpling of the breast.

A. Invasion of the lactiferous ducts will not produce dimpling of the breast.

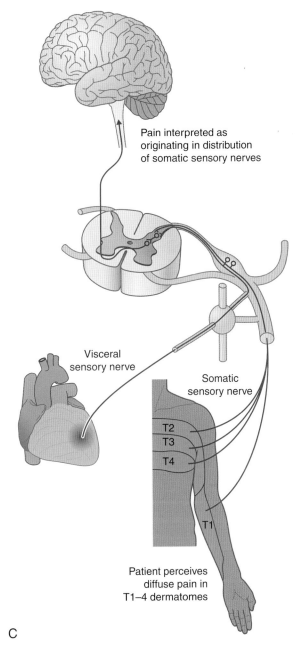

Pain interpreted as
originating in distribution
of somatic sensory nerves

Visceral
sensory nerve

Somatic
sensory nerve

T2
T3
T4

T1

Patient perceives
diffuse pain in
T1–4 dermatomes

C

GAS Fig. 3.114C

B. Invasion of the axillary lymph nodes results in stagnation and fibrosis of lymph resulting in the peau d'orange appearance of the overlying skin.

D. Invasion of the clavipectoral fascia will not produce the changes described here.

E. Invasion of the medial and lateral pectoral nerves will not result in dimpling of the breast tissue.
GAS 141–143; N 197; ABR/McM 196

152. E. The right coronary artery supplies the right ventricle, which lies immediately posterior to the sternum.

A. The circumflex artery supplies the left atrium, which is the most posterior cardiac chamber.

B. The anterior interventricular artery supplies the left ventricle and the anterior two thirds of the interventricular septum.

C. The inferior (posterior) interventricular artery supplies the posterior third of the interventricular septum.

D. The left marginal artery is a branch of the circumflex artery and supplies the obtuse margin of the heart.
GAS 207–213; N 230–231; ABR/McM 208–210

153. C. The CT scan shows an aneurysm of the arch of the aorta. The left recurrent laryngeal nerve loops around the arch of the aorta before traveling in the tracheoesophageal groove to supply the larynx.

A. The left vagus nerve travels lateral to the aortic arch and will not be compressed.

B. The phrenic nerve travels anterior to the root of the lung and will not be affected in this case.

D. The right recurrent laryngeal nerve loops around the right subclavian artery.

E. The greater thoracic splanchnic nerve originates in the thorax from the sympathetic trunk at the levels of T5–T9 and innervates abdominal structures (GAS Fig. 3.50).

GAS 233–235; N 243; ABR/McM 206

154. A. During development, the right subclavian artery forms from the fourth pharyngeal arch and seventh intersegmental arteries. If the fourth pharyngeal arch artery and the right dorsal aorta disappear cranial to the seventh segmental artery the right subclavian artery will be retroesophageal. In this case the right subclavian artery is formed by the right seventh intersegmental artery and the distal dorsal aorta, which does not regress.

B. This is incorrect as the deformity is described as occurring in the patient's right subclavian artery, not on the left side.

C. The deformity arose because the right dorsal aorta did not regress distal to the seventh intersegmental artery, but this option incorrectly states it was proximal to the seventh intersegmental artery.

D. The fifth arch artery is not involved in this deformity.

E. The ventral part of the first arch artery is not involved in this deformity.

GAS 225–226; ABR/McM 206

155. A. During embryonic development, the left dorsal aorta gives rise to the descending thoracic aorta. The aortic arch is formed by the aortic sac and the fourth pharyngeal arch artery. In this case the region of the arch of the aorta between the subclavian artery and the left common carotid artery is formed by the fourth aortic arch artery.

B. The third pharyngeal arch artery will give rise to the common carotid artery.

C. The left dorsal aorta contributes to the descending aorta but is not involved in this anomaly.

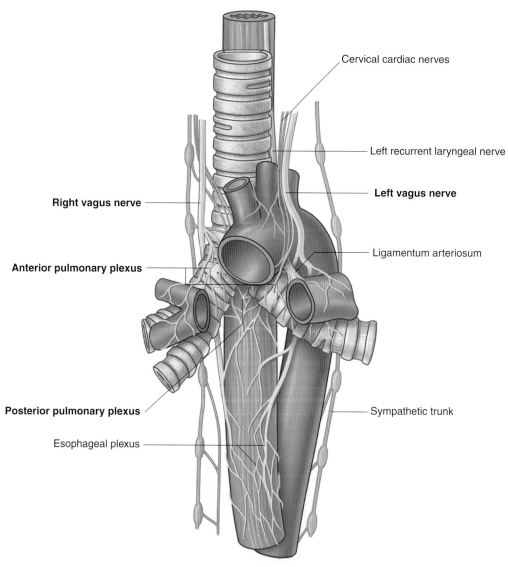

GAS Fig. 3.50

D. The fifth pharyngeal arch artery will disappear bilaterally and does not contribute to any significant structures.

E. The sixth pharyngeal arch artery will form the ductus arteriosus on the left and part of the pulmonary trunk.
GAS 220–226; ABR/McM 206

156. C. The septum secundum develops from the dorsal endocardial cushion and the wall of the primitive atria ventrally. It overgrows the septum primum, which becomes a right-to-left one way valve during intrauterine development.

A. The endocardial cushions are involved in formation of the AV septum, and deformities in their development may cause AV septal defects but are not associated with a patent foramen ovale.

B. The foramen primum is the space between the endocardial cushion and the developing septum primum. It is not involved in patent foramen ovale formation.

D. The truncus arteriosus will give rise to the ascending aorta and pulmonary trunk.

E. The bulbus cordis will give rise to the smooth parts (arterial outflow) of both the left and right ventricles.
GAS 213; N 232, 240; ABR/McM 211

157. A. The phrenic nerve passes anterior to the hilum of the lung on both the left and right sides and wraps around the hilar structures inferiorly. The phrenic nerve innervates the diaphragm and if damaged causes dyspnea.

B. The vagus nerves pass lateral to the esophagus and posterior to the lung roots on both sides.

C. The intercostal nerves are separated from the tumor by muscle, fat, and fascia.

D. Wrapping around the arch of the aorta on the left and the subclavian artery on the right, the recurrent laryngeal nerve is far too superior to be affected.

E. The thoracic visceral nerves join the cardiopulmonary plexus that is arranged around the trachea and is located along the roots of the lungs.
GAS 172; N 208; ABR/McM 205

158. C. The left atrium lies directly anterior to the esophagus and compresses it when enlarged, resulting in difficulty swallowing.

A. Nausea and vomiting may be present but are symptoms of a wide array of dysfunctions and are not a direct result of the enlarged atrium.

B. Pain and tenderness over the thoracic vertebral spinous processes will not result because there is no compression of sensory nerves.

D. Epigastric pain resulting from eating fatty foods is an indication of acute cholelithiasis, which is due to gallstones.

E. Increased coughing could only result from irritation of the vagus nerves above the larynx, which is above the level of the left atria.

GAS 228–229; N 223; ABR/McM 205

159. D. The apex of the heart is typically visualized and palpated in the left fifth intercostal space of the midclavicular line. This is termed the "apex beat" and is the result of blood being forced against it during atrial contraction.

A. The right atria should not give a visible pulsation on the thoracic wall unless there is atrial fibrillation.

B. The left atrium would not cause visible pulsations, even if there is atrial fibrillation in the left heart as it is too posteriorly located to cause pulsations on the thoracic wall.

C. Pulsations from the aortic arch will only be present if there is an aneurysm of the aortic arch.

E. The mitral valve may be auscultated at this location and is one of the reasons why the physician would locate the apex beat.
GAS 200–206, 243; N BP51; ABR/McM 190–191

160. B. The great cardiac vein accompanies the anterior interventricular artery and is the vessel which must be protected from iatrogenic injury.

A. The middle cardiac vein accompanies the inferior (posterior) interventricular artery and is therefore not implicated in procedures involving the anterior interventricular artery.

C. The small cardiac vein accompanies the right marginal artery as it passes along the acute margin of the heart and is not associated with the anterior interventricular artery.

D. The anterior cardiac veins are found on the anterior aspect of the right ventricles, and they accompany small unnamed branches off the right coronary artery.

E. The posterior vein of the left ventricle is found on the posterior aspect of the ventricle, and it accompanies the posterior artery of the left ventricle (GAS Fig. 3.82).
GAS 207–215; N 229; ABR/McM 208–210

161. B. The correct answer is performing thoracentesis at the seventh intercostal space as this question is referring to where it should be done in reference to the mid-clavicular line. The extent of the costodiaphragmatic recess of the pleural cavity at the midclavicular line is between ribs six and eight, which includes the sixth and seventh intercostal spaces. At the mid-axillary line, the costodiaphragmatic recess is between ribs eight and ten, which includes the eighth and ninth intercostal spaces. At the paravertebral line, the costodiaphragmatic recess is between ribs 10 and 12, which includes the tenth and eleventh intercostal spaces. All of the other levels stand the risk of damaging the lung and will not effectively extract all of the fluid from the space.
GAS 168–171; N 208

162. E. The esophageal hiatus creates a physiological sphincter during diaphragmatic contraction. As the

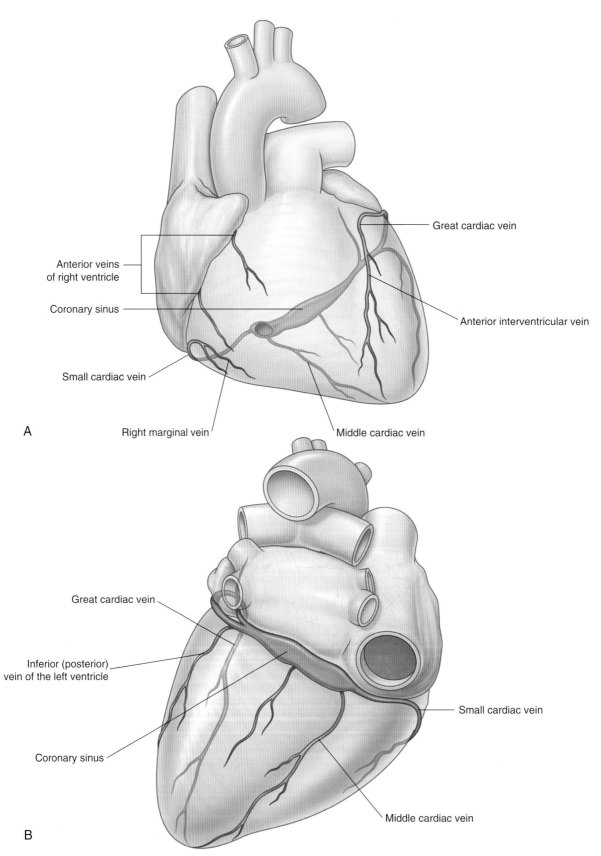

Great cardiac vein

Anterior veins
of right ventricle

Coronary sinus

Anterior interventricular vein

Small cardiac vein

A

Right marginal vein

Middle cardiac vein

Great cardiac vein

Inferior (posterior)
vein of the left ventricle

Small cardiac vein

Coronary sinus

Middle cardiac vein

B

GAS Fig. 3.82

esophagogastric junction does not have a valve either anatomically or physiologically this would be the last point of resistance.

A. The area posterior to the left atrium may be compressed slightly but would not give resistance to the passing of the tube.

B. At the level of the superior thoracic opening the pharyngoesophageal junction is located and will give resistance; however, this is the first resistance offered by the esophagus.

C. The area posteromedial to the aortic arch serves as the second site of resistance of the esophagus.

D. The area posterior to the left main bronchus acts as the third site of resistance to the nasogastric tube as it passes through the esophagus.

GAS 231–234; N 244

163. E. The question of dominance is determined by where the inferior (posterior) interventricular artery arises. If it arises from the right corona it is a right dominant heart; if from the circumflex of the left coronary it is left dominant.

A. The right marginal artery arises from the right coronary artery and plays no role in determining right or left dominance.

B. The anterior interventricular artery may anastomose with the posterior but is not a determinant of dominance.

C. The left marginal artery comes off the circumflex artery which arises from the left coronary artery. This does not determine dominance.

D. The artery to the sinuatrial node usually arises from the right coronary artery and does not contribute to dominance.

GAS 207–213; N 229; ABR/McM 210–212

164. A. Murmurs of the tricuspid valve can be best auscultated in the fourth intercostal space at the left border of the sternum.

B. The fifth intercostal space at the left midclavicular line is the best site to auscultate the mitral valve.

C. The fifth intercostal space at the right border of the sternum is not used to auscultate the tricuspid valve.

D and E. Second and third intercostal spaces on the right side of the sternum are the areas to listen to the aortic valve.

GAS 214, 243; N BP51;ABR/McM 190–191

165. E. The patient exhibits signs of cardiac tamponade, known as Beck's triad: hypotension, muffled or absent heart sounds, and jugular vein distention. As a result, a pericardiocentesis procedure should be performed. Pericardiocentesis is a procedure whereby a needle is inserted into the pericardial space to extract fluid.

A. Chest tube insertion will be done to alleviate a pneumothorax, not cardiac tamponade.

B. Central venous lines are utilized to deliver intravenous fluids, and not to alleviate a cardiac tamponade.

C. Nasogastric tube insertion will not alleviate any of the symptoms that occur secondary to cardiac tamponade.

D. Thoracocentesis may be done to resolve a pleural effusion, but it will not assist with management of cardiac tamponade.

GAS 190–194; N 223; ABR/McM 208

166. D. The sinuatrial node receives information from the sympathetic preganglionic fibers T1–T4 to increase the heart rate. If these fibers are damaged the preganglionic vagal fibers from the cardiac plexus are unopposed and will slow down the heart rate.

A. Preganglionic parasympathetic fibers arising from the vagus nerve within the cardiac plexus will not act to increase the heart rate.

B. Somatic efferents in the phrenic nerve supply the diaphragm and have no effect on cardiac function.

C. Visceral afferents in the thoracic visceral nerves carry pain fibers from the heart and bronchi.

E. T1–T4 ventral horn neurons are somatic motor nerves and have no effect on cardiac function.

GAS 216–219; N 236, 238; ABR/McM 211

167. A. The thoracic duct originates in the abdomen, sometimes as a dilation called the cisterna chyli, and ascends through the aortic hiatus in the diaphragm. It ascends in the posterior mediastinum with the descending thoracic aorta on its left, the azygos vein on its right, the esophagus anteriorly, and the vertebral bodies posteriorly. At the level of the sternal angle, the thoracic duct crosses to the left, posterior to the esophagus, and ascends into the superior mediastinum. Therefore, in this scenario, this vessel would most likely contain lymph.

B. The vessel will not contain deoxygenated blood as it is a lymphatic structure, not a vein.

C. The vessel will not contain saliva as it is a lymphatic structure.

D. The vessel will not contain urine as it is a lymphatic structure.

E. The vessel will not contain oxygenated blood as it is a lymphatic structure, not an artery.

GAS 236–238; N 242–243; ABR/McM 228

168. C. The major structures in the superior mediastinum, from anterior to posterior, are thymus, veins, arteries, airway, alimentary tract, and lymphatic trunks. The thymus develops from the third pharyngeal pouch as does the inferior parathyroid gland.

A. The first pharyngeal pouch derivatives are the endoderm lining the future auditory tube (pharyngotympanic, Eustachian tube), middle ear, mastoid antrum, and inner aspect of the tympanic membrane. This answer choice is therefore incorrect as the thymus comes from the third pharyngeal arch.

C. Although the second pharyngeal pouch is largely obliterated, it contributes to the palatine tonsils.

D. The fourth pharyngeal pouch forms the superior parathyroid gland and ultimobranchial body, which forms the parafollicular C-cells of the thyroid gland.

E. The fifth pharyngeal pouch is a rudimentary structure that has no contributions to significant structures.

GAS 220–222; N 222; ABR/McM 228

169. D. A tension pneumothorax occurs when intrapleural air accumulates progressively, exerting positive pressure on mediastinal and intrathoracic structures. It is a life-threatening occurrence requiring rapid recognition and treatment if cardiac arrest is to be avoided. Therefore, the needle must be inserted between the visceral and parietal layers of the pleura in order to relieve the tension pneumothorax.

A. The space between the visceral and parietal layers of the pericardium is where pericardiocentesis is performed and will not alleviate a pneumothorax.

B. Inserting the needle into the space between the serous and fibrous layers of the pericardium will not alleviate a pneumothorax.

C. Inserting the needle between the mediastinal pleura and fibrous pericardium will not relieve a pneumothorax.

E. Inserting the needle between the endothoracic fascia and parietal pleura will also not alleviate a pneumothorax.

GAS 164–165, 169–170; N 211; ABR/McM 218

170. C. With ectopia cordis, a rare condition, the heart is in an abnormal location. In the thoracic form of ectopia cordis, the heart is partly or completely exposed on the surface of the thorax. The pericardium and sternum do not develop properly because the lateral folds undergo incomplete fusion during thoracic wall formation.

A. The pleuropericardial folds form pleuropericardial membranes that unite to become the pericardial sac. Their incomplete fusion does not cause ectopia cordis.

B. Failed fusion of the septum transversum with the pleuropericardial folds does not lead to ectopia cordis.

D. Failure of fusion of the pleuroperitoneal folds will lead to a diaphragmatic hernia, not ectopia cordis.

E. Failure of fusion between the pericardial coelom and the peritoneal coelom will not lead to ectopia cordis.

GAS 195–199; N 222–223; ABR/McM 203

171. A. There are four clinically significant types of atrial septal defect: ostium secundum defect, endocardial cushion defect with ostium primum defect, sinus venosus defect, and common atrium. Endocardial cushion defects with ostium primum occur in approximately 20% of persons with trisomy 21 (Down syndrome); otherwise, it is a relatively uncommon cardiac defect. This specific defect arises due to failed fusion of the septum primum with the AV septum.

B. Atrial septal defect due to failed fusion of the septum primum with the septum secundum is also relatively common, but it is not specifically associated with trisomy 21 (Down syndrome).

C–E. These are relatively rare types of septal defects and show no association with trisomy 21 (Down syndrome).

GAS 213; N 233–235; ABR/McM 211–213

172. D. Ventricular septal defects are the most common type of heart malformation, accounting for approximately 25% of heart defects. A membranous ventricular septal defect is the most common type but it may occur at any part of the interventricular septum. It is most commonly caused by failed fusion of the interventricular septum and endocardial cushions.

A. A bulbus cordis partitioning defect may lead to persistent truncus arteriosus or transposition of the great vessels.

B. Ventricular septal defect initially causes a left to right shunt at birth due to pressure gradient between the left heart and the right heart.

C. Ventricular septal defect is an acyanotic heart disease.

E. Septum primum and septum secundum should fuse soon after birth. Failure of closure will lead to patent foramen ovale.

GAS 213; N 233–235; ABR/McM 211–213

173. D. With isolated dextrocardia, the abnormal position of the heart is not accompanied by displacement of other viscera. This defect is usually complicated by severe cardiac anomalies (e.g., single ventricle and transposition of the great vessels). This case most likely resulted from abnormal growth of the primordial heart tube to the left.

A. Posterior and superior growth of the primordial atrium will not lead to the dextrocardia seen in this patient.

B. Anterior and inferior growth of the primordial ventricle will not lead to isolated dextrocardia.

C. Defects of the bulbus cordis could lead to persistent truncus arteriosus or transposition of the great vessels.

E. Growth of the primordial heart tube to the right is part of the normal developmental process.

GAS 227; N 223; ABR/McM 203

Answers 174–189

174. A. The thoracic duct originates in the abdomen, sometimes as a dilation called the cisterna chyli, and ascends through the aortic hiatus in the diaphragm. It ascends in the posterior mediastinum with the thoracic aorta on its left, the azygos vein on its right, the esophagus anteriorly, and the vertebral bodies posteriorly. At the level of the sternal angle, the thoracic duct crosses to the left, posterior to the esophagus, and ascends into the superior mediastinum. Given its location, it is most likely responsible for the collection of fluid seen on chest CT.

B. The esophagus would not be responsible for the findings described in this patient.

C. Injury to the descending aorta might produce a collection of blood in the posterior mediastinum, but it would likely cause more immediate discomfort due to its high pressure.

D. The azygos vein would also not produce the collection described here.

E. The bronchial lymphatics would also not produce the collection seen in this patient.
GAS 236–238; N 242–243; ABR/McM 228

175. B. Congenital diaphragmatic hernia is usually unilateral and results from defective formation and/or fusion of the pleuroperitoneal membranes with the other three parts of the diaphragm. This results in a large opening in the posterolateral region of the diaphragm. As a result, the peritoneal and pleural cavities are continuous with one another along the posterior body wall.

A. In septum transversum defect the patient presents with midline diaphragmatic hernia.

C. Tracheoesophageal septum defects can lead to esophageal atresia or TEF.

D. The laryngotracheal groove is a rudimentary respiratory structure that contributes to development of the larynx and trachea. It would not be implicated in the changes described in this patient.

E. The lesser omentum and falciform ligament form from the ventral mesogastrium, which is formed by the septum transversum.
GAS 372; N 222

176. A. A tension pneumothorax occurs when intrapleural air accumulates progressively, exerting positive pressure on mediastinal structures and leading to mediastinal shift to the opposite side. It is a life-threatening occurrence requiring rapid recognition and treatment if cardiorespiratory arrest is to be avoided. In this patient, the most likely scenario is a right-sided tension pneumothorax as the mediastinal contents have shifted to the left.

B. Simple pneumothorax would not cause the trachea to shift to the left as it is a non-expanding collection of air around the lung that can be difficult to detect on physical exam.

C, D, and E. Cardiac tamponade is pressure on the heart that occurs when blood or fluid builds up in the pericardial cavity between the visceral and parietal layers of the pericardium. Classical cardiac tamponade includes three signs, known as Beck's triad: hypotension, muffled heart sounds, and jugular vein distention. These signs are not seen in this patient, so these options would be incorrect.
GAS 164–165, 169; N 211; ABR/McM 218

177. A. The patient has developed hemothorax that can be associated with delayed presentation of cyanosis as blood continues to pool in the thoracic cavity.

B. A flail chest by itself will just show minimal soft tissue opacification without any lung field involvement and will not cause cyanosis.

C. Paralysis of the diaphragm will likewise not cause opacification of the lung fields.

D. Tension pneumothorax will not result in opacification of lung fields and may be associated with shifting of mediastinal contents toward the opposite lung.

E. Spontaneous pneumothorax will also not cause opacification of the lung fields but loss of vascular markings and there is loss of pleural integrity even if not observable.
GAS 164–165, 169–170; N 211; ABR/McM 218

178. A. Pleuritic pain is due to inflammation of the parietal pleura which is mainly supplied by the intercostal nerves.

B. The phrenic nerve only supplies the central and diaphragmatic parts of the diaphragmatic parietal pleura which is not typically affected and not amenable to nerve blocks.

C. The vagus nerve supplies visceral efferents and afferents to the lungs and visceral pleura but not the parietal pleura.

D. The thoracic visceral (cardiopulmonary) nerves do not carry somatic afferent fibers and would not be targeted to alleviate the pleuritic pain seen in this patient.

E. The recurrent laryngeal nerve is a branch of the vagus nerve and does not innervate the lungs.
GAS 166–172; N 220; ABR/McM 200

179. E. Due to the long looping course of the left recurrent laryngeal nerve and its location in the superior mediastinum, it is more easily damaged during thoracoscopic procedures than the other nerves, which are more posterior and protected from introduction of the thoracoscope. Increased pulmonary vascular markings indicate the presence of a left-to-right shunt. A systolic murmur crossing the S_2 heart sound characterizes the continuous (machinery) murmur heard in patent ductus arteriosus. Prematurity increases the risk of a patent ductus arteriosus. The blood shunt through the patent duct increases with physiological decline in the pulmonary artery pressure toward the end of the first month of life.

A. The left vagus nerve runs deep and posterior to where the procedure would take place and would have a much less risk of injury.

B. The right vagus nerve would not be affected as this procedure does not involve structures of the right thorax.

C. The left phrenic nerve is not as likely to be affected as the left recurrent laryngeal nerve, which has a much more looping and variable course.

D. The right phrenic nerve will not be affected.
GAS 228–233; N 243; ABR/McM 202

180. B. Any pneumothorax may cause hyperresonance to percussion, decreased breath sounds, and reduce vascular markings, but tracheal deviation to the opposite side accompanied by distended jugular veins can only be caused by a tension pneumothorax. Tracheal deviation to the opposite side of the affected lung is a result of a tension pneumothorax. Tension pneumothorax is typically caused by injuries to the chest wall that cause defects in either the parietal or visceral pleura.

A. Spontaneous pneumothorax is incorrect as it will not shift the trachea and other mediastinal structures to the opposite side. Spontaneous pneumothorax normally causes tracheal deviation to the same side of the collapsed lung to fill the pleural space now unused by the lung.

C. Cardiac tamponade will cause muffled heart sounds, decreased blood pressure, and distended jugular veins.

D. Lung contusion will not cause any of the above signs but may produce some soft tissue edema and minor lung inflammation.

E. Pneumonia will not cause tracheal deviation or hyperresonance but lung dullness to percussion.
GAS 164–165, 169–170; N 211; ABR/McM 218

181. D. The right and left coronary arteries arise directly from the root of the ascending aorta. The right coronary artery gives rise to the artery to the sinuatrial node and artery to the AV node. It also supplies the area of the pulmonary infundibulum or anterior ventricular wall and to the right marginal artery that supplies the lower portion (closer to the diaphragm) of the anterior ventricular wall. In 85%–90% of individuals, the right coronary artery gives rise to the posterior (inferior) interventricular (posterior descending) artery. This artery supplies the posterior or diaphragmatic surface of the heart.

A. The anterior interventricular (LAD) artery comes off the left coronary artery and supplies the anterior two-thirds of the interventricular septum through septal perforating branches and the anterior wall of the left ventricle with diagonal branches.

B. The circumflex coronary artery comes off the left coronary artery and it supplies most of the anterior and left lateral surfaces of the heart via obtuse marginal branches.

C. The left coronary artery gives off the anterior interventricular artery (LAD) and the circumflex coronary artery. It does not give off branches that supply the diaphragmatic surface of the heart.

E. The right marginal branches of the heart come off the right coronary artery but do not contribute to structures found at the heart's diaphragmatic surface.
GAS 207–211; N 229–230; ABR/McM 208–210

182. A. The embryological basis of the combination of lesions is anterosuperior deviation (malalignment) of the developing outlet ventricular septum (pulmonary infundibulum) and hypertrophied septoparietal trabeculations. The deviation of the muscular outlet septum (not to be confused with the aorticopulmonary septum) is also responsible for creating the malalignment type of ventricular septal defect and results in the aortic override. The associated hypertrophy of the right ventricular myocardium is the hemodynamic consequence of the anatomical lesions created by the deviated outlet septum. The cause of the abnormal anterosuperior deviation of the outlet ventricular septum is abnormal neural crest cell migration.

B. Endocardial cushion defect will be responsible for defects in the AV septum and AV valves. The endocardial cushion defects do not produce cyanosis.

C. Aortic arch constriction would not produce the constellation of signs and symptoms observed in this patient.

D. Pulmonary hypertension would produce symptoms typical of right heart failure.

E. Abnormal primitive heart tube looping would not produce the symptoms seen in this patient.
GAS 213; N 233–235; ABR/McM 211–213

183. E. The main structure immediately posterior to the esophagus is the descending aorta, and therefore it would be seen immediately posterior to the ultrasound transducer.

A. The left atrium lies anterior to the esophagus, but it does form the majority of the posterior surface of the heart while residing adjacent to the esophagus. Enlargement of the left atrium can compress the esophagus and cause dysphagia.

B. The pulmonary veins are too lateral at this point to be seen posterior to the transducer.

C. The right atrium lies further anterior and will not be seen.

D. The right ventricle lies further anterior and will not be seen.
GAS 228–229; N 223, 244; ABR/McM 205

184. C. The esophageal hiatus within the diaphragm is found at the T10 vertebral level.

A. The T7 vertebral level is not usually associated with any diaphragmatic openings.

B. The diaphragmatic passage found at the T8 vertebral level is for the IVC/right phrenic nerve.

D. The T11 vertebral level is not associated with any significant diaphragmatic openings.

E. The T12 diaphragmatic hiatus is for the aorta and thoracic duct.
GAS 228–229; N 244

185. C. Cardiac tamponade will cause muffled heart sounds, decreased blood pressure, and distended jugular veins (Beck's triad).

A. Pneumothorax will cause hyperresonance to percussion, decreased breath sounds, reduced vascular markings, tracheal deviation to the opposite side, and distended jugular veins.

B and D. Deep vein thrombosis may lead to pulmonary embolism, which can cause shortness of breath and even death but not Beck's triad.

E. Hemothorax presents with dullness to percussion and lung field opacification but will not produce the described symptoms which make up Beck's triad.
GAS 188–194; N 223; ABR/McM 208

186. **A.** The pulmonic valve is auscultated at the left parasternal area in the second intercostal space and is the correct answer in this scenario.

B. The aortic valve is best heard at the right parasternal area in the second intercostal space.

C and E. The mitral (bicuspid) valve is auscultated at the apex of the heart, which is typically the fifth intercostal space at the midclavicular line, to the left of the sternum.

D. The tricuspid valve is auscultated at the fourth intercostal space along the left parasternal border.
GAS 243; N BP51; ABR/McM 190–191

187. **C.** Since the sternal angle (of Louis) is in the transverse plane, the best plane to view both the anterior and posterior mediastinum, as well as superior mediastinal structures, would be a lateral view.

A. The anteroposterior view alone would make it difficult to distinguish between anterior and posterior mediastinal structures.

B. The posteroanterior view alone would make it difficult to distinguish between posterior and anterior mediastinal structures.

D. The apical lordotic view is used to examine areas of the lung apices that may be missed on a A/P or P/A view. It would not ideally visualize the angle of Louis.

E. As the sternal angle (of Louis) lies within the axial plane, an axial cut may miss the level completely.
GAS 132–133; N 2192; ABR/McM 199, 201

188. **E.** The order traversed is skin, external intercostal muscles, internal intercostal muscles, innermost intercostal muscle, and parietal pleura. The chest tube should not traverse the visceral pleura because this could cause a pneumothorax when it is removed. Therefore, E is the most correct answer choice.

A. This answer is incorrect as the parietal pleura (4) would be one of the last structures traversed by the chest tube.

B. This answer is incorrect as the visceral pleura (6) would not be traversed before the parietal pleura (4).

C. This answer is incorrect as the visceral pleura (6) would not be traversed before the parietal pleura (4), and the innermost intercostal muscle (3) would not be traversed before the external intercostal muscle (5).

D. This answer is incorrect as the internal intercostal muscle (1) would not be traversed before the external intercostal muscle (5).
GAS 153–157; N 206; ABR/McM 199–200

189. **A.** Vagus nerve carries postganglionic parasympathetic fibers responsible for contracting the smooth muscles of the tracheobronchial tree. Since the patient suffers from asthma, a condition that the smooth muscles cells of the tracheobronchial tree are constricted, vagus nerve is the most likely correct answer. The vagus nerve is also responsible for innervating the mucous gland found in the submucosa of the tracheobronchial tree, as well as being responsible for pain sensation.

B, C, D, and E. Phrenic nerve will provide motor supply to muscle of the diaphragm, greater thoracic splanchnic nerve will carry preganglionic sympathetic fibers from T5 to T9 to the celiac ganglion in the abdomen, as well as carry visceral pain sensation from the abdomen back to the dorsal root ganglia of T5–T9, thoracic visceral nerves are mainly responsible for innervation of the heart, and finally, intercostal nerves are responsible for motor, sensory, and sympathetic innervation of the dermatome that they innervate.
GAS 358–364; N 214; ABR/McM 218

3

Abdomen

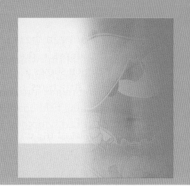

Questions

Questions 1–25

1. A 1-year-old girl is brought to the physician with a genital mass. She was born full term without complications and has achieved age-appropriate developmental milestones. Physical examination shows a mass at the right labium majus. The mass is reducible and nontender to palpation. An ultrasound of the right labium majus shows a herniated loop of intestine deep within it. This condition is because of failure of an embryonic structure to obliterate. From which of the following tissue layers is this structure derived?
   A. Parietal peritoneum
   B. Extraperitoneal tissue
   C. Transversalis fascia
   D. Dartos fascia
   E. Internal abdominal oblique aponeurosis

2. A 3-year-old boy is brought to the emergency department because of dark urine and abdominal pain. His vital signs are within normal limits. Physical examination of the eye shows aniridia. Masses are palpated in the left and right flanks. A computed tomography (CT) scan shows bilateral masses involving the kidneys. A renal biopsy confirms the diagnosis of Wilms tumor. Which of the following gene mutations is the most common for this condition?
   A. The gene responsible for *WT1*
   B. The gene responsible for *HGF*
   C. The gene responsible for *VEGF*
   D. The gene responsible for *GDNF*
   E. The gene responsible for *FGF-2*

3. A 10-year-old girl is brought to the physician for evaluation of recurrent urinary tract infections. She has a history of delayed developmental milestones. Her vital signs are within normal limits. Physical examination shows up-slanting palpebral fissures and simian creases in the palms of the hands. No masses are palpated in the flanks. A CT scan of the abdomen shows normal appearing renal tissue at the L3–L4 vertebral level with fusion of the left and right kidneys at the lower poles in the midline. Which of the following is the most likely diagnosis of the patient's congenital condition?
   A. Bicornuate uterus
   B. Cryptorchidism

C. Horseshoe kidney
D. Hypospadias
E. Renal agenesis

4. A 35-year-old woman, gravida 3, para 1, aborta 1, at 29 weeks' gestation comes to the physician for a prenatal visit. She has no medical history of chronic diseases. Her vital signs are within normal limits. Physical examination shows a uterine fundal height at the level of the umbilicus. An ultrasound of the abdomen shows amniotic fluid of less than 5 cm, consistent with oligohydramnios. Which of the following congenital malformations best explains the clinical findings of the ultrasound examination?
   A. Anencephaly
   B. Pyloric stenosis
   C. Renal agenesis
   D. Tracheoesophageal fistula (TEF)
   E. Urethral atresia

5. A 28-year-old woman, gravida 1, para 0, delivers a boy at 38 weeks via an induced labor. The physician induced labor due to severely low amniotic fluid levels. Shortly after the delivery, the infant develops respiratory distress requiring resuscitation and mechanical ventilation. An x-ray of the chest shows a correctly positioned endotracheal tube, reduced lung volumes bilaterally, and no signs of diaphragmatic hernias. It appears that the boy's respiratory difficulties were caused by an in utero problem that results in failure of the fetus to urinate. Which of the following relationships best describes this condition?
   A. Oligohydramnios linked with hypoplastic lungs
   B. Polycystic kidneys linked to TEF
   C. Polyhydramnios
   D. Renal agenesis linked to insufficient surfactant
   E. Urethral obstruction linked to ectopic viscera

6. A 2-year-old boy is brought to the emergency department with greenish-yellow vomiting for the past 2 days. The patient's mother says that his diet has not changed. He has not passed stool since the vomiting began. His medical history includes premature birth, low birth weight, and trisomy 21. His vital signs are within normal limits. Physical examination shows sunken eyes and loss of skin turgor, the abdomen is

soft but tender in the epigastric region. An x-ray of the abdomen shows a "double-bubble" sign. A CT scan of the abdomen shows an annular pancreas. Which of the following structures is most likely obstructed in this condition?

A. Pylorus of the stomach
B. First part of the duodenum
C. Second part of the duodenum
D. Third part of the duodenum
E. Jejunum

7. A 3-year-old boy is brought to the physician with a swollen scrotum. The patient was born at term by an uncomplicated spontaneous vaginal delivery. He has achieved age-appropriate developmental milestones. Physical examination shows a swollen, nontender right side of the scrotum. An ultrasound of the scrotum shows that the intermediate portion of the processus vaginalis is not obliterated. Which of the following is the most likely diagnosis for this patient?

A. Hypospadias
B. Sterility
C. Congenital hydrocele
D. Ectopic testis
E. Epispadias

8. A 1-year-old boy is brought to the physician for follow-up examination. The mother says that the child says "dada" and "mama" and is now pulling himself up to stand. The patient's vaccinations are up to date. Physical examination shows bilateral absence of the testes from the scrotum and the testes are palpated in the inguinal canals bilaterally. Which of the following is the most likely diagnosis?

A. Pseudohermaphroditism
B. True hermaphroditism
C. Cryptorchidism
D. Congenital suprarenal gland hyperplasia
E. Chordee

9. A 28-year-old woman, gravida 2, para 1, at 32 weeks' gestation comes to the physician for an initial prenatal examination. She has no past medical history and her last pregnancy resulted in a healthy baby girl born at term. Physical examination shows fundal height of 32 cm. An ultrasound of the fetus shows herniation of the small bowel into the amniotic cavity. Malformation of which of the following structures has resulted in the ultrasound findings?

A. Head fold
B. Tail fold
C. Neural folds
D. Lateral folds
E. Amnion

10. The embryonic development of the gastrointestinal tract involves a series of rotations that position the alimentary structures. Rotation of the stomach during development results in movement of the left vagus nerve from its original position. Through approximately how many degrees of rotation does the nerve move, and what is its final position?

A. 90 degrees to become the anterior vagal trunk
B. 90 degrees to become the posterior vagal trunk
C. 270 degrees to become the anterior vagal trunk
D. 270 degrees to become the posterior vagal trunk
E. 180 degrees to become the right vagal trunk

11. A newborn girl is brought to the emergency department because of difficulty breathing. A diagnosis of eventration of the diaphragm is made. Which of the following is the most likely mechanism of this congenital defect?

A. Absence of a pleuropericardial fold
B. Absence of musculature in one half of the diaphragm
C. Failure of migration of the diaphragm
D. Failure of development of the septum transversum
E. Absence of a pleuroperitoneal fold

12. A 2-day-old full term boy is brought to the emergency department because of developing cyanosis during multiple attempts of breastfeeding. His mother had polyhydramnios during the pregnancy. Physical examination shows crackles auscultated in the right lower lung field. A nasogastric tube is inserted, and an x-ray is done to evaluate the correct positioning of the tube. An x-ray shows that the tube is coiled in the proximal esophageal pouch. A TEF is suspected. Which of the following structures has most likely failed to develop properly?

A. Esophagus
B. Trachea
C. Tongue
D. Tracheoesophageal septum
E. Pharynx

13. A 3-day-old boy is admitted to the neonatal intensive care unit with difficulty breathing. The boy is currently afebrile. Physical examination shows a sunken abdomen, and bowel sounds are auscultated in the left chest. An x-ray of the chest shows bowel air-fluid levels in the left hemithorax. A CT scan of his chest and abdomen shows the absence of the central tendon of the diaphragm. Malformation of which of the following structures most likely occurred during embryogenesis?

A. Pleuroperitoneal folds
B. Pleuropericardial folds
C. Septum transversum
D. Cervical myotomes
E. Dorsal mesentery of the esophagus

14. A 1-month-old girl is brought to the emergency department because of greenish-yellow vomiting and feeding intolerance for the past day. Her temperature is 40°C (102°F). Physical examination shows a toxic-appearing infant with a tender abdomen and absent bowel sounds. An upper gastrointestinal contrast imaging study shows findings consistent with malrotation of the small intestine and the vessels around the duodenojejunal junction are obstructed, increasing the risk of the patient developing gangrenous intestines. Laboratory

studies show leukocytosis. Which of the following has occurred to cause the obstruction?

A. Diaphragmatic atresia

B. Subhepatic cecum

C. Midgut volvulus

D. Duplication of the intestine

E. Congenital megacolon

15. A 5-day-old boy is being evaluated for failure to pass meconium within the first 48 hours of life. Physical examination shows a distended abdomen that is soft and nontender. An x-ray of the abdomen with barium enema contrast shows dilation of the proximal colon and marked narrowing of the sigmoid colon. A rectal biopsy shows findings consistent with Hirschsprung disease. Which of the following most likely represents the embryologic mechanism responsible for the findings in this patient?

A. Failure of neural crest cells to migrate into the wall of the distal colon

B. Incomplete separation of the cloaca

C. Failure of recanalization of the colon

D. Defective rotation of the hindgut

E. Oligohydramnios

16. A 4-month-old girl is brought to the physician for a well-child follow up examination. She was delivered preterm by spontaneous vaginal delivery. Physical examination shows a 0.5 cm mass that pushes the umbilicus outwards. The mass is reducible and does not appear to cause her pain. As she cries the mass increases in size. An ultrasound of the abdomen shows that part of another organ is attached to the inner surface of the hernia. What portion of the gastrointestinal tract is most likely to be attached to the inner surface of the umbilical hernia?

A. Anal canal

B. Appendix

C. Cecum

D. Ileum

E. Stomach

17. A 38-year-old woman is brought to the emergency department with severe vaginal bleeding. She says that she is sexually active with her husband, and they have been trying to conceive for the past year. Her last menstrual period was 8 weeks ago. Physical examination shows tenderness in the right lower quadrant. Urine human chorionic gonadotropin (HCG) is positive. An ultrasound examination confirms the diagnosis of an ectopic pregnancy. Which of the following is the most likely site of this type of pregnancy?

A. Uterine tube

B. Cervix

C. Mesentery of the small intestine

D. Lower part of uterine body overlapping the internal cervical os

E. Fundus of the uterus

18. A 23-year-old woman is brought to the emergency department because of severe abdominal pain, nausea, and vomiting. The pain is severe and has been constant for 4 days. The pain began in the epigastric region and radiated bilaterally around the chest to just below the level of the scapulae. Currently the pain is localized in the right hypochondrium. A CT scan of the abdomen shows calcified stones in the gallbladder. Which of the following nerves carries the afferent fibers of the referred pain?

A. Greater thoracic splanchnic nerves

B. Dorsal rami of thoracic spinal nerves

C. Phrenic nerves

D. Vagus nerves

E. Pelvic splanchnic nerves

19. A 32-year-old man is brought to the emergency department because of groin pain. Physical examination shows the patient has a protrusion of the abdominal wall and a diagnosis of an indirect inguinal hernia is made. Which of the following nerves is compressed by the herniating structure in the inguinal canal to result in pain?

A. Iliohypogastric

B. Lateral femoral cutaneous

C. Ilioinguinal

D. Subcostal

E. Pudendal

20. A 54-year-old man is brought to the emergency department with severe upper abdominal pain. Gastroscopy shows a tumor in the antrum of the stomach. A CT scan of the abdomen is ordered to evaluate the lymphatic drainage of the stomach. Which of the following lymph nodes is most likely to be involved in a malignancy of the stomach?

A. Celiac

B. Superior mesenteric

C. Inferior mesenteric

D. Lumbar

E. Hepatic

21. A 47-year-old woman is brought to the emergency department with right upper abdominal pain. She has a history of similar pain after eating fatty meals. Physical examination shows a positive Murphy sign. An ultrasound of the abdomen shows findings consistent with acute cholecystitis. The patient undergoes a laparoscopic cholecystectomy. During the procedure the hepatoduodenal ligament is clamped instead of the cystic artery. Which of the following vessels was most likely occluded?

A. Superior mesenteric artery

B. Proper hepatic artery

C. Splenic artery

D. Common hepatic artery

E. Inferior vena cava

22. A 45-year-old man is brought to the emergency department with groin pain. His vital signs are within normal limits. Physical examination shows a palpable, nonreducible mass just superior to the inguinal ligament. The patient is diagnosed with an incarcerated inguinal

hernia and is scheduled for surgical repair. During the operation, a loop of intestine is observed passing through the deep inguinal ring. Which of the following types of hernias accurately represents the surgical findings?

A. Direct inguinal
B. Umbilical
C. Femoral
D. Lumbar
E. Indirect inguinal

23. A 55-year-old man comes to the emergency department with severe abdominal pain. The patient says that the pain began suddenly and is progressively worsening. His past medical history is significant for peptic ulcer disease. Physical examination shows diminished bowel sounds, and a rigid, tender abdomen that is tympanic to percussion. An x-ray of the abdomen shows free air within the abdominal cavity. A gastroscopy shows a perforating ulcer in the posterior wall of the stomach. Which of the following locations would peritonitis most likely develop initially?

A. Right subhepatic space
B. Hepatorenal space (of Morison)
C. Omental bursa (lesser sac)
D. Right subphrenic space
E. Greater sac

24. A 58-year-old man comes to the emergency department with one episode of vomiting dark red blood. The patient is drinking at least two pints of vodka every day. Medical history is significant for portal hypertension. As the patient is triaged, he continues to vomit blood. An intravenous access is established, broad-spectrum antibiotics and octreotide is started, and the patient is taken to the endoscopy suite. Esophagogastroduodenoscopy shows ruptured esophageal varices, most likely resulting from portal hypertension. Which of the following venous tributaries to the portal system anastomose with the caval veins to cause the varices?

A. Splenic
B. Left gastro-omental
C. Left gastric
D. Left hepatic
E. Right gastric

25. A 45-year-old man comes to the emergency department with severe lower abdominal pain and fever for the past 2 days. His medical history is significant for an unrepaired right indirect inguinal hernia. His temperature is 40°C (102.2°F), pulse is 100/min, respirations are 20/min, and blood pressure is 98/83 mm Hg. Physical examination shows dusky skin over the right side of the scrotum. The right side of the scrotum is tender to touch and the right cremasteric reflex is absent. A diagnosis of a strangulated hernia is made. Which of the following nerves is responsible for the efferent limb of the cremasteric reflex?

A. Ilioinguinal
B. Iliohypogastric

C. Genitofemoral
D. Pudendal
E. Ventral ramus of T12

Questions 26–50

26. A 32-year-old woman comes to the emergency department with severe abdominal pain and nausea. She has a medical history of gastroesophageal (GE) reflux disease (GERD) and peptic ulcer disease, for which she is not taking any medications. Her temperature is 36.9°C (98.4°F), pulse is 100/min, respirations are 20/min, and blood pressure is 135/85 mm Hg. Physical examination shows tenderness in the epigastrium. An x-ray shows free air under the diaphragm. An exploratory laparotomy is performed. During this procedure, where would the incision most likely be made to separate the left and right rectus sheaths?

A. Midaxillary line
B. Arcuate line
C. Semilunar line
D. Tendinous intersection
E. Linea alba

27. A 45-year-old man comes to the physician for surgical consultation. He recently lost 90 kg (200 lb) from his previous weight of 179 kg (395 lb). Physical examination shows loose skin around his abdomen that he would like to have removed. The patient's preoperative assessment indicates that he is fit for the surgery and is scheduled for an abdominoplasty ("tummy-tuck") the following week. The operation is performed without complications. As the physician closes the incision, which of the following layers of the abdominal wall will hold the sutures?

A. Scarpa fascia (membranous layer)
B. Camper fascia (fatty layer)
C. Transversalis fascia
D. Extraperitoneal tissue
E. External abdominal oblique aponeurosis

28. A 49-year-old man comes to physician to establish primary care contact. The patient says he does not have any chronic medical diseases but has a gnawing pain in his stomach that is gradually worsening. He says he is becoming full faster with reduced meal portions. The patient is a smoker and smokes two packs of cigarettes daily for the past 30 years. Physical examination shows yellowing of the eyes and skin, as well as epigastric tenderness. A CT scan of the abdomen shows 4-cm mass at the head of the pancreas. Laboratory studies show marked direct (conjugated) hyperbilirubinemia and elevated CA 19-9. Given the presentation of the patient, which of the following structures is most likely being obstructed?

A. Bile duct
B. Common hepatic duct
C. Cystic duct
D. Accessory pancreatic duct
E. Proper hepatic artery

29. A 44-year-old man comes to the emergency department with excessive nausea and vomiting. Physical examination shows sunken eyes and loss of skin turgor. The abdomen is soft, with minimal tenderness in the epigastric region without guarding or rigidity. Bowel sounds are heard in all four quadrants. There are no signs of organomegaly or ascites. A CT scan of the abdomen shows that part of the bowel is being compressed between the abdominal aorta and the superior mesenteric artery. The diagnosis of "nutcracker syndrome" is made. Which of the following intestinal structures is most likely being compressed?
    A. Second part of duodenum
    B. Transverse colon
    C. Third part of duodenum
    D. First part of duodenum
    E. Jejunum

30. A 47-year-old man is brought to the emergency department because of a 3-hour history of severe generalized abdominal pain. His temperature is 38.3°C (101°F), pulse is 100/min, respirations are 20/min, and blood pressure is 88/65 mm Hg. Physical examination shows board-like rigidity and obstipation. The patient undergoes an emergency surgical repair of a perforated duodenal ulcer. During the surgery the gastroduodenal artery is ligated. A branch of which of the following arteries will continue to provide blood supply to the pancreas in this patient?
    A. Inferior mesenteric
    B. Left gastric
    C. Right gastric
    D. Proper hepatic
    E. Superior mesenteric

31. A 70-year-old man comes to the emergency department with bloody diarrhea and severe abdominal pain. His history includes atherosclerosis, hypertension, and diabetes. He was discharged from the emergency department a week ago after having a myocardial infarction. His temperature is 36.9°C (98.4°F), pulse is 110/min, respirations are 22/min, and blood pressure is 95/85 mm Hg. Physical examination shows hypoactive bowel sounds, and the abdomen is tender to palpation. IV access is established, and a bolus of normal saline is administered. An arteriogram shows 90% blockage at the origin of the inferior mesenteric artery from the aorta. Which of the following arteries would most likely provide collateral supply to the descending colon?
    A. Left gastro-omental artery
    B. Middle colic artery
    C. Sigmoid artery
    D. Splenic artery
    E. Superior rectal artery

32. A 24-year-old woman comes to the emergency department with abdominal pain and nausea. She says that the pain is located around the umbilicus and is dull and achy in character. Her temperature is 40°C (104°F), pulse is 100/min, respirations are 20/min, and blood pressure is 135/85 mm Hg. Physical examination shows that flexion of the hip against resistance (psoas test) causes a sharp pain in the right lower abdominal quadrant. Which of the following structures is most likely inflamed to cause the pain?
    A. Appendix
    B. Urinary bladder
    C. Gallbladder
    D. Pancreas
    E. Uterus

33. A 35-year-old man comes to the emergency department because of fever, and excruciating pain in the back and left shoulder. His temperature is 40°C (104°F), pulse is 100/min, respirations are 20/min, and blood pressure is 100/95 mm Hg. Physical examination shows left costovertebral angle tenderness. A CT scan of the abdomen shows an abscess in the upper part of the left kidney. Urinalysis shows increased leukocytes. The patient's shoulder pain is most likely caused by the spread of the inflammation to which of the following neighboring structures?
    A. Descending colon
    B. Diaphragm
    C. Duodenum
    D. Spleen
    E. Pancreas

34. A 62-year-old man comes to the emergency department with dull, diffuse abdominal pain. The patient has a history history of chronic obstructive pulmonary disease (COPD) and alcoholism. He had smoked three packs of cigarettes per day since he was 20-year-old but has recently cut down to one pack. Physical examination shows a nondistended abdomen with normal bowel sounds auscultated in all quadrants. He has mild tenderness in the epigastric area upon palpation. A CT scan of the abdomen shows a tumor of the head of the pancreas. The abdominal pain in this patient is mediated by afferent fibers that travel initially with which of the following nerves?
    A. Greater thoracic splanchnic
    B. Intercostal
    C. Phrenic
    D. Vagus
    E. Subcostal

35. A 52-year-old man comes to the physician for infertility evaluation. He has a medical history of hypercholesterolemia, coronary artery disease, and peripheral vascular disease due to atherosclerosis. He has smoked two packs of cigarettes per day for the past 37 years. Physical examination shows normal external male genitalia. Laboratory studies show normal testosterone levels, normal GnRH, and normal LH levels. Semen analysis shows a low sperm count. Which of the following arteries is most likely occluded?
    A. External iliac
    B. Inferior epigastric
    C. Umbilical

D. Testicular

E. Deep circumflex iliac

36. A 42-year-old man comes to the physician for a routine examination. His vital signs are within normal limits. Physical examination shows a nontender mass palpated in the left side of the scrotum. An ultrasound examination of the abdomen shows that the mass does not involve the testes. What are the first group of lymph nodes to drain the affected area?

A. Superficial inguinal

B. Internal iliac

C. Lumbar

D. Presacral

E. Axillary

37. A 35-year-old man undergoes open hernioplasty for an incarcerated indirect inguinal hernia. During the operation, the spermatic cord and the internal abdominal oblique muscle is identified. Which covering of the spermatic cord is derived from the internal abdominal oblique muscle?

A. External spermatic fascia

B. Cremaster muscle

C. Tunica vaginalis

D. Internal spermatic fascia

E. Dartos fascia

38. A 63-year-old man comes to the emergency department because he is vomiting blood (hematemesis). He has a history of alcoholism. His vital signs are within normal limits. Physical examination shows a distended abdomen due to ascites with shifting fluid dullness. He undergoes an endoscopic examination that shows bleeding from esophageal varices. The varices are most likely a result of the anastomoses between the left gastric vein and tributaries to which other vessels?

A. Azygos system of veins

B. Inferior vena cava

C. Left umbilical vein

D. Superior mesenteric vein

E. Subcostal veins

39. A 34-year-old man comes to the emergency department because of vomiting and abdominal pain. The patient had an appendectomy at age 12, and an exploratory laparotomy after being involved in a motor vehicle collision 8 months ago. His vital signs are within normal limits. Physical examination shows hyperactive bowel sounds. An exploratory laparoscopy is performed for possible small bowel obstruction. During the surgery, which of the following anatomic features are the most useful to distinguish the jejunum from the ileum?

A. Jejunum has thinner walls compared with the ileum

B. Jejunum has less mesenteric fat compared with the ileum

C. Jejunum has more numerous vascular arcades compared with the ileum

D. Jejunum has more numerous lymphatic follicles beneath the mucosa compared with the ileum

E. Jejunum has fewer villi compared with the ileum

40. A 44-year-old woman is undergoing reconstructive breast surgery following a mastectomy. During the procedure, a musculocutaneous flap is used to restore the thoracic contour. The ipsilateral rectus abdominis muscle is detached carefully from the surrounding structures and transposed to the thoracic wall. Which of the following landmarks is most often used to locate the inferior end of the posterior tendinous layer of the rectus sheath?

A. Supracristal line

B. Linea alba

C. Arcuate line

D. Pectineal line

E. Semilunar line

41. A 31-year-old woman comes to the physician with abdominal pain. She was previously treated for tuberculous spondylitis involving vertebral levels T12–L1. She has been asymptomatic for 10 years. Her vital signs are within normal limits. Physical examination shows a nontender palpable mass in the right upper quadrant below the level of the lower costal margin. There is no costovertebral angle tenderness. An x-ray of the lumbar region shows a density suspicious for a calcified tuberculous abscess. Which of the following is the most likely site of the suspected abscess?

A. Body of pancreas

B. Cecum

C. Fundus of stomach

D. Psoas fascia

E. Suspensory muscle of the duodenum

42. A 45-year-old woman comes to the emergency department with nausea, vomiting, and abdominal pain. Physical examination shows normal bowel sounds in all four quadrants. There is minimal tenderness in the epigastric region without guarding or rigidity. A CT scan of the abdomen shows that the third (transverse) portion of the duodenum is being compressed by a vascular structure. Which of the following vessels will most likely be causing the compression?

A. Inferior mesenteric artery

B. Superior mesenteric artery

C. Inferior mesenteric vein

D. Hepatic portal vein

E. Splenic vein

43. A 61-year-old woman comes to the emergency department because of abdominal pain. The pain is associated with fatty foods. Ultrasound of the abdomen shows gallstones and she is scheduled for an elective cholecystectomy. During the operation the scissors of the physician enter the tissues immediately posterior to the omental (epiploic) foramen (its posterior boundary) and the surgical field is immediately filled with blood. Which of the following vessels is the most likely source of the bleeding?

A. Aorta

B. Inferior vena cava

C. Hepatic vein

    D. Right renal artery

    E. Superior mesenteric vein

44. A 32-year-old woman comes to the emergency department because of severe pain in the abdomen. Physical examination shows pain in the right lower quadrant with rebound tenderness. A CT scan of the abdomen shows acute appendicitis and the appendix is successfully removed in an emergency appendectomy. One week postoperatively, the patient experiences paresthesia of the skin over the pubic region and the anterior portion of her perineum. Which of the following nerves was most likely injured during the appendectomy?

    A. Genitofemoral

    B. Ilioinguinal

    C. Subcostal

    D. Iliohypogastric

    E. Spinal nerve T9

45. A 25-year-old man is brought to the emergency department after being involved in a motor vehicle collision. A Focused assessment with sonography in trauma (FAST) ultrasound examination shows fluid in the abdomen and he is taken to the operating room for an exploratory laparotomy. Which of the following anatomic relationships would be seen clearly without dissection when the physician exposes the initial aspect of the jejunum?

    A. The second portion of the duodenum is related anteriorly to the hilum of the right kidney.

    B. The superior mesenteric artery and vein pass posterior to the third part of the duodenum.

    C. The portal vein crosses anterior to the neck of the pancreas.

    D. The second part of the duodenum is crossed anteriorly by the attachment of the transverse mesocolon.

    E. The third part of the duodenum is related anteriorly to the hilum of the left kidney.

46. A 30-year-old woman comes to the physician because she has been weak and easily fatigued over the past 6 months. She has a 3-month history of severe hypertension that has required treatment with antihypertensive medications. She has recently gained 4.5 kg (10 lb) and currently weighs 75 kg (165 lb). Her blood pressure is 170/100 mm Hg. Physical examination shows purple striae over the abdomen and a "buffalo hump." Laboratory studies show fasting serum glucose concentration of 140 mg/dL. A CT scan of the abdomen shows a 6-cm mass immediately posterior to the inferior vena cava. Which of the following organs is the most likely origin of the mass?

    A. Suprarenal gland

    B. Appendix

    C. Gallbladder

    D. Ovary

    E. Uterus

47. A 45-year-old woman comes to the physician because of 2-day history of nausea and intermittent pain in the right upper quadrant of the abdomen. Physical examination shows an obese woman with scleral icterus and tenderness in the right upper quadrant. She has a history of gallstones. Which of the following structures has most likely been obstructed by a gallstone?

    A. Bile duct

    B. Cystic duct

    C. Left hepatic duct

    D. Pancreatic duct

    E. Right hepatic duct

48. A 67-year-old man comes to the physician because of abdominal discomfort. He has a history of alcohol abuse. Physical examination shows palmar erythema, female distribution of body hair, and ascites. A diagnosis of severe cirrhosis of the liver is made. He most likely has enlarged anastomoses between which of the following pairs of veins?

    A. Inferior phrenic and superior phrenic

    B. Left colic and middle colic

    C. Left gastric and esophageal

    D. Lumbar and renal

    E. Sigmoid and superior rectal

49. A 45-year-old man comes to the emergency department because of a massive hernia that passes through the inguinal triangle (of Hesselbach). Which of the following structures is used as a landmark to distinguish a direct inguinal hernia from an indirect inguinal hernia?

    A. Inferior epigastric vessels

    B. Femoral canal

    C. Inguinal ligament

    D. Rectus abdominis muscle (lateral border)

    E. Pectineal ligament

50. A 36-year-old man was brought to the emergency department with a bullet wound to the abdomen. Physical examination shows the bullet penetrated the anterior abdominal wall superior to the umbilicus. If the bullet passed directly posterior in the midline, which of the following structures was most likely to have been struck first by the bullet?

    A. Abdominal aorta

    B. Transverse colon

    C. Stomach

    D. Gallbladder

    E. Pancreas

Questions 51–75

51. A 48-year-old man comes to the emergency department because he is vomiting blood. He has had three episodes of hematemesis in the past 24 hours and has a history of chronic alcoholism but has recently been rehabilitated. Physical examination shows ascites and splenomegaly. A diagnosis of esophageal variceal bleeding is made. Which of the following surgical venous anastomoses is most commonly used to relieve these symptoms and signs before a liver transplant is attempted?

    A. Left gastric to splenic vein

    B. Right gastric to left gastric vein

    C. Right renal to right gonadal vein

D. Splenic to left renal vein

E. Superior mesenteric to inferior mesenteric vein

52. A 55-year-old man comes to the emergency department because of nausea, vomiting, and hematuria. A CT scan of the abdomen shows a neoplasm in the posterior surface of the inferior pole of the left kidney that has invaded through the renal pelvis, renal capsule, ureter, and fat. To which of the following regions will pain most likely be referred?

A. Skin of the anterior and lateral thighs and femoral triangle

B. Skin over the gluteal region and pubic areas

C. Skin over the medial, anterior, and lateral side of the thigh

D. Skin over the pubis and umbilicus

E. Skin over the pubis, umbilicus, and posterior abdominal wall muscles

53. A 30-year-old woman comes to the physician because of weakness and fatigue over the past 6 months. She has a 3-month history of severe hypertension that has not responded to antihypertensive medications. Fasting serum glucose concentration is 140 mg/dL. A CT scan of the abdomen shows a 6-cm mass in the suprarenal gland affecting secretory (chromaffin) cells of the adrenal medulla and a pheochromocytoma is suspected. Which of the following structures is most likely releasing products into the bloodstream leading to the sign and symptoms of this patient?

A. Preganglionic sympathetic axons in thoracic splanchnic nerves

B. Cells of neural crest origin that migrated to the suprarenal medulla

C. Preganglionic parasympathetic branches of the posterior vagal trunk

D. Postganglionic parasympathetic branches of the left or right vagus nerves

E. Postganglionic fibers from pelvic splanchnic nerves

54. A 48-year-old man comes to the emergency department because of vague abdominal pain for the past 6 months. Physical examination shows a cachexic man with mild abdominal tenderness. A CT scan of the abdomen shows a tumor in the tail of the pancreas. A diagnostic arteriogram shows that the tumor has compromised the blood supply to another organ. Which of the following organs is most likely to have its blood supply compromised by this tumor?

A. Duodenum

B. Gallbladder

C. Kidney

D. Liver

E. Spleen

55. A 57-year-old man comes to the emergency department because of pain in the left abdomen. A magnetic resonance imaging (MRI) of the abdomen shows that blood flow in the left renal vein is being occluded by an arterial aneurysm where the vein crosses the aorta. Laboratory studies show hematuria and anemia. The aneurysm is most likely located in which of the following arteries?

A. Celiac

B. Inferior mesenteric

C. Left colic

D. Middle colic

E. Superior mesenteric

56. A 57-year-old man comes to the emergency department with pain in his left flank and testes. A CT scan examination shows that blood flow in the left renal vein is being occluded where it crosses anterior to the aorta. Laboratory studies shows hematuria and anemia. Which of the following is the most likely cause of the testicular pain?

A. Compression of the testicular artery

B. Occlusion of flow of blood in the testicular vein

C. Compression of the afferent fibers in the lumbar splanchnic nerves

D. Compression of the sympathetic fibers in the preaortic plexus

E. Compression of the posterior vagus nerve

57. A 51-year-old woman comes to the emergency department because of severe pain in the abdomen. Physical examination shows rebound tenderness. An x-ray of the abdomen shows air under the diaphragm and an endoscopy shows penetration of the fundic region of the stomach by an ulcer, resulting in intra-abdominal bleeding. Which of the following arteries is the most likely source of the bleeding?

A. Common hepatic artery

B. Inferior phrenic artery

C. Left gastro-omental artery

D. Short gastric artery

E. Splenic artery

58. A 39-year-old woman comes to the emergency department with pain in the abdomen radiating to her inguinal region. Physical examination shows a hernia. Which of the following is the most common type of hernia in women?

A. Femoral

B. Umbilical

C. Direct inguinal

D. Indirect inguinal

E. Epigastric

59. A 42-year-old woman comes to the emergency department because of severe pain in the abdomen. Physical examination shows rebound tenderness and an x-ray shows air under the diaphragm. An endoscopy shows penetration of the duodenal bulb by an ulcer, resulting in profuse intra-abdominal bleeding. Which of the following arteries is the most likely source of the bleeding?

A. Posterior superior pancreaticoduodenal

B. Superior mesenteric

C. Inferior mesenteric

D. Inferior pancreaticoduodenal

E. Right gastric

60. A 23-year-old man comes to the physician because of a bulge in his scrotum. Physical examination shows an indirect inguinal hernia. During the open hernia repair the internal spermatic fascia is identified and reflected to expose the ductus deferens and testicular vessels. From which of the following does the internal spermatic fascial layer of the spermatic cord develop?
    A. External abdominal oblique aponeurosis
    B. Internal abdominal oblique aponeurosis
    C. Transversus abdominis aponeurosis
    D. Transversalis fascia
    E. Processus vaginalis

61. A 45-year-old woman comes to the emergency department because of severe abdominal pain. Physical examination shows scleral icterus and mild tenderness in the epigastric region. A CT scan of the abdomen shows a tumor of the head of the pancreas involving the uncinate process. Which of the following vessels is most likely to be occluded?
    A. Common hepatic artery
    B. Cystic artery and vein
    C. Superior mesenteric artery
    D. Inferior mesenteric artery
    E. Hepatic portal vein

62. A 35-year-old man comes to the emergency department because of jaundice and abdominal pain. Physical examination shows scleral icterus and tenderness in the right upper quadrant that migrates posteriorly toward the scapula. An ultrasound of the abdomen shows multiple gallstones. Which of the following structures is most likely obstructed by the gallstones?
    A. Bile duct
    B. Cystic duct
    C. Left hepatic duct
    D. Pancreatic duct
    E. Right hepatic duct

63. A 36-year-old woman G1, P0 comes to the emergency department because of contractions. The decision is made to perform an emergency cesarean section. A Pfannenstiel incision is used to reach the uterus by making a transverse incision through the external sheath of the rectus muscles, about 2 cm above the pubic bones. It follows natural folds of the skin and curves superior to the mons pubis. Which of the following nerves is most at risk when this incision is made?
    A. T10
    B. T11
    C. Iliohypogastric
    D. Ilioinguinal
    E. Lateral femoral cutaneous

64. A 37-year-old woman comes to the emergency department because of high fever, nausea, vomiting, and right lower quadrant abdominal pain. Physical examination shows rebound tenderness over McBurney point, and a positive psoas test. Laboratory studies show marked leukocytosis. Which of the following is the most likely diagnosis?
    A. Ectopic pregnancy
    B. Appendicitis
    C. Cholecystitis
    D. Kidney stone
    E. Perforation of the duodenum

65. A 56-year-old man comes to the emergency department because of severe abdominal pain. The patient has a history of "irritable bowel syndrome" affecting his rectum. Which of the following nerves will most likely be responsible for the transmission of pain in this case?
    A. Lumbar sympathetic trunks
    B. Pelvic splanchnic nerves
    C. Pudendal nerves
    D. Sacral sympathetic trunks
    E. Vagus nerves

66. A 42-year-old woman comes to the emergency department because of blood in her stools. Physical examination shows no signs of inflammation, infection, or tumor. An endoscopic examination of the distal segment of the ileum shows a lesion of the intestinal wall. A biopsy shows histologic evidence that the lesion contains gastric mucosa. Which of the following clinical conditions will most likely explain the symptoms and signs?
    A. Internal hemorrhoids
    B. External hemorrhoids
    C. Diverticulosis
    D. Meckel diverticulum
    E. Borborygmi

67. An 80-year-old man comes to the physician for a routine examination. He has had a poor appetite for some time. Physical examination shows that his blood pressure is 175/95 mm Hg and he has marked pulsation in his epigastric region. Which of the following diagnoses will most likely explain the symptoms and signs?
    A. Hiatal hernia
    B. Splenomegaly
    C. Cirrhosis of the liver
    D. Abdominal aortic aneurysm
    E. Kidney stone

68. A 48-year-old woman comes to the emergency department because of abdominal discomfort. Physical examination shows ascites which is confirmed by a CT scan (Fig. 3.1). In which of the following locations will an ultrasound examination most likely confirm the presence of the ascitic fluid with the patient in the supine position?
    A. Subphrenic recess
    B. Hepatorenal recess (pouch of Morison)
    C. Rectouterine recess (pouch of Douglas)
    D. Vesicouterine recess
    E. Costodiaphragmatic recess

69. A 19-year-old man is brought to the emergency department after a motor vehicle collision. An MRI of the abdomen shows that the spinal cord has been transected at the L4 cord level. Which of the following

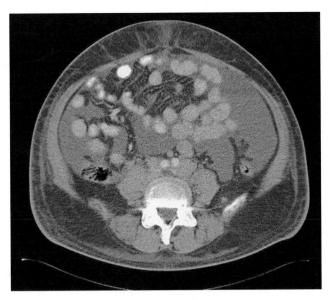

• Fig. 3.1

portions of the intestine will most predictably lose parasympathetic innervation from the central nervous system (CNS)?

A. Jejunum
B. Ascending colon
C. Ileum
D. Descending colon
E. Transverse colon

70. A 55-year-old man comes to the physician because of severe weight loss over the preceding 6 months. A CT scan of the abdomen shows that a tumor is causing portal hypertension. Laboratory studies show that the patient has fatty stool, malnutrition, and liver hypoxia. At which of the following locations is the tumor most likely located?

A. Right lobe of the liver
B. Left lobe of the liver
C. Porta hepatis
D. Falciform ligament
E. Hepatogastric ligament

71. A 61-year-old man comes to the emergency department because of pain in the abdomen. He says the pain occurs after eating and is intermittent. An ultrasound of the abdomen shows stones in the gallbladder and he is scheduled for an elective cholecystectomy. During a laparoscopic cholecystectomy which of the following arteries must be clamped to remove the gallbladder safely?

A. Common hepatic
B. Proper hepatic
C. Right hepatic
D. Left hepatic
E. Cystic

72. A 45-year-old woman is brought to the emergency department after her automobile left the highway in a rainstorm and hit a tree. She was wearing a seat belt. A FAST examination shows intra-abdominal bleeding and an x-ray of the abdomen shows that she has fractures of the ninth and tenth rib on her left side. Physical examination shows hypovolemic shock. Which of the following organs is most likely injured to result in these clinical signs?

A. Liver
B. Pancreas
C. Left kidney
D. Spleen
E. Ileum

73. A 45-year-old man comes to the emergency department because of severe pain in the right lower quadrant. A diagnosis of appendicitis is made, and he is taken for an appendectomy. Two days after the appendectomy, his temperature is 39°C (102.2), he is hypotensive, and has abdominal pain. An exploratory laparotomy shows large amounts of blood in the peritoneal cavity because of an injury to a vessel that occurred during the appendectomy. Which of the following vessels must be ligated to stop the bleeding?

A. Right colic artery
B. Right colic artery and superior rectal artery
C. Superior mesenteric artery
D. Ileocolic artery
E. Ileocolic artery and middle colic artery

74. A 42-year-old man comes to the emergency department because of severe hematemesis. Physical examination shows that the patient is icteric (jaundiced) and dilated veins ("caput medusae") are seen on his anterior abdominal wall. A CT scan of the abdomen shows hepatomegaly and an endoscopy shows esophageal varices. Which of the following venous structures is most likely obstructed for the development of caput medusae?

A. Hepatic portal vein
B. Inferior vena cava
C. Superior vena cava
D. Lateral thoracic vein
E. Superficial epigastric vein

75. A 58-year-old man comes to the physician because of pain in the right upper quadrant and fever. Physical examination shows a positive Murphy sign. Ultrasound examination of the abdomen shows numerous large gallstones in his gallbladder and pericholecystic fluid. Which of the following nerves transmits the pain of cholecystitis?

A. The right vagus nerve, with referral to the inferior angle of the scapula
B. Afferent fibers in spinal nerves T1–T4
C. Visceral afferent fibers in the greater thoracic splanchnic nerve, with referral to the dermatomes from T6 to T8
D. Sympathetic T10–T12 portions of greater thoracic splanchnic nerve via celiac ganglion and celiac plexus
E. Afferent fibers of dorsal rami of spinal nerves T6–T8, with referral to the epigastric region

Questions 76–100

76. A 15-year-old girl is brought to the emergency department because of fever, nausea, and diffuse periumbilical pain, which later becomes localized in the lower right quadrant. Physical examination shows rebound tenderness and a diagnosis of appendicitis is made. An appendectomy procedure is begun with an incision at McBurney point. Which of the following landmarks best describes McBurney point?
    A. The midpoint of the inguinal ligament in line with the right nipple
    B. Two-thirds of the distance from the umbilicus to the anterior superior iliac spine
    C. A line that intersects the upper one-third of the inguinal ligament
    D. A line that intersects the lower third of the inguinal ligament, about 2 cm from the pubic tubercle
    E. One-third of the distance from the anterior inferior iliac spine to the umbilicus

77. A 41-year-old woman comes to the physician because of an upper abdominal pain. She describes the pain as gnawing and occurs usually with food. An endoscopy shows multiple small ulcerations in the body of the stomach. Which of the following nerves transmits the sensation of pain from this region?
    A. Spinal nerves T5–T12
    B. Greater thoracic splanchnic nerves
    C. Vagus nerve
    D. Lumbar splanchnic nerves
    E. Spinal nerves T12–L2

78. A 68-year-old woman comes to the emergency department because of severe pain radiating from her lower back toward her pubic symphysis. Ultrasound examination of the abdomen shows that a renal calculus is partially obstructing her right ureter. At which of the following locations is the calculus most likely to lodge?
    A. Major calyx
    B. Minor calyx
    C. Pelvic brim
    D. Midportion of the ureter
    E. Between the pelvic brim and the uterine cervix

79. A 42-year-old woman is brought to the emergency department after a traumatic landing while skydiving. A FAST examination shows intra-abdominal bleeding and a CT scan shows a ruptured spleen. An emergency splenectomy is performed. Which of the following peritoneal structures must be carefully manipulated to prevent further intraperitoneal bleeding?
    A. Coronary ligament
    B. Gastrocolic ligament
    C. Splenorenal ligament
    D. Hepatogastric ligament
    E. Falciform ligament

80. A 74-year-old woman comes to the emergency department because of passing blood in the stool. A colonoscopy shows diverticulosis of the lower portion of the descending colon. It is determined that the involved area of the bowel should be removed. If the patient's anatomy follows the most typical pattern, which vessels and nerves will be cut during the operation?
    A. Branches of the vagus nerve and middle colic artery
    B. Superior mesenteric plexus and superior rectal artery
    C. Branches of pelvic splanchnic nerves and left colic artery
    D. Branches of vagus nerve and ileocolic artery
    E. Left lesser thoracic splanchnic nerve and inferior mesenteric artery

81. A 15-year-old girl is brought to the emergency department because of pain in the right lower quadrant. A diagnosis of appendicitis is made, and she undergoes an appendectomy. Two weeks postoperatively, she feels numbness of the skin over the pubic region and anterior portion of her genitals. Which of the following nerves was most likely injured during the operation?
    A. Pudendal
    B. Genitofemoral
    C. Spinal nerve T10
    D. Subcostal
    E. Ilioinguinal

82. A 5-year-old boy is brought to the emergency department because of dysphagia and a history of recurrent chest infections. Two days later, the boy develops aspiration pneumonia. An Esophagogastroduodenoscopy (EGD) shows webs and strictures in the distal third of the thoracic esophagus. Which of the following developmental conditions will most likely explain the symptoms?
    A. Incomplete recanalization of the esophagus during the 8th week
    B. TEF
    C. Esophageal atresia
    D. Duodenal atresia
    E. Duodenal stenosis

83. A 5-day-old girl is brought to the emergency department because of vomiting for the past 2 days. The vomitus contains stomach contents and bile. An x-ray of the abdomen shows stenosis of the fourth part of the duodenum. The child cries almost constantly, appearing to be hungry all of the time. The girl has not gained any weight since birth. Which of the following developmental conditions most likely explain the symptoms?
    A. Patent bile duct
    B. Duodenal stenosis
    C. Hypertrophic pyloric sphincter
    D. Atrophic gastric antrum
    E. TEF

84. A 4-day-old girl is brought to the emergency department because of vomiting. The vomiting is described as projectile and contains the contents of her stomach but does not appear to contain bile. The girl makes

sucking movements of her lips in response to offerings to suckle by her mother or of the bottle. She is failing to thrive. Physical examination shows an olive-like mass in the epigastric region. Which of the following conditions will best explain the symptoms?

A. Duodenal stenosis
B. Duodenal atresia
C. Hypertrophic pyloric sphincter
D. Atrophic gastric fundus
E. TEF

85. A 5-day-old girl is brought to the emergency department because of vomiting. The vomitus contains stomach contents and bile. The vomiting continues for 2 days. An x-ray of the abdomen shows stenosis of the third part of the duodenum. The child cries constantly and is hungry, but she does not gain any weight. Which of the following conditions will most likely explain her symptoms?

A. Incomplete recanalization of the esophagus during the 8th week
B. Incomplete recanalization of the duodenum
C. Esophageal atresia
D. Duodenal atresia
E. TEF

86. A 2-day-old boy was brought to the emergency department because of vomiting stomach contents and bile for 2 days. He was diagnosed in utero with polyhydramnios. An ultrasound examination of the abdomen shows a "double bubble" sign. The child cries constantly and is always hungry but has lost 300 g in weight since birth. Which of the following conditions will most likely explain the symptoms?

A. Duodenal stenosis
B. Duodenal atresia
C. Hypertrophied pyloric sphincter
D. Atrophied gastric antrum
E. TEF

87. A 4-year-old boy is admitted to the emergency department because of severe vomiting. A diagnosis of an annular pancreas is made. Which of the following mechanisms best describes the development of this condition?

A. The pancreatic duct persisted as an accessory duct that opened at the minor papilla.
B. Bile ducts failed to canalize.
C. The ventral pancreatic bud fused with the dorsal bud around the duodenum.
D. The dorsal pancreatic bud formed a ring of pancreatic tissue.
E. The dorsal pancreatic bud developed around the third part of the duodenum.

88. A 35-year-old-man is brought to the emergency department because of nausea, vomiting, and constipation for the past week. He also describes a periumbilical pain that localizes to the right lower quadrant of the abdomen. The patient undergoes an emergency appendectomy because of a ruptured appendix. A midline incision was made for greater access to the peritoneal cavity. Intraoperatively, a 5-cm-long finger-like pouch on the anterior border of the ileum about 60 cm away from the ileocecal junction is noted. Such a pouch is a remnant of which of the following developmental structures?

A. Omphaloenteric duct (yolk stalk)
B. Branch of superior mesenteric artery
C. Umbilical vesicle (yolk sac)
D. Cecal diverticulum
E. Umbilical cord

89. A 3-month-old boy is brought to the emergency department by his parents because of an abnormal mass of tissue protruding from his abdomen. An MRI examination shows that the mass contains some portions of the greater omentum and small intestine. The mass protrudes when the boy cries, strains, and coughs. Which of the following conditions will most likely explain the symptoms?

A. Umbilical hernia
B. Omphalocele
C. Gastroschisis
D. Epigastric hernia
E. Indirect inguinal hernia

90. A 24-year-old woman comes to the emergency department for her antenatal examination. Ultrasound examination indicates a defect on the right side of the fetus, lateral to the median plane, in which the viscera protrude into the amniotic cavity. Which of the following conditions will most likely explain these findings?

A. Nonrotation of the midgut
B. Patent urachus
C. Abdominal contents have not returned from the umbilical cord
D. Incomplete closure of the lateral folds
E. Persistent cloacal membrane

91. A 2-day-old boy is brought to the emergency department because of continuous vomiting of stomach contents and bile. The vomiting continues for 2 days. Physical examination shows abdominal distension, and he is unable to pass meconium (the earliest feces to be eliminated after birth). Vital signs are within normal limits. Which of the following is the most common cause of this condition?

A. Infarction of fetal bowel due to volvulus
B. Incomplete closure of the lateral folds
C. Failure of recanalization of the ileum
D. Remnant of the proximal portion of the omphaloenteric duct
E. Nonrotation of the midgut

92. A 5-year-old boy is brought to the emergency department because of sudden onset of nausea, vomiting, and periumbilical pain. A diagnosis of appendicitis is made and an appendectomy is performed. During this procedure, an ileal (Meckel) diverticulum is

discovered. Which of the following is the most common cause of this condition?

A. Infarction of fetal bowel due to volvulus

B. Incomplete closure of the lateral folds

C. Failure of recanalization of the ileum

D. Retention of the proximal portion of the omphaloenteric duct

E. Nonrotation of the midgut

93. A newborn boy fails to pass stool (meconium) in the first 48 hours after birth. Physical examination shows that the boy has anal agenesis with a perineal fistula. Which of the following is the most common cause of this condition?

A. Incomplete separation of the cloaca by the urorectal septum

B. Dorsal deviation of the urorectal septum

C. Failure of the anal membrane to perforate

D. Abnormal recanalization of the colon

E. Remnant of the proximal portion of the omphalo-enteric duct

94. A 3-month-old girl is brought to the emergency department by her parents because of several periods of stool infrequency, 2 of which lasted 10 days without a bowel movement. Physical examination shows narrowing of the anal canal and a diagnosis of anal stenosis is made. Which of the following is the most likely cause of this condition?

A. Incomplete separation of the cloaca by the urorectal septum

B. Dorsal deviation of the urorectal septum

C. Failure of the anal membrane to perforate

D. Abnormal recanalization of the colon

E. Remnant of the proximal portion of the omphalo-enteric duct

95. A 2-month-old infant is brought to the emergency department because of fecal discharge from his umbilicus. Which of the following diagnoses will best explain this condition?

A. Enterocystoma

B. Vitelline cyst

C. Ileal (Meckel) diverticulum

D. Vitelline fistula

E. Volvulus

96. A 5-day-old boy is diagnosed with anorectal agenesis. An ultrasound examination of the abdomen and pelvis shows the presence of a rectourethral fistula. Which of the following is the most likely embryological cause of this condition?

A. Failure of the proctodeum to develop

B. Agenesis of the urorectal septum

C. Failure of fixation of the hindgut

D. Abnormal partitioning of the cloaca

E. Premature rupture of the anal membrane

97. A 12-year-old boy is brought to the emergency department with massive rectal bleeding. Upon inspection, the color of the blood ranged from bright to dark red. The child appeared to be free of any pain.

A technetium-99m pertechnetate scan shows an ileal (Meckel) diverticulum. Which of the following is the underlying embryological cause of this condition?

A. Failure of yolk stalk to regress

B. Duplication of the intestine

C. Malrotation of the cecum and appendix

D. Nonrotation of the midgut

E. Herniation of the intestines

98. A 23-year-old primigravid woman comes to the physician for routine examination. Physical examination is within normal limits. Ultrasound examination of the fetus shows unilateral renal agenesis and oligohydramnios. Which of the following conditions most likely occurred?

A. Polycystic kidney disease

B. Degeneration of the mesonephros

C. Ureteric duplication

D. Failure of a ureteric bud to form

E. Wilms tumor

99. A 15-year-old girl was brought to the physician by her parents because of bilateral inguinal masses. She has not started to menstruate yes. Physical examination shows normal breast development for her age and female external genitalia. The vagina is shallow, and the uterus cannot be palpated. Laboratory studies shows a negative sex chromatin pattern. Which of the following is the most likely diagnosis?

A. Male pseudohermaphroditism

B. Female pseudohermaphroditism

C. Androgen insensitivity syndrome

D. Inguinal hernias

E. Turner syndrome

100. An 18-year-old woman is brought to the emergency department because of pelvic pain. The pain is cyclic and has been worsening over the past 6 months. The patient also has a history of primary amenorrhea. Physical examination shows a small suprapubic mass palpated on exam. A vaginal examination shows a bulging bluish membrane between the labia. A diagnosis of an imperforate hymen is made. Which of the following is the most likely explanation for this condition?

A. Failure of the vaginal plate to canalize

B. Cervical atresia

C. Patent processus vaginalis

D. Androgen insensitivity syndrome

E. Failure of the sinovaginal bulbs to develop

Questions 101–125

101. A 22-year-old woman comes to the physician because of dyspareunia. She has had one sexual partner and her last sexually transmitted disease screening, performed 1 month ago, was negative. A routine pelvic examination shows a 3 cm cystic mass detected on the lateral wall of the vagina. A transvaginal ultrasound examination shows that the abnormal structure is

likely a Gartner duct cyst. Which of the following embryonic structures does this cyst originate from?

A. Mesonephric tubules
B. Paramesonephric duct
C. Urogenital folds
D. Mesonephric duct
E. Sinovaginal bulbs

102. A 30-year-old woman, gravida 1, para 0, abort 0, at 30 weeks' gestation comes to the physician for a prenatal visit. Physical examination shows a uterus consistent with a 27-week gestation. Fetal ultrasonography shows a fetus with clubbed feet, broad nasal bridge, low-set ears, micrognathia, and oligohydramnios. Which of the following is the most likely explanation for these initial findings?

A. Multicystic dysplastic kidney
B. Polycystic kidney
C. Renal agenesis
D. Wilms tumor
E. Exstrophy of the urinary bladder

103. A 58-year-old man is brought to the emergency department by his wife because of severe pain that radiates from his lower back to the pubic region. He says the pain is colicky in character. His pulse is 86/min, respirations are 18/min, blood pressure 130/85 mm Hg, and he is afebrile. Physical examination shows right-sided costovertebral angle tenderness. An ultrasound of the abdomen shows that a kidney stone is partially obstructing his right ureter and the presence of a second ureter on the right side. Which of the following is the most likely cause of this latter finding?

A. Failure of ureteric bud to form
B. Early splitting of the ureteric bud
C. Failure of urorectal septum to develop
D. Persistent urachus
E. Failure of ureteric bud to branch

104. A 50-year-old woman is brought to the emergency department by her son because of sudden, severe epigastric pain. She has a history of chronic heartburn, which is self-treated with various over-the-counter medications. An upper endoscopy shows a small, perforated ulcer in the posterior wall of the stomach and the patient is taken for surgical repair. During the procedures, 150 mL of blood-tinged, frothy gray liquid is aspirated from the peritoneal cavity. Where in the peritoneal cavity would liquid most likely first collect when the patient is supine position?

A. Right subphrenic space
B. Hepatorenal pouch (of Morison)
C. Left paracolic gutter
D. Vesicouterine pouch
E. Rectouterine pouch (of Douglas)

105. A 43-year-old woman is brought to the emergency department because of sudden epigastric pain. The patient has a history of smoking and long-term Nonsteroidal anti-inflammatory drug (NSAID) use. Physical examination shows epigastric tenderness and

generalized rigidity. An upright chest x-ray shows a small amount of free air under the diaphragm. An upper endoscopy shows a small, perforated ulcer in the posterior wall of the greater curvature of the stomach. Where is the air most likely located?

A. Right subphrenic space
B. Supravesical space
C. Paracolic gutters
D. Vesicouterine pouch
E. Rectouterine pouch (of Douglas)

106. A 25-year-old woman is brought to the emergency department because of a sudden, sharp pain in the left lower quadrant. She says that her last menstrual period was 10 days ago. A pregnancy test is negative. A transvaginal ultrasound shows a ruptured cyst on the left ovary, which resulted in approximately 100 mL of fluid in the pelvis. In which of the following spaces would fluid most likely accumulate?

A. Right subphrenic space
B. Hepatorenal pouch (of Morison)
C. Paracolic gutters
D. Vesicouterine pouch
E. Rectouterine pouch (of Douglas)

107. A 60-year-old man is brought to the emergency department because of severe abdominal pain. He has a history of hypertension and atherosclerosis with noncompliance to medication. Physical examination shows severe tenderness, guarding, and rigidity in all quadrants of the abdomen. CT angiography of the abdomen shows a thrombus in the artery supplying the ileum. Which of the following layers of peritoneum will the physician enter to access the affected vessel?

A. Parietal peritoneum and the greater omentum
B. Greater and lesser omentum
C. Lesser omentum and the gastrosplenic ligament
D. Parietal peritoneum and the mesentery
E. Greater omentum and the transverse mesocolon

108. A 52-year-old man comes to the emergency department because of persistent severe right upper quadrant pain for the past 2 hours. The pain began shortly after greasy "fast food." Physical examination shows nausea, profuse sweating, and pain in the lower posterior aspect of his right shoulder. An ultrasound examination of the abdomen shows multiple stones in an inflamed gallbladder with normal bile duct. Which of the following spinal nerve segments are involved in the back pain associated with cholecystitis?

A. C3–C5
B. C5–C8
C. T1–T4
D. T5–T9
E. T10, T11

109. A 64-year-old woman comes to the emergency department because of severe abdominal pain. She has a history of gallstones. Her vital signs are within normal limits. Physical examination shows tenderness in the

right upper quadrant. The patient was taken for cholecystectomy and the right hepatic artery was injured during surgery. Which of the following procedures would most likely be performed by the physician to reduce the blood loss?

A. Pringle maneuver
B. Kocher maneuver
C. Valsalva maneuver
D. Heimlich maneuver
E. Placement of a vascular clamp on the porta hepatis

110. A 73-year-old man is brought to the emergency department because of painful rectal bleeding and severe abdominal pain. His temperature is 38°C (100.4°F), pulse is 100/min, respirations are 20/min, and blood pressure is 100/73 mm Hg. Physical examination shows abdominal distention, and lower left quadrant tenderness. Stool guaiac is negative. A CT scan of the abdomen shows massive bleeding from the descending colon. Which of the following arteries is the most likely source of the hemorrhage?

A. Left colic
B. Middle colic
C. Superior rectal
D. Inferior rectal
E. Left gastro-omental

111. A 51-year-old woman comes to the emergency department because of sudden abdominal pain, nausea, and vomiting. She says that the pain radiates from the abdomen to the back. Physical examination shows tenderness in the right upper quadrant. An ultrasound of the abdomen shows multiple gallstones, consistent with the diagnosis of cholecystitis. Which of the following would most likely be present on physical examination?

A. Rebound tenderness
B. Iliopsoas test
C. Obturator sign
D. Murphy sign
E. Cough tenderness

112. A 35-year-old man is brought to the emergency department after receiving a gunshot wound in the left upper quadrant. His temperature is 36.9°C (98.4°F), pulse is 120/min, respirations are 16/min, and blood pressure is 80/60 mm Hg. An ultrasound of the abdomen shows profuse intraperitoneal bleeding. An emergency laparotomy is performed, and the source of bleeding appears to be a vessel within the lesser sac. Which of the following ligaments would most likely be transected to gain adequate entry to the lesser sac?

A. Coronary
B. Gastrosplenic
C. Splenorenal
D. Gastrocolic
E. Hepatoduodenal

113. A 55-year-old woman is brought to the emergency department because of rectal bleeding and abdominal pain. She reports fatigue and unintentional weight loss for the past 6 months. Physical examination shows an abnormal mass of tissue protruding below the pectinate line. A biopsy confirms the presence of adenocarcinoma. Which of the following groups of lymph nodes would most likely first receive lymphatic drainage from the area of pathology?

A. Internal iliac
B. External iliac
C. Middle rectal
D. Superficial inguinal
E. Deep inguinal

114. A 53-year-old man is brought to the emergency department because of multiple episodes of rectal bleeding and abdominal pain. His vital signs are within normal limits. Physical examination shows an abnormal mass of tissue protruding from an area superior to the external anal sphincter, superior to the pectinate line. A diagnosis of internal hemorrhoids is made. Which of the following groups of lymph nodes would most likely first receive lymphatic drainage from this area?

A. Internal iliac
B. External iliac
C. Middle rectal
D. Superficial inguinal
E. Deep inguinal

115. A 32-year-old man comes to the emergency department with severe heartburn and abdominal pain. The patient has a long history of smoking. His vital signs are within normal limits. A CT scan of the abdomen shows that the patient has a hiatal hernia, and a surgical repair is scheduled. Which of the following landmarks would be the most useful to distinguish between sliding and paraesophageal hiatal hernias?

A. Sliding hernias possess a normal GE junction.
B. In sliding hernias, the GE junction is displaced.
C. Paraesophageal hernias have a displaced GE junction.
D. In paraesophageal hernias, the antrum moves into the stomach corpus.
E. In paraesophageal hernias, the antrum and the cardia move into the body of the stomach.

116. A 43-year-old man is brought to the emergency department because of severe abdominal pain and vomiting. He has a low-grade fever and nausea. Physical exam shows generalized abdominal tenderness. A CT scan of the abdomen shows a right subphrenic abscess that extends to the midline. Which of the following structures would most likely be in a position to prevent the spread of the abscess across the midline?

A. Round ligament
B. Falciform ligament
C. Coronary ligament
D. Hepatoduodenal ligament
E. Gastroduodenal ligament

117. A 21-year-old man is brought to the emergency department because of back pain after sustaining

an injury during football. He also has a sharp pain during breathing. Physical examination shows that his left lower back is bruised and swollen. An x-ray of thorax shows a fracture of the eleventh rib on the left side. Which of the following organs would be the most likely to sustain injury at this site?

A. Spleen
B. Lung
C. Kidney
D. Liver
E. Pancreas

118. A 46-year-old man comes to the emergency department because of a large mass in his right groin. He says that the mass is painless. Physical examination shows hard and palpable superficial inguinal lymph nodes. A lymph node biopsy shows the presence of malignant cells. Which of the following locations would be the most likely primary source of carcinoma?

A. Prostate
B. Urinary bladder
C. Testis
D. Anal canal
E. Sigmoid colon

119. A 54-year-old man comes to the emergency department because of vomiting and severe weight loss. Physical examination shows tenderness of the umbilical and epigastric regions. A CT scan of the abdomen shows a massive tumor originating from the third part of the duodenum. Which of the following structures is most likely to be compressed or invaded by the tumor?

A. Bile duct
B. Hepatic portal vein
C. Superior mesenteric artery
D. Gastroduodenal artery
E. Posterior superior pancreaticoduodenal artery

120. A 24-year-old woman comes to the emergency department because of lower abdominal pain. Physical examination shows tenderness of the left lower abdominal quadrant. A CT scan of the abdomen and pelvis shows an abnormal mass occupying the left adnexa in the pelvis. During the surgical procedure to remove the tumor, the ureter and the structures immediately medial to the ureter are identified. Which of the following vascular structures crosses the ureter just lateral to the cervix of the uterus?

A. Middle rectal artery
B. Superior vesical artery
C. Internal pudendal vein
D. Uterine artery
E. Gonadal vein

121. A 32-year-old woman comes to the emergency department because of cramping abdominal pain around her umbilicus and vomiting for the past 2 days. Physical examination shows a distressful patient with tenderness in the lower abdominal quadrants. An ultrasound of the abdomen shows numerous stones in the gallbladder and air accumulation in the gallbladder and biliary tree. At which of the following locations will an obstructive stone most likely be found?

A. Jejunum
B. Terminal ileum
C. Bile duct
D. Duodenum
E. Hepatic duct

122. A 37-year-old woman comes to the emergency department because of acute onset nausea, vomiting, and right upper quadrant abdominal pain. She says that the pain radiates to the right posterior shoulder. Physical examination confirms the diagnosis and a cholecystectomy is planned. Which of the following landmarks will best describe the precise location of the gallbladder with respect to the body wall?

A. The intersection of the right linea semilunaris with the ninth costal cartilage
B. The intersection of the right linea semilunaris with the intertubercular plane
C. To the right of the epigastric region
D. Superiorly to the umbilical region
E. Upper right quadrant

123. A 45-year-old man comes to the emergency department because of a palpable and painful mass at his groin that is exacerbated when he stands erect or physically exerts himself. Physical examination shows the probability of a direct inguinal hernia based on the location of the mass, and the diagnosis is confirmed laparoscopically. Which of the following is the most likely cause of this type of inguinal hernia?

A. Defective transversalis fascia around the deep inguinal ring
B. Defective peritoneum around the deep inguinal ring
C. Defective aponeurosis of external abdominal oblique muscle
D. Defective extraperitoneal connective tissue
E. Weakness of internal abdominal oblique and transversus abdominis muscles

124. A 22-year-old woman comes to the emergency department because of severe periumbilical pain. Physical examination shows a strong possibility of appendicitis. Shortly before an appendectomy is to be performed, the inflamed appendix ruptures. In which area would the extravasating blood and infectious fluids from the appendiceal region most likely tend to collect if the patient was sitting upright?

A. Subphrenic space
B. Hepatorenal recess (pouch of Morison)
C. Rectouterine recess (pouch of Douglas)
D. Vesicoutrine space
E. Right subhepatic space

125. A 22-year-old woman comes to the emergency department because of severe upper abdominal pain. A CT scan of the abdomen shows that the source of the pain is an inflamed appendix. Which of the

following structures contain the nerve cell bodies from the appendix that are causing the referred pain in the epigastrium?

A. Sympathetic trunk ganglia
B. Celiac ganglion
C. Lateral horn of the spinal cord
D. Dorsal root ganglia of spinal nerves T8–T10
E. Dorsal root ganglia of spinal nerves L2–L4

Questions 126–150

126. A 30-year-old woman comes to the physician because of a 6-month history of weakness and fatigue. She has a 3-month acute history of severe hypertension that has required treatment with antihypertensive medications. A CT scan of the abdomen shows a tumor of her right suprarenal gland. A diagnosis of a pheochromocytoma (tumor of the suprarenal medulla) is made, and is scheduled for a laparoscopic adrenalectomy. Which of the following nerve fibers will need to be cut when the suprarenal gland and tumor are removed?

A. Preganglionic sympathetic fibers
B. Postganglionic sympathetic fibers
C. Somatic motor fibers
D. Postganglionic parasympathetic fibers
E. Preganglionic parasympathetic fibers

127. A 72-year-old man is admitted to the emergency department after a chemotherapy treatment for prostatic cancer 6 months ago. A CT scan of the abdomen and pelvis shows a new tumor that has incorporated the proximal left common iliac artery and compressed the vein that lies inferior to it. An ultrasound shows the development of a deep venous thrombosis that could block venous return from the left lower limb, causing ischemia and pain. Which of the following vessels is most likely to be involved in the production of the deep venous thrombosis?

A. Inferior vena cava
B. Right renal vein
C. Left testicular vein
D. Left common iliac vein
E. Right common iliac vein

128. A 48-year-old woman comes to the emergency department because of severe abdominal pain. A CT of the abdomen shows carcinoma of the head of the pancreas. A celiac plexus block is performed to relieve her pain. Which of the following best describes the nerve structures that are most likely to be present in the celiac ganglion?

A. Preganglionic parasympathetic and somatic motor fibers
B. Postganglionic parasympathetic and visceral afferent fibers
C. Postganglionic sympathetic and visceral afferent fibers
D. Pre- and postganglionic sympathetic, preganglionic parasympathetic, and visceral afferent fibers

E. Preganglionic sympathetic, preganglionic parasympathetic, and visceral afferent fibers

129. A 21-year-old woman is brought to the emergency department because of severe pain radiating from her lower back toward her pelvis. She says that the pain comes in waves and describes the pain as sharp. Her vital signs are within normal limits. An ultrasound examination of the abdomen shows a kidney stone that is partially obstructing her right ureter. Which of the following nerves is most likely responsible for this referred sensation of pain?

A. Subcostal
B. Iliohypogastric
C. Ilioinguinal
D. Lateral femoral cutaneous
E. Obturator

130. A 42-year-old woman is brought to the emergency department because of sudden and severe abdominal pain accompanied by bloating. She has a history of long-term NSAID use. Physical exam shows tachycardia, diffuse abdominal tenderness, and rigidity. An x-ray of the chest shows air under the diaphragm. A diagnosis of perforated duodenal ulcer is made. Which of the following arteries is most commonly eroded by this type of ulcer?

A. Gastroduodenal artery
B. Superior mesenteric
C. Posterior superior pancreaticoduodenal
D. Posterior inferior pancreaticoduodenal
E. Right gastric

131. A 50-year-old man is brought to the emergency department because of abdominal pain and reflux for the past 2 months. He has a history of smoking and alcohol abuse. Physical exam shows tenderness and rigidity in the epigastric region. Upper endoscopy shows penetration of an anterior duodenal ulcer in the first part of the duodenum. Which of the following conditions will most likely occur?

A. Bleeding from gastroduodenal artery
B. Bleeding from superior mesenteric artery
C. Bleeding from posterior superior pancreaticoduodenal artery
D. Bleeding from posterior inferior pancreaticoduodenal artery
E. Peritonitis

132. A 56-year-old man is brought to the emergency department because of abdominal pain and multiple episodes of vomiting. The patient did not have a bowel movement in 3 days. Physical exam shows diffuse tenderness and moderate distention. An x-ray of the abdomen shows multiple dilated loops of bowel. A laparotomy is performed to release the obstruction of the intestines. Which of the following structures is used as a landmark to determine the position of the duodenojejunal junction?

A. Superior mesenteric artery
B. Inferior mesenteric artery

C. Vasa recta

D. Suspensory muscle of the duodenum (ligament of Treitz)

E. Ladd bands

133. A 4-month-old girl is brought to the emergency department by her parents because of decreased activity and difficulty breathing. Physical examination shows cyanosis, decreased breath sounds, bowel sounds in the thorax, and respiratory distress. An x-ray of the abdomen shows a posterolateral defect of the diaphragm and abdominal contents in the left pleural cavity. Which of the following is the most likely cause of this defect?

A. Absence of a pleuropericardial fold

B. Absence of musculature in one half of the diaphragm

C. Failure of migration of diaphragm

D. Failure of the septum transversum to develop

E. Failure of pleuroperitoneal fold to close

134. A 58-year-old man comes to the physician because of sharp epigastric pain. He says that he has exacerbation of the pain with food. Physical exam shows tenderness to palpation at the xiphisternal junction. Barium swallow and dye injections (Hepatobiliary iminodiacetic acid [HIDA] scan) to test gallbladder functions are negative. A CT scan of the abdomen shows that a portion of the greater omentum is trapped at its passage into the thorax between the xiphoid process and the costal margin on the right. What is the most likely diagnosis of this condition?

A. Bochdalek hernia

B. Sliding esophageal hernia

C. Morgagni hernia

D. Cholecystitis

E. Hiatal hernia

135. A 62-year-old woman is brought to the emergency department by her son because of severe abdominal pain and vomiting. Physical exam shows diffuse abdominal tenderness and rigidity. A CT scan of the abdomen shows an aortic aneurysm affecting the origin of the superior mesenteric artery resulting in ischemia to an abdominal organ. Which of the following organs is most likely affected?

A. Ileum

B. Transverse colon

C. Spleen

D. Stomach

E. Duodenum

136. A 41-year-old man comes to the physician for follow-up examination after sustaining abdominal trauma from a motor vehicle collision 2 months ago. A surgical repair was achieved without complications. During this visit, the patient experiences abdominal pain. A CT scan of the abdomen shows an internal hernia in which the hepatic flexure of the colon had herniated through the omental (epiploic) foramen (of Winslow). Gastrointestinal veins appear to be markedly dilated, including the veins forming anastomoses between the portal and caval systems (veins of Retzius). Which of the following structures is most likely compressed?

A. Hepatic portal vein

B. Inferior vena cava

C. Hepatic artery

D. Bile duct

E. Cystic duct

137. A 48-year-old woman is brought to the emergency department because of abdominal pain and painless rectal bleeding for the past 3 months. The patient also says she has constipation and bloating. Her vital signs are within normal limits. Physical exam shows tenderness in the left lower quadrant. A colonoscopy shows diverticulosis affecting the distal part of the descending colon. To which of the following dermatomes would pain have most likely been referred?

A. T5–T9

B. T10–L1

C. L1–L2

D. L1–L4

E. T10–L2

138. A 61-year-old man is brought to the emergency department because of abdominal pain and multiple episodes of vomiting for the past 2 days. Physical examination shows significant abdominal distention and diffuse tenderness to palpation. Auscultation shows episodes of pain associated abnormal bowel sounds. A CT scan of the abdomen shows gallstones and mechanical obstruction of the bowel. Which of the following parts of the gastrointestinal tract is most likely obstructed?

A. Hepatopancreatic ampulla (of Vater)

B. Duodenal bulb

C. Proximal ileum

D. Pyloric sphincter

E. Ileocecal junction

139. A 43-year-old woman is brought to the emergency department because of esophageal pain and odynophagia after swallowing a fish bone 2 hours ago. Her vital signs are within normal limits. Physical examination is within normal limits. Upper endoscopy shows a perforation of the lower esophagus by the fish bone. Which of the following arteries is most likely at risk of injury?

A. Branches of left gastric

B. Bronchial

C. Intercostal

D. Branches of right gastric

E. Right inferior phrenic

140. A 42-year-old man is brought to the emergency department after being involved in a motor vehicle collision. The man is stable but has severe pain that radiates to the left shoulder. Physical exam shows left upper quadrant tenderness. An ultrasound examination of the abdomen shows splenic hemorrhage.

Which of the following signs best describes the pain experienced by the patient?

A. Mittelschmerz
B. Kehr sign
C. Rovsing sign
D. Psoas sign
E. Obturator sign

141. A 43-year-old man is brought to the emergency department after sustaining a knife wound to the right lobe of the liver. After a laparotomy is performed, digital pressure (Pringle maneuver) is applied to the hepatoduodenal ligament, but brisk bleeding continues, indicating a variation in the origin of the right hepatic artery. Which of the following is the most common variation in the arterial supply to the right lobe of the liver?

A. The right hepatic originates from the gastroduodenal
B. The right hepatic originates from the superior mesenteric
C. The right hepatic originates from the left gastric
D. The right hepatic originates from the left hepatic
E. The right hepatic originates directly from the aorta

142. A 38-year-old woman comes to the emergency department because of right upper quadrant pain and nausea. The patient says that the pain is exacerbated after meals. Physical examination shows jaundice and tenderness in the right upper quadrant. During cholangiography, the catheter is inserted with difficulty into the gallbladder. Which of the following structures is most likely to interfere with the passage of the catheter into the cystic duct?

A. Cystic duct compression by a hepatic artery
B. Spiral valve (of Heister)
C. Tortuosity of the cystic duct
D. Adhesions from the hepatoduodenal ligament
E. Portal vein compression of the cystic duct

143. A 44-year-old woman is brought to the emergency department with sudden abdominal pain in the right upper quadrant. She describes the pain as colicky and accompanied with nausea and vomiting. Physical examination shows right upper quadrant tenderness and a positive Murphy sign. The patient undergoes a successful cholecystectomy but develops bile peritonitis on the fifth postoperative day. Which of the following conditions would most likely account for this complication?

A. The bile duct is leaking
B. The ducts of Luschka are leaking
C. The right hepatic duct is leaking
D. The cystic duct is leaking
E. The left hepatic duct is leaking

144. A 35-year-old man is brought to the emergency department with sudden abdominal pain and multiple episodes of vomiting. The patient has a long history of alcohol abuse. Physical exam shows epigastric tenderness and rigidity. Laboratory studies show elevated serum amylase and lipase. Which of the

following neural fibers would be the most likely to transmit pain sensation from the pancreas?

A. Sympathetic preganglionic
B. Sympathetic postganglionic
C. Visceral afferent
D. Preganglionic parasympathetics
E. Postganglionic parasympathetics

145. A 54-year-old man is brought to the emergency department because of abdominal pain, bloating, nausea, vomiting, and poor appetite for the past 2 days. The patient recently recovered from a pneumonia infection. Physical exam shows generalized abdominal tenderness. An x-ray of the abdomen shows paralytic ileus. Which of the following signs would most likely be present during physical examination?

A. Increased bowel sounds
B. Absent bowel sounds
C. Continuous borborygmi
D. Crampy abdominal pain
E. Localized tenderness

146. A 65-year-old man is brought to the emergency department because of abdominal pain and loss of appetite. He has a history of hypertension and diabetes. Physical examination shows severe tenderness and rigidity in all quadrants. Angiography shows intestinal ischemia due to atherosclerotic occlusion of the mid-proximal part of the superior mesenteric artery. Which of the following vessels will most likely provide collateral circulation between the celiac trunk and the superior mesenteric artery?

A. Superior and inferior pancreaticoduodenal
B. Left gastric and hepatic
C. Cystic and gastroduodenal
D. Right and left colic
E. Right and left gastro-omental

147. A 22-year-old man is brought to the emergency department because of abdominal pain, nausea, and vomiting for the past 2 days. Physical examination shows tachycardia, right lower quadrant tenderness, and rebound tenderness. An ultrasound of the abdomen shows evidence of acute appendicitis. The patient is taken for laparoscopic appendectomy. Through which of the following abdominal layers must the physician pass to reach the appendix through this incision?

A. External abdominal oblique muscle, internal abdominal oblique muscle, transversalis fascia, and parietal peritoneum
B. Aponeurosis of the external abdominal oblique muscle, internal abdominal oblique muscle, transversus abdominis muscle, transversalis fascia, and parietal peritoneum
C. Aponeurosis of the external abdominal oblique muscle, internal abdominal oblique muscle, transversus abdominis muscle, and parietal peritoneum
D. Aponeurosis of the external abdominal oblique muscle, aponeurosis of internal abdominal oblique

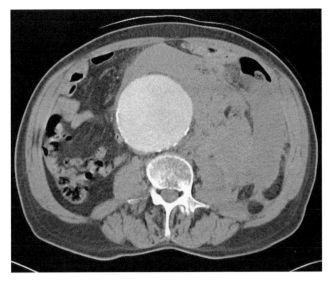

• Fig. 3.2

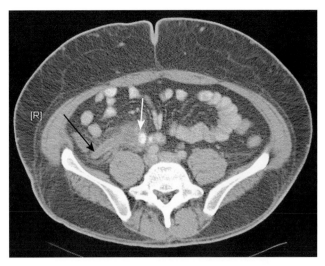

• Fig. 3.3

muscle, transversus abdominis muscle, transversalis fascia, and parietal peritoneum

E. Aponeurosis of the external abdominal oblique muscle, aponeurosis of internal abdominal oblique muscle, aponeurosis of transversus abdominis muscle, transversalis fascia, and parietal peritoneum

148. A 12-year-old boy is brought to the emergency department by his parents because of profuse and painless rectal bleeding. The patient is otherwise asymptomatic and his vitals are within normal limits. There is no history of recent travel, sick contacts, and vaccinations are up to date. Which of the following is the most common cause of severe rectal bleeding in the pediatric age group?
A. Internal hemorrhoids
B. External hemorrhoids
C. Diverticulosis
D. Ileal (Meckel) diverticulum
E. Borborygmi

149. A 48-year-old man comes to the emergency department because of abdominal pain and shortness of breath. The patient says that the symptoms have been progressively worsening over the past four months. He has a history of hypertension and smoking. The radiographic image is shown in Fig. 3.2. In which of the following locations will blood be detected with an ultrasound examination if the patient stands upright?
A. Subphrenic space
B. Hepatorenal space (pouch of Morison)
C. Rectouterine space (pouch of Douglas)
D. Rectovesical space
E. Subhepatic space

150. A 27-year-old woman is brought to the emergency department because of abdominal pain and vomiting for the past 2 days. She has a low-grade fever and loss of appetite. She says that the pain started in the middle of

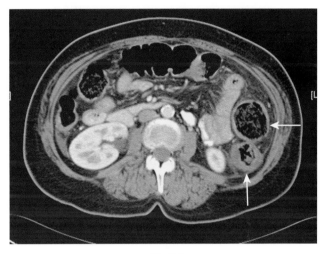

• Fig. 3.4

the abdomen then shifted to the right lower quadrant. A CT scan of the abdomen is shown in Fig. 3.3. Which of the following structures is most likely affected?
A. Right ovary
B. Appendix
C. Ileocecal junction
D. Ascending colon
E. Ileum

Questions 151–174

151. A 61-year-old man comes to the physician because of sudden and severe abdominal pain. He has a history of chronic abdominal pain, but today's episode is severe. Physical exam shows generalized abdominal tenderness and rigidity. A CT scan of the abdomen is shown in Fig. 3.4. An angiogram shows that several arteries of the gastrointestinal tract are occluded due to atherosclerosis, producing bowel ischemia. Which of the following arteries is most likely occluded in the CT scan?
A. Middle colic
B. Right colic

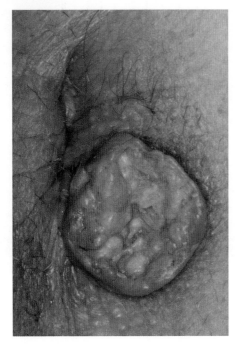

• **Fig. 3.5**

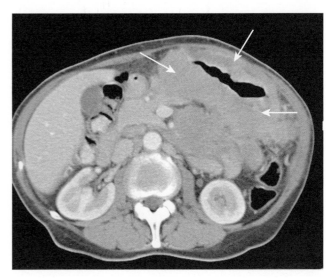

• **Fig. 3.6**

C. Left colic

D. Ileocolic

E. Marginal

152. A 53-year-old man comes to the physician because of an abnormal mass in his anal canal. An image from the physical examination is seen in Fig. 3.5. A biopsy of the tissue shows squamous cell carcinoma of the anus. Which of the following lymph nodes will most likely first receive cancerous cells from the anal tumor?

   A. Deep inguinal lymph nodes

   B. Superficial inguinal lymph nodes

   C. Internal iliac nodes

   D. External iliac nodes

   E. Lumbar nodes

153. A 49-year-old man comes to the physician because of 4-month history of bloating, nausea, and mild abdominal pain. He says that he uses long-term NSAIDs for joint pain. His vital signs and physical examination are within normal limits. A CT scan examination of the abdomen is shown in Fig. 3.6. Which of the following structures is most likely affected?

   A. Spleen

   B. Stomach

   C. Duodenum

   D. Pancreas

   E. Descending colon

154. 52-year-old man comes to the physician for follow-up examination after a gastric biopsy. The patient has a long history of abdominal pain related to food and acid reflux. An endoscopy is performed, and a biopsy is taken from an abnormal mass in the stomach. The biopsy shows a gastric adenocarcinoma, and a total gastrectomy is performed. Which of the following

lymph nodes will most likely first receive metastatic cells?

   A. Celiac

   B. Splenic

   C. Suprapancreatic

   D. Right gastric

   E. Cisterna chyli

155. A 28-year-old woman comes to the physician for a routine examination. The patient has no complaints and is otherwise healthy. Her vital signs are within normal limits. Physical examination and laboratory results are within normal limits. An x-ray of the abdomen in this patient is shown in Fig. 3.7. Which of the following is the most likely diagnosis?

   A. Cholecystitis

   B. Carcinoma of the liver

   C. A caudal extension of the right hepatic lobe (Riedel lobe)

   D. Pancreatic carcinoma

   E. Carcinoma of the stomach

156. A 35-year-old woman comes to the emergency department because of a mass protruding beneath her skin at the right lower quadrant. She says that the mass protrudes intermittently and is painless. Her vital signs are within normal limits. Physical examination shows intestinal herniation with no evidence of strangulation, as shown in Fig. 3.8. Which of the following is the most likely diagnosis?

   A. Richter hernia

   B. Spigelian hernia

   C. Paraumbilical hernia

   D. Incisional hernia

   E. Ventral hernia

157. A 3-year-old boy is brought to the emergency department by his parents because of a palpable mass in the right side of his scrotum. He is otherwise healthy and is not in pain. His vital signs are within normal limits. A preliminary diagnosis of a congenital, indirect

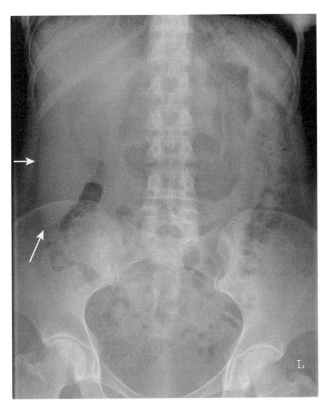

• Fig. 3.7

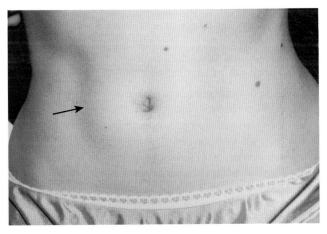

• Fig. 3.8

inguinal hernia is made. Which of the following is the most likely cause of an indirect inguinal hernia in this patient?

A. The deep inguinal ring opens into an intact processus vaginalis
B. Congenital hydrocele
C. Ectopic testis
D. Epispadias
E. Rupture of the transversalis fascia

158. A 43-year-old man comes to the physician because of chronic dysphagia and GE reflux. The patient says he has a progressive worsening dysphagia for the past 4 months. His vital signs are within normal limits. A barium study shows evidence of achalasia. Which of the following is the most likely cause of this condition?

A. Failure of relaxation of the lower esophageal sphincter
B. Dyspepsia
C. Gastritis
D. Gastroparesis
E. Peptic ulcer

159. A 3-year-old boy is brought to the emergency department by his parents because of abdominal pain and rectal bleeding. His parents say the boy had multiple episodes of vomiting. His vital signs are within normal limits. A CT scan of the abdomen shows a mass about 61 cm (2 ft) proximal to the ileocecal junction. Which of the following is the most likely diagnosis?

A. Ruptured appendix
B. Volvulus
C. Diverticulosis
D. Ileal (Meckel) diverticulum
E. Borborygmi

160. A 45-year-old man is brought to the emergency department because of pain in the right upper quadrant. Physical examination shows the pain radiates to the tip of his scapula and worsens after meals. An ultrasound of the abdomen shows gallbladder stones with associated cholecystitis. An open cholecystectomy using a Kocher incision (along the right costal margin) is performed. Which of the following nerves are most likely at risk during this incision?

A. T5–T6
B. T6–T7
C. T7–T8
D. T9–L1
E. T5–T9

161. A 3-year-old girl is brought to the physician by her mother because of a palpable right inguinal mass. Physical examination shows a nontender solitary fluctuant mass. The mass is not visible when the patient is standing. An open surgical repair is performed where digital pressure is used to return organ contents of the hernia to the abdomen. During the procedure, a sac of peritoneum can be seen clearly protruding from the deep inguinal ring. Which of the following terms is most accurately describing the origin of this structure?

A. A patent processus vaginalis (canal of Nuck)
B. Congenital hydrocele
C. Ectopic uterus
D. Femoral hernia
E. Rupture of the transversalis fascia

162. A 48-year-old woman is brought to the emergency department because of severe abdominal pain. She has a history of alcohol abuse and chronic pancreatitis. The pain has been worsening over the last 4 months. Physical examination shows a palpable upper abdominal mass. A CT scan of the abdomen shows a large cystic mass confirming a pancreatic pseudocyst.

Which of the following is the typical topographic location for this type of pseudocyst?

A. Right subhepatic space
B. Hepatorenal space
C. Omental bursa
D. Right subphrenic space
E. Greater sac

163. A 38-year-old man comes to the outpatient clinic because of mild abdominal pain for 2 years duration. Physical examination shows a dull pain located primarily in the left upper quadrant around the xiphoid process. An upper endoscopy confirms the diagnosis of gastric ulcer. At which of the following spinal nerve levels are the neuronal cell bodies located for the sensory fibers in such a case of gastric ulcer?

A. T5–T6
B. T6–T8
C. T7–T8
D. T9–L1
E. T5–T9

164. A 43-year-old man is brought to the emergency department by his wife because of abdominal pain and an episode of vomiting. A CT scan of the abdomen shows an internal hernia involving the duodenum at the left paraduodenal fossa (of Landzert). He undergoes an exploratory laparotomy, which shows a paraduodenal hernia. Which of the following arteries is most likely at risk during the repair of this hernia?

A. Middle colic
B. Sigmoidal
C. Ileocolic
D. Ileal
E. Ascending branches of left colic

165. A 62-year-old man is brought to the emergency department because of severe epigastric abdominal pain that radiates to his back. He has unintentionally lost 11.3 Kg (25 lb) over the last 3 months. He has at 40-year history of smoking two packs of cigarettes a day. Physical examination shows jaundice and a nontender palpable right upper quadrant mass. A CT scan of the abdomen shows a tumor at the neck of the pancreas. A biopsy confirms ductal adenocarcinoma. Which of the following structures will first receive metastatic cells?

A. Stomach
B. Spleen
C. Duodenum
D. Liver
E. Vertebral column

166. A 62-year-old man is brought to the emergency department because of worsening epigastric pain, clay-colored stool, and jaundice. He has diabetes and a 35-year smoking history. Physical examination shows a nontender palpable gallbladder. A CT scan of the abdomen shows pancreatic ductal adenocarcinoma at the neck of the pancreas. A major vessel also

appears to be nearly occluded. Which of the following vessels would be the most likely to be obstructed?

A. Inferior mesenteric vein
B. Hepatic portal vein
C. Celiac trunk
D. Posterior superior pancreaticoduodenal artery
E. Great pancreatic artery

167. A 49-year-old obese woman is brought to the emergency department because of a steady, aching right upper quadrant abdominal pain. Physical examination shows the pain radiates toward the patient's right side and posteriorly toward the scapula. There is no evidence of icterus of the skin or conjunctiva. An ultrasound of the abdomen shows cholecystitis with a large gallstone. In which of the following structures is the gallstone most likely located?

A. Bile duct
B. Hartmann pouch
C. Left hepatic duct
D. Pancreatic duct
E. Right hepatic duct

168. A 47-year-old woman is brought to the emergency department because of yellowing of the skin and severe aching epigastric pain. Physical examination shows the pain migrates toward the patient's right side and posteriorly toward the scapula. An ultrasound of the abdomen shows cholecystitis with a large gallstone. Which of the following is the most likely site for a gallstone to lodge?

A. Bile duct
B. Hepatopancreatic ampulla (of Vater)
C. Left hepatic duct
D. Pancreatic duct
E. Right hepatic duct

169. A 26-year-old woman comes to the physician because of a palpable mass in the midline of the abdominal wall several inches above the level of the umbilicus. Physical examination shows a nontender soft palpable mass which is reproducible with coughing and straining. Which of the following is the most likely diagnosis?

A. Umbilical hernia
B. Spigelian hernia
C. Epigastric hernia
D. Femoral hernia
E. Omphalocele

170. A 23-year-old man is brought to the emergency department after being stabbed in the epigastric region. His blood pressure is 96/60 mm Hg, pulse is 120/min, and respirations are 20/min. He is taken to surgery for an exploratory laparotomy. When the abdomen is opened for inspection, the liver is noted to be injured between the bed of the gallbladder and the falciform ligament, and is bleeding profusely. The Pringle maneuver is performed with a nontraumatic vascular clamp, but blood continues spurting from

the surface of the liver. Which part of the liver and which artery is most likely injured?

A. Lateral segment of the left lobe and the left hepatic artery

B. Caudate segment of the liver, with injury both to right and left hepatic arteries

C. Anterior segment of the right lobe, with injury to the right hepatic artery

D. Medial segment of the left lobe, with injury to an aberrant left hepatic artery

E. Quadrate lobe, with injury to the middle hepatic branch of the right hepatic artery

171. A 47-year-old man is brought to the physician because of severe epigastric pain for the last year. He has a history of peptic ulcer pain which improves with food and worsens few hours following a meal. Lifestyle modifications and pharmacologic treatment with proton pump inhibitors have not resolved his pain. In order to relieve his chronic refractory case of peptic ulcers, the patient undergoes bilateral vagotomy with division of both vagal trunks at the esophageal hiatus. Which of the following conditions will most likely occur?

A. Parasympathetic supply to the descending colon is lost.

B. The patient would no longer have contraction of the urinary bladder.

C. The patient would become impotent.

D. The patient would be sterile because of paralysis of the ductus deferens and ejaculatory duct.

E. Parasympathetic supply to the ascending colon would be reduced or absent.

172. A 35-year-old man is brought to the emergency department because of intense abdominal pain of 1-hour duration. He also has pain in his right shoulder. Physical examination shows a distended, rigid abdomen which is immobile during respiration, and tender to palpation. A diagnosis of adynamic (paralytic) ileus resulting from a ruptured peptic ulcer is made. An ultrasound examination of the abdomen shows very little bleeding into the peritoneal cavity. Which of the following conditions will most likely occur?

A. x-rays would not show the presence of air under his diaphragm.

B. Borborygmi would be decreased in frequency and amplitude.

C. He probably suffered from a posterior penetrating ulcer rather than from an anterior perforating ulcer.

D. The patient's ulcer probably occurred in the second part of the duodenum.

E. The patient probably had acute appendicitis.

173. A 68-year-old woman is brought to the emergency department with left lower quadrant pain. The patient has been experiencing long-term effects of diverticulosis and inflammation of the transverse colon. Physical

examination shows tenderness upon palpation at the left lower quadrant. To permit operating on a patient with severe diverticulosis of the transverse colon, it would be necessary to first ligate (tie off) or clamp the source of arterial supply. Which of the following arteries will most likely be ligated?

A. Middle colic

B. Right colic

C. Superior mesenteric

D. Ileocolic

E. Left colic

174. A 27-year-old man is brought to the emergency department by his girlfriend because of abdominal pain, nausea, and 2 episodes of vomiting. His blood pressure is 126/88 mm Hg, pulse is 105/min, respirations are 16/min, and temperature is 36.6°C (98°F). Physical examination shows tenderness to palpation in the periumbilical area. This region receives its sensory supply from which of the following spinal nerves?

A. T7

B. T8

C. T10

D. T12

E. L1

Questions 175–199

175. A 55-year-old man is brought to the emergency department by his daughter after he was found being belligerent and wandering on the street. His medical records show a history of alcohol abuse for the past 7 years. Physical examination shows a disoriented man who is slurring his words; his skin is yellow. His breath is found to have a strong odor. Laboratory studies show severe portal hypertension. Which of the following is a severe feature of the development of this condition?

A. Esophageal varices—from increased pressure in the right gastric vein

B. Ascites—from effusion of fluid from the inferior mesenteric vein

C. Internal hemorrhoids—from increased pressure within the superior mesenteric vein and its tributaries

D. Expansion of veins within the falciform ligament, which anastomose with veins of the umbilical region

E. Recanalization and expansion of the vessels within the medial umbilical ligaments

176. A 24-year-old woman comes to the emergency department because of pain and a bulge lateral to pubic tubercle. The patient is a gymnast and noticed the bulge while training. A diagnosis of a femoral hernia is made, and a laparoscopic repair is performed. During the procedure, the iliopubic tract is traced medially to the site of the femoral herniation. Which of the following best characterizes this structure?

A. The iliopubic tract represents the aponeurotic origin of the transversus abdominis.

B. The iliopubic tract forms the lateral border of the inguinal triangle (of Hesselbach).

C. The iliopubic tract forms the lateral border of the femoral ring.

D. The iliopubic tract is the part of the inguinal ligament that attaches to the pectineal ligament.

E. The iliopubic tract is the lateral extension of the pectineal ligament.

177. A 47-year-old man is brought to the emergency department because of abdominal pain, nausea, and constipation. He also has a loss of appetite. The pain was diffuse but is now more localized to the right lower quadrant. His blood pressure is 128/86 mm Hg, pulse is 108/min, respirations are 18/min, and temperature is 37.83°C (100.1°F). Physical examination shows tenderness to palpation, rebound tenderness, and positive Rovsing sign. A diagnosis of appendicitis is made, and an appendectomy is performed. During the open operative procedure atypical embryologic rotation of the intestine, adhesions, and adipose tissue made it difficult to identify the appendix. Most commonly, the vermiform appendix is best located by locating and tracing which of the following structures?

A. Anterior cecal artery

B. Descending branch of the right colic artery

C. Ileum to the ileocecal juncture

D. Posterior cecal artery

E. Taeniae coli of the ascending colon

178. A 2-day-old girl is brought to the physician after experiencing an episode of bilious vomiting. The girl has also failed to pass her first stool. Physical examination shows abdominal distention with no stool in the rectal vault. A CT scan of the abdomen shows an abnormally dilated descending colon and a diagnosis of Hirschsprung disease (megacolon) is made. What is the embryologic mechanism responsible for this disease?

A. Failure of neural crest cells to migrate into the walls of the colon

B. Incomplete separation of the cloaca

C. Failure of recanalization of the colon

D. Defective rotation of the hindgut

E. Oligohydramnios

179. A 32-year-old man comes to the physician because of left groin pain for the past 4 days. He was lifting weights at the gym when he had a sudden onset of pain in this left groin. He noticed a bulge in the same area and was able to reduce it. He says that the bulge comes and goes sporadically. Physical examination shows an indirect inguinal hernia due to its location on the abdominal wall. Which nerve is most likely responsible for the pain transmission?

A. Iliohypogastric

B. Lateral femoral cutaneous

C. Ilioinguinal

D. Lumbar splanchnic

E. Greater thoracic splanchnic

180. A 65-year-old man comes to the physician because of a rash on his abdomen for the past 2 days. He says the rash was first itchy and then the area erupted with vesicles and pain. He describes the pain as severe and characterizes it as sharp and burning. Physical examination shows a vesicular rash around the umbilicus. A diagnosis of herpes zoster (shingles) is made. Which of the following spinal nerves contributes to this dermatome?

A. T8

B. T9

C. T10

D. T11

E. T12

181. A 68-year-old woman comes to the physician because of localized swelling on the right side of her back. Physical examination shows a fixed nontender mass. An ultrasound and MRI of the abdomen show a large heterogeneous soft tissue tumor in the posterior abdominal wall that has invaded the superior mesenteric plexus. Which of the following structures will most likely be affected?

A. Ascending colon

B. Rectum

C. Stomach

D. Descending colon

E. Kidney

182. A 35-year-old woman comes to the emergency department with nausea and periumbilical pain that localized to the right lower abdominal quadrant. Physical examination shows guarding on palpation with rebound tenderness. A diagnosis of appendicitis is made and an appendectomy is performed. Two weeks following the surgery, the patient has paresthesia over the anterior part of her right labium majus. Which nerve was most likely injured during the procedure?

A. Iliohypogastric and ilioinguinal

B. Ilioinguinal

C. Genital branch of genitofemoral

D. Subcostal

E. Obturator

183. A 54-year-old man comes to the physician because of loss of appetite and epigastric pain. He has lost 4.5 kg (10 lb) in the last 2 months unintentionally. A gastroscopy shows a tumor in the pyloric antrum of the stomach. A CT scan of the abdomen is ordered to evaluate the lymph node involvement. Which of the following nodes initially drain the pyloric antrum?

A. Celiac

B. Superior mesenteric

C. Inferior mesenteric

D. Lumbar

E. Hepatic

184. A 21-year-old man is brought to the emergency department with severe back pain. The pain is sharp

and severe and worsens with deep inspirations. Physical examination shows bruising and tenderness along the left lateral side of the back. An x-ray of the back shows a fractured angle of the eleventh rib on the left side. Which of the following organs is most likely at risk for injury?

A. Stomach
B. Descending colon
C. Kidney
D. Liver
E. Pancreas

185. A 32-year-old woman is brought to the emergency department because of upper abdominal pain. Physical examination shows a dull and burning type of pain that improves with meals but worsens 2 hours after. A CT scan of the abdomen shows evidence of an ulcer in the posterior wall of the duodenal cap. Which structure will most likely be affected if this ulcer perforates?

A. Hepatic portal vein
B. Superior mesenteric artery
C. Bile duct
D. Proper hepatic artery
E. Gastroduodenal artery

186. A 45-year-old man is brought to the emergency department with groin pain and a palpable mass just superior to the inguinal ligament. Physical examination shows the mass is reducible with no evidence of incarceration. A diagnosis of a hernia is made, and a surgical repair is performed. During the procedure a loop of intestine is noticed in the deep inguinal ring. Which type of hernia is this?

A. Direct inguinal
B. Umbilical
C. Femoral
D. Lumbar
E. Indirect inguinal

187. A 67-year-old woman is brought to the emergency department because of a 2-hour history of severe abdominal pain and associated pain in the right shoulder. Physical examination shows guarding and rebound tenderness. An x-ray of the abdomen shows air under the diaphragm. A CT scan of the abdomen shows a perforating ulcer in the posterior wall of the stomach, spilling stomach contents and blood directly into which of the following areas?

A. Right subhepatic space
B. Hepatorenal space
C. Omental bursa (lesser sac)
D. Right subphrenic space
E. Greater sac

188. A 55-year-old woman is brought to the emergency department with severe abdominal pain. She has a history of peptic ulcer disease and recently resumed a course of NSAIDs for arthritis pain in her knees. Physical examination of the abdomen shows a non-distended firm abdomen with guarding and rebound

tenderness. An ultrasound of the abdomen shows intraperitoneal fluid. A diagnosis of perforated peptic ulcer is made. Which of the following sites is least likely to show fluid collection in this patient?

A. Pouch of Morison
B. The rectouterine pouch
C. The right paracolic gutter
D. The greater sac
E. The omental bursa

189. A 45-year-old woman is brought to the emergency department because of a 1-day history of severe right-side lower abdominal pain. Initially, the pain was poorly localized to the umbilical region, 2 days ago. Physical examination shows a nondistended abdomen with guarding and tenderness maximally at McBurney point. Bowel sounds are decreased upon auscultation. An ultrasound of the abdomen shows fluid in the right paracolic gutter. Which of the following mechanisms best explains the initial periumbilical pain this patient experienced?

A. Sympathetic supply to the appendix and somatic sensation to the umbilicus share the same spinal cord levels.
B. Parasympathetic supply to the appendix shares the same spinal cord levels with the umbilicus.
C. Somatic afferents of the peritoneum were stimulated by the inflamed appendix.
D. Somatic afferents travel with visceral afferents to T10 spinal cord level.
E. Somatic afferents synapse with visceral afferents of T10 spinal cord level.

190. A 45-year-old woman is brought to the emergency department because of a 1-day history of abdominal pain and vomiting. She has a history of GERD and was previously diagnosed with gallstones. Initially, her pain was poorly localized at the epigastric region, but became sharp and well localized in the right hypochondrium. Physical examination shows a positive Murphy sign. Which of the following mechanisms best explains the initial pattern of pain?

A. Visceral afferent fibers synapse with sympathetic fibers at T7–T9 spinal cord levels
B. Visceral afferent and sympathetic fibers to the gallbladder share T7–T9 spinal cord levels
C. Gallbladder inflammation spread to diaphragmatic peritoneum supplied by phrenic nerve
D. The inflamed gallbladder contacted the abdominal peritoneum at dermatomes T7–T9
E. Visceral afferents travel with intercostal nerves back to T7–T9 spinal cord levels

191. A 28-year-old woman delivers a healthy infant at term after an uncomplicated pregnancy. His birth weight was 3500 g (7 lb 11 oz), and Apgar scores were 8 and 10 at 1 and 5 minutes, respectively. Physical examination shows a clear fluid draining from the umbilicus of the infant. Fluid is collected and a urine dipstick test is performed on the sample. The fluid is determined

to be urine. Which of the following developmental defects best explains this finding?

A. Obliterated distal end of the urachus
B. Obliterated proximal end of the urachus
C. Completely patent urachus
D. Patent urachus at one point along its length
E. Completely obliterated urachus

192. A 33-year-old woman is brought to the emergency department because of sharp, well-demarcated, right-side abdominal pain of 1-day duration. She is also experiencing a low-grade fever, 2 episodes of vomiting, and loose stools. Physical examination shows tenderness on palpation at one-third of the distance from the anterior iliac spine to the umbilicus. There is also guarding and rebound tenderness. A urine HCG test is negative. Which of the following mechanisms best explains the distribution of pain in this patient?

A. Visceral afferents of the appendix travel with sympathetics to T10 spinal cord level
B. Inflamed visceral peritoneum stimulates somatic intercostal nerves
C. The appendix is a midgut structure, thus, pain is referred to T10 and T11 dermatomes
D. Contact of inflamed appendix with visceral peritoneum stimulates visceral afferents
E. Contact of inflamed appendix with parietal peritoneum stimulates somatic afferents

193. An 81-year-old man is brought to the emergency department because of left-side abdominal pain and fever for the past 2 days. Physical examination shows a soft and tender abdomen but in the left lumbar region there is a firm mass. The psoas sign is negative and bowel sounds are decreased upon auscultation. A CT scan of the abdomen shows evidence of a large perinephric abscess. Which of the following will most likely describe the fluid location?

A. Between renal fascia and transversalis fascia
B. Between the renal capsule and renal fascia
C. Between transversalis fascia and peritoneal fascia
D. Between the renal cortex and renal capsule
E. Within the paranephric fat

194. A 55-year-old woman is brought to the emergency department because of upper abdominal pain. Physical examination shows epigastric pain, burning in nature, that worsens after eating spicy or greasy foods. The pain improves with chewable antacids. She has no shortness of breath or diaphoresis. The patient is diagnosed with GERD and she is started on lifestyle modification and a trial of proton pump inhibitors. Which of the following organs is not derived from the same embryological structure as this patient's stomach?

A. Spleen
B. Right bronchus
C. Second part of the duodenum
D. Tail of the pancreas
E. Right lobe of the liver

195. A 45-year-old woman is brought to the emergency department by her husband because of severe abdominal pain, vomiting, and fever. The pain was initially poorly localized to the epigastrium but became sharp and settled to the right hypochondrium. The pain radiates to her right shoulder. Her temperature is 40°C (104°F), pulse is at 110/min and respirations are 18/min. Physical examination shows dry mucous membranes, icteric, with a soft and tender abdomen and a positive Murphy sign. An ultrasound of the abdomen shows thickening of the wall of the gallbladder but no free fluid in the abdomen. Laboratory studies show elevated serum bilirubin. An endoscopic retrograde cholangiopancreatography (ERCP) is performed and shows an obstruction along the extrahepatic biliary tree with normal pancreatic duct flow. Which structure is most likely obstructed?

A. The infundibulum of the gallbladder
B. The cystic duct
C. The bile duct
D. The hepatopancreatic ampulla
E. The left hepatic duct

196. A 72-year-old woman is brought to the emergency department because of a 3-day history of abdominal pain, fever, vomiting, diarrhea, and anorexia. She has a history of atrial fibrillation but refuses to take warfarin because it makes her feel unwell. Her pulse is 140/min, blood pressure 90/5 mm Hg, respirations are 20/min, and temperature is 40°C (104°F). Physical examination shows an ill appearing woman with pale skin and dry mucous membranes. Her abdomen is distended with tenderness upon palpation of the epigastric and umbilical regions. There is guarding and rebound tenderness. Bowel sounds are absent. An x-ray of the abdomen shows dilated small bowel with air-fluid levels displaying a "stacked coins" appearance. A diagnosis of mesenteric ischemia secondary to embolus to intestinal vessels is made. If the superior mesenteric artery is occluded, how could the midgut receive its blood supply?

A. Anastomosis between left and right gastric arteries
B. Anastomosis between left and right gastroepiploic arteries
C. Anastomosis between left and right gastro-omental arteries
D. Anastomosis between superior and inferior pancreaticoduodenal arteries
E. Anastomosis between adjacent short gastric arteries

197. A 72-year-old man is brought to the emergency department because of severe abdominal pain that started suddenly 1 hour ago. The patient has a history of diverticular disease, smokes a pack of cigarettes a week, and drinks 12 beers every weekend. His blood pressure is 100/50 mm Hg, pulse is 110/min, respirations are 30/min, and is afebrile. Physical examination shows a diaphoretic man with a firm abdomen

and tenderness in the epigastrium. He also has guarding and rebound tenderness. A CT of the abdomen shows pneumoperitoneum under the diaphragm. An exploratory laparotomy shows perforation of the posterior wall of the third part of the duodenum. Which of the following structures is most likely in immediate danger in this patient?

A. Aorta and inferior vena cava
B. Superior mesenteric artery and vein
C. Head of the pancreas
D. Transverse colon
E. Greater curvature of the stomach

198. A 51-year-old man is brought to the emergency department after a 2-month history of difficulty swallowing, vomiting, and weight loss. The patient has a history of GERD and was treated with antibiotics for *Helicobacter pylori* infection 10 years previously. He also has a 20-pack per year history of smoking. Physical examination shows a soft nontender abdomen. An ultrasound of the abdomen shows a 4 × 6 cm hard, irregular nonpulsatile and nontender mass resembling a Sister Mary Joseph nodule in the umbilical area. A CT scan of the abdomen shows a large mass involving the stomach in the region of the lesser curvature. Which of the following structures is most likely at immediate risk of damage by the tumor in this patient?

A. Right and left gastro-omental vessels
B. Right and left pancreaticoduodenal vessels
C. Right and left gastric vessels
D. The portal triad
E. Short gastric vessels

199. A 55-year-old woman comes to the physician because of 3-day history of pale colored stool and tea-colored urine. Physical examination shows yellowing of the sclerae. An ultrasound of the abdomen shows dilation of the biliary tree. Laboratory studies show:

Increased serum bilirubin to be elevated at 5 mg/dL,
Increased alanine aminotransferase (ALT),
Increased aspartate aminotransferase (AST),
Increased alkaline phosphatase (ALP),
Increased gamma-glutamyl transferase (GGT),
Increased prothrombin time.

She is diagnosed with cholestasis and scheduled for a laparoscopic cholecystectomy. During the procedure, she is found to have an aberrant cystic artery. What are the boundaries of the triangle of Calot?

A. Inferior border of the left ventricle (LV), cystic duct, common hepatic duct
B. Gallbladder, hepatic duct, bile duct
C. Inferior border of LV, bile duct, common hepatic duct
D. Cystic artery, inferior border of LV, bile duct
E. Cystic artery, common hepatic duct, bile duct

Questions 200–223

200. A 10-year-old boy is brought to the emergency department after falling down a hill and hitting a tree trunk while camping. Physical examination shows bruising and tenderness on the abdominal wall. A CT scan of the abdomen shows a laceration of the body of the pancreas with hemorrhaging around the vessel traveling along the superior border of the pancreas. This vessel is identified as which of the following?

A. Superior mesenteric artery
B. Hepatic portal vein
C. Left gastric artery
D. Splenic artery
E. Left gastro-omental artery

201. A 5-year-old girl is brought to the emergency department because of fever and severe abdominal pain. Her blood pressure is 130/85 mm Hg, pulse is 115/min, respirations are 20/min, and temperature is 38.8°C (102°F). She is suspected of having an acute appendicitis. During physical examination, she keeps her right thigh flexed and resists extension at the hip. If the thigh is extended there is severe pain caused by stretching the irritated parietal peritoneum lying over which of the following muscles?

A. Psoas major
B. External abdominal oblique
C. Obturator internus
D. Transversus abdominis
E. Quadratus lumborum

202. A 40-year-old obese woman is brought to the emergency department because of severe right upper abdominal pain. The pain radiates to the right shoulder and worsens after eating a meal. Physical examination shows cessation of breathing on deep palpation of the right upper quadrant. A diagnosis of acute cholecystitis is made and she undergoes a laparoscopic cholecystectomy. Which of the following structures would most likely be identified and ligated within the triangle of Calot?

A. Bile duct
B. Right hepatic duct
C. Cystic duct
D. Right hepatic artery
E. Cystic artery

203. A 34-year-old man is brought to the emergency department after a motor vehicle collision. His blood pressure is 90/50 mm Hg, pulse is 120/min, respirations are 30/min, and afebrile. An ultrasound of the abdomen shows a lacerated spleen requiring an urgent splenectomy. During the procedure, the blood supply of the spleen is ligated at its hilum. Improper placement of the ligature may occlude the arteries that supply which of the following structures?

A. Fundus of the stomach
B. Kidney
C. Pyloric sphincter
D. Head of the pancreas
E. Splenic flexure of the colon

204. A 55-year-old man is brought to the emergency department with severe abdominal pain. Physical

examination shows abdominal swelling, icterus of the skin, and vascular markings surrounding the umbilicus. The patient has a history of alcohol abuse with cirrhosis and a diagnosis of portal hypertension is made. A CT scan of the chest at the vertebra level T7 shows a circular grey structure immediately anterior to the vertebral bodies and just to the right of midline. The structure appears to be much larger than usual. Given the location and the patient's history what is this structure?

A. Inferior vena cava
B. Superior vena cava
C. Esophagus
D. Azygos vein
E. Pulmonary vein

205. A 65-year-old man comes to the emergency department because of pain at his right costovertebral angle and hematuria. He has a 40-pack-per-year smoking history and has one drink a week. A CT scan of the abdomen shows a mass confined within the renal fascia of the right kidney. The patient is scheduled for surgical removal of the mass. Using a posterolateral approach to reach the kidney, which of the following layers will most likely have to be incised?

A. Parietal pleura
B. Diaphragmatic pleura
C. Parietal peritoneum
D. Transversalis fascia
E. Visceral peritoneum

206. A 43-year-old obese woman is brought to the emergency department with a severe upper right quadrant abdominal pain. The pain started suddenly and worsens after meals. Physical examination shows tenderness upon palpation of the right upper quadrant. An ultrasound of the abdomen shows thickened inflamed gallbladder walls with several large echogenic gallstones. She has acute cholecystitis and is scheduled for a laparoscopic cholecystectomy. During the procedure, the scope is passed into the greater sac through a small port in the anterior abdominal wall. Which of the following organs is the physician unable to view directly?

A. Ileum
B. Jejunum
C. Pancreas
D. Stomach
E. Transverse colon

207. A 2-year-old boy is brought to the emergency department by his mother after an episode of bright red blood per rectum in his diaper. The boy does not appear to be in distress, but he cries during palpation of the right lower quadrant. A technetium-99 scan shows a 2-inch long spot of radioactive accumulation in the midabdomen. Which of the following is the most likely diagnosis?

A. Gastritis
B. Hirschsprung disease

C. Hemorrhoids
D. Meckel diverticulum
E. Anal fissure

208. A 21-year-old man is brought to the emergency department because of a 5-day history of high fever. He reports having a small stab wound in his back a few months ago; however, since it was a shallow wound, he did not seek medical attention. His pulse is 100/min, blood pressure 124/86 mm Hg, respirations are 22/min, and temperature 39.4°C (103°F). Blood chemistry shows a high white blood cell count. A diagnosis of a retroperitoneal abdominal infection is made. Which of the following structures is most likely to be affected?

A. Descending colon
B. Jejunum
C. Stomach
D. Transverse colon
E. Appendix

209. A 68-year-old man is brought to the emergency department because of a sudden onset of right lower back pain with associated loss of sensation in the right posterolateral gluteal and right anterior pubic regions. Physical examination shows tenderness to palpation at the region inferior to the twelfth rib at the right costovertebral angle. There is also weakness of the right internal abdominal oblique and transversus abdominis muscles. A CT scan of the abdomen shows a tumor that originates in the right kidney, breaks through the center of the posterior renal capsule and is pressing on the ipsilateral quadratus lumborum muscle. Which of the following nerves is most likely compressed by the tumor?

A. Subcostal
B. Lateral femoral cutaneous nerve
C. Ilioinguinal
D. Femoral
E. Iliohypogastric

210. A 15-year-old boy who is an amateur bodybuilder has begun an intensive abdominal workout routine. His goal is to develop a "6-pack" by incorporating sit-ups and crunches to his workout regimen. The muscle that this adolescent is isolating in his workout to get this "6-pack" attaches to which of the following skeletal areas?

A. Iliac crest
B. Ribs 10–12
C. Pubic crest
D. Costal cartilages 7–12
E. Xiphoid process

211. A 52-year-old man is brought to the emergency department by his wife because of severe difficulty in swallowing solids that has been getting worse over the last 5 years. He has a burning, retrosternal pain which no longer resolves with antacids. He is scheduled to undergo an esophagogastroduodenoscopy. During the procedure the endoscope is advanced until its tip

reached the esophageal hiatus of the diaphragm. At which of the following vertebral levels did the tip of the endoscope most likely end?

A. T7
B. T8
C. T10
D. T11
E. T12

212. A 65-year-old man comes to the emergency department because of a pulsatile mass in his abdomen. An ultrasound of the abdomen shows an abdominal aortic aneurysm and he is urgently taken to an operating room. At exploration, the patient's abdominal aortic aneurysm is repaired using an endovascular graft where the center of the graft was in-line with the subcostal plane. The center of the graft is most likely anterior to which of the following vertebrae?

A. L1
B. L2
C. L3
D. L4
E. L5

213. A 59-year-old man comes to the emergency department for an abdominal pain. The patient has a long history of alcoholism and cirrhosis. A CT scan shows a tumor in the liver, and the patient is scheduled to undergo right hepatectomy. During the surgery the liver is divided in the principal plane. Which of the following liver segments will most likely be removed?

A. V, VI, VII, VIII
B. IV, V, VI, VII
C. III, IV, V, VI
D. II, III, IV, V
E. I, II, III, IV

214. A 50-year-old man with a long history of alcohol abuse comes to the emergency department with a severe abdominal pain. Physical examination of his abdomen shows caput medusae. The blood vessel that is obstructed in this patient is most likely formed by the union of which of the following vessels?

A. Right and left common iliac arteries
B. Superior mesenteric and left gastric veins
C. Inferior mesenteric and left gastric veins
D. Inferior mesenteric and paraumbilical veins
E. Superior mesenteric and splenic veins

215. A 65-year-old man comes to the emergency department because of a dull abdominal pain. The patient is found to have a tumor in the middle of the posterior wall of the stomach that perforated the stomach at this location. A CT scan of the abdomen shows that the stomach fluid has traversed the resultant aperture. Which of the following spaces did the fluid most likely first enter after it traversed the aperture?

A. Supracolic compartment
B. Omental foramen
C. Infracolic compartment

D. Paracolic gutter
E. Omental bursa

216. A 68-year-old woman comes to the emergency department because of 2-hour history of a sharp abdominal pain. A CT scan of the abdomen shows complete occlusion of the inferior vena cava at the L3 vertebral level. As a result of the occlusion, which of the following veins most likely acted as collateral channels to allow blood to flow from the lower to upper parts of her body?

A. Left common iliac
B. Hemiazygos
C. Ascending lumbar
D. Azygos
E. Left renal

217. A 19-year-old man comes to the emergency department after a gang fight, sustaining a shot with a 9mm bullet to his right lower quadrant. The bullet entered and traversed the anterolateral abdominal wall. The following structures form the layers of this wall:

A. Internal abdominal oblique muscle
B. Transversalis fascia
C. Transversus abdominis muscle
D. Camper fascia
E. Scarpa fascia
F. External abdominal oblique muscle

Which of the following best represents the order of structures traversed by the bullet?

A. 4-5-6-1-3-2
B. 4-5-2-6-1-3
C. 4-5-1-6-3-2
D. 4-2-6-1-3-5
E. 5-4-6-1-3-2

218. A 72-year-old man comes to the emergency department because of 1-day history of bloody stools. The patient has a family history of colon cancer and is scheduled for colonoscopy the next day. The scope typically passes through the entire colon in order to examine for any abnormal surface changes in the lumen of the colon. Which of the following colonic landmarks is indicative that the end of the colon has been reached?

A. Hepatic flexure
B. Splenic flexure
C. Paracolic gutter
D. Ileocecal valve
E. GE junction

219. A 55-year-old man comes to the emergency department because of 2-hour history of vomiting blood. He has a history of cirrhosis of the liver due to a chronic hepatitis B infection. He also has a 2-month history of abdominal distention, dilated veins over the anterior abdominal wall, and rectal varices. The anastomosis of which portal system vein with the esophageal veins can result in the hematemesis?

A. Right gastric
B. Periumbilical

C. Left gastric

D. Splenic

E. Left gastro-omental

220. A 55-year-old man comes to the emergency department because of a 3-month history of nausea and abdominal pain around his umbilical area. Physical examination shows rebound tenderness in the right lower quadrant with involuntary guarding. A CT scan of the abdomen shows inflamed appendix that is 28 mm in diameter. Which nerve fibers carried the pain from the inflamed organ?

A. Somatic afferents

B. Preganglionic sympathetic

C. Preganglionic parasympathetic

D. Postganglionic sympathetic

E. Visceral afferent

221. A 32-year-old man comes to the emergency department with severe pain in the left lower quadrant radiating over his lower back. Physical examination shows bloody stains on his underwear and subsequent urinalysis showed positive blood. An ultrasound of the abdomen shows that the ureters are of normal size, but the left renal pelvis appears enlarged and the renal calyces were rounded and blunted because of a kidney stone. Where is the most likely location for this stone to be lodged?

A. Urethra

B. Urinary bladder

C. Ureter at the uretero-vesical junction

D. Ureter at the pelvic brim

E. Ureter at the uretero-pelvic junction

222. A 49-year-old man comes to the emergency department because of a 3-month history of worsening acute abdominal pain and jaundice. The patient has a history of chronic pancreatitis and had an unintentional weight loss of 9 kg (20 lb) for the past 3 months. A CT scan of the abdomen shows a 3 cm tumor at the head of the pancreas. The tumor will most likely obstruct which of the following structures?

A. Bile duct

B. Common hepatic duct

C. Left hepatic duct

D. Cystic duct

E. Right hepatic duct

223. A 47-year-old man comes to the emergency department because of severe abdominal pain and bloated abdomen. An upright x-ray shows a free air under the diaphragm and he is urgently taken to the operating room. At exploration, the patient was found to have a perforated duodenal ulcer and part of the small bowel was resected. During the procedure the gastroduodenal artery is ligated. A branch of which artery will continue to supply blood to the duodenum in this patient?

A. Splenic

B. Left gastric

C. Right gastric

D. Proper hepatic

E. Superior mesenteric

Questions 224–244

224. A 70-year-old woman comes to the emergency department because of 3-month history of intense abdominal pain. A CT scan of the abdomen shows a 2 cm tumor at the head of the pancreas. A neurectomy is performed to interrupt the neural pathway carrying pain from the pancreas. Which of the following neural structure was most likely severed?

A. Vagus nerve

B. Phrenic nerve

C. Celiac ganglion

D. Aorticorenal ganglion

E. Inferior mesenteric ganglion

225. A 39-year-old woman comes to the emergency department with pain in her right side that radiates to the suprapubic region. She also has hematuria and a history of urinary tract infections. A CT scan of the abdomen shows polycystic kidney disease and a stretched kidney capsule. Which nerve will transmit the pain to the CNS?

A. Greater thoracic splanchnic nerve

B. Lesser thoracic splanchnic nerve

C. Pelvic splanchnic nerve

D. Celiac plexus

E. Iliohypogastric nerve

226. A 21-year-old woman comes to the emergency department for an abdominal pain radiating from her lower back toward her pubic symphysis. A kidney stone is suspected, and an ultrasound of the abdomen shows a stone partially obstructing the lower part of her right ureter. The stone is probably lodged where the ureter crosses which of the following structures?

A. Inferior vena cava

B. Internal iliac artery

C. Common iliac artery

D. Fourth lumbar artery

E. Inferior mesenteric artery

227. A 40-year-old woman comes to the emergency department because of jaundice and epigastric pain. Upper right quadrant ultrasound shows stones in the bile duct and gallbladder. The patient is scheduled for a laparoscopic cholecystectomy the next day. During surgery, the cystic artery and is ligated and cut. A branch from which nervous structure traveling along the artery was also cut?

A. Inferior mesenteric plexus

B. Superior mesenteric plexus

C. Celiac plexus

D. Renal plexus

E. Superior hypogastric plexus

228. Seven hours after delivery, the baby girl began crying and started to vigorously bilious vomit. Physical examination shows distended abdomen and small amounts of meconium. Two abdominal x-rays are

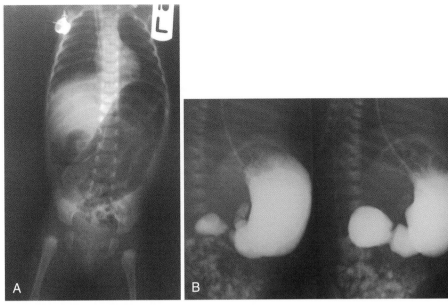

• **Fig. 3.9**

shown below (Fig. 3.9). Which of the following embryological abnormalities is the most likely cause of this condition?

A. Defect in the tracheoesophageal septum
B. Failure of the muscular tissue from the body wall to extend into the pleuroperitoneal membrane
C. Failure of recanalization of the duodenum
D. Malrotation of the intestines
E. Defective fusion of the pleuroperitoneal membranes

229. Autopsy of a newborn boy shows multiple congenital heart defects and absence of kidneys and poorly developed ureters bilaterally. Mother was 40 years old and had not had any prenatal care. If she had ultrasonography at 28 weeks' gestation, which of the following would most likely have shown?

A. Polyhydramnios
B. Annular pancreas
C. Malrotation of the gut
D. Bilateral gonadal dysgenesis
E. Oligohydramnios

230. A neonate was born at 34 weeks' gestation and was admitted to the emergency department for pneumonitis. A CT scan of the abdomen shows the upper segment of the esophagus ending blindly and the presence of an abnormal communication between trachea and the lower segment of esophagus. Which of the following clinical conditions is most likely seen with this congenital anomaly?

A. Polyhydramnios
B. Oligohydramnios
C. Anhydramnios
D. Umbilicoileal fistula
E. Down syndrome

231. A newborn boy has a foul-smelling yellow-brown discharge from his umbilicus. A catheter is inserted into a small opening in the umbilicus and contrast material is injected before acquiring an abdominal x-ray. An x-ray of the abdomen shows that the contrast material filled the loops of ileum through a small (4–5 cm) connection between the ileum and the umbilicus. Which of the following is the most likely diagnosis?

A. Ileal diverticulum
B. Ileal diverticulum with ulceration
C. Omphaloenteric fistula
D. Omphaloenteric cyst
E. Persistent vitelline artery

232. A 4-year-old boy comes to the emergency department for bile-stained vomiting. The patient does not have Down syndrome and was tolerating diet until a few weeks ago. He was followed up by the physician regularly and meeting all the developmental milestones. A CT scan of the abdomen shows an annular pancreas. Which structure is most likely obstructed by this condition?

A. Pylorus of the stomach
B. First part of the duodenum
C. Second part of the duodenum
D. Third part of the duodenum
E. Jejunum

233. A 2-year-old boy is brought to the physician because his parents noticed a gradually enlarging scrotal mass. Transillumination and scrotal ultrasound showed a large fluid collection around a normally developed testis. Which of the following structures has most likely developed abnormally?

A. Deep inguinal ring
B. Tunica albuginea
C. Processus vaginalis

    D. Gubernaculum

    E. Dartos tunic

234. A 25-year-old woman in the 8th month of pregnancy comes to the physician for a routine examination. An ultrasound examination of the abdomen of the fetus shows part of the small bowel herniating into the amniotic cavity due to failure of fusion of the lateral folds in the abdominal region. Which of the following conditions explains this presentation?

    A. Volvulus

    B. Nonrotated gut

    C. Situs inversus

    D. Gastroschisis

    E. Ileal diverticulum

235. A 35-year-old woman delivers a 4.5 kg (10 lb) girl with no complications. However, she had not had any prenatal care during pregnancy. The newborn girl had typical facial features of Down syndrome and she begins vomiting shortly after her first feeding. The vomitus is stained with bile. Which condition is most likely causing the vomiting?

    A. Atresia of the third part of the duodenum

    B. Atresia of the first part of the duodenum

    C. Congenital hypertrophic pyloric stenosis

    D. Esophageal stenosis

    E. TEF

236. A 2-day-old girl is brought to the physician because of a low-grade fever for 2 days. An x-ray of the abdomen shows malrotation of the small intestine with unfixed mesenteries. The vessels around the duodenojejunal junction are obstructed and there is progression to gangrene of the small intestine. Which of the following is the most likely diagnosis?

    A. Diaphragmatic atresia

    B. Subhepatic cecum

    C. Midgut volvulus

    D. Duplication of the intestine

    E. Congenital megacolon

237. A 32-year-old man comes to the physician because of groin pain after weightlifting and swelling in his scrotum. Physical examination shows that the patient has an indirect inguinal hernia. Which nerve is most likely responsible for the pain transmission?

    A. Iliohypogastric

    B. Lateral femoral cutaneous

    C. Ilioinguinal

    D. Lumbar splanchnic

    E. Greater thoracic splanchnic

238. A 26-year-old man comes to the physician complaining because of areas of thickened scaly skin on his abdominal wall below the level of the umbilicus. An actinic keratosis is a suspected, which is a premalignant condition and can progress to squamous cell carcinoma. Which lymph nodes will first receive drainage from this area of skin?

    A. Deep inguinal

    B. External iliac

    C. Internal iliac

    D. Lateral aortic

    E. Superficial inguinal

239. A 33-year-old man is admitted to the emergency department for a scheduled vasectomy. During the procedure the physician separates the various layers covering the spermatic cord to expose the ductus deferens so that it can be ligated and cut. From which of the following structures is the internal spermatic fascia derived?

    A. Internal abdominal oblique muscle

    B. Cremaster muscle

    C. External abdominal oblique muscle

    D. Transversus abdominis aponeurosis

    E. Transversalis fascia

240. A 45-year-old man comes to the emergency department with severe nausea and recurrent bilious vomiting. His symptoms initially began 1 month ago as postprandial epigastric pain, but have worsened during the past week. Physical examination shows a slightly tender and distended abdomen with high-pitched bowel sounds. A CT scan of the abdomen shows that the angle between the superior mesenteric artery and the aorta is significantly decreased. Which of the following structures is most likely to be obstructed by the artery?

    A. Ascending portion of the duodenum

    B. Descending portion of the duodenum

    C. Duodenal bulb

    D. Duodenojejunal flexure

    E. Transverse portion of the duodenum

241. A 70-year-old man is brought to the emergency department because of cramping mid-abdominal pain, abdominal distention, and vomiting for the past 24 hours. Physical examination shows positive Murphy sign and right upper quadrant ultrasound shows gallstones with gallbladder wall thickening. An x-ray of the abdomen shows air in the gallbladder and biliary tree. In which of the following sites is a gallstone most likely lodged?

    A. Cystic duct

    B. Bile duct

    C. Duodenum

    D. Jejunum

    E. Ileum

242. Which of the following age ranges best represents when the bones that form the acetabulum fuse?

    A. 13–15 years

    B. 16–18 years

    C. 19–21 years

    D. 22–24 years

    E. 25–27 years

243. A 68-year-old man comes to the emergency department because of pain during urination. Imaging and subsequent biopsy show a tumor that originated from the lining of the urinary bladder. During transurethral resection to remove the tumor, the cystoscope enters the urinary bladder. Which of the following structures will the cystoscope traverse immediately before entering the urinary bladder?

A. Intramural part of urethra
B. Membranous part of urethra
C. Prostatic urethra
D. Spongy urethra
E. Paraurethral part

244. A 38-year-old man is brought to the emergency department because of a swelling in his scrotum. The transillumination was negative for hydrocele and a diagnosis of metastatic cancer of the left testes is made. Which of the following most likely represents the route by which the cancer spread from the left testes to the rest of the body?

A. Left testicular vein; inferior vena cava; left renal vein
B. Right testicular vein; left testicular vein; inferior vena cava
C. Left testicular vein; left common iliac vein; inferior vena cava
D. Left testicular vein; median sacral vein; inferior vena cava
E. Left testicular vein; left renal vein; inferior vena cava

245. A 25-year-old woman comes to the physician for a routine examination. The patient is placed in the lithotomy position and a pelvic examination is performed. In order to palpate the patient's uterus, the index and middle fingers of the physicians' right hand were inside her vagina while he used his left hand to press on the abdomen inferior to the umbilicus. The physician concomitantly lowered his left palm onto the patient's skin and felt a bony structure in the lower midline. Which of the following structures did the physician most likely feel on the palm of his left hand?

A. Ilium
B. Coccyx
C. Sacrum
D. Ischium
E. Pubis

246. A 67-year-old man is brought to the emergency department because of an acute-onset right lower back pain with loss of sensation of the skin in the postero-lateral gluteal and anterior pubic regions on the right side. Physical examination shows severe tenderness inferior to the twelfth rib at the right costovertebral angle on palpation. The patient also has paralysis of the right internal abdominal oblique and transversus abdominis muscles. A CT scan of the abdomen shows a tumor that is originated from the right kidney, entering the posterior renal capsule, and pressing on the ipsilateral quadratus lumborum muscle. Which of the following nerves is most likely compressed by the tumor?

A. Subcostal
B. Lateral femoral cutaneous nerve
C. Ilioinguinal
D. Femoral
E. Iliohypogastric

Answers

Answers 1–25

1. A. The processus vaginalis (meaning sheath-like process) is composed of parietal peritoneum that precedes the testis as it "migrates" from a position in the upper lumbar wall to a position outside the abdomen. This process usually obliterates, leaving only a distal portion that surrounds most of the testis as the tunica vaginalis testis. Whereas these features are typical of development in males, females also have a processus vaginalis that extends into the labium majus, although congenital inguinal hernias are more common in men than in women. The other listed structures are not involved in congenital inguinal hernias.
   B, C, D, and E. These structures are not involved in the formation of the inguinal canal.
   GAS 289; N 264; ABR/McM 285, 288

2. A. Wilms tumor is a kidney malignancy that usually occurs in children. It has recently been shown that it can be caused by mutations in the *WT1* gene, behaving according to the Knudson 2-hit model for tumor suppressor genes.
   B, C, D, and E. These genes are not involved in the mutations involved Wilms Tumors.
   GAS 373–374; N 311; ABR/McM 265, 268

3. C. During development, the kidneys typically "ascend" from a position in the pelvis to a position high on the posterior abdominal wall. Although the kidneys are bilateral structures, occasionally the inferior poles of the 2 kidneys fuse. When this happens, the "ascent" of the fused kidneys is arrested by the first midline structure they encounter, the inferior mesenteric artery. The incidence of horseshoe kidney is about 0.25% of the population.
   A. Interruption of the Müllerian duct fusion process gives rise to bicornuate uterus
   B. Cryptorchidism occurs when one or both of the testes fail to descend from the abdomen into the scrotum.
   D. Hypospadias is a congenital malformation of the urethra, where in the opening is located at the ventral surface of the penis instead of its normal location at the head of the penis.
   E. Renal agenesis is the congenital absence of renal tissue resulting from failure of one or both kidneys to develop during embryogenesis.
   GAS 373–374; N 312; ABR/McM 269, 260

4. C. In normal kidney development the kidneys function during the fetal period with the resulting urine

contributing to the fluid in the amniotic cavity. When the kidneys fail to develop (renal agenesis), this contribution to the fluid is missing and decreased amniotic fluid (oligohydramnios) results. The amniotic fluid can be assessed by measuring the amniotic fluid index. A normal amniotic fluid index is considered 5–25 cm using the standard assessment method. Less than 5 cm amniotic fluid index is considered as oligohydramnios, while over 25 is considered as polyhydramnios.

A. Anencephaly is a part of the spectrum of neural tube defects (NTDs). Anencephaly occurs when the upper portions of the neural tube fails to develop. This defect can be noticed during pregnancy with an ultrasound; additionally, alpha fetoprotein (AFP) levels are elevated in anencephaly.

B. Pyloric stenosis, also known as infantile hypertrophic pyloric stenosis, is a relatively common condition occurring within four to 6 weeks of birth. Pyloric stenosis is an acquired obstruction of the gastric outlet due to progressive thickening of the circular muscle of the pylorus. Infants present with projectile vomiting.

D. TEF is the abnormal development of the trachea and esophagus. There are several types of this malformation; however, the most common anomaly consists of a blind esophageal pouch and a distal TEF.

E. Urethral atresia is the congenital absence of the urethra. This condition is incompatible with life.
GAS 373–374; N 311; ABR/McM 265, 266

5. A. There is some evidence that oligohydramnios is linked to hypoplastic lungs. This is apparently not a genetic link but rather related to the importance of adequate amniotic fluid in normal lung development.

B. Genitourinary congenital abnormalities including polycystic kidney disease are reported to be associated with TEFs. However, these congenital abnormalities are not linked with oligohydramnios or hypoplastic lungs.

C. There are several maternal factors and congenital defects that can result in polyhydramnios. One maternal cause of polyhydramnios is diabetes mellitus, which also results in fetal hyperglycemia and fetal polyuria. Fetal polyuria increases amniotic fluid, thus leading to polyhydramnios. Fetal conditions where swallowing may be impaired, for example, anencephaly or esophageal atresia, can also result in polyhydramnios.

D. Renal agenesis will impair urine excretion of the fetus, leading to decreased amniotic fluid (oligohydramnios). Surfactant production is affected by the maturity of the fetus, not by renal agenesis.

E. Ectopic viscera obstructing the urethra is highly unlikely.
GAS 170, 373–374; N 215; ABR/McM 211

6. C. In normal pancreatic development, the ventral pancreatic bud rotates around the dorsal side of the gut tube and fuses with the dorsal pancreatic bud. Rarely, a portion of the ventral bud rotates around the ventral side of the gut tube, resulting in an annular pancreas. The portion of the gut tube that is affected is the same as where the pancreatic duct enters: the second part of the duodenum (along with the bile duct). The incidence of annular pancreas is about 1 in 7000.

A, B, D, and E. These structures will not be compressed by an annular pancreas.
GAS 366 N 288; ABR/McM 245

7. C. The distal portion of the processus vaginalis contributes to the tunica vaginalis testis that is related to the testis. If an intermediate portion of the processus vaginalis persists, it often fills with fluid, creating a hydrocele. If the entire processus vaginalis persists, the patient is likely to develop a congenital inguinal hernia.

A. Hypospadias is a congenital malformation of the urethra, where in the opening is located at the ventral surface of the penis instead of its normal location at the head of the penis.

B. A patent processus vaginalis will not affect male sterility.

D. Ectopic testis occurs when a testis fails to descend (cryptorchidism). This process is not affected by a patent processus vaginalis.

E. Epispadias is a congenital malformation of the urethra, in which the opening is located on the dorsal surface of the penis instead of its normal location at the head of the penis.
GAS 265; N 369; ABR/McM 278, 279

8. C. Cryptorchism, often called an undescended testis, is the result of incomplete migration of the gonad from the abdomen to a location in the scrotum where it is exposed to temperatures slightly lower than core body temperature. This is important for spermatogenesis and testicular function. A testis that cannot be surgically relocated into the scrotum is usually removed because it would otherwise be prone to develop testicular cancer.

A. Pseudohermaphroditism occurs when the gonads represent the chromosomal sex, but external genitalia express features of the opposite sex.

B. True hermaphroditism is defined as the coexistence of seminiferous tubules and ovarian follicles.

D. Congenital suprarenal hyperplasia occurs when there are aberrations in the biochemical synthetic pathways of the suprarenal gland hormones.

E. Chordee is a condition wherein which the head of the penis is curved (either upward or downward) at the junction of the head and the shaft of the penis. This abnormal curvature is most obvious during erection.
GAS 289; N 368; ABR/McM 278, 279

9. D. The lateral folds are key structures in forming the muscular portion of the anterior abdominal wall. Failure of the lateral folds can cause a minor defect, such as an umbilical hernia, or a major defect, such as gastroschisis.

A, B, C, and E. These other folds and the amnion are not involved in formation of the anterior abdominal wall.
GAS 261, 308; N 254; ABR/McM 232

10. A. Rotation of the gut tube is a major event in the development of the gastrointestinal system. Parts of the tube rotate 270 degrees, but the proximal foregut, specifically that portion that forms the esophagus, rotates only 90 degrees. Looking from below (the standard CT or MRI view), this rotation is counterclockwise. This brings the left vagus nerve onto the anterior surface of the esophagus as it passes through the thorax.

B, C, D, and E. The other rotations and position of the vagus nerve do not accurately depict the rotation of the gut tube and orientation of the left vagus nerve. *GAS 261, 363–364; N 270; ABR/McM 251, 267*

11. B. The diaphragm develops from several components. Initially, the septum transversum (which will become the central tendon) forms in the cervical region, gaining innervation from C3, C4, and C5. Later, myoblasts migrate in from the body wall to form the muscular part of the diaphragm, often considered to be 2 bilateral hemidiaphragms. These muscles are innervated by the phrenic nerves that are derived from C3, C4, and C5. Eventration of the diaphragm occurs when one muscular hemidiaphragm fails to develop. With positive pressure in the abdominal cavity, and low or negative pressure in the thoracic cavity, abdominal organs are pushed into the thorax. The pleuroperitoneal folds contribute to a portion of the diaphragm posteriorly.

A, C, D, and E. The other mechanisms mentioned will not cause eventration of the diaphragm. *GAS 371; N 200, 201; ABR/McM 225, 270*

12. D. The tracheoesophageal septum is the downgrowth that separates the ventral wall of the foregut (esophagus) from the laryngotracheal tube. The presence of a fistula would result in passage of fluid from the esophagus into the trachea and could cause aspiration pneumonia.

A. If the esophagus did not develop correctly, as in esophageal atresia, it would end as a blind tube. This kind of defect, although associated with TEF, is not the result of an opening into the trachea, and pneumonia would not result.

B. Abnormal tracheal development can be associated with TEF, therefore, but it is not the direct cause of it.

C. Abnormal tongue development does not result in a TEF.

E. Abnormal development of the pharynx is not associated with a TEF. *GAS 172; N 237; ABR/McM 208*

13. C. The septum transversum forms the central tendon of the diaphragm.

A. The pleuroperitoneal folds form the posterolateral part of the diaphragm.

B. The pleuropericardial folds separate the pericardial cavity from the pleural cavity and form the fibrous pericardium.

D. The cervical myotomes form the musculature of the diaphragm.

E. The dorsal part of the dorsal mesentery of the esophagus forms the crura of the diaphragm. *GAS 163; N 200, 201; ABR/McM 225, 270*

14. C. Midgut volvulus is a possible complication of malrotation of the midgut loop without fixed mesentery. The small intestines twist around the vasculature that is providing support for them. This can cause ischemic necrosis of the intestine, resulting in gangrene. A. Diaphragmatic atresia is not a cause of volvulus.

B. Subhepatic cecum is due to failure of the descent of the cecal bud and results in the absence of an ascending colon.

D. Duplication of the intestine would not cause volvulus because there would still be a fixed mesentery and no free movement of the intestines.

E. Congenital aganglionic megacolon is due to faulty migration of neural crest cells into the wall of the colon, resulting in a lack of parasympathetic postganglionic neurons and creating a functional blockage and an enlarged colon proximal to the block. *GAS 308; N 270; ABR/McM 290*

15. A. Congenital megacolon (Hirschsprung disease) results from the failure of neural crest cells to migrate into the walls of the colon.

B. Incomplete separation of the cloaca would result in anal agenesis either with or without the presence of a fistula.

C. The failure of recanalization of the colon results in rectal atresia, wherein both the anal canal and rectum exist but are not connected due to incomplete canalization or no recanalization.

D. Defective rotation of the hindgut can cause volvulus or twisting of its contents.

E. Oligohydramnios is a deficiency of amniotic fluid, which can cause pulmonary hypoplasia but would not cause Hirschsprung disease. *GAS 321; N 271; ABR/McM 249*

16. D. The distal ileum approximately 2 feet from the cecum is the most common site of Meckel diverticulum. This outpouching is a persistence of the vitelline duct and it can be attached to the umbilicus.

A, B, C, and E. The parts of the abdominal viscera presented in these options are not derived from the vitelline duct. *GAS 315; N 281; ABR/McM 233*

17. A. The most common site of ectopic pregnancy is in the uterine (fallopian) tube. Implantation in the internal os of the cervix can result in placenta previa, but the internal os of the cervix is not the most common site.

B, C, D, and E. The other choices listed are not the most common sites of ectopic pregnancy. The endometrium in the fundus of the uterus is the normal site of implantation. *GAS 471, 524 N 304; ABR/McM 287*

18. A. The greater thoracic splanchnic nerve carries general visceral afferent fibers from abdominal organs, specifically the foregut, and can be involved in the occurrence of referred pain.

B. The dorsal rami of thoracic spinal nerves carry general somatic afferent fibers. Pain from these fibers would result in sharp, localized pain not dull and diffuse as occurs in referred pain.

C. Although the phrenic nerve carries visceral afferent fibers, it does not innervate the gallbladder.

D. The vagus nerve carries visceral afferent fibers that are important for visceral reflexes, but they do not transmit pain.

E. The pelvic splanchnic nerves are parasympathetic nerves from S2 to S4 and contain visceral afferent fibers that transmit pain from the pelvis but not from the gallbladder.
GAS 358–365, 38; N 306; ABR/McM 246

19. **C.** An indirect inguinal hernia occurs when a loop of bowel enters the inguinal canal through the deep inguinal ring (lateral to the inferior epigastric vessels). The ilioinguinal nerve runs through the inguinal canal to innervate the anterior portion of the labium majus or scrotum and proximal parts of the genitals and could be compressed during an indirect inguinal hernia. The other nerves listed are not likely to be compressed by the hernia.

A. The iliohypogastric nerve innervates the skin of the suprapubic region.

B. The lateral femoral cutaneous nerve innervates the skin over the lateral thigh.

D. The subcostal nerve innervates the band of skin superior to the iliac crest and inferior to the umbilicus.

E. The pudendal nerve innervates the musculature and skin of the perineum.
GAS 298–299; N 263; ABR/McM 234

20. **A.** The celiac lymph nodes receive lymph drainage directly from the stomach before they drain into the intestinal lymph trunk and the thoracic duct.

B and C. The superior and inferior mesenteric lymph nodes receive lymphatic drainage from organs below the level of stomach and not from the stomach itself.

D. The lumbar lymph nodes receive drainage from structures inferior to the stomach and not the stomach directly.

E. Hepatic lymph nodes are associated with liver drainage and not drainage from the stomach (*GAS* Fig. 4.168).
GAS 358; N 268; ABR/McM 245

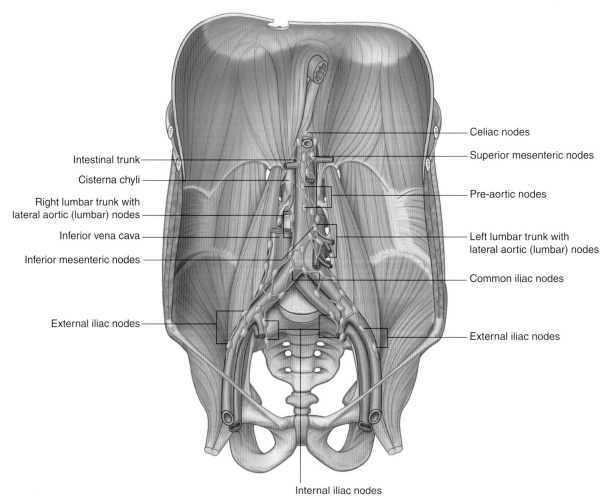

• *GAS* **Fig. 4.168**

21. B. The proper hepatic artery passes superiorly within the hepatoduodenal ligament and therefore would be occluded. This artery lies within the right anterior free margin of the omental (or epiploic) foramen (of Winslow).

A. The superior mesenteric artery branches from the abdominal aorta inferior to the hepatoduodenal ligament.

C. The splenic artery runs behind the stomach and is not located in the hepatoduodenal ligament.

D. The common hepatic artery gives origin to the proper hepatic artery but does not run within the hepatoduodenal ligament.

E. The inferior vena cava is located at the posterior margin of the omental foramen and therefore would not be clamped.
GAS 343; N 291; ABR/McM 234

22. E. Indirect hernias commonly result from herniation of the intestines through the deep inguinal ring.

A. Direct hernias penetrate the anterior abdominal wall medial to the inferior epigastric vessels through the inguinal triangle (of Hesselbach) and do not penetrate the deep inguinal ring.

B. Umbilical hernias exit through the umbilicus, not the deep inguinal ring.

C. Femoral hernias exit through the femoral ring posteroinferior to the inguinal ligament.

D. Lumbar hernias can penetrate through the superior (Grynfelt) or inferior (Petit) lumbar triangles.
(*GAS* Figs. 4.48 and 4.49)
GAS 298; N 263; ABR/McM 235

23. C. The omental bursa or lesser sac is located directly posterior to the stomach and therefore would be the most likely space to develop peritonitis initially.

A and B. The right subhepatic space (also called the hepatorenal space, or pouch of Morison) is the area posterior to the liver and anterior to the right kidney. This space can potentially accumulate fluid and may participate in peritonitis but primarily when the patient is in the supine position.

D. The right subphrenic space lies just inferior to the diaphragm on the right side and is not likely to accumulate fluid from a perforated stomach ulcer. Peritonitis could develop in this area only when the patient is in the supine position.

E. Fluid from a perforated ulcer on the posterior aspect of the stomach is not likely to enter the greater sac (*GAS* Fig 4.102).
GAS 304; N 273; ABR/McM 241

24. C. The left gastric vein carries blood from the stomach to the hepatic portal vein. Above the esophageal-gastric junction, the left gastric vein (portal system) anastomoses with esophageal veins (caval system). High blood pressure in the portal system causes high pressure in this anastomosis, causing the ruptured esophageal varices.

A. The splenic vein and its tributaries carry blood away from the spleen and do not form a caval-portal anastomosis.

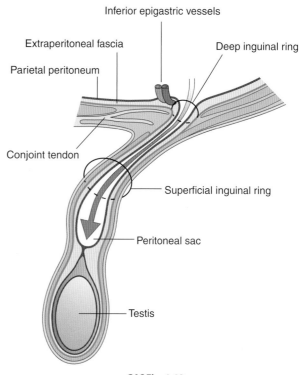

• *GAS* **Fig. 4.48**

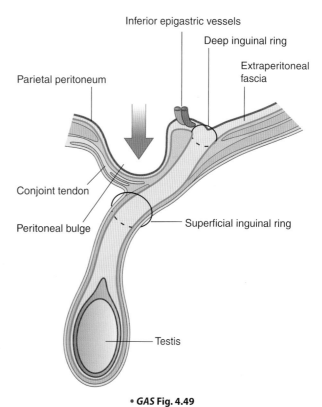

• *GAS* **Fig. 4.49**

B. The left gastro-omental vein accompanies the left gastro-omental artery and joins the splenic vein with no direct anastomosis with caval veins.

D. The left hepatic vein is a caval vein and empties into the inferior vena cava.

E. The right gastric vein drains the lesser curvature of the stomach and is part of the portal system but does not have any caval anastomosis (*GAS* Fig. 4.41). *GAS 269, 354; N 296; ABR/McM 258*

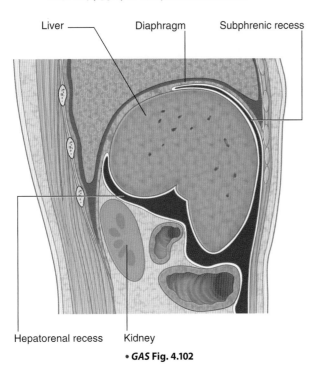

Liver — Diaphragm — Subphrenic recess

Hepatorenal recess — Kidney

• *GAS* **Fig. 4.102**

25. **C.** The genitofemoral nerve originates from the ventral rami of L1 and L2. The "femoral" part supplies skin to the femoral triangle area, whereas the "genito" part travels as part of the spermatic cord and supplies the cremaster muscle and labial or scrotal skin anteriorly.

A. The ilioinguinal nerve arises from L1 and supplies the skin over the root of the penis and anterior part of the scrotum in males.

B. The iliohypogastric nerve arises from L1 (and possibly fibers from T12) and supplies skin innervation over the hypogastric region and anterolateral gluteal region.

D. The pudendal nerve provides innervation to the external genitalia for both sexes but does not innervate the cremaster muscle in males.

E. The ventral ramus of T12 is also associated with the lower portion of the anterior abdominal wall; it does not contribute to the cremasteric reflex. *GAS 296–298; N 260; ABR/McM 271*

Answers 26–50

26. **E.** The linea alba is formed by the intersection of aponeurotic tissues between the right and left rectus abdominis muscles. It represents a midline union of the aponeuroses of the abdominal muscles.

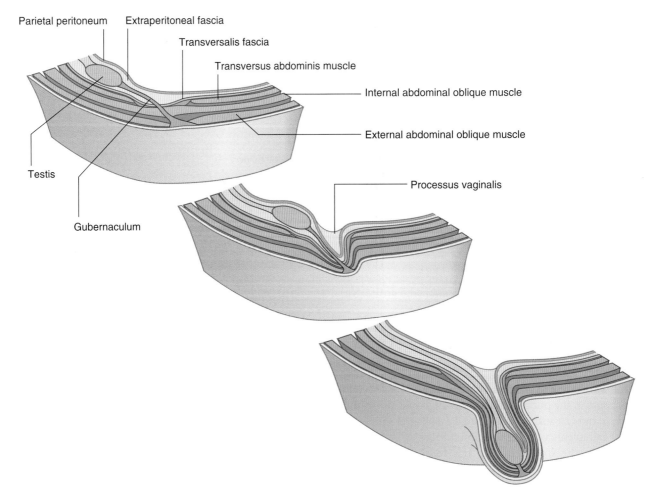

Parietal peritoneum — Extraperitoneal fascia

Transversalis fascia

Transversus abdominis muscle

Internal abdominal oblique muscle

External abdominal oblique muscle

Testis

Processus vaginalis

Gubernaculum

• *GAS* **Fig. 4.41**

A. The midaxillary line is oriented vertically in a straight line inferior to the shoulder joint and axilla.

B. The arcuate line (of Douglas) is a curved horizontal line that represents the lower edge of the posterior tendinous portion of the rectus abdominis sheath. An incision at this line will not separate the rectus abdominis sheaths.

C. The semilunar line is represented by an imaginary vertical line below the nipples and usually parallels the lateral edge of the rectus sheath.

D. The tendinous intersections of the rectus abdominis muscles divide the muscle into sections and are usually not well defined. An incision along these intersections would not divide the 2 rectus sheaths (*GAS* Fig. 4.27).
GAS 278; N 252; ABR/McM 229

27. **A.** Scarpa fascia is the thick, membranous layer deep to the Camper adipose fascia in the anterior abdominal wall (subcutaneous). Because of the relatively thick, tough nature of connective tissue that makes up Scarpa fascia, this layer is typically the site to maintain sutures.

B. Camper fascia is a fatty layer (subcutaneous) and tends not to hold sutures as well, due to the increased cellular content versus the connective tissue found in Scarpa layer.

C. Transversalis fascia is located deep to the abdominal musculature and associated aponeuroses.

D. Extraperitoneal fascia is the deepest layer, adjacent to the parietal peritoneum of the abdominal wall.

E. The anterior wall of the rectus sheath is the layer just deep to Scarpa fascia and superficial to the rectus abdominis muscle anteriorly.
GAS 276; N 324; ABR/McM 233

28. **A.** The bile duct is formed by the union of the cystic duct and common hepatic duct, and it passes inferiorly within the hepatoduodenal ligament and posterior to the first part of the duodenum to enter the head of the pancreas. An obstruction at this site causes a backup of bile back through the bile duct and common hepatic duct, with resulting pain and jaundice.

B. The common hepatic duct is located more superior to the head of the pancreas and unites with the cystic duct to form the bile duct.

C. The cystic duct allows bile to enter the gallbladder from the common hepatic duct (draining the liver) and releases bile to the bile duct.

D. The accessory pancreatic duct is not affected by an obstruction of the bile duct due to a lack of any connections between the two ducts.

E. The proper hepatic artery will not be obstructed, for it carries blood from the liver to the inferior vena cava.
GAS 292; N 287; ABR/McM 256

29. **C.** The third part of the duodenum takes a path anterior to the abdominal aorta and posteroinferior to the superior mesenteric artery (a major ventral branch of the abdominal aorta). Because the third part of the duodenum lies in the angle between ("sandwiched" between (as is a nut in a nutcracker) these two structures, constrictions of this portion of the duodenum can occur readily.

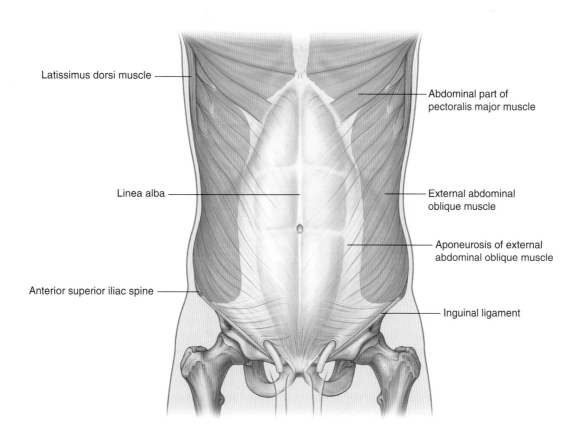

Latissimus dorsi muscle

Linea alba

Anterior superior iliac spine

Abdominal part of pectoralis major muscle

External abdominal oblique muscle

Aponeurosis of external abdominal oblique muscle

Inguinal ligament

• *GAS* **Fig. 4.27**

A. The second part of the duodenum lies parallel with, and to the right of, the abdominal aorta and is not normally in close proximity to the superior mesenteric artery.

B. The transverse colon takes a horizontal path through the anterior abdominal cavity but travels anterior to the superior mesenteric artery.

D. The first part of the duodenum continues from the pylorus, flexing to lead to the second part of the duodenum; thus, it is located anterosuperior to the origin of the superior mesenteric artery from the abdominal aorta.

E. The jejunum is an extension of the small intestine after the duodenum and is further removed from the superior mesenteric artery.
GAS 346; N 288; ABR/McM 248

30. E. The superior mesenteric artery will supply the pancreas if the gastroduodenal artery is ligated. It arises immediately inferior to the celiac trunk from the thoracic aorta. Its first branch is the inferior pancreaticoduodenal artery, which has anterior and posterior branches, and these anastomose with the anterior and posterior superior pancreaticoduodenal arteries (which take origin from the gastroduodenal branch of the common hepatic artery) in supplying the pancreas with oxygenated blood.

A. The inferior mesenteric artery is the most inferior of the three main arterial branches supplying the gastrointestinal tract. It supplies the hindgut from the left colic flexure to the rectum.

B. The left gastric artery is the smallest branch of the celiac trunk and supplies the GE junction, the inferior esophagus, and the lesser curvature of the stomach.

C. The right gastric artery arises from the proper hepatic artery, which is a branch of the common hepatic artery from the celiac trunk. It supplies the lesser curvature of the stomach and anastomoses with the left gastric artery.

D. The proper hepatic artery arises from the common hepatic artery and ascends to supply the liver and gallbladder. It is one of three structures forming the portal triad and is found in the free edge of the hepatoduodenal ligament.
GAS 348; N 291; ABR/McM 248

31. B. The middle colic artery can provide collateral supply to the descending colon when the inferior mesenteric artery is blocked or ligated. It is one of the first branches of the superior mesenteric artery and supplies the transverse colon. It provides collateral blood supply both to the ascending colon and descending colon by anastomosing with the right colic branch of the superior mesenteric artery and with the left colic artery, a branch from the inferior mesenteric artery. This anastomotic channel is referred to as the marginal artery.

A. The left gastro-omental artery, also known as the left gastroepiploic artery, is a branch of the splenic artery and supplies the greater curvature of the stomach along with the right gastro-omental branch of the gastroduodenal artery.

C. The sigmoid arteries are branches from the inferior mesenteric artery and supply the inferior portion of the descending colon, the sigmoid colon, and the rectum. The sigmoid arteries have no contributing branches to the foregut or midgut.

D. The splenic artery is the longest and often the largest artery arising from the celiac trunk. It supplies the spleen and the neck, body, and tail of the pancreas and also provides short gastric and left gastroomental branches to the stomach. It supplies no structures in the midgut or hindgut.

E. The superior rectal artery is the terminal branch of the inferior mesenteric artery and supplies only the rectum.
GAS 348; N 295; ABR/McM 248

32. A. The appendix is the most likely structure that is inflamed. It lies in the right lower quadrant, and of the choices provided, it is most closely associated with the umbilical region by way of referral of pain. The patient also exhibited a positive psoas sign when flexion of the hip against resistance was attempted. This is because the iliopsoas muscle lies directly beneath the appendix, and upon flexion of this muscle, contact and direct irritation to the appendix can occur.

B. The urinary bladder lies inferior to the umbilicus within the pelvis and is not related to the site of pain or with a positive psoas sign.

C. The gallbladder lies inferior to the liver and is positioned in the upper right abdominal quadrant, which is superior to the umbilicus. It is not associated with a positive psoas sign.

D. The pancreas lies behind the stomach and is positioned between the spleen and the duodenum. It therefore lies primarily in the upper left quadrant and is superior to the umbilicus.

E. The uterus is located within the pelvis and is positioned anteflexed and anteverted over the urinary bladder. It lies inferior and medial to the iliopsoas group and would not be affected by flexion of psoas muscle (*GAS* Fig. 4.22).
GAS 319–320; N 280; ABR/McM 271

33. B. The abscess may have spread to the diaphragm and be causing the referred shoulder pain. This is because the diaphragm lies in close proximity to the superior poles of the kidneys. The diaphragm is innervated by the phrenic nerves, bilaterally, which descend to the diaphragm from spinal nerve levels C3, C4, and C5. It is probably at the spinal cord that the referral of pain occurs between the phrenic nerve and somatic afferents entering at those levels.

A. The descending colon is innervated by parasympathetic nerves from S2 to S4 and visceral afferents, which do not carry pain.

C. The duodenum is innervated by the vagus nerve, which innervates the gastrointestinal tract to the left colic flexure. Sympathetic innervation to the duodenum is provided by the greater thoracic splanchnic nerves, from levels T5–T9. Innervation

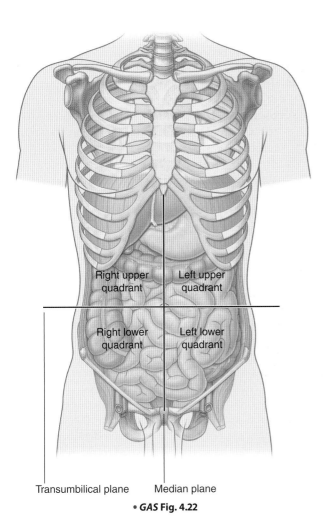

Right upper quadrant

Left upper quadrant

Right lower quadrant

Left lower quadrant

Transumbilical plane   Median plane

• *GAS* **Fig. 4.22**

of the duodenum does not enter the spinal cord at the level of afferents from the shoulder (C4–C5) and therefore will not result in referred pain to the shoulder.

D. The spleen is innervated sympathetically from the celiac ganglion; the parasympathetic nerves to the liver are by the vagus nerve. Innervation of the spleen does not enter the spinal cord at the level of the shoulder and therefore will not result in referred pain to the shoulder.

E. The pancreas is innervated by the vagus nerve, branches from the celiac ganglion, and the pancreatic plexus. None of these nerves enter the spinal cord at the level of the shoulder and therefore cannot facilitate referral of pain to the shoulder.
GAS 373–374; N 266; ABR/McM 270

34. A. The afferent fibers mediating the pain from the head of the pancreas run initially with the greater thoracic splanchnic nerves. The greater thoracic splanchnic nerves arise from sympathetic ganglia at the levels of T5–T9 and innervate structures of the foregut and thus the head of the pancreas. Running within these nerves are visceral afferent fibers that relay pain from foregut structures to the dorsal horn of the spinal cord. Also entering the dorsal horn are the somatic afferents from that vertebral level, which mediate pain from the body wall.

B. Intercostal nerves T1–T12 provide the terminal part of the pathway to the spinal cord of visceral afferents for pain from the thorax and much of the abdomen. Therefore, pain fibers from the pancreas pass by way of the thoracic splanchnic nerves to the sympathetic trunks and then, by way of communicating rami, to ventral rami of spinal nerves, finally entering the spinal cord by way of the dorsal roots.

C. The phrenic nerve innervates the diaphragm and also carries visceral afferents from mediastinal pleura and the pericardium, but it does not carry with it any visceral afferent fibers from the pancreas.

D. The vagus nerve innervates the pancreas with parasympathetic fibers and ascends all the way up to the medulla where it enters the brain. It has no visceral afferent fibers for pain.

E. The subcostal nerve is from the level of T12 and innervates structures below the pancreas and carries no visceral afferents from the pancreas.
GAS 332, 358–364; N 303; ABR/McM 247

35. D. The testicular artery originates from the abdominal aorta and is one of the components of the spermatic cord, supplying the testis.

A. The external iliac artery is located "downstream" to the origin of the testicular artery from the aorta and would not cause any problems in sperm count.

B. The inferior epigastric artery originates close to the deep inguinal ring (where the spermatic cord is formed) as a branch of the external iliac artery and is not associated with the testicular production of sperm.

C. The umbilical artery originates from the internal iliac artery and is divided in adults: its distal part is obliterated (medial umbilical ligament), and the proximal part gives origin to superior vesical arteries for the urinary bladder. The umbilical artery plays no role in sperm production.

E. The deep circumflex iliac artery arises from the external iliac artery and as such does not provide blood supply to the testes.
GAS 387–389; N 266; ABR/McM 271

36. A. The lymph drainage of the scrotum is into the superficial inguinal nodes, but the testis drains to lumbar lymph nodes.

B. The internal iliac lymph nodes drain the pelvis, deeper portions of the perineum, and the gluteal region.

C. The lumbar nodes drain lymph from the kidneys, the suprarenal glands, testis or ovaries, upper portions of the uterus, and uterine tubes. They also receive lymph from the common, internal, and external iliac nodes.

D. Presacral nodes are positioned immediately anterior to the sacrum and posterior to the mesorectal fascia. The presacral nodes drain lymph from the rectum and anal canal, in males the prostate, and in females the cervix, lower portion of the uterus, and upper part of the vagina.

E. Axillary lymph nodes drain the anterior abdominal wall above the umbilicus.

GAS 514; N 268; ABR/McM 278

37. B. The components of the spermatic cord include ductus deferens; testicular, cremasteric, and deferential arteries; the pampiniform plexus of veins; the genital branch of the genitofemoral nerve; and the testicular sympathetic plexus and also lymph vessels. The cremaster muscle and fascia originate from the internal abdominal oblique muscle.

A. The external spermatic fascia is derived from the fascia of the external abdominal oblique muscle.

C. The tunica vaginalis testis is a continuation of the processus vaginalis (from parietal peritoneum) that covers the anterior and lateral sides of the testis and epididymis.

D. The internal spermatic fascia is derived from the transversalis fascia.

E. The dartos tunic consists of a blending of the adipose (Camper) and membranous (Scarpa) layers of the superficial fascia, with interspersed smooth muscle fibers.

GAS 275; N 369; ABR/McM 278

38. A. Esophageal varices are dilated veins in the submucosa of the lower esophagus. They often result from portal hypertension due to liver cirrhosis. The left gastric vein and the esophageal veins of the azygos system form an important portal-caval anastomosis when pressure in the hepatic portal vein, and in turn the left gastric vein, is increased.

B, C, D, and E. None of the other choices forms important portal-caval anastomoses.

GAS 270, 356; N 241; ABR/McM 221

39. B. The jejunum makes up the proximal 2/5ths of the small intestine. There are several ways in which the ileum and jejunum differ. During surgery the easiest way to distinguish the two based on appearance is the relative amount of mesenteric fat. The jejunum has less mesenteric fat than the ileum. Although the jejunum does have thicker walls, more villi, and higher plicae circulares compared with the ileum, these distinctions are not visible unless the intestinal wall is incised. The jejunum has fewer vascular arcades in comparison with the ileum, and its vasa rectae tend to be longer than those in the ileum. Lymphatic follicles are visible, usually only histologically, in the ileum.

A, C, D, and E. The other option choices inaccurately depict the gross morphological differences of the jejunum compared to the ileum.

GAS 310; N 270; ABR/McM 262

40. C. The arcuate line is a curved horizontal line that demarcates the lower limit of the posterior aponeurotic portion of the rectus sheath. It is also where the inferior epigastric vessels enter the sheath to supply the rectus abdominis.

A. The supracristal line is an imaginary line drawn in the horizontal plane at the upper margin of the iliac crests.

B. The linea alba is a tendinous, median raphe running vertically between the two rectus abdominis muscles from the xiphoid process to the pubic symphysis.

D. The pectineal line is a feature of the superior ramus of the pubic bone; it provides an origin for the pectineus muscle of the thigh and medial insertions for the abdominal obliques and transversus abdominis muscles.

E. The semilunar line is the curved, vertical line along the lateral border of the sheath of the rectus abdominis.

GAS 283; N 254; ABR/McM 230

41. D. The psoas muscles (covered in psoas fascia) originate from the transverse processes, intervertebral disks, and bodies of the vertebral column at levels T12–L5. In the image, this fascia contains a calcified tuberculous abscess.

A. The pancreas is an elongated organ located across the back of the abdomen, behind the stomach. The tapering body extends horizontally and slightly upward to the left and ends near the spleen.

B. The cecum is the blind-ending pouch of the ascending colon, lying in the right iliac fossa.

C. The fundus of the stomach lies inferior to the apex of the heart at the level of the fifth rib.

E. The suspensory muscle of the duodenum is a fibromuscular band that is attached to the right crus of the diaphragm.

GAS 371; N 265; ABR/McM 267

42. B. The superior mesenteric artery arises from the aorta, behind the neck of the pancreas, and descends across the uncinate process of the pancreas and the third part of the duodenum before it enters the root of the mesentery behind the transverse colon. It can compress the third part of the duodenum.

A. The inferior mesenteric artery passes to the left behind the horizontal portion of the duodenum.

C. The inferior mesenteric vein is formed by the union of the superior rectal and sigmoid veins and it does not cross the third part of the duodenum.

D. The hepatic portal vein is formed by the union of the splenic vein and the superior mesenteric vein posterior to the neck of the pancreas. It ascends behind the bile duct and the proper hepatic artery within the hepatoduodenal ligament.

E. The splenic vein is formed by the tributaries from the spleen and is superior to the third part of the duodenum.

GAS 348; N 266; ABR/McM 245

43. B. The omental (epiploic) foramen (of Winslow) is the only natural opening between the lesser and greater sacs of the peritoneal cavity. It is bounded superiorly by the visceral peritoneum (liver capsule of Glisson) on the caudate lobe of the liver, inferiorly by the peritoneum on the first part of the duodenum, anteriorly by the free edge of the hepatoduodenal ligament, and posteriorly by the parietal peritoneum covering the inferior vena

cava. Therefore, the inferior vena cava would be the most likely source of bleeding.

   A. The aorta lies to the left of the inferior vena cava in the abdomen.

   C, D and E. The hepatic portal vein, right renal artery, and superior mesenteric vein are not borders of the omental foramen.
   GAS 301–304; N 273; ABR/McM 241

44. B. The ilioinguinal nerve, which arises from the ventral ramus of the L1 spinal nerve, innervates the skin on the medial aspect of the thigh, labium majus or scrotum, and the mons pubis. It has been injured in this patient.

   A. The genitofemoral nerve splits into two branches: The genital branch supplies the cremaster muscle and the skin of the anterior portion of the labium majus or scrotum whereas the femoral branch supplies the skin of the femoral triangle.

   C. The subcostal nerve has a lateral cutaneous branch that innervates skin in the upper gluteal region, in addition to distribution over the lower part of the anterior abdominal wall.

   D. The iliohypogastric nerve innervates the skin over the iliac crest and the hypogastric region.

   E. Spinal nerve T9 supplies sensory innervation to the dermatome at the level of T9, above the level of the umbilicus.
   GAS 398; N 260; ABR/McM 230

45. D. The second part of the duodenum is crossed anteriorly by the transverse mesocolon, a relationship that can be seen when the beginning of the jejunum is exposed by lifting the transverse colon superiorly.

   A and C. The posterior relationships of the second part of the duodenum and the hepatic portal vein cannot be seen without some dissection.

   B. The superior mesenteric artery and vein pass anterior to the third part of the duodenum.

   E. The third part of the duodenum is not related anteriorly to the hilum of the left kidney.
   GAS 309; N 278; ABR/McM 249

46. A. The right suprarenal gland is a retroperitoneal organ on the superomedial aspect of the right kidney, partially posterior to the inferior vena cava.

   B. The appendix is a narrow, hollow tube that is suspended from the cecum by a small mesoappendix.

   C. The gallbladder is located at the junction of the ninth costal cartilage and the lateral border of the rectus abdominis, quite anterior to the pathologic mass.

   D and E. The ovaries and uterus are both inferior to the confluence of the inferior vena cava, which begins as the union of the common iliac veins.
   GAS 386; N 324; ABR/McM 268

47. A. The symptoms of yellow eyes and jaundice would be caused by reversal of flow of bile into the bloodstream. The bile duct, if obstructed, allows no collateral pathway for drainage of bile from the liver or gallbladder.

   B. The cystic duct would block gallbladder drainage but allow for bile flow from the liver.

C and E. Obstruction of either the right or left hepatic duct would still allow for drainage from the liver as well as the gallbladder.

   D. The pancreatic duct is not involved in the path of bile flow from the liver to the duodenum. It drains pancreatic enzymes from the pancreas to the duodenum.
   GAS 330, 340–342; N 287; ABR/McM 256

48. C. Cirrhosis of the liver would lead to inability of the portal system to accommodate blood flow. Blood backs up toward systemic circulation, draining to the inferior vena cava, with pooling at areas of portal-caval anastomoses. The left gastric vein (portal) anastomoses with the esophageal vein (caval) and enlarges or expands in instances of cirrhosis.

   A. The inferior phrenic and superior phrenic veins are both systemic veins and would not be affected by portal hypertension.

   B and D. The left colic and middle colic veins are both tributaries to the portal system. The same can be said for the renal and lumbar veins, both components of the caval-systemic venous system.

   E. The sigmoidal and superior rectal veins are both components of the portal venous system and would not engorge due to the portal-caval hypertension experienced in cirrhosis. (The anastomoses between the superior rectal veins and middle or inferior rectal veins can expand in portal hypertension as rectal varices.)
   GAS 356; N 299; ABR/McM 247

49. A. The key distinguishing feature of a direct inguinal hernia is that it does not pass through the deep inguinal ring; it passes through the lower portion of the inguinal triangle (of Hesselbach). This triangle is bordered laterally by the inferior epigastric artery and vein; medially, it is bordered by the lateral edge of rectus abdominis; inferiorly, it is bordered by the iliopubic tract and inguinal ligament. An indirect hernia passes through the deep inguinal ring and into the inguinal canal. It often descends through the superficial ring into the scrotum or labium, a feature less common in a direct inguinal hernia. If the tip of the examiner's little finger is inserted into the superficial ring and the patient is asked to cough, an indirect inguinal hernia may be felt hitting the very tip of the examining finger. A direct inguinal hernia will be felt against the side of the digit. Both types of inguinal hernias occur above the inguinal ligament, and both are present lateral to the lateral border of the rectus abdominis – providing no information for distinguishing the type of hernias

   B, C. The femoral canal, a feature of the femoral sheath, passes beneath the inguinal ligament into the thigh, providing the pathway taken by a femoral hernia – not an inguinal hernia

   D. The pubic symphysis, a midline joint between the two pubic bones, provides no information for distinguishing types of hernias.

   E. The pectineal ligament lies behind, or deep to, the proximal end of the femoral canal. (GAS Fig. 4.50A).
   GAS 296–298; N 264; ABR/McM 230

Inferior epigastric vessels

Deep inguinal ring

Transversus abdominis muscle

Rectus abdominis muscle

Inguinal triangle

Superficial inguinal ring

Lacunar ligament

Anterior superior iliac spine

Iliopubic tract

Testicular vessels

External iliac artery

External iliac vein

Ductus deferens

• *GAS* **Fig. 4.50A**

50. B. The bullet would probably first penetrate the transverse colon because it is the most superficial structure located slightly superior to the umbilicus, although it may hang variably down toward the pelvic cavity in erect posture.
  A. The abdominal aorta is located deep, on the vertebral column, and would not be encountered first.
  C. The stomach is located more superior, to the left, and posterior to the transverse colon and would not be affected by the anterior-posterior trajectory of the bullet.
  D. The gallbladder is located superiorly in the upper right quadrant of the abdomen, largely under cover of the liver. This would exclude its possibility of being penetrated by the midline bullet.
  E. The pancreas is located deep to the stomach and its head is cradled by the duodenum.
  GAS 273, 320; N 298; ABR/McM 229

Answers 51–75

51. D. Surgical anastomosis to alleviate symptoms of portal hypertension are rooted in the premise that connection of a large hepatic portal vein to a large systemic vein allows for collateral drainage of the portal system.
  A, B and E. The splenic vein, a major tributary of the portal venous system, and the left renal vein, a component of the caval-systemic venous system, are ideally located to allow for a low-resistance, easily performed anastomosis. Anastomosing the left gastric vein to the splenic vein, the right gastric vein to the left gastric vein, or the superior mesenteric vein to the inferior mesenteric vein would all be

ineffectual because each of these veins is a component of just the portal venous system.
  C. The right renal and right gonadal veins are both tributaries of the caval system, and surgical connection would provide no benefit.
  GAS 356–357; N 299; ABR/McM 246

52. B. Visceral pain from the kidneys and the ureter at the point of the neoplasm is mediated via T11 and T12 spinal cord levels. Therefore, pain is referred to these dermatomes leading to pain in the upper gluteal and pubic areas (from the subcostal nerve, in particular).
  A and C. The dermatomes that supply the anterior and lateral thighs are of upper lumbar origin and would not receive pain referred from the kidneys.
  D and E. The umbilical region, the T10 dermatome, is supplied by the T10 spinal nerve.
  GAS 380–381; N 321; ABR/McM 271

53. B. The mass leads to increased stimulation and secretions of the chromaffin cells of the suprarenal medulla. These cells are modified postganglionic sympathetic neurons of neural crest origin, and the epinephrine (adrenaline) and norepinephrine (noradrenaline) released by these cells passes into the suprarenal (adrenal) veins.
  The suprarenal medulla receives stimulation from preganglionic sympathetic fibers carried by the greater thoracic splanchnic nerves.
  C and D. Parasympathetic neurons are not found in the suprarenal medulla and would have no participation in the effects of the tumor.
  E. The pelvic splanchnic nerves are parasympathetic and do not travel to the suprarenal medulla.
  GAS 386; N 322; ABR/McM 268

54. E. The splenic artery lies along the superior border of the pancreas. The organ it principally supplies is the spleen, which is located at the termination of the pancreatic tail. Blood supply to the spleen can therefore be affected in the event of a tumor in the tail of the pancreas.
  A. The duodenum receives blood from the gastroduodenal artery, located near the head of the pancreas.
  B. The gallbladder is supplied by the cystic artery, a branch of the right hepatic artery, and is not in contact with the pancreas.
  C. The kidneys are supplied by the right and left renal arteries. The left renal artery lies deep and medial to the pancreatic tumor, and blood supply would proceed uninterrupted.
  D. The liver is also supplied by the common and proper hepatic arteries.
    GAS 337–346; N 291; ABR/McM 244

55. E. The superior mesenteric artery lies just superior and anterior to the left renal vein as the vein passes to its termination in the inferior vena cava.
  A. The celiac artery is located superiorly and would not compress the left renal vein.
  B and C. The inferior mesenteric artery and its left colic branch are located too inferiorly to occlude the left renal vein.
  D. The middle colic artery arises from the anterior aspect of the superior mesenteric artery inferior to the position of the left renal vein. An aneurysm of the superior mesenteric artery would therefore be most likely to occlude the left renal vein.
    GAS 348, 379; N 295; ABR/McM 248

56. B. Blood flow would be impeded or greatly reduced in the left testicular vein because of the occlusion of the left renal vein—into which the left testicular vein drains. This would result in pain as the testicular venous vessels become swollen.
  The testicular artery originates from the abdominal aorta more inferiorly and is not being compressed.
  C. Pain mediated from the kidneys would pass to the T11 and T12 spinal cord levels via the lesser and least thoracic splanchnic nerves. There would be no compression of lumbar splanchnic nerves in this case.
  D. Compression of the preaortic sympathetics would not produce pain, nor would it cause referral of pain. Visceral afferents for pain terminate at the T7 level of the spinal cord.
  E. The vagus, a parasympathetic nerve, does not carry visceral pain fibers in the abdomen; pain is mediated by branches of the sympathetic trunks.
    GAS 511; N 313; ABR/McM 268

57. D. The most likely candidate for bleeding from the fundic region of the stomach in this case would be either the short gastric or dorsal gastric branches of the splenic artery. The short gastric arteries pass from the area of the splenic hilum to the fundus, supplying anterior and posterior branches to this part of the stomach.

The dorsal gastric artery, which arises from the midportion of the splenic artery, passes to the dorsal aspect of the fundus.
  A and B. The common hepatic artery and inferior phrenic artery are quite removed from the area of the ulcer.
  C. The left gastro-omental artery courses along the greater curvature of the body of the stomach, distal to the fundus.
  E. The main stem of the splenic artery would pass somewhat inferior to the location of the ulceration.
    GAS 346; N 290; ABR/McM 251

58. D. Indirect inguinal hernia is the most common groin hernia in women.
  A. Although femoral hernias occur more commonly in women than in men, the occurrence of indirect inguinal hernias in women is greater than femoral hernias. Inguinal hernias are much more common in men than in women.
  B and E. Epigastric and umbilical hernias would not present with pain to the inguinal region.
  C. Direct inguinal hernias, while exhibiting equal incidence in both sexes, are not the most common hernia in women.
    GAS 296–298; N 264; ABR/McM 235

59. A. The posterior superior pancreaticoduodenal artery arises from the gastroduodenal artery and travels behind the first part of the duodenum, supplying the proximal portion, with branches to the head of the pancreas. Duodenal ulcers commonly arise within the first portion of the duodenum, thus making the posterior superior pancreaticoduodenal artery one of the more frequently injured vessels.
  B. The superior mesenteric artery supplies derivatives of the midgut from the distal half of the duodenum to the left colic flexure. It lies inferior to the region of ulceration.
  C. The inferior mesenteric artery is responsible for supplying most of the hindgut derivatives, generally supplying intestine from the left colic flexure to the superior aspect of the rectum.
  D. The inferior pancreaticoduodenal artery arises from the superior mesenteric artery and supplies the distal portion of the second part of the duodenum, and anastomoses with its superior counterparts.
  E. The right gastric artery is responsible for supplying the pyloric portion of the lesser curvature of the stomach (*GAS* Fig. 4.67).
    GAS 347; N 291; ABR/McM 247

60. D. The transversalis fascial layer is the source of the internal spermatic fascia. The coverings of the spermatic cord consist of three layers: external spermatic fascia, cremaster muscle, and the internal spermatic fascia.
  A. The external spermatic fascia is an extension of the external abdominal oblique fascia and aponeurosis.
  B. The cremaster muscle is a derivative of the internal abdominal oblique muscle and its fascia.

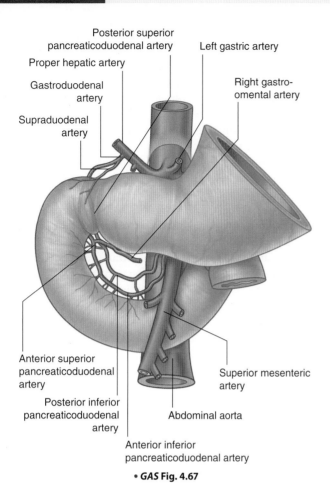

Posterior superior pancreaticoduodenal artery

Proper hepatic artery

Gastroduodenal artery

Supraduodenal artery

Left gastric artery

Right gastro-omental artery

Anterior superior pancreaticoduodenal artery

Posterior inferior pancreaticoduodenal artery

Superior mesenteric artery

Abdominal aorta

Anterior inferior pancreaticoduodenal artery

• *GAS* Fig. 4.67

C. The transversus abdominis aponeurosis inserts into the pubic crest and pectineal line and forms unites with the aponeurotic insertion of the internal abdominal oblique to form the conjoint tendon.

E. The processus vaginalis is a pouch of peritoneum that precedes the testis as it descends through the deep inguinal ring and inguinal canal in the 7th month of development. That portion of the processus that is normally retained forms the tunica vaginalis testis. Retention of the proximal part of the processus provides a pathway for a congenital indirect inguinal hernia. If a portion of the intermediate part of the processus remains, it can form a fluid-filled hydrocele.
GAS 292–293; N 264; ABR/McM 230

61. **C.** The superior mesenteric artery arises from the aorta, deep to the neck of the pancreas, then crosses the uncinate process and third part of the duodenum. An uncinate tumor can cause compression of the superior mesenteric artery.

A. The common hepatic artery passes superior to the body of the pancreas and is unlikely to be affected by a tumor in the uncinate region of the pancreas.

B. The cystic artery and vein, supplying the gallbladder, are also superior to the pancreas.

D. The inferior mesenteric artery arises at the level of L3, which is thus situated inferior to the head of the pancreas.

E. The hepatic portal vein, formed by the confluence of the superior mesenteric vein and splenic vein, passes deep to the neck of the pancreas.
GAS 348; N 266; ABR/McM 248

62. **A.** The bile duct is occluded. The pattern of pain combined with jaundice indicates blockage of release of bile into the duodenum.

B. The cystic duct joins the common hepatic duct to form the bile duct. Bile is released from the gallbladder into the cystic duct in response to cholecystokinin. From the cystic duct, bile flows normally through the bile duct and the hepatopancreatic ampulla (of Vater) to enter the descending duodenum. Patients will often present with multiple gallstones. Cholecystitis is an inflammation of the gallbladder, most frequently in association with the presence of gallstones, and often resulting from a blocked cystic duct. Increasing concentration of bile in the gallbladder can precipitate a bout of inflammation. Blockage of the cystic duct, with concomitant cholecystitis, is not necessarily associated with jaundice. An obstruction in the common hepatic duct and subsequently the bile duct would thus prevent communication between the duodenum and the liver, causing obstructive jaundice.

C and E. An occlusion in either the left or right hepatic duct might cause mild jaundice; however, gallstones might not be present.

D. An occlusion in the main or accessory pancreatic ducts would result in neither gallstones nor jaundice but may cause pancreatitis.
GAS 330, 340; N 287; ABR/McM 256

63. **C.** The anterior cutaneous branch of the iliohypogastric nerve is responsible for the innervation of the skin above the mons pubis. This nerve arises from the ventral ramus of the L1 spinal nerve and runs transversely around the abdominal wall and over the lowest portion of the rectus sheath. It is the first cutaneous nerve situated superior to the mons pubis.

A. T10 innervates the umbilical region.

B. Nerves from the T11 and the T12 ventral rami terminate below the umbilicus but superior to the mons pubis.

D. The ilioinguinal nerve courses through the inguinal canal, commonly on the lateral side of the spermatic cord and is therefore typically inferior to the incision.

E. The lateral femoral cutaneous nerve travels lateral to the psoas muscle and emerges from the abdomen about an inch medial to the anterior superior iliac spine, passing thereafter to the lateral aspect of the thigh.
GAS 398; N 260; ABR/McM 263

64. **B.** Appendicitis is often characterized by acute inflammation and is indicated with both a positive psoas test and rebound pain over McBurney point. McBurney point lies one-third of the distance from the anterior superior iliac spine to the umbilicus. In patients with

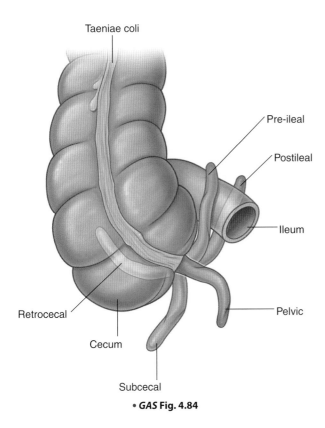

Taeniae coli

Pre-ileal

Postileal

Ileum

Pelvic

Retrocecal

Cecum

Subcecal

• *GAS* Fig. 4.84

appendicitis, rebound tenderness may be felt over McBurney point after quick, deep compression of the left lower quadrant.

A. An ectopic pregnancy would be associated with generalized abdominal pain instead of the localized pain felt over McBurney point.

C. Cholecystitis results from an inflammation of the gallbladder and would result in pain over the epigastric region shifting to the right hypochondriac region.

D. Kidney stones result in referred pain to the lumbar or possibly inguinal regions.

E. Perforation of the duodenum could result in pain on palpation of the abdomen, together with adynamic (paralytic) ileus, rigidity of the abdominal wall, and referral of pain to the shoulder (*GAS* Fig. 4.84).
GAS 319–320 N 280; ABR/McM 261

65. B. The visceral afferent innervation of the rectum is transmitted by way of the pelvic splanchnic nerves, which also provide the parasympathetic supply to this organ.

A. The lumbar sympathetic trunk receives sensory fibers from the fundus and body of the uterus.

C. The pudendal nerve provides origin for the inferior anal (rectal) nerve, the perineal nerve, and the dorsal nerve of the penis. The inferior anal nerve supplies somatosensory fibers to the anal canal below the pectinate line and the perianal skin; the perineal nerve and dorsal nerve of the penis innervate structures of the urogenital region.

D. The lumbar and sacral sympathetic trunks contribute sympathetic fibers for innervation of smooth muscle and glands of certain pelvic viscera, but not sensory fibers for the rectum.

E. The vagus nerve provides parasympathetic supply and afferent innervation (excluding pain) to the intestine proximal to the left colic flexure.
GAS 358–364; N 392; ABR/McM 281

66. D. Meckel diverticulum is a fingerlike projection of the ileum that is generally remembered by the "rule of 2s": It occurs in about 2% of the population, is approximately 2 feet proximal from the ileocecal junction, is about 2 inches long, occurs 2 times as often in men as in women, may contain 2 types of ectopic tissue, and may be confused often with 2 different clinical conditions. The two types of ectopic tissue are gastric mucosa and pancreatic tissue. These, along with bleeding and pain, may give indications of peptic ulcer or appendicitis.

A and B. Internal and external hemorrhoids involve the rectoanal area, not the ileum, in addition to which biopsy of hemorrhoids would not show the presence of gastric mucosa.

C. Diverticulosis or diverticular disease is a condition in which small outpouchings occur in the walls of the colon and would therefore be lined with colic mucosa.

E. Borborygmi are bowel sounds that occur with the passage of gas and bowel contents through the intestines.
GAS 315; N 281; ABR/McM 242

67. D. Abdominal aortic aneurysm often occurs between L3 and L4, below the bifurcation of the aorta, resulting in significant increase in pressure, creating the marked abdominal pulsation.

A, B, C, and E. The remaining answer choices would be associated with referred pain and would not be likely to result in elevated blood pressure.
GAS 388; N 266; ABR/McM 268

68. B. In a supine patient, fluid accumulation will often occur in the hepatorenal pouch (of Morison), which is the lowest space in the peritoneal cavity in the supine position. The hepatorenal space is located behind the liver and in front of the parietal peritoneum covering the right kidney.

A. The subphrenic space is between the right lobe of the liver and the diaphragm.

C and D. The vesicouterine and rectouterine spaces are also potential areas of fluid accumulation; however, fluid accumulation in these spaces occurs when the patient is in an erect position rather than a supine position.

E. The costodiaphragmatic recess is a space in the pleural cavity.
GAS 319 N 345; ABR/McM 279

69. D. Descending colon. Beginning at the left colic flexure, innervation of the hindgut portion of the gastrointestinal tract is supplied by parasympathetic

fibers of the pelvic splanchnic nerves. The parasympathetic innervation of the midgut up to the left colic flexure is supplied by the vagus nerve. A lesion of the spinal cord occurring below L4 would affect innervation of the descending colon because the pelvic splanchnic nerves arise from spinal nerve levels S2–S4.

A, B, C, and E. The jejunum, ascending colon, ileum, and transverse colon are all innervated by the vagus nerve.

GAS 319; N 306; ABR/McM 249

70. C. The porta hepatis (transverse fissure of liver) transmits the proper hepatic artery, hepatic portal vein, common hepatic duct, autonomic nerves, and lymph vessels. A tumor in this region would be most detrimental because of its abundance of vessels and lymphatics that could lead to all of these symptoms when they are compromised functionally.

A and B. A tumor in either the right or left lobes would not be as serious because it would not completely obstruct all of these vessels.

D. The falciform ligament does not carry any vessels (except some small paraumbilical veins), so a tumor in this area would not lead to the symptoms described.

E. The hepatogastric ligament is the bilaminar peritoneal connection between the liver and the lesser curvature of the stomach and is unrelated to the symptoms and signs here.

GAS 329; N 284; ABR/McM 255

71. E. The cystic artery is the only artery listed that goes directly to the gallbladder. It is often a branch of the right hepatic artery and must be clamped before the gallbladder is cut free from its attachments.

A, B, C, and D. The common hepatic artery provides origin to the proper hepatic artery, which divides into right and left hepatic arteries supplying the liver, gallbladder, and biliary tree (*GAS* Fig. 4.106A).

GAS 330; N 287; ABR/McM 256

72. D. The spleen is a large lymphatic organ that rests against the diaphragm and ribs 9, 10, and 11 in the left hypochondriac area. A laceration of this organ is often associated with severe blood loss and shock.

A. Almost all of the liver is located in the right hypochondrium and epigastrium, although some protrudes into the left hypochondrium below the diaphragm.

B. The pancreas lies behind the stomach and will not be injured in this case.

C. The left kidney lies retroperitoneally approximately at the level of the T11–L3 vertebrae on the left side of the body.

E. The ilium is the upper portion of the hip bone and contributes to the bony pelvis. Ileum is the distal portion of the small intestine and is pronounced the same as "ilium."

GAS 337; N 288; ABR/McM 245

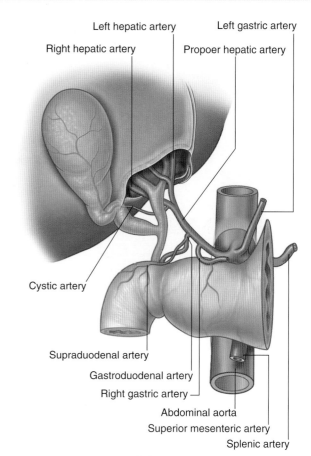

Left hepatic artery
Left gastric artery
Right hepatic artery
Propoer hepatic artery
Cystic artery
Supraduodenal artery
Gastroduodenal artery
Right gastric artery
Abdominal aorta
Superior mesenteric artery
Splenic artery

• *GAS* **Fig. 4.106A**

73. D. The ileocolic artery is the only artery listed that supplies the appendix, giving off an appendicular branch directly or from one of its branches.

A, B, C, and E. The superior mesenteric artery gives origin to the ileocolic, right colic, and middle colic arteries; however, the latter 2 lie superior to the site of the appendix. The superior rectal artery is the terminal branch of the inferior mesenteric artery and supplies the lower portion of the sigmoid colon and superior rectum.

GAS 350; N 294; ABR/McM 261

74. A. Caput medusae (referring to the head of Medusa, whose hair was formed by snakes) is caused by severely elevated portal pressure, with venous reflux from the liver to the paraumbilical veins, small veins within the falciform ligament. The presence of caput medusae is usually associated with end-stage disease. Caput medusae is identified by the appearance of engorged veins radiating toward the lower limbs. The hepatic portal vein is the central connection of these anastomoses.

B, C, and D. Obstruction of the inferior vena cava, superior vena cava, and lateral thoracic vein do not cause portal hypertension and would not produce these symptoms.

E. The superficial epigastric vein also is not associated with the development of portal hypertension but could provide a collateral channel for venous drainage.

GAS 271; N 299; ABR/McM 246

75. C. Cholecystitis is an inflammation of the gallbladder due to increased concentration of bile or obstruction of the cystic duct by gallstones. Pain is ultimately felt in the right hypochondriac region, which corresponds to the T6–T8 dermatomes. Sensory afferents from the viscera carry pain fibers as they travel with sympathetic axons in the greater thoracic splanchnic nerves. Pain cannot be felt in the viscera and is therefore referred to the body wall.

  A. The vagus nerve carries visceral sensory fibers from the head, neck, and trunk, but these do not include pain fibers.

  B. Spinal nerves of T1–T4 receive afferents for pain from thoracic viscera, including the heart, but not abdominal organs.

  D. Sympathetic neurons are autonomic motor nerves and therefore do not carry sensory information.

  E. Afferent fibers of the dorsal rami of spinal nerves T6–T8 convey sensory fibers from the back but not from internal organs.
  GAS 340; N 309; ABR/McM 247

Answers 76–100

76. B. McBurney point usually corresponds to the location of the base of the appendix where it attaches to the cecum. It is found on the right side of the abdomen, about two-thirds of the distance from the umbilicus to the anterior superior iliac spine.

  A, C, and D. The inguinal ligament is localized lateral and inferior to the appendix and hence would not be used as a landmark.

  E. McBurney point is two-thirds of the distance from the umbilicus.
  GAS 318; N 282; ABR/McM 231

77. B. The greater thoracic splanchnic nerves arise from the levels of the T5–T9 thoracic sympathetic ganglia and are responsible for carrying general visceral afferents from upper abdominal organs and, therefore, from the body of the stomach. The pain fibers pass from the sympathetic trunk to spinal nerves T5–T9, thereafter to the spinal cord.

  A. Spinal nerves T1–T5 do receive sensory afferents for pain, but these come from thoracic, not abdominal, organs.

  C. The vagus nerves do not carry afferents for pain.

  D. The lumbar splanchnic nerves are associated with the lower portion of the abdominopelvic area.

  E. Spinal nerves T12–L2 innervate the lower abdominal wall, anterior perineum, and anterior thigh.
  GAS 358–364; N 303; ABR/McM 222

78. C. The ureter is normally constricted to some degree as it crosses the pelvic brim from major to minor pelvis.

  A and B. The minor and major calyces are proximal to the ureter and not typical sites for obstruction by kidney stones.

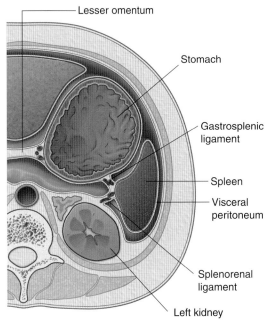

- Lesser omentum
- Stomach
- Gastrosplenic ligament
- Spleen
- Visceral peritoneum
- Splenorenal ligament
- Left kidney

• *GAS* Fig. 4.113

  D. The midportion of the ureter is not a typical site for obstruction. The site of oblique entrance of the ureter into the urinary bladder is a common site for obstruction because it is compressed by urinary bladder contents and the muscular wall as the urinary bladder fills.

  E. There are no common sites of obstruction between the pelvic brim and the uterine cervix.
  GAS 380; N 317; ABR/McM 269, 271

79. C. The splenorenal ligament is the attachment of the spleen to posterior abdominal wall anterior to the left kidney and is the only ligament that contains the major branches of the splenic artery to the spleen and greater curvature of the stomach.

  A. The coronary ligament is the peritoneal reflection from the diaphragmatic surface of the liver onto the diaphragm that encloses the bare area of liver; it is not attached to the spleen.

  B. The gastrocolic ligament contains branches of the gastro-omental vessels but should not be a factor in splenectomy.

  D. The hepatogastric ligament connects the liver to the stomach.

  E. The falciform ligament is a peritoneal fold connecting the liver to the inner aspect of the upper anterior abdominal wall (*GAS* Fig. 4.113).
  GAS 338; N 273; ABR/McM 260

80. C. Pelvic splanchnic nerves and the left colic artery supply the descending colon.

  A. The vagus nerve supplies the bowel only to the proximal ⅔ of the transverse colon, and the middle colic artery supplies the same portion of the transverse colon.

B. The superior rectal artery supplies the rectum.

D. The ileocolic artery supplies the terminal ileum, cecum, appendix, and ascending colon.

E. The left lesser thoracic splanchnic nerve has nothing to do with the descending colon.
GAS 350, 358–364; N 306; ABR/McM 282

81. **E.** The ilioinguinal nerve is a terminal branch of ventral ramus of spinal nerve L1. It innervates the skin overlying the iliac crest; the anterior portion of the urogenital region; and the upper, inner thigh. Its usual pathway takes it below McBurney point, but it can be injured with extension of an appendectomy incision.

A, B, and C. Spinal nerve T10, the genitofemoral nerve, and the pudendal nerve are not located in the area of the incision; what is more, the area of sensory deficit does not correlate well with their injury. The genital branch of the genitofemoral nerve leaves the body wall at the superficial inguinal ring, well below the appendectomy incision. The pudendal nerve is both motor and sensory to the perineum. The genital branch of genitofemoral nerve provides motor supply to the cremaster and sensory fibers to the labium majus or scrotum anteriorly, and a femoral branch innervating only the skin over the femoral triangle. Spinal nerve T10 innervates muscles and skin of the abdominal wall as far anteriorly as the umbilical region.

D. The subcostal nerve innervates the muscles and skin of the abdominal wall from below the 12th rib posteriorly to above the pubic region.
GAS 286, 317; N 260; ABR/McM 230

82. **A.** Esophageal stenosis results from a failure of esophageal recanalization in the 8th week of development, which may also cause esophageal atresia.

B. A TEF is an abnormal passage between the trachea and the esophagus and is associated with esophageal atresia; therefore, webs and strictures would not be seen.

C. Webs and strictures are found in an examination of the esophagus in cases of stenosis, but they are not noticed in cases of atresia.

D and E. Duodenal atresia and stenosis occur in the small intestine and would not cause aspiration pneumonia, and clinical manifestations would not be seen in the esophagus.
GAS 225; N 238; ABR/McM 226

83. **B.** Duodenal stenosis is caused by incomplete recanalization of the duodenum. The vomit contains bile in addition to the stomach contents because of the location of the occlusion, distal to the hepatopancreatic ampulla (of Vater) where the bile duct enters the small intestine. Lack of weight gain is due to constant vomiting.

A. A patent bile duct would not cause vomiting with bile.

C. A hypertrophic pyloric sphincter would cause projectile vomiting without the presence of bile.

D. An atrophic gastric antrum is caused by the removal of the membranous lining of the stomach and occurs proximal to the site of the entrance of the bile duct; therefore, the vomit would not contain bile.

E. A TEF would not cause vomiting of stomach contents and bile because it is a defect of the respiratory system and occurs proximal to the site at which bile is added to stomach contents.
GAS 309; N 279; ABR/McM 246

84. **C.** With hypertrophy of the pyloric sphincter and the associated narrowing of the pyloric canal, there is projectile vomiting of stomach contents, but without bile, because bile enters the duodenum distal to the pyloric constriction.

A and B. Duodenal atresia, like duodenal stenosis, causes vomiting of stomach contents and bile. Vomiting begins soon after birth in cases of atresia; vomiting due to stenosis does not begin necessarily immediately after birth and can occur days after delivery. Lack of weight gain is due to constant vomiting.

D. An atrophic gastric fundus would not produce the signs seen here.

E. A TEF would not cause vomiting of stomach contents and bile because it is a defect of the respiratory system and occurs proximal to the site at which bile is added to intestinal contents.
GAS 309; N 277; ABR/McM 246

85. **B.** Incomplete recanalization of the duodenum is caused either by duodenal stenosis or partial occlusion of the lumen of the duodenum and usually occurs in the distal third portion of the duodenum. This occlusion often results in vomiting of stomach contents plus bile later in life and is the reason the child was constantly hungry but did not gain weight.

A. Incomplete recanalization of the esophagus during the eighth week of development causes esophageal stenosis and presents as webs and strictures.

C. Esophageal atresia is generally seen with a TEF because it is caused by the tracheoesophageal septum deviating in the posterior direction. In some cases, it may result from a failure of recanalization during the eighth week of development and presents as a fetus with polyhydramnios due to an inability to swallow amniotic fluid.

D. Duodenal atresia is the result of a failed reformation of the lumen of the duodenum and is associated with vomiting within the first few days of birth, polyhydramnios, and the "double bubble" sign.

E. TEF is an abnormal passage between the trachea and esophagus and would not be a cause for vomiting because it is associated with the respiratory system and also occurs proximal to the site of the defect.
GAS 261; N 279; ABR/McM 246

86. B. Duodenal atresia is the result of a failed reformation of the lumen of the duodenum and is associated with vomiting within the first few days of birth. Polyhydramnios is seen due to abnormal absorption of amniotic fluid by the intestines. Finally, radiographic or ultrasound examination would show the "double bubble" sign because of distended, gas-filled stomach.

   A. Duodenal stenosis is caused by incomplete recanalization of the duodenum and often results in vomiting of stomach contents plus bile later in life.

   C. Hypertrophied pyloric sphincter would cause projectile vomiting.

   D. An atrophied gastric antrum is caused by the removal of the membranous lining of the stomach and occurs proximal to the site of the entrance of the common bile duct; therefore, vomit would not contain bile.

   E. TEF is an abnormal passage between the trachea and esophagus and would not be a cause for any of symptoms cited in the question.
   GAS 309; N 279; ABR/McM 246

87. C. Annular pancreas causes duodenal obstruction due to the thick band of pancreatic tissue that surrounds and constricts the second part of the duodenum. This obstruction can be found shortly after birth or much later. Annular pancreas can result from the *ventral* pancreatic bud wrapping around the duodenum during development and fusing with the dorsal pancreatic bud, thereafter, forming a ring. Both the dorsal and ventral pancreatic buds are involved in this process.

   B. As stated above, this anomaly is not involved with lack of canalization of the bile ducts.

   A. Accessory pancreatic duct at the minor papilla results from persistence of a distal segment of the *dorsal* bud duct.

   D. Annular pancreas results from fusion of the ventral *and* dorsal buds, not the dorsal alone.

   E. Annular pancreas results from *fusion* of the ventral and dorsal buds, not the dorsal alone.
   GAS 335; N BP80; ABR/McM 245

88. A. A remnant of the omphaloenteric duct generally presents as an ileal (Meckel) diverticulum in the proximal portion of the omphaloenteric duct. It normally arises as a fingerlike pouch about 3–6 cm long from the antimesenteric border of the ileum and 40–50 cm from the ileocecal junction.

   B. The ileal diverticulum is not a remnant of the superior mesenteric artery

   C. The umbilical vesicle normally turns into a pear-shaped remnant about 5 mm in diameter by week 20.

   D. The cecal diverticulum is the primordium of the cecum and appendix.

   A. A Meckel diverticulum is not a remnant of the umbilical cord.
   GAS 315; N 270; ABR/McM 248

89. A. An umbilical hernia results when the body wall does not close appropriately at the site of attachment of the umbilical cord. In such cases, part of the greater omentum and small intestine can herniate from the abdomen.

   B. Umbilical herniation differs from omphalocele. In congenital omphalocele, there is a failure of intestine to return to the abdominal cavity so that there is an apparent herniation of abdominal viscera into the proximal portion of the umbilical cord, without a covering of the hernia by skin. In umbilical hernia, the herniating structures are covered by subcutaneous tissue and skin.

   C. Gastroschisis is incomplete closure of the lateral folds, resulting in an epigastric hernia, in which the viscera protrude into the amniotic cavity, surrounded by amniotic fluid.

   D. An epigastric hernia occurs through a defect in the linea alba superior to the level of the umbilicus and occurs far more commonly in adults.

   E. An indirect inguinal hernia is when the communication between the tunica vaginalis and the peritoneal cavity does not close, and a loop of intestine or a portion of another organ such as the cecum herniates through the deep inguinal ring into the inguinal canal, with possible further descent through the superficial inguinal ring into the scrotum or labium majus.
   GAS 298–299 N 254; ABR/McM 233

90. D. Gastroschisis results from an incomplete closure of the lateral folds during the fourth week of development from a defect in the medial plane of the abdominal wall. This results in an epigastric hernia, with viscera that protrude into the amniotic cavity and amniotic fluid without a peritoneal covering.

   A. Nonrotation of the midgut results in the lower portion of the loop returning to the abdomen first, the small intestine passing to the right side of the abdomen, and the large intestine lying entirely on the left. Most cases are asymptomatic; however, obstruction of the superior mesenteric artery can cause infarction and gangrene of the part of the intestine it supplies.

   B. A patent urachus occurs when there is a communication between the umbilicus and the urinary bladder.

   C. An umbilical hernia results when an abdominal organ herniates through an umbilical ring that does not close completely. Such a hernia often contains part of the greater omentum and small intestine.

   E. The cloacal membrane usually ruptures during the eighth week of development, creating a communication between the anal canal and the amniotic cavity.
   GAS 261; N 254; ABR/McM 232

91. A. The inability to pass meconium denotes an obstruction of the fetal bowel. Midgut volvulus results in the twisting of the intestines and ultimately obstruction of the small and/or large intestines.

   B. Gastroschisis is caused by incomplete closure of the lateral folds during the fourth week of development and it creates a defect in the medial plane of the abdominal wall. This results in an epigastric hernia, with viscera that protrude into the amniotic cavity and are covered by amniotic fluid.

C. Failure of recanalization of the ileum is seen with 50% of obstructive lesions of the intestine. This obstruction is caused by stenosis or atresia of the intestines.

D. A remnant of the omphaloenteric duct generally presents as an ileal (Meckel) diverticulum in the proximal portion of the omphaloenteric duct. It normally arises as a fingerlike pouch about 3–6 cm long from the antimesenteric border of the ileum and 40–50 cm from the ileocecal junction.

E. Nonrotation of the midgut results in the lower portion of the loop returning to the abdomen first, the small intestine sitting on the right side of the abdomen, and the large intestine lying entirely on the left. Most cases are asymptomatic; however, obstruction of the superior mesenteric artery can cause infarction and gangrene of the part of the intestine it supplies.
GAS 323; N 324; ABR/McM 239

92. **D.** A remnant of the proximal portion of the omphaloenteric duct generally presents as an ileal (Meckel) diverticulum. It normally arises as a fingerlike pouch about 3–6 cm long from the antimesenteric border of the ileum and 40–50 cm from the ileocecal junction.

A. Midgut volvulus results from a twisting of the intestines and, ultimately, obstruction of the small and large intestines. Infarction of fetal bowel is seen and would not be the cause of the signs of appendicitis.

B. Gastroschisis is caused by incomplete closure of the lateral folds during the fourth week of development and it creates a defect in the medial plane of the abdominal wall. This results in an epigastric hernia, with viscera that protrude into the amniotic cavity and are covered by amniotic fluid.

C. Failure of recanalization of the ileum is seen in 50% of obstructive lesions of the intestine. This obstruction is caused by stenosis or atresia of the intestines.

E. Nonrotation of the midgut results in the lower portion of the loop returning to the abdomen first so that the small intestine becomes fixed on the right side of the abdomen, with the large intestine lying entirely on the left. Most cases are asymptomatic; however, obstruction of the superior mesenteric artery can cause infarction and gangrene of the part of the intestine it supplies.
GAS 311; N 270; ABR/McM 248

93. **A.** Incomplete separation of the cloaca by the urorectal septum results in anal agenesis.

B. Dorsal deviation of the urorectal septum would result in anal stenosis.

C. Failure of the anal membrane to perforate externally results in imperforate anus, not anal agenesis.

D. Abnormal recanalization of the colon results in rectal atresia, in which there is no connection between the rectum and anal canal.

E. Remnants of the proximal portion of the omphaloenteric duct would result in a Meckel diverticulum, not anal agenesis.
GAS 498; N 311; ABR/McM 280

94. **B.** Dorsal deviation of the urorectal septum results in anal stenosis.

A. Incomplete separation of the cloaca by the urorectal septum results in anal agenesis.

C. Failure of the anal membrane to perforate results in imperforate anus. The anal canal exists but is obstructed by a layer of tissue.

D. Abnormal recanalization of the colon results in rectal atresia, in which there is no connection between the rectum and anal canal.

E. Remnants of the proximal portion of the omphaloenteric duct would result in a Meckel diverticulum, not anal stenosis.
GAS 479; N 311; ABR/McM 280

95. **D.** A vitelline fistula is caused by the persistence of the vitelline duct, which can, by its connections with the umbilicus, cause the symptoms described.

A. An enterocystoma is a tumor and would not result in the symptoms described.

B. A vitelline cyst is a remnant of the vitelline duct; however, it would not open directly to the outside so would not cause the symptoms.

C. Meckel diverticulum can result in a vitelline fistula, but it is simply the persistence of a portion of the vitelline duct that can appear in different forms (such as cyst or fistula).

E. Volvulus is the twisting of the small intestines around their suspending vasculature. It can result from malrotation of the midgut loop and would not result in the symptoms described.
GAS 315; N 254; ABR/McM 233

96. **D.** Anorectal agenesis is due to abnormal partitioning of the cloaca and is often associated with a rectourethral, rectovaginal, or rectouterine fistula.

A. Failure of the proctodeum to develop will result in an imperforate anus.

B. Agenesis of the urorectal septum would most likely lead to a fistula but would not cause anorectal agenesis.

C. Failure of fixation of the hindgut can result in volvulus.

E. Premature rupture of the anal membrane would not cause anorectal agenesis.
GAS 498; N 311; ABR/McM 279

97. **A.** Meckel diverticulum is a remnant of the yolk stalk. It is usually 2 inches long and 2 feet proximal from the ileocecal junction. Meckel diverticulum is prone to ulceration (possibly leading to perforation) that can result in gastrointestinal bleeding.

B. Duplication of the intestine does not predispose the patient to GI bleeding.

C. A subhepatic cecum and appendix is due to failure of complete midgut rotation during development.

D. Nonrotation of the midgut could lead to volvulus but is not the most likely cause for GI bleeding.

E. Herniation of intestines can exist without any symptoms; however, if the loop of intestine becomes strangulated, it can lead to gangrene.
GAS 315; N 270; ABR/McM 242

98. **D.** Failure of the ureteric bud to form results in renal agenesis and oligohydramnios, that is, deficient production of amniotic fluid.

A. Polycystic kidney disease is an autosomal recessive disease characterized by spongy kidneys with a multitude of cysts.

B. Degeneration of the mesonephros occurs during normal development; however, a small portion of the mesonephric tubules may go on to form parts of the urogenital system.

C. Ureteric duplication occurs due to premature division of the ureteric bud and can result in either a double kidney or a duplication of the ureter.

E. Wilms tumor is a malignancy of the kidney that is more common in children than it is in adults; it does not cause renal agenesis.
GAS 373–374; N 311; ABR/McM 263

99. **C.** Androgen insensitivity syndrome involves the development of testes and female external genitalia, with a blind-ending vagina and absence of the uterus and uterine tubes. This is consistent with the presenting symptoms.

A and B. Male pseudohermaphroditism and female pseudohermaphroditism have different presentations from those described and result from 46XY and 46XX genotypes, respectively.

D. Inguinal hernias have nothing to do with absence of the uterus and a negative sex chromatin pattern.

E. Turner syndrome results from a 45X genotype and presents with short stature, webbed neck, congenital hypoplasia of the lymphatics, and shield chest—among other symptoms—and is not consistent with the symptoms described.
GAS 470; N 371; ABR/McM 285

100. **A.** The vaginal plate, which arises from the sinovaginal bulbs, undergoes canalization during embryonic development. Failure of canalization results in a persistent vaginal plate and thus imperforate hymen. The hymen is a fold of mucous membrane that covers the opening of the vaginal canal. It is often torn early in life.

A. The processus vaginalis is a tube-like projection of the peritoneum into the inguinal canal that precedes the descent of the testis.

B and D. Both cervical atresia and androgen insensitivity syndrome would result in amenorrhea; however, neither disorder would present with an imperforate hymen because the vaginal canal would still undergo canalization.

E. The sinovaginal bulbs are responsible for the development of the vaginal plate. Failure of development would result in complete absence of the vagina.
GAS 474; N 370; ABR/McM 285

Answers 101–125

101. **D.** Gartner duct cysts, which often appear in the lateral wall of the vagina, are the result of remnants of the mesonephric (Wolffian) duct. The mesonephric duct gives rise to a variety of structures, including the ureter and collecting tubules. In men, the duct eventually forms the ductus deferens and ejaculatory ducts, whereas it often disappears in women. The only remaining traces of the mesonephric ducts are the epoophoron, paroophoron, and Gartner duct, which can form a cyst.

A. The mesonephric tubules are elongations of the mesonephric vesicles. These tubules are subsequently invaginated by the glomeruli to form a component of the renal corpuscle.

B. The paramesonephric ducts are responsible for formation of the uterus, cervix, and uppermost aspect of the vagina.

C. The urogenital folds form the labia minora in women and the spongy urethra in men. E. Sinovaginal bulbs are responsible for the development of the vaginal plate in embryonic development.
GAS 474; N 371; ABR/McM 286

102. **C.** Potter sequence, or Potter syndrome, is a rare autosomal recessive trait and is associated with renal agenesis or hypoplasia. Altered facial characteristics include flattened nasal bridge, mandibular micrognathia, malformed low-set ears, etc. Absence or lack of proper development of the kidneys causes oligohydramnios, or possibly anhydramnios.

A and B. Multicystic dysplastic kidney and polycystic kidney are usually secondary to Potter sequence and are therefore not the cause of Potter sequence or oligohydramnios.

D. Wilms tumor is a relatively common renal tumor that presents in children; it is not associated with oligohydramnios and Potter sequence.

E. Exstrophy of the urinary bladder is a congenital defect that exposes the posterior surface of the urinary bladder on the exterior of the abdominal wall; there is no indication of this defect in the patient.
GAS 373–374; N 311; ABR/McM 268

103. **B.** The ureteric bud is responsible for the development of the ureter, and thus an early splitting of the ureteric bud would result in formation of a second ureter on the ipsilateral side.

A. Failure of the ureteric bud to form would cause a complete absence of the ureter.

C. The urorectal septum is a section of tissue of mesenchymal origin that develops between the allantois and hindgut. Failure of this structure to develop would not result in an additional ureter.

D. Persistent patent urachus acts as an abnormal fistula that runs from the urinary bladder to the umbilicus, resulting in urine leaking from the anterior abdominal wall.

E. Failure of the ureteric bud to branch occurs normally during embryonic development and results in one ureter joined to each kidney.

GAS 373–374; N 317; ABR/McM 271

104. B. The hepatorenal pouch (or recess or space of Morison) is situated between the liver and the parietal peritoneum covering both the right kidney and suprarenal gland. This recess is the lowest space in the peritoneal cavity in supine patients. Accumulation of fluid in the peritoneal cavity will ordinarily collect in this pouch.

A. The right subphrenic space is located between the liver and diaphragm. Although this recess is positioned in the appropriate abdominal quadrant, it is not the deepest space within the peritoneal cavity. Fluid may reach the right subphrenic space, but it will not accumulate in this region.

C. The paracolic gutters are grooves lateral to the ascending and descending colons. Though these recesses are potential spaces for fluid accumulation, they are located inferior to the hepatorenal recess and would not collect fluid while the patient is supine. D, E. The vesicouterine and rectouterine pouch would not be potential spaces for fluid accumulation in a supine patient, although they provide predictable sites when the patient is upright or ambulating.

GAS 328; N 276; ABR/McM 285

105. A. The right subphrenic space is located between the inferior aspect of the diaphragm and the superior surface of the liver. An ulceration in the posterior stomach wall would allow the passage of air from the stomach into the right subphrenic space through an open communication in the omental bursa.

B, C. These structures are located inferior to the site of ulceration and would not accumulate air. The paracolic gutters traverse lateral to the ascending and descending colons.

D, E. The vesicouterine and rectouterine pouches are located in the pelvic cavity; air would not accumulate in these spaces.

GAS 328; N 284; ABR/McM 254

106. E. The most likely location for fluid to accumulate is the rectouterine pouch (of Douglas) because it is the lowest point in the pelvis when a patient is standing erect. Additionally, fluid would accumulate here because the mesovarian ligament causes the ovary to be located on the posterior aspect of the broad ligament. This allows for communication between the fluid of the ovary and the rectouterine pouch.

A, C. The right subphrenic space is located inferior to the right side of the diaphragm and superior to the liver. The paracolic gutters are located lateral to the ascending and descending colons. Neither of these locations is a likely site of fluid accumulation when the patient is standing.

B. The hepatorenal recess is situated between the liver and both the right kidney and suprarenal gland. This recess, also known as Morison pouch, is the deepest space in the peritoneal cavity where fluid can collect in the supine position.

D. The vesicouterine pouch is located between the urinary bladder and uterus and is separated from the ovaries by a double layer of mesentery also known as the broad ligament of the uterus.

GAS 381–382; N 350; ABR/McM 285

107. D. The parietal peritoneum lines the abdominal wall, whereas the visceral peritoneum is in intimate contact with organs. The greater omentum extends from the greater curvature of the stomach and its omental apron portion hangs below the transverse colon. Access to the ileum would require penetration of the parietal peritoneum to enter the peritoneal cavity and interruption of the peritoneum of "the mesentery" covering the thrombosed vessel. Although it would probably be necessary to reflect the omental apron portion of the greater omentum for adequate exposure, it would not ordinarily require an incision.

A, B, C, E. These structures will not provide access to the affected vessel.

GAS 387; N 264; ABR/McM 239

108. D. Referred pain from cholecystitis is generally referred to the region of the inferior angle of the right scapula. These fibers are generally from T5 to T9 via the greater thoracic splanchnic nerve. These sensory fibers for pain are stimulated by the gallbladder inflammation because of the proximity of the adjacent structures.

A. C3–C5 spinal nerves provide sensory innervation to the upper shoulder area.

B. C5–C8 spinal nerves provide sensory innervation to primarily to the upper limb, to the level of the hand;

C. T1–T4 spinal nerves provide sensory innervation to the upper thoracic wall and medial arm; T1–T4 visceral fibers for pain are generally associated with referred pain from the heart.

E. T10–T11 spinal nerves provide sensory innervation to the abdominal wall at the level of the umbilicus.

GAS 340, 358–364; N 309; ABR/McM 246

109. A. The Pringle maneuver is a surgical technique employed when a hepatic artery has been accidentally ligated. The hepatoduodenal ligament is clamped off to prevent the passage of blood flow through both the proper hepatic artery and the hepatic portal vein.

B. The Kocher maneuver, in which the duodenum and head of the pancreas are reflected to the left, is often employed to expose and arrest a hemorrhage from the inferior vena cava.

C. The Valsalva maneuver involves stopping the passage of air with the vocal folds to build up intrathoracic pressure, as for coughing or vocalization.

D. The Heimlich maneuver involves sharp, rapid compressions of the xiphisternal region to expel foreign bodies from the trachea.

E. Putting a clamp on the porta hepatis would not stop the bleeding but could certainly produce major injury to the numerous vascular elements there.

GAS 304; N 276; ABR/McM 247

110. **A.** The most likely source of this hemorrhage is from the left colic artery, which is a branch of the inferior mesenteric artery. Colonic diverticular disease is the development of blind end sacs from the wall of the colon. Of the selected choices the left colic artery is the only artery supplying a portion of the descending colon.

B. The middle colic artery is a branch of the superior mesenteric artery and supplies the transverse colon.

C, D. The superior and inferior rectal (hemorrhoidal) arteries supply the rectum and anal canal.

E. The left gastro-omental artery arises from the splenic artery and supplies the greater curvature of the stomach (*GAS* Fig. 4.92).

GAS 350; N 295; ABR/McM 249

111. **D.** Murphy sign is a specific test designed to detect and diagnose problems in the upper right abdominal quadrant. It is classically used to diagnose diseases of the gallbladder: pressing deeply under the right costal margin, one asks the patient to breathe deeply. This causes sharp pain in the patient with cholecystitis.

A. Rebound tenderness is pain experienced when applied pressure is removed quickly from a location on the body. It is not specific to areas of the body and is not indicative of problems in the upper right quadrant.

B. The iliopsoas test is generally used to diagnose appendicitis because flexing the iliopsoas muscle group applies pressure to the cecum and appendix. When the appendix is inflamed, this pressure elicits pain.

C. The obturator sign is used to diagnose irritation of the obturator internus muscle and would not elicit a positive test with the patient's current symptoms.

E. Cough tenderness would not be present because it is generally associated with hernias and problems associated with rises in intra-abdominal pressure.

GAS 330, 340; N 309; ABR/McM 246

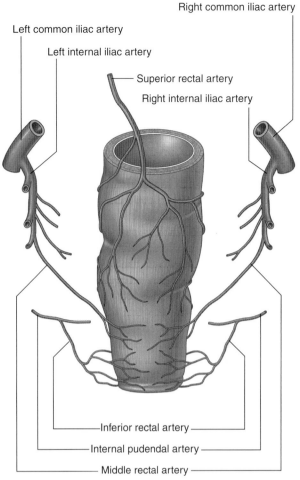

• *GAS* **Fig. 4.92**

112. **D.** The lowest point of the lesser sac occurs at the intersection of the gastrocolic ligament and transverse colon. Bleeding would travel to the lowest point of the lesser sac. Access to this area would require entry through the gastrocolic ligament, which is the portion of the greater omentum which extends from the greater curvature of the stomach to the transverse colon. The hepatogastric and hepatoduodenal ligaments attach between the liver and the lesser curvature of the stomach and the first part of the duodenum, respectively. Dividing the hepatogastric ligament provides entry through the lesser omentum, but this is not the most efficient access point because it does not provide the best exposure of the inferior aspect of the lesser sac (*GAS* Fig. 4.60).

A, B, C, and E. Transecting these ligaments will not provide adequate exposure to the lesser sac.

GAS 300–306; N 275; ABR/McM 240

113. **D.** Superficial inguinal nodes. The external anal sphincter is skeletal muscle of the anal canal. This suggests that the carcinoma is originating from the anal canal. The results of the biopsy support the finding that the carcinoma most likely occurred below the pectinate line where squamous cells of the anal

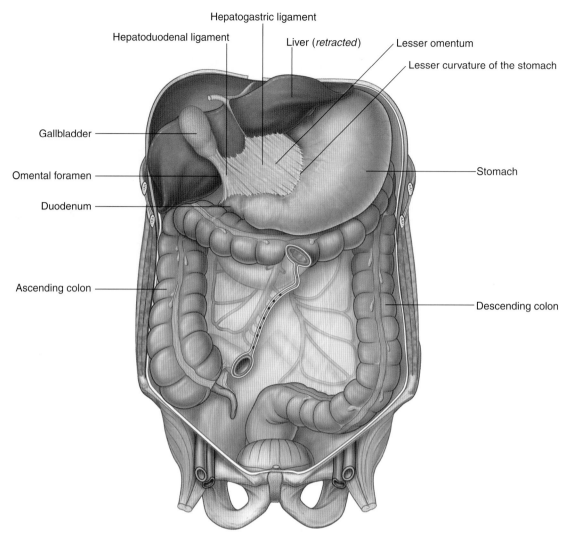

Hepatogastric ligament

Hepatoduodenal ligament

Liver (*retracted*)

Lesser omentum

Lesser curvature of the stomach

Gallbladder

Omental foramen

Duodenum

Stomach

Ascending colon

Descending colon

• *GAS* **Fig. 4.60**

canal are found. The anal canal primarily drains to the superficial inguinal lymph nodes.
- **A.** The inferior rectum above the pectinate line drains into the internal iliac nodes.
- **B.** The middle rectal lymph nodes drain the superior aspect of the rectum.
- **C.** The external iliac nodes primarily drain the lower limb, pelvic, and deep perineal structures.
- **E.** The deep inguinal lymph nodes drain the glands of the clitoris and penis and receive some of the lymph of the superficial inguinal nodes.
  GAS 514; N 268; ABR/McM 234

114. **A.** The lymphatics of the inferior rectum above the pectinate line drain into the internal iliac nodes. Below the pectinate line, lymphatics of the anal canal will primarily drain into the superficial inguinal (horizontal) nodes.
- **B.** The external iliac nodes primarily drain lower limb, pelvic, and deep perineal structures.
- **C.** The superior aspect of the rectum is drained by the middle rectal nodes, lymph from which eventually flows into the lumbar nodes.

- **D.** The superficial inguinal lymph nodes drain the area superior to the pectinate line.
- **E.** The deep inguinal lymph nodes primarily drain the glands of the clitoris and penis, receiving lymph also from the superficial inguinal nodes.
  GAS 514; N 390; ABR/McM 281

115. **B.** In sliding hernias, the GE junction is displaced. Diaphragmatic hernias of the esophagus can be characterized by analyzing the GE junction. In sliding hernias, the GE junction is displaced superiorly into the mediastinum.
- **A.** Sliding hernias do not possess a normal GE junction.
- **C–E.** A paraesophageal hernia is generally characterized by herniation of the stomach into the mediastinum; however, the GE junction remains fixed. In paraesophageal hernias the fundus herniates into the mediastinum, but the antrum does not.
  GAS 372; N 265; ABR/McM 270

116. **B.** The falciform ligament separates the subphrenic spaces into right and left recesses and extends between the liver and the anterior abdominal wall. Because of

its location and attachments, it would serve to stop the spread of such an abscess from one side to the other across the midline.

A. The round ligament of the liver is the obliterated remains of the umbilical vein and lies in the free margin of the falciform ligament ascending from the umbilicus to the inferior surface of the liver.

C. The coronary ligament encloses the bare area of the liver and forms the triangular ligaments.

D, E. The hepatoduodenal and hepatogastric ligaments attach the liver to the duodenum and stomach, respectively. Together they form the lesser omentum.
GAS 328; N 284; ABR/McM 254

117. A. The spleen lies under the left side of the liver superior to the kidneys, adjacent to ribs 9–11. It would be the most common organ to get injured.

B. The lungs are located completely within the thoracic cavity above the level of the twelfth rib.

C. The kidney lies at the twelfth rib, and problems with pain associated with respiratory processes would result from the ribs being injured.

D. The liver is located on the right side of the body and lies around the level of the fifth to tenth ribs.

E. The pancreas is predominantly located in the middle of the body more medial to the kidneys at the level of the eleventh to twelfth ribs.
GAS 373–374; N 311; ABR/McM 263

118. D. A malignancy of the anal canal would drain into the superficial inguinal lymph nodes.

A and B. The internal iliac lymph nodes receive drainage from the rectum, the uterus, the prostate, and the urinary bladder.

C. The testes, though located in the scrotum external to the abdominopelvic cavities, drain into the lumbar nodes located on the anterior aspect of the aorta.

E. The sigmoid colon drains into the inferior mesenteric lymph nodes.
GAS 514; N 390; ABR/McM 281

119. C. The superior mesenteric artery arises from the aorta behind the neck of the pancreas, at the L1 vertebral level, and passes inferiorly across the anterior surface of the third part of the duodenum. As it crosses the uncinate process of the pancreas and duodenum, this artery could readily be affected by a tumor in the immediate area.

A and B. The bile duct and the hepatic portal vein are associated with the first part of the duodenum.

B. The gastroduodenal artery supplies the duodenum, the head of the pancreas, and the greater curvature of the stomach and is a branch of the common hepatic artery. This artery does not cross the third part of the duodenum.

C. The posterior superior pancreaticoduodenal courses posteriorly over the head of the pancreas and supplies both the head of the pancreas and the second portion of the duodenum. It is

therefore more associated with the second part of the duodenum.
GAS 343, 353; N 295; ABR/McM 248

120. D. Vascular structures situated immediately medial to the ureter are often subject to ligation during surgical procedures. The ureter is crossed by the uterine artery an inch or so lateral to the cervix and must be identified and avoided when ligating the uterine vessels.

A. The middle rectal artery arises from the internal iliac artery and passes dorsal to the uterus and the rectum.

B. The superior vesical artery arises from the umbilical artery anteriorly in the pelvis.

C. The internal pudendal vein enters the pelvis through the greater sciatic foramen and terminates in the internal iliac vein, laterally at the pelvic wall.

E. The gonadal vein in females passes from the ovary by way of the suspensory ligament of the ovary or infundibulopelvic ligament, near the pelvic brim.
GAS 380; N 317; ABR/McM 271

121. B. Pain in the umbilical region can be indicative of referred pain from the large intestine. Gallstones can ulcerate through the wall of the fundus of the gallbladder and into the transverse colon, or through the wall of the body of the gallbladder into the duodenum. The stone would then most likely be entrapped at the ileocecal junction, possibly leading to an intestinal obstruction. This could lead predictably to the pain, cramping, and vomiting experienced by the patient.

A. Because the gallstones could pass freely through the intestine as far distally as the ileocecal junction, it would be unlikely that they would accumulate in the jejunum.

C and E. The radiographic results suggest that the biliary trees are clear (indicated by the presence of air) and rule out the bile duct or common hepatic duct as potential sites of gallstone obstruction.

D. Because the gallstones would pass thereafter through the duodenum, this would not be the site of blockage.
GAS 330, 340; N 309; ABR/McM 248

122. A. The intersection of the right linea semilunaris with the ninth costal cartilage in the right upper quadrant is associated typically with the point of contact of the gallbladder fundus with the anterior abdominal wall. The anatomic quadrants provide a useful tool for understanding the location of various anatomic structures and viscera located within the body. The linea semilunaris runs parallel with the lateral border of the rectus sheath and is a prominent landmark for surface anatomy.

B. The intersection of the right semilunaris with the right intertubercular plane is situated in the upper right quadrant; however, this is not the most precise location of the gallbladder.

C and D. The epigastric region is located superior to the umbilical region. The contents of the epigastric region are the left portion of the liver and a portion of the stomach. The right hypochondriac region, the anatomic region situated to the right of the epigastric region, is located superior and lateral to the gallbladder.

E. The upper right quadrant is the correct anatomic region for the location of the gallbladder as mentioned earlier; however, this is too general and would not be the best answer.
GAS 407; N 251; ABR/McM 227

123. **E.** The internal abdominal oblique and transversus abdominis muscles and aponeuroses form the falx inguinalis, which moves down to close off the posterior wall of the inguinal canal and the lower part of the inguinal triangle (of Hesselbach) when the muscles of the abdominal wall contract, such as when coughing or straining. Gradual weakness or attrition of these muscles provides the likelihood of egress of a direct inguinal hernia.

A and B. A patent processus vaginalis at the deep inguinal ring, or expansion of the deep inguinal ring, with stretching of the transversalis fascia there, can contribute to the formation of indirect inguinal hernias.

C and D. Weakness of the transversalis fascia by itself is not a key feature of inguinal herniation, nor is weakness of the peritoneum, or defects in the aponeuroses of the external or internal abdominal oblique muscles.
GAS 298; N 264; ABR/McM 232

124. **C.** The rectouterine pouch (of Douglas) is the lowest recess of the female abdominopelvic cavity when standing or sitting upright. Any fluid accumulation in this cavity will settle in the rectouterine pouch due to it being the most dependent or inferior space.

A. The subphrenic space would likely not collect fluid because of its location in the superior abdominal cavity, which does not tend to collect fluid from the pelvis when the body is in the upright position.

B and E. The hepatorenal pouch (of Morison), also known as the right subhepatic space, is located in the right posterosuperior aspect of the abdominal cavity, far from the pelvic cavity.

D. The vesicouterine space is a recess that is similarly located in the lower portion of the abdomen between the urinary bladder and uterus, but it is slightly superior to the rectouterine pouch (of Douglas) and is separated from it and the pathway of the leaking fluid by the broad ligament of the uterus. The broad ligament tends to prevent the collection of fluids in the vesicouterine pouch.
GAS 475; N 350; ABR/McM 285

125. **D.** The dorsal root ganglia contain all cell bodies of sensory neurons from the body wall and limbs.

Afferent fibers from the appendix travel in the dorsal root ganglia of T8–T10.

A. The sympathetic trunk contains postganglionic sympathetic cell bodies that are targeted to smooth muscle and glands of the viscera and heart muscle.

B. The greater thoracic splanchnic nerve (T5–T9) carries preganglionic sympathetic axons to the celiac ganglion, which is formed by postganglionic sympathetic neurons.

C. The lateral horn of the spinal cord is found in levels T1–L2 and contains preganglionic sympathetic cell bodies.

E. The dorsal root ganglia of L2–L4 are not indicated in appendicitis
GAS 311; N 306; ABR/McM 222

Answers 126–150

126. **A.** The preganglionic sympathetic fibers running to the suprarenal gland would be cut during adrenalectomy for they synapse on catecholamine-secreting cells within the suprarenal medulla. Unlike the normal route of sympathetic innervation, which is to first synapse in a sympathetic ganglion and then send postganglionic fibers to the target tissue, the chromaffin cells of the suprarenal gland are innervated directly by preganglionic sympathetic fibers. This is because the chromaffin cells are embryologically postganglionic neurons that migrate to the medulla and undergo differentiation.

B, C, D, and E. The suprarenal gland receives no other recognized types of innervation.
GAS 394; N 322; ABR/McM 268

127. **D.** The left common iliac vein passes inferior to the left common iliac artery. Compression of the vein in this location may cause of deep venous thrombosis of the left lower limb; that is, the venous drainage of the lower limb is obstructed. This can cause extreme pain, together with ischemia of the limb that, in some untreated cases, can lead to amputation of the limb or gangrene leading to death.

A. The inferior vena cava, which is formed by the union of the right and left common iliac veins at the L5 vertebral level, passes posterior to the right common iliac artery and would be compressed by enlargement of that artery.

B. The renal veins would not be compromised because these veins extend from the kidneys to the inferior vena cava quite far above the blockage.

C. The testicular veins pass lateral to the area of obstruction, with the right gonadal vein passing superiorly to join the inferior vena cava, and the left gonadal vein terminating in the left renal vein.

E. The right common iliac vein passes superiorly along the pelvic brim to unite with the left common iliac vein to form the inferior vena cava and

would not be subjected to compression by the left common iliac artery.
GAS 268; N 295; ABR/McM 271

128. **D.** Preganglionic and postganglionic sympathetics, preganglionic parasympathetic, and visceral afferent fibers are present within the celiac ganglion. The cell bodies of postganglionic sympathetic fibers are contained within the celiac ganglion and their axons pass to upper abdominal organs (foregut).

A, B, C, and E. Preganglionic parasympathetic nerves also run through the ganglion but do not synapse within the ganglion; therefore, there are no postganglionic parasympathetic nerves in the ganglion. The preganglionic parasympathetic fibers are extensions from the vagal trunks and run within the preaortic plexus. No somatic motor fibers are present within this ganglion. Running through all of the abdominal ganglia are also visceral afferent fibers passing superiorly to reach the spinal cord at spinal nerve levels T5–L2. There are no postganglionic parasympathetic fibers running within the ganglion or the celiac plexus. Postganglionic parasympathetic nerves arise from terminal ganglia located upon, or within the wall of, target organs. Answers C and E are incorrect because they do not include postganglionic sympathetic cell bodies and their axons, which also run through the celiac ganglion.
GAS 359; N 310; ABR/McM 252

129. **C.** The ureter is innervated by sympathetic and parasympathetic fibers in the ureteric plexus. General visceral afferent fibers in the ureteric plexus follow sympathetic fibers from spinal cord levels T11–L2; therefore, pain from these fibers will be referred to nerves at these levels. The ilioinguinal nerve is a branch of the L1 ventral ramus and it innervates muscles of the lower abdominal wall and the skin from the iliac crest to the anterior portions of the labium majus.

A. The subcostal nerve innervates skin at the T12 dermatome level.

B. The iliohypogastric nerve is a branch of the L1 ventral ramus, although it may also receive fibers from T12. It innervates abdominal muscles and skin superior to and parallel with the inguinal ligament, as well as skin over the pubic symphysis.

D. The lateral femoral cutaneous nerve contains fibers from L2 and L3 spinal cord levels and innervates the skin over the lateral thigh.

E. The obturator nerve contains fibers from L2 to L4 spinal cord levels and innervates the adductors of the thigh.
GAS 286, 381; N 321; ABR/McM 230

130. **A.** Perforation of a posterior duodenal ulcer most commonly damages the gastroduodenal artery.

C. The posterior superior pancreaticoduodenal artery is a branch of the gastroduodenal artery near its origin from the common hepatic artery.

B. The superior mesenteric artery does not lie directly beneath the duodenum and is not likely to be damaged.

D. The posterior inferior pancreaticoduodenal artery branches from the superior mesenteric artery and lies too far inferior to be damaged.

E. The right gastric artery branches from the proper hepatic artery and runs along the pyloric portion of the lesser curvature of the stomach.
GAS 312; N 291; ABR/McM 246

131. **E.** A perforating ulcer in the anterior wall of the duodenum is likely to cause peritonitis. The duodenum is covered anteriorly by a layer of peritoneum, and an erosion would allow intestinal contents into the greater peritoneal sac. Perforating ulcers pierce the duodenum or stomach anteriorly; penetrating ulcers pierce the duodenum or stomach posteriorly.

A, C. The gastroduodenal and posterior superior pancreaticoduodenal arteries lie posterior to the first part of the duodenum and are not likely to be damaged.

B. The superior mesenteric artery crosses the third or horizontal part of the duodenum anteriorly and is not likely to be damaged. E. The posterior inferior pancreaticoduodenal artery is a branch of the superior mesenteric artery and is not likely to be damaged because it passes posterior to the duodenum.
GAS 312; N 291; ABR/McM 246

132. **D.** The suspensory muscle of the duodenum (ligament of Treitz) originates from the right crus of the diaphragm and is attached to the fourth part of the duodenum at the duodenojejunal junction. This ligament is commonly used as a palpable landmark during abdominal surgeries.

A–C. The superior and inferior mesenteric arteries, and the vasa recta are highly variable and cannot be used as reliable landmarks.

E. Ladd bands connect the cecum to the abdominal wall and can obstruct the duodenum in cases of malrotation of the intestine. These bands can be surgically divided to treat malrotation of the intestine, but Ladd bands are not used as a common landmark (*GAS* Fig. 4.69).
GAS 310; N 271; ABR/McM 244

133. **E.** Failure of fusion of the pleuroperitoneal folds can cause herniation of abdominal contents into the thorax (congenital diaphragmatic hernia), most commonly on the left side. This defect can impair lung function, causing respiratory distress and cyanosis.

A. The absence of the pleuropericardial fold would cause communication between the pericardial sac and the pleural cavity of the lung and would not lead to the symptoms described.

B. The musculature of the diaphragm is derived from the third to fifth cervical myotomes. Absence of musculature in one half of the diaphragm (eventration of the diaphragm) would cause paradoxical respiration.

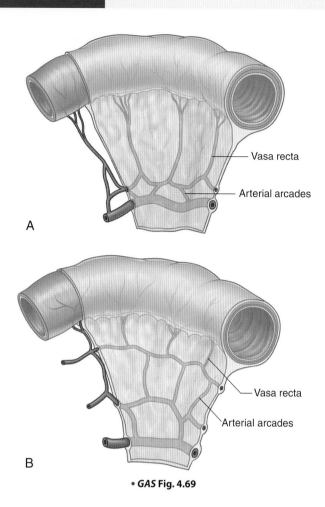

A

B

• **GAS** Fig. 4.69

C. The downward migration of the diaphragm is due to the elongation of the posterior body wall and is not likely to lead to this patient's condition.

D. Failure of the septum transversum to develop would cause an absence of the central tendon of the diaphragm and is not normally associated with congenital diaphragmatic hernia.
GAS 373–374; N 200; ABR/McM 270

134. C. Both Morgagni and Bochdalek hernias are due to defects in the pleuroperitoneal membrane. Morgagni hernia is normally found retrosternally just lateral to the xiphoid process and, if severe, can cause respiratory distress. More commonly, it is perceived as a sharp, epigastric pain that can be confused with several other maladies.

A. Bochdalek hernia can cause similar symptoms but is due to a posterolateral herniation and would not be near the xiphoid process.

B, D. In this case, the barium test rules out esophageal problems; the negative HIDA rules out cholecystitis.

E. A congenital hiatal hernia occurs when part of the stomach herniates into the thoracic cavity and can be caused by a shortened esophagus. This type of hernia would not present between the xiphoid process and costal margin.
GAS 372; N 200; ABR/McM 270

135. A. The ileum can become ischemic when arterial supply from the superior mesenteric artery is compromised. The superior mesenteric artery arises from the aorta posterior to the neck of the pancreas. It descends across the third part of the duodenum and enters the root of the mesentery behind the transverse colon. This artery gives origin to the following branches: inferior pancreaticoduodenal artery, middle colic artery, ileocolic artery, right colic artery, and intestinal arteries. The ileocolic artery descends behind the peritoneum toward the right and ends by dividing into the ascending colic artery, anterior and posterior cecal arteries, the appendicular artery, and ileal branches. The terminal ileum is supplied by the ileal branches, which do not have any anastomoses with another major source vessel.

B. The transverse colon is supplied by the marginal artery (of Drummond), which possesses anastomoses of the right colic artery arising from the superior mesenteric artery and the left colic artery arising from the inferior mesenteric artery.

C–E. The spleen, stomach, and duodenum are all supplied by branches of the celiac trunk, which arise from the abdominal aorta just below the aortic hiatus of the diaphragm.
GAS 354; N 294; ABR/McM 248

136. A. The hepatic portal vein is compressed in its passage through the hepatoduodenal ligament because it is the anterior border of the omental (epiploic) foramen (of Winslow). The veins of Retzius are located along the sides of the abdominal walls and communicate between tributaries of retroperitoneal parts of the gastrointestinal tract and veins of the body wall. In portal hypertension the portal blood cannot pass freely through the liver, and the portal-caval tributaries and their anastomoses become dilated. The superior and inferior epigastric veins anastomose with the paraumbilical veins, which are normally tributary to the hepatic portal vein. These would be the first affected in portal hypertension.

B. The inferior vena cava is the main route of blood return to the right atrium and is posterior to the omental (epiploic) foramen (of Winslow); it is not as likely to be compressed due to herniation through the foramen as the hepatic portal vein.

C. Compression of the proper hepatic artery in the hepatoduodenal ligament would not result in dilation of veins of Retzius but could conceivably diminish blood supply to the gallbladder and liver.

D. Bile duct compression would result in jaundice and increased serum bilirubin.

E. The cystic duct joins with the common hepatic duct to form the bile duct. Compression of this would lead to an inflamed gallbladder (cholecystitis).
GAS 354–357; N 296; ABR/McM 246

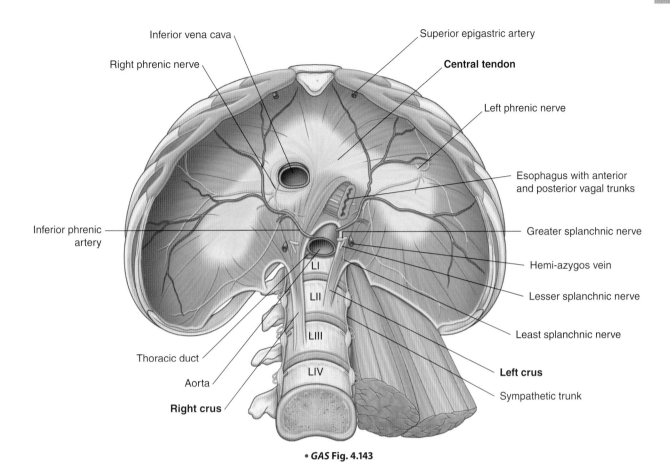

Inferior vena cava

Right phrenic nerve

Superior epigastric artery

Central tendon

Left phrenic nerve

Esophagus with anterior and posterior vagal trunks

Inferior phrenic artery

Greater splanchnic nerve

Hemi-azygos vein

Lesser splanchnic nerve

Least splanchnic nerve

LI

LII

LIII

LIV

Left crus

Sympathetic trunk

Thoracic duct

Aorta

Right crus

• *GAS* **Fig. 4.143**

137. C. A dermatome is an area of skin that is supplied by a single spinal nerve. The descending colon receives its visceral sensory supply for pain from spinal segments L1 and L2. Injury to the descending colon can cause referral of pain to the corresponding dermatomes.
A, B, D, E. Spinal segments T5–T9 supply upper abdominal organs, including the pancreas and the duodenum. L3–L4 supply the rectum, urinary bladder, and uterus. T10–L1 supply portions of abdominal viscera proximal to the descending colon.
GAS 405; N 306; ABR/McM 101

138. E. A gallstone ileus occurs when a gallstone (cholelith) ulcerates through the wall of the body of the gallbladder and into the duodenum. In this case, gallstones became lodged in the ileocecal region. Obstruction in the ileocecal junction can produce pain that mimics appendicitis. However, bowel sounds will be exaggerated above the obstruction and absent distal to the obstruction. This obstruction would require surgical correction.
A. The hepatopancreatic ampulla (of Vater) is the location where the pancreatic and bile ducts join before entering the duodenum. An obstruction here would cause jaundice, and radiating pain would be localized into the right upper quadrant, with referred pain to the scapula.
B. The duodenal cap, or bulb, is proximal to the entrance of the bile duct, and any obstruction would be distal to this point.

C. The proximal ileum is not a likely site for gallstone obstruction.
D. The pyloric sphincter surrounds the pyloric orifice and controls the rate of emptying of the stomach contents into the duodenum. This location is proximal to the entrance of gallbladder contents into the small intestine.
GAS 330, 340; N 280; ABR/McM 242

139. A. The upper and intermediate portions of the esophagus receive blood supply from three branches of the aorta: the inferior thyroid, bronchial, and esophageal arteries; the lower portion of the esophagus is supplied by the inferior phrenic and left gastric arteries. The lowest part of the esophagus, below the diaphragm, is supplied by the left gastric artery. Perforation to this area could easily injure this artery.
B. Bronchial arteries supply a small section of the esophagus inferior to the level of the carina (T4).
C. The intercostal arteries supply intercostal spaces and do not contribute to esophageal arterial supply.
D. The right gastric arises from the proper hepatic artery and supplies the pyloric part of the lesser curvature of the stomach.
E. The inferior phrenic supplies the portion of the esophagus just inferior to the diaphragm (*GAS* Fig. 4.143).
GAS 343–344; N 240; ABR/McM 251

140. B. Kehr sign is a clinical indication of a ruptured spleen and is characterized by intense radiating pain to the top of the left shoulder.

A. Mittelschmerz can occur in the middle of a woman's menstrual cycle when the graafian follicle ruptures and the ovum is released from the ovary.

C. Rovsing sign is a clinical indicator of gallbladder inflammation and pain referred to the right shoulder, also owing to diaphragmatic irritation.

D. The iliopsoas muscle has clinically important relations to the kidneys, ureters, cecum, appendix, sigmoid colon, pancreas, lumbar lymph nodes, and nerves of the posterior abdominal wall. If any of these structures is diseased, a positive psoas sign will be observed.

E. The obturator sign may cause painful spasms of the adductor muscles of the thigh and sensory deficits in the medial thigh.
GAS 342; N 291; ABR/McM 259

141. B. The most common variation in hepatic artery supply to the right lobe of the liver is the right hepatic artery, originating from the superior mesenteric artery occurring in approximately 18% of cases.

A, C, D, E. These are not common anatomical variations of the origin of the right hepatic artery.
GAS 347; N 291; ABR/McM 246

142. B. The gallbladder consists of a fundus, body, and neck. The fundus is the rounded, blind end that comes in contact with the transverse colon. The body is the major part and rests on the upper part of the duodenum and transverse colon. The neck is the narrowest part and gives rise to the cystic duct. This duct contains the spiral valve (of Heister), which is a redundant mucosal fold that maintains patency of the duct. This is not actually a valve and does not determine the direction of flow of bile. This could potentially be a point of constriction that could present difficulty with insertion of a catheter.

A, E. Though the cystic duct is in close relation to the hepatic portal vein and the hepatic artery, the most likely cause of difficulty would be potential constriction by the spiral valve.

C. The cystic duct comes into contact only with the cystic artery and is not particularly tortuous.

D. The hepatoduodenal ligament is the thickened free edge of the lesser omentum, and it conducts the portal triad (portal vein, hepatic artery, and bile duct) and other structures that pass through the porta hepatis. This ligament is unlikely to compress the cystic duct.
GAS 330; N 287; ABR/McM 256

143. B. The ducts of Luschka are accessory biliary ducts that are not present in all individuals. During a cholecystectomy, the cystic duct and cystic artery are ligated and the gallbladder is removed, using sharp dissection to separate the gallbladder from the liver. Routinely, the right hepatic duct and left hepatic duct are not encountered directly. If the physician was unaware that ducts of Luschka were present in the patient, they

would not have been ligated or clipped and their leakage would result in bile peritonitis.

A, C, E. The bile duct and hepatic ducts are left intact during the surgery and should not leak.

D. The cystic duct is ligated during the surgery and with proper ligation would not produce bile peritonitis.
GAS 334; N 287; ABR/McM 256

144. C. Visceral afferents are nerve fibers that transmit the sensation of visceral pain. The target of the neurectomy would be to eradicate visceral pain.

A, B, D, E. One would not want to interfere with sympathetic and parasympathetic nerves, as these provide motor innervation to viscera and vascular smooth muscle.
GAS 394; N 310; ABR/McM 245

145. B. Adynamic ileus entails paralysis of the bowel. It can result from many causes, including kidney stone, spinal injury, and peritonitis. Mechanical obstruction can be caused by blockage within the bowel or compression of the bowel from an external source. Typically, bowel obstruction is characterized initially by increased borborygmi (bowel sounds, particularly the stomach). Increased borborygmi usually follow such obstructions immediately. As the bowel muscle tires, however, bowel sounds can become reduced or absent.

A. Increased borborygmi usually follow such obstructions immediately. As the bowel muscle tires, however, bowel sounds can become reduced or absent and this patient is presenting two days after symptom onset.

C. Borborygmi would be diminished or absent in this patient who is presenting two days after symptom onset. Bowel sounds that are hyperactive to the extent of being continuous would not be present in a paralytic bowel days after onset.

D. Crampy pain may be noted as a symptom, not elicited as a sign on physical examination.

E. Although this patient might have peritonitis, with an abdomen tender to palpation, the data simply indicate generalized abdominal pain.
GAS 305; N 270; ABR/McM 262

146. A. Blood supply from the inferior pancreaticoduodenal artery via the superior mesenteric artery can provide collateral blood supply to the head of the pancreas and the first part of the duodenum in situations when the celiac trunk is occluded. Such anastomoses occur between the superior pancreaticoduodenal branches of the gastroduodenal artery (a derivative of the common hepatic branch of the celiac trunk) and the inferior pancreaticoduodenal (a branch of the superior mesenteric artery).

B. The left gastric artery and hepatic artery are derivatives of the celiac trunk and do not anastomose with the superior mesenteric artery.

C. The cystic artery and the gastroduodenal artery are derivatives of the common hepatic from the celiac trunk. They would not typically provide an anastomosis between the celiac trunk and superior mesenteric artery (unless there is an aberrant right hepatic branch from the superior mesenteric artery).

D. The right and left colic arteries anastomose via the marginal artery of the colon, but this provides collateral supply to the inferior mesenteric artery.

E. The right and left gastro-omental arteries anastomose and provide collateral supply to the greater curvature of the stomach but are derived from the celiac trunk and thus do not provide communication between the celiac trunk and superior mesenteric artery.
GAS 344–350; N 291; ABR/McM 247

147. **B.** The incision and tissue separation at McBurney point to reach the appendix will usually encounter the aponeurosis of the external abdominal oblique muscle, the internal abdominal oblique muscle, transversus abdominis muscle, transversalis fascia, and parietal peritoneum. Muscle fibers of the internal abdominal oblique and transversus can be separated bluntly, without cutting them. The appendix is located intraperitoneally within the abdomen, thus it is covered with visceral peritoneum. The transversalis fascia separates the internal surface of the transversus abdominis from the parietal peritoneum. Thus, five layers must be penetrated to access the inflamed appendix.

A, C, D, E. These are not the correct layers that need to be dissected to expose the appendix.
GAS 389; N 282; ABR/McM 231

148. **D.** Ileal (Meckel) diverticulum, which is an outpouching of the distal ileum, is twice as prevalent in men as in women. The diverticulum is clinically important because ulceration of the diverticulum with pain, bleeding, perforation, and obstruction is a complication that may require emergent surgery. Signs and symptoms frequently mimic appendicitis or peptic ulcer.

A. Internal hemorrhoids are thrombosed tributaries of the middle rectal vein, which can prolapse into the anal canal.

B. External hemorrhoids are thrombosed tributaries in the veins of the external rectal venous plexus.

C. Diverticulosis is ordinarily an outpouching of the wall of the large intestine. This primarily affects the elderly and does not cause bleeding in most cases.

E. Borborygmi are sounds created by gas and intestinal contents as they pass through the gastrointestinal tract.
GAS 315; N 280; ABR/McM 248

149. **D.** Fig. 3.2 is a CT scan that shows an abdominal aortic aneurysm with hemorrhage. If the man stands in an erect position, the blood will be detected in the rectovesical space, which is a peritoneal recess between the urinary bladder and the rectum in men and is the lowest space in the peritoneal cavity.

A. The subphrenic space is a peritoneal pouch between the diaphragm and the anterior and superior part of the liver.

B. The hepatorenal space (pouch of Morison) is a deep peritoneal pocket between the posterior surface of the liver and the right kidney and suprarenal gland.

C. The rectouterine space (pouch of Douglas) is a space in women formed by a peritoneal-lined recess between the rectum and uterus.

E. The subhepatic space is between the liver and the transverse colon.
GAS 473–474; N 373; ABR/McM 281

150. **B.** Paraumbilical pain progressing into the right iliac fossa is a sign of appendicitis. The CT scan is one of an inflamed appendix. The structures in the scan that lie to the right of the vertebral body are part of the psoas muscle. Transverse section of this muscle signifies that it is a cut from the lumbar region.

A, C, D, E. These structures will not explain the patient's symptoms
GAS 407; N 306; ABR/McM 261

Answers 151–174

151. **C.** The arrows in the CT scan point to the descending colon. Therefore, the left colic artery, which supplies the descending colon, is the one most likely occluded in the CT scan.

A, B, D, and E. The middle colic, right colic, and ileocolic artery supply the ascending colon, and the marginal artery provides an anastomosis between branches of the superior mesenteric artery and inferior mesenteric artery.
GAS 350; N 295; ABR/McM 239

152. **B.** The superficial inguinal lymph nodes are the first drainage site for superficial perineal structures like the skin of the perianal region, prepuce of penis, scrotum, and anal canal inferior to the pectinate line. The superficial inguinal nodes also drain structures of the inferolateral quadrant of the trunk, including the anterior abdominal wall inferior to the umbilicus, gluteal region, and the lower limb.

A. The deep inguinal lymph nodes drain the glans of the penis and the distal spongy urethra and receive drainage from the superficial inguinal lymph nodes.

C–D. The common iliac nodes drain the external and internal iliac lymph nodes. The internal iliac lymph nodes drain inferior pelvic structures and deep perineal structures and receive drainage from the sacral nodes.

E. The lumbar lymph nodes are the final drainage site for all the above lymph nodes before they drain to the thoracic duct by way of the lumbar lymph trunks.
GAS 392; N 268; ABR/McM 376

153. **B.** The white arrows in the CT scan in Fig. 3.6 point to the stomach, which fits with the patient's history of long-term NSAID use.

A. The spleen would not be in this CT image because it is located more superiorly in the body than this section. Also, note that the psoas muscles are seen lying on the sides of the vertebral body, meaning that the section is in the lumbar region of the body.

C. The duodenum is the structure located to the right of the stomach in the scan and is posterolateral to the aorta.

D. As a retroperitoneal organ, the pancreas would not be located this far anterior in the CT image.

E. The descending colon is located in the left anterior pararenal space, far posterior to the structure indicated in the CT scan.
GAS 302–303; N 276; ABR/McM 229, 238

154. A. Cancerous cells in the stomach would metastasize first to the celiac nodes.

B. The splenic nodes are located along the splenic artery and are related to drainage from the pancreas; therefore, they will not be the first to receive metastatic cells from a stomach cancer.

C. The suprapancreatic nodes would be associated with pancreatic carcinoma.

D. The right gastric lymph nodes may receive metastatic cells but would not be the first to receive this lymph because they are located along the lesser curvature of the stomach. E. The cisterna chyli, an occasional proximal expanded portion of the thoracic duct, receives lymph drainage from the entire abdomen; therefore, it would not be first to receive cancerous cells.
GAS 315, 358; N BP79; ABR/McM 246

155. C. Because physical examination and laboratory studies show a normal, healthy woman, the anomaly seen on the x-ray would be expected to be benign. Riedel lobe is a normal variation of the liver, often an inferior extension of the right lobe of the liver, lateral to the gallbladder that extends about 4 or 5 cm below the rib cage.

A–B, D–E. Carcinomas would present with abnormal laboratory examinations, and cholecystitis would present with an abnormal physical examination, as when the gallbladder is inflamed.
GAS 328; N 284; ABR/McM 245

156. B. A Spigelian hernia occurs along the semilunar line below the umbilical region and can protrude beneath the skin.

A. Richter hernia is a hernia that presents as a strangulated segment of part of the wall of an intestinal loop through any hernial opening.

C. A paraumbilical hernia occurs at the level of the umbilicus, near the midline.

D. An incisional hernia occurs with dehiscence (breakdown and reopening) of an operative incision after surgery.

E. A ventral hernia is a type of incisional hernia located on the ventral surface of the abdomen, occurring only after surgery.
GAS 298; N 258; ABR/McM 229

157. A. Congenital inguinal hernias occur when a large patency of the processus vaginalis remains so that a loop of intestine herniates into the inguinal canal.

B. A congenital hydrocele is also caused by a patent segment of a processus vaginalis filled with fluid, but it does not cause an indirect hernia.

C. Ectopic testes occur when the gubernaculum does not migrate correctly during development and the testis does not reach the scrotum, but this does not cause a hernia. D. Epispadias occurs when the external urethral orifice opens onto the dorsal surface of the penis and is generally associated with exstrophy of the urinary bladder.

E. A rupture, or tear, of the transversalis fascia would not cause the intestines to herniate through the deep inguinal ring and therefore would not cause an indirect inguinal hernia.
GAS 296–298; N 264; ABR/McM 233

158. A. Failure of relaxation of the lower esophageal sphincter (also known as the cardiac sphincter) causes an accumulation of food in the esophagus. Achalasia is the failure of motility of food through the esophagus into the stomach. A constricted lower esophageal sphincter is the cause of these conditions.

B. Dyspepsia is chronic pain or discomfort in the upper abdomen. This usually accompanies problems with digestion and is not associated with difficulty swallowing.

C. Gastritis is inflammation of the mucosal lining of the stomach and would also not contribute to dysphagia.

D. Gastroparesis is defined as delayed stomach emptying due to stomach paralysis, which would show chyme overloading in the stomach and esophagus (achalasia involves only the esophagus).

E. Peptic ulcers mostly result in pain in the stomach, more commonly the duodenum, due to erosion of the mucosal lining.
GAS 307; N 237; ABR/McM 225

159. D. Meckel diverticulum is an embryologic remnant of the vitelline duct in the embryo located on the distal ileum and proximal to the cecum. If this diverticulum becomes infected, it produces pain in the umbilical region of the abdomen, in addition to possible bleeding.

A. A ruptured appendix usually presents with pain in the lower right quadrant of the abdomen, when the infective processes come in contact with adjacent parietal peritoneum.

B. A volvulus is characterized by a twisted bowel, which causes obstruction of the bolus and/or ischemia as the blood supply is occluded.

C. Diverticulosis is a condition that causes outpouchings of the wall of the gut tube, usually found in the sigmoid colon. Pain from this condition would usually present in the lower left quadrant.

E. Borborygmi are sounds produced from gas and other contents moving through the bowels. This would not cause pain in one specific area because peristaltic activity moves the length of the GI tract.
GAS 315; N 280; ABR/McM 237

160. C. Pain from the gallbladder is sent to the spinal cord by visceral afferents and also is mediated (referred) by nerve fibers that provide pain sensation to the scapula. Open cholecystectomy would cause a risk to the T7 and T8 spinal nerves due to their close proximity to the gallbladder. These nerves are located below the associated rib and along the same horizontal plane as the gallbladder.

A. T5 and T6 nerves are located superior to an incision and thus are not affected.

B. For the same reason, nerves from T6 to T7 would not be the right choice due to T6 not being at risk during this procedure.

D. Nerves from T9 to L1 are located inferior to the incision during this procedure.

E. T5–T9 is a broad range that includes many nerves that would not be affected by the incision.
GAS 340, 358–364; N 309; ABR/McM 227

161. A. The processus vaginalis is formed as the parietal peritoneum layer of the abdominal wall (inguinal region) evaginates through the deep inguinal ring and continues through the superficial inguinal ring. Normally, this evagination or outpouching is obliterated during development. A cyst can develop in a segment of the processus (which is also referred to as the canal of Nuck) if this processus is not obliterated completely between the deep inguinal ring and the testis.

B. Congenital hydrocele would present at the base of the canal; in this case, the swelling would be in the labium majus.

C. An ectopic uterus would present as a mass in the pelvis and not the inguinal region.

D. A femoral hernia would be palpated below the inguinal ligament (usually) within the femoral triangle.

E. A defect of the transversalis fascia could result in inflammation in a specific area but would not be located along the inguinal ligament because this fascial layer is located deep to the inguinal ligament.
GAS 265; N 264; ABR/McM 233

162. C. The most likely place that a pancreatic pseudocyst will be formed is in the floor of the omental bursa, deep to the stomach. The omental bursa is a potential space behind the stomach and directly anterior to the pancreas. Pancreatic extravasations will fill this space.

A. The right subhepatic space is the space in the peritoneal cavity between the inferior visceral surface of the liver and the transverse colon.

B. The hepatorenal space of the subhepatic space, also known as the pouch of Morison, is located between the right lobe of the liver and the parietal peritoneum covering the superior pole of the right kidney and suprarenal gland.

D. The right subphrenic space is the space directly inferior to the diaphragm and above the diaphragmatic surface of the liver. It is above the pancreas; therefore, fluid from the pancreas could not accumulate there.

E. Finally, the greater sac is the general peritoneal cavity of the abdomen. The greater sac communicates with the omental bursa (lesser sac) by way of the omental (epiploic) foramen (of Winslow). The peritoneal cavity contains nothing except a very thin film of serous fluid that allows the organs to slip around relatively freely against one another and on the body wall.
GAS 304; N 288; ABR/McM 240

163. C. The spinal cord levels containing the soma of the sensory fibers transporting the sensation of pain are more than likely at the level of T7 and T8. This is because the xiphoid process is at these dermatome levels for somatic sensations of pain, and these same spinal nerves receive visceral afferents from the stomach.

A, B, D, E. These spinal nerves would not carry the sensory fibers for this patient's presentation.
GAS 358; N 303; ABR/McM 238

164. E. The left paraduodenal fossa (of Landzert) is formed by two peritoneal folds enclosing the ascending branch of the left colic artery and the inferior mesenteric vein, respectively, on the left side of the duodenum. Herniation into the left paraduodenal fossa (of Landzert) occurs more frequently than herniation into the right fossa (of Kolb). The ascending branches of the left colic artery are at risk during repair of a paraduodenal hernia because the location of this hernia is in the upper left quadrant, adjacent to the junction of the terminal duodenum and the jejunum. The ascending branches of the left colic artery supply the upper segment of the descending colon and the splenic flexure of the transverse colon.

A. The middle colic artery arises from the superior mesenteric artery and supplies the transverse colon and anastomoses with the left colic artery. The right colic artery is a more distal branch of the superior mesenteric artery and supplies the ascending colon.

B. The sigmoidal arteries supply the lower segment of the descending colon and the sigmoid colon.

C. The ileocolic artery supplies the cecum, appendix, terminal portion of the ileum, and proximal portion of the ascending colon.

D. Finally, the ileal arteries are the small terminal branches of the superior mesenteric artery supplying blood to the ileum.
GAS 352–353; N 295; ABR/McM 249

165. D. The liver would be the first structure to receive these metastatic cells because they would flow through the portal venous system from the pancreas to the liver.

A. The stomach would not receive these cells because there is no communication between the stomach and pancreas through circulatory or ductal pathways.

B. The spleen also does not have direct communication with the pancreas and would not receive metastatic cells first.

C. The duodenum is the site for pancreatic emptying, but as these metastases pass through venous circulation they would not pass into the duodenum.

E. The vertebral column would not receive the metastases because they would not enter the vertebral venous plexus.

GAS 328, 354; N BP80; ABR/McM 258

166. B. The hepatic portal vein is the most likely structure to be occluded by a large tumor at the neck of the pancreas due to its proximity. The most of the pancreas is drained via the splenic vein which empties into the hepatic portal vein.

A. The inferior mesenteric vein drains the distal part of the large intestine and is inferior to the tumor.

C. The celiac trunk is superior to the tumor.

D, E. The posterior superior pancreaticoduodenal artery would never receive these metastases, nor would the great pancreatic artery. Similarly, the celiac trunk is outside the plane of the tumor.

GAS 354; N 299; ABR/McM 253

167. B. Hartmann pouch is located in the gallbladder at the junction of the neck and the cystic duct. When a gallstone is located in this area, the patient will present with pain but usually no jaundice because the cystic duct is not occluded.

A, C, E. A bile duct and/or left and right hepatic duct obstruction would cause posthepatic jaundice due to bile obstructed in the duct system.

D. Obstruction of the pancreatic duct would cause pain in the umbilical region, not in the right upper quadrant.

GAS 340; N 287; ABR/McM 256

168. B. The hepatopancreatic ampulla is also known as the ampulla of Vater and is located at the junction of the pancreatic duct and bile duct. It is the narrowest part of the biliary duct system.

A, C, D, E. The bile duct, left hepatic duct, pancreatic duct, and right hepatic duct all have larger diameters than the hepatopancreatic ampulla (of Vater) (*GAS* Fig. 4.109).

GAS 332–336; N 287; ABR/McM 257

169. C. An epigastric hernia is formed by a weakness in the intersecting fibers of the linea alba superior to the umbilicus. In most cases, herniation of fat and other tissue through the defect causes a palpable, but painless, mass. If a nerve branch also passes through the defect, it can be associated with local pain.

A. Umbilical hernias are common in newborn babies and pregnant women in the third trimester of pregnancy. This kind of hernia usually represents a weakness in the wall structure at the level of the umbilicus.

B. Spigelian hernias occur through the semilunar lines, lateral to the rectus sheath.

D. Femoral hernias pass through the femoral canal, deep to the inguinal ligament.

E. Omphaloceles are a more serious (but less common) defect, representing failure of the intestines to return to the abdominal cavity, associated with lack of proper growth of the body wall.

GAS 298; N 258; ABR/McM 228

170. D. The knife injured the medial segment of the functional left lobe of the liver, located between the falciform ligament and the gallbladder. This area of the liver is usually supplied by the left hepatic artery, an indirect branch of the celiac trunk. If this were the case, the Pringle maneuver (compression of the hepatoduodenal ligament) would slow or stop the bleeding. An aberrant hepatic branch of the left gastric artery can replace the left hepatic artery; however, it passes through the hepatogastric ligament rather than the hepatoduodenal ligament and is therefore not compressed in a Pringle maneuver. Thus the bleeding is not reduced by that technique.

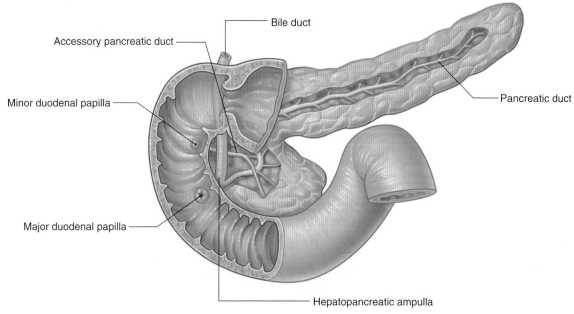

Bile duct

Accessory pancreatic duct

Minor duodenal papilla

Major duodenal papilla

Pancreatic duct

Hepatopancreatic ampulla

• *GAS* **Fig. 4.109**

A. The lateral segment of the left lobe is located to the left of the falciform ligament.

B. The caudate segment of the liver is located in the inferior aspect of the upper portion of the liver, well above the site of injury.

C. The anterior segment of the right lobe is located to the right of the gallbladder.

E. The quadrate lobe is the medial segment of the functional left lobe of the liver, and it receives its arterial supply from the left hepatic artery.
GAS 328–331; N 251; ABR/McM 255

171. **E.** Interruption of both vagal trunks would deprive the abdominal viscera (foregut and midgut) of parasympathetic supply, that is, to the level of the splenic flexure of the colon. Parasympathetic supply to the ascending colon is carried by the vagus nerves and vagal trunks and would be lost.

A, B, C. Distal to the splenic flexure, the colon receives parasympathetic nerves from pelvic splanchnic nerves. Pelvic splanchnic nerves supply the splenic flexure, the descending and sigmoid colon, the rectum and anal canal, the urinary bladder, and the erectile tissues of the penis.

D. The innervation of the ductus deferens and ejaculatory duct is carried by sympathetic nerve supply through the pelvic plexuses.
GAS 363; N 306; ABR/McM 251

172. **B.** Adynamic ileus is paralysis of the bowel. Peristaltic activity ceases. Borborygmi (bowel sounds) are absent when this occurs, as in peritonitis. Pain in the shoulder is due to air under the diaphragm from the perforated anterior duodenal wall; this air irritates somatic afferent pain fibers of the diaphragm, carried by the right phrenic nerve to spinal nerve levels C3–C5. Referral of pain to the shoulder occurs because somatic sensory fibers from the shoulder enter the spinal cord at similar levels.

A. an x-ray would indicate the presence of air under the diaphragm.

D, C. A posterior penetrating ulcer would be associated usually with profuse bleeding, mostly from branches of the gastroduodenal artery that supply the duodenal bulb, the first part of the duodenum.

E. Acute appendicitis is not associated with shoulder pain and adynamic ileus. A perforated appendix, however, will produce symptoms of peritonitis.
GAS 408; N 276; ABR/McM 241

173. **A.** The middle colic artery is the principal source of arterial supply to the transverse colon.

B. The right colic artery, an infrequent branch of the superior mesenteric artery, supplies the ascending colon.

C. The superior mesenteric artery supplies the lower duodenum to ⅔ of the transverse colon, including the lower portions of the pancreas.

D. The ileocolic branch of the superior mesenteric artery supplies the distal ileum, cecum, and ascending colon.

E. The left colic artery provides blood supply to the left colic flexure and descending colon.
GAS 348; N 295; ABR/McM 248

174. **C.** The dermatome of spinal nerve level T10 crosses the level of the umbilicus. Pain from appendicitis is most often perceived at first in the periumbilical region, reflecting the level of embryologic spinal nerve supply to the appendix, which is from T10. When the appendix swells and/or ruptures and contacts the body wall, somatic sensory fibers of the adjacent body wall cause the apparent site of pain to shift to the lower right abdominal quadrant.

A. T7 is at the level of the xiphoid process.

B. T8 and T9 dermatomes lie between the two preceding spinal nerve levels.

D. T12 innervates the lowest portion of the rectus abdominis and overlying skin with motor and sensory supply, respectively.

E. L1 distribution by iliohypogastric and ilioinguinal nerves supplies the suprapubic region, the pubic area, and anterior portions of the urogenital region.
GAS 285–286; N 306, 162; ABR/McM 215 (no clinical thumbnails in new edition)

Answers 175–199

175. **D.** Caput medusae is an end-stage characteristic of liver cirrhosis. The snakelike appearance of veins on the body wall results from anastomoses between small veins called paraumbilical veins that accompany the round ligament (ligamentum teres hepatis) (within the falciform ligament) with veins of the anterior abdominal body wall. The body wall veins become dilated and tortuous, due to portal hypertension.

A. Esophageal varices result from portal-systemic anastomoses between the left gastric vein and esophageal tributaries to the azygos system of veins.

B. Ascites is formed by fluid transudate from thin-walled and dilated anastomotic vessels joining retroperitoneal veins of the gastrointestinal tract with veins of the body wall.

C. Internal hemorrhoids result from expansion of anastomoses between superior rectal tributaries to the inferior mesenteric vein and middle rectal branches of the internal iliac vein.

E. The medial umbilical ligaments do not recanalize in response to portal hypertension.
GAS 356; N 299; ABR/McM 280 (no clinical thumbnails in new edition)

176. **A.** The iliopubic tract is a reflective band of aponeurotic tissue at the origin of the transversus abdominis, when visualized with the laparoscope.

B. The lateral border of the inguinal triangle (of Hesselbach) is provided by the inferior epigastric artery and vein.

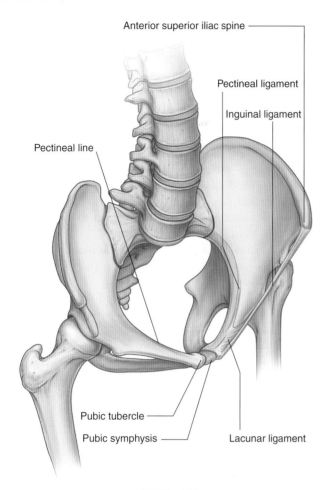

Anterior superior iliac spine

Pectineal ligament

Inguinal ligament

Pectineal line

Pubic tubercle

Pubic symphysis

Lacunar ligament

• *GAS* **Fig. 4.29**

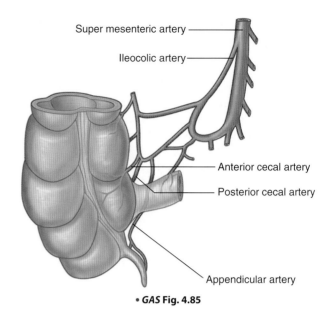

Super mesenteric artery

Ileocolic artery

Anterior cecal artery

Posterior cecal artery

Appendicular artery

• *GAS* **Fig. 4.85**

C. The lateral border of the femoral ring is the femoral vein and connective tissue separating the vein from the femoral canal.

D. The part of the inguinal ligament that attaches to the pectineal ligament is the lacunar ligament (of Gimbernat).

E. The pectineal ligament becomes less dense and thinner as it is traced laterally from the femoral artery toward the iliopectineal portion of the inguinal ligament (*GAS* Fig. 4.29).
GAS 298; N 264; ABR/McM 235

177. **E.** Taeniae coli are three conspicuous longitudinal bands that are a characteristic feature of the colon. Those of the ascending colon extend to the cecum and can be traced inferiorly to the base of the appendix, even when the appendix is retrocolic or retroileal in position, and therefore hidden.

D. The posterior cecal artery, although it often provides origin to the appendicular artery, is very difficult to find quickly, especially in the presence of malrotation and much adipose tissue. The other structures listed do not lead easily to the location of the appendix (*GAS* Fig. 4.85).

A, B, C. These structures would not be the best for tracing and locating the vermiform appendix.
GAS 316; N 283; ABR/McM 261

178. **A.** Infants with congenital aganglionic megacolon, or Hirschsprung disease, lack autonomic ganglion cells in the myenteric plexus distal to the dilated segment of colon. The enlarged colon—megacolon—has the normal number of ganglion cells. The dilation results from failure of relaxation of the aganglionic segment, which prevents movement of the intestinal contents, resulting in a functional obstruction and dilation of the colon proximal to it. Megacolon results from failure of neural crest cells to migrate into the wall of the colon during the fifth to seventh weeks. This results in failure of parasympathetic ganglion cells to develop in the Auerbach and Meissner plexuses.

B. Incomplete separation of the cloaca causes malformation of the hindgut like imperforate anus or absent anus, insufficient anus and ectopic sinus.

C. The cause of rectal atresia may be abnormal recanalization of the colon.

D. The rotation happens at the midgut.

E. Oligohydramnios can be associated with Hirschsprung disease, but it's not one of the causes of it.
GAS 316; N 283; ABR/McM 250

179. **C.** The ilioinguinal nerve is a branch of the ventral ramus of the first lumbar nerve (L1). It pierces the internal abdominal oblique muscle, distributing filaments to it, and then accompanies the spermatic cord through the superficial inguinal ring. Its fibers are then distributed to the skin of the upper and medial parts of the thigh, and the skin over the mons pubis and labium majus in women or the root of the penis and upper part of the scrotum in men.

A. The iliohypogastric nerve is the superior branch of the ventral ramus of spinal nerve L1 that perforates the transversus abdominis and internal abdominal oblique muscles, and divides into a lateral and an anterior cutaneous branch.

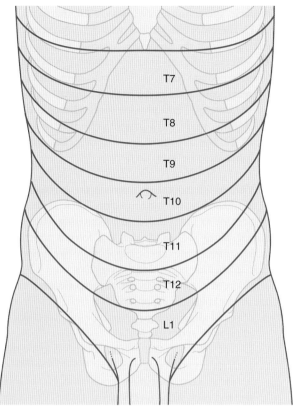

• *GAS* **Fig. 4.38**

B. The anterior cutaneous branch pierces the internal abdominal oblique, becomes cutaneous by perforating the aponeurosis of the external abdominal oblique muscle about 2.5 cm above the superficial inguinal ring, and is distributed to the skin of the hypogastric region. Lateral femoral cutaneous nerve innervates the skin on the lateral part of the thigh.

D, E. The lumbar and greater thoracic splanchnic nerves do not give off cutaneous branches.
    GAS 398; N 260; ABR/McM 271

180. C. The unilateral area of skin innervated by the sensory fibers of a single spinal nerve is called a dermatome. The anterior cutaneous branch of the 10th thoracoabdominal nerve supplies the area around the umbilicus.

A, B, D, E. The anterior cutaneous branches of the ventral rami of the 7th thoracic spinal nerves supply the area of the xiphoid process, while those of the 12th thoracic spinal nerves supply the hypogastric area (*GAS* Fig. 4.38).
    GAS 287–288; N 171; ABR/McM 215 (no clinical thumbnails in new edition)

181. A. The foregut is innervated mainly by the celiac plexus. The superior mesenteric plexus supplies the intestines as far as the splenic flexure and to the some of the pancreas.

B, D. The descending colon and the rectum are supplied by the inferior mesenteric and intermesenteric plexuses, as well as by branches of the pelvic splanchnic nerves.

C, E. These regions are not supplied by the superior mesenteric plexus.
    GAS 358–364; N 301; ABR/McM 244

182. B. The ilioinguinal nerve is a branch of ventral ramus of the the first lumbar nerve (L1). It pierces the internal abdominal oblique muscle, distributing filaments to it, and then accompanies the spermatic cord through the superficial inguinal ring. Its fibers are then distributed to the skin of the upper and medial part of the thigh, and the skin of the mons pubis and labia majora in women and over the root of the penis and upper part of the scrotum in men.

C. The genital branch of the genitofemoral nerve will supply the labium majus with the ilioinguinal nerve but the ilioinguinal nerve is more commonly damaged during appendectomy.

A, D, E. These structures do not supply the labium majus and injury to these nerves would not produce the symptoms seen in the patient.
    GAS 398; N 260; ABR/McM 271

183. A. The lymphatic drainage follows the arterial supply in the abdomen. The stomach is supplied by the celiac trunk, so the lymph will drain to the celiac lymph nodes.

B, C, D, E. These structures are not the initial nodes for drainage of the stomach.
    GAS 358; N BP79; ABR/McM 247

184. C. The kidneys lie retroperitoneally on the posterior abdominal wall, one on each side of the vertebral column at the level of the T12–L3 vertebrae. The left kidney lies slightly higher than the right, and its upper pole reaches the level of the 11th rib.

A. A fracture through the angle of the rib would be unlikely to injure the stomach, which can have a varied level.

B, E. The pancreas and the descending colon are at a level below L1.

D. The liver is found primarily on the right side.
    GAS 373–374; N 311; ABR/McM 265

185. E. The duodenal cap or the first part of the duodenum is supplied by the gastroduodenal artery, which arises from the common hepatic artery, and its supraduodenal and retroduodenal branches. The gastroduodenal artery descends retroperitoneally, posterior to the first part of the duodenum, and divides into the right gastro-omental artery and anterior superior pancreaticoduodenal artery.

A. The hepatic portal vein is formed behind the neck of the pancreas.

B. The superior mesenteric artery usually arises from the abdominal aorta at the level of the L1 vertebra, approximately 1 cm inferior to the celiac trunk, and will supply the derivatives of the midgut.

C. The bile duct is joined by the pancreatic duct to form the hepatopancreatic ampulla (of Vater) at the second the part of the duodenum.

D. The proper hepatic artery branches from the common hepatic artery and travels with the hepatic portal vein and the bile duct within the hepatoduodenal ligament. It gives off the right gastric artery before dividing into the right and left hepatic arteries.
GAS 309, 344; N 291; ABR/McM 246

186. E. The indirect inguinal hernia is the most common form of hernia and is believed to be congenital in origin. The hernia sac enters the inguinal canal through the deep inguinal ring lateral to the inferior epigastric vessels.
   A. Direct inguinal hernias make up about 15% of all inguinal hernias. The sac of a direct hernia bulges directly anteriorly through the posterior wall of the inguinal canal medial to the inferior epigastric vessels.
   B. The hernia sac does not protrude through the umbilical scar, but through the linea alba in the region of the umbilicus. Acquired umbilical hernia of adults is more correctly referred to as a paraumbilical hernia.
   C. The hernia sac descends through the femoral canal within the femoral sheath, creating a femoral hernia.
   D. The lumbar hernia occurs through the lumbar triangle and is rare. The lumbar triangle (Petit triangle) is a weak area in the posterior part of the abdominal wall.
   GAS 296–298; N 264; ABR/McM 235

187. C. The omental bursa is a potential space that lies posterior to the stomach, lesser omentum, and adjacent structures. The omental bursa has a superior recess, limited superiorly by the diaphragm and the posterior layers of the coronary ligament of the liver, and an inferior recess between the superior parts of the layers of the greater omentum.
   A, B. The hepatorenal space or subhepatic space is the space that separates the liver from the right kidney.
   E. The omental bursa communicates with the greater sac through the omental foramen (epiploic foramen of Winslow).
   D. Right and left subphrenic spaces lie between the diaphragm and liver and are separated by the falciform ligament.
   GAS 304; N 273; ABR/McM 240

188. D. The greater peritoneal sac encompasses the most space in the peritoneal cavity, beginning with the diaphragm and ending at the pelvic cavity.
   A, B, C, E. Pouch Morison, the rectouterine pouch (of Douglas), the right paracolic gutter, and the omental bursa are all dependent areas in the peritoneal sac, where fluid will collect if the patient is supine or standing.
   GAS 304; N 324; ABR/McM 238

189. A. Visceral afferents that innervate the appendix will be stimulated by the inflammation. These visceral afferents return to the spinal cord by traveling with sympathetics. Since the appendix is a midgut structure, it receives major sympathetic supply from the lesser thoracic splanchnic nerve, which originates at T10–T11. Therefore the patient will initially experience a visceral pain at the umbilicus, which is at the T10 level.
   B. Visceral afferents that travel with parasympathetics mediate unconscious sensations (that may reach conscious levels, such as nausea and the urge the defecate) and physiological reflexes and so are not involved in this patient's condition.
   C, D, E. The appendix is a visceral organ and is not innervated by somatic nerves.
   GAS 358–364; N 306; ABR/McM 261

190. B. Visceral afferents that innervate the gallbladder will be stimulated by the inflammation. These visceral afferents return to the spinal cord by traveling with sympathetics. Since the gallbladder is a foregut structure, it receives major sympathetic supply from the greater thoracic splanchnic nerve, which originates from T5 to T9. Therefore the patient will initially experience a visceral pain at the epigastric region, which is at the T7–T9 levels.
   A. Visceral afferents return to the spinal cord by traveling with sympathetics.
   C, D The phrenic nerve innervates the diaphragmatic peritoneum and originates from C3, C4 and C5. If it were affected, the patient would complain of shoulder and neck pain corresponding to the dermatomes innervated by this spinal nerve. The sharp and well-localized pain in the right hypogastrium corresponds to the inflammation spreading to the abdominal peritoneum but does not explain the initial epigastric pain.
   E. The gallbladder receives major sympathetic supply from the greater thoracic splanchnic nerve, which originates from T5 to T9.
   GAS 354–364; N 309; ABR/McM 243

191. C. The urachus is a thick fibrous cord that is a remnant of the allantois (a tube connecting the urinary bladder to the umbilicus in the fetus. It is involved in the processing of nutrition and the excretion of waste products in the embryo). In some cases a remnant of the lumen can persist, leading to the development of urachal cyst and/or sinus.
   A, B, D, E. If the entire urachus remains patent, it forms a urachal fistula connecting the urinary bladder to the umbilicus. This allows urine to escape from the umbilical orifice.
   GAS 301; N 324; ABR/McM 233

192. E. The anatomical location of the appendix is in the right lower quadrant at McBurney point. When the inflamed appendix contacts the parietal peritoneum, it stimulates the somatic afferents that innervate the body wall. This results in sharp, localized pain in the right lower quadrant.
   A, B, C, D. Visceral afferents are stimulated by inflammation, not contact. They travel back to the spinal cord with sympathetics of the T10 dermatome. The patient will experience dull periumbilical pain, which is usually a prelude to the somatic pain.
   GAS 320; N 306, N 282; ABR/McM 231

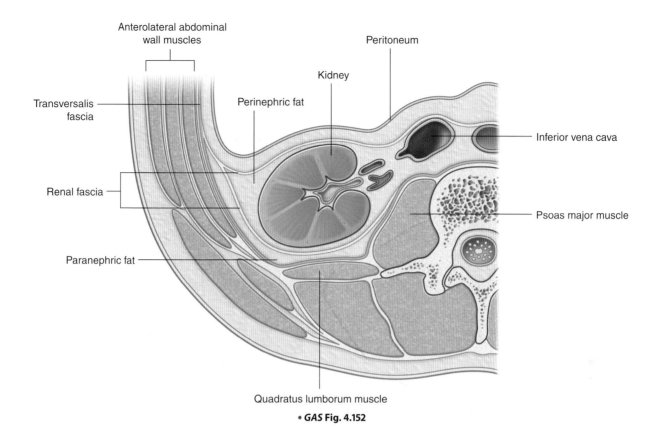

Anterolateral abdominal
wall muscles

Peritoneum

Kidney

Transversalis
fascia

Perinephric fat

Inferior vena cava

Renal fascia

Psoas major muscle

Paranephric fat

Quadratus lumborum muscle

• *GAS* **Fig. 4.152**

193. B. Immediately external to the renal capsule is an accumulation of extraperitoneal fat called the perinephric fat. This fat variably surrounds the kidney but is especially abundant near the renal hilum and within the renal sinus. Surrounding the perinephric fat is a membranous condensation of extraperitoneal fascia called the renal fascia (of Gerota). A final external layer of paranephric fat completes the renal fat and fasciae. The patient is suffering from a perinephric abscess, which would be located in the perinephric fat between the renal capsule and renal fascia (*GAS* Fig. 4.152).
A, C, D, E. These regions do not indicate a perinephric abscess.
GAS 377; N 318; ABR/McM 267

194. A. The stomach is derived from the foregut. Other derivatives of the foregut include the upper and lower respiratory system, the pharynx, esophagus, the first and second parts of the duodenum up to the major duodenal papillae, the liver, the pancreas and the gallbladder. The spleen is derived from the dorsal mesogastrium of the stomach.
B, C, D, E. These structures are derivatives of the foregut.
GAS 307; N 324; ABR/McM 246

195. C. Obstruction of the bile duct will result in stasis of bile. The bile duct receives the cystic duct from the gallbladder and the common hepatic duct from the liver. Therefore there will be backflow into the gallbladder leading to the symptoms of cholecystitis (fever, positive Murphy sign, pain that began at

the epigastrium then moved to the right hypogastrium). There will also be backflow into the liver leading to the increase in serum bilirubin.
A. Obstruction of the infundibulum of the gallbladder or the cystic duct will affect the gallbladder but not the liver.
B. There is backflow into the liver leading to the increase in serum bilirubin, which cannot be explained if the obstruction was solely in the bile duct.
D. Obstruction of the hepatopancreatic ampulla will not only lead to symptoms from the gallbladder and the liver, but also to the pancreas as the pancreatic duct will also be obstructed (*GAS* Fig. 4.111).
E. Obstruction of the left hepatic duct will only affect the liver.
GAS 340; N 287; ABR/McM 256

196. D. The superior pancreaticoduodenal arteries are branches of the gastroduodenal artery, which is a branch of the celiac trunk. The inferior pancreaticoduodenal artery is a branch of the superior mesenteric artery. If the superior mesenteric artery was occluded, the anastomosis between these two vessels will allow blood to flow from the celiac trunk to the midgut to provide blood supply.
A, B, C, E. The right and left gastric arteries, the left and right gastro-omental arteries (formerly called gastro-epiploic arteries), the short gastric arteries all provide blood supply to the stomach (*GAS* Fig. 4.115).
GAS 347–348; N 291; ABR/McM 244

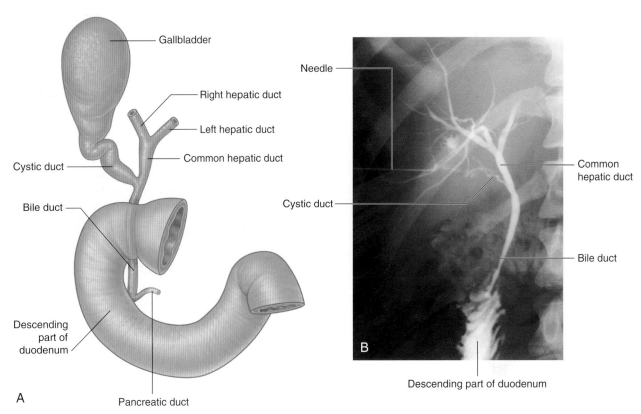

• *GAS* Fig. 4.111

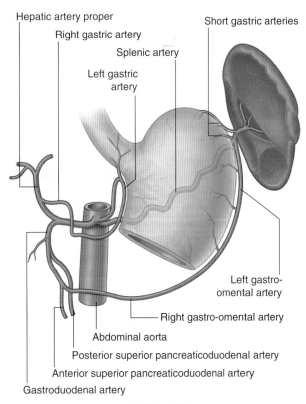

• *GAS* Fig. 4.115

197. A. The third part (inferior) of the duodenum is the longest section. It crosses over the inferior vena cava, aorta, and vertebral column. Any perforation to the posterior wall will jeopardize these structures.
B. It is crossed anteriorly by the superior mesenteric artery and vein (*GAS* Fig. 4.66).
C, D, E. These structures will not be affected when there is a perforation at the posterior wall of the third part of the duodenum
GAS 346–347; N 291; ABR/McM 245

198. C. The left gastric is a branch of the celiac trunk while the right gastric is usually a branch of the proper hepatic artery. They anastomose on the lesser curvature and provide it with arterial supply.
A. The right and left gastro-omental vessels anastomose on the greater curvature and provide its blood supply.
B. The pancreaticoduoduodenal vessels form an anastomosis between the celiac trunk and the superior mesenteric artery and supplies the pancreas and the duodenum.
D. The portal triad is located at the porta hepatis of the liver.
E. The short gastric vessel supplies the fundus of the stomach.
GAS 344; N 291; ABR/McM 244

199. A. The borders of the cystohepatic triangle (of Calot) are the cystic duct inferiorly, the common hepatic duct medially and the inferior border of the liver

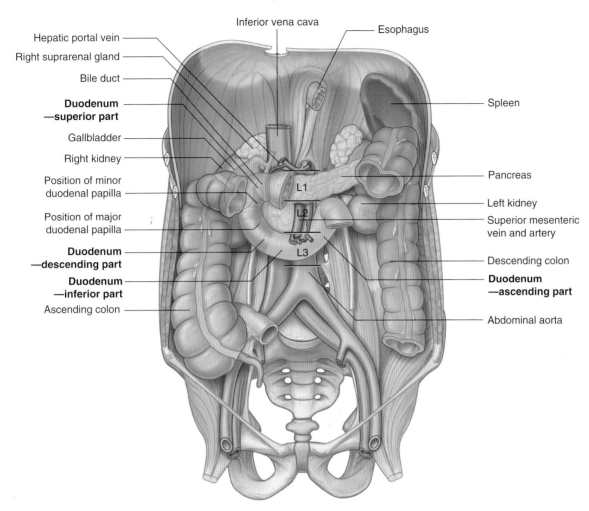

Inferior vena cava

Hepatic portal vein

Right suprarenal gland

Bile duct

Duodenum —superior part

Gallbladder

Right kidney

Position of minor duodenal papilla

Position of major duodenal papilla

Duodenum —descending part

Duodenum —inferior part

Ascending colon

Esophagus

Spleen

Pancreas

Left kidney

Superior mesenteric vein and artery

Descending colon

Duodenum —ascending part

Abdominal aorta

L1

L2

L3

• *GAS* **Fig. 4.66**

superiorly. It is currently used clinically to locate the cystic artery in cases where a cholecystectomy is performed. It is also the location of the node of Calot, which directly drains the gallbladder. (Of note: Jean-Francois Calot originally described the cystic artery as one of the boundaries of the triangle.).

B, C, D, E. These structures do not make up the triangle of Calot.
GAS 331, 347; N 291; ABR/McM 246

Answers 200–223

200. D. The splenic artery is the longest and often the largest branch of the celiac trunk. It takes a tortuous course to the left along the superior border of the pancreas. As it passes along the superior border of the pancreas it gives off branches to the neck, body, and tail of the pancreas.

A. The superior mesenteric artery is a direct branch of the abdominal aorta and runs anterior to the uncinate process of the pancreas before giving branches to the intestines.

B. The hepatic portal vein is formed by the union of the splenic and superior mesenteric veins posterior to the neck of the pancreas before ascending to the liver.

C. The left gastric artery is located on and supplies the lesser curvature of the stomach.

E. The left gastro-omental artery is located on and supplies the greater curvature of the stomach.
GAS 347; N 291; ABR/McM 245

201. A. The retrocecal appendix (the most common position) is located posterior to the cecum. The right psoas major muscle lies directly posterior to it. By keeping her right thigh flexed, the patient prevents any excessive contact of the inflamed appendix and the underlying parietal peritoneum covering the psoas muscle. If the thigh is extended, this causes the inflamed appendix to rub against the parietal peritoneum resulting sharp somatic pain for the patient.

B, C, D, E. These muscles are not in contact with the appendix to cause the resulting sharp somatic pain during thigh extension.
GAS 318–319; N 282; ABR/McM 261

202. E. The borders of the cystohepatic triangle (of Calot) are the cystic duct inferiorly, the common hepatic duct medially and the inferior border of the liver superiorly. It is currently used clinically to locate the cystic artery in cases where a cholecystectomy is performed.

A, B, C, D. These structures are not associated with the triangle of Calot.

GAS 330–331, 347; N 291; ABR/McM 246

203. A. The rich arterial supply of the stomach arises from the celiac trunk and its branches. Most blood is supplied by anastomoses formed along the lesser curvature by the right and left gastric arteries, and along the greater curvature by the right and left gastro-omental (gastroepiploic) arteries. The short gastric arteries arise from the splenic artery at the hilum of the spleen and pass forward in the gastrosplenic ligament to supply the fundus. B. The kidney is supplied by the renal arteries, which are branches of the abdominal aorta.
   C. The pyloric sphincter is supplied by the gastro-duodenal artery and the supraduodenal artery.
   D. The head of the pancreas is supplied by superior and inferior pancreaticoduodenal arteries, which are branches of the gastroduodenal and superior mesenteric arteries.
   E. The left colic artery, which is a branch of the inferior mesenteric artery, supplies the splenic flexure of the colon and the descending colon.

GAS 344; N 290; ABR/McM 244

204. D. The azygos vein ascends in the posterior mediastinum, passing close to the right sides of the bodies of the inferior 8 thoracic vertebrae. It arches over the superior aspect of the root of the right lung to join the superior vena cava (SVC), similar to the way the arch of the aorta passes over the root of the left lung. In portal hypertension (an abnormally increased blood pressure in the portal venous system), blood is unable to pass through the liver via the hepatic portal vein, causing a reversal of flow into the systemic tributaries of the azygos veins at the lower third of the esophagus. The large volume of blood causes the submucosal veins to enlarge markedly, forming esophageal varices.
   A, B, C, E. These structures are not associated with esophageal varices due to portal hypertension.

GAS 356; N 210; ABR/McM 221

205. D. The kidneys lie retroperitoneally and therefore, of the layers listed, a posterior approach will only require transection of the transversalis fascia.
   A, B. The diaphragmatic pleura is located in the thoracic cavity and is a subdivision of the parietal pleura.
   C, E. The parietal peritoneum lies anterior to the kidneys and the visceral peritoneum covers the gastrointestinal tract forming the peritoneal cavity between them.

GAS 374–375; N 312; ABR/McM 260

206. C. The pancreas is located retroperitoneally and may only be visualized directly if the posterior parietal peritoneum is divided.
   A, B, D, E. The ileum, jejunum, stomach, and transverse colon are all intraperitoneal and therefore easily visualized with the scope.

GAS 332; N 273; ABR/McM 237

207. D. Meckel diverticulum is a congenital condition where the proximal portion of the omphaloenteric (vitelline) duct does not completely regress, so it forms a fingerlike projection from the ileum. It may become filled with fecal material and subsequently obstructed with resulting inflammation.
   A. Gastritis is inflammation of the lining of the stomach and will not give the appearance of a 2-inch long structure in the midabdomen on radiographic studies.
   B. Hirschsprung disease is a congenital disorder marked by difficulty in passing stool and may as a result produce a bloody sample. The blood will be bright red and the 2-inch structure will not be present on radiography.
   C. Hemorrhoids are varicose veins in the anal canal and rectum, which may protrude from the canal if very large and are typically the result of excessive straining while trying to pass stool.
   E. Anal fissures are tears that may result from straining excessively and trying to pass hard or dry stools.

GAS 315; N 280; ABR/McM 237

208. A. The descending colon is the only option listed which is a retroperitoneal organ.
   B, C, D, E. All the other organs are intraperitoneal and will therefore not be affected by a retroperitoneal infection.

GAS 320; N 295; ABR/McM 236

209. E. The ilioinguinal and iliohypogastric nerves are located directly posterior to the kidney. Much of the sensory distribution of the iliohypogastric nerve is to the skin over the posterolateral gluteal and pubic regions.
   A. The subcostal nerve runs just inferior to the 12th rib and supplies the muscles and skin of the surrounding area.
   B. The lateral femoral cutaneous nerve gives sensory innervation to the lateral thigh.
   C. The ilioinguinal nerve supplies the upper medial thigh and, specifically, the skin over the mons pubis and labium majus anteriorly in women or skin over the root of the penis and anterior scrotum in men.
   D. The femoral nerve is the nerve of the anterior thigh and supplies muscles and skin of this region.

GAS 398; N 260; ABR/McM 263

210. C. The muscle that will provide the "6-pack" look is the rectus abdominis, which runs between the pubic crest and the costal margin in the midline of the abdominal wall.
   A, B. Ribs 10–12 and the iliac crest are too far lateral for rectus abdominis to attach to it.
   D. The upper attachment is the lower border of the 7th costal cartilage and the muscle often covers the costal cartilages for a short distance anteriorly.

E. The xiphoid process may be covered by the muscle but does not serve as an attachment.
GAS 282–283; N 253; ABR/McM 228

211. C. There are three major structures that pass through the diaphragm. At the level of T10 the esophagus will pass through, while the inferior vena cava (B) will traverse at T8 and the aorta at T12 (E).

A, D. The levels T7 and 11 are not associated with any particular structures passing through the diaphragm.

212. C. The ribs slope vertically downward as they move to attach to the sternum in the midline. This produces a thoracic cage with lowermost anterior point being several vertebral levels lower than that of the posterior part of the rib. The costal margin therefore corresponds with the L3 vertebra.

A, B. Vertebrae L1 and 2 are too high and correspond to the lower margin of the 11th and 12th ribs respectively.

D, E. Levels L4 and 5 are close to the pelvic area and are therefore too low.
GAS 258, 269, 307; N 265; ABR/McM 225

213. A. The principal plane also known as Cantlie line divides the liver into functional right and left lobes. This division makes the caudate and quadrate lobes part of the left lobe of the liver. The caudate lobe is segment I, the quadrate lobe segment IV and the left lobe consisting of segments II and III. Removing the right lobe according to this resection will therefore remove segments; V, VI, VII and VIII (*GAS* Fig. 4.116).

B, C, D, E. Incorrect set of lobes from right hepatectomy when resected along the principal plane.
GAS 338; N 284; ABR/McM 255

214. E. Caput medusae is the appearance of enlarged veins radiating outward from the umbilical area and is a sign of increased pressure in the hepatic portal vein. The hepatic portal vein takes nutrient rich blood from the intestines to the liver and is formed by the fusion of the superior mesenteric and splenic veins. The right and left common iliac arteries are the terminal branches of the abdominal aorta and carry oxygen rich blood toward the lower

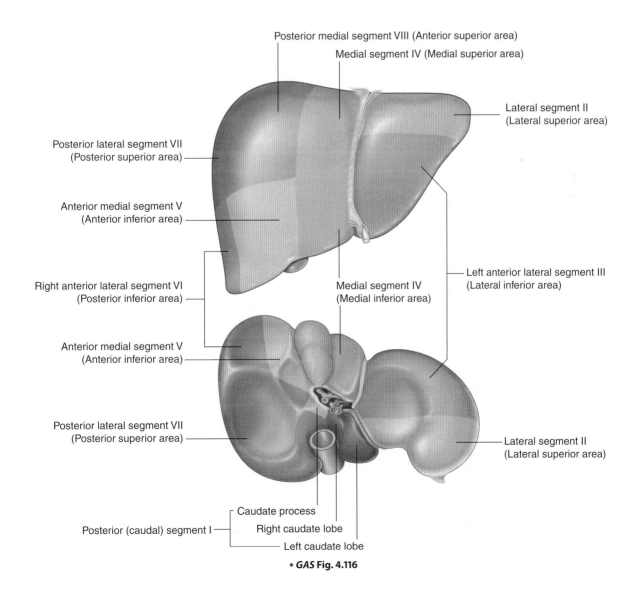

Posterior medial segment VIII (Anterior superior area)

Medial segment IV (Medial superior area)

Lateral segment II (Lateral superior area)

Posterior lateral segment VII (Posterior superior area)

Anterior medial segment V (Anterior inferior area)

Right anterior lateral segment VI (Posterior inferior area)

Anterior medial segment V (Anterior inferior area)

Posterior lateral segment VII (Posterior superior area)

Medial segment IV (Medial inferior area)

Left anterior lateral segment III (Lateral inferior area)

Lateral segment II (Lateral superior area)

Posterior (caudal) segment I

Caudate process

Right caudate lobe

Left caudate lobe

• *GAS* **Fig. 4.116**

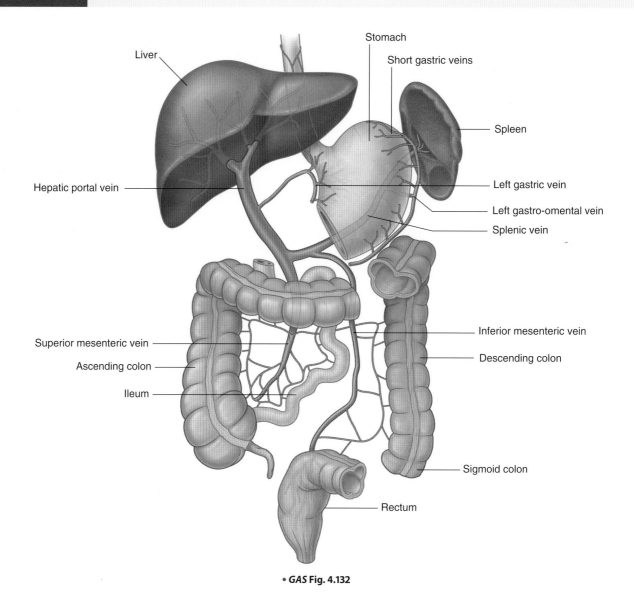

• *GAS* Fig. 4.132

limbs. The gastric veins drain into the splenic, superior mesenteric, and hepatic portal veins and do not contribute to the formation of the hepatic portal vein. The inferior mesenteric vein drains typically into the splenic vein. The paraumbilical veins are the ones that take the blood toward the umbilicus as an alternative direction of blood flow back to the heart. This alternative route will bypass the liver entirely (*GAS* Fig. 4.132).
A, B, C, D. They do not form union responsible for caput medusa.
GAS 356; N 299; ABR/McM 258

215. E. The stomach forms part of the anterior boundary of the omental bursa. A perforated lesion in the posterior wall will result in stomach contents being expelled into the omental bursa, also referred to as the lesser peritoneal sac. The omental (epiploic) foramen (of Winslow) is the space bounded by the portal triad and inferior vena cava, which is the only communication between the greater and lesser sacs. The paracolic gutters are spaces lateral to the ascending

and descending colons in which fluid may accumulate when the patient is supine. The supracolic and infracolic compartments are spaces above and below the transverse colon and are located in the greater sac.
A, B, C, D. The fluid will not flow into those spaces after traversing the aperture.
GAS 301; N 285; ABR/McM 240

216. C. The ascending lumbar vein connects the common iliac veins to the azygos system bilaterally and would provide an additional pathway for blood.
A. The left common iliac will join with the right common iliac to give rise to the inferior vena cava.
B, D. The azygos and hemiazygos veins drain the posterior thoracic walls of the right and left sides respectively and will receive the ascending lumbar and subcostal veins in most instances.
E. The left renal vein drains into the inferior vena cava superior to the L3 vertebra, and although it receives the left gonadal vein it cannot provide an alternative pathway for blood.
GAS 390–391; N 198; ABR/McM 221

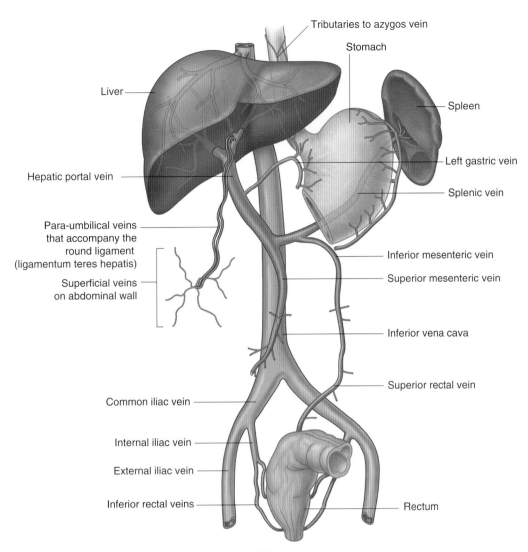

Tributaries to azygos vein

Stomach

Liver

Spleen

Hepatic portal vein

Left gastric vein

Splenic vein

Para-umbilical veins
that accompany the
round ligament
(ligamentum teres hepatis)

Inferior mesenteric vein

Superior mesenteric vein

Superficial veins
on abdominal wall

Inferior vena cava

Superior rectal vein

Common iliac vein

Internal iliac vein

External iliac vein

Inferior rectal veins

Rectum

• *GAS* **Fig. 4.133**

217. A. The layers of the anterior abdominal wall in the right lower quadrant from superficial to deep are: skin, Camper fascia, Scarpa fascia, external abdominal oblique, internal abdominal oblique, transversus abdominis, transversalis fascia, extraperitoneal fat, and parietal peritoneum.
  B. Moving superficial to deep, Scarpa's fascia is immediately followed by the external abdominal oblique muscle - not transversalis fascia.
  C. Moving superficial to deep, Scarpa's fascia is immediately followed by the external abdominal oblique muscle - not the internal abdominal oblique muscle.
  D. Moving superficial to deep, Camper's fascia is immediately followed by Scarpa's fascia - not transversalis fascia.
  E. In the right lower quadrant Scarpa's fascia is deep, not superficial, to Camper's fascia.
  GAS 276; N 258; ABR/McM 230
218. D. The ileocecal valve is a narrowing in the medial wall of the cecum. This indicates the junction of the small intestine and the colon.
  A. The hepatic flexure indicates the junction between the transverse colon and the descending colon.

  B. The splenic flexure indicates the transition between the ascending and transverse colons.
  C. The paracolic gutters are external to the colon.
  D. The GE junction is located at the point where the esophagus joins the stomach and is not located in the colon (*GAS* Fig. 4.89).
  GAS 317–318; N 281; ABR/McM 261
219. C. Left gastric vein anastomoses with the esophageal branches of the azygos vein. Distension of this network in cases of obstruction results in esophageal varices at lower esophagus.
  A. The right gastric vein drains directly to the hepatic portal vein and forms no communication with a systemic vein.
  B. The paraumbilical veins anastomose with the superficial epigastric vessels around the umbilicus. They form caput medusae when distended.
  D. The splenic vein joins the superior mesenteric vein and forms no clinically described disorder.
  E. The left gastro-omental vein drains into the superior mesenteric vein and is therefore not involved in hematemesis.
  GAS 354, 356; N 299; ABR/McM 251

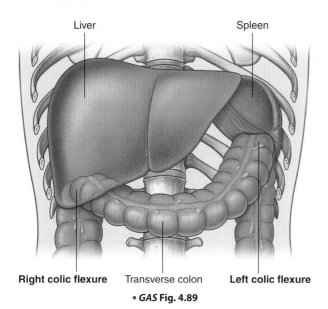

Liver   Spleen

Right colic flexure   Transverse colon   Left colic flexure
• **GAS Fig. 4.89**

220. E. Pain from the appendix is originally felt as a visceral pain. This pain is initially felt around the umbilical area (at about T10 region) because the appendix is a midgut structure and embryologically related to the umbilical area (during physiological hernia and reduction of the hernia). Subsequently during gut rotation, the appendix, which is located at the base of the cecum, rests in the right iliac fossa. However, it maintains its innervation (this is a rule in embryology).

A. Somatic afferent carries pain sensation from body wall structures. This will be the case if the inflammation of the appendix spreads to the peritoneum.

B. Preganglionic sympathetic fibers to the midgut will synapse in the aorticorenal ganglion (the lesser thoracic splanchnic nerve) before postganglionic fibers will accompany blood vessels to the appendix.

C. Preganglionic parasympathetic fibers to the appendix perform motor function

D. Postganglionic sympathetic fibers to the appendix perform visceral motor functions, for example, secretion by intestinal glands.
GAS 317, 358–364; N 306; ABR/McM 261

221. E. The abnormality seen on ultrasound was proximal to the ureters. Renal stones have propensity to be lodged at the 3 narrow areas of the ureters of which the ureteropelvic junction is the most superior.

A. The urethra is not involved in urinary stones, and stones in the urinary bladder rarely lead to obstruction that will result in pelvic or calyceal enlargement.

B. Stones are not formed in the urinary bladder.

C, D. Stone obstruction at the ureterovesical junction will likely lead to enlargement of the ureters, and stone obstruction at the pelvic brim will most likely result in enlargement of the ureters.
GAS 381; N 317; ABR/McM 265, 269

222. A. The pancreatic head is related to the concavity of the duodenum. The bile duct and the pancreatic duct join at the hepatopancreatic ampulla (of Vater) to open into the beginning portion of the second part of the duodenum. Carcinoma of the head of the pancreas can therefore obstruct the bile duct at this region.

B, C. The common hepatic duct is proximal to the duodenum and not likely to be compressed by carcinoma of the pancreatic head. Similarly, the left hepatic duct is also proximal to the duodenal concavity and will not be obstructed in cancer of the head of pancreas.

D. The cystic duct is above and to the right of the duodenum and pancreatic head and not likely to be compressed in cancer of the head of the pancreas.

E. The right hepatic artery is proximal and above the duodenum and the head of the pancreas.
GAS 332; N BP80; ABR/McM 257

223. E. The inferior pancreaticoduodenal artery will continue to supply the pancreas, particularly the head of the pancreas, if the gastroduodenal artery is compromised. This artery is a branch of the superior mesenteric artery.

A. The splenic artery does not supply the head of the pancreas.

B. The left gastric artery gives off branches to the inferior esophagus and supplies the lesser curvature of the stomach together with the right gastric artery.

C, D. The right gastric artery supplies the lesser curvature of the stomach, and the proper hepatic artery provides blood supply to the liver.
GAS 348; N 291; ABR/McM 253

Answers 224–244

224. C. The visceral afferent fibers from the pancreas accompany sympathetic nerves. Postganglionic sympathetic nerves to the foregut, including the pancreas, are located in the celiac ganglion, as are visceral afferent fibers. Neurectomy of this ganglion will therefore interrupt the pain pathway from the pancreas by disrupting the afferent fibers. The nerve cell bodies of these fibers are located in the dorsal root ganglia of T5–T9.

A. Visceral pain fibers from the pancreas do not travel with the vagus nerve.

B. The phrenic nerve supplies motor innervations to the diaphragm.

D. The aorticorenal ganglion is the location of the postganglionic cell bodies of the least thoracic splanchnic nerve, which supplies sympathetic innervation to the midgut.

E. The inferior mesenteric ganglion receives fibers from the intermesenteric plexus. This ganglion mainly supplies postganglionic sympathetic fibers to the hindgut (Fig. 4.137).
GAS 358–364; N 310; ABR/McM 245

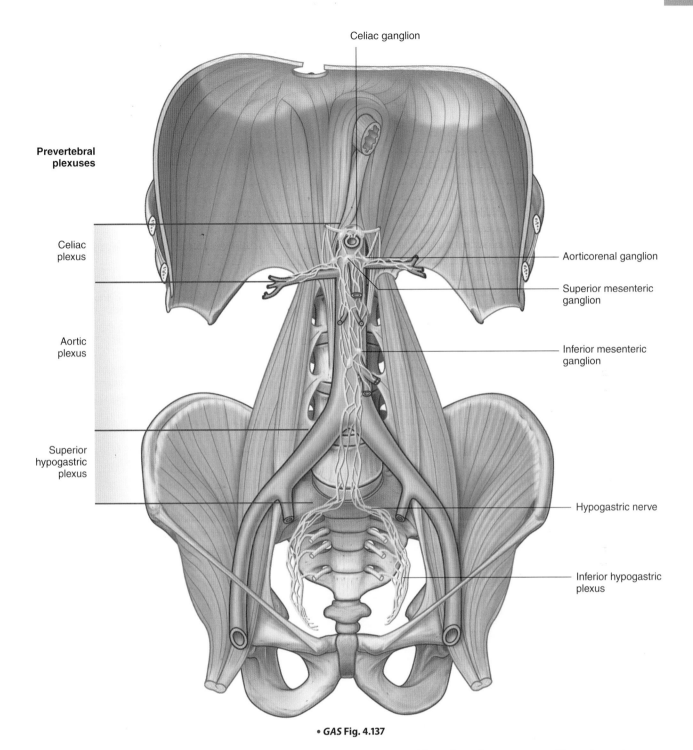

Celiac ganglion

Prevertebral plexuses

Celiac plexus

Aortic plexus

Superior hypogastric plexus

Aorticorenal ganglion

Superior mesenteric ganglion

Inferior mesenteric ganglion

Hypogastric nerve

Inferior hypogastric plexus

• *GAS* **Fig. 4.137**

225. E. The iliohypogastric nerve will receive sensation from the capsule of the kidney and is typically innervating the dermatome over the pubic symphysis. The skin below the pubic symphysis is innervated by the ilioinguinal nerve

  A. Greater thoracic splanchnic nerves provide sympathetic innervation to foregut structures and the adrenal medulla.

  B. Lesser thoracic splanchnic nerves provide sympathetic innervation to midgut structures.

  C. Pelvic splanchnic nerves provide parasympathetic innervation for pelvic organs such as the urinary bladder, ureter, prostate, and urethra.

  D. The celiac plexus receives fibers from the greater thoracic splanchnic nerves and the lesser thoracic splanchnic nerves.

GAS 373–374, 394–401; N 260; ABR/McM 270

226. C. The ureter is narrowed at some regions, hence stones are more likely to be trapped at these areas of constriction. At the lower part of the ureter, the ureter is narrowed at the point where it crosses the bifurcation of the common iliac artery and where it opens into the urinary bladder at the vesicoureteral junction.

  A, B, D. The ureters do not cross the inferior vena cava in its path; they cross the common iliac artery where it divides into internal and external

Esophagus

Anterior and posterior vagal trunks

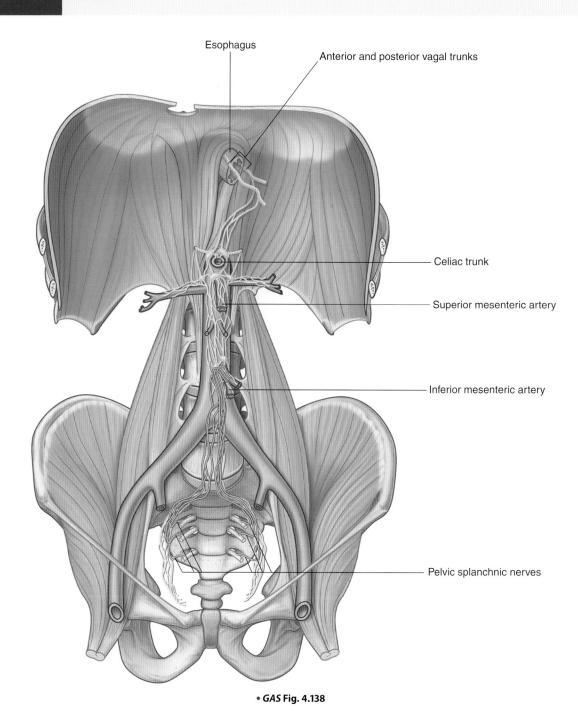

Celiac trunk

Superior mesenteric artery

Inferior mesenteric artery

Pelvic splanchnic nerves

• **GAS Fig. 4.138**

iliac arteries. The 4th lumbar artery and in fact all lumbar arteries are located medial and posterior to the ureters and therefore are not crossed by the ureters.

E. The inferior mesenteric artery is a midline and unpaired branch of the abdominal aorta. The ureters are more laterally located and do not cross the inferior mesenteric artery.
GAS 332, 358–364; N 317; ABR/McM 271

227. C. The gallbladder and its biliary trees are foregut structures. The celiac ganglion contains cell bodies of postganglionic sympathetic fibers from the greater thoracic splanchnic nerve that innervate these structures. A branch of this nerve travels with the cystic artery to supply the gallbladder.

A. The inferior mesenteric plexus contains mostly postganglionic sympathetic fibers to the midgut, mostly from the lesser and then least thoracic splanchnic nerves.

B. The superior mesenteric plexus contains postganglionic sympathetic fibers from the lesser thoracic splanchnic nerve to the midgut.

D. The renal plexus contains postganglionic fibers from the least thoracic splanchnic nerve to the kidney to regulate local blood supply.

E. The superior hypogastric plexus contains postganglionic sympathetic fibers to the pelvic and perineal regions (*GAS* Figs. 4.137, 4.138 and 4.170).
GAS 358–364; N 301; ABR/McM 256

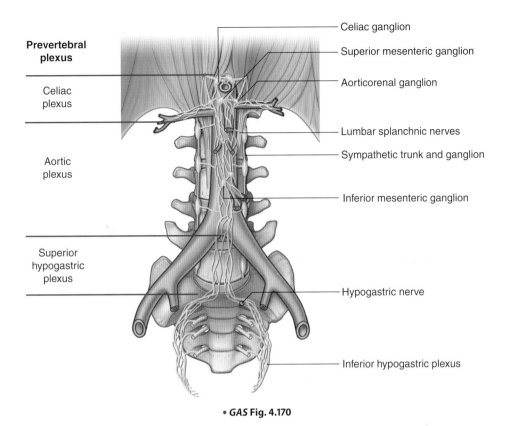

Prevertebral plexus

Celiac plexus

Aortic plexus

Superior hypogastric plexus

Celiac ganglion

Superior mesenteric ganglion

Aorticorenal ganglion

Lumbar splanchnic nerves

Sympathetic trunk and ganglion

Inferior mesenteric ganglion

Hypogastric nerve

Inferior hypogastric plexus

• *GAS* Fig. 4.170

228. C. Duodenal atresia presents with a distended epigastrium, bilious vomiting, and double-bubble sign on radiography. Atresia results from failure of recanalization of the duodenum.

A. Defects of the tracheoesophageal septum lead to TEFs with nonbilious vomiting.

B, D, E. Defects of the pleuroperitoneal folds lead to diaphragmatic hernias whereas malrotation without a concomitant volvulus will not present with bile tainted vomiting or the above x-ray.

GAS 309; N 279; ABR/McM 245

229. E. Bilateral renal agenesis or obstructive uropathy is associated with oligohydramnios because little or no urine is excreted into the amniotic cavity.

A. Polyhydramnios conversely is associated with esophageal atresia and CNS defects.

B. An annular pancreas causes duodenal obstruction. The gonads are not a derivative of the metanephros or its diverticulum.

C, D. Malrotation of the gut and bilateral gonadal dysgenesis would not be shown in Potter syndrome.

GAS 374; N 311; ABR/McM 267

230. A. Polyhydramnios is associated with esophageal atresia, TEFs and CNS defects due to lack of circulation and absorption of the amniotic fluid, which occurs in the respiratory and digestive tracts.

B, C, D. Bilateral renal agenesis or obstructive uropathy is associated with oligohydramnios because little or no urine is excreted into the amniotic cavity.

E. Down syndrome not directly related to tracheoesophageal fistulae.

GAS 374; N 238; ABR/McM 230

231. C. Omphaloenteric (vitelline) fistula is an abnormal patent connection between the umbilical surface and terminal ileal lumen, whereas the omphaloenteric (vitelline) cyst is a cyst connected to the ileum and umbilicus by a fibrous band, which is the remnant of the yolk stalk.

A, B. An ileal diverticulum is an outpouching of the ileal lumen at the antemesenteric border, which can become ulcerated.

D, E. Omphaloenteric cyst and persistent vitelline artery would not be a diagnosis in this case.

GAS 315; N 324; ABR/McM 237

232. C. An annular pancreas, which probably develops from a bifid ventral pancreatic bud, may obstruct the second part of the duodenum either at birth or much later following inflammation or fibrosis. Since the pancreatic buds all develop at the caudal part of the foregut, which forms the second part of the duodenum, B, C, D, E: the other answer can be excluded.

GAS 335; N BP80; ABR/McM 245

233. C. A persistent processus vaginalis may be too small for bowel but may allow peritoneal fluid passing through the abdominal end into the scrotum, forming a hydrocele of the testis. The gubernaculum aids in testicular descent into the scrotum (*GAS* Fig. 4.41).

A, B, D, E. They would not be involved in hydrocele.

GAS 289–294; N 324; ABR/McM 278

234. D. Gastroschisis is congenital failure of closure of the anterior abdominal wall due to incomplete closure of lateral folds.
  A. Volvulus is twisting around of the bowel and may be a result of a diverticulum.
  C. Situs inversus is when all the internal organs are situated in the opposite side of the body.
  B, E. These will not present as small bowel herniation.
  GAS 256–257; N 258; ABR/McM 237

235. A. Down syndrome is associated with increased incidence of duodenal atresia but to get bilious vomiting the atresia will have to be distal to the 1st part of the duodenum.
  B, C, D, E. All the other conditions occur proximal to the major duodenal papilla.
  GAS 309; N 279; ABR/McM 241

236. C. Midgut volvulus occurs following failure of the small intestines to enter the abdominal cavity for fixation following rotation of the midgut loop. The resultant twisting of the gut usually occurs and affects the vasculature at the duodenojejunal junction.
  A, B, D. These conditions are not related to Down syndrome and will not present as malrotation of small bowel.
  E. Congenital megacolon is due to failure of neural crest migration and occurs in the distal colon.
  GAS 309–310; N 324; ABR/McM 250

237. C. The ilioinguinal nerve supplies skin of the lower inguinal region, mons pubis, anterior scrotum or labium majus, and adjacent medial thigh, as well as the inferiormost internal abdominal oblique and transversus abdominis muscles.
  B, C, D, E. These nerves are not responsible for transmitting pain signal in an indirect hernia.
  GAS 398–401; N 260; ABR/McM 230

238. E. The superficial inguinal nodes receive lymph drainage from the abdominal wall below the level of the umbilicus, from the back below the iliac crest, and from superficial structures of the perineum and buttock.
  A. The deep inguinal nodes receive some of the lymph from superficial lymph nodes and the lower limbs.
  B. The external iliac nodes receive lymphatics from deep structures, such as the prostate, fundus of the urinary bladder, cervix, glans penis, and adductor region of the thigh.
  C. The internal iliac nodes receive lymphatics that run with the branches of the internal iliac artery, receiving lymph from pelvic viscera and deep perineum.
  D. The lateral aortic nodes receive lymph from the kidneys and suprarenal glands, ovaries, uterine tubes, body of the uterus, testis, and the lateral abdominal muscles that run with the lumbar veins.
  GAS 288, 514; N 319; ABR/McM 230

239. E. The internal spermatic fascia is an extension of the transversalis fascia.
  A. The internal abdominal oblique muscle lies superficial to the transversus abdominis muscle and gives origin to the cremaster muscle.
  B. The cremaster muscle covers the testis and spermatic cord. It is found between the external and internal spermatic fascia.
  C, D. These structures do not give rise to the internal spermatic fascia (*GAS* Fig. 4.47).
  GAS 289–294; N 264; ABR/McM 235, 278

240. E. The superior mesenteric artery leaves the aorta at the level of L1 and supplies the intestine from the duodenum and pancreas to the left colic flexure. The transverse portion of the duodenum lies horizontally at the level of L3, between the aorta and superior mesenteric artery. Normally, the superior mesenteric artery and aorta form an approximately 45-degree angle. If this angle diminishes to less than 20 degrees, the transverse portion of the duodenum can get entrapped between the superior mesenteric artery and aorta, leading to symptoms of partial small bowel obstruction. This condition is called superior mesenteric artery, or "nutcracker," syndrome.
  A, B, C, D. These parts are not located between the superior mesenteric artery and aorta at the level of L3.
  GAS 348; N 291; ABR/McM 245

241. E. This patient is most likely suffering from gallstone ileus, a condition that occurs in patients with long-standing cholelithiasis (often middle-aged to elderly women). A large (typically 2.5 cm or greater) gallstone causes the formation of a cholecystenteric fistula between the gallbladder and adjoining gut tissue due to persistent pressure on these tissues. The fistula ultimately allows passage of the gallstone into the small bowel, and the resulting communication between the gallbladder and small bowel allows intestinal gas to enter the gallbladder and biliary tree. Often this gas can be observed on abdominal x-ray.
  A, B. Obstruction of the cystic duct or bile duct by a gallstone leads to biliary colic, jaundice, and cholangitis.
  C, D. Gallstones usually don't lodge at duodenum or jejunum.
  GAS 340–341; N 287; ABR/McM 240, 256

242. B. At 16–18 years of age the hipbone is ossified from eight centers, three primary and five secondary. These centers appear from about the eighth or ninth week of fetal life, and at birth the three primary centers are separate. By age 7–9 the inferior rami of pubis and ischium are almost completely fused.
  A, C. By age 13 or 14 the 3 growth centers grow toward the base of the acetabulum, and at around puberty the remaining portions ossify. At 13–15 years the 3 primary growth centers have only just extended toward the base of the acetabulum.

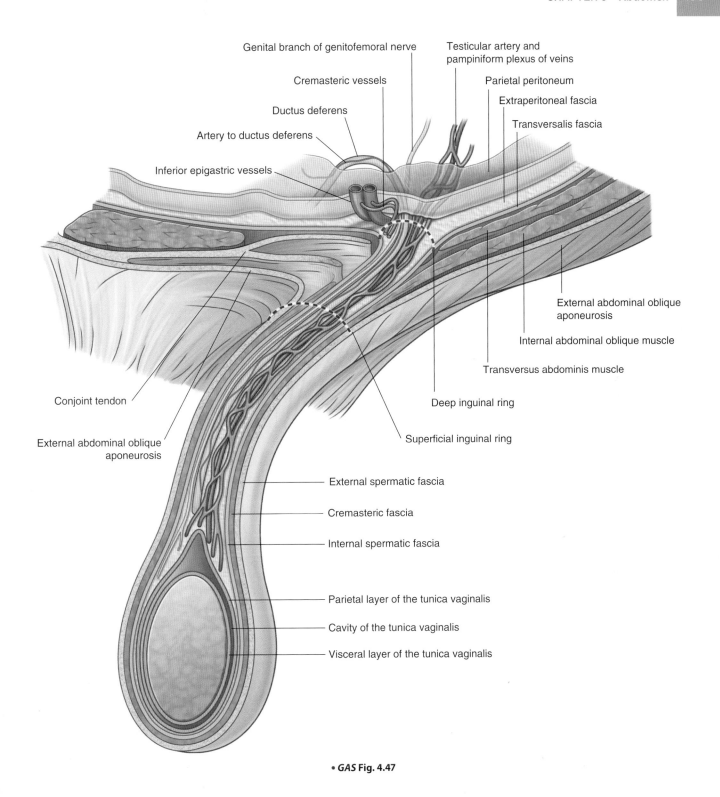

Genital branch of genitofemoral nerve

Cremasteric vessels

Ductus deferens

Artery to ductus deferens

Inferior epigastric vessels

Testicular artery and
pampiniform plexus of veins

Parietal peritoneum

Extraperitoneal fascia

Transversalis fascia

External abdominal oblique
aponeurosis

Internal abdominal oblique muscle

Transversus abdominis muscle

Deep inguinal ring

Superficial inguinal ring

Conjoint tendon

External abdominal oblique
aponeurosis

External spermatic fascia

Cremasteric fascia

Internal spermatic fascia

Parietal layer of the tunica vaginalis

Cavity of the tunica vaginalis

Visceral layer of the tunica vaginalis

• *GAS* **Fig. 4.47**

D. Between 22 and 24 years old, ossification takes place in the remaining centers, and they fuse with the remaining bone.

E. At 25–27 years, these bones should have already fused.
GAS 434–435; N 250; ABR/McM 295

243. A. The intramural part of the urethra is the most proximal part of the urethra, with the initial part traversing the wall of the urinary bladder.

B. The membranous part of the urethra, also called the intermediate portion, is the shortest and one of the narrowest segments, which leads from the prostate to the penile bulb.

C. Prostatic urethra is the segment passing through the prostate. Perforation of this segment leads to damage to the prostatic parenchyma.

D. The spongy urethra runs along the length of the penis through the corpus spongiosum.

Left kidney

Right kidney

Rib XI

Diaphragm

Rib XII

Rib XII

Psoas major muscle

Quadratus lumborum muscle

Transversus abdominis muscle

• • *GAS* **Fig. 4.151**

E. Paraurethral part will not traversed by the cystoscope.
GAS 459–462; N 349; ABR/McM 279

244. E. The left testicular vein, after draining the testis and epididymis, joins the left renal vein, which later joins the inferior vena cava.

A, B, C, D. The testicular veins drain ipsilateral structures, so the right testicular vein should not be involved in the drainage of the left testis. The right testicular vein drains directly into the inferior vena cava. The left testicular vein has no direct connection with the left common iliac vein. The median sacral vein receives blood from the sacral region and drains into the left common iliac vein.
GAS 266, 516; N 313; ABR/McM 271

Answers 245–246

245. E. The pubis is described as the anteroinferior part of the pelvis. The mons pubis is a fatty pad that rests above the pubis and the pubis can be palpated as a bony prominence below.

A. The ilium articulates posteriorly with the sacrum and terminates anteriorly as the anterior superior iliac spine, which is located lateral to the pubic symphysis away from the midline.

B. The coccyx is the terminal part of the vertebral column. As such, it is too posterior a structure to be palpated through the anterior abdominal wall.

C. The sacrum is formed by the fusion of five sacral vertebrae and similar to the coccyx, it cannot be palpated through the anterior abdominal wall.

D. The ischium makes up the posterior inferior part of the pelvic bone. Its most prominent feature is the ischial tuberosity located on the posteroinferior part of the bone, again making palpation as described in this case impossible.
GAS 433–436; N 250; ABR/McM 285

246. E. The iliohypogastric nerve emerges from the upper part of the lateral border of the psoas major muscle and crosses the quadratus lumborum to the iliac crest running just posterior to the kidneys. It perforates the transversus abdominis and internal abdominal oblique muscles and divides into lateral and anterior cutaneous branches.

A. The subcostal nerve does not innervate the skin of the posterolateral gluteal region, which does not correspond to the area with sensory deficits described in this case.

B. The lateral femoral cutaneous nerve does not relate to quadratus lumborum.

C. The ilioinguinal nerve innervates the skin over the inguinal canal and anterior part of the labium majus or scrotum.

D. The femoral nerve innervates the muscles of the anterior compartment of the thigh and the skin on the anterior aspect of the thigh and medial leg (*GAS* Fig. 4.151).
GAS 398; N 260; ABR/McM 263

4

Pelvis and Perineum

Questions

Questions 1–24

1. A 29-year-old woman delivers a 4.5 kg (9.8 lb) boy via an uncomplicated vaginal birth. Antenatal examinations showed no abnormalities. Physical examination shows downward curvature of the glans penis with an incomplete prepuce ventrally and the external urethral orifice opening immediately superior to the anus. Which of the following embryologic structures most likely failed to fuse, resulting in the ectopic location of the urethral orifice?
   A. Labioscrotal folds
   B. Cloacal membrane
   C. Urogenital folds
   D. Genital tubercle
   E. Urogenital membrane

2. A 5-hour-old girl is brought to the emergency department by her father with frothing and rapid breathing. She was delivered at term via a vaginal home birth. Antenatal records are unavailable. Physical examination shows respiratory distress and an imperforate anus. An x-ray of the abdomen shows dilation of the descending and sigmoid colon, with no gas shadow seen in the distal rectum. An invertogram shows that the rectum, vagina, and colon join into a single channel. Which of the following structures is directly involved in this malformation?
   A. Labioscrotal folds
   B. Persistent cloaca
   C. Urogenital folds
   D. Genital tubercle
   E. Urogenital membrane

3. A 4-year-old boy is brought to the physician by his mother because of a swelling in the abdomen. All developmental milestones have been met. Physical examination shows a palpable mass located external to the aponeurosis of the external abdominal oblique and a nonpalpable right testis. Examination of the left testis shows no abnormalities. Ultrasonography of the abdomen shows that the mass is an ectopic testis, classified as interstitial. Which of the following embryological structures most likely failed to develop resulting in the clinical presentation?
   A. Gubernaculum
   B. Processus vaginalis

C. Genital tubercle
   D. Seminiferous cords
   E. Labioscrotal swellings

4. A 32-year-old primigravida at 20 weeks' gestation comes to the physician for her prenatal visit. Her pregnancy has no abnormalities. Ultrasonography of the abdomen shows an abdominal mass in the lower part of the fetal abdominal wall. The scan failed to visualize the urinary bladder. A prenatal diagnosis of bladder exstrophy is made. Which of the following is the most likely cause of this condition?
   A. Failure of the primitive streak mesoderm to migrate around the cloacal membrane
   B. Failure of urethral folds to fuse
   C. Insufficient androgen stimulation
   D. Klinefelter syndrome
   E. Persistent allantois

5. A 6-year-old boy is brought to the physician by his mother because of crying during urination. Physical examination shows suprapubic tenderness. Urine dipstick shows leukocytes and nitrites. A diagnosis of urinary tract infection is made, and further workup is indicated. Ultrasonography of the kidneys shows a left bifid ureter. Which of the following embryological structures is most likely abnormally divided resulting in this clinical condition?
   A. Ureteric bud/metanephric diverticulum
   B. Mesonephric duct
   C. Paramesonephric duct
   D. Metanephric mesoderm
   E. Pronephros

6. A 31-year-old man comes to the physician because of a 1-week history of painful urination and pain below the umbilicus. One year ago, he was treated for a urinary tract infection. Physical examination shows suprapubic tenderness and a tender infraumbilical mass. Ultrasonography of the abdomen shows the presence of a 1.5 cm cystic structure along the anterior aspect of the urinary bladder. Which of the following is the most likely diagnosis?
   A. Hydrocele
   B. Epidermoid cyst
   C. Meckel diverticulum
   D. Omphalocele
   E. Urachal cyst

7. A 30-year-old woman, gravida 3, para 2, at 35 weeks' gestation is brought to the emergency department by her partner because of severe contractions lasting an average of 10 seconds. The patient received no antenatal care. Her first pregnancy was a normal vaginal birth. Her second pregnancy resulted in an emergency cesarean section secondary to failure to progress. The notes for this pregnancy were unavailable. Twenty-four hours after admission, the patient's cervix failed to dilate fully, and she was taken for an emergency cesarean section. Intraoperatively, the patient has adhesions and a uterus didelphys. Which of the following is the most likely embryological explanation of this condition?
   A. A complete fusion of the paramesonephric ducts
   B. An incomplete fusion of the paramesonephric ducts
   C. Failure of the mesonephric ducts to degenerate
   D. Failure of recanalization of the Müllerian ducts
   E. Regression of the pronephros

8. A 7-year-old boy is brought to the physician because of an inability to control his urinary bladder, despite being toilet trained at the age of 5. Five months ago, he was treated for a urinary tract infection. Ultrasonography of the abdomen shows a mild dilatation of the left pelvicalyceal system. Diagnostic cystoscopy shows a ureteral orifice inserting directly into the urethra. A diagnosis of ectopic ureter is made. An ureteroureterostomy is performed to correct the defect. Which of the following landmarks is used to identify the position of left ureter during the procedure?
   A. Anterior to the left common iliac artery
   B. Medial to the left inferior epigastric artery
   C. Anterior to the left gonadal artery
   D. Anterior to the left renal vein
   E. Anterior to the left inferior epigastric artery

9. A 15-day-old boy is brought to the physician by his mother for a circumcision. He has no abnormalities and developmental milestones are currently being met. During the circumcision, the urethra was noticed to be malpositioned as shown in Fig. 4.1. Which of the following embryological structures most likely failed to fuse, resulting in this malposition?
   A. Processus vaginalis
   B. Labioscrotal folds
   C. Urethral folds
   D. Urogenital folds
   E. Genital tubercle

10. A 6-month-old boy is brought to the physician by his mother for a follow-up examination. Developmental milestones and immunizations are up to date. Physical examination shows no other abnormality except for the defect noted in Fig. 4.1. Which of the following embryologic structures most likely developed abnormally, resulting in this clinical presentation?
   A. Spongy urethra
   B. Labioscrotal folds
   C. Cloacal membrane
   D. Urogenital folds
   E. Genital tubercle

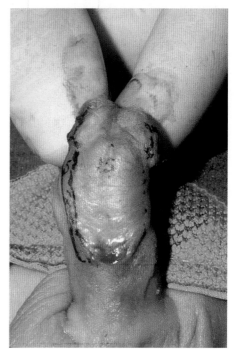

• Fig. 4.1

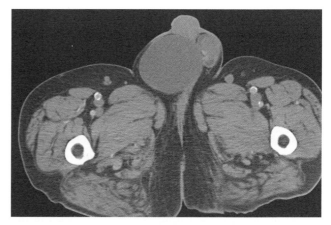

• Fig. 4.2

11. A 25-year-old man comes to the physician with a 3-month history of an enlarged scrotum on the right. Physical examination shows the right side of the scrotum is remarkably larger compared to the left. On palpation, the scrotum is soft and nontender and a fluid-filled mass is felt anterior to the testis. A CT scan shows abnormal accumulation of fluid in the cavity of the tunica vaginalis testis (Fig. 4.2). Which of the following is the most likely diagnosis?
   A. Varicocele
   B. Rectocele
   C. Cystocele
   D. Hydrocele
   E. Hypospadias

12. A 54-year-old man comes to the physician because of 3-week history of blood in his urine. He also has a persistent feeling of generalized tiredness and 2.2 kg (5 lb)

weight loss. Urine analysis shows the presence of red blood cells. A CT scan of the abdomen shows the presence of a renal mass extending into the left renal vein. Which of the following conditions is most likely to be associated with this disease?

A. Varicocele

B. Rectocele

C. Cystocele

D. Hydrocele

E. Hypospadias

13. A 30-year-old man comes to the physician because of inability to conceive for the past 2 years. Physical examination shows the left side of the scrotum feels like a bag of worms on palpation. The right side of the scrotum shows a similar finding when the patient is asked to bear down. An x-ray with contrast is shown in Fig. 4.3. Which of the following conditions will be most likely associated with this radiographic picture?

A. Varicocele

B. Rectocele

C. Cystocele

D. Hydrocele

E. Hypospadias

14. A 16-year-old woman is brought to the emergency department because of the sudden onset of severe abdominal pain and fever. Laboratory studies show a leukocyte count of 20,000/mm^3 and a positive pregnancy test. Colpocentesis shows the presence of blood in the pelvis confirming the diagnosis of a ruptured ectopic pregnancy. Which of the following structures was the needle most likely inserted through to perform the colpocentesis?

A. perineal body into the vesicouterine space

B. posterior part of the vaginal fornix into the recto-uterine pouch

C. anterior part of the vaginal fornix into the endocervical canal

D. vaginal orifice into the greater vestibular gland

E. perineal membrane into the external urethral sphincter

15. A 46-year-old woman comes to the physician because of 1-month history of a feeling of heaviness in the pelvic region and constipation. She has 5 children, all of whom were delivered via normal vaginal deliveries. Physical examination shows a noticeable bulge of tissue through her vaginal opening, which increases in size when she is asked to bear down. A diagnosis of rectocele is made. Which of the following is most likely responsible for this condition?

A. Compromised rectovaginal septum

B. Weakened superficial and deep transverse perineal muscles

C. Paralyzed ischiocavernosus muscle

D. Loose sacrospinous ligament

E. Ruptured external urethral sphincter

16. A 68-year-old man comes to the physician because of an inability to pass urine for the past 2 days. He has been

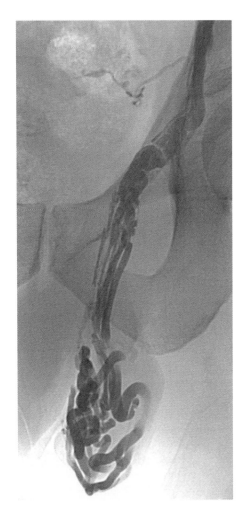

• **Fig. 4.3**

experiencing painful urination and nocturia for the past 6 months. Ultrasonography of the pelvis shows enlargement and irregularity of the uvula. Which of the following lobes of the prostate will most likely be hypertrophied?

A. Anterior

B. Median

C. Lateral

D. Posterior

E. Lateral and posterior

17. A 19-year-old woman comes to the physician with painful swelling of the clitoris for the past 14 days. A course of antibiotics was previously prescribed, but it has had no effect. Physical examination shows a firm, tender mass arising from the clitoris. Laboratory studies show no abnormalities. Fine needle aspiration shows the presence of cells suggestive of an aggressive sarcoma. A decision to perform a wide excision along with lymph node clearance is made. Which of the following lymph nodes is this cancer likely to have drained to first?

A. Superficial and deep inguinal lymph nodes

B. External iliac nodes

C. Para-aortic lymph nodes

D. Presacral lymph nodes

E. Axillary lymph nodes

18. A 45-year-old man is brought to the emergency department after falling 4.5 m (15 ft) during a mountain climbing expedition. Physical examination shows paralysis of the lower limbs bilaterally and a distended urinary bladder. A diagnosis of sacral cord injury is made. During insertion of the catheter to relieve the urinary retention, too much force is used, and the membranous urethra is ruptured. Which of the following structures would most likely be traumatized at this location?
    A. Bulbospongiosus muscle
    B. External urethral sphincter
    C. Corpus cavernosus
    D. Ischiocavernosus muscle
    E. Opening of the bulbourethral duct

19. A 22-year-old woman comes to the physician because of intermittent suprapubic pain and urinary frequency for the past 3 months. The pain varies from a 5 to 9 out of 10 without any particular triggers. During a diagnostic cystography, the woman experiences pain on filling of the urinary bladder. A diagnosis of interstitial cystitis is made. What is the location of the neural cell bodies responsible for pain sensation in this patient?
    A. Dorsal root ganglia of spinal cord levels S2, S3, and S4
    B. The intermediolateral cell column of spinal cord levels S2, S3, and S4
    C. The sensory ganglia of spinal nerves T5–T9
    D. The preaortic ganglia at the site of origin of the testicular arteries
    E. Dorsal root ganglia of spinal levels T10–L2

20. A 55-year-old woman comes to the physician because of an inability to control her bowel movements for the past year. She is particularly embarrassed and avoids going out into social settings. She has five children, all of whom were delivered vaginally. Her last pregnancy required a forceps delivery and resulted in a grade IV tear (perineal tear extending into the anus). Which of the following structures is defective and thus, most likely responsible for this patient's presentation?
    A. Pubococcygeus muscle
    B. Iliococcygeus muscle
    C. Coccygeus muscle
    D. Pubovesicocervical fascia
    E. External urethral sphincter

21. A 40-year-old obese woman comes to the physician because of pain in her leg for the past 3 months. The pain is worsened by standing and alleviated by sitting. Physical examination shows tenderness in the anterolateral thigh of the right lower limb. Tapping over the lateral aspect of the inguinal ligament just medial to the anterior superior iliac spine reproduces the pain. Which of the following nerves was most likely affected in this patient?
    A. Femoral branch of the genitofemoral nerve
    B. Femoral nerve
    C. Iliohypogastric nerve
    D. Ilioinguinal nerve
    E. Lateral femoral cutaneous nerve

22. A 24-year-old woman comes to the physician for a routine cervical cancer screening. Her previous screening was 3 years prior, during her first pregnancy. This pregnancy ended in a cesarean section due to failure to progress. Bimanual examination of the vagina shows a retroverted and retroflexed uterus. Which of the following is the most common position of the uterus?
    A. Anteflexed and retroverted
    B. Retroflexed and anteverted
    C. Anteflexed and anteverted
    D. Retroflexed and retroverted
    E. In the pouch of Douglas

23. A 55-year-old woman comes to the physician because of 5-month history of a pelvic discomfort. She recently has had difficulty passing urine. She has five children, all of whom were birthed via uncomplicated vaginal deliveries. Physical examination shows a uterine prolapse extending to the level of the hymen, which increases on straining. Which of the following ligaments is most likely defective resulting in this condition?
    A. Mesosalpinx and mesometrium
    B. Infundibulopelvic ligament
    C. Round ligament of the uterus
    D. Lateral cervical (cardinal) ligament
    E. Broad ligament of the uterus

24. A 60-year-old woman comes to the physician because of a 6-month history of abdominal pain and bloating. She says she feels fatigued and has a 4.5 kg (10 lb) weight loss in the last 3 months. She has never had any children. Physical examination shows a pelvic mass. A CT scan of the abdomen and pelvis shows bilateral ovarian masses with spread to the lymph nodes. Which of the following lymph nodes would most likely be the first to receive lymph from the diseased ovaries?
    A. Superficial and deep inguinal lymph nodes
    B. External iliac nodes
    C. Para-aortic nodes at the level of the renal vessels
    D. Node of Cloquet
    E. Internal iliac nodes accompanying the uterine artery and vein

Questions 25–49

25. A 29-year-old woman at 39 weeks' gestation comes to the hospital in labor. She was diagnosed with diabetes mellitus during an antenatal examination. During the vaginal delivery, a midline episiotomy is performed which extends from the hymen ring to the perineal body. Three months after the delivery, the woman experiences frequent episodes of "soiling her underwear." Which of the following structures was most likely damaged during the episiotomy leading to this presentation?
    A. Superficial and deep transverse perineal muscles
    B. External anal sphincter
    C. Ischiocavernosus muscle
    D. Sacrospinous ligament
    E. External urethral sphincter

26. A 41-year-old woman comes to the physician with multiple episodes of urine leakage for the past 2 months. She says that the episodes mainly occur during physical activity or while coughing. She has 5 children, all of whom were delivered vaginally. A diagnosis of stress incontinence is made, and the defect is scheduled to be surgically corrected. Ultrasonography of the perineum shows altered position of the neck of the urinary bladder and the urethra. Which of the following structures has most likely been injured during the multiple deliveries resulting in this presentation?
    A. Tendinous arch of levator ani
    B. Coccygeus
    C. Tendinous arch of pelvic fascia
    D. Obturator internus
    E. Rectovaginal septum

27. A 58-year-old woman undergoes a colectomy for carcinoma of the distal gastrointestinal tract. During surgery, lymph nodes from the sacral, internal iliac, and inguinal lymph node groups are removed and sent for histopathologic examination. Biopsy specimen shows positive cancerous cells only at the superficial inguinal lymph nodes. Which of the following parts of the gastrointestinal tract was most likely primarily affected by this cancer?
    A. Cutaneous portion of anal canal
    B. Distal rectum
    C. Mucosal zone of anal canal
    D. Pectinate line of anal canal
    E. Proximal rectum at the inferior valve (of Houston)

28. A 50-year-old woman comes to the physician because of worsening urine leakage for the past 3 months. She was diagnosed with urinary stress incontinence 1.5 years ago for which lifestyle and medical treatment has not been effective. A decision is made to perform a Burch colposuspension. During the operation, a low midline incision is made into the rectus abdominis fascia and muscle splitting it in half to visualize the pubic symphysis. The space posterior to the pubic symphysis is then dissected to visualize the urinary bladder neck, anterior vaginal wall, and urethra. Which of the following spaces was dissected to expose the urinary bladder neck?
    A. Ischioanal fossa
    B. Perineal body
    C. Retropubic space (of Retzius)
    D. Superficial perineal cleft
    E. Deep perineal space

29. A 13-year-old girl is brought to the emergency department by her parents because of a severe, deep pelvic discomfort which started a few hours ago. Her mother says that she has experienced similar episodes for the last 3 months all lasting a few days. Physical examination shows normal breast development and pubic hair. A bulging blueish membrane is observed across the vestibule. Incision of the hymen shows hematocolpos.

Which of the following conditions is most likely associated with this diagnosis?
    A. Cyst of greater vestibular (Bartholin) gland
    B. Bleeding from an ectopic pregnancy
    C. Imperforate hymen
    D. Indirect inguinal hernia with cremasteric artery bleeding
    E. Iatrogenic bleeding from the uterine veins

30. A 55-year-old woman comes to the physician because of dull, poorly localized pain in the deep pelvis for the past 6 months. Her father passed away from a rectal cancer. Physical examination shows a 2 cm descent of the vaginal wall towards the hymenal ring which is only evident during Valsalva maneuver. An MRI of her pelvis shows a tear of the rectovaginal septum and is negative for any masses. Which of the following is the most likely diagnosis?
    A. Cystocele
    B. Urethrocele
    C. Enterocele
    D. Urinary incontinence
    E. Prolapsed uterus

31. A 34-year-old woman comes to the physician because of a 4-month history of repeated episodes of urinary leakage during her weightlifting sessions. She had her uterus removed one year ago due to the presence of multiple fibroids which were causing significant menorrhagia and dysmenorrhea. Cystourethroscopy shows urethral hypermobility with a normal internal sphincter functionality. Which of the following muscles is most likely dysfunctional?
    A. Pubococcygeus
    B. Obturator internus
    C. Piriformis
    D. Coccygeus
    E. Iliococcygeus

32. A 42-year-old woman comes to the physician because of a dull left-sided abdominal pain lasting for the past 5 months. She says she is always bloated and that the pain is getting worse. Physical examination shows a distended abdomen with a palpable left-sided mass. An MRI of the pelvis shows a mass in the organ at the arrow (Fig. 4.4). A frozen biopsy confirms the presence of a malignancy. Which of the following structures can be ligated to reduce the pain from this malignancy?
    A. Infundibulopelvic ligament
    B. Pelvic sympathetic trunk
    C. Clunial nerves
    D. Pudendal nerve
    E. Broad ligament

33. A 45-year-old man is brought to the emergency department after falling on to the crossbar of his bicycle. Physical examination shows a man in obvious painful distress with pronounced swelling in the perineal region. An MRI of the pelvis shows a torn spongy urethra, along with a rupture of the deep (Buck) fascia of the penis, resulting in extravasation of urine and blood

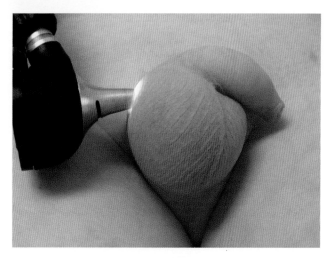

• **Fig. 4.4**

into the surrounding area. Which of the following fasciae most likely provide boundaries for the space into which urine has extravasated?

A. Camper fascia and Scarpa fascia
B. Perineal membrane and external perineal fascia of Gallaudet
C. Colles fascia and external perineal fascia of Gallaudet
D. Perineal membrane and the superior fascia of the external urethral sphincter
E. The external urethral sphincter and the apex of the prostate

34. A 34-year-old woman is brought to the emergency department after falling 1.5 m (5 ft) onto her back during a mountain-climbing expedition. Physical examination shows loss of anal tone and perianal numbness. A catheter is inserted to treat her urinary retention. A CT scan shows multiple fractures of her pelvis and her lower lumbar spine. Which of the following nerves was most likely traumatized leading to this patient's urinary symptoms?

A. Superior hypogastric
B. Pelvic splanchnic
C. Sacral splanchnic
D. Lumbar splanchnic
E. Pudendal

35. A 34-year-old woman is hospitalized because of an enlarged, painful abdomen. An ultrasound examination is performed and the presence of ascites (fluid) in the peritoneal cavity is confirmed. A needle is placed through the posterior part of the vaginal fornix to drain the fluid. Which space must the needle enter to drain the fluid?

A. Rectouterine pouch
B. Pararectal fossa
C. Paravesical space
D. Uterovesical pouch
E. Superficial perineal space

36. A 36-year-old man is brought to the emergency department with a painful, swollen penis. During intercourse he struck his erect penis against his partner's pelvis.

He heard a popping sound and rapid detumescence resulted. Physical examinations show a 3 cm preputial hematoma. During surgical exploration shows rupture of the distal spongy urethra and deep penile (Buck) fascia. Which of the following is the most likely place into which urine would have extravasated?

A. Ischioanal fossa
B. Rectovesical pouch
C. Deep perineal space
D. Retropubic space
E. Superficial perineal cleft

37. A 68-year-old man comes to the physician because of a 2-month history of with dysuria, nocturia, and urgency. An MRI of the pelvis shows an enlarged prostate and a needle biopsy shows a prostate malignancy. Subsequently, he undergoes a radical prostatectomy. Postoperatively, he has urinary incontinence secondary to paralysis of the external urethral sphincter. Which of the following nerves was most likely injured during the operation?

A. Pelvic splanchnic
B. Sacral splanchnic
C. Pudendal
D. Superior gluteal
E. Inferior gluteal

38. A 50-year-old man comes to the physician because of erectile dysfunction. He has a history of smoking 1 pack a day for the last 40 years. He was diagnosed with hypercholesterolemia 10 years prior. Duplex ultrasonography of the penis shows arterial insufficiency. Which of the following arteries is most likely compromised leading to this condition?

A. External iliac
B. Inferior epigastric
C. Umbilical
D. Internal pudendal
E. Superficial and deep circumflex

39. A 58-year-old postmenopausal woman comes to the physician because of a 2-month history of pelvic discomfort and dull pain. Physical examination shows a distended abdomen with palpable superficial inguinal nodes. The vulva and anal canal show no abnormalities. A CT scan of the pelvis shows a mass with lymph node spread. Lymph nodes from the sacral, internal iliac, and superficial inguinal lymph node groups are surgically removed for histopathologic examination. The biopsies show cancerous cells only in the inguinal lymph nodes. Which of the following pelvic organs was more than likely the site of the primary tumor?

A. The body of the uterus
B. Distal rectum
C. One or both of her ovaries
D. Proximal rectum
E. Anal canal superior to the pectinate line

40. A 34-year-old woman comes to the physician because of pelvic and abdominal pain, bloating, increased urination, and constipation. A CT scan of her pelvis

shows an ovarian tumor. Which of the following lymph nodes will most likely become invaded by cancerous cells?

A. Superficial inguinal
B. External iliac
C. Lumbar/lateral aortic
D. Deep inguinal
E. Internal iliac

41. A 62-year-old woman comes to the physician with painless vaginal bleeding for the past 2 weeks. Physical examination shows an erythematous, ulcerating nodule in the vestibule of her vagina. A biopsy of the lesion is performed. A diagnosis of squamous cell carcinoma is made. Which are the first lymph nodes most likely to filter lymph drainage from this area?

A. Superficial inguinal
B. Internal iliac
C. Lumbar/lateral aortic
D. Presacral lymph
E. Axillary lymph

42. A 34-year-old woman at 38 weeks' gestation comes to the physician to be induced for her scheduled delivery. During the course of her pregnancy, her diabetes mellitus has been uncontrolled. A pudendal nerve block is performed using a transvaginal approach. Which bony structure would most likely be palpated as a landmark to block this nerve?

A. Ischial spine
B. Posterior inferior iliac spine
C. Ischial tuberosity
D. Posterior superior iliac spine
E. Coccyx

43. A 55-year-old man comes to the physician because of rectal bleeding and pain at his anus for the past week. He says that he is generally in good health, except for an episode of constipation for the past 1 month. Physical examination shows a tender, blueish mass perianally. Which of the following nerves is responsible for the transmission of pain sensation from this region?

A. Sacral splanchnic
B. Superior hypogastric
C. Pelvic splanchnic
D. Pudendal
E. Ilioinguinal

44. A 26-year-old woman comes to the physician because of burning upon urination for the past 3 days. She recently returned from her honeymoon. Physical examination shows no abnormalities. A urine dipstick shows leukocytosis and the presence of nitrites. A diagnosis of urinary tract infection is made. Which of the following is the best anatomical explanation for the fact that women are more susceptible than men to these kinds of infections?

A. The vagina contains less bacterial flora than the penis
B. The prostate produces antibacterial prostatic fluids
C. The urethra is much shorter in women

D. The paraurethral gland produces mucus
E. The seminal glands produce fluids resistant to bacteria

45. A 52-year-old woman comes to the physician because of difficulty passing urine. Physical examination shows a mass extending through the vaginal orifice past the hymenal ring. A cystogram shows a prolapse of the urinary bladder through the anterior wall of the vagina. Which of the following structures is more than likely defective leading to this problem?

A. Pubovesical and vesicocervical fasciae
B. Cardinal ligament
C. Uterosacral ligament
D. Levator ani
E. Median umbilical ligament

46. A 40-year-old woman comes to the physician to undergo a hysterectomy for leiomyoma uteri. She has extremely heavy periods, which have resulted in a chronic anemia despite the use of iron supplements. In the past month, she has also experienced significant abdominal pain. During surgery, the uterine artery is identified. Which of the following adjacent structures is most susceptible to potential iatrogenic injury during ligation of this artery?

A. Ureter
B. Internal iliac artery
C. Internal iliac lymph nodes
D. Obturator nerve
E. Lumbosacral trunk

47. A 32-year-old woman comes to the physician because of painful intercourse. She is from a very conservative family and has recently begun engaging in sexual activities. Physical examination shows involuntary contractions of the vaginal musculature on attempted manual examination of the vagina. Laboratory studies for sexually transmitted diseases are negative. Which of the following conditions is the most likely diagnosis of this patient?

A. Vaginismus
B. Pudendal nerve compression in the pudendal (Alcock) canal
C. Disruption of the perineal body
D. Endometriosis
E. Fibroma of the uterus

48. A 46-year-old man is brought to the emergency department after being involved in a motor vehicle collision. His blood pressure is 90/80 mm Hg and pulse is 102/min. Physical examination shows multiple ecchymosis of the pelvis, and an intact pelvic girdle. There is also periurethral ecchymosis. A retrograde cystourethrogram shows extravasation of the contrast into the abdominal wall beneath the superficial fascia. Where would the contrast initially extravasate?

A. Between the superior aspect of the external urethral sphincter muscle and the pelvic diaphragm
B. Between the perineal membrane and the fascia of Gallaudet
C. Between Camper fascia and Scarpa fascia
D. Between Colles' fascia and Gallaudet fascia
E. Between Buck fascia and the dartos layer

49. A 45-year-old woman comes to the physician because of a 4-month history of lower back pain and a sensation of vaginal fullness. In the last month she has noticed difficulty voiding. Physical examination shows descent of the cervix to the level of the vaginal orifice. An abdominal sacrocolpopexy is planned to treat this condition. During this procedure, the vaginal vault is suspended from the sacral promontory to create the natural anatomical support that is usually provided by ligaments. Which of the following ligaments provides the natural anatomical support that this procedure tries to reestablish?
    A. Uterosacral
    B. Round ligament of the uterus
    C. Broad ligament
    D. Arcus tendineus fasciae pelvis
    E. Levator ani

Questions 50–74

50. A 68-year-old man comes to the physician because of 1-month history of dysuria, nocturia, and urgency. The patient has 9.1 kg (20 lb) weight loss over the past 4 months. Laboratory studies show high levels of PSA. A transurethral biopsy is performed and a diagnosis of prostate cancer is made. A CT scan of the abdomen shows regional lymphatic metastasis and a prostatectomy is performed. Which of the following lymph nodes should be removed during prostatectomy?
    A. Internal iliac and sacral
    B. External iliac
    C. Superficial inguinal
    D. Deep inguinal
    E. Gluteal

51. A 22-year-old man comes to the physician with a painless enlargement of the right groin for the past 3 months. Physical examination shows a nontender, palpable nodule on the right testis. Ultrasonography examination of the scrotum shows an intrinsic testicular lesion. An abdominal and pelvic CT examination shows regional lymphatic spread. Which of the following lymph nodes is most likely to be involved in this metastasis?
    A. Internal iliac
    B. External iliac
    C. Superficial inguinal
    D. Deep inguinal
    E. Para-aortic or lumbar

52. A 50-year-old man comes to the physician for a follow-up examination after a radical prostatectomy. Preoperatively, he was placed on sildenafil (Viagra) in an attempt to maintain his sexual functionality. One month postoperatively, he says he is incapable of penile erection without the use of sildenafil. He also has no nocturnal penile tumescence. Which nerve was most probably damaged during the operation?
    A. Pudendal
    B. Perineal
    C. Pelvic splanchnic

D. Sacral splanchnic
E. Dorsal nerve of penis

53. A 15-year-old boy is admitted to the emergency department 2 days after crashing his bicycle. MRI examination shows severe edema of the boy's scrotum and abdominal wall and extravasated urine. Which of the following structures is most likely ruptured?
    A. Spongy urethra
    B. Preprostatic urethra
    C. Prostatic urethra
    D. Urinary bladder
    E. Ureter

54. A 35-year-old man comes to the physician for a follow-up examination, 1 month after an elective hernia repair. He says for the past 2 weeks he has been experiencing a burning sensation which spreads from his lower abdomen to the medial aspect of his left inner thigh and sometimes to the scrotum. Physical examination shows tenderness on palpation of the left inguinal region below the midpoint of the inguinal ligament and an absent cremasteric reflex on the left side is noticed. Which of the following nerves is responsible for this reflex?
    A. Ilioinguinal nerve
    B. Genital branch of genitofemoral
    C. Iliohypogastric nerve
    D. Pudendal nerve
    E. Obturator nerve

55. A 19-year-old woman comes to the physician because of pain during sexual intercourse for the past 2 weeks. She says that she does not have a stable sexual partner. Speculum examination shows an inflamed cervix with a mucopurulent discharge. Bimanual examination shows cervical motion tenderness. Which of the following nerves conveys sensory fibers from this inflamed structure?
    A. Pudendal
    B. Superior hypogastric
    C. Pelvic splanchnic
    D. Sacral splanchnic
    E. Lesser splanchnic

56. A 24-year-old woman comes to the physician for a routine pap smear examination. She had one done 3 years prior which showed no abnormality. Physical examination of the cervix shows a smooth, pink surface with a clear mucoid secretion. During the collection of cells from her uterine cervix she feels a mild pain. Which of the following areas is most likely to experience "referred pain" during this procedure?
    A. Perineum and posterior portion of the thigh
    B. Suprapubic region
    C. Umbilical region
    D. Inguinal region
    E. Epigastric region

57. A 35-year-old man comes to the emergency department after being kicked in the groin while playing football.

Physical examination shows a swollen left scrotum. An MRI examination shows coagulation of blood in the veins draining the testis. Into which of the following veins would a thrombus most likely pass first from the injured area?

A. Inferior vena cava
B. Left renal vein
C. Left inferior epigastric
D. Left internal pudendal
E. Left iliac vein

58. A 1-year-old girl is brought to the emergency department by her mother because of vomiting and inconsolable crying for the past hour. The mother also noticed a swelling in the groin area. Her mother was diagnosed and treated for a CNS tumor when she was 10 years old. Physical examination shows a palpable mass superior to the inguinal ligament. The mass is nonreducible. Which of the following structures would the surgeon expect to find in the canal?

A. Round ligament of uterus
B. Urachus
C. Suspensory ligament of the ovary
D. Uterine tube
E. Mesosalpinx

59. A 25-year-old woman is brought to the emergency department by her mother because of intense lower abdominal pain which started 1 hour ago. She is unable to recall the date of her last menstrual period. Her temperature is 37.9°C (100.22°F), pulse is 112/min, blood pressure is 95/80 mm Hg and respirations are 20/min. Physical examination shows a rigid abdomen with rebound tenderness. Laboratory studies show a declining hemoglobin with leukocytosis and a positive pregnancy test. Which of the following is the most common site of the inciting etiology?

A. Over the internal cervical os
B. Wall of the bowel
C. Uterine tube
D. Mesentery of the bowel
E. Surface of the ovary

60. A 32-year-woman is brought to the emergency department after she reported being raped 2 hours ago. Fluids from her vagina are collected for DNA and fructose examination. Which of the following organs is responsible for fructose production?

A. Prostate
B. Seminal glands
C. Kidneys
D. Testis
E. Bulbourethral (Cowper) glands

61. A 6-month-old boy is brought to the physician by his mother for a follow-up examination. The boy was delivered via a normal vaginal birth at term. At birth, it was noted that his left testis was not palpable. Physical examination shows absence of a palpable testis in the left scrotal sac. A mass is palpated

in the left inguinal canal. Which of the following is the most likely diagnosis?

A. Pseudohermaphroditism
B. True hermaphroditism
C. Cryptorchidism
D. Congenital suprarenal gland hyperplasia
E. Chordee

62. A 38-year-old woman at 35 weeks' gestation is brought to the emergency department by her spouse because of vaginal bleeding which started 10 minutes ago and spontaneously stopped. She denies any abdominal pain. She has not been to any of her prenatal checkups. Ultrasonography of the abdomen shows a low-lying placenta. A diagnosis of placenta previa is made. What is the most likely site of implantation of the placenta in this disorder?

A. Uterine (fallopian) tubes
B. Cervix
C. Mesentery of the abdominal wall
D. Distal part of uterine body, overlapping the internal cervical os
E. Fundus of the uterus

63. A 63-year-old man comes to the physician because of bright red blood per rectum for the past week. He is currently a recovering alcoholic in a 12-step program. Physical examination shows a distended abdomen with a positive shifting dullness. Multiple tender, intrarectal masses projecting into the anal orifice are palpated on digital rectal examination. A diagnosis of grade 1 hemorrhoids is made. Which of the following best describes the nerves responsible for the transmission of pain fibers from this region?

A. Inferior anal (rectal) nerve
B. Perineal nerve
C. Hypogastric plexus
D. Visceral afferent fibers
E. Pelvic splanchnic nerves

64. A 34-year-old man is admitted to the emergency department after a traumatic landing into a swimming pool from a high diving platform. The patient has multiple traumas in his abdominal cavity. After a reconstructive operation of his abdominal organs the patient develops a high fever. A CT scan examination shows that the lower portion of the descending colon and rectum has become septic and must be excised. Six months postoperatively the patient experiences impotence. Which of the following structures was most likely injured during the second operation?

A. Pudendal nerve
B. Sacral splanchnic nerves
C. Pelvic splanchnic nerves
D. Sympathetic trunk
E. Vagus nerve

65. A 27-year-old woman comes to the physician for a follow-up examination. Two weeks ago, she underwent a loop electrosurgical excision because of an abnormal pap smear.

A biopsy specimen shows an invasive carcinoma with positive margins. A CT scan of the abdomen shows local lymphatic spread. Which of the following lymph nodes is most likely to have received metastasis from this malignancy?

A. Internal iliac
B. External iliac
C. Superficial inguinal
D. Deep inguinal
E. Sacral

66. A 2-year-old boy is brought to the physician because of a swollen left scrotum for the past week. Physical examination shows an enlarged left scrotum with a nontender flocculent mass. The testis are palpable on the posterior aspect of the mass. The remainder of the examination shows no other abnormalities. An otoscope is placed beneath on the right side of the scrotum and the testis is transilluminated through the scrotum (see Fig. 4.4). Which of the following is the most likely diagnosis in this patient?

A. Varicocele
B. Rectocele
C. Cystocele
D. Hydrocele
E. Hypospadias

67. A 34-year-old man comes to the physician because of a 1-week history of worsening perirectal pain. For the past 2 days, he has experienced chills. His temperature is 38°C (100.4°F), pulse is 83/min, respirations are 16/min, and blood pressure is 115/86mm/Hg. Laboratory studies shows leukocyte count of 15,000/mm^3 (with 85% neutrophils). Physical examination shows an extremely tender, indurated mass in the ischioanal fossa. To facilitate a complete physical examination the decision is made to anesthetize the area. Which of the following nerves will most likely need to be anesthetized?

A. Dorsal nerve of the clitoris
B. Superficial branch of perineal nerve
C. Perineal nerve
D. Inferior rectal nerve
E. Pudendal nerve

68. A 40-year-old man comes to the physician because of a 1-week history of painful defecation. His temperature is 39°C (100.4°F), pulse is 90/min, respirations are 16/min, and blood pressure is 120/78 mm/Hg. Laboratory studies show a leukocyte count of 20,000/mm^3. Physical examination shows perforation of the wall of the anal canal at the level of the anal valves. Anoscopic examination shows an opening with pus draining at the posterior midline of the level of the anal valves. Which of the following nerves is most likely responsible for the pain experienced by this patient upon defecation?

A. Dorsal nerve of the clitoris
B. Superficial branch of perineal nerve
C. Perineal nerve
D. Inferior rectal nerve
E. Pudendal nerve

69. A 35-year-old woman undergoes a tension-free vaginal tape procedure for a stress urinary incontinence.

Two days postoperatively, her temperature is 36.8°C (98.24°F), pulse is 105/min, respirations are 20/min and blood pressure is 90/80 mm Hg. Ultrasonography of the pelvis shows free fluid in the rectouterine pouch (of Douglas). She is taken to operating room for an emergency laparotomy. During surgery, the vessel crossing the pectineal (Cooper) ligament as it descends into the pelvis was injured by a staple, confirming the presence of the so-called "arterial circle of death." Which of the following arteries is most likely injured?

A. Obturator artery
B. Aberrant obturator artery
C. Superior vesical artery
D. Middle rectal
E. Inferior vesical

70. A 41-year-old man comes to the physician because of a 1-month history of testicular pain and pain upon ejaculation. He underwent a vasectomy 7 months ago. Physical examination shows fullness of the ductus deferens, which is tender to palpation. A diagnosis of postvasectomy pain syndrome is made. Which of the following nerves was most likely injured?

A. Sympathetic fibers to ductus deferens
B. Ilioinguinal
C. Iliohypogastric
D. Genital branch of genitofemoral
E. Visceral afferents from T10 to L2

71. A 41-year-old woman undergoes a scheduled tubal ligation. Two days postoperatively, her temperature is 37°C (98.6°F), pulse is 100/min, respirations are 18/min, and blood pressure is 96/80 mm Hg. Ultrasonography of the pelvis shows a large hematoma adjacent to the external iliac artery. Which of the following vessels was most likely injured during this procedure?

A. Ovarian arteries
B. Ascending branch of uterine arteries
C. Descending branch of uterine arteries
D. Superior vesical artery
E. Inferior vesical artery

72. A 31-year-old woman comes to the physician because of a 1-month history of pelvic pain. Physical examination shows a palpable mass in the right lower quadrant. Ultrasonography of the abdomen and pelvis shows a partially echogenic mass with posterior sound attenuation. A diagnosis of a teratoma is made. An ovariectomy is performed and the ovarian vessels are ligated. Which of the following structures is most likely at risk of injury when the ovarian vessels are ligated?

A. Uterine artery
B. Vaginal artery
C. Ureter
D. Internal pudendal artery
E. Pudendal nerve

73. A 23-year-old woman at 30 weeks' gestation comes to the physician because of a 2-week history of pelvic pain which is exacerbated on walking. Physical examination shows tenderness over the pubic symphysis. An x-ray of

the pelvis shows a 20 mm diastasis of the pubic symphysis. A diagnosis of peripartum diastasis of the pubic symphysis is made. The patient is informed that a hormone called relaxin is responsible for the separation of the sacroiliac joint and pubic symphysis. Which of the following pelvic distances will most likely remain unaffected?

A. Transverse diameter
B. Interspinous distance
C. True conjugate diameter
D. Diagonal conjugate
E. Oblique diameter

74. A 63-year-old woman undergoes an ovariectomy for an ovarian malignancy. During the procedure, the lymphatics of the lateral pelvic wall are also removed. Four days postoperatively, the patient has painful spasms of the muscles of the innermost aspect of the thigh. Physical examination shows a sensory deficit in the distal medial thigh. Which of the following nerves was most likely injured?

A. Genitofemoral
B. Ilioinguinal
C. Iliohypogastric
D. Obturator
E. Lumbosacral trunk

Questions 75–98

75. A 68-year-old man undergoes a radical prostatectomy. Preoperatively, he was placed on sildenafil (Viagra) in an attempt to maintain his sexual functionality. One month postoperatively, the patient is incapable of penile erection without the use of sildenafil (Viagra). He also denies nocturnal penile tumescence. Where are the cell bodies most likely located for the nerve that was damaged during the procedure?

A. Sacral parasympathetic nucleus
B. Sacral sympathetic trunk ganglia
C. Inferior mesenteric ganglion
D. Superior hypogastric plexus
E. Intermediolateral nuclei of L1, L2

76. A 32-year-old woman at 32 weeks' gestation comes to the physician for a follow-up examination. Her previous pregnancy required a cesarean section due to cephalopelvic disproportion. She was diagnosed with gestational diabetes in her previous pregnancy. Laboratory studies show uncontrolled blood sugar levels. She is scheduled for a cesarean section due to the high risk of cephalopelvic disproportion. Which of the following dimensions is the most likely reason this patient requires a cesarean section?

A. Transverse diameter
B. Interspinous distance
C. True conjugate diameter
D. Diagonal conjugate
E. Oblique diameter

77. A 20-year-old man comes to the physician because of a 2-month history of a painless swelling in his right scrotum. Physical examination shows a nontender, palpable mass which is indistinguishable from the testis.

Ultrasonography of the scrotum shows a homogeneous hypoechoic intratesticular mass. A radical orchiectomy is performed. A diagnosis of testicular seminoma is made. Which of the following are the most likely lymph nodes this cancer will metastasize to first?

A. Deep inguinal
B. External iliac
C. Internal iliac
D. Lumbar
E. Superficial inguinal

78. A 42-year-old woman comes to the physician because of a 5-month history of heavy menstrual bleeding. For the past month, she has also experienced intermenstrual bleeding and she has noticed her "heart racing." Physical examination shows a uterine mass on bimanual palpation. Ultrasonography of the pelvis shows a concentric, hypoechoic intramural mass of dimensions 7.2 × 8 cm. A uterine artery embolization is performed. Which of the following arteries most likely provides collateral supply to this organ?

A. External iliac
B. Inferior mesenteric
C. Ovarian
D. Internal pudendal
E. Superior mesenteric

79. A 34-year-old woman at 40 weeks' gestation goes into labor. Fifteen hours later, her cervix is fully dilated, but the descent of the fetus has arrested as the head fails to progress through the vaginal orifice. In an attempt to decrease the risk of tearing, an oblique surgical incision of the perineum is made to the right of the midline. Which of the following structures is most likely maintained?

A. External anal sphincter
B. External urethral sphincter
C. Right superficial transverse perineal muscle
D. Right ischiocavernosus muscle
E. Perineal body

80. A 34-year-old woman at 36 weeks' gestation is brought to the emergency department because of severe abdominal pain every 3 minutes, each lasting more than 10 seconds. Each contraction was associated with the urge to "push." Physical examination shows strong uterine contractions on palpation of the abdomen. The cervix is fully dilated, and the fetal membranes have ruptured. The woman requests pain relief. A pudendal nerve block is performed. Which of the following best describes this nerve block?

A. Injection near ischial tuberosity anesthetizes the mons pubis and anterior labia majora
B. Injection near ischial tuberosity anesthetizes and prevents pain from the uterus
C. Injection superomedial to the anterior superior iliac spine anesthetizes most perineal skin
D. Injection near ischial spines prevents pain from the uterus, cervix and upper $\frac{2}{3}$ vagina
E. Injection near ischial spines anesthetizes the posterior labia majora and inferior vagina

81. A 75-year-old man comes to the physician because of a 5-month history of generalized fatigue, weight loss, and anorexia. He has difficulty urinating, dysuria, hesitancy, and feelings of incomplete emptying with urination. Physical examination shows an emaciated man with a soft, flat nontender abdomen. Digital rectal examination shows a hard, nontender nodule on palpation of the prostate. Which of the following aspect of this organ is most likely implicated in this patient's condition?
    A. Posterior lobe
    B. Fibromuscular zone
    C. Median zone
    D. Lateral zone
    E. Lateral capsule

82. A 5-year-old boy is complaining of pain of the penis after falling off his bicycle seat and striking himself between the legs with the bicycle bar. When he attempted to urinate, he could produce only small amounts of urine and his mother noticed that the penis and scrotum were swollen. During physical examination, there was blood at the external urethral meatus, and the penis, scrotum, and lower anterior abdominal wall were swollen. A CT scan showed that the prostate was in its normal position, and no bony fractures were observed. An MRI identified fluid around the penis and into the scrotum. Which of the following has occurred in this patient?
    A. Deep (Buck) fascia of the penis was intact
    B. The membranous urethra was injured
    C. The attachment of superficial perineal fascia limited urine flow into the thigh
    D. The attachment of the superficial penile (Colles) fascia prevented urine flow into the anorectal triangle
    E. There was urine between the fatty and membranous layers of superficial fascia (Camper and Scarpa fasciae) over the lower abdomen

83. After studying several hours straight in a seated position for an upcoming anatomy examination, a medical student experienced focal (nonradiating) pain in the buttocks. The pain immediately resolved when the student stood up. Which of the following bony features was most likely responsible for the student's pain?
    A. Inferior pubic ramus
    B. Posterior superior iliac spine
    C. Ischial tuberosity
    D. Pubic tubercle
    E. Ischial spine

84. A radiologist observed a pelvic MRI of a 22-year-old pregnant woman and measured the distance between the sacral promontory and the superior margin of the pubic symphysis. Which of the following was most likely measured by the radiologist?
    A. Bispinous outlet
    B. Maximum transverse diameter of inlet
    C. Sagittal inlet
    D. Sagittal outlet
    E. Bispinous inlet

85. A 35-year-old woman at 40 weeks' gestation gives birth vaginally to a macrosomic infant. She was diagnosed with diabetes at 16 weeks of gestation, which was uncontrolled throughout her pregnancy. After repair of the episiotomy, she continues to bleed profusely. An emergency hysterectomy is performed. Which of the following is the most likely abdominal surgical incision used to perform this procedure?
    A. Right subcostal incision
    B. Median longitudinal incision
    C. Transverse incision just below the umbilicus
    D. McBurney point incision
    E. Suprapubic incision

86. A 36-year-old man comes to the physician because of the inability to have an erection for the past 2 weeks. He says that during his last intercourse he experienced significant pain which subsided on its own. He does not have any issues passing urine. Physical examination shows a palpable gap between the penis and pubis. Penile instability is also noted. A diagnosis of penile suspensory ligament disruption is made. During surgery, it is observed that the structure that "slings" around the base of the body of penis and helps support it is damaged. Which of the following structures was most likely damaged?
    A. Pubic symphysis
    B. Suspensory ligament of penis
    C. Midline raphe
    D. Fundiform ligament of penis
    E. Bulb of penis

87. A 35-year old-man comes to the physician because of a 2-week history of itching and severe pain of the left scrotum. He tried an antifungal cream for the past week ago but there have been no improvements of his symptoms. Physical examination shows a swollen scrotum with ulcerations oozing a serosanguinous fluid, which is particularly pronounced on the anterolateral surface of the scrotum. Which of the following nerves is most likely responsible for painful stimuli from the anterolateral surface of this organ?
    A. Ilioinguinal nerve (L1)
    B. Iliohypogastric nerve (L1)
    C. The anterior cutaneous branch
    D. Lateral femoral cutaneous nerve
    E. Pudendal nerve (S3)

88. A 13-year-old girl is brought to the emergency department because of severe, deep pelvic discomfort which started a few hours ago and has persisted. Her mother says that she has experienced similar episodes for the last 3 months all lasting a few days. She has never had a menstrual period. Physical examination shows normal breast development and pubic hair. A bulging blueish membrane is observed across the vestibule. Which of the following embryologic structures/ processes most likely failed resulting in this presentation?
    A. Cervical atresia
    B. Patent processus vaginalis
    C. Failure of the urorectal septum to develop
    D. Failure of the vaginal plate to canalize
    E. Incomplete fusion of the paramesonephric ducts

89. A 60-year-old woman comes to the physician because of abdominal pain and bloating of 6 months duration. She says she has been feeling fatigued and has noticed a 4.5 kg (10 lb) weight loss in the last 3 months. She does not have any children. Physical examination shows a pelvic mass. A CT scan of the abdomen and pelvis shows a left ovarian mass without local spread. An ovariectomy is performed. Which of the following structures should be ligated in order to avoid excessive bleeding during the surgery?
    A. Round ligament
    B. Suspensory ligament
    C. Ovarian ligament
    D. Transverse cervical ligament
    E. Mesosalpinx

90. A 60-year-old woman comes to the physician because of abdominal pain and bloating of 6 months duration. She is fatigued and has a 4.5 kg (10 lb) weight loss in the last 3 months. She does not have any children. Physical examination shows a pelvic mass. A CT scan of the abdomen and pelvis shows a left ovarian mass without local spread. An ovariectomy is performed. During the procedure, the left ureter is palpated immediately medial to which of the following vessels?
    A. Gonadal vein
    B. External iliac artery
    C. Inferior vena cava
    D. Internal iliac artery
    E. Uterine artery

91. A 23-year-old woman at 25 weeks' gestation gives birth via an unplanned cesarean section because of fetal distress. She did not receive any antenatal care. Physical examination shows an imperforate anus with the left foot rotated inward and downward. Skeletal survey shows a hemivertebra. Which of the following additional defects is most likely to be found in the patient?
    A. Tracheoesophageal fistula
    B. Vertebral abnormalities
    C. Urinary tract defects
    D. Cardiac abnormalities
    E. Ileal atresia

92. A 20-year-old, gravida 1, para 0, aborta 0, woman at 38 weeks' gestation goes into labor. She appears to be in painful distress and requests anesthesia. The physician palpated the ischial spine transvaginally and then injected a local anesthetic. Which of the following ventral rami segments did the nerve that was most likely blocked by anesthetic originate from?
    A. S2, S3, S4
    B. L4, L5, S1
    C. L5, S1, S2
    D. S1, S2, S3
    E. S3, S4, S5

93. A 30-year-old woman undergoes bilateral autogenous breast surgery. Six months ago, she had a prophylactic bilateral mastectomy due to a recent BRCA1 diagnosis. Both her mother and older sister have been diagnosed with breast cancer. The decision is made to utilize a gluteal myocutaneous flap. During the harvesting of this flap, a blood vessel that courses between the lumbosacral trunk and ventral ramus of S1 and exits the pelvic cavity through the greater sciatic foramen is identified and preserved. Which of the following arteries is this?
    A. Inferior gluteal
    B. Superior vesical
    C. Iliolumbar
    D. Lateral sacral
    E. Superior gluteal

94. A 69-year-old woman complained of fecal incontinence that was found to be due to dysfunction of a muscle. Dysfunction of which of the following muscles most likely caused this patient's condition?
    A. Puborectalis
    B. Pubococcygeus
    C. Iliococcygeus
    D. Coccygeus
    E. Obturator internus

95. A 28-year-old pregnant woman delivers her baby before reaching the hospital and incurs a posterior vaginal tear. A pudendal nerve block is necessary to adequately anesthetize the area to facilitate proper closure of the wound. If this block is performed transvaginally, which landmark can be palpated to determine the proper site of anesthetic injection?
    A. Ischial spine
    B. Posterior inferior iliac spine
    C. Ischial tuberosity
    D. Posterior superior iliac spine
    E. Coccyx

96. A 30-year-old man comes to the physician because of a 1-week history of pain during defecation which lasts several minutes afterward. He says that in the past 2 days he has also noticed bright red blood on the toilet paper upon wiping. Physical examination shows slit-like openings in the anal mucosa. A diagnosis of anal fissures is made. Which of the following nerves most likely innervates this region affected by anal fissures?
    A. Sacral splanchnic
    B. Superior hypogastric
    C. Pelvic splanchnic
    D. Pudendal
    E. Ilioinguinal

97. A 69-year-old man comes to the physician because of a 2-week history of a painful lesion on the glans penis. He says that he first noticed the lesion 1 year ago, but it only recently became painful. Physical examination shows an ulcerated lesion with rolled edges. A biopsy of the lesion is done and a diagnosis of squamous cell carcinoma is made. Which lymph nodes will most likely be affected first if metastatic spread of the cancer occurs?
    A. External iliac
    B. Internal iliac
    C. Deep inguinal
    D. Lumbar/lateral aortic
    E. Axillary

98. A 4-month-old boy is brought to the physician by his parents because urine is leaking through an opening on the dorsal surface of the penis. What is the most likely diagnosis?

A. Epispadias
B. Hermaphrodism
C. Hydrocele
D. Hypospadias
E. Ectopic ureter

Questions 99–105

99. A 6-year-old girl is admitted to the hospital with fever, malaise, and painful voiding. She is treated with antibiotics for a urinary tract infection, but the symptoms persist. An abdominal CT scan shows a suprapubic cystic mass attached to the umbilicus and the apex of the urinary bladder. What is the most likely diagnosis?

A. Hydrocele
B. Meckel cyst
C. Meckel diverticulum
D. Omphalocele
E. Urachal cyst

100. A 72-year-old man undergoes radical prostatectomy for a cancerous prostatic mass. Following the operation, he is unable to achieve erection. The nerve fibers that were injured during the procedure are carried by which nerve(s)?

A. Superior hypogastric
B. Pelvic splanchnics
C. Sacral splanchnics
D. Lumbar splanchnics

101. A 55-year-old man comes to the physician for a follow-up examination. He received radiotherapy 3 months ago for prostate cancer. He has been unable to have an erection ever since. He also denies nocturnal tumescence. A diagnosis of cavernous nerve damage secondary to radiation therapy is made. Which of the following structures receive efferent fibers from these nerves?

A. Erectile bodies of the penis
B. Glans penis
C. External urethral sphincter
D. Internal urethral sphincter
E. Seminal gland

102. A 34-year-old man comes to the physician because of a 6-week history of a painful left scrotum. His temperature is 37°C (98.6°F), pulse is 90/min, blood pressure is 124/80 mm Hg and respirations are 13/min. Physical examination shows a grossly enlarged left scrotum, which is tender to palpation. Ultrasonography of the scrotum shows a complex echoic mass connected to the testis. A diagnosis of scrotal abscess is made. Which of the following lymph nodes is most likely to be tender and swollen?

A. External iliac
B. Internal iliac
C. Lateral aortic/lumbar
D. Sacral
E. Superficial inguinal

103. A 48-year-old woman undergoes an abdominal hysterectomy for leiomyomata uteri. One day after the procedure, physical examination shows tenderness over the right lower quadrant. She also has a low urine output. A retrograde pyelogram shows contrast material in the left renal pelvis and none in the right, and it is suspected that the right ureter has been damaged. That structure passes inferior to which of the following?

A. Ovarian artery
B. Ovarian ligament
C. Mesosalpinx
D. Round ligament of the uterus
E. Uterine artery

104. A 55-year-old woman comes to the physician because of 5-day history of blood in her stools. Physical exam shows firm, enlarged superficial inguinal lymph nodes. A CT scan shows a cancerous mass in the lower part of the gastrointestinal tract. In which of the following locations is the mass most likely located?

A. Anal canal inferior to the pectinate line
B. Distal rectum
C. Sigmoid colon
D. Proximal rectum
E. Anal canal superior to the pectinate line

105. A 35-year-old woman with a malignancy involving the lower part of her vagina is admitted to the hospital to undergo chemotherapy. In the image above (Fig. 4.5) which of the following nodes would first receive drainage from this area?

A. A
B. B
C. C
D. D
E. E

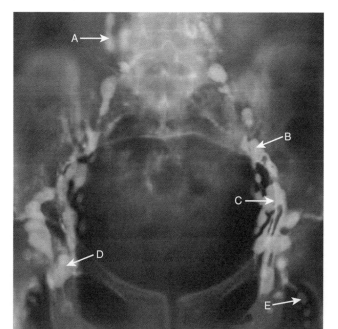

• **Fig. 4.5**

Answers

Answers 1–24

1. A. Perineal hypospadias is also referred to as third-degree hypospadias. Similar to penile hypospadias, it also results from failure of fusion of the urogenital (urethral) folds.

C. In perineal hypospadias, the labioscrotal folds also fail to fuse resulting in the halves of the scrotum being unfused. The failure of the labioscrotal folds fusion is secondary to the initial failure of the urogenital folds. Thus, it is the urogenital folds which are ultimately responsible for this defect.

B. The cloacal membrane is formed from endoderm of the cloaca and ectoderm of the proctodeum and forms the future anus.

D. The genital tubercle is formed in the 4th week at the anterior end of the cloacal folds. The tubercle matures into the body and glans penis. The dorsal displacement of this tubercle results in the development of epispadias.

E. The urogenital membrane is bounded by the urogenital folds and ruptures to form the urogenital orifice.
GAS 459–461, 512; N 370; ABR/McM 278

2. B. Most anorectal anomalies result from abnormal development of the urorectal septum, ultimately resulting in nondivision of the cloaca into urogenital and anorectal parts. The common outlet of the intestinal, urinary, and reproductive tracts is specifically associated with a persistent cloaca.

A. The labioscrotal folds are involved in forming the external urethral orifice only.

C. The urogenital folds normally fuse along the ventral side of the penis to form the spongy urethra.

D. The genital tubercle is responsible for the development of the body and glans penis.

E. The urogenital membrane is bounded by the urogenital folds and ruptures to form the urogenital orifice.
GAS 422, 452; N 370; ABR/McM 279

3. A. The gubernaculum arises in the upper abdomen from the lower end of the gonadal ridge and helps guide the testis in its descent through the abdominal wall and then into the scrotum. Several competing theories exist with regard to the exact embryologic origin of testicular ectopia; all of which recognize the integral role of the gubernaculum. One popular theory postulates that ectopic testes occur when a portion of the gubernaculum passes to an abnormal position or otherwise fails to descend or become fixed to the skin of the scrotum.

B. The processus vaginalis is an extension of the peritoneum into the scrotum which arises as the gubernaculum traverse the abdominal wall muscles. The processus vaginalis usually obliterates and the distal portion is retained as the tunica vaginalis testis. Failure of the processus vaginalis to completely obliterate results in conditions such as hydrocele of the testis or spermatic cord or an indirect inguinal hernia.

C. The genital tubercle forms the primordial phallus and is associated with epispadias.

D. The seminiferous cords form the primordia of the seminiferous tubules.

E. The labioscrotal swellings approach each other and fuse to form the scrotum.
GAS 289–298, 463; N 368; ABR/McM 279

4. A. When the urinary bladder mucosa is open to the outside in the fetus or newborn, the condition is referred to as exstrophy of the urinary bladder. The exstrophy results from failure of the primitive streak mesoderm to migrate around the cloacal membrane, and it occurs often in combination with epispadias.

B. Penile hypospadias is characterized by a failure of fusion of the labioscrotal folds, with the external urethral orifice located between the two unfused halves of the scrotum.

C. Androgens are responsible for development of the external genitalia in utero. Insufficient androgen stimulation of a 46 XY fetus results in varying degrees of pseudohermaphroditism.

D. Klinefelter syndrome is a condition in which the male has 47,XXY chromosomes.

E. A persistent allantois is associated with a patent urachus and an allantoic cyst.
GAS 456 ; N 352; ABR/McM 279

5. A. The ureteric bud, or metanephric diverticulum, is an outgrowth from the mesonephric duct. It is the primordium of the ureter, renal pelvis, the calyces, and the collecting tubules. Incomplete division results in a divided kidney with a bifid ureter. Complete division results in a double kidney with a bifid ureter, or separate ureters.

B. The mesonephric duct, also known as the Wolffian duct, results in the formation of the male internal sexual organs.

C. The paramesonephric duct results in the formation of the female internal sexual organs.

D. The metanephric mesoderm gives rise to components of the nephron extending to the distal convoluted tubules.

E. The pronephros are transitory structures which initially open into the cloaca and regress by the 5th week.
GAS 380, 455; N 317; ABR/McM 280

6. A. Hydrocele is fluid accumulation between the visceral and parietal layers of the tunica vaginalis of the testis. Thus, it presents as a nontender swelling of the scrotum.

B. An epidermoid cyst is a rare lesion which originates from ectodermal tissue. It may occur in any location of the body. Epidermoid cysts tend to result after trauma or surgical implantation of ectodermal tissue.

Thus, the patient's clinical presentation makes this diagnosis unlikely.

C. A Meckel diverticulum is located in the ileum of the small intestine. It tends to be discovered incidentally in the majority of patients. On the other hand, patients with symptomatic Meckel diverticulum tends to present with complication such as hemorrhage or bowel obstruction.

D. An omphalocele is the persistence of the herniation of the abdominal contents into the umbilical cord. This presents at birth with as a centrally located abdominal wall defect

E. The persistence of the epithelial lining of the urachus can give rise to a urachal cyst. This swelling is found in the midline in the umbilical region. Patients with urachal cyst are often asymptomatic until it becomes infected. Presenting symptoms include palpable mass with overlying erythema, recurrent UTIs and lower abdominal pain.
GAS 456; N 352; ABR/McM 233

7. A. A complete fusion results in abnormal development of the uterine tubes because the uterine tubes form from the unfused portions of the cranial parts of the paramesonephric ducts.

B. A double uterus is caused by failure of inferior parts of the paramesonephric ducts.

C. Failure of the mesonephric ducts to degenerate in a woman may result in a Gartner duct cyst.

D. Failure of the paramesonephric (Müllerian) ducts to recanalize completely may lead to a blockage in the female genital tract.

E. The pronephros is part of the primordial urinary system and generally degenerates in the first 4 weeks of development.
GAS 380, 455; N 371; ABR/McM 287

8. A. The ureters cross the pelvic brim anterior to the bifurcation of the common iliac artery bilaterally. Thus, it can serve as a landmark for the identification of the ureters. Because of the proximity of this artery to the ureter, it is in danger of being damaged during surgery.

B, C, D, E. There is no reliable association of the ureters and these other structures.
GAS 459–461; N 382; ABR/McM 271

9. C. Hypospadias is a developmental defect which results in the urethra opening on the ventral surface of the penis. This ectopic malformation occurs when the urethral folds fail to completely fuse.

A. The processus vaginalis is an extension of the peritoneum into the scrotum which arises as the gubernaculum traverse the inguinal muscles. The processus vaginalis usually obliterates and the distal portion is retained as the tunica vaginalis testis. Failure of the processus vaginalis to completely obliterate results in conditions such as hydrocele of the testis or spermatic cord or an indirect inguinal hernia.

B. A failure of the labioscrotal folds to fuse will cause the external urethral orifice to be situated between the two scrotal halves. This is referred to as penile hypospadias.

D. Failure of the urogenital folds to fuse would lead to agenesis of the external urethral folds.

E. In the male fetus, the body of the penis is derived from the genital tubercle. Failure of the genital tubercle to develop results in aphallia, that is, congenital absence of the penis.
GAS 459–461, 507; N 370; ABR/McM 278

10. A. Epispadias is a developmental defect in the spongy urethra resulting in urine being expelled from the dorsal aspect of the penis.

B. A failure of the labioscrotal folds to fuse will cause the external urethral orifice to be situated between the two scrotal halves. This is referred to as penile hypospadias.

C. The cloacal membrane is formed by ectoderm and endoderm and typically this membrane covers the embryonic cloaca.

D. Failure of the urogenital folds to fuse would lead to agenesis of the external urethral folds.

E. The genital tubercle would not directly cause epispadias, as the tubercle still continues to develop, but it is located more dorsally.
GAS 459–461, 507; N 370; ABR/McM 279

11. D. Hydrocele results from an excess amount of fluid within a persistent processus vaginalis. Hydrocele can result from injury to the testis or by retention of a processus that fills with fluid in infants. The tunica vaginalis testis consists of parietal and visceral layers, the latter of which is closely attached to the testis and epididymis. The fluid buildup occurs within the cavity between these layers.

A. A varicocele consists of varicosed veins of the pampiniform plexus and is associated with increased venous pressure in the testicular vein, followed by the accumulation and coagulation of venous blood.

B. A rectocele is a herniation of the rectum through the posterior vaginal wall.

C. A cystocele is the herniation of the posterior wall of the urinary bladder through the anterior vaginal wall.

E. Hypospadias refers to the displacement of urethral meatus on to the ventral surface of the body of the penis.
GAS 463 ; N 372; ABR/McM 279

12. A. Varicose veins occur with loss of elasticity within the walls of the vessels. As the veins weaken, they consequently dilate under pressure. A varicocele often occurs with a varicosity of the veins of the pampiniform venous plexus, resulting in a swelling of the veins. This condition can arise from a tumor in the left kidney, which occludes the testicular vein due to an anatomical constriction and increased pressure in veins draining the testis.

B. A rectocele is a herniation of the rectum into the posterior vaginal wall.

C. A cystocele is the herniation of posterior wall of the urinary bladder into the anterior vaginal wall.

D. A hydrocele is an accumulation of excess fluid within the cavity of the tunica vaginalis testis. E. Hypospadias occurs from failure of fusion of the urethral or labioscrotal folds, resulting in an external urethral opening on the ventral surface of the penis or in the perineum, respectively.
GAS 511–512, 522; N 383; ABR/McM 278

13. **A.** When veins lose their elasticity, they can become weak and often dilate. This causes the veins to become swollen and oftentimes tortuous, as a result of incompetent valves. The appearance of a "bag of worms" on the x-ray is characteristic of a varicosity of the pampiniform venous plexus the image shows a selective venography of the left testicular vein demonstrating dilatation of the pampiniform venous plexus around the left testes.
    B. A rectocele is a herniation of the rectum into the posterior vaginal wall.
    C. A cystocele is the herniation of posterior wall of the urinary bladder into the anterior vaginal wall.
    D. A hydrocele is an accumulation of excess fluid within the tunica vaginalis testis cavity.
    E. Hypospadias occurs from failure of fusion of the urethral and labioscrotal folds, resulting in an external urethral opening on the ventral surface of the penis or in the perineum.
    GAS 511–512, 522; N 385; ABR/McM 278

14. **B.** In the women, the rectouterine pouch, also known as the pouch of Douglas, represents the lowest point of the peritoneal cavity. Thus, it is the most gravity dependent allowing fluid to accumulate. The most direct route to the rectouterine pouch is through the posterior part of the vaginal fornix.
    A. The vesicouterine space, which is located between the urinary bladder and uterus, is superior to the rectouterine space. Thus, fluid is unlikely to accumulate there first. Therefore, it would not be advisable to attempt initially to insert a needle into the vesicouterine space.
    C. Inserting a needle through the anterior part of the vaginal fornix into the endocervical canal would lead one into the uterine cavity, with the probability of other undesirable consequences.
    D. The greater vestibular gland is located in the perineum. Thus, entering this gland with a needle would not be diagnostically useful in the presence of an ectopic pregnancy.
    E. The external urethral sphincter muscle lies postero-superior to the perineal membrane. Thus, one is unable to assess fluid in the pelvic cavity by examining this.
    GAS 477; N 345; ABR/McM 285

15. **A.** A break or tear in the rectovaginal septum (fascia of Denonvilliers) can allow small intestine (in an enterocele) or rectum (in a rectocele) to herniate into the posterior vaginal wall, even to the point of protrusion through the vaginal orifice.

B, C, E. The muscles listed are all in the anterior region of the perineum and have no association with an enterocele or rectocele. D. The sacrospinous ligament is unrelated to this condition.
GAS 475; N 345; ABR/McM 285

16. **B.** When the internal urethral orifice is obstructed, it is most likely due to an enlargement of the median (or middle) lobe of the prostate. The prostate is located at the base of the urinary bladder and is often described as possessing five ill-defined lobes, although this is not accepted by most urologists. The middle lobe consists of glandular tissue dorsal to the uvula of the urethral meatus of the urinary bladder, adjacent to the beginning of the urethra. This glandular tissue is most frequently involved in benign hypertrophy.
    A. The anterior lobe is not associated with benign prostatic hyperplasia.
    C. The lateral lobe roughly corresponds to what is referred to as the peripheral zone, where most adenocarcinomas of the prostate are found.
    D and **E.** The posterior lobe is the portion that is most readily palpated by digital rectal exam.
    GAS 459–461, 466; N 366; ABR/McM 281

17. **A.** The lymphatics from the skin of the clitoris drain first into the superficial inguinal nodes. The deep inguinal lymph nodes drain the glans clitoris and receive lymph also from superficial nodes.
    B. The external iliac nodes drain the upper vagina and body of the cervix.
    C. The para-aortic lymph nodes, or lumbar nodes, receive drainage from the fundus of the uterus along with the uterine tubes and ovaries. Lymph from the common iliac nodes also drain into these nodes.
    D. The drainage of presacral lymph nodes can pass to the common or internal iliac nodes.
    E. Axillary nodes drain body wall structures above the T10 dermatome (or the umbilicus).
    GAS 495; N 389; ABR/McM 376

18. **B.** The membranous urethra is located in the deep perineal space. Within this space, the urethra is surrounded by a sheet of skeletal muscle (compressor urethrae) which collectively form the external urethral sphincter. Thus, this muscle is susceptible to damage in the event of damage to the membranous urethra. If the membranous portion of the urethra is injured, urine and blood can leak upward into the retropubic space (of Retzius) limited inferiorly by the external urethral sphincter and perineal membrane.
    A, C, D. The bulbospongiosus muscle and other perineal muscles, the corpus cavernosum and the ischiocavernosus muscle, are located in the superficial perineal space.
    E. While the bulbourethral glands are located in the deep perineal space, the ducts of the bulbourethral ducts pierce the perineal membrane to open in the proximal spongy urethra.
    GAS 459–461; N 367; ABR/McM 279

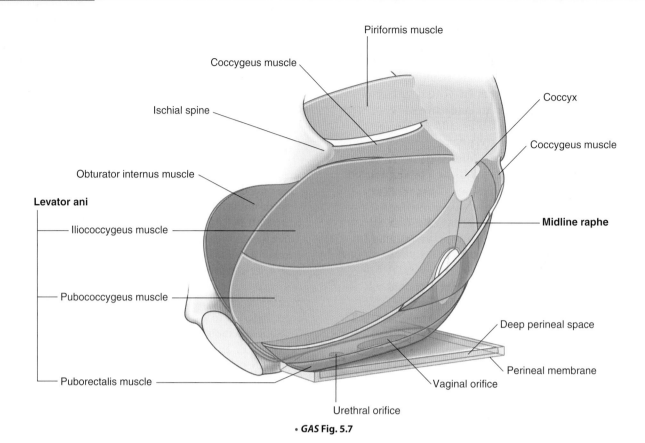

Piriformis muscle

Coccygeus muscle

Ischial spine

Obturator internus muscle

Levator ani

Iliococcygeus muscle

Pubococcygeus muscle

Puborectalis muscle

Urethral orifice

Coccyx

Coccygeus muscle

Midline raphe

Deep perineal space

Perineal membrane

Vaginal orifice

• *GAS* **Fig. 5.7**

19. A. Conscious pain due to urinary bladder fullness results from the excitation of stretch receptors in the bladder wall. These pain fibers are carried through the pelvic nerve plexuses and into the pelvic splanchnic nerves. The sensory fibers enter the dorsal root ganglia of spinal nerves S2, S3, and S4. Sensory fibers enter the spinal cord via these ganglia. Spinal cord levels S2, S3, and S4 contain parasympathetic soma. The levels T5–T9, T10–L2, and preaortic ganglia are well above where sensory fibers from the urinary bladder are located.
   B. The intermediolateral cell column of spinal cord levels S2, S3, and S4 is not responsible for pelvic pain.
   C. The sensory ganglia of spinal nerves T5–T9 are not responsible for pelvic pain.
   D. The preaortic ganglia at the site of origin of the testicular arteries are not responsible for pelvic pain.
   E. Dorsal root ganglia of spinal levels T10–L2 not responsible for pelvic pain.
   GAS 456, 488; N 399; ABR/McM 271
20. A. The pubococcygeus muscle, especially its most medial portion, the puborectalis, is of prime importance in fecal continence. The levator ani consists of two major portions, the pubococcygeus and iliococcygeus, which help support pelvic viscera and resist increases in intra-abdominal pressure. The puborectalis muscle is most medial and inferior portion of the pubococcygeus. The puborectalis forms a loop

around the anorectal junction, which should keep the anorectal angle to around 90 degrees; the integrity of this muscle is critical in the maintenance of fecal continence.
   B. The iliococcygeus forms part of the levator ani. Its main function is to elevate the pelvic floor and the anorectal canal. The puborectalis is the main muscle responsible for fecal continence.
   C, D. The coccygeus and pubovesicocervical fascia are not in direct contact with the rectum.
   E. Damage to the external urethral sphincter can contribute to urinary incontinence but not fecal incontinence (*GAS* Fig. 5.7).
   GAS 446–448; N 340; ABR/McM 277
21. E. The lateral femoral cutaneous nerve (L2, L3) emerges from the lateral side of the psoas muscle and runs in front of the iliacus and through, or behind, the inguinal ligament and innervates the skin of the lateral aspect of the thigh to the level of the knee. This nerve has been constricted in this case of "Calvin Klein syndrome" (in this case from the patient's obesity, not their too-tight jeans) causing pain, tingling, or burning sensations in the lateral thigh.
   A. The femoral branch of the genitofemoral nerve (L1, L2) supplies a small area of skin (over the femoral triangle), just inferior to the midpoint of the inguinal ligament.
   B. The femoral nerve (L2–L4) is motor to the quadriceps and sartorius muscles and sensory to the anterior thigh and the medial thigh and leg.

C. The ilioinguinal supplies the suprapubic region; part of the genitalia and anterior perineum; and the upper, medial thigh.

D. Cutaneous branches of the iliohypogastric nerve innervate skin of the anterolateral gluteal area and suprapubic region.
GAS 398; N 395; ABR/McM 271

22. **C.** Normally, the uterus is anteflexed at the junction of the cervix and the body and anteverted at the junction of the vagina and the cervical canal.

A. The anteflexed, retroverted uterus is now regarded as a normal variant. It is frequently encountered in early pregnancy. However, persistence into the second trimester has been associated with uterine incarceration.

B. An anteverted retroflexed uterus is generally a rare finding. However, this lie is more frequently observed in women who have undergone a cesarean delivery.

D. The retroflexed, retroverted uterus is particularly rare. It is associated with dyspareunia and dysmenorrhea, difficulty estimating gestational age by palpation, and obstetric complications.

E. The pouch of Douglas or rectouterine pouch lies between the uterus and the rectum.
GAS 471; N 353; ABR/McM 286

23. **D.** The cardinal ligament, also known as Mackenrodt ligament or lateral or transverse cervical ligament, is composed of condensations of fibromuscular tissues that accompany the uterine vessels. These bands of pelvic fascia provide direct support to the uterus.

A. The mesosalpinx and mesometrium are parts of the broad ligament which drape the uterine tube and uterus, respectively.

B. The infundibulopelvic ligament is also known as the suspensory ligament of the ovary. The suspensory ligament extends from the ovaries to the lateral abdominal wall. Its main function is to contain the ovarian vessels and nerve.

C. The round ligament of the uterus is a remnant of the gubernaculum. It attaches from the uterus to the labia majora.

E. The broad ligament extends from the uterus to the lateral wall and functions to hold the uterus in position.
GAS 475; N 354; ABR/McM 287

24. **C.** Ovarian lymph first drains into the para-aortic nodes at the level of the renal vessels.

A. The superficial and deep inguinal nodes drain the body wall below the umbilicus, the lower limbs, and the cutaneous portion of the anal canal and parts of the perineum.

B. The external iliac nodes receive the lymph from the inguinal nodes. The upper vagina, body of the uterus, and the cervix drains directly into this node.

D. The node of Cloquet is a deep inguinal lymph node that is located in the femoral ring, adjacent to the external iliac vein and beneath the inguinal ligament. The node of Cloquet drains into the external iliac nodes.

E. The internal iliac nodes accompany the uterine artery and vein. These nodes receive lymph from much of the uterus but not the ovaries.
GAS 495; N 388; ABR/McM 368

Answers 25–49

25. **B.** The external anal sphincter is important for maintaining fecal continence. The external anal sphincter is located immediately posterior to the perineal body (central tendon) and would be susceptible to damage during a midline episiotomy.

A. The superficial and deep transverse perineal muscles is found in the superficial and deep perineal spaces, respectively. The superficial transverse perineal muscle overlies the deep transverse perineal muscle. This muscle extends to the perineal body to which it provides support. While this muscle is cut during a midline episiotomy, it does not function in fecal continence.

C. In the woman the ischiocavernosus muscle covers the crura of the clitoris. It traverses laterally from the base of the crura to attach to the ischiopubic ramus. Thus, it is not susceptible to injury during the procedure.

D. The sacrospinous ligament attaches from the ischial spine to the sacrum and coccyx. It is an integral part of the wall of the lesser pelvis. Thus, it is not at risk of injury.

E. external urethral sphincter is a component of the deep perineal space. Thus, it is unlikely to be injured during an episiotomy which targets structure in the superficial perineal space (*GAS* Fig. 5.17).
GAS 452–453; N 351; ABR/McM 290

26. **C.** The tendinous arch of pelvic fascia is a dense band of connective tissue that joins the fascia of the levator ani to the feltlike pubocervical fascia that covers the anterior wall of the vagina. If this fascial band is torn, the ipsilateral side of the vagina falls, carrying with it the urinary bladder and urethra, often leading to urinary incontinence.

A. The tendinous arch of the levator ani is a thickened portion of the fascia of the obturator internus and provides part of the origin of the levator ani, but it plays no direct role in incontinence.

B. The coccygeus muscle supports and raises the pelvic floor but is not directly associated with urinary incontinence.

D. The obturator internus is involved with lateral rotation of the thigh.

Bulbospongiosus muscle
Ischiocavernous muscle
Superficial transverse perineal muscle
Levator ani muscle
External anal sphincter
Perineal body

• *GAS* Fig. 5.17

E. If the rectovaginal septum is torn, the patient can be subject to the occurrence of rectocele or enterocele, as the lower portion of the gastrointestinal tract prolapses into the posterior wall of the vagina (*GAS* Fig. 5.34). *GAS 447–450; N 360; ABR/McM 288*

27. **A.** Lymph from the cutaneous portion of the anal canal (below the pectinate line) drains into the superficial inguinal nodes.
    B, C, D, E. Lymph from most parts of the rectum and from the mucosal zone of the anal canal (above the pectinate line) drains into the internal iliac nodes. Lymph from some parts of the rectum also drains into the sacral nodes. *GAS 495; N 388; ABR/McM 376*

28. **C.** The retropubic space (of Retzius) is the extraperitoneal space between the pubic symphysis and the urinary bladder.
    A. The ischioanal fossa surrounds the anal sphincters. It is not located immediately posterior to the pubic symphysis.
    B. The perineal body represents a central tendinous structure through which muscles of the pelvis and perineum merge. It is located in the superficial perineal space.
    D. The superficial perineal space is bounded superiorly by the perineal membrane and inferiorly by the superficial perineal fascia. It is therefore located inferior to the urinary bladder.
    E. The deep perineal space is bounded inferiorly by the perineal membrane and superior fascia of the external urethral sphincter muscle. It is therefore located inferiorly to the urinary bladder. *GAS 456, 459; N 378; ABR/McM 279*

29. **C.** Hematocolpos is characterized by filling of the vagina with menstrual blood. This commonly occurs due to the presence of an imperforate hymen.
    A. Bartholin or greater vestibular gland ducts open into the vestibule of the vagina; therefore, a cyst in Bartholin gland would not cause hematocolpos.
    B. Blood from a ruptured ectopic pregnancy most often drains into the rectouterine pouch (of Douglas).
    D. Women often have a diminutive cremaster muscle and cremasteric artery and vein, but none of these are associated with hematocolpos. The cremasteric artery provides a small branch to the round ligament of the uterus (sometimes called "Samson's artery"), which must be kept in mind during a hysterectomy, with division of the round ligament.
    E. Bleeding from the uterine veins would not flow into the vagina. *GAS 474; N 358; ABR/McM 285*

30. **C.** An enterocele (herniation of small intestine into the posterior wall of the vagina) is caused by a tear of the rectovaginal septum that weakens the pelvic floor.
    A. A cystocele is characterized by the prolapse of the urinary bladder through the anterior vaginal wall.
    B. An urethrocele is characterized by prolapse of the urethra into the vagina. It is usually associated with a cystocele (prolapse of the urinary bladder into the urethra). Cystocele or urethrocele are associated with defects in the pubocervical fascia that covers the anterior wall of the vagina and assists in supporting the urinary bladder.

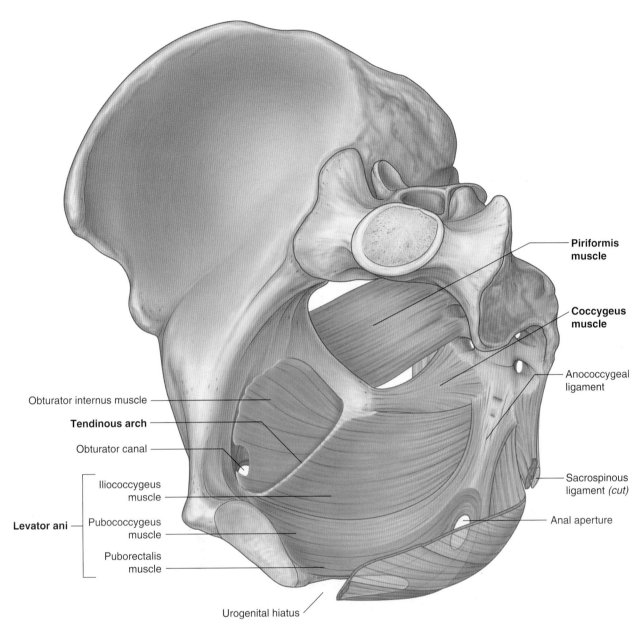

Piriformis
muscle

Coccygeus
muscle

Anococcygeal
ligament

Sacrospinous
ligament *(cut)*

Anal aperture

Obturator internus muscle

Tendinous arch

Obturator canal

Iliococcygeus
muscle

Levator ani

Pubococcygeus
muscle

Puborectalis
muscle

Urogenital hiatus

• *GAS* **Fig. 5.34**

D. Urinary incontinence can result from weakening of the muscles that surround the urethra but would not be caused by a tear of the rectovaginal septum.

E. Prolapse of the uterus is caused by weakening or tearing of the ligaments that support the uterus (especially the cardinal and/or uterosacral ligaments).

GAS 474; N 347; ABR/McM 285

31. A. Of the answer choices listed, the pubococcygeus is the only muscle that is directly associated with the arcus tendineus pelvic fascia and connective tissues of the vagina and the support of the urinary bladder.

B, C, D. The obturator internus, piriformis, and coccygeus do not form parts of the levator ani and provide no direct support to the urogenital organs, nor do they have any role in urinary incontinence.

E. The iliococcygeus does form part of the levator ani, but it is located lateral to the pubococcygeus and therefore does not play a direct role in maintaining urinary continence.

GAS 447–448; N 340; ABR/McM 277

32. A. The ovarian vessels and nerves lie within the infundibulopelvic ligament (suspensory ligament of the ovary); therefore, cutting this ligament interrupts pain fibers from the ovary.

B. Cutting the sympathetic trunk might help to reduce some of the pain from the ovary, but the results of such a procedure are rather unpredictable, plus locating the lumbar sympathetic trunk is more of a surgical challenge.

C. The clunial nerves are cutaneous nerves that innervate parts of the buttocks. They are not associated with the ovaries.

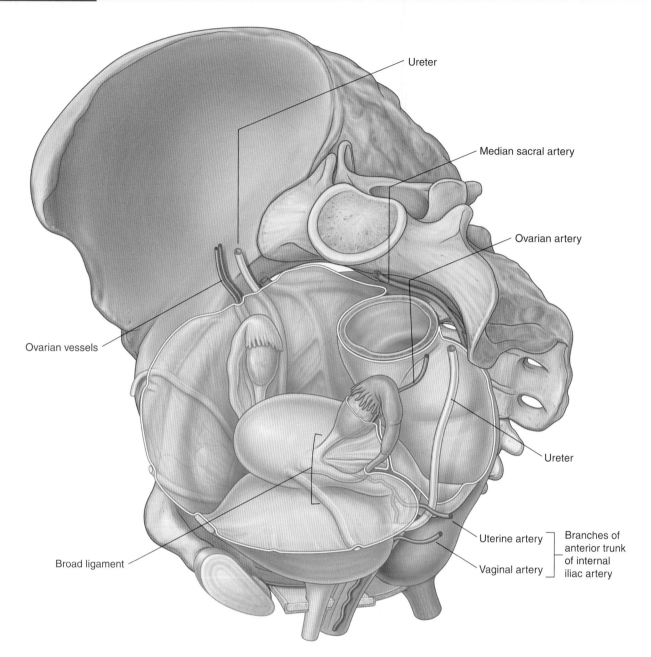

Ureter

Median sacral artery

Ovarian artery

Ovarian vessels

Ureter

Broad ligament

Uterine artery

Vaginal artery

Branches of anterior trunk of internal iliac artery

• *GAS* **Fig. 5.66**

D. The pudendal nerve innervates the perineum and does not carry afferent pain fibers from the ovary.

E. The broad ligament contains only the uterovaginal vessels and nerve plexus and does not carry any nerve fibers from the ovary (*GAS* Fig. 5.66). *GAS 492; N 346; ABR/McM 287*

33. C. The superficial perineal space or cleft lies between the external perineal fascia of Gallaudet (fascia of inferior perineal muscles in the superficial perineal compartment) and the membranous layer of Colles fascia.

A. Camper fascia is the superficial fatty layer of the anterior abdominal wall and the perineum; Scarpa fascia is the deep membranous layer of the abdominal wall.

B. The perineal membrane is the inferior fascia of the external urethral sphincter that forms the inferior boundary of the deep perineal compartment.

D. The superior fascia of the external urethral sphincter muscle bounds the inferior border of the anterior recess of the ischioanal fossa.

E. There is no space between the external urethral sphincter muscle and the apex of the prostate (*GAS* Fig. 5.70). *GAS 500–507; N 378; ABR/McM 279*

34. B. The urinary bladder wall includes the detrusor muscle, and it receives both its motor and sensory innervation from parasympathetic nerve fibers transmitted by way of the pelvic splanchnic nerves from S2 to S4.

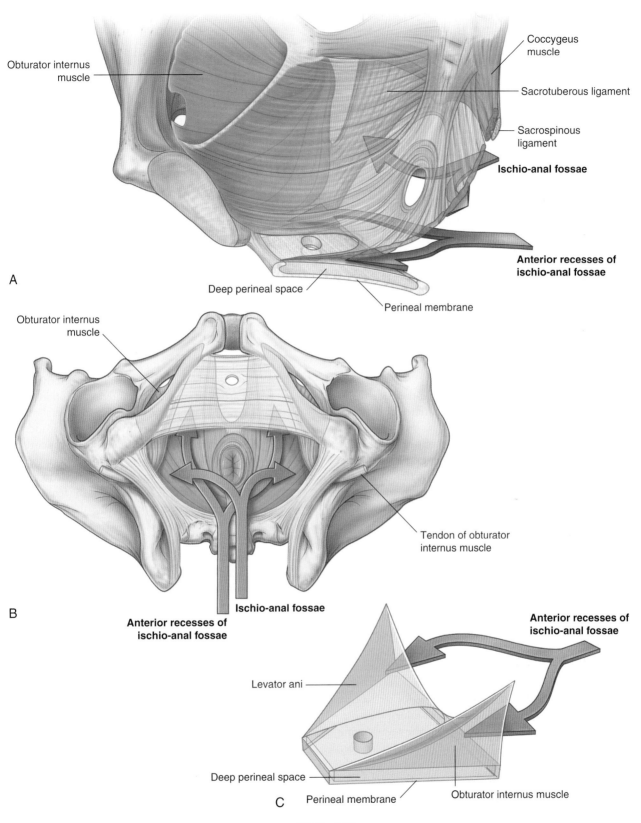

Obturator internus muscle

Coccygeus muscle

Sacrotuberous ligament

Sacrospinous ligament

Ischio-anal fossae

Anterior recesses of ischio-anal fossae

A

Deep perineal space

Perineal membrane

Obturator internus muscle

Tendon of obturator internus muscle

B

Ischio-anal fossae

Anterior recesses of ischio-anal fossae

Anterior recesses of ischio-anal fossae

Levator ani

Deep perineal space

Perineal membrane

Obturator internus muscle

C

• *GAS* Fig. 5.70

A. The superior hypogastric plexus provides sympathetic innervation to the urinary bladder. This results in constriction of the internal urethral sphincter and relaxation of the detrusor muscle.

C. The sacral splanchnics arise from the sacral aspect of the sympathetic trunk and join the inferior hypogastric plexus to provide sympathetic innervation to the pelvic organs.

D. The lumbar splanchnics arise from the lumbar sympathetic trunk and provide innervation to the pelvic organs via the superior hypogastric plexus.

E. The pudendal nerve arises from sacral segments S2–24. It is the main nerve of the pelvis and perineum providing both somatic motor and sensory innervation, in addition to sympathetic innervation to the skin.

GAS 486–488; N 399; ABR/McM 281

35. A. The rectouterine pouch (of Douglas) is the lowest point of the woman's peritoneal cavity. Therefore, a fluid collection within the peritoneal cavity accumulates here when the patient is standing or sitting. It is accessible transvaginally through the posterior part of the vaginal fornix, with the patient positioned upright.

B. The pararectal fossa is formed on either side of the rectum. The needle will not penetrate this space to collect pelvic fluid space.

C. The paravesical space is the extraperitoneal space around the urinary bladder. The needle should not penetrate this space to collect pelvic fluid samples.

D. The uterovesical pouch lies between the uterus and the urinary bladder. Entrance into this space is via the anterior fornix of the vagina.

E. The superficial perineal pouch is an anatomic space located below the perineal membrane in the urogenital triangle of the perineum. During the colpocentesis procedure the needle will not penetrate this space.

GAS 477; N 345; ABR/McM 285 (GAS Fig. 5.59)

36. E. Because the spongy urethra and deep penile (Buck) fascia are both located in the superficial perineal space, rupture will occur here, with extravasation of fluids into the superficial perineal cleft.

A. The ischioanal fossa is located posterior to the urogenital triangle, behind the area of injury.

B. The rectovesical pouch represents the lowest point of the peritoneal cavity in men. It is located between the urinary bladder and the lower one-third of the rectum.

C. The deep perineal space is a space between the perineal membrane and the superior fascia of the external urethral sphincter muscle. It is deep to the superficial perineal space where the erectile bodies and spongy urethra is found.

D. The retropublic space, also known as the cave of Retzius, is located posterior to the pubic symphysis and anterior to the urinary bladder.

GAS 459–461, 507; N 378; ABR/McM 279

37. C. The perineal branch of the pudendal nerve is responsible for the innervation of the external urethral sphincter, and injury to this nerve can result in paralysis of the sphincter and urinary incontinence.

A. Pelvic splanchnics supply parasympathetic innervation to the pelvis.

B. Sacral splanchnic nerves are autonomic nerves that do not supply skeletal muscle. Instead, they join the inferior hypogastric nerves to supply the pelvis with sympathetic innervation.

D. The superior gluteal nerve provides motor innervation to the gluteus minimus, gluteus medius, and tensor fasciae latae.

E. The inferior gluteal nerve innervates the gluteus maximus.

GAS 483, 485; N 393; ABR/McM 279

38. D. The internal pudendal artery gives rise to both the dorsal artery and deep artery of the penis. The deep artery is the main supply for erectile tissue; therefore, significant atherosclerosis of the internal pudendal artery may result in impotence (erectile dysfunction).

A. The external iliac artery gives rise to the femoral artery which is responsible for supplying the lower limb.

B. The inferior epigastric artery arises from the external iliac artery. It supplies the anterior abdominal wall.

C. The umbilical artery gives rise to several superior vesical arteries that supply the urinary bladder and then becomes the medial umbilical ligament.

E. The deep circumflex artery originates from the external iliac artery and the superficial circumflex iliac artery arises from the beginning of the femoral artery. Both provide blood supply to the abdominal wall.

GAS 490–491; N 387; ABR/McM 280

39. A. Cancer present in the superficial inguinal nodes can be indicative of cancer of the uterus at the level of the round ligaments, by which the cancerous cells drain to the inguinal region. Uterine cancer must be especially suspected if the tissues of the lower limb, vulva, and anal canal appear normal.

B. Lymph from the lower two-thirds of the rectum flows to the internal iliac lymph nodes.

C. Lymph from the ovaries flows to the para-aortic nodes at the level of the kidneys.

D. Lymph from the proximal one thirds of the rectum drain to the inferior mesenteric group of lymph nodes.

E. The pectinate line marks the end of the mucosal lining of the anal canal, below which the canal is lined with nonkeratinized, stratified squamous epithelium. The pectinate line is also associated with the distal ends of the anal columns and anal valves. Lymphatic vessels inferior to the pectinate line of the anal canal will drain into the superficial inguinal nodes, but those above the pectinate line flow to internal iliac nodes.

GAS 495; N 388; ABR/McM 287

40. C. The lymphatic vessels of the ovaries join with lymphatics from the uterine tubes and the fundus of the uterus. These ascend to the right and left lumbar (caval/

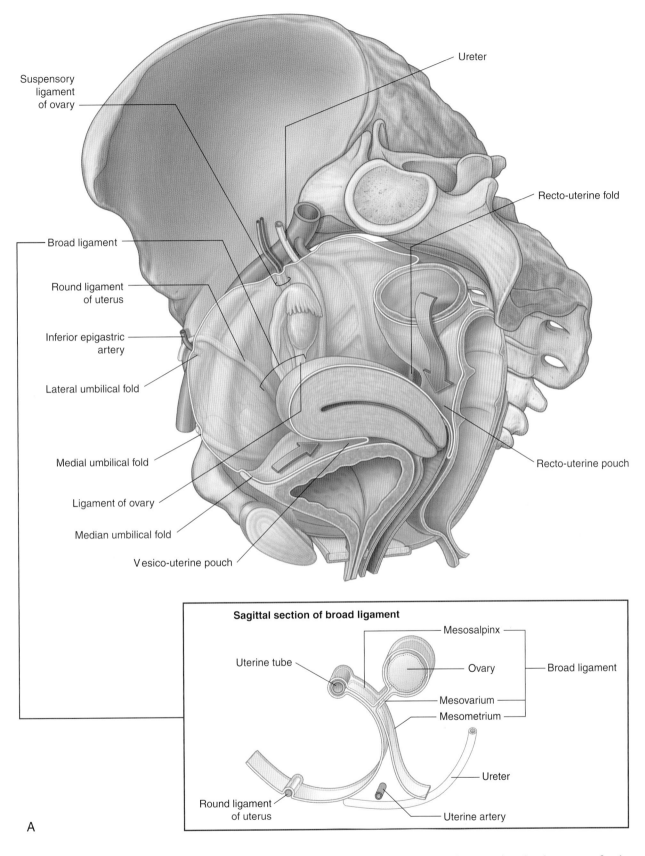

Suspensory ligament of ovary

Ureter

Broad ligament

Round ligament of uterus

Inferior epigastric artery

Lateral umbilical fold

Medial umbilical fold

Ligament of ovary

Median umbilical fold

Vesico-uterine pouch

Recto-uterine fold

Recto-uterine pouch

Sagittal section of broad ligament

Uterine tube

Mesosalpinx

Ovary

Broad ligament

Mesovarium

Mesometrium

Ureter

Uterine artery

Round ligament of uterus

A

aortic) lymph nodes. These lymph nodes are the first to receive cancerous cells from the ovaries. Superficial inguinal nodes drain the lower limb, the anterior abdominal wall inferior to the umbilicus, and superficial perineal structures.

A. The superficial inguinal nodes drain superficial perineal structures, including the superolateral uterine body near attachment of the round ligament, skin of the perineum (including the vulva), and the orifice of the vagina inferior to the hymen.

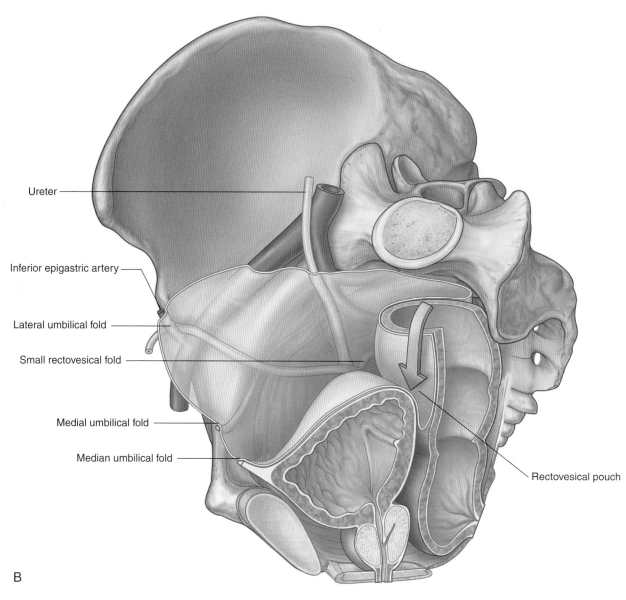

Ureter

Inferior epigastric artery

Lateral umbilical fold

Small rectovesical fold

Medial umbilical fold

Median umbilical fold

Rectovesical pouch

B

• *GAS* **Fig. 5.59**

B, D. The external iliac nodes drain the deep inguinal nodes that drain the clitoris and superficial inguinal nodes.

E. The internal iliac nodes drain inferior pelvic structures and deep perineal structures.
GAS 493–495, 509; N 388; ABR/McM 368, 374–375

41. B. The internal iliac nodes drain the middle and upper vagina, cervix, and body of the uterus.

C. The lumbar/lateral aortic lymph nodes drain the ovaries.

D. The presacral node which is found in the mesorectum receives drainage from the rectum, anal canal, and the prostate in men.

E. The axillary lymph nodes drain the upper limb and chest wall, including the breasts.
GAS 494- 495, 509; N 389; ABR/McM 376

42. A. The ischial spine is the correct bony landmark used to administer a pudendal nerve block. The pudendal nerve crosses the sacrospinous ligament, which attaches to the ischial spine. Accessing the ischial spine and thus the pudendal nerve is done most easily using a transvaginal approach.

B, D. The posterior superior and inferior iliac spines are located on the posterior aspect of the pelvis and articulate with the lateral aspect of the sacrum. They do not relate to the course of the pudendal nerve.

C. The ischial tuberosities are the most inferior aspect of the bony pelvis. The skin and soft tissues around the ischial tuberosities receive sensory supply from the pudendal nerve and perineal branches of the posterior femoral cutaneous nerve. Injections into the area around the tuberosities are less certain, however, than

injections at the sacrospinous ligament and often fail to anesthetize the anal triangle well.
 E. The coccyx is a poor target for locating and anesthetizing the pudendal nerve.
 GAS 433–437; N 395; ABR/McM 96

43. D. Hemorrhoids are divided into two categories: internal and external. Pain due to external hemorrhoids is mediated by the pudendal nerve (somatosensory), which serves the majority of the perineum.
 A. The sacral splanchnic nerves transmit postganglionic sympathetic fibers from the sacral sympathetic trunk to the abdominal vessels and the organs they supply.
 B. Superior hypogastric nerves are mixed nerves located anterior to the sacral promontory and do not mediate pain information from the perineum
 C. The pelvic splanchnic nerves carry preganglionic parasympathetic fibers to the pelvic organs. Additionally, pain from the pelvic organs below the pelvic pain line travel retrogradely with the pelvic splanchnic nerves.
 E. The ilioinguinal nerve provides sensory innervation to the skin at the base of the penis/clitoris; the scrotum/labium majus; and upper inner thigh.
 GAS 498; N 398; ABR/McM 279

44. C. The urethra is shorter in women than in men. Because of its close proximity to the vestibule in women, it commonly leads to infections of the urinary tract. The vagina contains more bacterial flora than the penis.
 B. The prostate produces a clear, alkaline fluid, but it has not been proven that it protects against bacterial infections.
 C. The uterus has no known antibacterial functions.
 D. The paraurethral glands are responsible for the secretion of mucus during sexual activity. This mucus has no impact on UTI.
 E. The seminal glands produce a fructose-containing fluid that provides nutrients to the sperm for the journey through the female genital tract.
 GAS 459–461, 507; N 352; ABR/McM 285

45. A. The uterus is stabilized and anchored to the urinary bladder by the pubovesical and vesicocervical fasciae on its anterior surface. During pregnancy and childbirth this connective tissue can be torn, allowing the urinary bladder to herniate into the anterior vaginal wall, with prolapse possible through the vaginal orifice.
 B. The transverse cervical (cardinal) ligament is located within the base of the broad ligament and is a major ligament of the uterus but would offer no support if the urinary bladder herniates through the vagina.
 C. The uterosacral ligament serves to anchor the uterus to the sacrum for support.
 D. Injury to the levator ani would not cause the urinary bladder to herniate through the vagina.
 E. The median umbilical ligament or urachus and is located on the posterior aspect of the linea alba; the ligament is an embryologic remnant of the allantois.
 GAS 457, 471; N 347; ABR/McM 288

46. A. During a hysterectomy, ligation of or injury to the ureter can happen relatively easily because it is the most susceptible structure due to its location. The ureter is located immediately inferior to the uterine vessels ("water passes under the bridge") in the pelvic cavity approximately 1 cm lateral to the supravaginal cervix.
 B. and C. The internal iliac artery bifurcates near the pelvic brim but is not in close proximity to the uterine vessels in the vicinity of the cervix.
 D. The obturator nerve travels along the pelvic sidewall and is not close to the site of ligation of the uterine vessels. E. The lumbosacral trunk is located on the lateral side of the sacrum and the pelvic sidewall, not in close proximity to the uterine vessels.
 GAS 472, N 382; ABR/McM 288

47. A. Vaginismus is a painful, psychosomatic gynecologic disorder; it is described as involving distension of the cavernous tissues and the bulbospongiosus and transverse perineal muscles, the stimulation of which triggers the involuntary spasms of the perivaginal and levator ani muscles. This can in turn lead to dyspareunia.
 B, C, D, E. These conditions would not cause involuntary contractions of the vaginal musculature during manual examination of the vagina.
 GAS 474; N 353; ABR/McM 289

48. E. This is a classic example of extravasation of blood and urine from the superficial perineal space. This usually is a result of rupture of the spongy urethra. The extravasation of the fluid (urine) will begin to invade the layer between the deep penile (Buck) fascia and the dartos layer. This extravasation example is evident due to the fluid invading up to the abdomen between the subcutaneous tissues and muscle fascia.
 A, B, C, D. If the fluid collects between the other layers of the perineum, the clinical evidence will present differently in the perineum and abdominal area.
 GAS 459–461, 496–498; N 378; ABR/McM 279

49. A. The uterosacral ligaments and the transverse cervical (cardinal) ligaments are the two main ligaments stabilizing the uterus. They help to inhibit the uterus from prolapsing into the vagina.
 B. round ligament of the uterus is related to the descent of the ovaries in embryologic development and continues into the inguinal canal. This ligament is the remnant of the gubernaculum ovary.
 C. The broad ligament is the peritoneal covering over the ovaries, uterine tubes, uterus, and vessels.
 D. The arcus tendineus fasciae pelvis joins the muscle fascia of the levator ani to the pubocervical fascia on the vagina and is not directly associated with the uterus or its ligaments.
 E. The levator ani muscles contribute to the floor of the pelvis and support all of the pelvic viscera indirectly; it does not, however, prevent prolapse of the uterus into the vagina (*GAS* Fig. 5.58).
 GAS 475; N 355; ABR/McM 288

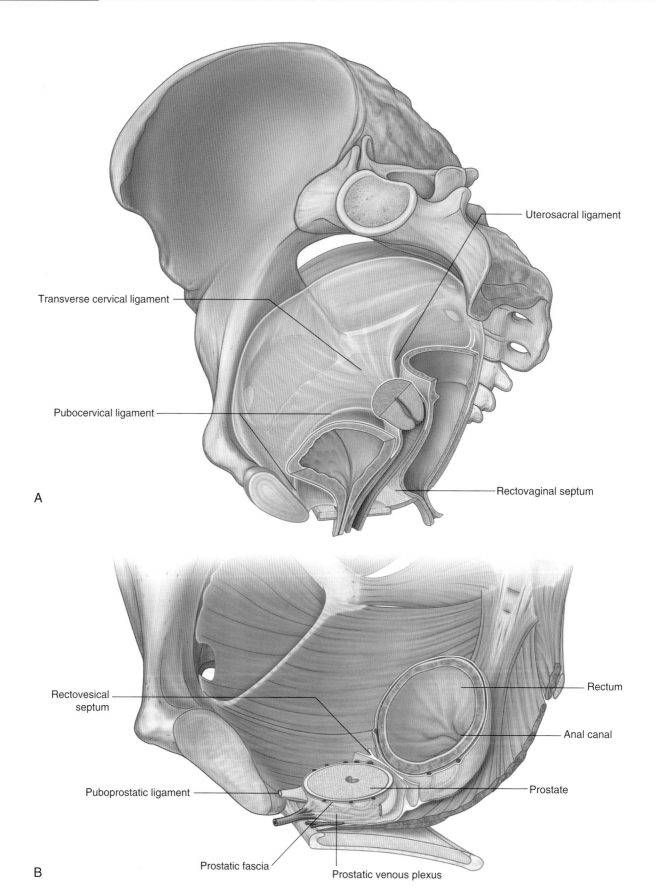

A

Uterosacral ligament

Transverse cervical ligament

Pubocervical ligament

Rectovaginal septum

B

Rectovesical septum

Puboprostatic ligament

Prostatic fascia

Prostatic venous plexus

Rectum

Anal canal

Prostate

• *GAS* **Fig. 5.58**

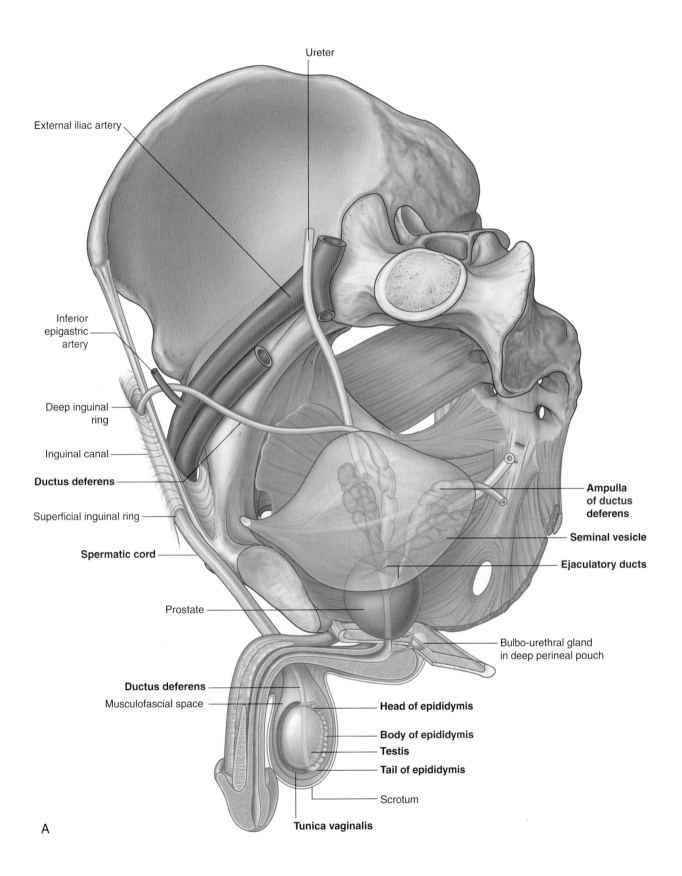

Ureter

External iliac artery

Inferior epigastric artery

Deep inguinal ring

Inguinal canal

Ductus deferens

Superficial inguinal ring

Spermatic cord

Prostate

Ductus deferens

Musculofascial space

Ampulla of ductus deferens

Seminal vesicle

Ejaculatory ducts

Bulbo-urethral gland in deep perineal pouch

Head of epididymis

Body of epididymis

Testis

Tail of epididymis

Scrotum

Tunica vaginalis

A

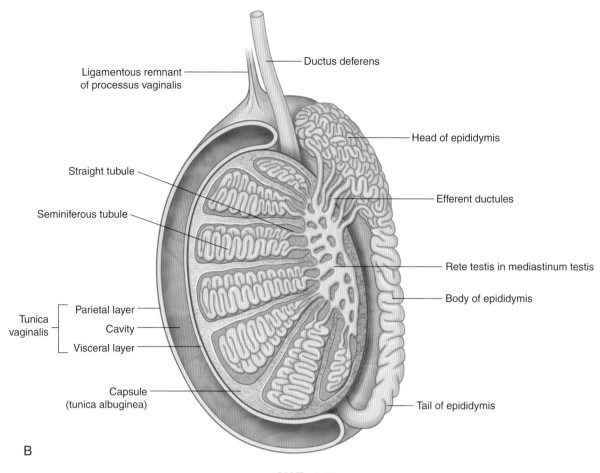

Ligamentous remnant of processus vaginalis

Ductus deferens

Head of epididymis

Straight tubule

Efferent ductules

Seminiferous tubule

Rete testis in mediastinum testis

Body of epididymis

Tunica vaginalis
— Parietal layer
— Cavity
— Visceral layer

Capsule (tunica albuginea)

Tail of epididymis

B

• **GAS Fig. 5.47**

Answers 50–74

50. A. The internal iliac lymph nodes and sacral nodes would be involved in a pelvic lymphadenectomy, which often would be desired in surgical resection for prostate cancer. Sacral lymphatics can communicate with lymphatics within the vertebral canal and thus metastasize cranially.
B. The external iliac nodes drain all of the anterosuperior pelvic structures, the lower limb and perineum, and the body wall to the level of the umbilicus.
C. The superficial inguinal nodes drain all of the superficial structures below the umbilicus.
D. The deep inguinal nodes drain the glans penis in the men.
E. The gluteal nodes are subdivided into the superior and inferior gluteal nodes, which are found along its respective vessels.
GAS 495, 514; N 390; ABR/McM 281

51. E. The para-aortic or lumbar nodes at the level of the kidneys will most likely be infiltrated by metastasis of testicular cancer because testicular lymphatics run in close association with the testicular vessels and drain the testes and epididymis. Testicular cancer is a disease that is especially dangerous for young men, as intraabdominal lymph node swelling is often a late clinical presentation.
A. The internal iliac nodes drain the inferior pelvis and deep perineal structures.

B. The external iliac nodes drain all anterosuperior pelvic structures.
C. The superficial inguinal nodes drain all of the superficial structures below the umbilicus.
D. The deep inguinal nodes receive more superficial vessels and drain the glans penis in men.
GAS 495, 514; N 390; ABR/McM 368

52. C. Penile erection is a parasympathetically mediated response that is delivered via the pelvic splanchnic nerves that pass through nerve bundles on the posterolateral aspect of the prostate. (In prostatectomy, these bundles should be left intact, if at all possible, to avoid erectile dysfunction, also known as impotence.)
A, B, E. The pudendal nerve and its terminal branch, the dorsal nerve of penis, carry the primary skeletal motor and sensory innervation to the external genitalia, and also sympathetic fibers.
D. Sacral splanchnic nerves contain sympathetic fibers.
GAS 486–488, 510; N 398; ABR/McM 282

53. A. Rupture of the spongy urethra leads to accumulation of fluid (edema) in the superficial perineal cleft. The continuity of Colles fascia (superficial membranous layer of the superficial perineal fascia) with Scarpa fascia of the abdominal wall (the membranous layer of superficial fascia) allows for fluid spread upward upon the body wall.
B, C, D. Rupture of the preprostatic urethra, prostatic urethra, or urinary bladder would lead to internal fluid

accumulation within the pelvis because they are not located in the perineum.

    E. Damage to the ureter would manifest within the abdomen or pelvis, depending upon the level of rupture (*GAS* Fig. 5.47).
GAS 459–461, 507; N 373; ABR/McM 279

54. B. The cremasteric reflex afferents are carried by the ilioinguinal nerve; the motor (efferent) output is by the genitofemoral nerve. The sensory fibers of the genitofemoral nerve are to skin over the femoral triangle and scrotum.

    A. The ilioinguinal nerve is sensory to parts of the suprapubic region, anterior perineum, and inner thigh.

    C. The iliohypogastric nerve provides sensation for the abdominal wall and suprapubic area.

    D, E. The pudendal and obturator nerves do not travel through the inguinal canal and would not be damaged by the hernia. In addition, they play no role in the cremasteric reflex.
GAS 486–488, 510; N 391; ABR/McM 275

55. C. Pain from the cervix is transmitted via the pelvic splanchnic nerves because the cervix is below the inferior limit of the peritoneum, which is also known as the pelvic pain line.

    B. Pain above the pelvic pain line is carried via nerves that are primarily sympathetic in function. The superior hypogastric nerves carry pain fibers from the upper portions of the uterus. Sacral splanchnic nerves are principally sympathetic in function.

    A. The pudendal nerve contains skeletal motor, sensory, and sympathetic fibers and provides primary sensory innervation to external genitalia, including the distal third of the vagina.

    D. Sacral splanchnic nerves are principally sympathetic in function.

    E. The lesser splanchnic nerves carry afferent fibers.
GAS 486–488, 510; N 397; ABR/McM 282

56. A. Pain from this area is mediated via parasympathetic responses and would thus travel to the S2–S4 levels through the pelvic splanchnic nerves. The S2, S3, and S4 spinal cord levels also provide sensory innervation of the perineum and posterior thigh.

    B, D. The suprapubic and inguinal regions are supplied by ilioinguinal and iliohypogastric nerves (L1).

    C. The umbilical region receives sensory innervation from the T10 level. In the epigastric region the sensory innervation is provided by T7–T10.

    E. In the epigastric region the sensory innervation is provided by T7–T10.
GAS 486–488, 510; N 397; ABR/McM 285

57. B. The left testicular vein drains directly into the left renal vein, which then crosses over the midline to enter the inferior vena cava (choice A).

    C, D, E. The left inferior epigastric, left internal pudendal, and left iliac veins are not involved in the drainage of the testes.
GAS 266, 493, N 383; ABR/McM 271

58. A. During repair, the round ligament of the uterus may be seen within the inguinal canal, although it is often a small, fibrous strand that is easily overlooked. The remaining choices are not found in this region.

    B. The urachus is a fibrous remnant embryologic of the allantois which drain's the fetus's urinary bladder.

    C. The ovarian ligament connects the ovary to the uterus, whereas the suspensory (infundibulopelvic) ligament contains the ovarian vessels, nerves, and lymphatic.

    D. The uterine tubes are lateral projections of the uterus toward the ovaries.

    E. The mesosalpinx is a portion of the peritoneum of the broad ligament that attaches to the uterine tubes.
GAS 470–473; N 353, 354; ABR/McM 285

59. C. The most common site of ectopic pregnancy is the uterine (Fallopian) tube.

    A. Implantation at the internal cervical os would be within the uterus and lead to placenta previa.

    B, D, E. The other choices are less common sites of ectopic pregnancies.
GAS 471; N 355; ABR/McM 287

60. B. Seminal glands produce the alkaline portion of the ejaculate. This includes fructose and choline.

    A. The prostate secretes prostaglandins, citric acid, and acid phosphatase.

    C. The kidneys are the sites of urine production.

    D. The testes produce spermatozoa and sex hormones.

    E. The bulbourethral glands (Cowper glands) produce mucous secretions that enter the penile bulb.
GAS 467; N 366; ABR/McM 281

61. C. In cryptorchidism, the testis has failed to descend into its proper location in the scrotum and may be found within the abdomen or in the inguinal canal.

    A, B, D, E. These conditions do not correlate with the presenting signs or symptoms.
GAS 463; N 368; ABR/McM 279

62. D. By definition, the site of implantation in placenta previa overlaps the internal cervical os.

    A. Ectopic pregnancy in the uterine (fallopian) tubes results in tubal pregnancy.

    B. The cervix is not a notable site of ectopic implantation.

    C. Implantation within the mesenteries of the abdomen will result in an abdominal pregnancy.

    E. The fundus of the uterus is the normal site of implantation.
GAS 471–473; N 355; ABR/McM 285

63. D. Internal hemorrhoids are located above the pectinate line. This tissue is derived from the hindgut and innervated by visceral nerves. Pain is not a common symptom of internal hemorrhoids.

    A, B, C, E. these nerves do not carry pain fibers above the pectinate line.
GAS 498; N 381; ABR/McM 281

64. C. The pelvic splanchnic nerves (nervi erigentes) contain parasympathetic efferent fibers that mediate erection. These same nerves innervate the derivatives of the hindgut, the portions of the large intestine that were removed in this patient.

A, B, D, E. Lesions in these structures would not cause this patient's symptoms.
GAS 486–488, 515; N 398; ABR/McM 282

65. A. The internal iliac nodes are the first in a trunk of lymph nodes that receive lymph from the uterine cervix. Cancerous cells from the cervix are likely to involve the internal iliac nodes first. If these nodes do not have cancerous cells, this indicates that the tumor has not spread, at least through lymphatic channels. Presacral nodes are also sometimes involved and can be felt during a digital rectal examination.

B, C, D, E. The internal iliac lymph nodes are the first to receive lymph from the uterine cervix, the other structures are not.
GAS 495, 514; N 388; ABR/McM 373

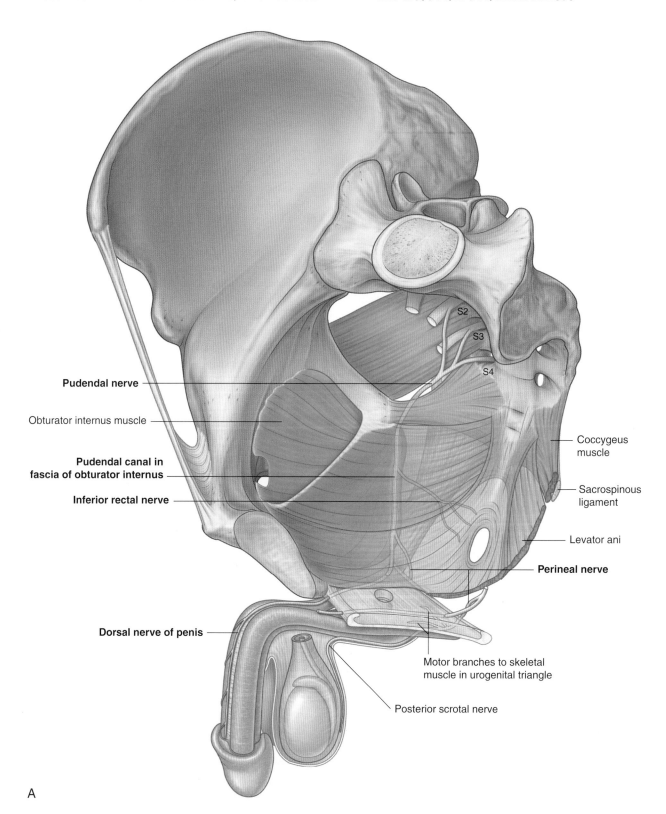

Pudendal nerve

Obturator internus muscle

Pudendal canal in
fascia of obturator internus

Inferior rectal nerve

Dorsal nerve of penis

S2

S3

S4

Coccygeus
muscle

Sacrospinous
ligament

Levator ani

Perineal nerve

Motor branches to skeletal
muscle in urogenital triangle

Posterior scrotal nerve

A

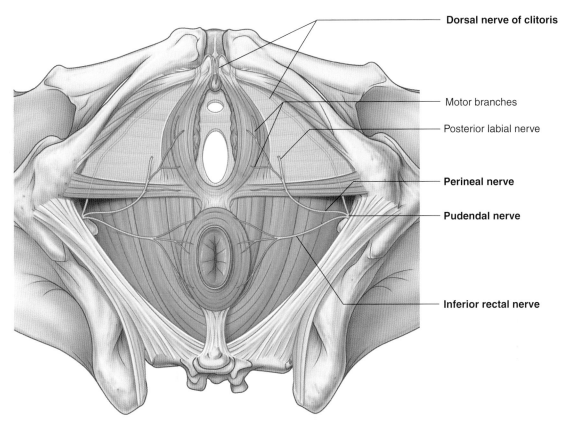

Dorsal nerve of clitoris

Motor branches

Posterior labial nerve

Perineal nerve

Pudendal nerve

Inferior rectal nerve

B

• *GAS* Fig. 5.76

66. D. As seen in the photograph, the swollen scrotum contains mostly a clear fluid. Since hydrocele is the accumulation of fluid between the visceral and parietal layers of the tunica vaginalis testis, this condition best accounts for the findings in this patient.

  A. Varicocele is caused when there is an increased venous pressure in the venous plexus causing dilatation of these veins.

  B. Rectocele is when the anterior wall of the rectum projects towards the vagina.

  C. Cystocele, known as a prolapsed urinary bladder, is when the urinary bladder protrudes into the vagina.

  E. Hypospadias is a congenital condition where the urethral opening is on the ventral surface of the penis.

  GAS 463–468; N 369; ABR/McM 279

67. C. The perineal nerve would need to be anesthetized because it supplies the area described.

  A. The dorsal nerve of the clitoris pierces the perineal membrane and innervates the clitoris and not the anterior recess of the ischioanal fossa.

  B. The superficial branch of the perineal nerve supplies only the posterior skin of the labium majus.

  D. The inferior anal (rectal) nerve innervates the skin around the anus and the external anal sphincter muscle.

  E. The pudendal nerve is the main nerve of the perineum and gives rise to all of the aforementioned nerves; therefore, anesthetizing it would result in

widespread effects that would be superfluous to what is actually needed for drainage of the abscess. *GAS 480–488; 510; N 395; ABR/McM 292*

68. D. The inferior rectal nerve supplies the external anal sphincter muscle and the skin around the anus. Therefore, this would be the best nerve to anesthetize for abscess drainage in this area.

  A. The dorsal nerve of the clitoris does not innervate the posterior recess of the perineum.

  B. The superficial branch of the perineal nerve supplies the posterior skin of the labium majus and would not need to be anesthetized in the event of a horseshoe anal abscess.

  C. The perineal nerve supplies all the perineal muscles and the labia majora, but for the area in question it does not have as direct a supply as the inferior rectal nerve.

  E. The pudendal nerve gives off all the branches above and thus anesthetizing it would result in additional unwanted side effects (*GAS* Fig. 5.76).

  GAS 510; N 395; ABR/McM 292

69. B. An aberrant obturator artery arising from the inferior epigastric artery can be found in 20% to 30% of the population. Patients with this variation are more susceptible to inadvertent damage during certain surgeries if the surgeon is not aware of presence of the aberrant artery. This artery is alternatively called the "corona mortis," which translates as "crown of death," relating to the result of cutting this artery without realizing the seriousness of the error.

A, C, D, E. The other arteries listed would be less likely to be injured because the surgeon would assume they are present and will thus take great care in making sure not to staple them.
GAS 489–490; N 382; ABR/McM 285

70. E. The afferents of the testis and most of the ductus accompany sympathetics to enter the trunk at T10–L2, with cell bodies in the dorsal root ganglia of those spinal nerves. (Which is why a forceful kick to the testes seems to hurt so severely in the periumbilical region of the abdomen.) The more proximal portion of the ductus has sensory fibers in the pelvic splanchnics.
  A. This answer choice refers to the sympathetic nerves which do not carry sensory information.
  B. The ilioinguinal nerve is somatic and innervates the upper and medial thigh as well as the anterior scrotum and skin at the root of the penis, not the ductus deferens.
  C. The iliohypogastric nerve is an anterior abdominal wall nerve that innervates transverse and oblique abdominal muscles, supplies skin above the pubis, and has cutaneous supply to the lateral buttocks.
  D. The genital branch of the genitofemoral nerve supplies the cremaster muscle and skin of the anterior scrotum.
  GAS 480, 510; N 398; ABR/McM 279

71. A. The ovarian arteries arise from the abdominal aorta, descend retroperitoneally along the posterior abdominal wall, and cross just anterior to the external iliac vessels. The ovarian arteries are the most likely source of blood from a hematoma following a tubal ligation.
  B, C, D, E. The uterine and inferior vesical arteries branch from the internal iliac arteries and superior vesical arteries branch from umbilical artery, also from the internal iliac. These arteries are not likely to be the source of blood in this situation.
  GAS 489–492; N 382; ABR/McM 285

72. C. When an ovariectomy (also called oophorectomy) is performed, the ovarian vessels must be ligated. The ovarian vessels lie anterior to the ureter just proximal to the bifurcation of the aorta. The ureter is the structure that is at the most risk when ligating the ovarian vessels. The vaginal artery is a branch of the internal iliac artery and lies well inferior to the ovary.
  A. The uterine artery does anastomose with the ovarian vessels via the ascending uterine artery; however, it lies too far distally to be at risk during ligation of the ovarian vessels.
  B. The vaginal artery is a branch of the uterine artery. D and E. The internal pudendal artery and pudendal nerve mostly lie in the perineum and are not at risk.
  GAS 489–492; N 382; ABR/McM 285

73. C. The conjugate diameter of the pelvis (anteroposterior) is not altered by relaxation of the pelvic joints.

  A. The transverse diameter is the longest distance extending from the middle of one pelvic brim to the other.
  B. The interspinous distance is the distance between the ischial spines and changes dramatically during pregnancy due to relaxation of the joints.
  D and E. The diagonal conjugate and oblique diameters are slightly increased during pregnancy due to the effects of the hormone relaxin.
  GAS 438–445; N 336; ABR/McM 290

74. D. The obturator nerve runs a course along the lateral pelvic wall and innervates the adductors of the thigh and the skin on the medial aspect of the distal thigh. Damage to the obturator nerve is the most likely cause for the sensory and motor deficit experienced by the patient.
  A. The genitofemoral nerve is motor to the cremaster muscle and sensory to the skin over the femoral triangle.
  B. The ilioinguinal nerve innervates the skin over the labium majus and upper, inner thigh.
  C. The iliohypogastric nerve supplies skin over the anterolateral gluteal region and the area above the pubis.
  E. The lumbosacral trunk contains motor and sensory fibers from L4 and L5 and is the lumbar contribution to the lumbosacral plexus.
  GAS 480–488, 510; N 392; ABR/McM 285

Answers 75–98

75. A. The neural cell bodies responsible for erection are located in the sacral parasympathetic nucleus (intermediomedial cell column). The parasympathetic nervous system is responsible for producing an erection.
  B. The sacral sympathetic trunk ganglia would not be responsible for the action of erection but rather the action of ejaculation. (Mnemonic: "Point and Shoot": parasympathetics for erection, sympathetics for ejaculation.).
  C. The inferior mesenteric ganglion would not contain parasympathetic neural cell bodies responsible for erection because they travel to derivatives of the hindgut.
  D. The superior hypogastric plexus contains few if any parasympathetic fibers and is not the primary location for the parasympathetic neural cell bodies.
  E. The intermediolateral nuclei of L1 and L2 contains nerve cell bodies of preganglionic sympathetic neurons and therefore would not contribute to producing an erection.
  GAS 480–488, 510; N 399; ABR/McM 279

76. B. The interspinous distance is the distance between the ischial spines. The interspinous distance is usually the shortest distance, therefore it is the minimum dimension along the birth canal.
  C. The true conjugate diameter is the anteroposterior distance and does not change.
  A, D, E. The transverse diameter, oblique diameter, and diagonal conjugate diameter can change slightly

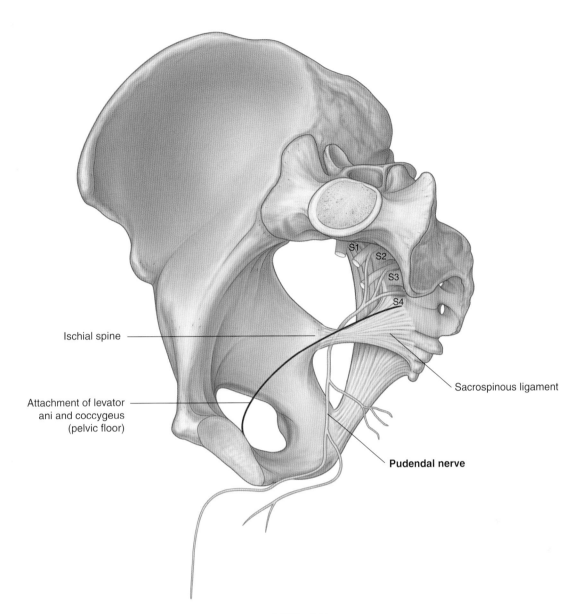

Ischial spine

Attachment of levator
ani and coccygeus
(pelvic floor)

S1
S2
S3
S4

Sacrospinous ligament

Pudendal nerve

• *GAS* Fig. 5.15

during pregnancy, but the interspinous distance changes the most during birth; it is also more easily measured.
GAS 438–445; N 336; ABR/McM 289

77. D. Lymph vessels from the testes follow the path of the testicular blood supply (abdominal aorta), and therefore lymph from the testes drains into the lumbar nodes. The superficial inguinal lymph nodes drain lymph from the lower limb, lower abdominal wall, and superficial perineal structures.

A. The deep inguinal nodes drain lymph from popliteal nodes and deep lymphatics of the lower limb, and receive a small portion of drainage from the superficial inguinal nodes, the glans penis, and spongy urethra.

B. The external iliac nodes drain lymph from anterosuperior pelvic structures and receive lymph from the superficial and deep inguinal nodes.

C. The internal iliac nodes drain lymph from inferior pelvic structures and receive lymph from the sacral nodes.

E. The superficial inguinal lymph nodes drain lymph from the lower limb, lower abdominal wall, and superficial perineal structures.
GAS 495, 514; N 390; ABR/McM 365

78. C. Uterine artery embolization is performed to starve uterine fibroids of their blood supply resulting in a decrease in size of these benign tumors. Following the procedure, the uterus receives collateral blood supply from the ovarian artery (a direct branch of the abdominal aorta).

A, B, D, E. The external iliac, inferior mesenteric, internal pudendal, and superior mesenteric arteries do not provide adequate collateral blood supply to the uterus.
GAS 489; N 386; ABR/McM 283, 288

79. E. The perineal body is a condensed mass of connective tissue to which the muscles of the pelvic floor and the muscles of the perineum attach. In many cases during childbirth, if the fetus' head is arrested, there is a high likelihood of perineal tears. In this situation an episiotomy is performed. This is usually done in an incision 45 degrees away from the midline in order to avoid damaging the perineal body. Damage to this tissue destabilizes the muscles that attach to it and can lead to urinary and fecal incontinence as well as uterine, urinary bladder, and rectal prolapse.
A, B, C, D. The aim of this procedure does not involve maintaining the integrity of these structures.
GAS 451; N 360; ABR/McM 289

80. E. The pudendal nerve is a somatic nerve that innervates the perineum with exception of the anterior part of the labium majus (innervated by the ilioinguinal and genitofemoral nerves). The pudendal nerve forms from S2 to S4 ventral rami. It leaves the pelvis via the greater sciatic foramen and enters into the perineum via the lesser sciatic foramen by coursing around the sacrospinous ligament where it attaches to the ischial spine. This pudendal nerve block will anesthetize the area of distribution of the pudendal nerve. It will not anesthetize the uterus or cervix as these are visceral organs (*GAS* Fig. 5.15).
A, B, C, D. These answer choices do not describe the pudendal nerve block.
GAS 480–488; N 395; ABR/McM 284, 289

81. A. The prostate is a walnut-shaped accessory organ of the reproductive system in men that lies immediately below the urinary bladder and surrounds the exiting urethra. Anatomically, the prostate has four lobes: two lateral lobes, a posterior lobe, and a median lobe that directly surrounds the urethra. A tumor of the posterior lobe does not necessarily obstruct the urethra but it is frequently cancerous.
C and D. Benign prostatic hyperplasia usually affects the median and lateral lobes. Micturition (urination) will be obstructed and patients present with a variety of symptoms including difficulty in initiating the urinary stream, a slow stream of urine, urinary frequency, and urinary urgency.
B, E. These structures are not involved in this condition.
GAS 467; N 366; ABR/McM 279, 281

82. D. The patient has a tear in the spongy (penile) urethra. This commonly occurs when force is applied to the bulb of the penis. If there is an accompanying tear of the erectile bodies and the deep penile (Buck) fascia that surrounds it, urine can spill into the superficial perineal space. This area is bound by the superficial penile (Colles) fascia inferiorly, the perineal body posteriorly, and the perineal membrane superiorly. The attachment of Colles fascia to the perineal body prevents the urine from spreading posteriorly to the anorectal triangle. The attachment of Colles fascia to the ischiopubic ramus prevents urine from entering into the thigh.
A. Urine and blood would not spill into the superficial perineal space if the deep fascia were intact.

B. Membranous urethra injury is associated with pelvic fractures, which was ruled out on CT.
C. The attachment of Colles fascia to the ischiopubic ramus prevents urine from entering into the thigh.
E. In this patient fluid collected around the penis and scrotum, not in the lower abdomen between.
GAS 459–461; N 378; ABR/McM 279, 281

83. C. The rough bony projection at the junction of the inferior end of the body of the ischium and its ramus is the large ischial tuberosity. Much of the upper body's weight rests on these tuberosities when sitting, and it provides the proximal, tendinous attachment of posterior thigh muscles (hamstring muscles and a portion of the adductor magnus).
A. The inferior pubic ramus is thin and flat and does not bear weight.
B. The iliac crest extends posteriorly, terminating at the posterior superior iliac spine.
D. The pubic tubercle is a prominent forward projecting tubercle on the lateral end of the pubic crest.
E. The small pointed posteromedial projection near the junction of the ramus and body of the ischium is the ischial spine.
GAS 433–437; N 338; ABR/McM 294, 300

84. C. The pelvic inlet or pelvic brim (sagittal inlet) is bounded posteriorly by the sacral promontory, laterally by the iliopectineal lines, and anteriorly by the pubic symphysis. The pelvic outlet (sagittal outlet) is bounded posteriorly by the coccyx, laterally by the ischial tuberosities, and anteriorly by the pubic arch. Bispinous (interspinous) outlet is the distance between the ischial spines. Maximum transverse diameter of inlet extends across the greatest width of the superior aperture, from the middle of the brim on one side to the same point on the opposite side.
A. Bispinous (interspinous) outlet is the distance between the ischial spines.
B. Maximum transverse diameter of inlet extends across the greatest width of the superior aperture, from the middle of the brim on one side to the same point on the opposite side.
D. The pelvic outlet (sagittal outlet) is bounded posteriorly by the coccyx, laterally by the ischial tuberosities, and anteriorly by the pubic arch.
E. Bispinous (pelvic) inlet determines the size and shape of the birth canal and is bordered by the sacral promontory posteriorly, the pubic symphysis anteriorly, and the iliopectineal line laterally.
GAS 440–445; N 336; ABR/McM 96, 233

85. E. Suprapubic (Pfannenstiel) incisions are made 5 cm superior to the pubis symphysis. They are used when access to the pelvic organs is needed. When performing this incision, care must be taken not the perforate the urinary bladder, as the fascia thins around the urinary urinary bladder area.
A. Subcostal incisions begin inferior to the xiphoid process, and extend inferior parallel to the costal

margin. They are mainly used on the right side to operate on the gallbladder and the liver.

B. Median incisions are made through the linea alba. They can be extended the whole length of the abdomen, by curving around the umbilicus. The linea alba is poorly vascularized, so blood loss is minimal, and major nerves are avoided. However, because it is poorly vascularized it heals slowly.

C. A transverse incision just below the umbilicus is made inferior and lateral to the umbilicus. This is a commonly used procedure, as it causes the least damage to the nerve supply to the abdominal muscles, and heals well.

D. McBurney incision is performed at McBurney point (one-third of the distance between the ASIS and the umbilicus). It is mostly used in appendectomies.
GAS 459; N 345; ABR/McM 279

86. D. The fundiform ligament of the penis is a thickening of the superficial fascia, and is superficial to the suspensory ligament that descends in the midline from the linea alba anterior to the pubic symphysis. The ligament splits to surround the penis and then unites and blends inferiorly with the dartos fascia forming the scrotal septum.

A, B, C, E. These structures are not damaged in this case.
GAS 502; N 349; ABR/McM 230

87. A. The ilioinguinal nerve is a branch of the first lumbar nerve (L1). Its fibers are distributed to the skin of the upper and medial part of the thigh, and the skin over the root of the penis and anterior part of the scrotum in men and the skin covering the mons pubis and labium majus in women.

B. The iliohypogastric nerve is the superior branch of the ventral ramus of spinal nerve L1, which perforates the transversus abdominis, and divides into lateral and anterior cutaneous branches.

C. The anterior cutaneous branch pierces the internal oblique, becomes cutaneous by perforating the aponeurosis of the external oblique about 2.5 cm above the superficial inguinal ring, and is distributed to the skin of the suprapubic region.

D. The lateral femoral cutaneous nerve innervates the skin on the lateral upper part of the thigh.

E. The skin of the penis (or clitoris) is mainly supplied by the dorsal nerve (S2), a branch of the pudendal nerve.
GAS 480–488, N 391; ABR/McM 228, 230

88. D. Failure of canalization of the vaginal plate results in atresia (blockage) of the vagina. A transverse vaginal septum occurs in approximately 1 in 80,000 women. Usually, the septum is located at the junction of the middle and superior thirds of the vagina. Failure of the inferior end of the vaginal plate to perforate results in an imperforate hymen. Variations in the appearance of the hymen are common. The vaginal orifice varies in diameter from very small to large, and there may be more than one orifice.

A. Cervical atresia is a rare Mullerian duct anomaly of the female reproductive tract, causing acute or chronic abdominal pain and reproductive problems.

B. The most common cause of indirect inguinal hernia is patent processus vaginalis.

C. Most anorectal anomalies result from abnormal development of the urorectal septum, resulting in incomplete separation of the cloaca into urogenital and anorectal parts.

E. Growth of one paramesonephric duct is retarded and does not fuse with the other one, a bicornuate uterus with a rudimentary horn (cornu) will develop.
GAS 474; N 353; ABR/McM 285, 286

89. B. The ovaries are supplied by ovarian vessels that originate from the abdominal aorta. Ovarian vessels cross the pelvic brim and descend in the suspensory ligament (B) of the ovary to supply the ovaries, fimbrial end of the uterine (Fallopian) tube, and portions of the abdominal/pelvic ureter.

A. The round ligament is a cord-like structure that passes from the uterus through the inguinal ring and attaches to the labia majora. No blood vessels pass through this ligament.

C. The ovarian ligament is a fibrous band of tissue that connects the uterus to the ovary. It joins the uterus just below the origin of the Fallopian tubes. No blood vessels pass through this ligament.

D. The transverse cervical ligaments, also known as the cardinal ligaments, are located at the base of the broad ligament and contain the uterine artery and vein.

E. The mesosalpinx is part of the broad ligament, along with the mesometrium and mesovarium. It originates superiorly to the mesovarium, enclosing the Fallopian tubes. No blood vessels pass through this ligament.
GAS 470; N 355; ABR/McM 287

90. A. The ureter, which is located retroperitoneally, originates from the renal pelvis and runs inferiorly crossing the pelvic brim close to the bifurcation of the common iliac artery. At this important landmark the ureter is medial to the gonadal vessels as it enters into the pelvis. It is lateral to the internal iliac artery as it descends past the pelvic brim.

B, C, E. Although not immediately adjacent, the ureter is medial in relation to the external iliac artery but not close to the inferior vena cava or uterine artery at this location.

D. The ureter is lateral to the internal iliac artery as it descends past the pelvic brim
GAS 380, 455; N 382; ABR/McM 270, 288

91. C. Most anorectal abnormalities including imperforate anus occur from abnormal development of the urorectal septum leading to abnormal or incomplete cloacal separation. This results in abnormal urogenital and anorectal compartments and as such imperforate anus is usually associated with urinary tract defects.

A, B, D. VATER syndrome may include tracheoesophageal, vertebral, renal, limb, and cardiac defects but this association is not as common as that between urogenital and anorectal defects. There is no association with ileal atresia. E. There is no association with ileal atresia.
GAS 452; N 376; ABR/McM 292

92. **A.** Pudendal or saddle block is less common than an epidural anesthesia but still used clinically to obtain perineal anesthesia during the final stages of labor or preceding an episiotomy. It is done by locating the pudendal nerve in or as it exits the pudendal canal and anesthetizing either transcutaneously or transvaginally by locating the ischial spine or tuberosity, respectively. The source for the pudendal nerve is S2–S4 ventral rami. **B, C, D, E.** The pudendal nerve does not originate from any of these other locations.
GAS 480–488; N 395; ABR/McM 289, 290

93. **E.** The superior gluteal artery, which is the largest branch of the posterior division of the internal iliac artery, provides spinal branches as it passes between the lumbosacral trunk and ventral ramus of S1 and exits the pelvis via the greater sciatic foramen superior to the piriformis and supplying piriformis, the gluteal muscles, and tensor fasciae latae. **A.** Inferior gluteal artery, an anterior division of the internal iliac, runs inferior to the first sacral nerve and it exits the pelvis through the infrapiriform part of the greater sciatic foramen. **B, C, D.** None of the remaining vessels traverses the greater sciatic foramen.
GAS 489; N 384; ABR/McM 281, 289

94. **A.** Puborectalis, a part of the levator ani group, is crucial to maintaining the anorectal angle and thereby maintaining fecal continence. Relaxation or injury to this muscle decreases the angle between the ampulla of the rectum and the proximal portion of the anal canal thus aiding in defecation or incontinence, respectively. None of the remaining muscles functions in maintaining the anorectal angle.
   B. The pubococcygeus part of the levator ani group originates from the body of the pubis, extending posteriorly and obliquely to the puborectalis muscle, and inserts on the coccyx. The puborectalis muscle is more directly involved in maintaining the anorectal angle and maintaining fecal continence.
   C. The iliococcygeus part of the levator ani group originates from the anterior ischial spines and inserts on the coccyx. This muscle group works to elevate the pelvic floor and the anorectal canal.
   D. The coccygeus muscles originate from the tips of the ischial spines and insert to the lateral margins of the coccyx and adjacent margins of the sacrum. These muscles aid in supporting the posterior aspect of the pelvic floor.
   E. The obturator internus muscle originates from the medial surface of the obturator foramen and inserts on the greater trochanter of the femur. It laterally rotates and abducts the femur at the hip joint.
   GAS 446–448; N 343; ABR/McM 281

95. **A.** The pudendal nerve passes between the sacrospinous and sacrotuberous ligaments. When performing this block with an internal approach, the ischial spine is used as a landmark as it is easily palpated transvaginally.
   C. The ischial tuberosity is used when the procedure is performed externally as it can be easily palpated in the ischioanal fossa.

B, D. The posterior inferior and the posterior superior iliac spines are posterior; they cannot be palpated transvaginally and are not associated with the pudendal nerve. **E.** The coccyx is the most inferior portion of the vertebral column, cannot be palpated transvaginally, and is not near the pudendal nerve.
GAS 480–488; N 393; ABR/McM 289, 290

96. **D.** Nerve supply to the perineum including the anal canal is via the pudendal nerve. **A.** The sacral splanchnic nerves carry postganglionic sympathetic nerve fibers to the pelvic organs.
   B. The pelvic splanchnic nerves carry preganglionic parasympathetic nerves to the pelvic organs.
   C. The superior hypogastric plexus is an autonomic plexus carrying sympathetic innervation to the pelvic region. **E.** The ilioinguinal nerve supplies the skin of the upper medial thigh and anterior perineal area.
   GAS 486–488, 510; N 398; ABR/McM 289, 290

97. **C.** In the perineum, lymph drains according to arteries that supply the area, and so the glans penis drains to the deep inguinal nodes. Superficial skin of the penis and scrotum would drain to the superficial inguinal nodes.
   A, B. External iliac nodes receive lymph from the deep inguinal, and the internal iliac from the pelvic organs.
   D. The lumbar/lateral aortic nodes receive lymph from the abdominal organs and the external, internal, and common iliac nodes.
   E. The axillary nodes drain the upper limb and chest wall.
   GAS 446–448; N 343; ABR/McM 281

98. **A.** Epispadias is the correct option. Epispadias describes the abnormal opening of the urethra on the dorsal side of the penis. During the development of the genital tubercle defective or inadequate interaction between the ectoderm and mesoderm leads to the genital tubercle developing more dorsally. As a consequence, when the more dorsally located urogenital membrane ruptures, the urogenital sinus will open on the dorsal aspect of the penis. Exstrophy of the urinary urinary bladder is a condition in which there is a defect in the anterior abdominal wall with the bladder and part of the urethra are protruding.
   B. Hermaphrodism is a condition in which the individual possesses the reproductive organs of both sexes.
   C. An hydrocele is an accumulation of serous fluid between the tunica vaginalis parietal layer and the testis.
   D. Hypospadias is a urethral opening on the ventral surface of the penis. **E.** Ectopic ureter occurs when the ureter terminates at another location other than the urinary bladder.
   GAS 459–461, 512; N 363; ABR/McM 278

Answers 99–105

99. **E.** Urachal cysts are embryological remnants of the epithelium of the urachus occurring between the umbilicus and urinary bladder. It presents as an extraperitoneal mass in the umbilical region. Urachal cysts are generally asymptomatic; however, if infected, they present with abdominal pain and fever. If fistulation occurs, it may drain through the umbilicus or rupture, leading to peritonitis.

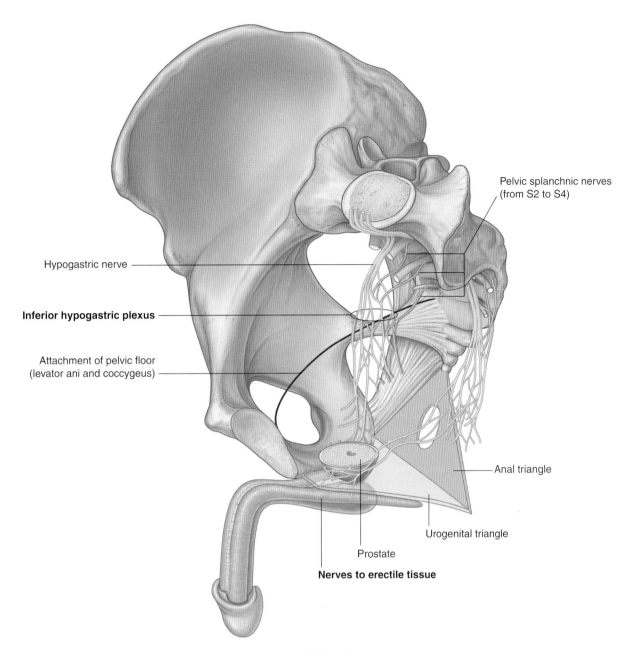

Pelvic splanchnic nerves
(from S2 to S4)

Hypogastric nerve

Inferior hypogastric plexus

Attachment of pelvic floor
(levator ani and coccygeus)

Anal triangle

Urogenital triangle

Prostate

Nerves to erectile tissue

• *GAS* Fig. 5.16

A. Hydroceles are the accumulation of fluids between the two layers of the tunica vaginalis testis surrounding the testes.

B and C. Meckel cyst and Meckel diverticulum are formed on the distal ileum and do not have the anatomical relations described in the CT findings.

D. Omphaloceles result from defective development of the muscles of the anterior abdominal wall where abdominal viscera herniate into the umbilical cord where they are outside of the abdomen.
GAS 456; N 344; ABR/McM 233, 285

100. B. The sacral components of the craniosacral outflow (parasympathetics) are the pelvic splanchnic nerves. These nerves take their origin from the ventral rami of the S2–S4 spinal segments and enter the sacral plexus. They carry both preganglionic parasympathetic fibers

as well as visceral afferent fibers. The pelvic splanchnics provide innervation to pelvic viscera and genitals regulating the voiding of the urinary bladder, controlling the internal urethral sphincter, rectal motility, as well as sexual functions such as erection.

A. The superior hypogastric plexus lies anterior to vertebra L5 between the promontory of the sacrum and the bifurcation of the aorta. It is joined by the pelvic splanchnic nerves carrying preganglionic fibers from S2-S4, forming the inferior hypogastric plexuses.

C, D. The pelvic splanchnic should not be confused with the lumbar splanchnics or sacral splanchnics which carry pre- and postganglionic sympathetics and general visceral afferents.
GAS 486–488, 510; N 398; ABR/McM 271, 282

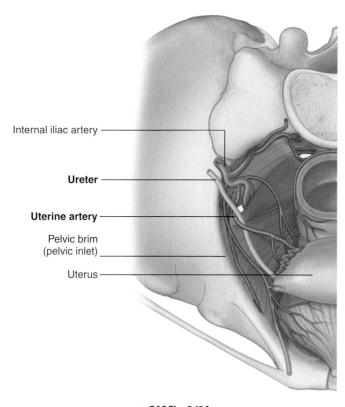

• *GAS* Fig. 5.12A

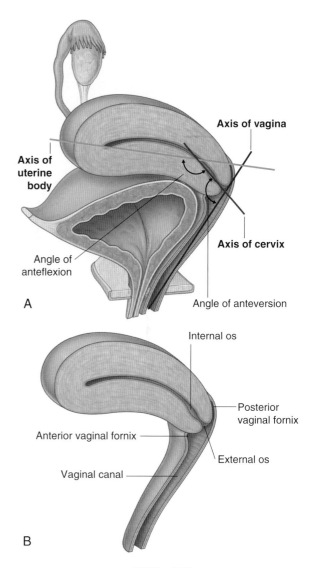

• *GAS* Fig. 5.55

101. A. Cavernous nerves are preganglionic parasympathetic fibers that mediate penile erection. Its preganglionic fibers derive from the pelvic splanchnic nerve (S2–S4).
B. The glans penis receives its supply from the pudendal nerve.
C. The external urethral sphincter is innervated by a voluntary, somatic nerve called the pudendal nerve.
D. The internal urethral sphincter receives parasympathetic fibers also from the inferior hypogastric plexus, which are very different from the cavernous nerves.
E. The seminal glands are innervated by the sympathetic nervous system via the inferior hypogastric plexus (*GAS* Fig. 5.16).
GAS 486–488, 510; N 398; ABR/McM 291, 292

102. E. The scrotal skin is drained by superficial lymphatics that will first empty into the horizontal group of superficial inguinal nodes.
A. The external iliac nodes are deep lymph nodes receiving lymphatics from deep abdominal wall structures below the umbilicus, the pelvic viscera as well as from superficial and deep inguinal lymph nodes.

B. The internal iliac nodes are also deep nodes that drain pelvic viscera, deeper parts of the perineum, and parts of the urethra. The testes and ovaries drain into lumbar lymph nodes, while the sacral nodes drain the rectum and posterior pelvic wall.
C. The lateral aortic/lumbar lymph nodes drains the iliac lymph nodes, ovaries and other pelvic organs.
D. The sacral nodes drain the rectum and posterior pelvic wall.
GAS 495, 514; N 390; ABR/McM 376

103. E. During hysterectomy, hemostasis may be ensured by proper ligation of the arteries that supply the uterus. The uterine artery, a branch of the internal iliac artery, is anterior to the ureter in the broad ligament of the uterus. During surgeries, the ureter may be ligated mistakenly in the place of the uterine artery.
A. The infundibulopelvic ligament, also known as the suspensory ligament, contains the ovarian vessels and is located lateral to the ureter in the pelvis.

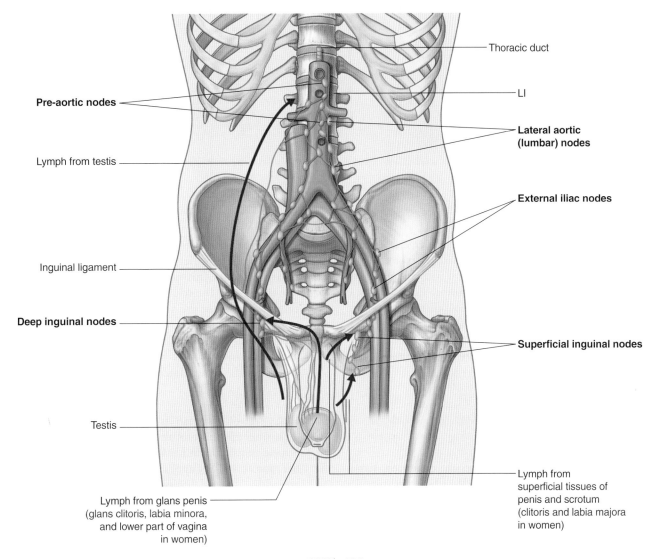

Thoracic duct

LI

Pre-aortic nodes

Lateral aortic
(lumbar) nodes

Lymph from testis

External iliac nodes

Inguinal ligament

Deep inguinal nodes

Superficial inguinal nodes

Testis

Lymph from
superficial tissues of
penis and scrotum
(clitoris and labia majora
in women)

Lymph from glans penis
(glans clitoris, labia minora,
and lower part of vagina
in women)

• *GAS* **Fig. 5.79**

B. The ovarian ligament attaches the ovary to the lateral and superior part of the uterus. It is a fibrous cord that is contained in the broad ligament of the uterus and has no direct relationship with the ureters.

C. The mesosalpinx is the part of the broad ligament that stretches from the ovary to the uterine tube above.

D. The round ligament of the uterus is an embryologic remnant of the gubernaculum ovary and has no direct relationship with the ureters (*GAS* Fig. 5.12A).
GAS 472; N 382; ABR/McM 287, 288

104. A. The lymph from the inferior part of the anal canal drains to the superficial inguinal nodes.

B. The lymph from the distal rectum drains to the sacral nodes.

C. The lymph from the sigmoid colon drains to the inferior mesenteric nodes and then to the lumbar nodes.

D. The lymph from the proximal rectum drains to the sacral nodes

E. The lymph from the anal canal above the pectinate line drains to the internal iliac nodes.
GAS 495, 514; N 388; ABR/McM 376

105. E. Fig. 4.5 depicts a lymphangiogram showing several lymphatic groups at the pelvic and inguinal region. The lymphatic groups are as follows A=Lumbar, B=Common iliac, C=External iliac, D=Deep iliac, and E=Superficial inguinal. Malignancies involving the lower part of the vagina typically involve the superficial inguinal lymph nodes, so E is the correct answer (*GAS* Fig. 5.79).
GAS 495, 514, N 388; ABR/McM 376

5

Lower Limb

Introduction

First Order Question

1. A 22-year-old woman is brought to the emergency department 30 minutes after she was involved in a motor vehicle collision. She appears to be well and without any major injuries. Vital signs are within normal limits. Physical examination shows no abnormalities other than a couple of lacerations over the quadriceps femoris muscle. Which of the following nerves innervates this muscle?
   A. Sciatic
   B. Femoral
   C. Obturator
   D. Saphenous
   E. Tibial

Explanation

B: Only the femoral nerve innervates the quadriceps femoris. The sciatic nerve, specifically the tibial part, supplies the posterior thigh muscles not the anterior compartment. The obturator nerve supplies the medial compartment and the saphenous nerve does not supply any muscles.

Second Order Question

2. A 22-year-old woman is brought to the emergency department 30 minutes after she was involved in a motor vehicle collision with her left and right leg pinned under her motorcycle. She appears to be well, and her vital signs are within normal limits. Physical examination shows that she cannot extend her right knee. Which of the following nerves is most likely affected?
   A. Sciatic nerve
   B. Femoral nerve
   C. Obturator nerve
   D. Saphenous nerve
   E. Tibial nerve

Explanation

B: Extension of the knee is carried out by the quadriceps femoris muscle, which attaches to the tibia via the patellar ligament. This muscle group is supplied by the femoral nerve. The sciatic nerve supplies the posterior thigh muscles not the anterior compartment. The obturator nerve supplies the medial compartment and the saphenous nerve does not supply motor innervation to any muscles but is a sensory (cutaneous) branch of the femoral nerve.

Third Order Question

3. A 22-year-old woman is brought to the emergency department 30 minutes after she was involved in a motor vehicle collision with her left and right leg pinned under her motorcycle. She appears to be well, and her vital signs are within normal limits. Physical examination shows that she cannot extend her right knee. The affected nerve gives rise to which of the following cutaneous nerves?
   A. Middle clunial
   B. Lateral femoral cutaneous
   C. Superficial fibular
   D. Saphenous
   E. Deep fibular

Explanation

D: The saphenous nerve is a cutaneous branch of the femoral nerve and supplies the skin on the medial leg along the great saphenous vein. Middle clunial nerves are branches of posterior rami of S1 to S3. Lateral femoral cutaneous is from L2 to L3 and the lumbar plexus but is not a femoral nerve branch. Superficial and deep fibular nerves are branches of the common fibular nerve.

Main Questions

Questions 1–24

1. A 42-year-old man is brought to the emergency department 30 minutes after he was involved in a motor vehicle collision. He is treated for a pelvic fracture and several deep lacerations. Physical examination shows that dorsiflexion and inversion of the left foot and extension of the great toe are very weak. Sensation from the dorsum of the foot, skin of the sole, and the lateral aspect of the foot has been lost and the patellar reflex is normal. The foot is everted and plantar flexed. Which of the following structures is most likely injured?
   A. The lumbosacral trunk at the linea terminalis
   B. L5 and S1 spinal nerves torn at the intervertebral foramina

C. Fibular (peroneal) division of the sciatic nerve at the neck of the fibula

D. Sciatic nerve injury at the greater sciatic foramen ("doorway to the gluteal region")

E. Tibial nerve in the popliteal fossa

2. A 23-year-old man is brought to the emergency department with a deep, bleeding stab wound of the pelvis. After the bleeding has been stopped, MRI of his pelvis shows that the right ventral ramus of L4 has been transected. Which of the following will most likely be seen during physical examination?

A. Reduction or loss of sensation from the medial aspect of the leg

B. Loss of sensation over the right little toe

C. Loss of sensation over the upper medial thigh

D. Loss of sensation over the middle toe

E. Loss of sensation over the posterior aspect of the knee

3. A 30-year-old man is brought to the emergency department 20 minutes after he was involved in a motor vehicle collision with his right hip caught beneath the motorcycle at the scene. Physical examination shows a deep laceration of the upper part of the right hip. A few days after stabilization and treatment, the patient is asked to walk, and he exhibits a waddling gait and the inability to perform abduction and medial rotation of the right thigh. The patient is most likely to show which of the following?

A. Difficulty in standing from a sitting position

B. Sagging of the left pelvis while standing only on the right lower limb

C. Drooping of the right pelvis while standing only on the left limb

D. Weakened flexion at the right hip joint

E. Difficulty in sitting from a standing position

4. A 45-year-old man is brought to the emergency department 40 minutes after he was involved in a motor vehicle collision. Physical examination shows he is not able to bear weight on the affected limb. In a supine position, the left foot is plantarflexed (Fig. 5.1). Eversion of the affected foot is intact. An x-ray examination of his left leg shows a fracture distal to the neck of the fibula. Which of the following nerves is most likely injured?

A. Tibial

B. Common fibular

C. Superficial fibular

D. Saphenous

E. Deep fibular

5. A 55-year-old woman comes to the physician because of 2-week history of a painful lump in her groin. Physical examination of the abdomen shows a herniation of abdominal viscera beneath the inguinal ligament into the medial aspect of the anterior thigh. The herniation of the bowel appears to be irreducible. Which of the following openings will the hernia initially pass through to extend from the abdomen into the thigh?

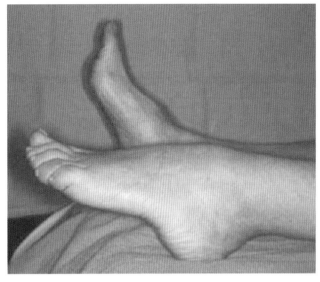

• Fig. 5.1

A. Femoral ring

B. Superficial inguinal ring

C. Deep inguinal ring

D. Saphenous opening

E. Obturator canal

6. A 16-year-old boy is brought to the physician by his mother because of an ankle sprain. While playing flag football, he jumped over other players and landed with his right foot over an unexpected pit. The ankle rolled outward. Since then, bearing weight on the affected foot has not been possible because of severe pain. Physical examination shows swelling of the medial aspect of the ankle with severe tenderness. If a related bone is fractured, which of the following nerves would most likely be injured?

A. Superficial fibular

B. Lateral sural

C. Deep fibular

D. Tibial

E. Sural

7. A 68-year-old woman is brought to the emergency department after she fell from a bicycle and landed hard on the lateral aspect of the left pelvis and thigh. Physical examination shows lateral rotation of the left leg with some shortening in the supine position. An x-ray of her thigh and pelvis show an intracapsular fracture of the neck of the left femur. A total hip arthroplasty is performed. An initial division of the overlying superficial tissues and gluteal musculature is performed, and the procedure continues to reach the neck of the femur. Which of the following muscles is considered as a landmark in surgical exploration of this area?

A. Gluteus medius

B. Superior gemellus

C. Inferior gemellus

D. Piriformis

E. Quadratus femoris

8. A 16-year-old boy is brought to the emergency department because of a superficial cut on the lateral side of his foot while playing football. The wound is sutured, and then the patient is discharged. Four days later the patient returns to the hospital with high fever and swollen lymph nodes in the affected lower limb. The wound appears to be infected. Which group of lymph nodes will first receive lymph from the infected wound?
   A. Popliteal
   B. Vertical group of superficial inguinal
   C. Deep inguinal
   D. Horizontal group of superficial inguinal
   E. Internal iliac

9. A 45-year-old man comes to the physician because of a 3-month history of posterior right knee pain and tightness, and difficulty in walking. He has a long history of chronic osteoarthritis. Physical examination shows the presence of a lump in the popliteal fossa in a supine position that disappears when the knee is flexed. An ultrasound examination of the popliteal fossa shows a large pure cystic structure compressing an adjacent nerve descending the fossa vertically. Which of the following movements will most likely be affected?
   A. Dorsiflexion of the foot
   B. Flexion of the thigh
   C. Extension of the digits
   D. Extension of the leg
   E. Plantar flexion of the foot

10. A 19-year-old football player is brought to the emergency department because of knee pain. In a mock practice, he was hit on the lateral side of his knee just as he put that foot on the ground. He felt a popping sensation. Since then, he is unable to walk without assistance. Physical examination shows a positive valgus stress test. Which structure would most likely also be injured due to its attachment to this ligament?
   A. Medial meniscus
   B. Anterior cruciate ligament
   C. Lateral meniscus
   D. Posterior cruciate ligament
   E. Tendon of semitendinosus

11. A 69-year-old man is brought to the emergency department because of a 30-minute history of chest pain. A coronary arterial angiography shows myocardial infarction due to complete occlusion of the anterior interventricular (left anterior descending) artery. The patient undergoes a coronary bypass graft procedure using the great saphenous vein. Postoperatively, the patient has pain and loss of sensation on the medial surface of the leg and foot on the limb from which the graft was harvested. Which nerve was most likely injured during the bypass surgery?
   A. Common fibular
   B. Superficial fibular
   C. Lateral sural
   D. Saphenous
   E. Tibial

12. A 22-year-old football player comes to the physician because of pain in his left ankle after he fell on the ground with his left foot inverted while trying to avoid a tackle by an opponent in practice. Physical examination shows tenderness and swelling over the lateral aspect of the affected ankle. An x-ray of the ankle shows no fracture but soft tissue swelling. Which of the following ligaments is most likely injured?
   A. Plantar calcaneonavicular (spring)
   B. Anterior talofibular
   C. Long plantar
   D. Short plantar
   E. Medial collateral (deltoid)

13. A 72-year-old woman comes to the physician because of a 6-week history of pain in her right foot. Physical examination shows weak dorsalis pedis pulse and cold right foot. A computed tomography (CT) angiography shows a thrombotic occlusion of the femoral artery in the proximal part of the adductor canal. Which artery will most likely provide blood supply to the leg through the genicular anastomosis?
   A. Medial circumflex femoral
   B. Descending branch of the lateral circumflex femoral
   C. First perforating branch of the deep femoral
   D. Inferior gluteal
   E. Descending genicular branch of femoral

14. A 75-year-old woman is brought to the emergency department after falling in her bathroom. The patient says that she was not able to bear weight on the affected lower limb after the incident. Physical examination shows an externally rotated left leg, and the left lower limb appears to be shorter than the right lower limb. A series of plain x-rays of the hip show an extracapsular fracture of the femoral neck. Which artery is most likely at risk for injury?
   A. Inferior gluteal
   B. First perforating branch of deep femoral
   C. Medial circumflex femoral
   D. Obturator
   E. Superior gluteal

15. A 56-year-old man with advanced bladder carcinoma is admitted to the hospital because of difficulty walking. Physical examination shows numbness on the medial aspect of the right thigh and weakness in adduction of the right lower limb. An MRI shows metastasis of the bladder carcinoma in the right lower limb. Which nerve is most likely being affected by the tumor to result in walking difficulty and the sensory deficit?
   A. Femoral
   B. Obturator
   C. Common fibular
   D. Tibial
   E. Sciatic

16. A 15-year-old boy is brought to the emergency department by his mother because of a lower limb injury. An x-ray of his leg shows a fracture of the left tibia, and a knee-high leg cast is placed. Several

weeks later, upon removal of the cast, the patient has numbness of the dorsum of his right foot and inability to dorsiflex and evert his foot. Which is the most probable site of the nerve compression that resulted in these symptoms?

A. Popliteal fossa
B. Neck of the fibula
C. Lateral compartment of the leg
D. Anterior compartment of the leg
E. Medial malleolus

17. A 32-year-old man comes to the physician for a follow-up examination of his mental disorder. The patient agrees to start an antipsychotic medication and receives an intramuscular injection to his gluteal region. A week later, he comes back to the physician because he has difficulty rising to a standing position from a seated position. Which nerve is most likely affected by the injection?

A. Inferior gluteal
B. Superior gluteal
C. Obturator
D. Nerve to piriformis
E. Nerve to quadratus femoris

18. A 23-year-old woman comes to the physician because of a foot injury. During the preparation of an evening meal, she dropped a sharp, slender kitchen knife. The blade pierced the first web space of her right foot. Physical examination shows a deep laceration on the web space between the first and second toes and numbness of the web space. If the affected nerve were to be injured just distal to its origin, which of the following movements at the ankle joint is most likely impaired?

A. Dorsiflexion and eversion
B. Dorsiflexion and inversion
C. Inversion only
D. Plantar flexion and inversion
E. Plantar flexion only

19. A 32-year-old woman comes to the physician following an injury of the knee during a soccer match. Physical examination shows that holding the right tibia with both hands, the tibia can be pressed backward under the distal part of her femur. The left tibia cannot be displaced in this way. Which ligament was most likely damaged in the right knee?

A. Anterior cruciate
B. Fibular collateral
C. Tibial collateral
D. Patellar
E. Posterior cruciate

20. A 24-year-old woman is brought to the emergency department 30 minutes after she was involved in a motor vehicle collision. She was the unrestrained driver. Physical examination shows a large bruise and severe tenderness on the lateral aspect of her hip. An x-ray of the hip shows an avulsion fracture of the greater trochanter. Which of the following muscles

would continue to function normally if such an injury occurred?

A. Piriformis
B. Obturator internus
C. Gluteus medius
D. Gluteus maximus
E. Gluteus minimus

21. A 58-year-old man is brought to the emergency department for a massive bleeding from his lower limb. Despite appropriate life-saving measures, he dies. Autopsy shows a slashing laceration on the right medial thigh, which resulted in rapid and significant exsanguination followed by hypovolemic shock and circulatory collapse. Based on the results of the autopsy, what is the most likely nature of his injury?

A. The femoral artery was cut at the inguinal ligament
B. A vessel or vessels were injured at the apex of the femoral triangle
C. The femoral vein was transected at its junction with the saphenous vein
D. The medial circumflex femoral was severed at its origin
E. The deep femoral artery was divided at its origin

22. A 72-year-old woman comes to the physician for a follow-up examination. Two months ago, the patient had a femoral neck fracture when she fell down the steps to her garage. During physical therapy, the therapist provides resistance against the patient pulling her thigh backward as much as possible. Which of the following structures is most significant in resisting hyperextension of the hip joint?

A. Pubofemoral ligament
B. Ischiofemoral ligament
C. Iliofemoral ligament
D. Transverse acetabular ligament
E. Ligament of the head of the femur

23. A 75-year-old man is brought to the emergency department after he was rescued by a police officer in an abandoned house. The man is not able to ambulate without assistance. Physical examination shows limited range of motion at the right hip joint because of pain and a laterally rotated right leg with some shortening in a supine position. An x-ray is shown in Fig. 5.2. Based on findings on the imaging, which of the following conditions most likely occurred to him?

A. Dislocation of the hip with tearing of the ligament of the head of the femur
B. Intertrochanteric fracture of the femur
C. Intracapsular femoral neck fracture
D. Thrombosis of the obturator artery
E. Comminuted fracture of the extracapsular femoral neck

24. A 45-year-old man comes to the physician because of 10-day history of sharp back pain while he was lifting a box of books. He told the physician that he "felt the pain in my backside, the back of my thigh, my leg, and the side of my foot." Physical examination shows

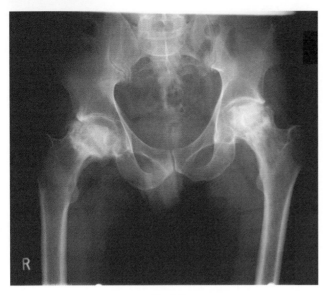

• Fig. 5.2

weakened calcaneal (Achilles) tendon jerk on the affected side. Which of the following is the most likely cause of the finding?

A. Disc herniation at L3–4
B. Disc herniation at L4–5
C. Disc herniation at L5–S1
D. Disc herniation at S1–2
E. Gluteal crush syndrome of the sciatic nerve or piriformis syndrome

Questions 25–47

25. A 55-year-old woman is brought to the emergency department 30 minutes after she was involved in a motor vehicle collision. She was the unrestrained driver. Physical examination shows that the patient's foot is everted and she cannot easily invert it. A weakness in dorsiflexion and inversion of the foot is noted. Her ipsilateral patellar reflex is reduced in quality, although the calcaneal (Achilles) tendon reflex is brisk. Knee extension is almost normal, as are all hip movements and knee flexion. Sensation is greatly reduced on the dorsum of the foot. Which of the following nerves is most likely injured?
A. L2 and L3 spinal nerves
B. L4 spinal nerve
C. L5 spinal nerve
D. S1 spinal nerve
E. S2 spinal nerve

26. A 46-year-old woman is brought to the emergency department after stepping on a broken wine bottle on the sidewalk. A close observation of the wound shows that the sharp glass has entered the posterior part of her foot. It is suspected that her lateral plantar nerve may have been transected. Loss of which of the following will most likely be found by further examination if the assumption is right?
A. Sensation over the plantar surface of the third toe
B. Abduction of the great toe

C. Abduction and adduction of the digits (lateral four toes)
D. Flexion of the great toe
E. Flexion of the digits (lateral four toes)

27. A 22-year-old man who practices martial arts comes to the physician because of left knee pain and serious disability that took place from a kick to the side of his left knee in a competition a week ago. Physical examination shows a large bruise just distal to the head of the fibula. An x-ray of the leg shows a comminuted fracture. Which of the following muscles will most likely be paralyzed?
A. Tibialis anterior and extensor digitorum longus
B. Tibialis posterior
C. Soleus and gastrocnemius
D. Plantaris and popliteus
E. Flexor digitorum longus and flexor hallucis longus

28. A 24-year-old woman comes to the physician because of a swelling in her groin and persistent low-grade fever. She was diagnosed with tuberculosis a year ago but has not been compliant with medicine. Physical examination shows a nontender, fluctuant swelling in her left groin. A CT scan shows a spread of a large abscess at lumbar vertebrae within the fascia of a muscle with which of the following actions at the hip?
A. Abduction
B. Adduction
C. Extension
D. Flexion
E. Medial rotation

29. A 32-year-old worker is brought to the emergency department because of an ankle injury. He says that during cleanup of an old residential area of the city, he accidentally cut the back of his right ankle with the blade of a brush cutter. Examination shows that a tendon lying posterior to the medial and lateral malleoli of the right ankle is severely transected obliquely. Which of the following bones serves as an insertion for the tendon?
A. Calcaneus
B. Fibula
C. Cuboid
D. Talus
E. Navicular

30. A 41-year-old woman comes to the physician for evaluation of her right foot. The patient has a long history of activity-related right sole pain and the pain now comes along with swelling and stiffness of the foot. A CT scan shows that the head of the talus has become displaced inferiorly, thereby causing the medial longitudinal arch of the foot to fall. What would be the most likely cause in this case?
A. Tearing of the plantar calcaneonavicular (spring) ligament
B. Fracture of the cuboid bone
C. Interruption of the plantar aponeurosis
D. Sprain of the anterior talofibular ligament
E. Sprain of the medial collateral (deltoid) ligament

31. A 21-year-old man is brought to the emergency department because of severe knee pain. During a football game, he was blocked by a linebacker, who threw himself against the lateral aspect of the receiver's left knee. The receiver grasped his knee in obvious pain. Physical examination shows swelling and tenderness over the knee joint. Which of the following structures is frequently subject to injury from this type of force against the knee?

A. Fibular collateral ligament
B. Anterior cruciate ligament
C. Lateral meniscus and posterior cruciate ligament
D. Fibular collateral and posterior cruciate ligament
E. All the ligaments of the knee will be affected

32. An 82-year-old woman comes to the physician because of a 3-month history of pain in her right leg below the knee. She says that her limb pain gets worse during her workout routines in the health spa. An angiography of the lower limbs shows minimal flow through the artery passing through the aperture present in the proximal part of the leg, between the tibia and fibula. Which of the following arteries is most likely affected?

A. Deep femoral
B. Popliteal
C. Posterior tibial
D. Fibular
E. Anterior tibial

33. A 43-year-old man comes to the physician because of a painful, swollen knee joint. The patient's history shows chronic gonococcal arthritis. A knee aspiration is ordered for bacterial culture of the synovial fluid. A standard suprapatellar approach is used, and the needle passes from the lateral aspect of the thigh into the region immediately proximal to and deep to the patella. Through which of the following muscles would the needle pass?

A. Adductor magnus
B. Short head of biceps femoris
C. Rectus femoris
D. Sartorius
E. Vastus lateralis

34. A 34-year-old man comes to the physician because of difficulty walking and pain at the back of the knee. Physical examination shows that the patient has a problem initiating gait from a standing position. A muscle injury responsible for unlocking the knee joint to permit flexion of the leg is suspected, and an imaging study is ordered. Which of the following nerves innervates the affected muscle?

A. Common fibular
B. Deep fibular
C. Superficial fibular
D. Tibial
E. Femoral

35. A 32-year-old man comes to the physician because of an ankle sprain. Yesterday, the patient, a basketball player, came down hard on his ankle during the match. Physical examination shows soft tissue swelling and severe tenderness on the medial aspect of the ankle. The patient is not able to put weight on the affected leg. An x-ray shows a bimalleolar fracture. Which of the following ligaments is most likely injured?

A. Talonavicular
B. medial collateral (deltoid)
C. Spring
D. Plantar
E. Long plantar

36. A 23-year-old man is brought to the emergency department because of severe pain and coldness of his right leg. Physical examination shows cyanosis and tenderness of the right leg. Doppler ultrasound shows that the femoral artery of the affected limb terminates midthigh. A thrombotic occlusion is seen in an unusual, rather tortuous, large vessel in the posterior compartment of the thigh, arising in the gluteal area and continuous inferiorly with a normal appearing popliteal artery. What is the identity of the aberrant artery?

A. A large, fifth perforating branch of the deep femoral artery
B. A sciatic branch of the inferior gluteal artery
C. Transverse branch of the medial circumflex femoral artery
D. Superficial branch of the superior gluteal artery
E. An enlarged descending branch of the lateral circumflex femoral artery

37. A 51-year-old man comes to the emergency department because of weakness of the right lower limb. He says that while he was attempting to lift one side of his new electric automobile from the ground to demonstrate his strength, he felt a sharp pain in his back and quickly dropped the vehicle. Physical examination shows deficits in sensation on the middorsum of his foot and sole and marked weakness in dorsiflexion and ankle inversion. What is most likely nature of his injury?

A. Disc herniation at L1–2
B. Disc herniation at L2–3
C. Disc herniation at L3–4
D. Disc herniation at L4–5
E. Disc herniation at L5–S1

38. A 43-year-old woman comes to the physician because of 6-month history of pain in her lower limb. She says she has pain in the hip, thigh, and leg of the affected limb and pain during sexual intercourse. Physical examination shows reduced sensation over the first web space, dorsum, and lateral side and weakness in eversion of the involved foot. A diagnosis of a piriformis entrapment syndrome is made, with compression of the common fibular division of the sciatic nerve. Which of the following conditions is also most likely found during physical examination?

A. Inability to plantar flex
B. Weakness in leg extension at the knee
C. Foot drop
D. Weakness in adduction of the thigh
E. Loss of sensation in the medial aspect of the leg

39. Three years following a 62-year-old man's hip replacement, his CT scans indicated that two of his larger hip muscles had been replaced by adipose tissue. The opinion is offered that his superior gluteal nerve could have been injured during the replacement procedure, and the muscles supplied by that nerve had atrophied and been replaced by fat. Which of the following muscles receives its innervation from the superior gluteal nerve?
A. Tensor fasciae latae
B. Rectus femoris
C. Gluteus maximus
D. Piriformis
E. Quadratus femoris

40. A popliteal arterial aneurysm can be very fragile, bursting with great loss of blood and the potential loss of the leg if it is not dealt with safely and effectively. In the 18th century, Dr. John Hunter (1728–1793) discovered that if a primary artery of the thigh is temporarily compressed, blood flow in the popliteal artery can be reduced long enough to treat the aneurysm in the popliteal fossa surgically, with safety. What structure is indicated in Fig. 5.3 that is related to his surgical procedure?
A. Sartorius
B. Femoral vein
C. Femoral artery
D. Gracilis
E. Adductor brevis

41. A 49-year-old man is brought to the emergency department after falling from a ladder, with his weight impacting on the heels of his feet. Physical examination shows tenderness and swelling of the bilateral heels and inability to stand on the feet. X-rays of his feet show bilateral comminuted calcaneal fractures. After the injury, the contraction of which one of the following muscles most likely aggravates the pain in the injured feet?
A. Flexor digitorum profundus
B. Gastrocnemius
C. Tibialis posterior
D. Tibialis anterior
E. Fibularis longus

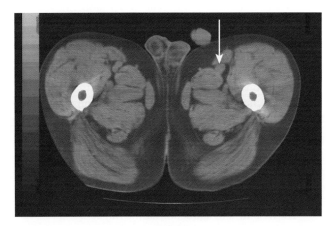

• **Fig. 5.3**

42. A 24-year-old woman is brought to the emergency department because of a small-caliber bullet wound to the knee from a drive-by assailant. Physical examination shows a penetrating wound to the popliteal fossa. The patient is immediately transferred to the operating room. The bullet had severed the nerve superficial to and coursing along the popliteal vein. Such an injury would most likely result in which of the following?
A. Inability to extend the leg at the knee
B. Foot drop
C. Dorsiflexed and everted foot
D. Plantar flexed and inverted foot
E. Total inability to flex the leg at the knee joint

43. An 82-year-old woman is brought to the emergency department by her son because of great pain in her right lower limb. Her son says that she was not able to get up after slipping on the polished floor in her front hall. Physical examination shows that the right lower limb is laterally rotated and noticeably shorter than her left limb. X-rays of the hip joint shows a disrupted Shenton line by subcapital fracture. Which of the following arteries supplying the head of the femur in early childhood but no longer in this patient?
A. Superior gluteal
B. Lateral circumflex femoral
C. A branch of the obturator artery
D. Inferior gluteal
E. Medial circumflex femoral

44. A 29-year-old man comes to the physician because of a 3-month history of discomfort in the lateral thigh. Physical examination shows a rather overweight man, wearing a heavy leather belt, to which numerous objects are attached, including his empty holster. After a thorough examination, a diagnosis of meralgia paresthetica is made. Which of the following nerves is most likely involved?
A. Superior gluteal
B. Femoral
C. Obturator
D. Fibular division of sciatic
E. Lateral femoral cutaneous

45. A 23-year-old female long distance runner is brought to the emergency department after she sprained her left ankle while running. An x-ray of the ankle shows a medial malleolus fracture of the left foot with the distal part of the malleolus displaced posteroinferiorly. Which of the following structures is most likely compressed by the displaced fragment of the bone?
A. Flexor hallucis longus tendon
B. Plantaris tendon
C. Tibialis anterior tendon
D. Tibialis posterior tendon
E. Tibial nerve

46. A 42-year-old man is brought to the emergency department after falling to the sidewalk from his ladder. Physical examination shows the patient is not able to put weight on his left leg. There is a swelling and bruises around the left midthigh, as well as multiple lacerations on his left arm and leg. An x-ray of the femur shows a fracture of the proximal shaft of the left femur. Which of the following arteries supplies the affected part of the femur?

A. Deep circumflex iliac
B. Acetabular branch of obturator
C. Lateral circumflex femoral
D. A branch of deep femoral
E. Medial circumflex femoral

47. A 22-year-old man is brought to the emergency department after falling from his bicycle. During physical examination, the patient is not able to put weight on the right leg and is unable to perform certain movements. An x-ray of the leg shows a fracture of the right tibia above the ankle. An MRI shows that the major nerve in the posterior compartment of the leg is severed by the fracture. Which of the following signs would have been most likely found during the physical examination?

A. Sensory loss of the dorsum of the foot
B. Sensory loss on the sole of the foot
C. Foot drop
D. Paralysis of the extensor digitorum brevis
E. Sensory loss of the entire foot

Questions 48–71

48. A 24-year-old man is brought to the emergency department 30 minutes after he was involved in a motor vehicle collision. An x-ray of the femur shows a fracture at the junction of the middle and lower thirds of the femur with the distal fragment of the fracture being pulled posteriorly. An angiogram of the lower limb shows that the popliteal vessels are compressed by the distal fragment of the fracture. Which of the following muscles is most likely to displace the distal fracture fragment?

A. Soleus
B. Gastrocnemius
C. Semitendinosus
D. Gracilis
E. Tibialis anterior

49. A 65-year-old man is brought to the emergency department after falling from his roof while cleaning leaves and pine needles from the gutters. An x-ray of the right foot shows a fracture of the talus. Much of the blood supply of this bone can be lost in such an injury and can result in osteonecrosis. From what artery does this bone receive its primary vascular supply?

A. Medial plantar
B. Lateral plantar
C. Dorsalis pedis
D. Anterior tibial
E. Posterior tibial

50. A 58-year-old woman comes to the physician because of 6-month history of pain during her work because of bilateral bunions. Physical examination shows

swelling, redness, and calluses at the lateral base of the proximal phalanx of the great toes. During the operation, the protruding bony and soft tissues of the toe are excised, and then a muscle is reflected from the lateral side of the proximal phalanx, together with a sesamoid bone, upon which the muscle also inserts. What muscle is this?

A. Adductor hallucis
B. Abductor hallucis
C. First dorsal interosseous
D. First lumbrical
E. Quadratus plantae

51. A 7-year-old girl is brought to the physician after she accidentally stepped on a sharp snail shell while walking to the beach. She receives a tetanus shot, and the wound is cleaned thoroughly and sutured. One week later, during a follow-up examination, she has great difficulty in flexing her great toe, even though there is no inflammation present in the sole of the foot. Which nerve is most likely damaged by the piercing of the shell?

A. Lateral plantar
B. Medial plantar
C. Sural
D. Superficial fibular
E. Deep fibular

52. A 73-year-old man comes to the physician because of 6-month history of progressive cold and pale foot. Physical examination shows a nontender, cyanotic cold foot. The pulse of the posterior tibial artery is absent. A Doppler ultrasound of the leg indicates a thrombotic occlusion of his popliteal artery. Absence of pulse during physical examination will most likely be found in which of the following locations?

A. Lateral to the muscular belly of the abductor hallucis
B. Posteroinferior to the medial femoral condyle
C. Groove midway between the lateral malleolus and the calcaneus
D. Groove midway between the medial malleolus and the calcaneus
E. Medially, between the two heads of the gastrocnemius

53. Young parents are concerned that their 14-month-old daughter has not yet begun walking. Their pediatrician reassures them, saying that one of the muscles of the leg, the fibularis tertius, has to complete its central neurologic development before the child could lift the outer corner of the foot and walk without stumbling over her toes. What is the most common nerve supply of this muscle?

A. Sural
B. Lateral plantar
C. Deep fibular
D. Superficial fibular
E. Tibial

54. A 22-year-old woman comes to the physician because of 5-day history of high fever and vaginal discharge. Her temperature is 39°C (102.2°F), and pulse is 105/

min. Laboratory studies confirm gonorrheal infection. A series of intramuscular antibiotic injections are ordered. Into which of the following parts of the gluteal region should the antibiotic be injected to avoid nerve injury?

A. Anterior and superior to a line between the posterior superior iliac spine and the greater trochanter

B. In the middle of a line between the anterior superior iliac spine and the ischial tuberosity

C. Inferolateral to a line between the posterior superior iliac spine and the greater trochanter

D. Inferomedial to a line between the posterior superior iliac spine and the greater trochanter

E. Halfway between the iliac tuberosity and the greater trochanter

55. A 45-year-old intoxicated man is brought to the emergency department 30 minutes after being struck by a tour bus while walking in the middle of the street. He is able to ambulate without an assistance. Physical examination shows "adductor gait," crossing one limb in front of the other due to unopposed hip adductors. Which of the following nerves most likely supply these muscles?

A. Tibial

B. Obturator

C. Inferior gluteal

D. Superior gluteal

E. Femoral

56. While a 27-year-old woman is trying to deliver her baby vaginally, the decision to inject local anesthetic into the perineum is made because of severe pain. A deep injection is made medial to the ischial tuberosity to anesthetize the pudendal nerve, which supplies much of the perineum in most cases. A few minutes later, it becomes very obvious to those in attendance that the injection has not been effective enough in the central and posterior parts of the perineum. A separate injection is therefore inserted lateral to the ischial tuberosity. What other nerve(s) can provide much of the sensory supply to the perineum in some individuals?

A. Posterior femoral cutaneous

B. Inferior clunial

C. Iliohypogastric

D. Inferior gluteal

E. Middle clunial

57. A 65-year-old man is admitted to the hospital to undergo an iliofemoral bypass because of an occlusion of the proximal aspect of the femoral artery. The operation is performed successfully and the blood flow between the iliac and femoral arteries is restored. During rehabilitation, which of the following arteries should be palpated to monitor good circulation of the lower limb?

A. Anterior tibial

B. Deep fibular

C. Deep plantar

D. Dorsalis pedis

E. Dorsal metatarsal

58. A 55-year-old woman is brought to the emergency department after being bitten by a stray dog on the dorsum of the foot. The wound is cleaned thoroughly, during which it is seen that no tendons have been cut, but the dorsalis pedis artery and the accompanying nerve have been injured. Which of the following conditions would be expected during physical examination?

A. Clubfoot

B. Foot drop

C. Inability to extend the great toe

D. Numbness between the first and second toes

E. Weakness in inversion of the foot

59. A 31-year-old woman comes to the physician because of a 5-week history of facial paralysis of one side of her face. Plastic surgery of a nerve graft, taking a cutaneous nerve from the lower limb to replace the defective facial nerve, is planned. Six months after the successful procedure, there is restoration of function of previously paralyzed facial muscles. There is an area of skin on the back of the leg laterally and also on the lateral side of the foot that has no sensation. What nerve was used in the grafting procedure?

A. Superficial fibular

B. Tibial

C. Common fibular

D. Sural

E. Saphenous

60. A 10-year-old girl is brought to the emergency department by her parent after falling from a tree while she was playing with her friends. She is able to walk, but she has severe knee pain. Physical examination shows tenderness at the distal aspect of the knee and swelling. An x-ray of the knee shows Osgood-Schlatter disease (Fig. 5.4). Which of the following bony structures is most likely affected?

A. Medial condyle of tibia

B. Posterior intercondylar area

C. Intercondylar eminence

D. Tibial tuberosity

E. Anterolateral tibial tubercle (Gerdy tubercle)

61. An 81-year-old man comes to the physician with severe pain in his knees. The patient has a long history of osteoarthritis. Physical examination shows swelling and tenderness of the knee bilaterally. An x-ray of the knee shows degeneration of the knee joints. The degeneration is more severe on the medial side of the knees, causing his knees to be bowed outward when he stands upright. Which of the following terms best describes the condition of his knees?

A. Genu varus

B. Genu valgus

C. Coxa varus

D. Coxa valgus

E. Hallux valgus

62. A 57-year-old diabetic woman comes to the physician because of a 6-month history of low energy level, weight gain, and constipation. Physical examination shows

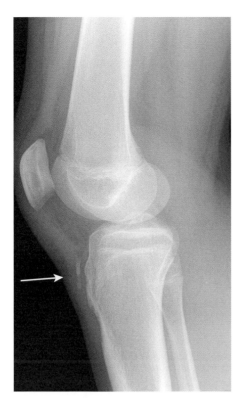

• Fig. 5.4

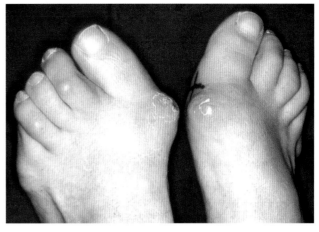

• Fig. 5.5

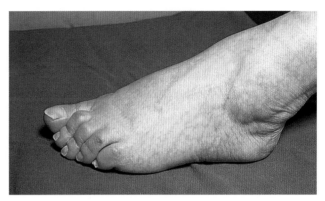

• Fig. 5.6

markedly reduced patellar reflex and slight swelling of the neck. Laboratory studies confirm hypothyroidism and appropriate treatment is initiated. The tendon of which of the following muscles is stretched during the reflex test?

A. Quadriceps femoris
B. Quadratus femoris
C. Sartorius
D. Pectineus
E. Biceps femoris

63. A 52-year-old woman is brought to the emergency department after severely injuring her right lower limb when she fell from a trampoline. She is not able to put weight on the affected foot. Physical examination shows swelling and bruises around the ankle of the right foot. X-ray of the ankle shows a trimalleolar fracture of the ankle involving the lateral malleolus, medial malleolus, and the posterior process of the tibia. Which of the following bones will also most likely be affected?

A. Navicular
B. Calcaneus
C. Cuneiform
D. Cuboid
E. Talus

64. A 72-year-old man comes to the physician because of a 3-year history of severe pain when walking. Physical examination shows the problems in his feet as shown in Fig. 5.5. What is the most likely diagnosis?

A. Coxa varus
B. Coxa valgus
C. Genu valgus
D. Genu vara
E. Hallux valgus

65. A 63-year-old woman comes to the physician because of a 1-year history of pain in her foot. The pain gets worse when she wears shoes. Physical examination shows constant extension at the metatarsophalangeal joints, hyperflexion at the proximal interphalangeal joints, and extension of distal interphalangeal joints (Fig. 5.6). Which of the following terms is most accurate to describe the signs of physical examination?

A. Pes planus
B. Pes cavus
C. Hammer toes
D. Claw toes
E. Hallux valgus

66. A 58-year-old man comes to the physician because of pain in his lower limb for the past 2 months. Physical examination shows point tenderness in the region of his greater sciatic foramen, with pain radiating down the posterior aspect of his thigh. An MRI of his pelvis and lower limb shows that the patient suffers from piriformis entrapment syndrome. He is directed to treatment by a physical therapist for stretching and relaxation of the muscle. Entrapment of which of the following nerves most likely mimicks the syndrome?

A. L4
B. L5
C. S1
D. S2
E. S3

67. A 22-year-old woman is brought to the emergency department after being found in a comatose condition, having lain for an unknown length of time on the tile floor of the courtyard. Cocaine is found in her possession. Physical examination shows signs of ischemia in the gluteal region. After regaining consciousness, she exhibits paralysis of knee flexion and dorsal and plantar flexion and sensory loss in the limb. What is the most likely diagnosis?
    A. Tibial nerve injury
    B. S1–2 nerve compression
    C. Gluteal crush injury
    D. Piriformis entrapment syndrome
    E. Femoral nerve entrapment

68. A 45-year-old woman is brought to the emergency department because of severe pain at her right hip and thigh. She has a history of multiple sclerosis (MS) and was recently treated with corticosteroids following an MS exacerbation. Physical examination shows reduced passive and active range of motion of the hip. An MRI examination shows avascular necrosis of the femoral head (Fig. 5.7). Which of the following arteries is most likely injured, resulting in avascular necrosis?
    A. Deep circumflex iliac
    B. Acetabular branch of obturator
    C. Descending branch of lateral circumflex femoral
    D. Second perforating branch of deep femoral
    E. Ascending branch of medial circumflex femoral

69. A 27-year-old woman is brought to the emergency department because of a penetrating injury in the popliteal region by an object thrown from a riding lawnmower. Physical examination shows no motor and sensory loss below the knee. During the operation, after making a midline incision in the skin of the popliteal fossa, a vein of moderate size is shown in the superficial tissues. What vein would be expected at this location?
    A. Popliteal
    B. Perforating tributary to the deep femoral
    C. Great saphenous
    D. Small saphenous
    E. Superior medial genicular

70. A 58-year-old diabetic patient comes to the physician because of a 2-year history of a painful foot. Physical examination shows that the patient has peripheral vascular disease. There is no detectable dorsalis pedis arterial pulse, but the posterior tibial pulse is strong. Which of the following arteries will most likely provide adequate collateral supply from the plantar surface to the toes and dorsum of the foot?
    A. Anterior tibial
    B. Fibular
    C. Arcuate
    D. Medial plantar
    E. Lateral plantar

71. A 32-year-old man is brought to the emergency department after an injury to his foot while playing football with his college friends. When the injury occurred, he heard a popping sound at the ankle joint. Physical examination shows an inability to stand on the toes

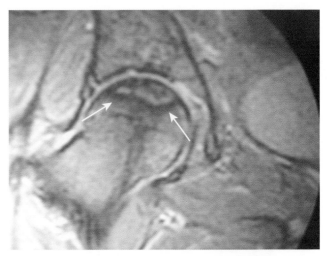

• Fig. 5.7

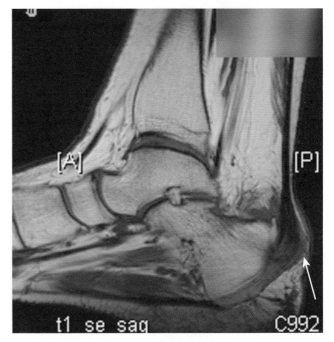

• Fig. 5.8

on the affected leg and tenderness with severe swelling near the heel. An MRI of the ankle shows multiple tendinous tears (Fig. 5.8). Which of the following bones is associated with the muscle tears?
    A. Navicular
    B. Cuboid
    C. Calcaneus
    D. Sustentaculum tali
    E. Talus

Questions 72–95

72. An 18-year-old woman is brought to the emergency department after she fell when she leaped for an overhead shot during her tennis practice and landed with her foot inverted. Physical examination shows swelling of the lateral aspect of the foot. An x-ray of the foot shows an avulsion fracture of the tuberosity of the fifth

metatarsal. Part of the tuberosity is pulled off, producing pain and edema. Which of the following muscles is pulling on the fractured fragment?

A. Fibularis longus
B. Tibialis posterior
C. Fibularis brevis
D. Extensor digitorum brevis
E. Adductor hallucis

73. A 58-year-old female employee of a housecleaning business comes to the physician with a 2-day history of a constant burning pain in her knees. She has no history of arthritis. Pain usually gets worse with activities. Physical examination shows severe swelling, warm to touch, and tenderness of the affected knee (Fig. 5.9). Which of the following structures is most likely affected?

A. Prepatellar bursa
B. Infrapatellar bursa
C. Semimembranosus bursa
D. Suprapatellar bursa
E. Subsartorial bursa (anserine bursa)

74. A 42-year-old mother of three children comes to the physician with her youngest son because he cannot walk yet even though he is 4 years old. Physical examinations show an unstable hip joint. An x-ray of the hip joint shows no deformity. The stability of the joint in childhood is most likely provided by which of the following ligaments?

A. Iliofemoral
B. Pubofemoral
C. Ischiofemoral
D. Ligament of the head of the femur
E. Transverse acetabular

75. A 45-year-old is brought to the emergency department by an ambulance after his left leg impacted a fence post when he was thrown from a powerful four-wheel all-terrain vehicle. Physical examination shows minor lacerations and swelling of the left knee and positive posterior drawer test. Which of the following structures was most likely injured?

A. Anterior cruciate ligament
B. Posterior cruciate ligament
C. Fibular collateral ligament
D. Lateral meniscus
E. Patellar ligament

76. A 55-year-old man comes to the physician because he cannot walk more than 5 minutes without feeling severe pain in his feet. The pain has caused an inability to perform daily activities over the past 6 months. Physical examination shows the feet of the patient shown in Fig. 5.10 and pain upon trying to perform a single-leg heel rise test. What is the most common cause of this condition?

A. Collapse of medial longitudinal arch, with eversion and abduction of the forefoot
B. Exaggerated height of the medial longitudinal arch of the foot
C. Collapse of long plantar ligament
D. Collapse of medial collateral (deltoid) ligament
E. Collapse of plantar calcaneonavicular ligament

77. A 32-year-old woman is brought to the emergency department 30 minutes after she was involved in a motor vehicle collision. Physical examination shows swelling, multiple bruises, and minor lacerations over the lateral aspect of the left midthigh. X-rays of the lower limb show a distal fracture of the femur. The patient is in severe pain, and a nerve block proximal to the injury is administered. What landmark is accurate for localizing the nerve for injection of anesthetics?

A. 1.5 cm superolateral to the pubic tubercle
B. 1.5 cm medial to the anterior superior iliac spine
C. 1.5 cm lateral to the femoral pulse
D. 1.5 cm medial to the femoral pulse
E. Midway between the anterior superior iliac spine and pubic symphysis

78. A 39-year-old woman comes to the physician because of a painful foot. The pain started a couple of months ago, and it has been gradually worsening especially with wearing narrow-toed shoes. She also has a tingling

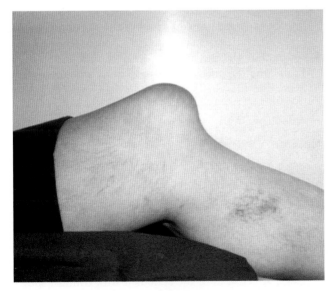

• **Fig. 5.9**

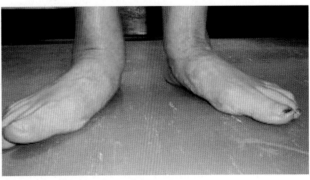

Pes planus

• **Fig. 5.10**

sensation of the foot. An MRI of the foot shows a Morton neuroma. Physical examination most likely showed a palpable mass between which of the following space?

A. Between the third and fourth metatarsophalangeal joints

B. Between the second and third metatarsophalangeal joints

C. Between the first and second metatarsophalangeal joints

D. Between the fourth and fifth metatarsophalangeal joints

E. In the region of the second, third, and fourth metatarsophalangeal joints

79. A 34-year-old man comes to the physician because of a 1-week history of pain in his foot. The pain is intense with the first few steps in the morning. Physical examination shows tenderness and warm skin over the plantar surface of the foot indicating an inflammation of the tough band of tissue stretching from the calcaneus to the ball of the foot. Which of the following conditions is most characteristic of these symptoms?

A. Morton neuroma

B. Ankle eversion sprain

C. Tarsal tunnel syndrome

D. Plantar fasciitis

E. Inversion sprain of the ankle

80. An otherwise healthy 2-week-old boy is brought to the physician by his father because of an atypical appearance of his feet. He is a full-term and his mother had received regular prenatal care. Physical examination shows that he has inversion and adduction of the forefoot relative to the hindfoot and plantar flexion. No other deformity is found. Which of the following terms is diagnostic for the signs observed on physical examination?

A. Coxa vara

B. Talipes equinovarus

C. Hallux valgus

D. Hallux varus

E. Plantar fasciitis

81. A 71-year-old man with a past history of polio comes to the physician because of difficulty in walking. Physical examination shows extension at the metatarsophalangeal joints with flexion of both the proximal and distal interphalangeal joints. Which of the following descriptions is most appropriate for this patient's condition?

A. Hallux valgus

B. Pes planus

C. Hammertoes

D. Claw toes

E. Pes cavus

82. An otherwise healthy 62-year-old man is brought by his son to the emergency department 20 minutes after he experienced an inability to walk by himself properly while he was walking with his dog. Physical examination shows a very brisk reaction in the deep tendon reflex test of the ankle. A CT scan of the head shows a stroke. Which of the following nerves is most likely responsible for the reflex arc?

A. Common fibular

B. Superficial fibular

C. Deep fibular

D. Tibial

E. Superficial and deep fibular

83. A 72-year-old man is brought to the emergency department after he fell. Physical examination shows that the left leg is shorter than the right leg and it is laterally rotated on a supine position. An x-ray of the hip shows a femoral neck fracture. Two months after a successful hip replacement, the patient has diminished sensation in the region of distribution of the posterior femoral cutaneous nerve. Which of the following is characteristic of this nerve?

A. Cutaneous supply of the superior aspect of the gluteal region

B. Arises from sacral spinal nerve levels S1, S2, and S3

C. Motor innervation of the obturator internus and gemelli muscles

D. Injury results in meralgia paresthetica

E. Provides origin of the sural nerve

84. A 34-year-old woman is brought to the emergency department 30 minutes after she was involved in a motor vehicle collision. She sustained a direct blow to the medial aspect of the right knee by the dashboard of the vehicle. Physical and radiologic examinations show the lateral dislocation of the patella. Which of the following structures requires strengthening by physical rehabilitation to prevent future dislocation of the patella?

A. Vastus lateralis

B. Vastus medialis

C. Vastus intermedius

D. Rectus femoris

E. Patellar ligament

85. A 15-year-old football player comes to the physician because of a small cut over the knee he had during training. Physical examination shows a 2 cm long superficial laceration over the lateral aspect of the left knee. While palpating the knee joint, a small bony structure is felt lateral to the patella. An x-ray of the knee is shown in Fig. 5.11. The patient has no past history of any knee problems. What is the most likely diagnosis?

A. Enlarged prepatellar bursa

B. Osgood-Schlatter disease

C. Normal intercondylar eminence

D. Bipartite patella

E. Injury to lateral meniscus

86. A 48-year-old woman comes to the emergency department because of a 30-minute history of severe abdominal pain. Physical examination shows that the pain is disproportionate to physical examination findings. A CT scan of the abdomen with contrast shows reduced blood flow to the superior mesenteric artery.

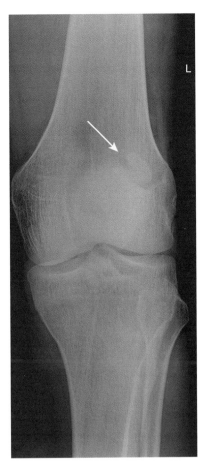

• Fig. 5.11

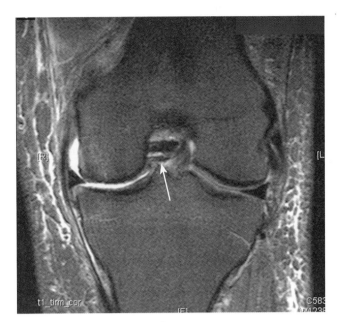

• Fig. 5.12

An abdominopelvic catheterization via femoral access is ordered for antegrade angiography. Which of the following landmarks is most likely used to guide the puncture of the artery?

A. Halfway between anterior superior iliac spine and pubic symphysis
B. 4.5 cm lateral to the pubic tubercle
C. Midpoint of the inguinal skin crease
D. Medial aspect of femoral head
E. Lateral to the fossa ovalis

87. A 23-year-old man is brought to the emergency department after injuring his knee while playing football. Physical examination shows tenderness and swelling of the knee. The knee is being locked in a flexed position. An MRI of the knee shows a bucket-handle meniscal tear (Fig. 5.12). Which of the following ligaments is most likely injured?

A. Posterior cruciate
B. Tibial collateral
C. Fibular collateral
D. Anterior cruciate
E. Coronary

88. A 27-year-old man triathlon competitor comes to the physician because he often experiences deep pain in one calf. A week ago, the pain almost caused him to drop out of a regional track-and-field event. An ultrasound of the

popliteal fossa shows the existence of an accessory portion of the medial head of the gastrocnemius, compressing the popliteal artery. Above the medial head of the gastrocnemius, the superior medial border of the fossa is formed by which of the following structures?

A. Tendon of biceps femoris
B. Tendons of semitendinosus and semimembranosus
C. Tendon of plantaris
D. Adductor hiatus
E. Popliteus

89. A 45-year-old woman comes to the physician because of severe headaches for the past 2 months. Imaging shows a tumor of the brain. During the surgical procedure a portion of the dura mater covering the brain is removed together with the tumor that has invaded the skull. To replace this important tissue covering of the brain, a band of the aponeurotic tissue of the lateral aspect of the thigh, covering the vastus lateralis muscle, is used. What muscle, supplied by the inferior gluteal nerve, inserts into this band of dense tissue as part of its insertion?

A. Gluteus medius
B. Gluteus minimus
C. Gluteus maximus
D. Tensor fasciae latae
E. Rectus femoris

90. A 28-year-old basketball player is brought to the emergency department because of a knee injury. Physical examination shows swelling of the medial aspect of the knee and tenderness. An MRI of the knee shows a tear in a medial ligament of the knee, the tubercle on the superior aspect of the medial femoral condyle could be seen more clearly than in most individuals. What muscle attaches to this tubercle?

A. Semimembranosus
B. Gracilis
C. Popliteus

D. Adductor magnus

E. Vastus medialis

91. A 65-year-old man is admitted to the hospital to undergo an iliofemoral bypass because of an occlusion of the proximal aspect of the femoral artery. The operation is performed successfully and the blood flow between the iliac and femoral arteries is restored. During the procedure the proximal portion of the femoral artery is isolated and gently separated it from surrounding tissues. Posterior to the femoral sheath, what muscle forms the lateral portion of the floor of the femoral triangle?

A. Adductor longus

B. Iliopsoas

C. Sartorius

D. Pectineus

E. Rectus femoris

92. A 37-year-old woman had been in pain for months from piriformis entrapment syndrome, which was not relieved by physical therapy. Part of the sciatic nerve passed through the piriformis, and a decision was made for surgical resection of the muscle. When the area of entrapment was identified and cleared, a tendon could be seen emerging through the lesser sciatic foramen, at first hidden by two smaller muscles and several nerves and vessels destined for the region of the perineum. The tendon of which of the following muscles pass through this opening?

A. Obturator internus

B. Obturator externus

C. Quadratus femoris

D. Gluteus minimus

E. Gluteus medius

93. A 67-year-old woman comes to the physician because of a 1-year history of osteoporosis. An x-ray of the lower limb shows an angle of 160 degrees made by the axis of the femoral neck to the axis of the femoral shaft. Which of the following conditions is associated with these examination findings?

A. Coxa vara

B. Coxa valga

C. Genu valgum

D. Genu varum

E. Hallux valgus

94. A 34-year-old man comes to the physician because of a 1-week history of pain in his foot. Physical examination shows inflammation of the tough band of tissue stretching from the calcaneus to the ball of the foot. Which of the following conditions is characteristic of these symptoms?

A. Pott fracture

B. Dupuytren fracture

C. Tarsal tunnel

D. Plantar fasciitis

E. Rupture of spring ligament

95. A 50-year-old woman is brought to the emergency department 30 minutes after she was involved in a motor vehicle collision. An MRI of the knee shows an injured anterior cruciate ligament. Physical examination shows a positive drawer sign. Which of the following signs is expected to be present during physical examination?

A. The tibia can be slightly displaced anteriorly

B. The tibia can be slightly displaced posteriorly

C. The fibula can be slightly displaced posteriorly

D. The fibula can be slightly displaced anteriorly

E. The tibia and fibula can be slightly displaced anteriorly

Questions 96–120

96. A 23-year-old male basketball player injured his foot during training and is admitted to the emergency department. An MRI examination shows a hematoma around the medial malleolus. Physical examination shows excessive eversion of the foot. Which of the following ligaments most likely has a tear?

A. Plantar calcaneonavicular (spring)

B. Calcaneofibular

C. Long plantar

D. Short plantar

E. medial collateral (deltoid)

97. A 5-year-old boy is brought to the emergency department 30 minutes after he was involved in a motor vehicle collision. An x-ray shows a fracture of the head of the femur. An MRI examination shows a large hematoma. Which of the following arteries is most likely injured?

A. Deep circumflex iliac

B. Acetabular branch of obturator

C. Descending branch of lateral circumflex femoral

D. Medial circumflex femoral

E. Retinacular branches of lateral circumflex femoral arteries

98. A 72-year-old woman is brought to the emergency department because she lost consciousness. A CT scan of the brain shows an area of ischemic stroke. Neurologic examination shows no response to the ankle reflex test. Which of the following nerve roots is most likely responsible for this reflex?

A. L2

B. L3

C. L4

D. L5

E. S1

99. A 20-year-old man comes to the physician because of a 3-month history of progressive difficulty to flexing and medially rotating his thigh while running and climbing. Which of the following muscles is most likely damaged?

A. Rectus femoris

B. Tensor fasciae latae

C. Vastus intermedius

D. Semimembranosus

E. Sartorius

100. A 69-year-old man comes to the physician because of a 6-month history of progressive worsening cold and pale foot. Physical examination shows no pulse in the popliteal artery. An ultrasound of the popliteal artery shows an occlusion of the artery and a diagnosis of peripheral vascular disease is made. An ultrasound of the femoral and tibial arteries is also performed. What is the landmark to feel the pulse of the femoral artery?
A. Adductor canal
B. Femoral triangle
C. Popliteal fossa
D. Inguinal canal
E. Pubic symphysis

101. A 49-year-old man comes to the physician because of a 6-month history of progressive difficulty in walking. Physical examination shows absence of pulses in the arteries of the lower limb. An ultrasound examination of the lower limb shows an occlusion of his femoral artery at the proximal portion of the adductor canal. A diagnosis of peripheral vascular disease is made. Which of the following arteries will most likely provide collateral circulation to the thigh?
A. Descending branch of the lateral circumflex femoral
B. Descending genicular
C. Medial circumflex femoral
D. First perforating branch of deep femoral
E. Obturator artery

102. A 34-year-old man comes to the physician because of a 2-day history of increased pain at the area of the lower abdomen and upper thigh. He has been lifting heavy weights for 10 years. Two days ago, while making a maximal effort, he drops the weight and immediately grabbed at his upper thigh, writhing in pain. Physical examination shows a femoral hernia. What reference structure would be found immediately lateral to the herniated structures?
A. Femoral vein
B. Femoral artery
C. Pectineus muscle
D. Femoral nerve
E. Adductor longus muscle

103. A 25-year-old man is admitted to the hospital for a detoxification program. He has been an intravenous drug abuser injecting himself with temazepam (a powerful intermediate acting drug in the same group as diazepam [Valium]) and heroin for 5 years, leaving much residual scar tissue over points of vascular access. The femoral veins in his groin are the only accessible and patent veins for intravenous use. Which of the following landmarks is the most reliable to identify these veins?
A. The femoral vein lies medial to the femoral artery.
B. The femoral vein lies within the femoral canal.
C. The femoral vein lies lateral to the femoral artery.
D. The femoral vein lies directly medial to the femoral nerve.
E. The femoral vein lies lateral to the femoral nerve.

104. A 42-year-old man is admitted to the emergency department because he was bitten on his posterior thigh by a dog 2 hours ago. The superficial wound is sutured, an antirabies shot is administered, and the patient is released. Four days later the patient returns to the emergency department because of high fever and swollen lymph nodes. Which group of nodes first receives lymph from the infected wound?
A. External iliac
B. Vertical group of superficial inguinal
C. Deep inguinal
D. Horizontal group of superficial inguinal
E. Internal iliac

105. A 19-year-old man is brought to the hospital because of a 2-hour history of being shot in the lateral aspect of the right foot by a bullet. The patient is hemodynamically stabilized, and his vital signs are within normal limits. An x-ray of the foot shows that the base of the fifth metatarsal is completely obliterated. Which of the following muscles is most likely affected by this injury?
A. Tibialis anterior
B. Fibularis longus
C. Gastrocnemius
D. Fibularis brevis
E. Extensor hallucis longus

106. A 22-year-old woman is brought to the emergency department 30 minutes after she was involved in a motor vehicle collision with her left and right leg pinned under her motorcycle. She appears to be well, and her vital signs are within normal limits. An x-ray shows a fracture of her pelvis that does not require surgery. During healing of the pelvic fracture, a nerve becomes entrapped in the bone callus. Six months after the incident, physical examination shows inability to adduct her thigh. Which of the following nerves is most likely affected?
A. Obturator
B. Femoral
C. Inferior gluteal
D. Superior gluteal
E. Tibial

107. A 29-year-old man is brought to the physician for removal of a cast from his left leg. He had sustained a fracture of the left lower limb 6 weeks prior, which was immobilized in a cast that extended from just below the knee to the foot. At the time of injury, there was severe pain but normal strength in the lower limb. When the cast was removed, physical examination showed a pronounced left foot drop with paresthesia and sensory loss over the dorsum of the left foot and lateral leg. Injury to which of the following nerves is the most likely cause of this patient's symptoms?
A. Common fibular
B. Superficial fibular
C. Deep fibular
D. Sciatic
E. Tibial

108. A 12-year-old boy is brought to the physician by his father because of redness and swelling of his left foot for 24 hours. Three days earlier he had scraped his foot while wading in a drainage ditch. Physical examination of the foot shows a purulent abrasion with edema, erythema, and tenderness on the lateral side. Infection will most likely spread from the lateral side of the foot to the regional lymph nodes in which of the following areas?
    A. Lateral surface of the thigh
    B. Medial malleolus, posteriorly
    C. Popliteal fossa
    D. Sole of the foot
    E. Superficial inguinal area

109. A 22-year-old man is brought to the emergency department because he collided with one of his teammates and is unable to walk. Physical examination shows when the posterior drawer test is performed the tibia moves backward in relation to his femur. Injury to which structure is confirmed by performing this test?
    A. Anterior cruciate ligament
    B. Fibular collateral ligament
    C. Tibial collateral ligament
    D. Medial meniscus
    E. Posterior cruciate ligament

110. A 16-year-old boy is brought to the emergency department by his parents because of pain in his right foot. An x-ray of the foot shows a fracture of the first and second toes. He receives a local anesthetic (lidocaine) injection in the first web space of his foot, to permit easy manipulation and correction. Which of the following nerves is most likely blocked by the local anesthetic?
    A. Saphenous
    B. Cutaneous branch of deep fibular
    C. Cutaneous branch of superficial fibular
    D. Sural
    E. Common fibular

111. During an interview, a 30-year-old man who is a psychiatric patient suddenly becomes aggressive. To calm him down, the patient is given an intramuscular injection in the upper lateral quadrant of the buttock. The injection is given at this specific location to prevent damage to which of the following nerves?
    A. Lateral femoral cutaneous
    B. Sciatic
    C. Superior gluteal
    D. Obturator
    E. Inferior gluteal

112. A 24-year-old woman is brought to the emergency department because of inability to walk after she received a lateral blow to the knee during a tackle in a football game. Physical examination shows positive anterior drawer sign. An MRI shows injury to several structures of the knee, including her medial meniscus.

Which of the following structures is also likely injured by the tackle?
    A. Tibial collateral ligament
    B. Fibular collateral ligament
    C. Lateral meniscus
    D. Posterior cruciate ligament
    E. Tendon of the semitendinosus

113. A 58-year-old woman comes to the physician because of a 5-year history of varicose veins on the medial aspect of her foot. A varicose vein striping procedure is performed, and the veins are removed. One month later the patient returns to the physician because of loss of sensation over the medial aspect of her leg and foot. Which of the following nerves is most likely injured during the procedure?
    A. Saphenous
    B. Obturator
    C. Lateral femoral cutaneous
    D. Tibial
    E. Femoral

114. A 16-year-old girl is brought to the physician by her mother because of a 2-day history of an inversion sprain of her ankle during dance class. Physical examination most likely will shows tenderness over which of the following ligaments?
    A. Plantar calcaneonavicular (spring)
    B. Calcaneofibular
    C. Long plantar
    D. Short plantar
    E. medial collateral (deltoid)

115. A 58-year-old man comes to the physician for a routine examination. Physical examination shows a hyperreflexive patellar reflex. Which of the following muscles contribute to the tendon that is struck when testing this reflex?
    A. Quadriceps femoris
    B. Quadratus femoris
    C. Sartorius
    D. Pectineus
    E. Biceps femoris

116. A 22-year-old woman is brought to the emergency department 30 minutes after she was involved in a motor vehicle collision with her left and right leg pinned under her motorcycle. She appears to be well, and her vital signs are within normal limits. Physical examination shows bruising, and an obvious deformity is seen over her left knee joint. An x-ray shows a posteriorly dislocated supracondylar fracture. An ultrasound of the knee shows severe compression of the popliteal artery. Which of the following arteries would ensure adequate blood supply to the leg and foot in this patient?
    A. Medial circumflex femoral
    B. Lateral circumflex femoral
    C. Anterior tibial artery
    D. Posterior tibial artery
    E. Fibular artery

117. A 68-year-old man comes to the physician because of a 6-month history of progressive difficulty with walking. Physical examination shows a nontender, cold lower limb. The pulse of the posterior tibial artery is absent. A Doppler ultrasound of the leg indicates a thrombotic occlusion of his femoral artery. A revascularization procedure involving the common iliac artery is performed. Postoperatively, nerve conduction studies show decreased activity in the nerve that innervates the adductors of the thigh. Which of the following nerves is this?
A. Femoral
B. Obturator
C. Common fibular
D. Tibial
E. Sciatic

118. A 30-year-old woman is brought to the emergency department 20 minutes after she was involved in a motor vehicle collision with her right hip caught beneath the motorcycle at the scene. She is hypovolemic and appears to be in a shock. An ultrasound examination shows massive hematoma in the medial thigh. A CT scan shows a fracture of the femur with a ruptured femoral artery. She is taken to the operating room for repair of the damaged structures. Two days postoperatively, the patient has loss of sensation to the anteromedial thigh and medial side of her leg and foot. Branches of which of the following nerves were most likely injured in the repair of the fracture?
A. Femoral
B. Saphenous
C. Obturator
D. Tibial
E. Fibular

119. A 57-year-old man comes to the physician because of a 6-month history of increasing difficulty walking and an area of numbness on the dorsum of his right foot. Physical examination shows a hard mass at the anterolateral aspect of his right leg just below the knee. A CT scan of the leg shows a large bone tumor between the fibula and tibia that is compressing a nerve, accounting for his neurological symptoms. Which of the following is the most likely description of abnormalities on neurologic examination?
A. Decreased/absent knee jerk reflex and decreased sensation on the medial aspect of the leg
B. Weakness of flexion at the knee and decreased sensation of the plantar aspect of the foot
C. Weakness of eversion at the ankle and decreased sensation between the first and second toes
D. Weakness of inversion, dorsiflexion at the ankle, and decreased sensation between the first and second toes
E. Weakness of plantar flexion at the ankle, weakness of toe flexion, decreased sensation of the plantar aspect of the foot

120. A 60-year-old man comes to the physician because of a 3-month history of bouts of numbness and tingling on the medial aspect of his heel during exercise. Physical examination shows trouble tiptoeing and positive Tinel sign. Which of the following conditions is most characteristic of these symptoms?
A. Plantar fasciitis
B. Ankle inversion sprain
C. Morton neuroma
D. Lateral ligament
E. Tarsal tunnel syndrome

Questions 121–143

121. A 50-year-old man comes to the physician for a follow-up examination. He has been diabetic and hypertensive for the past 20 years. Physical examination shows paresthesia in a classic glove and stocking distribution and low pulse of the dorsalis pedis artery. Which of the following locations is typically this artery palpated?
A. Between the tendons of extensor hallucis longus and extensor digitorum longus on the dorsum of the foot
B. Superior to flexor hallucis longus just distal to the tarsal tunnel
C. Inferolateral to the pubic symphysis and medial to the deep dorsal vein of the penis
D. 2 cm anterior to the medial malleolus
E. 2 cm posterior to the medial malleolus

122. A 35-year-old man is brought to the emergency department 20 minutes after he was involved in a motor vehicle collision. The patient is undergoing reconstructive arm surgery with an autograft using a weak adductor of the leg located superficially on the medial side of the thigh. Which muscle is most likely being harvested to perform this reconstruction?
A. Gracilis
B. Sartorius
C. Rectus femoris
D. Vastus lateralis
E. Vastus medialis

123. A 39-year-old woman comes to the physician because of a 3-day history of painful left buttock. She is a schoolteacher, and unwittingly she sat on a thumbtack that a student placed on her chair. Physical examination shows a left inflamed painful buttock. Which group of nodes will first receive lymph from the infected wound?
A. Superficial inguinal horizontal group
B. Superficial inguinal vertical group
C. Superior and inferior gluteal nodes
D. External iliac
E. Deep inguinal

124. A 25-year-old man comes to the physician because of a 2-week history of pain at his knee joint. He exercises regularly, and 2 weeks ago he injured himself as he was running in the open stadium. Physical examination shows a "tearing" pain sensation as he is trying to flex his knee. Based on these symptoms which of the following actions are affected due to this injury?

A. Flexion of the hip and extension of the knee

B. Extension of the hip and dorsiflexion

C. Medial rotation of the hip

D. Lateral rotation of the hip

E. Hip extension and knee flexion

125. A 24-year-old woman is brought to the emergency department because of excruciating pain in her thigh. She was exercising at the local gym, and she fell suddenly and developed pain and swelling on the right buttock. This happened following a forceful thigh movement. Physical examination shows severe weakness of right hip extension and knee flexion. Adduction of the thigh is also slightly weak. An x-ray shows an avulsion fracture of the ischial tuberosity. Which of the following group of muscles has most likely been involved in this process?

A. Adductor brevis, adductor longus, adductor magnus, pectineus, and gracilis

B. Biceps femoris, semimembranosus, semitendinosus, and adductor magnus

C. Iliacus and psoas major

D. Gluteus medius and gluteus minimus

E. Gluteus maximus and adductor magnus

F. Iliacus, psoas major, rectus femoris, and sartorius

126. A 6-year-old boy is brought to the physician by his parents for a follow-up examination. He has a family history of muscular disease leading to wheelchair dependency. Physical examination shows difficulty in standing from the seated position. He bends forward, uses his hands to help him push up from the floor, and then straightens his knees to stand. Which of the following muscles is most likely involved by this disease process?

A. Tibialis posterior and gastrocnemius

B. Quadratus femoris

C. Gluteus medius and gluteus minimus

D. Gluteus maximus

E. Hamstrings

F. Iliopsoas

127. A 43-year-old woman receives deep intramuscular injections for the past week for treatment of a sexually transmitted disease. She complains to her doctor that she has difficulty walking. During physical examination her right hip drops every time she raises her right foot. Which of the following injection locations will most likely correspond with the physical presentation of this patient?

A. Superomedial quadrant of the buttock

B. Superolateral quadrant of the buttock

C. Inferomedial quadrant of the buttock

D. Inferolateral quadrant of the buttock

E. Posterior thigh

128. A 22-year-old man is admitted to the emergency department because of a 30-minute history of acute right knee pain after sustaining a kick injury to an extended leg. An MRI of the lower limb showed that the trauma caused anterior displacement of the tibia with respect to his femur. Which of the following ligaments was most likely injured?

A. Fibular (lateral) collateral

B. Tibial (medial) collateral

C. Patellar

D. Anterior cruciate

E. Posterior cruciate

F. Oblique popliteal

129. A 51-year-old man is brought to the emergency department because of a 2-month history of progressively worsening cough and growing mass in his right groin. He was treated for tuberculosis last year, and a large flocculent mass was found over the lateral lumbar spine. Physical examination shows increased tenderness just medial to the ipsilateral anterior superior iliac spine. This pattern of involvement most likely suggests an abscess tracking along which of the following muscles?

A. Piriformis

B. Psoas major

C. Adductor longus

D. Gluteus maximus

E. Obturator internus

130. A 23-year-old man is taken to the emergency department because of anorexia, nausea, vomiting, and severe abdominal pain in the right lower quadrant. Physical examination shows tenderness in the right lower quadrant with rebound tenderness. A suspicion of diagnosis of appendicitis is made. To confirm this diagnosis, an attempt to straighten the patient's flexed thigh is made. This causes the patient to wince with pain. Which of the following muscles most likely caused this symptom?

A. Adductor magnus

B. Psoas major

C. Biceps femoris

D. Obturator internus

E. Gluteus maximus

131. A 60-year-old man comes to the physician because of a 3-day history of pain on the medial aspect of his thigh. He describes the pain to be constant and nonradiating. Physical examination shows numbness on the medial aspect of his leg and medial plantar arch. The nerve involved in this patient's numbness is closely associated with a structure with which of the following characteristics?

A. Empties into the popliteal vein

B. In its ascent in the medial aspect of the leg, it travels posterior to the medial condyle of the femur

C. In its ascent in the medial aspect of the leg, it travels anterior to the medial condyle of the femur

D. It arches posterior to the medial malleolus

E. It is associated with nodes that drain to the horizontal group of superficial inguinal nodes

132. A 56-year-old man comes to the physician for a follow-up examination of repeated injury and ulcers to his great toe. He has diabetes and hypertension for the past 10 years and finds it difficult maintaining his shoes because the tips of the shoes around the toe area easily wear down. He used to enjoy playing soccer on weekends but has found it difficult to be involved. Physical examination shows numbness of the first two toes. Which of the following nerves is most likely affected?
A. Superior gluteal nerve injury
B. Inferior gluteal nerve injury
C. Deep fibular nerve injury
D. Superficial fibular nerve injury
E. Common fibular nerve injury

133. A 34-year-old man comes to the physician because of a 2-day history of increased pain at the area of the lower abdomen and upper thigh. He has been lifting heavy weights for 10 years. Two days ago, while making a maximal effort, he dropped the weight and immediately grabbed at his upper thigh, writhing in pain. Physical examination shows pain and tingling sensation radiating down the inside of his thigh that is exacerbated upon thigh movement. A hernia through which opening would most likely cause this presentation?
A. Femoral ring
B. Superficial inguinal ring
C. Deep inguinal ring
D. Fossa ovalis
E. Obturator canal

134. A 22-year-old woman comes to the emergency department because of a deep stab wound to her posterior thigh. The wound is sutured with two layers of sutures, deep and superficial, and the patient is discharged. Three days later she develops a wound infection, and the lymphatics that first receive drainage from the deep wound area are enlarged. Which of the following group of lymph nodes is this?
A. External iliac
B. Superficial inguinal
C. Deep inguinal
D. Common iliac
E. Internal iliac

135. A 69-year-old woman is brought to the emergency department because she fell down the stairs. An x-ray of her foot shows a fracture of the talocrural (tibiotalar) joint. Which of the following movements are taking place at this joint?
A. Plantar flexion and dorsiflexion
B. Inversion and eversion
C. Plantar flexion, dorsiflexion, inversion, and eversion
D. Plantar flexion and inversion
E. Dorsiflexion and eversion

136. A 22-year-old woman is brought to the emergency department 30 minutes after she was involved in a motor vehicle collision with her left and right leg pinned under her motorcycle. She appears to be well, and her vital signs are within normal limits. Physical examination shows a swelling of her right knee. An ultrasound examination shows a large hematoma of the popliteal artery compressing her tibial nerve. Neurologic examination will show diminished in strength which of the following movements?
A. Dorsiflexion of the foot
B. Flexion of the thigh
C. Extension of the digits
D. Extension of the leg
E. Plantar flexion of the foot

137. A 50-year-old woman is brought to the emergency department because of a 2-day history of painful swelling to the left leg, fever, and malaise. The patient has a history of type 2 diabetes mellitus, and she was bitten on the left leg by an insect a week ago. She scratched the pruritic area and applied alcohol to the site when the swelling increased. A purulent fluid began to drain from it 2 days later. Physical examination shows a 5 × 5 cm tender, fluctuant swelling over the anterolateral aspect of the middle third of the left leg, which drained copious amounts of purulent fluid. Which of the following findings is most likely to be also present during physical examination of this patient?
A. Tender vertical group of superficial inguinal lymph nodes
B. Enlarged horizontal group of superficial inguinal lymph nodes
C. Enlarged group of deep inguinal lymph nodes
D. Enlarged popliteal lymph nodes
E. Enlarged iliac nodes

138. A 22-year-old woman is brought to the emergency department 30 minutes after she was involved in a motor vehicle collision with her left and right leg pinned under her motorcycle. She appears to be well, and her vital signs are within normal limits. Physical examination shows no deformity of the lower limb, but there is tenderness over the right ischiopubic ramus. An x-ray of the pelvis shows an inferiorly displaced fracture of the right superior and inferior pubic rami with dislocation of the right sacroiliac joint and pubic symphysis. An MRI examination confirms the diagnosis and shows rupture of the right obturator membrane. Which of the following physical examination findings are most likely to be seen in this patient?
A. Urinary and fecal incontinence and diminished sensation over the perineum
B. Weak adduction of the hip and diminished sensation over the lower medial thigh
C. Weak abduction of the hip and positive Trendelenburg sign
D. Weak flexion of the hip and diminished sensation over the anterior thigh and medial leg
E. Weak extension of the hip and diminished sensation over the posterior thigh

139. A 32-year-old man comes to the physician because of pain in the left ankle and foot. The patient recalls that during a football game, his left foot landed in a hole as he was running on an uneven dirt field. The ankle was externally rotated and everted while the knee twisted medially. He was unable to bear weight subsequently. Physical examination shows the left ankle is swollen and there is exquisite tenderness over the left medial malleolus and the proximal lateral leg. An x-ray of the left lower limb shows a displaced fracture of the neck of left fibula and a comminuted fracture of the tibial plafond and medial malleolus. Which of the following describes the most likely consequences of this injury?

A. Weak "push-off" while walking and numbness over the posteromedial leg

B. Weak ankle eversion and numbness over the dorsum of the foot

C. High stepping gait and numbness over the dorsum and first web space of the foot

D. Waddling gait and inability to feel a pin prick over the anterolateral leg

E. Swing-out gait and numbness over the medial leg

140. A 22-year-old woman is brought to the emergency department 30 minutes after she was involved in a motor vehicle collision with her left and right leg pinned under her motorcycle. She appears to be well, and her vital signs are within normal limits. Physical examination shows a painful left knee and leg and inability to bear weight on the affected limb. There is a joint effusion of the left knee, and tenderness over the medial and lateral side of the joint. A valgus stress test is positive, and the varus stress test is negative. An MRI of the left knee shows complete disruption of multiple ligament support structures of the knee. Which of the following symptoms will most likely be seen in physical examination?

A. Inability to extend the knee

B. Inability to flex the knee

C. Instability of the knee when walking down a flight of stairs

D. Instability of the knee when walking up a flight of stairs

E. Excessive extension of the knee and difficulty walking downstairs

141. A 22-year-old woman is brought to the emergency department because of pain and swelling to the right ankle. In a recent soccer game, she jumped to spike the ball then landed on the opponent's shoe with her right foot. She recalls hearing a loud "pop" and felt immediate pain to the ankle. She was unable to bear weight subsequently. Physical examination shows a right swollen ankle, with maximal tenderness inferior and anterior to the lateral malleolus. An x-ray of the foot and ankle showed no fractures. Which of the following ligaments were most likely teared?

A. Posterior talofibular

B. Plantar calcaneonavicular

C. Tibionavicular

D. Anterior talofibular

E. Calcaneofibular

142. A 30-year-old woman comes to the physician because of pain to the anterior left thigh. While participating in a 100-m race, she felt a sudden onset of pain in the anterior midthigh area and could only limp to the finish line. Physical examination shows a swollen, tender right thigh anteriorly. Extension of the knee is limited because of pain. An ultrasound examination of the thigh shows a defect in the fibers of the quadriceps femoris muscle. Which of the following is the embryologic origin of the affected structure?

A. Lateral plate mesoderm

B. Dorsolateral migration of neural crest cells

C. Preceded the development of chondrification centers

D. Intermediate mesoderm

E. Migration of cells from paraxial mesoderm

143. A 23-year-old woman delivers a boy at 37 weeks' gestation after an uneventful pregnancy. Physical examination shows the right second and third toes are fused. An x-ray of the right foot shows 14 phalanges in their correct position. Which of the following embryologic conditions explains the patient's deformity?

A. The digital ray for the third toe did not develop

B. Excessive neural crest cell migration into the foot

C. Incomplete apoptosis of tissue between digital rays

D. Lack of signal from the zone of polarizing activity (ZPA)

E. Faulty development of chondrification centers

Questions 144–148

144. A 22-year-old woman is brought to the emergency department 30 minutes after she was involved in a motor vehicle collision with her left and right leg pinned under her motorcycle. She appears to be well, and her vital signs are within normal limits. Physical examination shows pain in the right knee and an inability to bear weight. There are also several lacerations and a deep, 5-cm oblique laceration over the anterior right knee, which exposes the patella. She is unable to extend the right knee. An x-ray of the knee shows a displaced transverse fracture of the inferior pole of the patella. The superior fragment of the patella appears to be "high riding" over the anterior surface of the femur. Which of the following may most likely occur?

A. Blood and fat from the injury can enter the popliteus bursa

B. Blood and fat from the injury can enter the suprapatellar bursa

C. Joint fluid can enter the subcutaneous infrapatellar bursa

D. The deep infrapatellar bursa will be affected

E. The gastrocnemius bursa will not be affected

145. A 53-year-old woman comes to the physician because of a 6-month history of progressive difficulty in walking. Physical examination shows a positive Trendelenburg sign when she is asked to stand on her right leg. Which of the following nerve has been affected to produce the positive sign?

A. Sciatic
B. Right superior gluteal
C. Left inferior gluteal
D. Left superior gluteal
E. Right inferior gluteal

146. A 55-year-old man comes to the physician because of severe back pain for the past 2 days. The pain radiates down to the buttock, posterior thigh, and posterolateral leg. He also has numbness on the lateral side of his left foot. Physical examination shows decreased sensation to pain over the lateral side of the left foot. Deep tendon reflexes are absent at the left ankle, and there is a weakness of dorsiflexion of the left foot. Compression of which of the following nerve roots is the most likely cause of these findings?

A. T12
B. L2
C. L4
D. S1
E. S3

147. A 32-year-old man is brought to the emergency department because of severe pain to the left ankle and leg. During a game of football, his left foot landed in a hole as he was running on an uneven dirt field. He was unable subsequently to bear weight on his left limb. Physical examination shows a left swollen ankle, with exquisite tenderness over the left medial malleolus and over the distal third of lateral surface of the left leg. An x-ray of the left lower limb shows an inferiorly displaced fracture of the left medial malleolus and a spiral fracture of the distal third of the left fibula. Which of the following describes the most likely mechanism of this injury?

A. Forceful inversion of the ankle
B. Direct upward force from the talus into the tibial plafond
C. Forceful lateral rotation and eversion of the ankle
D. Forceful dorsiflexion of the foot
E. Extreme plantar flexion of the foot

148. A 15-year-old boy is brought to the emergency department by his parents after he falls and injures his ankle while skateboarding. Physical examination shows that his ankle is mildly sprained, and it is wrapped with an elastic bandage. The boy still has pain in his ankle. Which of the following peripheral nerves is involved in carrying pain sensation from the ankle joint?

A. Deep fibular
B. Femoral
C. Obturator
D. Posterior femoral cutaneous
E. Sural

Answers

Answers 1–24

1. A. The lumbosacral trunk consists of fibers from a portion of the ventral ramus of L4 and the entirety of the ventral ramus of L5 to provide continuity between the lumbar and sacral plexuses. The deep fibular nerve receives supply from segments of L4, L5, and S1. It supplies the extensor hallucis longus, tibialis anterior, extensor digitorum longus, and fibularis tertius, the main functions of which are extension of the toes and dorsiflexion of the ankle. L5 is responsible for cutaneous innervation of the dorsum of the foot. Injury to L4 would affect foot inversion by the tibialis anterior. Injury to L4 in the lumbosacral trunk would not affect the patellar tendon reflex because these fibers are delivered by the femoral nerve. Therefore an injury to the lumbosacral trunk would result in all of the patient's symptoms.

B. Nerve root injury at L5 and S1 would result in loss of sensation of the plantar aspect of the foot and motor loss of plantar flexion, with weakness of hip extension and abduction. The fibularis longus and brevis are supplied by the superficial fibular nerve, which is composed of fibers from segments L5, S1, and S2; these are responsible for eversion of the foot (especially S1).

C. Transection of the fibular division of the sciatic nerve would result in loss of function of all the muscles of the anterior and lateral compartments of the leg.

D. Injury to the sciatic nerve will affect hamstring muscles and all of the muscles below the knee.

E. Injury to the tibial nerve causes loss of plantar flexion and impaired inversion.
GAS 486–487; N 487–489; ABR/McM 275

2. A. The ventral ramus of L4 contains both sensory and motor nerve fibers. Injury from a stab wound could result in loss of sensation from the dermatome supplied by this segment. A dermatome is an area of skin supplied by a single spinal nerve; L4 supplies the medial aspect of the leg and foot.

B. The sensation of the little toe and lateral aspect of the foot including the heel are innervated by S1.

C. The upper medial thigh is innervated by L3.

D. The second, third, and fourth toes and lateral aspect of the leg are innervated by L5. E. S2 provides the sensation to the posterior aspect of the thigh, knee, and upper half of the leg (GAS Fig. 6.16).
GAS 35; N 398; ABR/McM 293

3. B. Injury to the superior gluteal nerve results in a characteristic motor loss, with paralysis of the gluteus medius

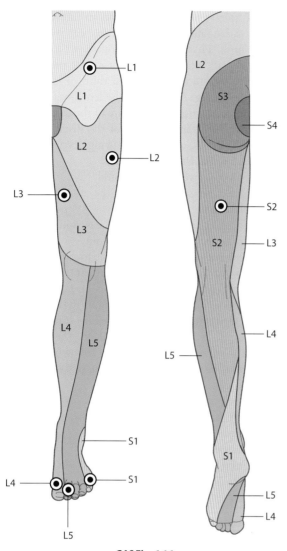

• *GAS* Fig. 6.16

and minimus. In addition to their role in abducting the thigh, the gluteus medius and minimus function to stabilize the pelvis. For example, the gluteus medius and gluteus minimus contract while the contralateral foot is lifted, preventing the contralateral pelvis from dropping. When the patient with a superior gluteal nerve injury is asked to stand on the affected limb, the pelvis descends on the opposite side. This is called positive Trendelenburg sign. In stepping forward, the affected individual leans over the injured side when lifting the good limb off the ground. The uninjured limb is then swung forward.

A. The gluteus maximus, supplied by the inferior gluteal nerve, is the main muscle responsible for allowing a person to rise from a sitting position to a standing position (extending the flexed hip).

C. Tipping of the pelvis to the right side while standing on the left foot indicates the injury to the left superior gluteal nerve.

D. Spinal nerve roots L1 and L2 and the femoral nerve are responsible for hip flexion.

E. The hamstring muscles, mainly responsible for flexing the knees to allow a person to sit down from a standing position, are innervated by the tibial division of the sciatic nerve.
GAS 569, 492, 564, 579; N 489; ABR/McM 325

4. **E.** The deep fibular nerve is responsible for innervating the muscles of the anterior compartment of the leg, which are responsible for toe extension, foot dorsiflexion, and inversion. Injury to this nerve will result in a foot drop and also loss of sensation of the first web space between the first and second toes. Unopposed (plantar) flexors of the foot, innervated by branches of the tibial nerve, will result in the plantar flexion of the foot in this patient. The ability to evert the affected foot indicates that the superficial fibular nerve is intact

A. Injury to the tibial nerve affects the posterior compartment muscles of the leg. The muscles in the posterior compartment are responsible for plantar flexion and toe flexion.

B and C. The common fibular nerve splits into the superficial and deep fibular nerves as it enters the lateral compartment of the foot, and these supply muscles in both the lateral and anterior compartments, respectively. The superficial fibular nerve innervates the fibularis longus and the fibularis brevis, which provide eversion of the foot. If the common fibular nerve were injured in this case, eversion of the foot would also be lost in addition to dorsiflexion and inversion.

D. The saphenous nerve, a continuation of the femoral nerve, is a cutaneous pure sensory nerve that supplies the medial side of the leg and foot.
GAS 627, 660; N 531; ABR/McM 344

5. **A.** In the subinguinal space, the femoral sheath is divided into three compartments: lateral, intermediate, and medial compartment. The medial compartment is also known as the femoral canal. The canal contains lymph nodes and adipose tissue. The femoral ring is the opening of the femoral canal, bounded medially by the lacunar ligament, laterally by the femoral vein, anteriorly by the inguinal ligament, and posteriorly by the pectineal ligament. The ring is closed by connective tissue. When the connective becomes weakened, part of the small intestine may protrude through the femoral ring, which is anterolateral aspect of the pubic tubercle.

B. The superficial inguinal ring is located superior to the pubic tubercle and the inguinal ligament. It is the opening of the medial end of the inguinal canal through which the spermatic cord or round ligament of the uterus exits.

C. The deep inguinal ring is located above the inguinal ligament and lateral to the inferior epigastric vessels, which is approximately a midpoint between the pubic tubercle and the anterior superior iliac spine.

D. The saphenous opening is an aperture of the fascia lata on the anterior aspect of the thigh. The opening is just lateral to the pubic tubercle and inferior to the inguinal ligament. The great saphenous vein passes through the saphenous opening to join the femoral vein.

E. The obturator canal is an opening of the obturator foramen bordered by the obturator membrane. The obturator vessels and nerve exit the pelvis to the thigh through the obturator canal.

GAS 298; N 256; ABR/McM 235

6. **D.** When the foot is rolled outward with eversion and abduction forces, the medial malleolus and medial collateral (deltoid) ligaments may become injured. The strength of the medial collateral (deltoid) ligaments may be stronger than the bone, which, with continuous force, may result in avulsion of the medial malleolus. The medial malleolus of the tibia is in close proximity of structures passing through the tarsal tunnel, including tendons of tibialis posterior, flexor digitorum longus, and flexor hallucis longus, the posterior tibial vessels, and the tibial nerve. Therefore the fracture of the medial malleolus may cause injury to the tibial nerve. Among the options, the tibial nerve is most likely injured in this case.

A. The superficial fibular nerve, which is a branch of the common fibular nerve, courses downward in the lateral compartment of the leg, innervating the fibularis longus and fibularis brevis. It enters the foot by piercing deep fascia and innervates the dorsum of the foot.

B. The lateral sural cutaneous nerve is a cutaneous branch of the common fibular nerve, and it provides the sensory to skin over the upper lateral leg

C. The deep fibular nerve is a branch of the common fibular nerve. After the common fibular nerve courses around the neck of the fibular, it enters the lateral compartment of the leg and divides into the superficial fibular nerve and the deep fibular nerve. Then the deep fibular nerve enters the anterior compartment of the leg by coursing through the anterior crural intermuscular septum. It innervates muscles in the anterior compartment and skin over the first web space of the foot.

E. The sural nerve is a cutaneous nerve of the lateral aspect of the calf area. The medial sural cutaneous branch from the tibial nerve and the lateral sural cutaneous branch from the common fibular nerve join together to form the sural nerve.

GAS 635–645; N 535; ABR/McM 364

7. **D.** The piriformis muscle arises from the anterior surface of the sacrum, passes laterally through the greater sciatic foramen, and inserts to the greater trochanter of the femur. It is considered the "anatomic key" to gluteal anatomy because major nerves in the gluteal region can be located relative to the piriformis. The sciatic nerve, the inferior gluteal nerve, the pudendal nerve, the posterior femoral cutaneous nerve, the nerve to quadratus femoris, and the nerve to obturator internus travel

under the inferior border of the piriformis, whereas the superior gluteal nerve courses over the superior border of the piriformis.

A. The gluteus medius lies posterior to the piriformis.

B. Superior gemellus arises from the external surface of the ischial spine and attaches to the greater trochanter of the femur. It is located just anteroinferior to the piriformis.

C. The base of the inferior gemellus arises from the upper side of the ischial tuberosity and attaches to the medial aspect of the greater trochanter of the femur. The inferior gemellus is located inferior to the obturator internus and superior to the quadratus femoris.

E. The quadratus femoris is the most inferior muscle in the deep gluteal region and is inferior to the obturator internus and the inferior gemellus.

GAS 426, 554, 575; N 492; ABR/McM 325

8. **A.** Lymphatics from the superficial lateral foot and posterolateral leg drain first into the popliteal lymph nodes, which will carry the lymph into the deep and superficial inguinal nodes.

B and E. Superficial thigh and superficial anteromedial foot and leg drain lymph into the vertical group of superficial inguinal node. The superficial inguinal nodes drain into external iliac nodes.

C. Deep drainage of the leg and foot takes lymph into popliteal nodes first, whereas deep lymphatics in the thigh drain into the deep inguinal nodes. The deep inguinal nodes drain into the external iliac nodes. Superficial inguinal lymph nodes are divided into two groups: the horizontal group and the vertical group.

D. The horizontal group lies parallel to and below the inguinal ligament, receiving lymph from the anterior abdominal wall below umbilicus, the perineum, and back and buttocks below the level of the iliac crest. The vertical group lies along the terminal part of the great saphenous vein. Most of superficial lymphatics of the lower limb drain into the vertical group except those draining into the popliteal nodes and gluteal region draining into the horizontal group.

GAS 562; N 475; ABR/McM 348

9. **E.** The affected nerve is most likely the tibial nerve as it descends vertically through the popliteal fossa. It is responsible for innervating muscles in the posterior compartment of the leg. These muscles are responsible for knee flexion, plantar flexion, and intrinsic muscle functions of the foot. Compression of this nerve by the cyst can affect plantar flexion of the foot and flexion of the toes. The cystic structure found is most likely a Baker cyst. Knee joint conditions such as arthritis and cartilage tears can result in excessive fluid production, typically, in the semimembranosus bursa, leading to the formation of a cyst.

A. Dorsiflexion of the foot would be compromised if the deep fibular nerve were compressed by this Baker cyst.

B. Flexion of the thigh is a function of muscles supplied by lumbar nerves and the femoral nerve.

C and D. The deep fibular nerve is responsible for extension of the digits whereas the femoral nerve is responsible for extension of the leg.

GAS 598; N 507; ABR/McM 352

10. A. The positive valgus stress test of the knee indicates injury to the tibial collateral ligament. The medial meniscus is firmly attached to the tibial collateral ligament. Damage to the tibial collateral ligament often causes concomitant damage to the medial meniscus because of this relationship. ABR/McMurray click test will be positive in injury to medial and lateral meniscus.

B. The anterior cruciate ligament lies inside the knee joint capsule but outside the synovial cavity. It is taut during extension of the knee and may be torn when the knee is hyperextended. Anterior drawer test will be positive in injury to anterior cruciate ligament. If this were damaged along with the medial meniscus and medial cruciate ligament, an "unhappy triad" (of O'Donoghue or Donahue [both spellings are correct]; also called a "blow knee") injury would result.

C. The lateral meniscus is not attached to the tibial collateral ligament but receives muscular attachment to the popliteus muscle.

D. The posterior cruciate ligament also lies outside of the synovial cavity and limits hyperflexion of the knee. Damage to the posterior cruciate ligament will result in a positive posterior drawer test.

E. The tendon of the semitendinosus forms one third of the pes anserinus, with the tendons of the sartorius and gracilis making up the other two-thirds. The pes anserinus (goose foot) is located at the medial border of the tibial tuberosity, and a portion can be used for surgical repair of the anterior cruciate ligament.

GAS 607–609; N 498; ABR/McM 339

11. D. The great saphenous vein is commonly used in coronary artery bypass grafts. Because branches of the saphenous nerve cross the vein in the distal part of the leg, the nerve can be damaged if the vein is stripped from the ankle to the knee. Stripping the vein in the opposite direction can protect the nerve and lessen the postoperative discomfort of patients. The saphenous nerve is responsible for cutaneous innervations on the medial surface of the leg and the medial side of the foot. Injury to this nerve will result in a loss of sensation and also can create chronic dysesthesias in the area.

A and B. The common fibular nerve bifurcates at the neck of the fibula into the superficial and deep fibular nerves, which continue on to innervate the lateral and anterior compartments of the leg, respectively. These nerves are lateral and therefore not associated with the great saphenous vein.

C. The sural nerve is a cutaneous nerve that arises from the junction of branches from the common fibular nerve and tibial nerve and innervates the skin on the lower posterior aspect of the leg and lateral side of the foot. This nerve is often harvested for nerve grafts elsewhere in the body.

E. The tibial nerve is a terminal branch of the sciatic nerve that continues deep in the posterior compartment of the leg.

GAS 560; N 513; ABR/McM 347

12. B. The calcaneofibular ligament is also commonly injured in the inversion sprain of the ankle.

A. The plantar calcaneonavicular ligament supports the head of the talus and resists depression of the medial arch of the foot.

C. The long plantar ligament passes from the plantar surface of the calcaneus to the tuberosity of the cuboid and the bases of metatarsals 3 to 5, and it is important in maintaining the longitudinal arch of the foot.

D. The short plantar ligament is located deep (superior) to the long plantar ligament and extends from the calcaneus to the cuboid and is also involved in maintaining the longitudinal arch of the foot.

E. The medial collateral (deltoid) attaches proximally to the medial malleolus and fans out to reinforce the joint capsule of the ankle. It is involved in an eversion ankle sp rain.

GAS 638; N 517; ABR/McM 359

13. B. The lateral circumflex femoral artery arises from the deep femoral (profunda femoris) artery and sends a descending branch down the length of the femur to anastomose with the superior medial genicular artery and the superior lateral genicular artery.

A. The medial circumflex femoral artery is responsible for supplying blood to the head and neck of the femur, and it does not anastomose with distal vessels at the knee.

C. The first perforating artery sends an ascending branch that anastomoses with the medial circumflex femoral and the inferior gluteal artery in the buttock.

D. The inferior gluteal artery is a branch of the internal iliac; it has important anastomotic supply to the hip joint.

E. The typically small descending genicular branch of the femoral artery is given off just proximal to the continuation of the femoral artery as the popliteal. Because the artery is distal to the occlusion, it will not be helpful.

GAS 592; N 490; ABR/McM 327

14. C. The medial circumflex femoral artery is responsible for supplying blood to the head and neck of the femur by a number of branches that pass under the edge of the ischiofemoral ligament. This artery is most likely at risk for injury in an extracapsular fracture of the femoral neck.

A. The inferior gluteal artery arises from the internal iliac and enters the gluteal region through the greater sciatic foramen, below the piriformis.

B. The first perforating artery sends an ascending branch that anastomoses with the inferior gluteal artery in the buttock.

D. The obturator artery arises from the internal iliac artery and passes through the obturator foramen. It commonly supplies the artery within the ligament of the head of the femur but is not likely to be patent in a person of this age since it is usually not patent by the teenage years.

E. The superior gluteal artery arises from the internal iliac artery and enters through the greater sciatic foramen above the piriformis.

GAS 589–592; N 491; ABR/McM 327

15. B. The obturator nerve arises from the lumbar plexus (L2–L4) and enters the thigh through the obturator canal. This nerve is responsible for innervation of the medial compartment of the thigh (adductor compartment) and innervates skin on the medial side of the thigh. Injury to this nerve can result in weakened adduction and difficulty walking and sensory deficit on the medial aspect of the thigh.

A. The femoral nerve innervates muscles of the anterior compartment of the thigh that are responsible for hip flexion and leg extension.

E. The sciatic nerve branches into the common fibular and tibial nerves.

C. The common fibular nerve branches into the deep and superficial branches of the fibular nerve responsible for innervation of the anterior and lateral compartments of the leg, respectively.

D. The tibial nerve innervates the muscles of the posterior compartment of the thigh and leg, which are responsible for extension of the hip, flexion of the leg, and plantar flexion of the foot.

GAS 486, 500, 563–565; N 529; ABR/McM 271

16. B. The common fibular nerve winds around the neck of the fibula before dividing into superficial and deep branches that go on to innervate the lateral and anterior compartments of the leg, respectively. The anterior and lateral compartments are responsible for dorsiflexion and eversion of the foot, respectively, and injury to these nerves would result in deficits in these movements.

A. The tibial nerve lies superficially in the popliteal fossa. This nerve innervates the posterior compartment of the leg, so compression in this area would result in a loss of plantar flexion and weakness of inversion.

C. The lateral compartment of the leg is innervated by the superficial fibular nerve and is mainly involved in eversion of the foot. The cutaneous branches of the superficial fibular nerve emerge through the deep fascia in the anterolateral aspect of the leg and supply the dorsum of the foot.

D. The anterior compartment of the leg is innervated by the deep fibular nerve and is mainly involved in dorsiflexion of the foot.

E. The medial malleolus is an inferiorly directed projection from the medial side of the distal end of the tibia. The tibial nerve runs near the groove behind the medial malleolus, and compression at this location would result in loss of toe flexion, adduction, and abduction.

GAS 538–541; N 531; ABR/McM 346

17. A. The gluteus maximus is innervated by the inferior gluteal nerve, and this muscle is responsible for extension and lateral rotation of the thigh. It is the primary muscle that extends the flexed hip and is used to rise from a seated position.

B. Superior gluteal nerve innervates the gluteus minimus and the gluteus medius that are responsible for abduction of the thigh.

C. The obturator nerve innervates the medial compartments including adductor longus, adductor brevis, and adductor magnus. The adductor muscles adduct and medially rotate the thigh.

D. Piriformis is innervated by nerve to piriformis, and the muscle rotates the thigh laterally and abducts the flexed femur.

E. The inferior gemellus and quadratus femoris are innervated by nerve to quadratus femoris. These muscles rotate the thigh laterally. The inferior gemellus also abducts the flexed femur.

GAS 572; N 395; ABR/McM 324

18. B. After the common fibular nerve courses around the neck of the fibular, it enters the lateral compartment of the leg and divides into the superficial fibular nerve and the deep fibular nerve. The deep fibular nerve then enters the anterior compartment of the leg by coursing through the anterior crural intermuscular septum. It innervates muscles in the anterior compartment responsible for toe extension, foot dorsiflexion, and inversion of the foot and skin over the first web space of the foot. The patient most likely injured the distal part of the deep fibular nerve affecting its sensory function only. If the injury to the nerve occurs at its origin, its motor function will be affected as well.

A. Dorsiflexion of the foot is carried by the deep fibular nerve; however, eversion of the foot is by the superficial fibular nerve.

C. Injury to the deep fibular nerve at its origin will affect both dorsiflexion and inversion of the foot.

D and E. Tibial nerve mediates plantar flexion of the foot.

GAS 622–623; N 511; ABR/McM 346

19. E. The posterior cruciate ligament is responsible for preventing the forward sliding of the femur on the tibia. In other words, the ligament prevents posterior displacement of the tibia relative to the fixed femur.

A. The anterior cruciate ligament prevents posterior displacement of the femur on the tibia, much like a drawer (hence the drawer test and drawer sign).

B. The fibular collateral ligament prevents varus forces on the knee, pushing the knee laterally.

C. The tibial collateral ligament resist valgus forces on the knee, pushing the knee medially.

D. Patellar ligament, with the quadriceps femoris muscle, straighten the knee.

GAS 606; N 500; ABR/McM 339

20. D. The gluteus maximus inserts into the gluteal tuberosity and the iliotibial tract. Although the gluteus maximus would continue to contract at the regions of insertion, their orientation would be displaced by the fracture.

A, B, C, and E. The gluteus medius, gluteus minimus, obturator internus, and piriformis all insert on some aspect of the greater trochanter of the femur.

GAS 566–567; N 479; ABR/McM 305

21. B. The apex of the femoral triangle occurs at the junction of the adductor longus and sartorius muscles. The adductor canal (subsartorial, Hunter canal) begins at this location. Immediately deep to this anatomic point lie the femoral artery, femoral vein, deep femoral artery, and deep femoral vein, often overlying one another in that sequence. This has historically been a site of injuries caused by slipping while handling sharp objects (such as a butcher's knife). For this reason, injuries at this location are referred to as the "butcher's block" injury. Fatal loss of blood can occur in just a few minutes if pressure, or a tourniquet, is not applied immediately.

A. The external iliac artery becomes the femoral artery at the inguinal ligament.

C. The great saphenous vein joins the femoral vein at the saphenous opening or hiatus, also known as fossa ovalis.

D and E. The medial circumflex femoral usually arises from the deep femoral artery approximately 3 to 5 inches inferior to the inguinal ligament, near the origin of the deep femoral artery from the femoral. Serious blood loss can occur with injury to any of these vessels, although injury to them is not often fatal.

GAS 564; N 475; ABR/McM 329

22. C. The iliofemoral ligament ("inverted Y ligament of Bigelow") is the most important ligament reinforcing the joint anteriorly that would resist both hyperextension and lateral rotation at the hip joint.

A. The pubofemoral ligament reinforces the joint inferiorly and prevents hyperabduction.

B. The ischiofemoral ligament reinforces the joint posteriorly and limits extension and medial rotation.

D. The transverse acetabular ligament bridges across the acetabular notch, converting the notch into an acetabular foramen.

E. The ligament of the head of the femur is a delicate connective tissue band. It connects the fovea on the femoral head to the acetabular fossa. The band carries the acetabular branch of the obturator artery that is a major blood supply to the femoral head in young people.

GAS 553; N 477; ABR/McM 333

23. C. The x-ray shows the fracture of the femoral neck, which is most likely an intracapsular fracture. In addition, the superior articular surface of the right femoral head is flattened, indicating avascular necrosis. Therefore it can be concluded that the intracapsular femoral neck fracture has most likely caused the avascular necrosis of the femoral head because the fracture damages the retinacular branches of the medial and lateral circumflex arteries that pass beneath the ischiofemoral ligament and pierce the femoral neck. Until an individual reaches approximately 6 to 10 years of age, blood supply to the head of the femur is provided by a branch of the obturator artery that runs with the ligament of the head of the femur. Thereafter the artery of the ligament of the head of the femur is insignificant.

A. The x-ray shows the femoral neck fracture not the dislocation of the hip. In addition, vascular injury is rare in the hip dislocation.

B. Intertrochanteric fracture of the femur would not damage the blood supply to the head of the femur but would cause complications because the greater trochanter is an attachment site for several gluteal muscles.

D. Thrombosis of the obturator artery could result in muscular symptoms, although there are several collateral sources of blood supply in the thigh.

E. Comminuted fracture of the extracapsular femoral neck would not ordinarily imperil the vascular supply.

GAS 558–561, 670; N 495; ABR/McM 335

24. C. The Achilles tendon reflex is a function of the triceps surae muscle, composed of the two heads of gastrocnemius and soleus muscles that insert on the calcaneus. The innervation is provided primarily by spinal nerve S1. The S1 root leaves the vertebral column at the S1 foramen of the sacrum, but a herniated disc at the L5–S1 intervertebral space puts the S1 root under tension, resulting in pain and possible weakness or paralysis of S1-supplied muscles, especially the plantar flexors.

A. A disc lesion at L3–4 would affect the L4 spinal nerve (hip flexion and knee extension);

B. A lesion at L4–5 would cause problems with L5 (affecting foot inversion and extension).

D. A disc lesion at S1–2 in the sacrum is improbable, unless there was lumbarization of the S1 vertebra.

E. The gluteal crush syndrome usually occurs when a patient has been lying unconscious and unmoving on a hard surface for an extended period of time.

GAS 619; N 531; ABR/McM 355

Answers 25–47

25. C. With L5 damage, ankle inversion would be weakened, and foot dorsiflexion is weakened because of partial denervation of the muscles of the anterior compartment of the leg. B. An injury to L4 would cause weakness in the patellar reflex and loss of cutaneous

innervation to the medial side of the leg. The patellar reflex is used to test L2 to L4 nerve integrity.

A. The motor side of the reflex is primarily derived from spinal nerves L2 and L3, whereas the sensory side of the arc is said to be principally from L4. The L4 spinal nerve supplies the L4 dermatome on the medial side of the leg and foot, by way of the saphenous nerve. It also supplies the quadriceps femoris muscle which extends the knee.

D. The foot is everted because the S1-supplied (by the superficial fibular nerve) fibularis longus and brevis are unopposed. The Achilles reflex is also primarily supplied by S1. Hip movements are produced primarily by L5- and S1-supplied muscles, as is knee flexion.

E. S2 spinal nerve innervates many muscles in the lower limbs including gluteus maximus, piriformis, obturator internus, semitendinosus, flexor hallucis longus, and so on; however, none of the muscles is solely innervated by S2. No direct effect of S2's deficit would be found on the extension of the knee or eversion and inversion of the foot.
GAS 626–627, 657; N 531; ABR/McM 337

26. C. The lateral plantar nerve innervates the dorsal and plantar interossei, adductor hallucis, flexor digiti minimi, quadratus plantae, abductor digiti minimi, and second, third, and fourth lumbricals. Sensation would be absent over the lateral side of the sole, the fifth and half of the fourth toes.

A, B, D and E. The medial plantar nerve provides sensation over the plantar surface of the first, second, third, and half of the fourth toe as well as function of the so-called LAFF muscles: first lumbrical, abductor hallucis, flexor hallucis brevis, and flexor digitorum brevis.
GAS 651; N 532; ABR/McM 361

27. A. The common fibular nerve passes around the neck of the fibula and gives off deep (L4–5) and superficial fibular nerve (L5, S1–2) branches. The two nerves supply the dorsiflexors and evertors of the foot, respectively. In this case the tibialis anterior and extensor digitorum longus are the only muscles listed that are supplied by either of these nerve branches, and both are innervated by the deep fibular nerve.

B, C, D, and E. Each of the other muscles listed is innervated by the tibial nerve.
GAS 621–622; N 531; ABR/McM 346

28. D. Tuberculosis can spread to any level of spinal vertebrae (which is called spinal tuberculosis) and form an abscess. The abscess is called cold abscess because it lacks signs of acute inflammation (red and hot) typically found when abscess is being formed. When lumbar vertebrae are involved, abscess can spread within the sheath of the psoas major to its insertion with the iliacus upon the lesser trochanter, presenting there with no tenderness. The iliopsoas muscle is the principal flexor of the hip joint.

A. Abduction of the hips is performed by the gluteus medius and minimus with assistance from piriformis.

B. Adductor longus, brevis, and magnus are major adductors of the thigh.

C. Extension of the hip is a function of the gluteus maximus, together with the hamstring muscles.

E. Internal (medial) rotation is performed by the adductor muscle group.
GAS 535–536; N 486; ABR/McM 335

29. A. The tendon lying posterior to the lateral and medial malleoli is most likely the calcaneal (Achilles) tendon. The calcaneal tendon connects the soleus and gastrocnemius muscles to the calcaneal tuberosity. The tendon of the plantaris inserts with the calcaneal tendon.

B. Fibula: The biceps femoris tendon attaches to the fibular head. The fibularis longus and fibularis brevis tendons attach to the lateral fibula. The extensor digitorum longus and extensor hallucis longis tendons attach to the medial fibula. The fibularis tertius attaches to the anterior surface of the distal fibula.

C. Cuboid: The tibialis posterior attaches to the plantar surface of the cuboid.

D. Talus: No tendons attach to the talus, however many ligaments do attach creating stability in the ankle joint.

E. Navicular: The tibialis posterior attaches to the navicular tuberosity.
GAS 616; N 506; ABR/McM 355

30. A. The plantar calcaneonavicular (spring) ligament is a fibrocartilaginous band and connects the anterior aspect of the sustentaculum tali and the plantar surface of the navicular bone. The spring ligament supports the head of the talus and maintains the medial longitudinal arch of the foot by providing resistance against depression of the medial arch of the foot. Tearing of the plantar calcaneonavicular ligament destabilizes the medial longitudinal arch that may result in flatfoot deformity with pain, stiffness, and swelling of the affected foot.

B. A fracture of the cuboid bone would not disrupt the longitudinal arch of the foot.

C. Interruption of the plantar aponeurosis is not the best answer because this aponeurosis provides only passive support, unlike the spring ligament.

D. A sprain of the anterior talofibular ligament would result from an inversion injury of the ankle and would not disrupt the medial longitudinal arch of the foot.

E. A sprain of the medial collateral (deltoid) ligament results from eversion of the ankle joint and would not disrupt the medial longitudinal arch of the foot (GAS Fig. 6.103).
GAS 635; N 518; ABR/McM 359

31. B. This type of injury can result in the "unhappy triad" (of O'Donoghue) injury, with damage to the tibial (medial) collateral ligament (MCL), anterior cruciate

Medial collateral ligament

Tibiocalcaneal part

Tibionavicular part

Anterior tibiotalar part

Posterior tibiotalar part

Medial tubercle of talus

Tuberosity of navicular bone

Sustentaculum tali of calcaneus bone

Plantar calcaneonavicular ligament

• *GAS* **Fig. 6.103**

ligament (ACL), and medial meniscus. A blow to the lateral side of the knee stretches and tears the MCL, which is attached to the medial meniscus. The ACL is tensed during knee extension and can tear subsequent to the rupture of the MCL.

A, C, D, and E. The remaining answer choices describe structures on the lateral surface of the knee, which are not usually injured by this type of trauma.
GAS 606; N 500; ABR/McM 339

32. E. The popliteal artery is the continuation of the femoral artery after it passes through the hiatus of the adductor magnus. The popliteal artery divides into the anterior and posterior tibial arteries. The anterior tibial artery courses into the anterior compartment through the aperture in the interosseous membrane between the tibia and fibula, whereas the posterior tibial artery continues in the posterior compartment of the leg, to its division into medial and lateral plantar arteries. The posterior tibial artery provides origin for the fibular artery, which supplies the lateral compartment of the leg. The deep femoral artery provides origin for the three or four perforating branches that supply the posterior compartment of the thigh.

A, B, C, and D. All the other options do not match the description.
GAS 620, 617; N 503; ABR/McM 345

33. E. The vastus lateralis muscle is located on the lateral aspect of the thigh. The distal portion of this muscle lies superficial to the proximal part of the lateral aspect of the joint capsule of the knee. When a needle is inserted superiorly and laterally to the patella, it penetrates the vastus lateralis muscle on its course to the internal capsule.

A. The adductor magnus is the deepest muscle in the medial thigh, not lateral.
B. The short head of biceps femoris has its origin on the posterior aspect of the femur, merges with the long head of the biceps femoris, and inserts on the head of the fibula. C. The rectus femoris passes longitudinally anterior to the femur and inserts on the tibial tuberosity, via the patellar tendon, or quadriceps femoris tendon. A needle inserted laterally to the patella would not penetrate this muscle.
D. The sartorius originates on the anterior superior iliac spine and forms part of the pes anserinus, which inserts on the medial aspect of the proximal part of the tibia. A needle inserted laterally to the patella would not penetrate this muscle.
GAS 584; N 529; ABR/McM 328

34. D. When the popliteus contracts, it rotates the distal portion of the femur in a lateral direction. It also draws the lateral meniscus posteriorly, thereby protecting this cartilage as the distal femoral condyle glides and rolls backward, as the knee is flexed. This allows unlocking the knee joint to initiate gate. The popliteus is innervated by the tibial nerve. Overuse of the popliteus (e.g., runners) may result in damage to the popliteus. A great force to the knee (e.g., motor vehicle collision, and lifting weights) can result in an acute injury to the popliteus.
A. Common fibular: The common fibular nerve innervates the short head of the biceps
B. Deep fibular: The deep fibular nerve innervates muscles of the anterior compartment of the leg including the tibialis anterior, the extensor digitorum longus, the extensor hallucis longus, and the fibularis tertius.
C. Superficial fibular: The superficial fibular nerve innervates the fibularis longus and brevis.
E. Femoral: The femoral nerve innervates muscles that act to flex the hip, including pectineus, iliacus, and sartorius, as well as muscles that act to extend the knee, including the quadriceps femoris.
GAS 617; N 500; ABR/McM 339

35. B. Pott fracture is a rather archaic term for a fracture of the fibula at the ankle. The term is often used to indicate a bimalleolar fracture of fibula and tibia, perhaps with a tear in the medial collateral (deltoid) or tibial collateral ligament, allowing the foot to be deviated laterally. (The medial malleolus will often break before the medial collateral (deltoid) ligament tears.) This fracture is also known as Dupuytren fracture. The fracture results from abduction and lateral rotation of the foot in extreme eversion. There can also be fracture of the posterior aspect of the distal tibia.
A. Talonavicular ligament reinforces the capsule of the talocalcaneonavicular joint. It passes from the neck of the talus to posterior aspect of the navicular bone. The ligament has no direct contact with medial malleolus.

C. The spring ligament, also known as the plantar calcaneonavicular ligament, extends from the calcaneus to the navicular bone and is a part of the medial longitudinal arch. This ligament would not be affected in eversion or inversion of the ankle.

D and E. The plantar ligament, which is composed of the long and short plantar ligaments, supports the lateral longitudinal arch of the foot and would therefore not be affected by inversion or eversion of the foot. The calcaneofibular ligament runs from the calcaneus to the fibula.

GAS 635; N 517; ABR/McM 359

36. B. The original axial vessel of the lower limb is retained as the (usually tiny) sciatic branch of the inferior gluteal artery. In some cases, this vessel is retained as the primary proximal vessel to the limb, wherein there is hypoplastic development of the femoral artery. Aneurysms of the enlarged sciatic artery in the gluteal region are relatively common, as is rupture of the vessel (with profuse bleeding) if they are exposed in the gluteal area.

A. The profunda femoris or deep femoral branch of the femoral artery usually provides three perforating branches to the posterior compartment but not a branch such as that described.

C. The transverse branch of the medial circumflex femoral anastomoses with the first perforating branch of the deep femoral artery.

D. The superior gluteal artery anastomoses with the inferior gluteal by a superficial branch or branches.

E. The descending branch of the lateral circumflex femoral anastomoses with the superior lateral genicular branch of the popliteal artery.

GAS 491, 582; N 489; ABR/McM 325

37. D. Sensory deficits on the middorsum and sole of the affected foot indicate L5 spinal nerve injury, which also explains weakness in dorsiflexion and ankle inversion due to partial denervation of the muscles of the anterior leg compartment. Herniation of the intervertebral disc at L4–5 results typically in compression of the L5 spinal nerve. The L4 spinal nerve exits at the L3–4 intervertebral foramen, but the L5 spinal nerve is put under tension as it passes the herniation to reach the L5–1 foramen.

A. Disc herniation at L1–2 most likely affects the L2 spinal nerve. Sensory deficit will be just below the inguinal ligament.

B. When the L3 spinal nerve is compressed by disc herniation between L2 and L3 vertebral body, sensory deficits will be over the medial side of the thigh.

C. Disc lesion at L3–4 would most likely affect the L4 spinal nerve. Sensory deficit over the anterior thigh and patellar region, medial side of the leg and medial aspect of the great toe is expected. **E.** Disc herniation at L5–S1 will affect S1 spinal nerve. Sensory deficit will be found over the heel of the foot.

GAS 80; N 529; ABR/McM 101

38. C. Entrapment compression of all or part of the sciatic nerve by the piriformis can mimic disc herniation. Foot drop would be anticipated with fibular nerve involvement. Compression of the common fibular division of the sciatic nerve by the piriformis may produce point pain in the gluteal area, pain in the posterior part of the limb, and possible weakness of muscles in the lateral and anterior compartments of the leg.

A. Paralysis of plantar flexion occurs with a lesion of the tibial division of the sciatic nerve or the tibial nerve.

B. Weakness in leg extension at the knee is associated with pathology of the femoral nerve.

D. The obturator nerve injury results in weakness in adduction of the thigh.

E. Skin of the medial side of the leg is innervated by the saphenous nerve which is a branch of the femoral nerve.

GAS 444; N 482, 490; ABR/McM 325

39. A. The superior gluteal nerve innervates the gluteus medius, gluteus minimus, and tensor fasciae latae muscles. The tensor fasciae latae arises from the iliac crest, inserts into the iliotibial tract of the lateral aspect of the thigh, and assists in flexion and abduction of the hip and medial rotation of the thigh. B. The rectus femoris is innervated by the femoral nerve; it flexes the hip and extends the knee, thus acting upon two major joints. It arises in part from the anterior inferior iliac spine and the rim of the acetabulum and inserts into the quadriceps femoris tendon.

C. The gluteus maximus is supplied by the inferior gluteal nerve.

D. The piriformis and quadratus femoris are both short lateral rotators of the hip and are supplied by branches of the sacral plexus.

E. The quadratus femoris is a muscle of the posterior hip that is innervated, along with the inferior gemellus, by the nerve to quadratus femoris.

GAS 485; N 496; ABR/McM 328

40. A. The sartorius is indicated by the arrow in Fig. 5.3. This muscle forms the roof of the adductor or subsartorial canal (Hunter canal), with the adductor longus and vastus medialis forming other muscular borders. The femoral artery and vein, the saphenous nerve, and the nerve to the vastus medialis all pass into this canal. The femoral artery leaves the canal by passing through the adductor hiatus, through the adductor magnus. The saphenous nerve emerges from the canal and from beneath the sartorius on the medial side of the lower limb proximally, thereafter providing sensory branches to the medial side of the leg and foot. Dr. Hunter mobilized the sartorius, thereby exposing the femoral artery (which continues as the popliteal artery beyond the adductor hiatus), which could be clamped while an aneurysmal popliteal artery was treated surgically.

B. Femoral vein: The femoral artery and vein pass through the adductor/subsartorial canal, which is

inferior to the Sartorius muscle. The image is referring to a muscle, rather than a vessel

C. Femoral artery: The femoral artery and vein pass
through the adductor/subsartorial canal, which is
inferior to the Sartorius muscle. The image is referring to a muscle, rather than a vessel

D. Gracilis: The gracilis is the most superficial and
medial muscle in the medial compartment of the
thigh. It is not involved in this procedure.

E. Adductor brevis: The adductor brevis is a short
muscle found inferior to the adductor longus,
between the anterior and posterior compartment of
the thigh. It is not involved in this procedure.

GAS 585; N 496; ABR/McM 328

41. B. Contraction of the gastrocnemius on the fractured
calcaneus would augment the pain because the gastrocnemius inserts with the soleus upon that bone, via the
calcaneal tendon, or tendon Achilles.

A. The flexor digitorum longus passes the ankle medially to enter the sole of the foot, where it inserts
upon the distal phalanges.

C. The tibialis posterior, likewise, passes behind the
medial malleolus, with complex insertions upon the
navicular bone, cuneiform bones, metatarsal bases,
and the cuboid bone.

D. The tibialis anterior, a muscle of the anterior leg
compartment, inserts upon the medial side of the
medial cuneiform and the base of the first metatarsal bone, and, with the tibialis posterior, is a strong
inverter of the foot.

E. The fibularis longus is a muscle of the lateral compartment of the leg. It passes behind the lateral malleolus, entering the sole of the foot by crossing the
lateral and inferior surface of the cuboid, and inserts
primarily into the medial cuneiform and base of the
first metatarsal bone laterally.

GAS 615; N 511; ABR/McM 350

42. C. The nerve superficial to and running along the popliteal vein is the tibial nerve. The common fibular nerve
is adjacent to the popliteal vein and the tibial nerve;
however, it typically courses laterally as it enters the
popliteal fossa. Therefore in this case the tibial nerve
is most likely the one severed by the bullet. A severe
injury of the tibial nerve in the popliteal fossa would
result in a dorsiflexed and everted foot because of the
intact muscles of the extensor (anterior) and evertor
(lateral) compartments of the leg. It would result also
in some weakening of knee flexion because of loss of
the gastrocnemius muscle, which flexes the knee and
plantar flexes the foot. The hamstrings also flex the
knee, so this function would not be lost.

A. The function of the quadriceps femoris is intact as
the femoral nerve is not affected.

B. Foot drop results from loss of the anterior compartment of the leg, innervated by the deep fibular
nerve. If the common fibular nerve is injured, foot

drop will be observed, but the tibial nerve is the
most likely one affected in this case.

D. Plantar flexion at the ankle is observed when the
common fibular nerve is injured.

E. The hamstrings are the major flexors of the knee.
The innervation of the hamstrings is made proximal
to the popliteal fossa; therefore their function will
be intact.

GAS 621; N 514; ABR/McM 355

43. C. Disruption of the Shenton line and subcapital fracture on the imaging indicate that the patient suffers an
intracapsular fracture of the femoral neck. The blood
supply to the femoral head is disrupted by subcapital
or intracapsular fracture of the femoral neck disrupts,
which may result in avascular necrosis of the femoral head. Primarily during childhood, the acetabular
branch of the obturator artery coursing within the ligament of the head of the femur (in approximately 60%
of cases), later becoming atretic. Therefore the acetabular branch is a least concern in the surgical intervention. In the adult the arterial supply of the neck and
head is provided by retinacular branches of the medial
circumflex femoral and lateral circumflex femoral arteries that pierce the neck of the femur, with some supply also from the gluteal arteries. The lateral circumflex
femoral artery arises from the deep femoral and supplies the vastus intermedius and lateralis muscles.

A. Superior gluteal: The superior gluteal artery supplies the gluteus maximus, gluteus medius, gluteus
minimus, and the tensor fascia lata.

B. Lateral circumflex femoral: In the adult, the arterial supply of the neck and head is provided by retinacular branches of the medial circumflex femoral
and lateral circumflex femoral arteries that pierce
the neck of the femur.

D. Inferior gluteal: The inferior gluteal artery supplies
adjacent structures in the gluteal region and posterior thigh such as gluteus maximus, piriformis,
ischiococcygeus, iliococcygeus, obturator internus, superior and inferior gemelli, and quadratus
femoris.

E. Medial circumflex femoral: In the adult the arterial supply of the neck and head is provided by retinacular branches of the medial circumflex femoral
and lateral circumflex femoral arteries that pierce
the neck of the femur.

GAS 549; N 495; ABR/McM 335

44. E. The lateral femoral cutaneous nerve leaves the pelvis laterally, approximately 1 cm medial to the anterior superior iliac spine, passing beneath, or through,
the inguinal ligament. As a consequence of its site of
exit, any tension upon or compression of the inguinal
ligament can affect the nerve. If it is thus affected, the
individual may feel burning sensations or pain along
the lateral aspect of the thigh, which is the region of
distribution of the nerve. Obesity, sudden weight loss,
wearing a heavy gun belt, wearing trousers that are too

tight (Calvin Klein syndrome), or having someone sitting on another's lap for an extended period of time can lead to meralgia paresthetica, the painful lateral thigh.

A. The superior gluteal nerve provides motor supply to the gluteus medius and minimus and tensor fasciae latae muscles.

B. The femoral nerve emerges from beneath the middle of the inguinal ligament and is not usually affected by similar traction or compression.

C. The obturator nerve leaves the pelvis through the obturator canal and enters the thigh deeply in a protected location. It innervates the adductor muscles and supplies sensation on the medial aspect of the thigh.

D. The fibular division of the sciatic nerve supplies the muscles of the anterior and lateral compartments of the leg and provides sensory fibers for the dorsum and lateral side of the foot.

GAS 398; N 486; ABR/McM 330

45. D. Posterior to the medial malleolus, the medial tarsal tunnel is found on the posteromedial aspect of the ankle. The tunnel is formed by the inferior surface of the sustentaculum tali of the calcaneus, medial surface of the calcaneus, medial and posterior surfaces of the talus, and medial malleolus of the tibia. Lastly, it is covered by the flexor retinaculum as a roof. Through this tunnel, several structures course to the sole of the foot. They are, from anterior to posterior, tibialis posterior tendon, flexor digitorum longus tendon, posterior tibial artery and veins, tibial nerve, and flexor hallucis longus tendon, which lies most posteriorly among the contents. (This is the basis of the mnemonic: "Tom, Dick,

and a Very Nervous Harry.") As most anteriorly located, the tibialis posterior tendon, is most likely compressed by the displaced fragment of the medial malleolus. Increases of pressure within the tissues of the plantar aspect of the foot, usually due to increased fluid from hemorrhage, inflammatory processes, or infections, can also affect the contents in the tarsal tunnel (tarsal tunnel syndrome). The plantar aponeurosis and other fibrous and osseous tissues of the plantar surface cause this area to be relatively nondistensible; therefore it takes little increase of fluid content to result in pressures adequate to restrict venous drainage and, thereafter, arterial inflow to the region. Fasciotomy of the medial skin and fascia of the foot and the posterior compartment of the leg can be required to reduce the pressure and allow healing to take place. (GAS Figs. 6.110 and 6.115).

A. Flexor hallucis longus tendon: The flexor hallucis longus tendon travels through the medial tarsal tunnel, however the tibialis posterior tendon is more anterior and therefore more likely to be compromised by the displaced fragment of the medial malleolus.

B. Plantaris tendon: This tendon does not travel through the medial tarsal tunnel.

C. Tibialis anterior tendon: This tendon does not pass through the medical tarsal tunnel.

GAS 645; N 520; ABR/McM 356

46. D. The second perforating branch of the profunda femoris (deep femoral) artery commonly provides the nutrient artery to the femur, a vessel that passes through a rather large foramen to enter the proximal part of the shaft.

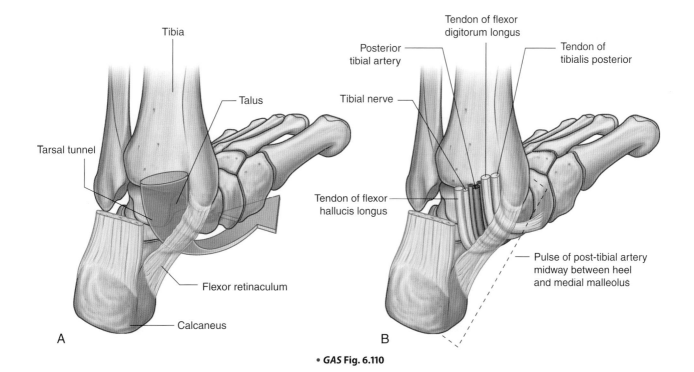

• *GAS* **Fig. 6.110**

- Superficial transverse metatarsal ligaments
- Anterior part of inferior extensor retinaculum
- Plantar aponeurosis
- Medial process of calcaneal tuberosity

• **GAS Fig. 6.115**

A. The deep circumflex iliac branch of the external iliac passes around the medial aspect of the iliac crest, also supplying the lower lateral part of the anterior abdominal wall.

B. The acetabular branch of the obturator artery supplies tissues in the hip socket, usually including a branch to the ligament of the head of the femur.

C. The lateral circumflex femoral branch of the deep femoral artery supplies the vastus lateralis muscle.

E. The medial circumflex femoral branch of the deep femoral artery supplies proximal adductor musculature and the region of the hip joint, including the neck and head of the femur.
GAS 592; N 495; ABR/McM 330

47. B. The tibial nerve divides into the medial and lateral plantar nerves on the medial side of the ankle. These two nerves provide sensation for the sole of the foot.

A. Sensory supply to the dorsum of the foot is provided mostly by the superficial fibular nerve, with the deep fibular nerve providing sensation for the skin between the first and second toes.

C. Foot drop would be caused by interruption of the common fibular or deep fibular nerve. Sensory loss to the lateral side of the foot results from loss of the

sural nerve. D. Paralysis of the extensor digitorum brevis would be attributed to injury to the terminal motor branch of the deep fibular nerve.

E. Sensory loss of the entire foot would result from the spinal cord injury.
GAS 656; N 531; ABR/McM 356

Answers 48–71

48. B. The gastrocnemius muscle arises from the femur just proximal to the femoral condyles. This strong muscle could displace the distal fragment of the fractured femur posteriorly. In addition, the popliteal artery is the deepest structure in the popliteal fossa (right against the popliteal surface of the distal femur) and is susceptible to laceration in this scenario as the fractured end of the distal femoral fragment is pulled against the popliteal artery. Orthopedic surgeons always look for damage to the popliteal artery in a patient with a supra-condylar fracture.

A. The soleus arises from the tibia and would have no effect upon the femur.

C. The semitendinosus arises from the ischial tuberosity and inserts medially on the proximal tibia, via the pes anserinus.

D. The gracilis arises from the pubic bone to the tibia.

E. The tibialis anterior arises from the tibia and inserts mostly onto the medial surface of the medial cuneiform and base of the first metatarsal.
GAS 621–623; N 506; ABR/McM 309

49. E. The posterior tibial artery provides most of the arterial supply for the neck and body of the talus bone. The fibular artery and anterior tibial artery also provide a vascular supply. A and B. The medial and lateral plantar branches of the posterior tibial artery are distributed to tissues in the plantar surface of the foot.

C. The dorsalis pedis is the continuation of the anterior tibial artery on the dorsum of the foot.

D. The anterior tibial artery ends at the ankle by becoming the dorsalis pedis artery.
GAS 653–654; N 509; ABR/McM 354

50. A. The adductor hallucis muscle inserts on the lateral side of the proximal phalanx of the great toe and also the lateral sesamoid bone, by way of its oblique and transverse heads. It is supplied by the lateral plantar nerve.

B. The abductor hallucis inserts upon the medial side of the proximal phalanx and the medial sesamoid bone of the great toe. The sesamoid bones are within the tendons of the flexor hallucis brevis and assist it in its function at the first metatarsophalangeal joint. The abductor and flexor hallucis brevis are innervated by the medial plantar nerve.

C and D. The first dorsal interosseous muscle and the first lumbrical both insert on the medial side of the extensor expansion of the second toe.

E. The quadratus plantae arises from the calcaneus and inserts on the tendon of the flexor digitorum

longus muscle. The first lumbrical is supplied by the medial plantar nerve. The quadratus plantae, the lumbricals 2 to 4, and all interossei are innervated by the lateral plantar nerve.
GAS 651; N 524; ABR/McM 360

51. B. The medial plantar nerve innervates the abductor hallucis, flexor digitorum brevis, flexor hallucis brevis, and the first lumbrical.
   A. The lateral plantar nerve innervates ll other intrinsic muscles in the plantar region of the foot.
   C. The sural nerve is sensory to the lateral posterior leg and lateral side of the foot; it arises from a combination of branches of the tibial nerve and common fibular nerve. D. The superficial fibular nerve innervates the fibularis longus and fibularis brevis in the lateral compartment of the leg.
   E. The deep fibular nerve supplies dorsiflexors, toe extensors, and invertors of the foot.
   GAS 656; N 532; ABR/McM 361

52. D. The posterior tibial artery passes behind the medial malleolus, approximately halfway between that bony landmark and the heel, or the calcaneus.
   A. The medial edge of the plantar aponeurosis can be palpated just medial to the muscular belly of the abductor hallucis.
   B. The sartorius passes behind the medial femoral condyle to insert on the proximal, medial aspect of the tibia via the pes anserinus; usually no pulse can be felt clearly there.
   C. The sural nerve and the small (lesser) saphenous vein pass around the lateral side of the foot, approximately halfway between the lateral malleolus and the calcaneus.
   E. The popliteal artery passes between the two heads of the gastrocnemius, where the arterial pulse may be felt very deeply, medial to the midline.
   GAS 620, 653; N 513; ABR/McM 354

53. C. The deep fibular nerve supplies the fibularis tertius muscle. Although its name might lead one to think that this muscle is in the lateral compartment with the other two fibularis muscles, it is in the anterior (extensor) compartment of the leg. It is named for its origin from the fibula. It inserts upon the dorsum of the base of the fifth metatarsal bone and assists in extension and eversion of the foot.
   A. The sural nerve is a cutaneous nerve, formed by contributions from the tibial and common fibular nerves; it supplies the posterolateral leg and the lateral side of the foot.
   B. The lateral plantar nerve is a branch of the tibial nerve; it innervates the quadratus plantae, muscles of the little toe, the adductor hallucis, lumbricals 2 to 4, and all of the interossei. It is sensory to the lateral side of the sole and the lateral three and a half digits
   D. The superficial fibular nerve supplies the fibularis longus and brevis and innervates the skin on most of the dorsum of the foot.

   E. The tibial nerve supplies the calf muscles and divides into the medial and lateral plantar nerves.
   GAS 622–625; N 512; ABR/McM 357

54. A. Gluteal injections should be given anterior and superior to a line drawn between the posterior superior iliac spine and the greater trochanter to avoid the sciatic nerve and other important nerves and vessels. Occasionally, one can encounter the lateral cutaneous branch of the iliohypogastric nerve, but this usually causes no serious problem.
   B, C, D, E. One must stay anterior to a vertical line dropped from the highest point of the ilium. If the injected material is too near the sciatic nerve or other motor nerves, it can infiltrate the connective tissue sheath of the nerve, following the nerve, and result in major insult to the neural elements. The needle can cause trauma to this, or other nerves, likewise. Precautions to avoid the sciatic nerve are especially important in injecting the gluteal area in babies. The reduced dimensions are less "forgiving" in babies.
   GAS 659; N 474; ABR/McM 324

55. B. The obturator nerve innervates the adductor muscles, including the gracilis, pectineus, and obturator externus. This gait pattern is characteristic of hypertonia in the lower limb. As a result these areas become flexed to various degrees, giving the appearance of crouching, while tight adductors produce extreme adduction.
   A. The tibial nerve supplies the calf muscles and intrinsic muscles in the plantar portion of the foot.
   C. The inferior gluteal nerve innervates the gluteus maximus.
   D. The superior gluteal nerve supplies the gluteus medius and minimus and tensor fasciae latae.
   E. The femoral nerve provides motor supply to the quadriceps femoris, sartorius, and, in most cases, the pectineus.
   GAS 556–557; N 488; ABR/McM 327

56. A. The perineal branch of the posterior femoral cutaneous nerve provides a significant portion of the cutaneous innervation of the perineum in some individuals and can require separate anesthetic blockade during childbirth or perineal surgery, if other types of anesthesia are not used.
   B. The inferior clunial branches of the posterior femoral cutaneous nerve supply the lower part of the skin of the buttocks.
   C. The lateral cutaneous branch of the iliohypogastric nerve provides sensation for the anterior superior aspect of the gluteal area.
   D. The inferior gluteal nerve innervates the gluteus maximus muscle.
   E. The middle cluneal nerves arise from the dorsal rami of S1 to S3 and supply skin over the middle of the gluteal region.
   GAS 485; N 531; ABR/McM 289

57. D. The dorsalis pedis is the continuation of the anterior tibial artery into the foot, as it passes the distal

end of the tibia and the ankle joint. The pulse of the dorsalis pedis can be felt between the tendon of the extensor hallucis longus and the tendon of the extensor digitorum longus to the second toe. A strong pulse is a positive indicator of circulation through the limb. (*GAS* Fig. 6.125).

A. Since the dorsalis pedis is a continuation of the anterior tibial artery, pulsations in the dorsalis pedis would also signify patency in the anterior tibial artery. The artery is also easier to palpate at the level of the dorsalis pedis.

B. The fibular artery is a branch of the posterior tibial artery and passes in the calf between the flexor hallucis longus and tibialis posterior, making it difficult to palpate.

C. The deep plantar artery passes deep to the aponeurotic tissues and central muscles of the foot, making palpation unlikely.

E. The dorsal metatarsal branches of the dorsalis pedis pass under cover of the extensor digitorum longus

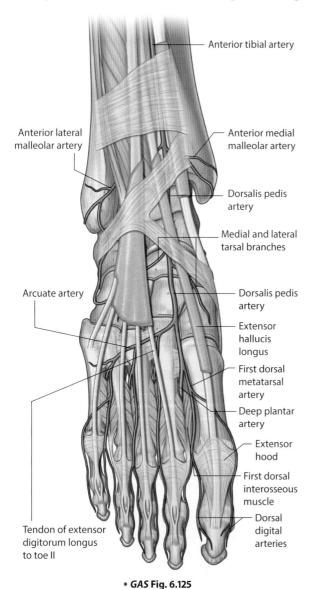

Anterior tibial artery

Anterior lateral malleolar artery

Anterior medial malleolar artery

Dorsalis pedis artery

Medial and lateral tarsal branches

Arcuate artery

Dorsalis pedis artery

Extensor hallucis longus

First dorsal metatarsal artery

Deep plantar artery

Extensor hood

First dorsal interosseous muscle

Dorsal digital arteries

Tendon of extensor digitorum longus to toe II

• **GAS Fig. 6.125**

and brevis tendons. Palpable pulses of the first or other dorsal metatarsal arteries can therefore be difficult to detect.
GAS 654; N 521; ABR/McM 354

58. D. Injury to the dorsalis pedis artery on the dorsum of the foot can also cause trauma to the terminal portion of the deep fibular nerve. This could result in loss of sensation between the first and second toes.

A. Clubfoot. Clubfoot is a congenital malformation observed in pediatric patients. This syndrome combines plantar flexion, inversion, and adduction of the foot. Neither extension of the great toe by the extensor hallucis longus nor paralysis of the tibialis anterior (weakness of foot inversion) would occur by this injury because both of these muscles are innervated by the deep fibular nerve much more proximally in the leg.

B, C, E. If the injury occurs in the proximal part of the foot, this could result in loss of sensation between the first and second toes and paralysis of the extensor digitorum brevis and the extensor hallucis brevis muscles. However, in the distal part of the foot, as in this patient, only sensory loss may be apparent.
GAS 654; N 533; ABR/McM 358

59. D. The sural nerve is formed by contributions from the tibial nerve and a branch from the common fibular nerve. It provides sensation for the lower lateral portion of the calf and continues beneath the lateral malleolus as the lateral cutaneous nerve of the foot. It is often used for nerve-grafting procedures and biopsied for diagnostic purposes. When it is grafted to the "living end" of a cut motor or sensory nerve, the severed nerve processes within the "living" nerve grow into the sural nerve sheath, using it as a guide to the distal, surgically anastomosed nerve. Thus axons from a branch of a functional motor nerve can grow to reinnervate paralyzed muscles. In this case the surgeon would connect portions of the sural nerve to the functional facial nerve, tunnel it to the opposite side of the face, and join it surgically to the branches of the paralyzed nerve, where it would grow through the now empty nerve sheaths (due to wallerian degeneration) to the muscles. Growth and reinnervation usually occur at a rate of 1 mm/day (or 1 inch/month) so the time estimated before reinnervation is based on the distance the regenerating fibers need to traverse.

A. Superficial fibular nerve supplies the fibularis longus and brevis which are the evertors of the foot.

B. The tibial nerve supplies muscles and sensation to the calf and plantar surface of the foot.

C. The common fibular nerve innervates the lateral and anterior compartment muscles and sensation to the dorsum of the foot.

E. The saphenous nerve accompanies the great saphenous vein on the medial side of the leg and foot.
GAS 624, 658; N 531; ABR/McM 348

60. D. Osgood-Schlatter disease is also called tibial tuberosity apophysitis and affects the area of the tibial tuberosity. It is not a disease but a problem of overuse, typically in boys of 12 to 14 years or girls 10 to 12 years of age. Very active boys and girls, usually during a growth spurt, are subject to the pain and swelling that occur at the site of attachment of the patellar ligament. The ligament can tear, resulting in a long period of healing following treatment.

A. The medial femoral condyle is the area of attachment of the tibial collateral ligament and medial meniscus of the knee joint.

B. The posterior intercondylar eminence is the location of origin of the posterior cruciate ligament.

C. The intercondylar eminence is a bony protuberance on the tibial plateau to which the cruciate ligaments and menisci are attached.

E. The anterolateral tibial tubercle, or Gerdy tubercle, is the attachment of the iliotibial tract; thus it connects the femur and tibia laterally.

GAS 578, 660; N 480; ABR/McM 342

61. A. The patient has bowlegs, or genu varus.

B. The contrary positioning of genu varus is genu valgus, or knock knee.

C. The normal angle between the femoral shaft and femoral neck is between 120 and 135 degrees. In coxa vara the angle between the shaft and neck of the femur is less than 120 degrees. This can result from fractures, other injuries, or congenital softness of the bone of the femoral neck. This defect results in limb shortening and limping.

D. In coxa valga there is an increase in femoral shaft neck angulation, which can lead to hip subluxation or dislocation. Coxa valga results from weakness of the adductor musculature.

E. Hallux valgus is commonly known as bunion. In this deformity the great toe points toward the little toe and may override the second toe; the base of the first metatarsal points medially, with a swollen bursal sac at the metatarsophalangeal joint. Excess bony growth of the distal protruding part of the metatarsal bone can also occur. Bunions occur only rarely in people who do not routinely wear shoes.

GAS 546; N 478; ABR/McM 339

62. A. The patellar ligament is a very strong ligament that connects the patella to the tibial tuberosity; it provides the insertion of the quadriceps femoris tendon upon the tibia. The patella can be thought of as a sesamoid bone that develops within the tendon of the quadriceps femoris muscle. When the reflex hammer strikes the patellar ligament, it stretches the ligament slightly for a brief time, resulting in reflex contraction of the quadriceps femoris muscles. This reflex arc is elicited by the femoral nerve (L4 sensory input component and L2, L3 motor output). The quadriceps femoris includes the rectus femoris and the vastus lateralis, intermedius, and medialis. The patella is the largest sesamoid bone in the body. A sesamoid bone is a bone that develops within a tendon.

B. The quadratus femoris muscle of the gluteal area arises from the ischial tuberosity and inserts on the femur proximally.

C. The sartorius arises from the anterior superior iliac spine and inserts on the proximal, medial aspect of the tibia as one of the three tendinous components of the pes anserinus (goose foot).

D. Pectineus is an adductor muscle found in the anteromedial superior thigh.

E. The biceps femoris of the posterior thigh has a long head that arises from the ischial tuberosity and a short head that arises from the femur; they unite to insert on the head of the fibula.

GAS 578; N 482; ABR/McM 342

63. E. The talus can be rotated externally when the ankle sustains a trimalleolar fracture, also called a Henderson fracture. The fracture may be caused by eversion and posterior displacement of the talus. This injury involves the fracture of the distal fibula (lateral malleolus); the medial malleolus of the tibia; and the posterior portion, or lip, of the tibial plafond (the distal articular portion of the tibia, sometimes referred to as the posterior malleolus). The posterior part of the plafond is not truly a malleolus but acts this way in this type of twisting fracture of the ankle. The talus can be forced from its normal position in this fracture, adding to the instability of the ankle.

A, B, D, C. The other bones listed are relatively far from the site of the fractures. The calcaneus resides beneath the talus and articulates distally with the cuboid bone. The head of the talus articulates also with the navicular bone. The navicular bone articulates distally with the three cuneiform bones.

GAS 629–640; N 517; ABR/McM 357

64. E. Hallux valgus, or lateral displacement of the great toe, usually comes as pain over the prominent metatarsal head, due to rubbing from shoes, and it can be associated with deformity of the second toe, which then tends to override the great toe. Hallux valgus is commonly known as bunion. In this deformity the great toe points toward the little toe; the base of the first metatarsal points medially, with a swollen bursal sac at the metatarsophalangeal joint. Excess bony growth of the distal protruding part of the metatarsal bone can also occur. Bunions occur only rarely in people who do not routinely wear shoes.

A. The normal angle between the femoral shaft and femoral neck is between 120 and 135 degrees. In coxa vara the angle between the shaft and neck of the femur is less than 120 degrees. This can result from fractures, other injuries, or congenital softness of the bone of the femoral neck. This defect results in limb shortening and limping.

B. In coxa valga there is an increase in femoral shaft neck angulation, which can lead to hip subluxation or dislocation. Coxa valga results from weakness of the adductor musculature.

C. The contrary positioning of genu varus is genu valgus, or knock knee.

D. Genu varus is also referred to as bowlegs, or bandy legs, in which the knees are bowed outward.
GAS 625, 629, 640; N 515; ABR/McM 360

65. C. The patient's complaint is due to her case of hammertoes. Hammer toe can affect any toe but most commonly the second toe, then the third or fourth toes. It results most commonly from wearing shoes that are too short or shoes with heels that are too high. In hammer toe, the metatarsophalangeal joint is extended, the proximal interphalangeal joint is flexed, and the distal phalanx points downward, looking like a hammer. Hammer toe can occur as a result of a bunion. Calluses, or painful corns, can form on the dorsal surface of the joints.

A. In pes planus the patient lacks an appropriately flexed plantar arch, which is not the presentation here.

B. In pes cavus the patient has a high, flexed plantar arch. This occurs as a result of hereditary motor and sensory neural problems. The condition may be painful because of metatarsal compression.

D. In claw toe, both the proximal and distal interphalangeal joints are strongly flexed, the result of muscle imbalance in the foot. Either hammer toe or claw toe can occur from arthritic changes.

E. Hallux valgus is also commonly known as a bunion. In this deformity the great toe points toward the little toe; the base of the first metatarsal points medially, with a swollen bursal sac at the metatarsophalangeal joint. Excess bony growth of the distal protruding part of the metatarsal bone can also occur. Bunions occur only rarely in people who do not routinely wear shoes.
GAS 632–635; N 515; ABR/McM 358

66. C. In piriformis syndrome or entrapment, the sciatic nerve can be compressed when the piriformis is contracted, leading to painful sensations in the lower limb. These usually involve pain in the gluteal area, posterior thigh, and leg, most frequently resembling a disc lesion at L5 -S1, with compression of the S1 spinal nerve.

A. L4 compression would involve the quadriceps femoris knee extension, foot inversion, and sensory loss on the medial side of the leg.

B. L5 compression would be indicated by weakness in dorsiflexion and foot inversion, and sensory loss on the dorsal surface of the foot.

C. S1 compression would weaken plantar flexion and foot eversion.

D, E. Pudendal nerve (S2-S4) entrapment would affect the perineal region. The fibular division of the sciatic nerve passes through the piriformis in some individuals, leading to L5, S1–S3 nerve compression.
GAS 524.e1, 557; N 489; ABR/McM 325

67. C. Incapacitation and unconsciousness from use of cocaine and other powerful narcotics have led to numerous cases of the "gluteal crush syndrome." Compression of the gluteal region while supine for extended periods of time can lead to gluteal crush injury, in which the nerves and vessels of the gluteal area are compressed. This can result in loss of gluteal muscles and other soft tissues and sciatic nerve compression. The nerve compression can cause paralysis of knee flexors and muscles of the anterior and lateral compartments of the leg, with sensory loss in the posterior thigh and leg and sensory loss in the foot.

A, B, D, E. Tibial nerve loss would not result in loss of dorsiflexion of the foot nor generalized sensory loss. Compression of nerves would be more extensive than S1-S2 by the injury in this case. Neither piriformis entrapment nor femoral nerve entrapment is associated with loss of gluteal musculature, nor loss of knee flexion or plantar flexion of the foot, nor do they lead to general sensory loss in the limb.
GAS 527–528, 566; N 489; ABR/McM 325

68. E. In infants and children until approximately the age of 8 years, the head of the femur gets its arterial supply by a direct branch of the obturator artery (variably, the medial circumflex femoral). The arterial supply reaches the head of the femur at the fovea capitis by traveling within the ligament of the head of the femur. This source of supply is replaced later by vessels such as branches of the ascending branch of the medial circumflex femoral that pass into foramina of the neck of the femur within the capsule of the hip joint. Similar branches can arise from the lateral circumflex femoral and gluteal arteries. (*GAS Fig. 6.31*).

A. The deep circumflex iliac artery arises from the external iliac artery and supplies branches to the ilium, the iliacus muscle, and lower portions of the abdominal wall.

B. The acetabular branch of the obturator artery often provides the branch to the head of the femur, an artery that normally regresses early in life, so that it supplies only the immediate area of the fovea capitis.

C. The descending branch of the lateral circumflex femoral supplies the vastus lateralis muscle and participates in anastomoses at the knee.

D. The second perforating branch of the deep femoral artery often supplies the nutrient artery of the shaft of the femur
GAS 550–553, 670.e3; N 495; ABR/McM 330

69. D. The lesser (small) saphenous vein ascends up the middle of the calf from beneath the lateral malleolus, most commonly terminating at the popliteal fossa by piercing the deep fascia and joining the popliteal vein.

A. The popliteal vein lies deep to the tibial nerve, which is the most superficial of major structures deep to the deep popliteal fascia.

B. The superior medial genicular vein is a tributary to the popliteal vein.

C. The great saphenous runs on the medial side of the leg and eventually empties into the femoral vein.

E. Superior medial genicular. The superior medial genicular vein is a tributary to the popliteal vein.
GAS 542, 560, 609, 655; N 513; ABR/McM 344

70. E. The lateral plantar artery provides origin to the deep plantar arterial arch. Medially, the vascular arch anastomoses with the distal portion of the dorsalis pedis by way of the deep plantar artery.

A. The anterior tibial artery continues as the dorsalis pedis at the ankle joint.

B. The fibular artery, by way of a perforating branch, replaces the dorsal pedis in some individuals.

C. The arcuate artery, a branch of the dorsalis pedis, provides origin for the dorsal metatarsal arteries to the lateral toes.

D. The medial plantar artery runs along the medial arch of the foot and mainly supplies to hallucis nerves and plantar aspect of the feet.
GAS 653; N 513; ABR/McM 361

71. C. The bone to which the injured ligament attaches is the calcaneus.

A. The navicular bone, located medially in the foot, articulates posteriorly with the head of the talus and anteriorly with the cuneiform bones.

B. The cuboid bone of the lateral longitudinal arch articulates posteriorly with the calcaneus.

D. Arises from the anteromedial portion of the calcaneus and not the posterior segment of the calcaneus.

E. The talus articulates with the tibia and fibula in the ankle joint mortise.
GAS 627–640; N 518; ABR/McM 355

Answers 72–95

72. C. The fibularis brevis arises from the fibula and inserts upon the tuberosity at the base of the fifth metatarsal bone. Its attachment is often involved in an inversion fracture of the foot. This common fracture can often be overlooked when it is combined with an inversion sprain of the ankle.

A. The fibularis longus arises from the fibula, passes under the lateral malleolus, and then turns medially into the plantar surface of the foot, where it inserts upon the medial cuneiform and first metatarsal bones.

B. The tibialis posterior arises from the tibia in the posterior compartment of the leg; it passes under the medial malleolus and inserts upon the navicular and metatarsal bones.

D. The extensor digitorum brevis arises dorsally from the calcaneus and inserts upon the proximal phalanges of the lateral toes.

E. The adductor hallucis arises from the lateral metatarsals and transverse tarsal ligament and inserts upon the proximal phalanx and lateral sesamoid bone of the great toe.
GAS 622–623, 642, 664; N 510; ABR/McM 363

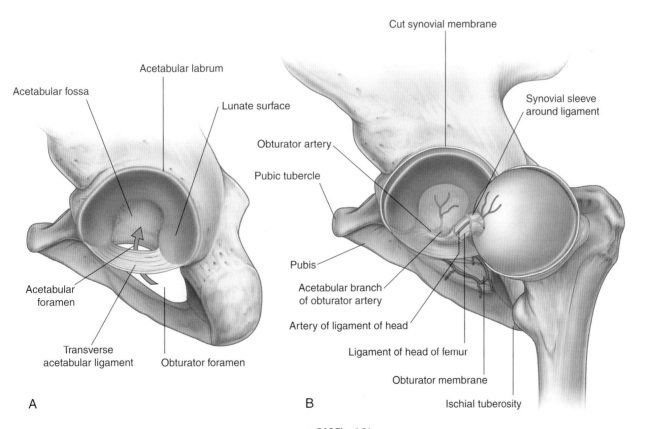

A

B

• *GAS* **Fig. 6.31**

73. A. Excessive compression of the prepatellar bursa, as in working on bended knees, can result in pain and swelling of the prepatellar bursa, the so-called housemaid's knee. Prepatellar bursitis affects plumbers, carpet layers, and other people who spend a lot of time working on their knees. The bursa normally enables the patella to move smoothly under the skin. The constant friction of these occupations irritates this small lubricating sac (bursa) located just in front of the patella, resulting in a deformable tense cushion of fluid. Treatment usually requires simple drainage, but this may need to be repeated and occasionally steroids introduced.

    B. Infrapatellar bursa. Excessive irritation of the infrapatellar bursa in kneeling for frequent and long periods of time (as in prayer) can result in "parson's knee."

    C. Semimembranosus bursa is located at the posteromedial aspect of the knee, on the medial aspect of the semimembranosus tendon.

    D. Suprapatellar bursa is located superior to the patellar, at the distal end of the femur posterior to the quadriceps tendon. Due to its location it would be less likely to become irritated by kneeling but may become inflamed due to direct trauma to the area.

    E. Pes anserine describes the region on the medial proximal end of the knee where the gracilis, sartorius and semitendinosus tendons attach. The bursa in this region (anserine bursa) may become inflamed due to repeated knee joint movements or due to direct trauma to the region.

GAS 598–603; N 502; ABR/McM 342

74. D. The ligament of the head of the femur conveys a small blood vessel for supply of the head of the femur (primarily in childhood). The ligament is stretched during abduction and lateral rotation of the hip joint and has an important role in stabilizing an infant's hip joint before walking. It has the potential to increase stability of the joint in hip reconstruction in developmental hip dysplasia in the pediatric population. The strength of this ligament is comparable to the anterior cruciate ligament of the knee.

    A. The iliofemoral ligament (the inverted "Y-shaped ligament of Bigelow") on the anterior aspect of the hip bone resists hyperextension of the hip joint.

    B. The pubofemoral ligament arises from the pubic bone and is located on the inferior side of the hip joint; it resists abduction of the joint.

    C. The ischiofemoral ligament is a triangular band of strong fibers that arises from the ischium and winds upward and laterally over the femoral neck, strengthening the capsule posteriorly.

    E. The transverse acetabular ligament attaches to the margins of the acetabular notch and provides origin for the ligament of the head of the femur. The transverse acetabular ligament is fibrous, not cartilaginous, but is regarded as part of the acetabular labrum.

GAS550–553; N 477; ABR/McM 334

75. B. The posterior cruciate ligament tightens in flexion of the knee. It can be damaged by posterior displacement of the tibia upon the femur. With the patient seated, a rupture of the ligament can be demonstrated by the ability to push the tibia posteriorly under the femur. This is called the posterior drawer sign because it is similar to pushing in a desk drawer.

    A. The anterior cruciate ligament resists knee hyperextension and integrity would be tested for by doing the anterior draw test which tests for the ability to displace the tibia anterior to the femur. If the tibia can be displaced anterior to the femur this signals a positive anterior draw test and may signify rupture of the anterior cruciate ligament.

    C. The fibular collateral ligament is a thick, cordlike band that passes from the lateral femoral condyle to the head of the fibula. It is located external to the capsule of the knee joint.

    D. The lateral meniscus is a nearly circular band of fibrocartilage that is located laterally within the knee joint. It is less frequently injured than the medial meniscus because it is not attached to the joint capsule or other ligaments.

    E. The patellar ligament is the strong, ligamentous band of insertion of the quadriceps femoris muscle to the tibial tuberosity.

GAS 576–578; N 500; ABR/McM 339

76. A. Flat foot (pes planus) is due to flattening of the medial longitudinal arch. Often congenital, it may be associated with minor structural anomalies of the tarsal bones. This condition can be seen in wet footprints in which the medial surface of the sole (normally raised in an arch) is visible. Treatment may include intensive foot exercises or arch supports worn in the shoes. Occasionally, surgery is needed in the form of arthrodesis (fusion of the tarsal bones).

    B. Pes cavus is a deformity of the foot characterized by a very high medial arch and hyperextension of the toes.

    C. Collapse of long plantar ligament. The long plantar ligament is a passive ligament of the longitudinal arch. The long plantar ligament connects the calcaneus and cuboid bones. It can be involved with the plantar aponeurosis in plantar fasciitis. The long plantar ligament converts the cuboid groove into a canal for the tendon of the fibularis longus

    D. The medial collateral (deltoid) ligament is a very strong ligament that interconnects the tibia with the navicular, calcaneus, and talus bones. The medial malleolus will usually fracture before this ligament tears.

    E. The plantar calcaneonavicular, or spring, ligament is a key element in the medial longitudinal arch; it supports the head of the talus bone and thereby is subject to vertical forces exerted through the lower limbs. In the present case, the bilateral pes planus appears to be the result of gradual weakening and failure of the arches.

GAS 534, 644; N 519; ABR/McM 320

77. C. If the needle is inserted approximately 1.5 cm lateral to the maximal femoral pulse, it will intersect the femoral nerve in most cases. (Fluoroscopic or ultrasound guidance is advisable to avoid iatrogenic errors.)

A. The deep inguinal ring is located approximately 4 cm superolateral to the pubic tubercle and very close to the origin of the inferior epigastric vessels from the external iliac artery and vein.

B. The approximate site of exit of the lateral femoral cutaneous nerve from the abdomen is 1.5 cm medial to the anterior superior iliac spine

D. 1.5 cm medial to the femoral pulse. Injections 1.5 cm medial to the femoral artery pulse will enter the femoral vein.

E. Midway between the anterior superior iliac spine and the pubic symphysis can vary approximately 1.5 cm either medial or lateral from the femoral artery.

GAS 660, 666; N 490; ABR/McM 328

78. A. Morton neuroma most commonly involves compression (and possible enlargement) of an anastomosing branch that connects the medial and lateral plantar nerves between the third and fourth toes. The pain can be severe. The medial plantar nerve provides sensation for the medial three and a half toes; the lateral plantar nerve supplies the little toe and half of the fourth toe. The neural interconnection can be compressed between the transverse metatarsal ligament and the floor. Women are 10 times more likely than men to be afflicted with this problem, most likely due to wearing shoes that put excessive stress on the forefoot. In approximately 80% of cases the pain can be eased with different (less-confining) shoes or cortisone injections.

B, C, D, E. Morton neuroma occurs between the third and fourth toes about 80% of the time but can also occur in other regions. This neuroma is less likely to occur in these other regions.

GAS 656–657; N 532; ABR/McM 361

79. D. Inflammation of the plantar aponeurosis is referred to as plantar fasciitis. Plantar fasciitis is a common physical condition that results from tearing or inflammation of the tough band of tissue stretching from the calcaneus to the ball of the foot (the plantar aponeurosis). It happens frequently to people who are on their feet all day, such as mail carriers, or engaged in athletics, especially in running and jumping. The pain of plantar fasciitis is usually most significant in the morning, just after you get up from bed and begin to walk. Rest, orthotics, night splints, and antiinflammatory medications are used in treatment.

A. Morton neuroma is a painful lesion of the neural interconnection of the medial and lateral plantar nerves between the third and fourth toes.

B. An eversion sprain of the ankle can break the medial malleolus or tear the medial collateral (deltoid) ligament.

C. Occurs due to compression of the tibial nerve by the flexor retinaculum in the tarsal tunnel. This may cause pain and numbness to the medial aspect of the feet and along the soles. This is pain caused by nerve compression versus the pain caused by inflammation of the plantar aponeurosis

E. An inversion sprain commonly injures the calcaneofibular ligament or anterior talofibular ligament.

GAS 647; N 523; ABR/McM 361

80. B. The child has the problem of talipes equinovarus, or clubfoot. Clubfoot is a congenital malformation observed in approximately 1 in 1000 pediatric patients and first appears in the first trimester of pregnancy. This syndrome combines plantar flexion, inversion, and adduction of the foot. The heel is drawn upward by the tendo calcaneus and turned inward; the forefoot is also adducted, or turned inward. The foot usually is smaller than normal.

A. In coxa vara, the angle between the femoral shaft and neck is reduced to less than 120 degrees, often due to excessive activity of the adductor musculature.

C. Hallux valgus is also known as bunion, in which the great toe points laterally.

D. Hallux varus involves a medial deviation of the first metatarsal or great toe, sometimes the result of attempted correction of bunions. It can also result from arthritis or muscular problems.

E. Plantar fasciitis is caused by inflammation of the plantar aponeurosis, not resulting in the malformation seen here.

GAS 534–535, 628, 656; N 516; ABR/McM 364

81. D. In claw toes, both the proximal and distal interphalangeal joints are strongly flexed as a result of muscle imbalance in the foot. With muscular imbalance, the extensors of the interphalangeal joints are overpowered by the long flexors. The metatarsophalangeal joint is extended, whereas in hammer toe it can be in a neutral position. Either hammer toe or claw toe can occur from arthritic changes.

A. Hallux valgus is more commonly referred to as a bunion. The great toe is angulated toward the little toe and may override the second toe. The base of the first metatarsal bone is directed medially and is subject, painfully, to compression.

B. Pes planus is flat foot and the patient has low plantar arch. Is due to flattening of the medial longitudinal arch. Often congenital, it may be associated with minor structural anomalies of the tarsal bones.

C. Hammertoes. Hammer toe can affect any toe, but it most commonly affects the second toe, then the third or fourth toes. It results most commonly from wearing shoes that are too short or shoes with heels that are too high. In hammer toe the metatarsophalangeal joint is extended, the proximal interphalangeal joint is flexed, and the distal phalanx may be dorsiflexed, or it may point downward, looking like a hammer. Hammer toe can occur as a result of a bunion. Calluses, or painful corns, can form on the dorsal surface of the joints.

E. Pes cavus. Pes cavus is the opposite of flat foot; the patient has a high, flexed plantar arch. Pes cavus occurs as a result of hereditary motor and sensory neural problems. It is painful because of metatarsal compression.

GAS 534, 636–641; N 515; ABR/McM 318

82. D. The ankle jerk reflex, elicited by tapping the calcaneal tendon (Achilles tendon) with the reflex hammer, is mediated by the tibial nerve. The medial plantar nerve innervates the abductor and flexor muscles of the great toe, the first lumbrical muscle, and flexor digitorum brevis muscle and provides sensation for the medial plantar surface and three and a half toes.

A. The common fibular nerve combines the functions of the superficial and deep branches.

B, E. The superficial fibular nerve supplies the foot evertor muscles of the lateral compartment of the leg and provides sensory supply for the dorsum of the foot.

C, E. The deep fibular nerve innervates the foot extensor and invertor muscles in the anterior compartment of the leg and dorsum of the foot and supplies skin between the first and second toes.

GAS 615–619; N 514; ABR/McM 355

83. B. The posterior femoral cutaneous nerve arises from ventral rami of S1 to S3. It provides inferior clunial branches to the lower portion of the gluteal region and a perineal branch to the perineum and supplies sensation to the posterior thigh to the level of the popliteal fossa.

A. Superior gluteal region innervation arises from the dorsal rami of L1 to L3 (superior cluneal nerves).

C. The posterior femoral cutaneous is a cutaneous (sensory) nerve and does not innervate muscles.

D. Meralgia paresthetica is the occurrence of pain or burning sensations on the lateral thigh, from compression of the lateral femoral cutaneous nerve.

E. The sural nerve provides sensation to the lower calf and lateral foot. It arises from contributions from the tibial nerve and common fibular nerve.

GAS 480, 554; N 531; ABR/McM 325

84. B. The lower portion of the vastus medialis inserts upon the medial aspect of the patella and draws it medially, especially in the last quarter of extension --during which it is especially palpable in contraction. This lower portion of the muscle is referred to as the vastus medialis obliquus (VMO). Increasing the strength of this muscle can lessen the lateral dislocation of the patella. The rectus femoris arises from the anterior inferior iliac spine and superior rim of the acetabulum and draws the patella vertically upward, as does the vastus intermedius.

A. The vastus lateralis attaches to the lateral portion of the patella and may contribute to lateral displacement of the bone.

C, D. The rectus femoris arises from the anterior inferior iliac spine and superior rim of the acetabulum and draws the patella vertically upward, as does the vastus intermedius.

E. The patellar ligament attaches the inferior portion of the patellar to the proximal part tibia this anchors the patellar inferiorly.

GAS 582; N 511; ABR/McM 337

85. D. Bipartite patella is a normal variant of an unfused superolateral secondary ossification center, which can easily be mistaken for a fracture on a x-ray. The subcutaneous prepatellar bursa can become painfully enlarged with acute or chronic compression, as in crawling about on the knees. The medial patellar retinaculum is an expanded portion of the vastus medialis tendon toward the patella.

A. The subcutaneous prepatellar bursa can become painfully enlarged with acute or chronic compression, as in crawling about on the knees.

B. Osgood-Schlatter disease is painful involvement of the patellar ligament on the tibial tuberosity, commonly in children 10 to 14 years of age.

C. The intercondylar eminence is part of the tibia and lies in between the interarticular facets of the proximal tibia.

E. Injury to lateral meniscus would occur in the knee joint itself and would not be seen so far proximally on the femur. They are usually caused by twisting injury with the feet anchored.

GAS 578; N 498; ABR/McM 342

86. D. Femoral artery puncture is one of the most common vascular procedures. The femoral artery can be localized often by simply feeling for the femoral pulse just inferior to the inguinal ligament. The femoral artery can be accessed with fluoroscopic assistance at the medial edge of the upper portion of the head of the femur. It is easily localized by Doppler ultrasound if the pulse is difficult to detect, such as in an obese patient. It is here that catheters are passed into the femoral artery for catheterization of abdominopelvic and thoracic structures and for antegrade angiography. It is also a site where arterial blood can be obtained for gas analysis.

A. The midinguinal point, halfway between the anterior superior iliac spine and the pubic symphysis, can be either medial or lateral to the femoral artery and is not a dependable landmark.

B. Four centimeters lateral to the pubic tubercle overlies the deep inguinal ring, with potential entry to spermatic cord, femoral vein, or artery.

C. A needle inserted at the level of the inguinal crease, or inferior to the femoral head, can enter the femoral artery distal to the origin of the deep femoral artery, presenting more risk for accidental vascular injury.

E. The fossa ovalis is the opening in the fascia lata for the termination of the great saphenous vein into the femoral vein.
GAS 660, 667; N 490; ABR/McM 328

87. D. Commonly seen in football players' knees, meniscal tears are usually diagnosed by MRI or arthroscopy. The presenting symptoms of tearing may be pain and swelling, or locking of the knee. Locking of the knee suggests a bucket-handle tear, in which a partly detached cartilage wedges between the tibia and femur, inhibiting further movement. A bucket-handle tear is often associated with rupture of the anterior cruciate ligament. Sometimes a momentary click can be heard in flexion/extension movements of the knee. Meniscectomy is usually successful operation, but currently there is greater emphasis on repairing small tears. Meniscal cysts can form secondary to meniscal tears and some of these can also be treated arthroscopically. Bucket handle tears and overall meniscal tears are more commonly associated with anterior cruciate ligament injury.

A. Posterior cruciate ligament injury is more commonly associated with posterior medial meniscus avulsion tear.

B, C. Both the medial and lateral menisci are subject to rotational injuries and may be torn. The medial meniscus is much more liable to injury because it is attached to the fused deep layer of the tibial collateral ligament and joint capsule. The lateral meniscus is separated from the lateral or fibular collateral ligament and is external to the capsule of the knee joint.

E. Coronary ligaments are part of the fibrous capsule of the knee joint.
GAS 579, 598; N 500; ABR/McM 339

88. B. The tendons of the semitendinosus and semimembranosus provide the superior medial border of the popliteal fossa. The semitendinosus inserts with the pes anserinus on the proximal, medial tibia. The semimembranosus inserts on the tibia posteriorly

A. The biceps femoris forms the superior lateral border of the fossa, as the tendon passes to insertion on the fibula.

C. Tendon of plantaris. The plantaris arises from the femur just above the lateral head of the gastrocnemius, passing distally to insert on the calcaneus beside the calcaneal tendon.

D. The adductor hiatus is a gap between the adductor magnus and the femur which allows for passage of the femoral vessels from the anterior to posterior thigh.

E. The popliteus arises from the tibia and passes superiorly and laterally to insert on the lateral condyle of the femur, with a connection to the lateral meniscus.
GAS 590, 610; N 507; ABR/McM 345

89. C. The iliotibial tract is a dense, wide aponeurosis that receives the insertion of the tensor fasciae latae and

approximately 75% of the gluteus maximus. The gluteus maximus is the only one of the muscles listed that is supplied by the inferior gluteal nerve.

A, B, C. Gluteus medius and gluteus minimus insert on the greater trochanter and are innervated by the superior gluteal nerve, as is the tensor fasciae latae.

E. The rectus femoris, supplied by the femoral nerve, inserts via the quadriceps femoris tendon on the patella and tibial tuberosity.
GAS 570; N 490; ABR/McM 329

90. D. The tendinous distal portion of the adductor magnus inserts on the adductor tubercle on the upper border of the medial condyle of the femur. The femoral artery passes through the adductor hiatus proximal to this tendinous band, continuing as the popliteal artery.

A. The semimembranosus inserts on the proximal, posterior portion of the tibia.

B. The gracilis inserts with the pes anserinus on the proximal, medial aspect of the tibia.

C. The popliteus inserts on the distal lateral portion of the femur, just above the origin of the lateral head of gastrocnemius.

E. The vastus medialis inserts with other quadriceps femoris muscle components on the patella and then on to the tibial tuberosity.
GAS 586–590; N 481; ABR/McM 305

91. B. The iliopsoas forms the lateral portion of the trough-like floor of the femoral triangle. (GAS Fig. 6.42).

A, C. The adductor longus provides a medial border for the femoral triangle and meets the sartorius, the lateral border of the triangle, at the apex.

D. The pectineus forms the middle portion of this floor.

E. The rectus femoris is a superficial contributor to the quadriceps femoris, lateral to the femoral triangle.
GAS 564; N 482; ABR/McM 329

92. A. The tendon of the obturator internus leaves the pelvic cavity by passing through the lesser sciatic foramen, wrapping around the lesser sciatic notch, changing direction by approximately 90 degrees. It is joined there by the superior and inferior gemelli and inserts with them on the medial surface of the greater trochanter.

B. The obturator externus arises on the external surface of the margins of the obturator foramen and obturator membrane and inserts in the intertrochanteric fossa.

C. The quadratus femoris arises from the ischial tuberosity and inserts on the quadrate line below the intertrochanteric crest of the femur.

D, E. The gluteus medius and gluteus minimus insert together on the lateral aspect of the greater trochanter.
GAS 440–443; N 485; ABR/McM 289

93. B. In general, the angle of inclination between the neck and shaft of the femur in older age decreases to approximately 120 degrees. However, in pathologic conditions it can either increase or decrease from the predicted

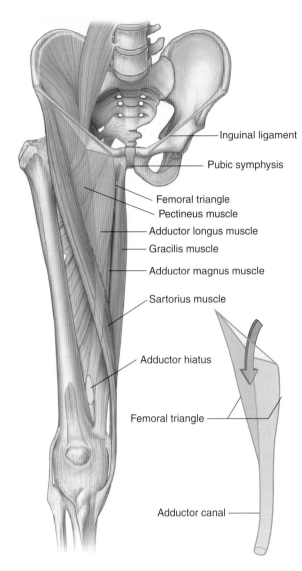

Inguinal ligament

Pubic symphysis

Femoral triangle
Pectineus muscle

Adductor longus muscle

Gracilis muscle

Adductor magnus muscle

Sartorius muscle

Adductor hiatus

Femoral triangle

Adductor canal

• *GAS* **Fig. 6.42**

value. When the angle of inclination increases, it is referred to as coxa valga.

A. In contrast, coxa vara is a condition characterized by a decreased angle of inclination.

C, D. Genu varum and genu valgum are deformities characterized by a decreased Q-angle and increased Q-angle, respectively. The Q-angle refers to the angle between the femur and tibia.

E. Hallux valgus is a condition that comes with a lateral deviation of the large toe.

GAS 546, 576; N 478; ABR/McM 302

94. D. Plantar fasciitis is a common physical condition that results from tearing or inflammation of the tough band of tissue stretching from the calcaneus to the ball of the foot (the plantar aponeurosis). It usually happens to people who are on their feet frequently or engaged in athletics, especially running and jumping. Plantar fasciitis is usually most painful in the morning, just after getting up from bed and beginning to

walk. Rest, orthotics, night splints, and antiinflammatory medications are used in treatment. Each of these fractures occurs due to sudden and forceful eversion of the foot.

A. A Pott fracture is a bimalleolar fracture, specifically a fracture of the distal end of the fibula (lateral malleolus) and medial malleolus, with outward displacement of the foot.

B. Dupuytren fracture involves fracture of the distal fibula with dislocation of the foot.

C. Compression of the tibial nerve by the flexor retinaculum in the tarsal tunnel may cause pain and numbness to the medial aspect of the feet and along the soles.

E. The plantar calcaneonavicular, or spring, ligament is a key element in the medial longitudinal arch; it supports the head of the talus bone and thereby is subject to vertical forces exerted through the lower limbs.

GAS 645; N 523; ABR/McM 360

95. A. When the anterior cruciate ligament is torn, the tibia can be slightly displaced anteriorly from the area of the knee joint by pulling firmly with both hands upon the leg, with the patient in a seated position. This is a positive anterior drawer sign.

B. Posterior displacement of the tibia from a posterior drawer test that signifies damage to the posterior cruciate ligament.

C, D, E. The anterior and posterior drawer tests focus on the displacement of the tibia in relation to the femur. The fibula is not the focus of either examination.

GAS 605–608; N 500; ABR/McM 339

Answers 96–120

96. E. One important function of the medial collateral (deltoid) ligament is the prevention of excessive extension of the ankle. The ligament is so strong that excessive eversion can cause the medial malleolus to be pulled off (an avulsion fracture) rather than tearing the medial collateral (deltoid) ligament.

A. The plantar calcaneonavicular, or spring, ligament is a key element in the medial longitudinal arch; it supports the head of the talus bone.

B. Calcaneofibular ligament extends from the distal tip of the fibular to the lateral aspect of the calcaneous and this supports the lateral aspect of the ankle joint.

C. The long plantar ligament is the longest and strongest ligament of the foot. It runs from the calcaneus to the base of the metatarsal bones and assists in forming the longitudinal arch of the foot.

D. The short plantar ligament or the plantar calcaneocuboid ligament stabilizes the calcaneocuboid joint. It attaches proximally to the inferomedial aspect of the calcaneus, and attaches distally to the plantar aspect of the cuboid bone.

GAS 634; N 518; ABR/McM 359

97. B. In infants and children up to approximately 8 years of age, the head of the femur gets its arterial supply by a direct branch (the acetabular branch) of the obturator artery (variably, the medial circumflex femoral). The arterial supply reaches the head of the femur at the fovea capitis by traveling within the ligament of the head of the femur. Probably due to repeated torsion on the ligament and therefore on the artery, this artery occludes early in life.

  A. The deep circumflex iliac artery arises from the external iliac artery and supplies branches to the ilium, the iliacus muscle, and lower portions of the abdominal wall.

  C. The descending branch of the lateral circumflex femoral supplies the vastus lateralis muscle and participates in anastomoses at the knee.

  D. In turn, this source of supply is replaced by branches of the medial femoral circumflex artery, primarily.

  E. These vessels extend to the head of the femur to also provide blood supply.

  GAS 551–554; N 495; ABR/McM 330

98. E. The ankle jerk reflex involves S1 and S2 levels.

  A, B, C. L2 -L4 are involved in the patellar reflex.

  D. L5 is not a component of a deep tendon reflex.

  GAS 615; N 532; ABR/McM 355

99 B. The tensor fasciae latae assists in flexion of the thigh, as well as medial rotation and abduction. Damage to this muscle would adversely affect these motions.

  A. The rectus femoris flexes the hip and extends the knee.

  C. The vastus intermedius extends the knee.

  D. The semimembranosus extends the hip and flexes and medially rotates the knee.

  E. The sartorius assists in flexion and lateral rotation of the hip, as well as in flexion of the knee.

  GAS 570; N 484; ABR/McM 329

100. B. The femoral triangle is the best place to palpate the femoral pulse. It is bounded by the sartorius muscle laterally, adductor longus medially, and the inguinal ligament superiorly. It contains the femoral vein, artery, and nerve (from medial to lateral, respectively).

  A. The adductor canal lies deep between the anterior and medial compartments of the thigh and therefore cannot be palpated.

  C. The popliteal fossa is the fossa at the back of the knee and contains the popliteal artery and vein, tibial nerve, and common fibular nerve. The femoral pulse cannot be palpated here.

  D. The inguinal canal is in the lower anterior abdominal wall. It contains the spermatic cord in men and round ligament of the uterus in women.

  E. Pubic symphysis is a cartilaginous structure that holds the pubic bones together. The femoral pulse would not be felt here.

  GAS 564; N 482; ABR/McM 329

101. A. If the femoral artery is occluded, the descending branch of the lateral circumflex femoral will provide collateral circulation to the thigh.

  B. The descending genicular artery is a branch of the femoral and therefore would also be occluded.

  C. The medial circumflex femoral artery is a proximal branch of the deep femoral artery and supplies retinacular branches to the head of the femur.

  D. The first perforating branch of the deep femoral artery supplies a small portion of the muscles of the posterior thigh.

  E. The obturator artery supplies a very small artery and vascularizes only the most proximal part of the head of the femur and usually only during the early years of life.

  GAS 553, 558, 574; N 495; ABR/McM 330

102. A. In a femoral hernia, abdominal contents are forced through the femoral ring, which is just lateral to the lacunar ligament (of Gimbernat) and just medial to the femoral vein. The femoral vein would be found immediately lateral to the femoral hernia.

  B, D. In the majority of people, the femoral vein is found more medial to both the femoral artery and nerve in the femoral triangle.

  C, E. The adductor longus muscle as well as the pectineus muscle would be found deep and medial to the hernia.

  GAS 564; N 256; ABR/McM 235

103. A. The femoral vein lies medial to the femoral artery in the femoral sheath. The femoral sheath is broken into three compartments: lateral, intermediate, and medial. The lateral compartment contains the femoral artery.

  B. The medial compartment encloses the femoral canal and consists of lymphatic tissue and a deep inguinal lymph node, plus areolar tissue. The intermediate contains the femoral vein.

  C. In most cases the femoral vein lies medial to the femoral artery.

  D. The femoral vein in most cases lies directly medial to the femoral artery and the femoral nerve lies lateral to the femoral artery.

  E. The femoral nerve lies lateral to the femoral vein in most cases.

  GAS 560, 575; N 490; ABR/McM 329

104. B. The superficial inguinal nodes are located near the saphenofemoral junction and drain the superficial lower limb and perineum.

  A, E. The external and internal iliac nodes first receive lymph from pelvic and perineal structures

  C. The deep inguinal lymph nodes lie deep to the fascia lata and receive lymph from deep lymph vessels (popliteal nodes).

  D. The vertical group receives lymph from the superficial thigh, and the horizontal group receives lymph from the gluteal regions and the anterolateral abdominal wall (*GAS Fig. 6.39*).

  GAS 562; N 475; ABR/McM 376

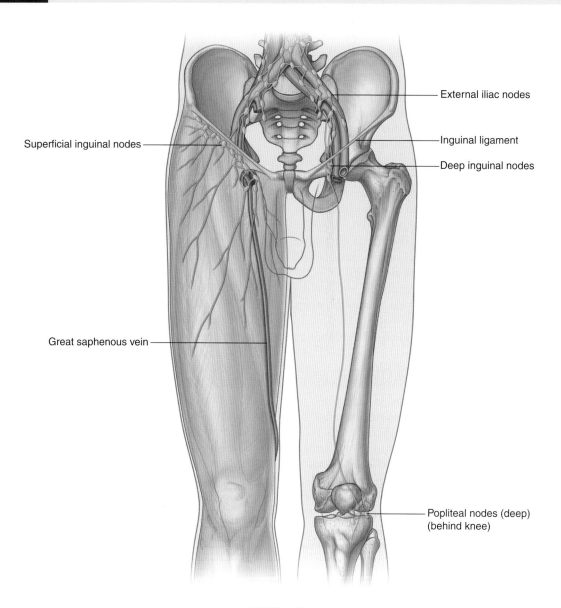

External iliac nodes

Superficial inguinal nodes

Inguinal ligament

Deep inguinal nodes

Great saphenous vein

Popliteal nodes (deep)
(behind knee)

• *GAS* **Fig. 6.39**

105. D. The fibularis brevis muscle originates from the lateral lower two-thirds of the shaft of the fibula and inserts on the tubercle at the base of the fifth metatarsal. Any injury to this area will affect this muscle. Patients will present with a weakness in eversion of the foot. The gastrocnemius inserts via the calcaneal (Achilles) tendon on the posterior surface of the calcaneus.

A, B, E. The fibularis longus, extensor hallucis longus, and tibialis anterior insert on the medial side of the foot and will not be affected in this patient.

C. The gastrocnemius inserts via the calcaneal (Achilles) tendon on the posterior surface of the calcaneus.

GAS 622–625; N 506; ABR/McM 351

106. A. The obturator nerve is a branch of the lumbar plexus that originates from L2 to L4. It descends medial to the psoas major, over the sacroiliac joint, and into the pelvis, where it runs along the lateral wall of the lesser pelvis, above and anterior to the obturator vessels. It enters into the medial thigh via the obturator canal (an opening above the obturator membrane) to supply the obturator externus muscle and the adductors of the thigh.

B. The femoral nerve innervates the anterior compartment of the thigh.

C. The inferior gluteal nerve innervates the gluteus maximus muscle.

D. The superior gluteal nerve innervates the gluteus minimus, gluteus medius, and tensor fasciae latae.

E. The tibial nerve innervates the posterior compartment of the lower limb and the muscles of the plantar foot.

GAS 555–558; N 486; ABR/McM 271

107. A, D. The common fibular nerve is a branch of the sciatic nerve. It descends on the lateral side of the popliteal fossa before winding around the head of the fibula. Due to its superficial course, it is easily injured in patients with long leg casts (which run from just below the knee). The nerve supplies the dorsiflexors of the leg, the skin of the first web space (via the deep fibular), the evertors of the foot, and the skin of the lateral side of the leg and dorsum of the foot (via the superficial fibular).

B, C. The common fibular nerve divides into superficial and deep nerves that supply the lateral and anterior compartments of the leg respectively.

E. Tibial nerve injury would present with issues with plantarflexion of the feet and not foot drop. There may also be sensory loss to distal part of the posterior leg.

GAS 624–626; N 531; ABR/McM 325

108. **C.** The lymphatic drainage of the foot follows its venous drainage. The small saphenous vein drains the lateral side of the foot and the posterolateral leg. It drains into the popliteal vein in the popliteal fossa. Therefore, a lesion on the lateral side of the foot will drain to the popliteal nodes in the popliteal fossa.

E. Lymphatic drainage of the medial foot follow the great saphenous vein and drain at the superficial inguinal lymph nodes.

A, B, D. The lower limb drains into either the lymph nodes in the popliteal region or in the inguinal region, not to the lateral surface of the thigh, posterior aspect of the medial malleolus, or the sole of the foot.

GAS 562–563; N 475; ABR/McM 365

109. **E.** The posterior cruciate ligament runs from the posterior aspect of the intercondylar area of the tibia to the medial wall of the intercondylar fossa. It prevents posterior displacement of the tibia relative to the femur. This is usually tested with the posterior drawer test, in which the physician pushes the tibia backward while the knee is flexed in an attempt to displace it posteriorly. This is called the positive posterior drawer sign.

A. The anterior cruciate ligament prevents anterior displacement of the tibia on the femur.

B. The fibular collateral ligament stabilizes the lateral side of the knee joint.

C. The tibial collateral ligament stabilizes the medial side of the knee joint.

D. The medial meniscus is an intracapsular fibrocartilage that improves the articulation of the femur and tibia.

GAS 605–608; N 500; ABR/McM 339

110. **B.** The deep fibular nerve innervates the anterior compartment of the leg and provides cutaneous innervation to the skin of the first web space.

A. The saphenous nerve is the terminal branch of the femoral nerve. It provides sensory innervation to the medial aspect of the lower leg and the medial foot as far as first metatarsal phalangeal joint.

C. The cutaneous branch of superficial fibular nerve innervates the anterior part of the lower leg and the dorsum of the foot.

D. The sural nerve provides sensation to the lower lateral leg, lateral heel, ankle, and dorsal lateral foot.

E. The deep fibular nerve is a branch of the common fibular nerve. Anesthesia to the common fibular nerve is not recommended as it would affect far more than targeting pain of the fracture region, such as motor innervation to anterior and lateral leg muscles as well as dorsal foot muscles.

GAS 626; N 512; ABR/McM 346

111. **B.** The gluteal region can be divided into quadrants by two lines positioned using palpable bony landmarks. One line runs inferiorly from the highest point of the iliac crest. The second line runs horizontally midway between the iliac crests and the ischial tuberosity. This divides the gluteal region into four quadrants. The sciatic nerve runs through the lower medial quadrant and must be avoided during intragluteal injections.

A. The lateral femoral cutaneous arises from the lumbar plexus. It provides sensory innervation to the skin of the anterior, lateral and posterior surfaces of the thigh.

C. The superior gluteal nerve is a branch of the sacral plexus (L4, 5, S1) and provides motor innervation to the gluteus medius and minimus muscles and the tensor fascia lata muscles. Injury to this nerve will result in the characteristic Trendenlenburg sign.

D. The obturator nerve originates from the lumbar plexus roots L2, L3 and L4. Injury to the obturator nerve classically presents with weakness upon hip adduction and loss of sensation to the medial part of the mid and lower-third parts of the thigh.

E. The inferior gluteal nerve originates from the sacral plexus (L5, S1, S2) and supplies motor innervation to the gluteus maximus muscle. Injury to this results in impaired leg extension.

GAS 573; N 485; ABR/McM 324

112. **A.** A lateral blow to the knee often produces a trio of injuries referred to as the "unhappy triad." This involves damage to the anterior cruciate ligament, medial meniscus, and tibial collateral ligament. The medial meniscus and tibial collateral ligament are often damaged together because they are tightly attached to each other.

B, C. The fibular collateral ligament and lateral meniscus would not be damaged because a blow to the lateral knee would not put strain on these structures.

D. Damage to the posterior cruciate ligament would produce a positive "posterior drawer sign" and is typically damaged during a blow to the medial side of the knee. The posterior cruciate ligament is stronger than the anterior and is only typically damaged when a person falls on the tibial tuberosity of a flexed knee.

E. Tendon of the semitendinosus is on the medial side of the knee but is not attached closely to the other structures or taut in this injury type.
GAS 598–605; N 499; ABR/McM 330

113. **A.** The saphenous nerve runs with the great saphenous nerve which was being removed from patient. Sensory innervation to the areas of loss described is by the L4 root, which is carried by the saphenous nerve.
B. The obturator nerve innervates the skin on the inferior medial thigh.
C. Lateral femoral cutaneous innervates the lateral aspect of the thigh.
D. The tibial nerve supplies cutaneous innervation to the posterior aspect of the leg and if damaged would also produce muscular dysfunction.
E. The femoral nerve is a motor and sensory nerve and is the origin of the saphenous nerve.
GAS 596; N 513; ABR/McM 356

114. **B.** Ligaments act to prevent excessive movement of joints. When a joint is forced into a position, that ligament is stretched and will be tender or rupture if the force is severe enough. Inversion is when the sole of the foot is turned medially and therefore will stretch ligaments that oppose this action. The calcaneofibular ligament is on the lateral side and stretches between the fibula and the calcaneus. It is the only ligament that would be damaged during such an action.
A, C, D. The plantar calcaneonavicular, long plantar, and short plantar ligaments are located on the plantar surface of the foot and will not be damaged during inversion injuries.
E. The medial collateral (deltoid) ligament is located medially and will not be affected.
GAS 634–643; N 518; ABR/McM 359

115. **A.** The patellar reflex causes extension of the knee and is produced by the quadriceps femoris muscle group which consist of rectus femoris and vastus lateralis, medialis, and intermedius.
B. Quadratus femoris is a lateral rotator of the thigh.
C. The sartorius is a flexor of the hip and knee.
D. The pectineus is an adductor and flexor of the hip.
E. The biceps femoris muscle is flexor muscle mainly responsible for flexion of the knee.
GAS 578, 598; N 490; ABR/McM 332

116. **B.** The lateral circumflex femoral artery is a branch of the deep femoral artery close to the hip joint. It gives a branch that runs down the lateral aspect of the thigh and joins the genicular anastomosis via the superior lateral genicular artery.
A. The medial circumflex femoral artery does not provide any branches that descend toward the knee.
C, D. The anterior and posterior tibial arteries are the terminal branches of the popliteal artery and would not receive any blood if the popliteal is damaged.
E. The fibular artery is a branch of the posterior tibial artery.
GAS 558, 574; N 495; ABR/McM 330

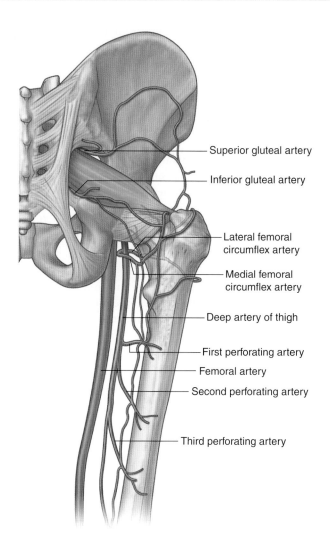

- *GAS* **Fig. 6.51**

117. **B.** The obturator nerve is responsible for innervation of the thigh adductors which form the medial compartment of the thigh.
A. The femoral nerve innervates the anterior compartment and is responsible for extension of the knee.
C, D, E. Common fibular nerve supplies the anterior and lateral compartments of the leg while the tibial nerve supplies the posterior compartments of the leg and thigh. Both the common fibular and tibial nerves are branches of the sciatic nerve.
GAS 480, 494, 555–557; N 486; ABR/McM 271

118. **A.** The skin of the anterior thigh and medial leg and foot is supplied by the femoral nerve.
B. The saphenous nerve is a branch of the femoral and supplies only the medial leg and foot.
C. The obturator supplies the lower medial aspect of the thigh.
D. The tibial nerve supplies the skin of the posterolateral leg, lateral ankle, foot, and sole of the foot.
E. The superficial fibular nerve supplies the skin over the lateral aspect of the leg and dorsal aspect of the foot.
GAS 537–541, 615; N 529; ABR/McM 328

119. A. Injury to the femoral nerve would result in decreased knee jerk reflex and decreased sensation on the medial aspect of the leg.

B. Weakened flexion at the knee and decreased sensation of the plantar aspect of the foot describes an injury to the posterior tibial nerve.

C. Injury to the superficial peroneal nerve would result in weakened eversion at the ankle and decreased sensation of the plantar aspect of the foot.

D. The deep fibular nerve is responsible for sensation over the first web space of the foot. Dorsiflexion and inversion of the ankle is produced by the muscles supplied by the deep fibular nerve. The nerves responsible for the knee jerk reflex, knee flexion, eversion, and plantar flexion are all located superior to the location of the tumor and will not be damaged. The nerve located in the space between the tibia and fibula is the deep fibular nerve.

E. Common peroneal nerve injury would result in weakened plantarflexion and toe flexion, as well as decreased sensation on the plantar aspect of the foot.

GAS 611, 626; N 533; ABR/McM 357

120. E. Tarsal tunnel syndrome is a compression neuropathy resulting from the compression of the tibial nerve in the tarsal tunnel. The tarsal tunnel is located between the medial malleolus, the inferomedial surface of the calcaneus, and the flexor retinaculum. The contents are the tibial nerve and its plantar branches, the tendons of the tibialis posterior, flexor digitorum longus, and the flexor hallucis longus muscles together with the posterior tibial vessels. Any inflammation or swelling in the area will compress on these structures, most significantly the tibial nerve. The posterior tibial vein will be most easily compressed, but the nerve is most significant. This syndrome is diagnosed with the patient's history and physical examination findings including a positive Tinel sign (lightly tapping over the flexor retinaculum elicits numbness and tingling in the skin over the calcaneus and the sole of the foot).

A. Plantar fasciitis is characterized by sharp pain on the bottom of the foot specially in the morning or after a period of rest which then improves with walking or activity. It may be worse at the end of the day after prolonged weight-bearing.

B. Ankle inversion sprain would show up acutely after hyper-inversion of the ankle.

C. Morton (interdigital) neuroma is a neuropathy of the interdigital nerve that commonly occurs after chronic compression. It causes plantar forefoot pain.

D. The lateral ligament at the knee may be torn when receiving lateral blows towards the knee. It would present acutely and not in a chronic fashion.

GAS 615–622; N 520; ABR/McM 355

121. A. Dorsalis pedis pulse is palpated at the prominent arch of the top of the foot between the first and second metatarsal bones between the tendon of the extensor hallucis longus and extensor digitorum longus for the second toe.

B, E. The posterior tibial artery pulse can be located superior to flexor hallucis longus just distal to the tarsal tunnel, 2 cm posterior to the medial malleolus.

D. The dorsal pedis pulse is not usually 2 cm anterior to the medial malleolus.

C. The femoral pulse is located inferolateral to the pubic symphysis and medial to the deep dorsal vein of the penis.

GAS 654; N 521; ABR/McM 358

122. A. Gracilis, due to its shape, size, and more importantly the nature of neurovascular supply, is used very commonly in reconstructive surgery as a free functioning autograft. In addition, the other adductors of the thigh compensate for the absence of the gracilis. For similar reasons the remaining muscles are not good candidates during reconstructive surgery of the upper limb.

B, C, D, E. The sartorius, recuts femoris, vastus lateralis, and vastus medialis muscles are not commonly used as reconstructive surgery grafts given how convenient the gracilis is for this purpose.

GAS 586; N 490; ABR/McM 332

123. A. Any superficial inflammation in the gluteal region drains into the horizontal group of superficial inguinal nodes. The vertical group drains the lower limbs, whereas deep gluteal injuries drain into the superior and inferior gluteal nodes.

B. The vertical group of superficial inguinal nodes receives superficial lymphatics from the medial side of the foot, leg, and all the superficial lymph from the thigh.

C. The superior and inferior gluteal nodes receive lymph from the deeper tissues of the pelvis, then drain into the internal and common iliac nodes before entering the lateral caval lumbar nodes.

D. The external iliac nodes drain the inguinal lymph nodes and drain into the common iliac lymph nodes.

E. The deep inguinal nodes receive drain nodes from the clitoris and glans of the penis.

GAS 514; N 475; ABR/McM 376

124. E. Because the hamstrings cross two joints and are very crucial during all phases of running, but especially during the late swing through midstance phase of running, they are easily injured. Their normal action includes hip extension and knee flexion.

A. The quadriceps femoris muscles consist of three vastus muscles and the rectus femoris. They are responsible for flexion of the hip and extension of the knee.

B. Anterior leg compartment muscles lead to dorsiflexion and would not be painful while initiating knee flexion.

C. Medial rotation of the hip is performed mainly by the gluteus medius, gluteus minimus, and the tensor fasciae latae.

D. Lateral rotation of the hips is performed mainly by the piriformis muscle.

GAS 590; N 482; ABR/McM 327

125. **B.** The rough bony projection at the junction of the inferior end of the body of the ischium and its ramus is the large ischial tuberosity. Much of the body's weight rests on these tuberosities when sitting, and it provides the proximal, tendinous attachment of the posterior thigh muscles (hamstring muscles and the hamstring portion of adductor magnus). The hamstring muscles are associated with hip extension and knee flexion. The adduction of the hip joint will be affected slightly because the hamstring portion of adductor magnus is affected, although the rest of the adductor muscles are intact.

A. The adductor brevis, adductor longus, adductor magnus, pectineus, and gracilis are the main muscles responsible for adduction of the hip. Additionally, these muscles attach to the more medial aspect of the ischium as opposed to the inferior part. Injury to these muscles would greatly affect adduction of the hip; this patient has only slight weakening.

C. The iliacus originates from the ilium of the pelvis and inserts into the neck of the femur. The psoas originates from the transverse processes, the sides of the vertebral bodies, and the intervertebral discs, from the twelfth thoracic to the fifth lumbar vertebrae and insert into the lesser trochanter of the femur. Therefore, a fracture of the ischial tuberosity would not affect these muscles.

D. The gluteus maximus originates from the posterior aspect of the dorsal ilium and inserts into the iliotibial band. The adductor magnus originates from the inferior pubic ramus and inserts into the gluteum tuberosity of the femur. Therefore, an avulsion fracture of the ischial tuberosity would not affect these muscles.

E. The iliacus, psoas major, recuts femoris and sartorius muscles are muscles closely associated with the femur but not the ischial tuberosity, therefore, they would not be affected by an avulsion fracture at the ischial tuberosity.

GAS 543–545, 567, 582, 586; N 476; ABR/McM 300

126. **D.** Duchenne muscular dystrophy is a condition that causes muscle weakness. It starts in childhood and may be noticed when a child has difficulty standing up, climbing, or running, which requires extension of the hip. This patient has the classic Gower sign. The gluteus maximus functions primarily between the flexed and standing (straight) positions of the thigh, as when rising from the sitting position, straightening from the bending position, walking uphill and upstairs, and running.

A. The tibialis posterior and gastrocnemius both function primarily to plantar flex, this patient's condition has limited his hip extension.

B. The quadratus femoris is a paired muscle in the gluteal region. Its primary function is for external thigh rotation. This patient is not presenting with abnormal thigh rotation.

C. The gluteus medius and gluteus minimus both stabilize the pelvis while walking or standing. Injury to either would present with abnormal gait and/or abnormal posture.

E. The iliopsoas also functions in flexion of the hip but mainly in activities such as running, walking, and rising from a chair. Injury would not cause the classic Gower sign seen in patients with Duchenne muscular dystrophy.

GAS 567, 582, 586; N 485; ABR/McM 326

127. **A.** The gluteal region (buttocks) is a common site for intramuscular injection of drugs, particularly if the volume of the injection is large. To avoid injury to the underlying sciatic nerve, the injection should be given well forward on the upper outer quadrant of the buttock (superolateral quadrant). The patient is showing the Trendelenburg gait pattern (or gluteus medius lurch), which is caused by weakness of the gluteus medius and minimus muscles. These muscles are supplied by the superior gluteal nerve (L4, L5, S1), which emerges from the greater sciatic notch above the upper border of the piriformis and immediately disappears beneath the posterior border of the gluteus medius and runs forward between the gluteus medius and minimus. Intramuscular injection in the upper inner quadrant (superomedially) is most likely to damage this nerve. The sciatic nerve is most likely damaged in the inferomedial quadrant of the buttock.

B, C, D, E. An intramuscular injection could be safely administered in the superolateral quadrant of the buttock, inferomedial quadrant of the buttock, inferolateral quadrant of the buttock, and posterior thigh with less concern for injuring the sciatic nerve.

GAS 573; N 485; ABR/McM 324

128. **D.** The anterior cruciate ligament (ACL) is attached to the anterior intercondylar area and the posterior part of the medial surface of the lateral femoral condyle. Posterior displacement of the femur on the tibia is prevented by the ACL. With the knee joint flexed, the ACL prevents the tibia from being pulled anteriorly.

A. The fibular (lateral) collateral ligaments are cord-like and attached prosimally to the lateral side of the head of the fibula overlapped by the tendon of biceps femoris.

B. The tibial (medial) collateral ligament is a flat band and is attached above to the medial condyle of the femur and below to the medial surface of the shaft of the tibia. It is firmly attached to the edge of the medial meniscus and consequently is more prone to be injured.

C. The patellar ligament (tendon) connects the lower border of the patella with the smooth convexity on the tuberosity of the tibia. It becomes the continuation of the quadriceps femoris tendon.

E. The posterior cruciate ligament is stronger, shorter, broader, and less oblique and prevents anterior displacement of the femur on the tibia.

F. The oblique popliteal ligament is a tendinous expansion derived from the semimembranosus muscle. It strengthens the posterior aspect of the knee joint capsule.

GAS 578–580, 605; N 500; ABR/McM 339

129. B. The psoas major muscle arises from the transverse processes, the sides of the vertebral bodies, and the intervertebral discs, from the twelfth thoracic to the fifth lumbar vertebrae and inserts into the lesser trochanter of the femur. The sheath of the psoas retains the pus of a psoas abscess, and spinal tuberculosis may present as a cold abscess in the groin (in the vicinity of the lesser trochanter). The psoas is enclosed in a fibrous sheath that is derived from the lumbar fascia. The sheath is not part of the lumbar fascia, but the lateral edge blends with the anterior layer of that fascia.

A. The piriformis is a gluteal muscle that originates from the ilium and sacrum and inserts into the greater trochanter of the femur. Therefore, it would not give the described lumbar flocculent mass and pain described.

C. The adductor longus functions primarily to adduct the hip. It originates from the body of the pubis and inserts into the femur. Therefore, it would not give the described lumbar flocculent mass and pain described.

D. The gluteus maximus functions primarily in thigh extension, rotation, adduction and abduction. It originates from the sacrum and coccyx and the gluteal surface of the the ilium. Therefore, it would not give the described lumbar flocculent mass and pain described.

E. The obturator internus functions primarily in external rotation of the extended thigh and abduction of the flexed thigh. It originates from the bony boundaries of the obturator foramen and inserts into the medial part of the greater trochanter of the femur.

GAS 582–583; N 486; ABR/McM 276

130. B. The psoas major muscle arises from the transverse processes, the sides of the vertebral bodies, and the intervertebral discs, from the twelfth thoracic to the fifth lumbar vertebrae and inserts into the lesser trochanter of the femur. The psoas flexes the thigh at the hip joint on the trunk, or if the thigh is fixed, it flexes the trunk on the thigh, as in sitting up from a lying

position. The inflamed appendix is pushed up against the peritoneum from the contracted psoas. As a result, it is in touch with the parietal peritoneum, producing acute pain. In some other cases it may retain the purulence of a psoas abscess, and spinal tuberculosis may present as a cold abscess in the groin. The psoas is enclosed in a fibrous sheath that is derived from the lumbar fascia. The sheath is not part of the lumbar fascia but the lateral edge blends with the anterior layer of that fascia.

A. The adductor magnus originates from the ischial tuberosity and inserts into the linea aspera and femur. It is not proximal enough to the appendix to lead to irritation during thigh flexion.

C. The biceps femoris originates from the ischial tuberosity and inserts into the fibular head. It is not proximal enough to the appendix to lead to irritation during thigh flexion.

D. The obturator internus originates from the ischiopubic ramus and inserts into the greater trochanter. It is not proximal enough to the appendix to lead to irritation during thigh flexion.

E. The gluteus maximus is located on the posterior aspect of the lower limb. It is not proximal enough to the appendix to lead to irritation during thigh flexion.

GAS 582–583; N 486; ABR/McM 277

131. B. The saphenous nerve is the longest and most widely distributed cutaneous branch of the femoral nerve; it is the only nerve branch in the lower limb not from the sciatic nerve to extend beyond the knee. It gives sensory innervations to the medial aspect of the leg and foot. It accompanies the great saphenous vein over the medial side of the leg.

A. The posterior tibial vein rises behind the lateral malleolus and enter the posterior compartment of the leg to end at the distal margin of the popliteus muscle. At the popliteus muscle, it converges with the anterior tibial veins to form the popliteal vein.

C. The great saphenous vein is formed by the union of the dorsal vein of the great toe and the dorsal venous arch of the foot. It ascends anterior to the medial malleolus and passes posterior to the medial condyle of the femur and ends when it joins the femoral vein.

D. The tibial nerve arises from the posterior thigh as a branch of the sciatic nerve at the apex of the popliteal fossa. It courses deep to the gastrocnemius muscle then exits the posterior compartment of the leg at the ankle passing posterior to the medial malleolus. It provides motor input to the posterior compartment muscles of the leg as well as sensation to the postcrolateral leg, the lateral foot, and the sole.

E. The lymph nodes draining the perineum drain to the horizontal group of the superficial inguinal nodes that run along the inguinal ligament.

GAS 615, 658; N 529; ABR/McM 338

132. C. The deep fibular nerve passes deep to the extensor retinaculum and supplies the intrinsic muscles on the dorsum of the foot (extensors digitorum and hallucis longus) and the tarsal and tarsometatarsal joints. When it finally emerges as a cutaneous nerve, it is so far distal in the foot that only a small area of skin remains available for innervation: the web of skin between and contiguous sides of the first and second toes. The superficial fibular nerve supplies the skin on the anterolateral aspect of the leg and divides into the medial and intermediate dorsal cutaneous nerves, which continue across the ankle to supply most of the skin on the dorsum of the foot.

A. Injury to the superior gluteal nerve would result in paralysis of the gluteus medius. This would result in changes in gait and posture consistent with the Trendelenburg gait.

B. Injury to the inferior gluteal nerve would result in paralysis of the gluteus maximus. This would result in impaired leg extension and would result in changes in gait and posture consistent with the Trendelenburg gait.

D. Injury to the superficial fibular nerve would result in pain or loss of sensation to the skin of the dorsum of the foot apart from the webbing between the great toe and the second digit as well as the anterior and lateral parts of the lower leg.

E. Injury to the common fibular nerve would result in pain or loss of sensation to the skin of the dorsum of the foot as well as the later part of the lateral leg. It would also result in weakness of the muscles of the anterior compartment of the leg.

GAS 625–626; N 533; ABR/McM 357

133. E. The obturator membrane is a fibrous sheet that almost completely closes the obturator foramen, leaving a small gap beneath the superior pubic ramus, the obturator canal, for the passage of the obturator nerve and vessels as they leave the pelvis to enter the medial thigh.

A. The femoral canal is the small medial compartment of the femoral sheath for the lymph vessels and nodes. It is approximately 0.5 in (1.3 cm) long, and its upper opening is called the femoral ring. It has the following borders: anteriorly the inguinal ligament; posteriorly the superior ramus of the pubis; medially the lacunar ligament; and laterally the femoral vein

B. A triangular-shaped defect in the external abdominal oblique aponeurosis lies immediately above and medial to the pubic tubercle. This is known as the superficial inguinal ring.

C. The deep inguinal ring is an oval opening in the transversalis fascia and lies approximately 0.5 in (1.3 cm) above the inguinal ligament, midway between the anterior superior iliac spine and the pubic symphysis.

D. Fossa ovalis, also called the saphenous opening, refers to an oval opening in the superomedial part of the fascia lata of the thigh. It lies 3 to 4 cm inferolateral to the pubic tubercle.

GAS 433, 486, 557, 572; N 477; ABR/McM 284

134. C. The deep inguinal lymph nodes are located beneath the deep fascia (fascia cribrosa) and lie along the medial side of the femoral vein. The presence of swollen inguinal lymph nodes is an important sign because swelling may indicate an infection in the lower extremities. They then drain superiorly to the external iliac lymph nodes. The superficial inguinal nodes lie in the superficial fascia below the inguinal ligament and can be divided into horizontal and vertical groups. External iliac nodes lie along the external iliac vessels; they are arranged in groups of three (anteriorly, medially, and lateral to vessels).

A. The external iliac nodes lie along the external iliac artery above the inguinal ligament. They are the primary drainage for the inguinal nodes.

B. The superficial inguinal nodes are located below the inguinal ligament. They drain skin from the penis, clitoris, lower abdomen, scrotum, and parts of the buttock area.

D. The common iliac nodes are located surrounding the common iliac artery and vein above the bifurcation of the external and internal iliac vessels. They drain the external and internal iliac nodes.

E. Internal iliac nodes are located adjacent to the internal iliac artery. They drain the genitalia anteriorly, the psoas muscle posteriorly and the medial thigh inferiorly.

GAS 562–563; N 475; ABR/McM 376

135. A. The talocrural joint is a synovial hinge joint that connects the distal end of the tibia and fibula with the proximal end of the talus. The articulation between the tibia and the talus bears more weight than other joints. Dorsiflexion (toes pointing upward) and plantar flexion (toes pointing downward) are possible. Dorsiflexion is performed by the tibialis anterior, extensor hallucis longus, extensor digitorum longus, and fibularis tertius. Plantar flexion is performed by the gastrocnemius, soleus, plantaris, fibularis longus, fibularis brevis, tibialis posterior, flexor digitorum longus, and flexor hallucis longus.

B, C, D, E. The movements of inversion and eversion take place at the talocalcaneal joint.

GAS 634; N 518; ABR/McM 359

136. E. Plantar flexion is mostly due to the gastrocnemius and soleus muscles, which are supplied by the tibial nerve. The tibial nerve leaves the popliteal fossa by passing deep to the gastrocnemius and soleus muscles and lies posterior to the popliteal vessels. Therefore a hematoma of the popliteal artery will also compress the nerve. Dorsiflexion of the foot is due to contraction of the muscles in the anterior compartment of the leg.

A. Dorsiflexion of the foot is a movement completed primarily by the common peroneal nerve.

B, D. Flexion of the thigh and extension of the leg are primarily performed by innervation from the femoral nerve.

C. Extension of the lower digits is primarily performed by innervation from the deep fibular nerve.

GAS 615; N 508; ABR/McM 344

137. C. The lymphatic drainage of the leg is such that superficial lymphatics on the anterolateral side of the foot and leg and all the deep lymphatics in the foot and leg first drain into the popliteal nodes and then to the deep inguinal nodes. This patient has an infected anterolateral midleg injury, which will first drain into the popliteal nodes.

   A. The vertical group of superficial inguinal nodes receives superficial lymphatics from the medial side of the foot, leg, and all the superficial lymph from the thigh.

   B. The horizontal group of superficial lymphatics receives lymph from the anterior abdominal wall below the umbilicus, perineum (except the glans penis in men and clitoris in women), and lower third of the anal canal.

   D. The popliteal nodes eventually drain to the deep inguinal nodes but are usually not palpable.

   E. The iliac nodes are deep structures and are not palpable during physical examination.

GAS 562–563; N 475; ABR/McM 365

138. B. The obturator membrane is a thin membrane that covers the obturator foramen except at its superior part. The obturator nerve exits the pelvis and enters into the medial compartment of the thigh by passing through the obturator canal with the obturator vessels. Traumatic injuries to the membrane will most likely lead to obturator nerve damage. The obturator nerve supplies motor innervations to the adductor muscles of the thigh (gracilis, obturator externus, adductor longus, adductor brevis and a portion of the adductor magnus). It also provides sensory innervation to the medial aspect of the thigh.

   A. Urinary and fecal incontinence is mediated by autonomic nerves and the pudendal nerve. Both nerves have no relationship with the obturator membrane.

   C. The gluteus medius and minimus muscles are the main hip abductors. They also stabilize the hip on the swing-side during motion. These muscles are supplied by the superior gluteal nerve, which leaves the pelvis through the greater sciatic foramen above the piriformis muscle.

   D. Flexors of the hip found in the anterior compartment of the thigh are innervated by the femoral nerve, which has no relationship with the obturator membrane.

   E. The sciatic nerve supplies the muscles in the posterior compartment of the thigh and also sends cutaneous innervations to the skin of the posterolateral leg and most of the foot. It enters the posterior compartment of the thigh from the gluteal region.

GAS 433, 486, 557, 572; N 477; ABR/McM 284

139. C. The deep fibular nerve is a branch of the common fibular nerve and begins at about the level of the neck of the fibula, between it and the fibularis longus. This nerve supplies the extensors of the foot (extensor digitorum longus, fibularis tertius, extensor hallucis longus, tibialis anterior, extensor digitorum brevis, and extensor hallucis brevis). It innervates the first web space of the foot. Fracture of the head of the fibula can damage this nerve, resulting in foot drop and a high stepping gait, as well as numbness over the dorsum and first web space of the foot.

   A. Muscles in the posterior compartment of the leg are involved in plantar flexion. These muscles are innervated by the tibial nerve, which is a branch of the sciatic nerve; its medial sural cutaneous branch supplies sensation to the posterior side of the leg.

   B. The superficial peroneal (fibular) nerve is a branch of the common peroneal (fibular) nerve. This nerve supplies the muscles of the lateral compartment (peroneus longus, peroneus brevis). It innervates the dorsum of the foot, excluding the webspace between the great toe and the second toe. Injury would cause pain and paresthesia of the dorsum of the foot as well as loss of foot eversion.

   D. Waddling gait and numbness at the anterolateral side of the leg are associated with the superficial fibular and the lateral sural cutaneous nerve.

   E. Swing out gait is associated with weakness of hip abductors and lesions of the superior gluteal nerve.

GAS 625–626; N 533; ABR/McM 346

140. D. A positive valgus stress test indicates injury to the tibial collateral ligament. Injuries to this ligament usually involve the anterior cruciate ligament. The femur is usually pushed posteriorly during stair climbing, an action that is opposed by a normal anterior cruciate ligament. Injury to the anterior cruciate ligament results in posterior displacement of the femur in relation to the tibia with difficulty climbing stairs.

   A. Extension of the knee is done mainly by the quadriceps femoris muscle.

   B. The posterior thigh muscles provide flexion of the knee.

   C, E. Gravity pushes the femur forward while walking down a flight, which is stabilized by the posterior cruciate ligament, which is not damaged in this case.

GAS 603–608; N 500; ABR/McM 339

141. E. The calcaneofibular ligament is located inferior to the lateral malleolus and connects the lateral malleolus to the calcaneus.

A. The posterior talofibular ligament only has a secondary role in ankle joint stability and is the least commonly injured ankle ligament.

B. The plantar calcaneonavicular ligament is located on the plantar surface of the foot deeply (*GAS* Fig. 6.104)

C. The tibionavicular ligaments are located on the medial side of the ankle joint, and the point of injury and tenderness is at the lateral side.

D. The anterior tibiofibular ligament is located anterior to the ankle joint, away from the point of injury.
GAS 634–641; N 518; ABR/McM 359

142. **E.** The paraxial mesoderm develops into somites. Limb muscles develop from the ventral myotome of the somites in response to molecular signals. (GAS Fig. 6.104).

A. Embryologic derivatives of the lateral plate mesoderm include the circulatory and gut wall, body wall lining, and dermis.

B. Derivative of the neural crest cells does not include the limb muscles.

C. Chondrification is associated with cartilage formation and not muscles.

D. The intermediate mesoderm eventually thins out laterally and becomes the mesoderm, which gives the circulatory and gut walls, plus the lining of the body wall and dermis.
GAS 29–32

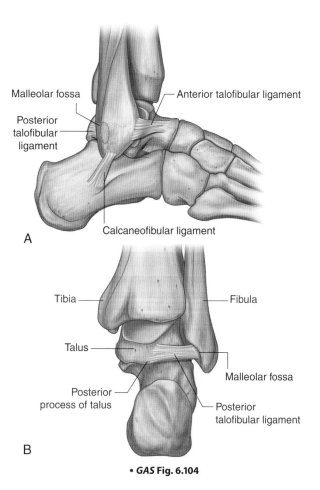

Malleolar fossa

Anterior talofibular ligament

Posterior talofibular ligament

Calcaneofibular ligament

A

Tibia

Fibula

Talus

Malleolar fossa

Posterior process of talus

Posterior talofibular ligament

B

• *GAS* **Fig. 6.104**

143. C. Mesenchyme between digital rays undergoes apoptosis for the digits to form. Failure or incomplete apoptosis usually results in fused digits (syndactyly). This may involve the skin and soft tissues alone or may include the bone.

A. Digital rays form from the hand plate. Failure of development of any digital ray results in underdevelopment of a finger or toe.

B. Neural crest cells do not contribute to the formation of the foot.

D. The ZPA modulates the patterning of the limb in the anteroposterior diameter.

E. The abnormality described did not involve the phalanges, as shown by x-ray and thus could not have been caused by faulty chondrification.
GAS 14

Answers 144–148

144. B. The suprapatellar bursa is found in the anterior surface of the inferior part of the femur under the quadriceps femoris muscle. A high-riding superior patellar fragment leads to the exposure of this bursa. In traumatic episodes following this condition, blood and fat from the knee can enter the suprapatellar bursa.

A. The popliteal bursa is located behind the knee, away from the site of injury.

C. The subcutaneous infrapatellar bursa is superficially located between the skin and the patellar tendon insertion point on the tibial tuberosity.

D. The deep infrapatellar bursa is located below the site of the injury, between the upper part of the tibia and the patella ligament.

E. The gastrocnemius bursa is at the back of the knee, as well as below the level of the injury.
GAS 602; N 502; ABR/McM 342

145. B. The superior gluteal nerve arises from the L4-S1 nerve roots. When a person stands on one leg or walks, the gluteus medius, gluteus minimus, and tensor fasciae latae act in synergy to stabilize the hip joint by abducting the hip (pelvic tilt). These muscles receive their innervation from the superior gluteal nerve. The abductors of the hip, as they contract to maintain the stability of the hip joint, draw the pelvis forcefully toward the weigh-bearing leg, causing the opposite side of the pelvis to tilt in that same direction. The right superior gluteal nerve innervates its ipsilateral gluteus medius, gluteus minimus, and tensor fasciae latae. Loss of these muscles results in a positive Trendelenburg sign with the pelvis dropping on the left side.

A. The sciatic nerve arises from the L4-S3 nerve roots. Injury to the sciatic nerve results in paralysis of the hamstring muscles and adductor magnus causing impaired knee flexion and hip adduction. It provides sensory innervation to the lower leg and foot.

C, E. The inferior gluteal nerve arises from L5-S2 nerve roots. Injury to this nerve results in paralysis of the gluteus maximus muscle causing impaired thigh extension.

D. Injury to the left superior gluteal nerve would present with weakness and elicitation of the Trendelenburg sign when standing on the left leg, not right, as in this case.

GAS 557, 567; N 493; ABR/McM 326

146. D. The S1 nerve root provides cutaneous innervation to the lateral aspect of the ankle, the lateral sides of the dorsum and sole of foot, and motor innervation to the gastrocnemius muscle, which plantar flexes the foot and contracts during the ankle jerk reflex. It receives its innervation from the S1, S2 nerve roots via the tibial nerve, making D the correct choice.

A. T12 roots do not reach the foot.

B. L2 roots will reach the hip region and thigh.

C. L4 innervates the invertors of the foot and skin over medial leg, ankle, and side of foot.

E. S3 innervates the sitting area of the buttocks, posterior scrotum or labia, and the small muscles of the foot.

GAS 537–542; N 533; ABR/McM 355

147. C. Forceful external rotation and eversion of the ankle often leads to this type of injury as the bony components are pushed apart forcefully. It is commonly referred to as a Pott fracture (the medial malleolus is pulled forcefully by the strong medial collateral (deltoid) ligament as the talus moves laterally, causing a fracture of the lateral malleolus).

A, D, E. Forceful inversion, dorsiflexion, or plantarflexion will more commonly lead to ligament rupture than fractures as seen in this patient.

B. Direct upward force of the talus is usually due to a fall from a considerable height and will damage the calcaneus.

GAS 637; N 518; ABR/McM 359

148. A. Knowledge of Hilton's Law would lead to this correct answer. This law in a modified form, can be remembered as "a joint is innervated by the same nerves that innervate the muscles that move that joint." A complete explanation of this law can be found in an article by Hebert-Blouin et al., Physical Anatomy 27:548 -555, 2013. The deep fibular nerve is the only nerve listed that innervates muscles that move the ankle joint.

B. The femoral nerve arises from nerve roots L2-L4. It innervates anterior compartment thigh muscles to facilitate the hip joint and extend the knee. It also provides sensory innervation to the anteromedial thigh down to the medial leg and foot.

C. The obturator nerve arises from nerve roots L2-L4. It innervates muscles of the medial compartment of the thigh. It also provides sensory innervation to the medial thigh.

D. The posterior femoral cutaneous nerve arises from nerve roots S2-S3. It provides sensory innervation to the posterior thigh, buttock, and posterior scrotum/labia.

E. The sural nerve arises from nerve roots S1-S2. It provides sensory innervation to posterolateral part of the lower leg, the ankle, foot and heel.

GAS 611, 626; N 533; ABR/McM 346

6

Upper Limb

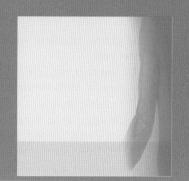

Introduction

First Order Question

1. A 25-year-old man is brought to the emergency department because he fell on a slippery trail and injured his right upper limb. Physical examination shows abrasions over his triceps brachii muscle. Which of the following nerves innervates the triceps brachii muscle?
  A. Radial
  B. Axillary
  C. Median
  D. Ulnar
  E. Musculocutaneous

Explanation

A: The nerve most likely affected is the radial nerve which innervates the triceps brachii muscle. The median and ulnar nerves do not innervate any muscles in the arm. The axillary nerve innervates the deltoid and teres minor. The musculocutaneous nerve innervates the coracobrachialis, biceps brachii, and brachialis muscles in the anterior compartment of the arm.

First Order Question

2. A 25-year-old man is brought to the emergency department because he fell on a slippery trail and injured his right upper limb. Physical examination shows abrasions over his triceps brachii muscle. An x-ray of his arm shows a fracture at the mid-body of the humerus. Which of the following nerves is most likely injured?
  A. Radial
  B. Axillary
  C. Median
  D. Ulnar
  E. Musculocutaneous

Explanation

A: The nerve most likely affected is the radial nerve as it travels in the radial groove and descends along the posterior surface of the humerus to the forearm. The axillary nerve runs around the surgical neck of the humerus, the median nerve passes in the neurovascular compartment medial to the muscles of the arm, the ulnar nerve runs medially toward the medial epicondyle, and the musculocutaneous nerve usually pierces the coracobrachialis muscle and then runs between the brachialis and biceps brachii muscles.

Second Order Question

3. A 25-year-old man is brought to the emergency department because he fell on a slippery trail and injured his right upper limb. Physical examination shows abrasions over his triceps brachii muscle. An x-ray of his arm shows a fracture at the mid-body of the humerus. Which of the following muscles is most likely paralyzed?
  A. Triceps brachii
  B. Biceps brachii
  C. Coracobrachialis
  D. Brachialis
  E. Deltoid

Explanation

A: The nerve most likely affected in the x-ray is the radial nerve as it travels in the radial groove along the posterior surface of the humerus and descends to the forearm. The radial nerve innervates the triceps brachii muscle (and wrist extensors in the forearm), whereas the biceps brachii, coracobrachialis, and brachialis muscles are innervated by the musculocutaneous nerve and the deltoid and teres minor muscles are innervated by the axillary nerve.

Third Order Question

4. A 25-year-old man is brought to the emergency department because he fell on a slippery trail and injured his right upper limb. Physical examination shows abrasions over his triceps brachii muscle. An x-ray of his arm shows a fracture at the mid-body of the humerus. Which of the following will most likely be present during physical examination?
  A. Wrist drop
  B. Inability to flex his wrist and loss of pronation
  C. Inability to flex the index and middle fingers at the distal interphalangeal (DIP) and proximal interphalangeal (PIP) joints
  D. Inability to flex the ring and little fingers at DIP
  E. Paralysis of the lumbricals and interosseous muscles

Explanation

A: The nerve likely affected is the radial nerve as it travels in the radial groove and descends along the posterior surface of the humerus to the forearm. The radial nerve innervates the wrist extensor muscles of the forearm. If these muscles are paralyzed because the radial nerve is injured, the wrist cannot be extended. This is referred to as wrist drop (*GAS* Fig. 7.69).

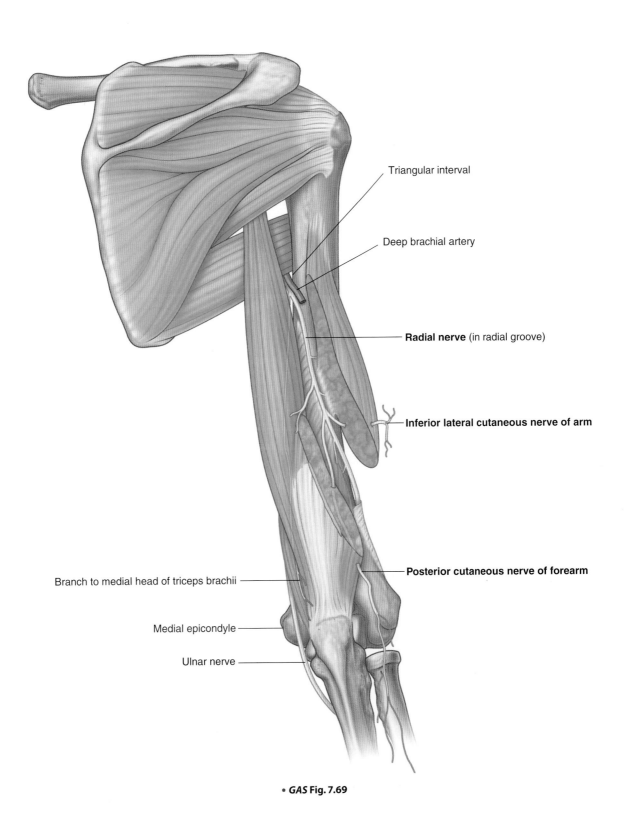

• *GAS* Fig. 7.69

Fourth Order Question

5. A 25-year-old man is brought to the emergency department because he fell on a slippery trail and injured his right upper limb. Physical examination shows abrasions over his arm. An x-ray of his arm is shown in Fig. 6.1. Which of the following deficits will most likely be encountered during physical examination?
   A. Inability to make a fist
   B. Inability to flex his wrist and loss of pronation
   C. Inability to flex the index and middle fingers at the DIP and PIP joints
   D. Inability to flex ring and little fingers at the DIP
   E. Paralysis of the lumbricals and interosseous muscles of the hand

Explanation

A: The nerve likely affected is the radial nerve as it travels in the radial groove as it descends along the posterior surface of the humerus to the forearm. Although the radial nerve does not provide innervation to muscles that help make a fist, it does innervate the extensor carpi radialis longus and brevis muscles. These muscles act as wrist extensors and are necessary for making a fist, as they contract synergistically with the flexors of the fingers to keep the wrist extended, making it indispensable while performing this action. The "position of function" of the hand is with the wrist extended about 30 degrees (see Fig. 7.22 from *GAS* 3e).

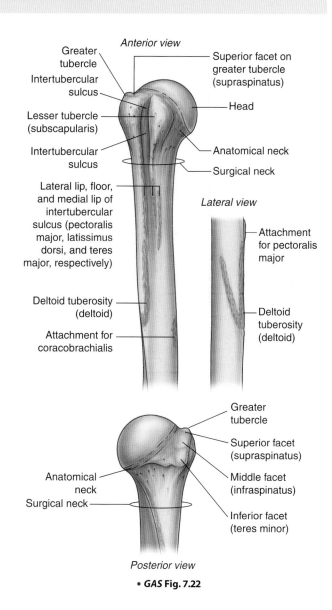

Anterior view

Greater tubercle
Intertubercular sulcus
Lesser tubercle (subscapularis)
Intertubercular sulcus
Lateral lip, floor, and medial lip of intertubercular sulcus (pectoralis major, latissimus dorsi, and teres major, respectively)
Deltoid tuberosity (deltoid)
Attachment for coracobrachialis

Superior facet on greater tubercle (supraspinatus)
Head
Anatomical neck
Surgical neck

Lateral view

Attachment for pectoralis major
Deltoid tuberosity (deltoid)

Greater tubercle
Superior facet (supraspinatus)
Middle facet (infraspinatus)
Inferior facet (teres minor)
Anatomical neck
Surgical neck

Posterior view

• **GAS Fig. 7.22**

Main Questions

Questions 1–25

1. A 45-year-old woman comes to the physician for a cosmetic breast surgery consultation. Physical examination shows that the areola falls below the inframammary fold at the level of the T8 dermatome. There is no erythema, fluctuance, swelling, dimpling, or lumps on either breast. The integrity of which of the following structure(s) is compromised?
   A. Scarpa fascia
   B. Pectoralis major muscle
   C. Pectoralis minor muscle
   D. Suspensory (Cooper) ligaments
   E. Serratus anterior muscle

2. A 27-year-old man was brought to the emergency department after he was involved in a motor vehicle collision. An x-ray of the right shoulder shows a fracture of the lateral border of the scapula. Six weeks later, the patient comes to the physician because of pain and weakness in the right shoulder while performing his daily activities. Physical examination shows weakness and pain on medial rotation and adduction of the humerus. Which of the following nerves is most likely injured?
   A. Lower subscapular
   B. Axillary
   C. Radial
   D. Accessory
   E. Suprascapular

3. A 48-year-old woman comes to the physician because of a 1-year history of pain and paresthesia in her right hand that has increased in severity during the past month. The pain has been persistent after falling on

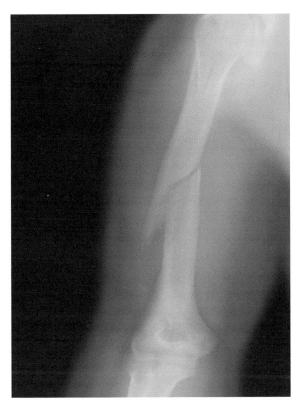

• **Fig. 6.1**

her outstretched hand one year ago. Physical examination shows loss of sensation in the radial 3½ digits of her right hand. Her left hand shows no abnormalities. Which muscle(s) is most likely weakened in this condition?

A. Dorsal interossei
B. Lumbricals III and IV
C. Thenar
D. Palmar interossei
E. Hypothenar

4. A 45-year-old man comes to the emergency department after sustaining an injury to his left arm during a bicycle race. The patient has pain and swelling of his left elbow. Physical examination shows warmth, swelling, and tenderness of the left elbow with decreased sensation over the medial 1½ digits. An x-ray of the left upper limb is shown. Which of the following muscles is most likely paralyzed?

A. Flexor digitorum superficialis
B. Biceps brachii
C. Brachioradialis
D. Flexor carpi ulnaris
E. Supinator

5. A 24-year old woman is brought to the emergency department after she slipped on wet pavement and fell against the curb, injuring her right arm. Physical examination shows loss of sensation of the posterior forearm

and dorsal hand. An x-ray of the right upper limb shows a mid-body fracture of the humerus. Which pair of structures is most likely injured at the fracture site?

A. Median nerve and brachial artery
B. Axillary nerve and posterior circumflex humeral artery
C. Radial nerve and deep brachial artery
D. Suprascapular nerve and artery
E. Long thoracic nerve and lateral thoracic artery

6. An 18-year-old man is brought to the emergency department because of left arm pain after an injury while playing rugby. Physical examination shows significant bruising over the left arm. An x-ray of the arm shows a transverse fracture of the humerus about 1 inch proximal to the epicondyles. Which of the following nerves is most likely injured by the jagged edges of the broken bone at this location?

A. Axillary
B. Median
C. Musculocutaneous
D. Radial
E. Ulnar

7. A 52-year-old man comes to the physician because of a 3-day history of pain in his right arm after strenuous field exercise for a major athletic tournament. Physical examination shows loss of extension of the wrist and decreased grip strength. There is no loss of sensation in the affected limb. An x-ray of the right upper limb shows no fractures. Which of the following nerves is most likely injured?

A. Ulnar
B. Anterior interosseous
C. Deep radial
D. Median
E. Superficial radial

8. A 32-year-old woman is brought to the emergency department 1 hour after a motor vehicle collision. She is awake and alert upon arrival. Her temperature is 37°C (98.6°F), pulse is 90/min, respirations are 16/min, and blood pressure is 118/72 mm Hg. Physical examination shows tenderness and bruising over the left arm. Flexion and supination of the forearm are severely weakened and she has loss of sensation on the lateral surface of the forearm. An x-ray of the upper limb shows multiple fractures of the humerus. Which of the following nerves is most likely injured?

A. Radial
B. Musculocutaneous
C. Median
D. Lateral cord of the brachial plexus
E. Lateral antebrachial cutaneous nerve

9. A 24-year-old woman comes to the emergency department after being bitten on her hand by a dog. She washed the wound with copious amounts of water, but the wound has progressively worsened in the last

6 hours. Physical examination shows tenderness and swelling at the base of the thumb, and difficulty with grasping and pinching movements. The infection eventually spreads to the radial bursa. The tendon(s) of which muscle will most likely be affected?

A. Flexor digitorum profundus
B. Flexor digitorum superficialis
C. Flexor pollicis longus
D. Flexor carpi radialis
E. Flexor pollicis brevis

10. Laboratory studies in the outpatient clinic on a 24-year-old woman included assessment of circulating blood chemistry. Which of the following arteries is most likely at-risk during venipuncture in the cubital fossa?

A. Brachial
B. Common interosseous
C. Ulnar
D. Anterior interosseous
E. Radial

11. A 52-year-old man comes to the physician because of a change in size and shape of a mole over his xiphoid process. He has a long history of sun exposure as a farmer of 30 years. A punch biopsy shows cellular changes consistent with a diagnosis of malignant melanoma which has metastasized. Which of the following lymph nodes are most likely to be palpable in this patient?

A. Deep inguinal
B. Vertical group of superficial inguinal
C. Horizontal group of superficial inguinal
D. Axillary
E. Deep and superficial inguinal

12. A 49-year-old man comes to the physician because of worsening fatigue and increasing difficulty performing daily tasks due to chest pain on exertion. After a positive stress test, a coronary angiography is performed and shows coronary artery stenosis. He is scheduled to undergo a coronary artery bypass graft procedure using the internal thoracic artery. Which of the following vessels will most likely continue to supply blood to the anterior part of the upper intercostal spaces after the procedure?

A. Musculophrenic
B. Superior epigastric
C. Posterior intercostal
D. Lateral thoracic
E. Thoracodorsal

13. A 22-year-old woman is brought to the emergency department 30 minutes after a motor vehicle collision. On arrival, she is unconscious. Her respirations are 30/min, and blood pressure is 100/50 mm Hg. The radial pulse is checked to determine the heart rate of the patient. This pulse is felt lateral to which of the following tendon?

A. Palmaris longus
B. Flexor pollicis longus
C. Flexor digitorum profundus
D. Flexor carpi radialis
E. Flexor digitorum superficialis

14. A 20-year-old man is brought to the emergency department 2 hours after sustaining an injury to his left hand during a rugby game. The injury occurred when the athlete gripped his opponent's jersey resulting in a forceful extension of his flexed digit. Physical examination shows inability to flex the DIP joints of the fourth and fifth digits. Which of the following muscles is most likely affected?

A. Flexor digitorum profundus
B. Flexor digitorum superficialis
C. Lumbricals
D. Flexor carpi ulnaris
E. Interossei

15. A 24-year-old man comes to the emergency department with a wound to the palm of his hand. On physical examination, he cannot touch the pad of his index finger with his thumb but can grip a sheet of paper between all fingers and has no loss of sensation on the skin of his hand. Which of the following nerves is most likely injured?

A. Deep branch of ulnar
B. Anterior interosseous
C. Median
D. Recurrent branch of median
E. Deep branch of radial

16. A 55-year-old man comes to the physician after receiving a blunt trauma to his right axilla during a fall. He has difficulty elevating the right arm above the level of his shoulder. Physical examination shows the inferior angle of his right scapula protrudes more than the lower part of the left scapula. The protrusion is more prominent when the patient pushes against a wall. Which of the following neural structures is most likely injured?

A. The posterior cord of the brachial plexus
B. The long thoracic nerve
C. The upper trunk of the brachial plexus
D. The site of origin of the middle and lower subscapular nerves
E. Spinal nerve ventral rami C7, C8, and T1

17. A 4-year-old boy is brought to the emergency department by his mother for refusal to move his left arm. His mother recalls that he screamed out in pain after she tugged violently on her son's hand to pull him out of the way of an oncoming car this morning. Physical examination shows no swelling or bruising, but the child cannot extend his elbow. An x-ray of the upper extremity shows dislocation of the head of the radius. Which of the following ligaments is most likely associated with this injury?

A. Annular
B. Joint capsular
C. Interosseous
D. Radial collateral
E. Ulnar collateral

18. A 28-year-old nulligravida woman gives birth to a 3500 g (7 lb 11 oz) baby boy by forceps delivery. The pregnancy was complicated by gestational diabetes. Physical

examination of the neonate finds an adducted, medially rotated left arm that is flexed at the wrist. Which part of the brachial plexus was most likely injured during the delivery?

A. Lateral cord
B. Medial cord
C. Ventral rami of the lower trunk
D. Ventral ramus of the middle trunk
E. Ventral rami of the upper trunk

19. A 35-year-old man comes to the physician because of a 2 cm, red, blanchable nodule under the nail of his fifth digit. The patient has sudden severe attacks of pain localized to the area of the lesion, that are exacerbated by cold temperatures and pressure. Total surgical excision is recommended. Which of the following nerves would have to be anesthetized for painless removal of the tumor?

A. Superficial radial
B. Common palmar digital branch of median
C. Superficial branch of ulnar
D. Deep radial
E. Recurrent branch of median

20. A 25-year-old man is brought to the emergency department because of pain in his right wrist 2 hours after falling on an outstretched hand while performing the pole vault. Physical examination shows mild swelling on the dorsal wrist and tenderness upon palpation of the anatomical snuffbox. An x-ray of his hand shows no abnormalities. If a fracture is suspected, which bone is most likely involved?

A. Lunate
B. Scaphoid
C. Capitate
D. Hamate
E. Trapezoid

21. A 36-year-old man is brought to the emergency department after sustaining a deep knife wound on the medial side of his distal forearm in a fight. Neurologic examination finds that he is unable to hold a piece of paper between his fingers and has a loss of sensation on the medial aspect of his hand and medial 1½ digits. The site of injury is extremely tender on palpation. Which of the following nerves is most likely injured?

A. Axillary
B. Median
C. Musculocutaneous
D. Radial
E. Ulnar

22. A 19-year-old man is brought to the emergency department after falling painfully onto his right shoulder in a soccer game. A diagnosis of a dislocated right shoulder is made. After reduction of the shoulder dislocation, he has persistent pain over the dorsal region of the shoulder. Physical examination shows no obvious bone deformities but he is unable to abduct the arm normally. A magnetic resonance imaging (MRI) of the shoulder shows a torn muscle. Which of the following muscles is most likely damaged by this injury?

A. Coracobrachialis
B. Long head of the triceps brachii
C. Pectoralis minor
D. Supraspinatus
E. Teres major

23. A 32-year-old man comes to the physician because of a 3-day history of right shoulder pain after taking part in a tennis competition. An MRI in the oblique sagittal plane shows thickening and hypertrophy of a shoulder ligament. The physician explains that over the years of playing tennis, a shoulder ligament has gradually caused severe damage to the underlying muscle. Which of the following ligaments is the physician most likely referring to?

A. Acromioclavicular (AC) ligament
B. Coracohumeral ligament
C. Transverse scapular ligament
D. Glenohumeral ligament
E. Coracoacromial ligament

24. A 79-year-old man comes to the physician because of numbness in the medial three digits of his right hand. He has difficulty grasping objects with that hand. He retired 9 years earlier, after working as a carpenter for 50 years. Physical examination shows atrophy of the thenar eminence (Fig. 6.2). Which of the following conditions is the most likely cause of the problems in his hand?

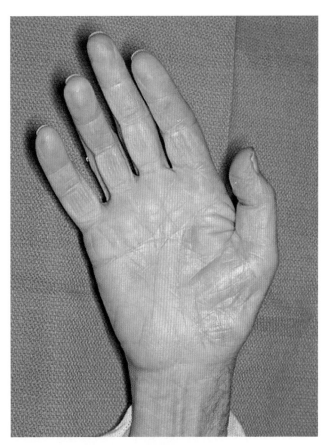

• **Fig. 6.2**

A. Compression of the median nerve in the carpal tunnel

B. Formation of osteophytes that compress the ulnar nerve at the medial epicondyle

C. Hypertrophy of the triceps brachii muscle compressing the brachial plexus

D. Osteoarthritis of the cervical spine

E. Repeated trauma to the ulnar nerve

25. A 20-year-old man is brought to the emergency department after a motorbike collision. He is awake, alert, and oriented and his vital signs are within normal limits. Physical examination shows several cuts and bruises on his body. He is unable to extend the left wrist. Extension of the elbow is normal bilaterally. Sensation is lost in the lateral half of the dorsum of the left hand. Which of the following nerves is most likely injured, and in what part of the arm is the injury located?

A. Median nerve, anterior wrist

B. Median nerve, arm

C. Radial nerve, mid humerus

D. Radial nerve, mid lateral forearm

E. Ulnar nerve, midpalmar region

Questions 26–50

26. A 17-year-old is brought to the emergency department after sustaining a knife wound to his left arm in a street fight. Physical examination shows a 4 cm wound on the proximal medial arm. He has weakness of elbow flexion and supination of the left hand. Extension at the elbow and wrist is normal. Which of the following additional findings would be present on physical examination?

A. Inability to adduct and abduct his fingers

B. Inability to flex his fingers

C. Inability to flex his thumb

D. Sensory loss over the lateral surface of his forearm

E. Sensory loss over the medial surface of his forearm

27. A 52-year-old man comes to the emergency department with excruciating pain in the posterior aspect of his right forearm. For the past several days he has been rehearsing with the symphony orchestra as a conductor. Physical examination shows excruciating pain upon palpation 2 cm distal and posteromedial to the lateral epicondyle. Intramuscular steroids are administered. Which of the following is the most likely mechanism of injury?

A. Compression of the ulnar nerve by the flexor carpi ulnaris

B. Compression of the median nerve by the pronator teres

C. Compression of the median nerve by the flexor digitorum superficialis

D. Compression of the superficial radial nerve by the brachioradialis

E. Compression of the deep radial nerve by the supinator

28. A 30-year-old woman comes to the physician with pain in her right wrist after falling with force onto her outstretched hand. Physical examination shows restricted movement of the wrist due to pain and decreased sensation on the palmar aspect of the lateral 3½ digits. An x-ray of the wrist shows an anterior dislocation of a carpal bone (Fig. 6.3). Which of the following bones is most likely dislocated?

A. Capitate

B. Lunate

C. Scaphoid

D. Trapezoid

E. Triquetrum

29. A 45-year-old man is brought to the emergency department after a motor vehicle collision. The patient is alert and vital signs are within normal limits. Physical examination shows lacerations of the scalp and neurologic examination finds sensory deficit of the C8 and T1 dermatomes. An x-ray of the cervical spine shows mild disc herniations of C7–T1 and T1–T2. The dorsal root ganglia of C8 and T1 would contain cell bodies of sensory fibers carried by which of the following nerves?

A. Medial antebrachial cutaneous nerve

B. Long thoracic nerve

C. Lateral antebrachial cutaneous nerve

D. Deep branch of ulnar nerve

E. Anterior interosseous nerve

30. A 23-year-old woman comes to the physician because of sudden severe pain over the base of the terminal phalanx of the index finger. Two days ago, she was making a bed in a hotel and caught the end of the index finger in a fold as she straightened the sheet. Physical examination shows the right index finger is swollen and she is unable to completely extend the DIP joint. Which one of the following structures within the digit was most likely injured?

A. The proper palmar digital branch of the median nerve

B. The vinculum longum

C. The insertion of the tendon of extensor digitorum onto the base of the distal phalanx

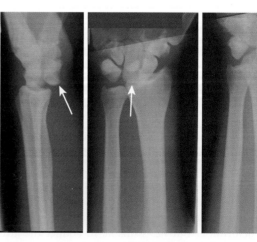

• Fig. 6.3

D. The insertion of the flexor digitorum profundus tendon

E. The insertion of the flexor digitorum superficialis tendon

31. A 16-year-old man is brought to the emergency department with pain and swelling of his right wrist after falling from his bike onto a flexed, outstretched hand. An x-ray of the forearm shows a fracture of the distal radius. The fractured bone displaced a carpal bone in the palmar direction, resulting in nerve compression within the carpal tunnel. Which of the following carpal bones is most likely dislocated?

A. Scaphoid

B. Trapezium

C. Capitate

D. Hamate

E. Lunate

32. A 15-year-old girl was brought to the emergency department after a severe bite by a dog on the dorsolateral aspect of her right hand. She has increasingly severe pain and swelling of her right hand. Physical examination shows symmetric enlargement of the first digit with severe pain on passive extension. An x-ray of the hand shows no abnormalities. The injured tendons in this compartment would include which of the following muscles?

A. Extensor carpi radialis longus and brevis

B. Abductor pollicis longus and extensor pollicis brevis

C. Extensor digitorum

D. Extensor indicis

E. Extensor carpi ulnaris

33. A 17-year-old girl is brought to the emergency department after falling from uneven parallel bars during a gymnastic routine. Neurologic examination finds altered sensation of the medial 1½ digits of her right hand. An MRI examination finds an injury to the medial cord of the brachial plexus. Which of the following spinal nerve levels is most likely affected?

A. C5, C6

B. C6, C7

C. C7, C8

D. C7, C8, T1

E. C8, T1

34. A 21-year-old woman comes to the emergency department after she was struck in the arm by a line drive during a softball game. Physical examination shows weakness on abduction and extension of the thumb. There is also weakness on extension of the wrist and metacarpophalangeal (MCP) joints. An x-ray of the arm shows no abnormalities. An MRI shows soft tissue injury to the central aspect of the lateral humerus. Which of the following muscles is most likely spared from injury?

A. Flexor carpi ulnaris

B. Extensor indicis

C. Brachioradialis

D. Extensor carpi radialis longus

E. Supinator

35. A 21-year-old woman comes to the physician after sustaining an injury of her left proximal arm with a baseball bat in a fight. Physical examination shows inability to extend her hand at the wrist. An x-ray shows a fracture of the mid-body of the humerus. Injury of the radial nerve in the radial groove is suspected. Which of the following signs would be present on physical examination?

A. Weakness of thumb abduction and thumb extension

B. Weakness of thumb opposition

C. Inability to extend the elbow

D. Paralysis of pronation of the hand

E. Paralysis of abduction and adduction of the arm

36. A 58-year-old man is brought to the emergency department after an attempted robbery in which he sustained a bullet wound to the medial side of the elbow. His vital signs are within normal limits. A major nerve was repaired at the site where it passed behind the medial epicondyle. Bleeding was stopped from an artery which plays an important role in supplying blood supply to the nerve. Which of the following arteries was most likely repaired?

A. The deep brachial artery

B. The radial collateral artery

C. The superior ulnar collateral artery

D. The inferior ulnar collateral artery

E. The anterior ulnar recurrent artery

37. A 60-year-old man is brought to the emergency department after he accidentally slashed his left wrist with his butcher's knife. Vital signs are within normal limits. Physical examination shows loss of sensation on the medial 1½ digits and decreased grip strength of the left hand. An x-ray of the wrist shows no other abnormalities. Which of the following actions would most likely be lost as a result of this injury?

A. Flexion of the PIP joint of the fifth digit (little finger)

B. Extension of the thumb

C. Adduction of the fifth digit

D. Abduction of the thumb

E. Opposition of the thumb

38. A 23-year-old man comes to the emergency department because he is unable to move his arm after he fell asleep in his chair with a book wedged into his axilla. Physical examination shows inability to extend his wrist and fingers and numbness of the lateral side of the dorsal aspect of the affected hand. Which of the following nerves is most likely compressed?

A. Lateral cord of the brachial plexus

B. Medial cord of the brachial plexus

C. Radial nerve

D. Median nerve

E. Lateral and medial pectoral nerves

39. A 32-year-old woman comes to the hospital for hemodialysis. Physical examination shows venous access in her upper limb was unexpectedly difficult as the caliber of the major vein on the lateral aspect her arm was too

small. A vein was found on the medial side of the arm that passed through the superficial and deep fascia to join veins beside the brachial artery. Which of the following veins is most likely located?

A. Basilic
B. Lateral cubital
C. Cephalic
D. Median cubital
E. Median antebrachial

40. A 29-year-old woman is brought to the emergency department after sustaining a deep laceration in the proximal part of the forearm. Physical examination shows normal flexion of the fourth and fifth digits at the interphalangeal (IP) joints. She is unable to extend the fourth and fifth digits at the MCP joints and is unable to flex the first three digits of her right hand. Sensation is absent on the lateral side of the palm and the palmar surfaces of the first 3½ digits. Which of the following nerve(s) is most likely injured?

A. Median nerve
B. Ulnar and median nerves
C. Ulnar nerve
D. Radial and ulnar nerves
E. Radial nerve

41. A 25-year-old man is brought to the emergency department because of excruciating pain in his right shoulder and proximal arm after a wrestling match. Physical examination shows that the arm is slightly abducted and externally rotated. The patient resists when passive medial rotation is attempted. Radial pulses are palpated bilaterally. An x-ray of the shoulder shows a dislocation of the humerus at the glenohumeral joint. Which of the following is the most likely mechanism of injury?

A. The head of the humerus is displaced laterally
B. The head of the humerus is displaced posteriorly
C. The head of the humerus is displaced inferiorly
D. The head of the humerus is displaced superiorly
E. The head of the humerus is displaced medially

42. The 35-year-old woman comes to the physician because of a breast lump that she noticed 1 month ago on self-breast examination. Physical examination shows a 1 cm hard nodule located just above and lateral to the areola of her right breast. A radioactive dye is injected into the tissue around the tumor, and an incision is made to expose the lymphatic vessels draining the area. Which of the following groups of lymph nodes will be first to receive the dye from the tumor?

A. Anterior axillary (pectoral) nodes
B. Rotter's interpectoral nodes
C. Parasternal nodes along the internal thoracic artery and vein
D. Central axillary nodes
E. Apical axillary or infraclavicular nodes

43. A 45-year-old man comes to the emergency department 1 hour after sustaining a shallow stab wound in the neck. He has neck pain that radiates to the left shoulder and upper back. Physical examination shows

a 4 cm laceration located in the posterior triangle of the left side of his neck. Asymmetry of the shoulders is noted. The superior angle of the left scapula protrudes slightly. Neurologic examination finds 5/5 power bilaterally when turning the head. Which of the following nerves is most likely injured?

A. Suprascapular nerve in the supraspinous fossa
B. The terminal segment of the dorsal scapular nerve
C. The upper trunk of the brachial plexus
D. The accessory nerve in the posterior cervical triangle
E. The thoracodorsal nerve in the axilla

44. A 65-year-old woman comes to the physician for a follow-up examination. Two months ago, she was diagnosed with late-onset radial nerve palsy after closed reduction of a mid-body humeral fracture. What findings are most likely to be present during physical examination?

A. Inability to abduct the digits at the MCP joint
B. Inability to adduct the digits at the MCP joint
C. Inability to extend the MCP joints only
D. Inability to extend the MCP, PIP, and DIP joints
E. Inability to extend the PIP and DIP joints

45. A 27-year-old man is brought to the emergency department because of pain and swelling of his right arm after falling from a ladder. He is unable to abduct his right arm more than 15 degrees and resists lateral rotation due to pain. The patient also has a loss of sensation over the right shoulder. An x-ray of the arm shows an oblique fracture of the humerus. The most likely cause of these symptoms is a fracture affecting which of the following locations?

A. Fracture of the medial epicondyle
B. Fracture of the glenoid fossa
C. Fracture of the surgical neck of the humerus
D. Fracture of the anatomical neck of the humerus
E. Fracture of the middle third of the humerus

46. A 47-year-old woman comes to the physician because of a 3-month history of skin changes of her right breast. Physical examination shows warmth, erythema, and skin dimpling of the right breast. A mammogram shows suspicious findings of breast cancer and a full-thickness skin biopsy is performed to confirm the diagnosis. This condition is primarily the result of which of the following?

A. Shortening of the suspensory ligaments by cancer in the axillary tail (of Spence) of the breast
B. Blockage of cutaneous lymphatic vessels
C. Contraction of the retinacula cutis of the areola and nipple
D. Invasion of the pectoralis major by the cancer
E. Ipsilateral (same side) inversion of the periareolar skin from ductular cancer

47. A 29-year-old woman is brought to the emergency department 2 hours after falling from her balcony. Physical examination shows noticeable swelling and bruising over the clavicle. There is tenderness, crepitus on palpation, and decreased range of motion of her

left upper limb. An x-ray of the left shoulder shows a fracture of the clavicle and internal bleeding is strongly suspected. Which of the following vessels is most likely to be injured in a clavicular fracture?

A. Subclavian artery
B. Cephalic vein
C. Lateral thoracic artery
D. Subclavian vein
E. Internal thoracic artery

48. A 68-year-old woman is brought to the emergency department 3 hours after she fell on the wet bathroom floor of her home. Physical examination shows a posterior displacement of the left distal wrist and hand. An x-ray of the wrist shows an oblique fracture of the radius. Which of the following types of fracture most likely occurred in this patient?

A. Colles fracture
B. Scaphoid fracture
C. Bennett fracture
D. Volkmann ischemic contracture
E. Boxer's fracture

49. A 34-year-old woman is brought to the emergency department with left shoulder pain for 2 hours after she struck a tree on a ski slope. Physical examination shows swelling and bruising of the left shoulder. The patient has tenderness to palpation and a "step-off" of the left clavicle is noted. An x-ray shows a high-grade left shoulder separation. Which of the following typically occurs in this type of injury?

A. Displacement of the head of the humerus from the glenoid cavity
B. Partial or complete tearing of the coracoclavicular ligament
C. Partial or complete tearing of the coracoacromial ligament
D. Rupture of the transverse scapular ligament
E. Disruption of the glenoid labrum

50. A 22-year-old man is brought to the emergency department after he sustains a penetrating injury to his left upper limb from a nail gun. His temperature is 37.6°C (99.68°F), pulse is 107/min, respirations are 22/min, and blood pressure is 108/65 mm Hg. He is unable to flex the DIP joints of the fourth and fifth digits of the left hand. An x-ray shows no fractures. What is the most likely cause of his injury?

A. Trauma to the ulnar nerve near the trochlea
B. Trauma to the ulnar nerve at the wrist
C. Median nerve damage proximal to the pronator teres
D. Median nerve damage at the wrist
E. Trauma to spinal nerve root C8

Questions 51–75

51. A 44-year-old man comes to the physician after sustaining a penetrating wound to his shoulder from a crossbow bolt. Physical examination shows a deep, 4 cm laceration of the anterior shoulder and asymmetry of the radial artery. A compress is placed on the wound and deep pressure is applied. An angiogram shows transection of the axillary artery just distal to the origin of the subscapular artery. What collateral arterial pathways are available to bypass the site of injury?

A. Suprascapular with circumflex scapular artery
B. Dorsal scapular with thoracodorsal artery
C. Posterior circumflex humeral artery with deep brachial artery
D. Lateral thoracic with brachial artery
E. Superior thoracic artery with thoracoacromial artery

52. A 17-year-old boy suffered the most common of fractures of the carpal bones when he fell on his outstretched hand. Which bone would this be?

A. Trapezium
B. Lunate
C. Pisiform
D. Hamate
E. Scaphoid

53. A 54-year-old man comes to the emergency department because of a penetrating injury to his forearm from a baling hook while farming. His temperature is 37°C (98.6°F), pulse is 117/min, respirations are 22/min, and blood pressure is 100/70 mm Hg. Physical examination of the upper limb shows the patient is unable to oppose the tip of the thumb to the tip of the index finger. He is able to touch the tips of the ring and little fingers to the pad of his thumb. Which of the following nerves is most likely injured?

A. Median
B. Deep branch of radial
C. Radial
D. Recurrent median
E. Anterior interosseous

54. A 62-year-old woman visits her physician because of 3-year history of worsening bilateral shoulder pain. The pain worsens when the arm is lifted overhead. She has a 40-year history of rheumatoid arthritis. Physical examination of the shoulder shows a positive Yergason test of the right shoulder. An ultrasound of the right shoulder joint shows findings consistent with tendinopathy. Arthroscopic examination of the right shoulder shows an erosion of a tendon within the glenohumeral joint. Which of the following tendons was most likely observed?

A. Glenohumeral
B. Long head of triceps brachii
C. Long head of biceps brachii
D. Infraspinatus
E. Coracobrachialis

55. A 26-year-old man comes to the physician because of a 1-week history of pain and weakness in the right shoulder after a tennis match. The pain is exacerbated by movement. He is referred to an orthopedic surgeon. During surgery, the supraspinatus muscle is reflected from its bed. Which artery was seen crossing the

ligament that bridges the notch of the superior border of the scapula?

A. Subscapular
B. Transverse cervical
C. Dorsal scapular
D. Posterior circumflex humeral
E. Suprascapular

56. A 61-year-old man is brought to the emergency department 2 hours after he was hit in the left arm by a cricket bat. His only medication is acetaminophen. He is 180 cm (5 ft 11 in) tall and weighs 82 kg (180 lb); BMI is 25 kg/m². His vital signs are within normal limits. Physical examination shows bruising and tenderness to palpation over the mid-humeral region of the left upper limb. Upper limb pulses are palpable bilaterally. Sensation is decreased over a small area of the dorsum of the left hand proximal to the lateral two digits. The patient is unable to extend the left wrist. Which of the following nerves is most likely injured?

A. Radial
B. Posterior interosseous
C. Lateral antebrachial cutaneous
D. Medial antebrachial cutaneous
E. Dorsal cutaneous of ulnar

57. A 45-year-old woman comes to the emergency department with a 2-week history of neck pain radiating to the left shoulder. Physical examination shows weakness in wrist extension and paresthesia on the back of her arm and forearm. An MRI examination finds a herniated disc in the cervical region. Which of the following spinal nerves is most likely injured?

A. C5
B. C6
C. C7
D. C8
E. T1

58. A 22-year-old man comes to the emergency department because of wrist pain after falling on his outstretched right hand. Physical examination shows bruising of the wrist and tenderness in the anatomical snuffbox. An x-ray of the wrist shows a displaced fracture of the scaphoid bone. A surgical intervention is recommended. When the anatomical snuffbox is exposed, which artery is seen crossing the fractured bone?

A. Ulnar
B. Radial
C. Anterior interosseous
D. Posterior interosseous
E. Deep palmar arch

59. A 78-year-old woman comes to the physician with worsening right shoulder pain over the past 6 months. She has severe pain when placing books on the overhead bookshelf at work and pain in her shoulder while combing her hair. Abduction of the right arm and palpation of the deltoid muscle produces exquisite pain. An MRI of the upper limb shows hyperintense focal

lesions of intermuscular inflammation extending over the head of the humerus. Which of the following structures is most likely inflamed?

A. Subscapular bursa
B. Infraspinatus muscle
C. Glenohumeral joint cavity
D. Subacromial bursa
E. Teres minor muscle

60. A 60-year old woman comes to the physician because of intermittent numbness and tingling sensation of her right hand, which often wakes her up at night. Physical examination shows flexion of the wrist for 60 seconds reproduces the painful symptoms. A 3-month trial of wrist splinting and non-steroidal anti-inflammatory drugs therapy did not relieve the pain. During surgery, an anesthetic injection into the axillary sheath is administered. The axillary sheath takes its origin from which of the following structures?

A. Superficial fascia of the neck
B. Superficial cervical investing fascia
C. Buccopharyngeal fascia
D. Clavipectoral fascia
E. Prevertebral fascia

61. A 45-year-old woman comes to the emergency department because of neck pain for 2 months. A computed tomography (CT) shows a single 5 × 7 cm tumor with an irregular border on the left side of her oral cavity. A radical neck surgical procedure is performed and the tumor, deep cervical lymph nodes, and related tissues are removed. Two months postoperatively the patient's left shoulder droops and she has weakness on turning her head to the right. Which of the following structures was most likely injured during the radical neck surgery?

A. Suprascapular nerve
B. Long thoracic nerve
C. Accessory nerve
D. C5 and C6 spinal nerves
E. Radial nerve

62. A 23-year-old man is brought to the emergency department 3 hours after injuring his shoulder playing basketball with his friends. Physical examination shows a step-off at the shoulder on palpation. An x-ray shows a total separation of the shoulder (Fig. 6.4). Which of the following structures has most likely been torn?

A. Glenohumeral ligament
B. Coracoacromial ligament
C. Tendon of long head of biceps brachii
D. AC ligament
E. Transverse scapular ligament

63. A 30-year-old man comes to the physician because of a 2-week history of dull, intermittent pain of the posterolateral right shoulder. The pain is exacerbated by overhead activities. Physical examination shows enlarged shoulder muscles that reduces the size of the quadrangular space. There is point tenderness over the quadrangular space and weakness on lateral rotation of the abducted humerus. An MRI of the shoulder shows

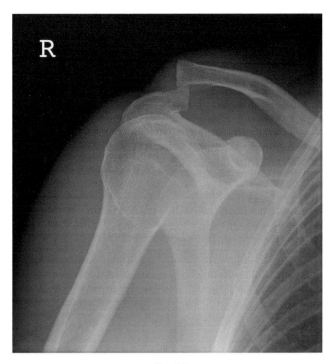

• Fig. 6.4

atrophy of the teres minor. Which of the following structures would most likely be compressed?

A. Axillary nerve
B. Anterior circumflex humeral artery
C. Cephalic vein
D. Radial nerve
E. Subscapular artery

64. A 43-year-old woman comes to the office because she cannot hold a piece of paper between her thumb and the lateral side of her index finger without flexing the distal joint of her thumb. This is a positive Froment sign, which is consistent with ulnar neuropathy. Weakness of which specific muscle causes this sign to appear?

A. Flexor pollicis longus
B. Adductor pollicis
C. Flexor digiti minimi
D. Flexor carpi radialis
E. Extensor indicis

65. A 48-year-old woman comes to the physician because of a 1-month history of intermittent numbness and tingling in her right hand. The symptoms awake her from sleep at night and are relieved by shaking her hand. A diagnosis of nerve compression in the carpal tunnel was made, and the patient underwent an endoscopic nerve release. Two weeks postoperatively, the patient has weakness in the thumb, with loss of thumb opposition. Sensation to the hand is normal. Which of the following nerves was injured during the operation?

A. The first common palmar digital branch of the median nerve
B. The second common palmar digital branch of the median nerve

C. Recurrent branch of median nerve
D. Deep branch of the ulnar nerve
E. Anterior interosseous nerve

66. A 19-year-old man is brought to the emergency department after sustaining a deep laceration of his right upper limb when he stumbled and fell onto a broken bottle. His temperature is 37°C (98.6°F), pulse is 92/min, respirations are 18/min, and blood pressure is 128/75 mm Hg. Neurological examination finds he is able to extend the MCP joints of all his fingers in the right limb. He is unable to extend the IP joints of the fourth and fifth digits, and extension of the IP joints of the second and third digits is weak. Sensation of the hand is normal. Which of the following nerves is most likely injured?

A. Radial nerve at the elbow
B. Median nerve at the wrist
C. Ulnar nerve in the mid forearm
D. Deep branch of ulnar nerve
E. Recurrent branch of the median nerve

67. A 41-year-old woman comes to the physician for a follow-up examination. One year ago, she underwent a mastectomy of her left breast. She is scheduled for a latissimus dorsi muscle flap to cosmetically augment the site of her absent left breast. During surgery, part of the latissimus dorsi muscle is advanced to the anterior thoracic wall. Which artery forms the vascular base of this flap?

A. Thoracodorsal artery
B. Dorsal scapular artery
C. Transverse cervical artery
D. Lateral thoracic artery
E. Thoracoacromial artery

68. A 31-year-old man is brought to the emergency department 1 hour after falling onto his elbow during a hockey game. He has a restricted range of motion of his left arm due to pain. His temperature is 37°C (98.6°F), pulse is 90/min and regular, respirations are 18/min, and blood pressure is 128/76 mm Hg. Physical examination shows swelling and ecchymosis at the proximal shoulder. An x-ray of the shoulder shows a fracture of the surgical neck of the humerus with elevation and adduction of the distal fragment. Which of the following muscles most likely caused the adduction of the distal fragment?

A. Brachialis
B. Teres minor
C. Pectoralis major
D. Supraspinatus
E. Pectoralis minor

69. A 74-year-old woman is brought to the emergency department because of pain and swelling of her forearm after stumbling and falling over her pet dog. Physical examination of the forearm shows no open wounds and the neurovascular examination is within normal limits. The patient holds her left forearm in the pronated position and is unable to supinate the left hand. An x-ray

of the right forearm shows a fracture of the upper third of the radius. The proximal end of the fracture deviates laterally. Which of the following muscles is primarily responsible for the lateral deviation?

A. Pronator teres

B. Supinator

C. Pronator quadratus

D. Brachioradialis

E. Brachialis

70. A 12-year-old boy is brought to the emergency department 30 minutes after he lacerated the palmar surface of his wrist while playing with a sharp knife. His temperature is 37°C (98.6°F), pulse is 116/min, respirations are 20/min, and blood pressure is 100/70 mm Hg. Physical examination shows a 2 cm wound at the midline of the wrist. The cut ends of a tendon are exposed within the wound. The flexor retinaculum is intact. Which tendon most commonly lies in this position?

A. Palmaris longus

B. Flexor carpi radialis

C. Abductor pollicis longus

D. Flexor carpi ulnaris

E. Flexor pollicis longus

71. A 22-year-old man comes to the emergency department because of pain and swelling of the fifth digit of his right hand. Two hours ago, he hit a vending machine in the hospital when he did not receive his drink after inserting money twice. Physical examination shows swelling of the medial aspect of the dorsum of the hand. When the patient is asked to make a fist, one of his knuckles cannot be seen. Which of the following most likely best explains the knuckle deformity?

A. Fracture of the styloid process of the ulna

B. Fracture of the neck of the fifth metacarpal

C. Colles fracture of the radius

D. Smith fracture of the radius

E. Bennett fracture of the thumb

72. A 14-year-old girl is brought to the physician because of difficulty holding a pen in her right hand. The patient is unable to perform opposition of the thumb, abduction and adduction of the digits, and IP joint extension of the right hand. There is notable anesthesia of the skin on the medial side of the forearm. Long flexor and extensor muscles of the hand and wrist appear to be functioning within normal limits. An x-ray shows marked elevation of the right first rib due to scoliosis. Which of the following neural structures is most likely impaired?

A. Median nerve

B. Middle trunk of the brachial plexus

C. Radial nerve

D. Lower trunk of the brachial plexus

E. T1 ventral ramus

73. A 23-year-old woman is brought to the emergency department 4 hours after she had a painful injury to her hand in a dry ski-slope competition. The patient caught her thumb in the matting as she fell. Physical examination shows pain and swelling at the ulnar aspect of the MCP joint of the first digit. Lidocaine is injected into the MCP joint and increased laxity of the thumb is noted during flexion and extension at the MCP joint. An MRI shows a rupture of the ulnar collateral ligament. She is scheduled for surgical repair. Which of the following is the most likely diagnosis?

A. De Quervain syndrome (tenosynovitis)

B. Navicular bone fracture

C. Boxer's thumb

D. Gamekeeper's thumb

E. Bennett thumb

74. A 26-year-old man comes to the office because of a 2-week history of left shoulder pain. The pain is dull and is exacerbated when the patient lifts his arm overhead. An x-ray of the shoulder shows no abnormalities. An MRI shows tendinopathy of the long head of the biceps brachii muscle. Which of the following findings will most likely be present on physical examination?

A. Pain is felt in the anterior shoulder during forced contraction

B. Pain is felt in the lateral shoulder during forced contraction

C. Pain is felt during abduction and flexion of the shoulder joint

D. Pain is felt during extension and adduction of the shoulder joint

E. Pain is felt in the lateral shoulder during flexion of the shoulder joint

75. A 43-year-old woman comes to the physician because of a 1-week history of elbow pain. She has pain over the lateral aspect of the right elbow that radiates to the posterior forearm. Physical examination shows tenderness distal to the origin of the extensor carpi radialis brevis. A diagnosis of lateral epicondylitis is made. Which of the following tests should be performed during physical examination to confirm the diagnosis?

A. Nerve conduction studies (nerve conduction velocity test)

B. Evaluation of pain experienced during flexion and extension of the elbow joint

C. Observing the presence of pain when the wrist is extended against resistance

D. Observing the presence of numbness and tingling in the ring and little fingers when the wrist is flexed against resistance

E. Evaluation of pain felt over the styloid process of radius during brachioradialis contraction

Questions 76–100

76. A 29-year-old man is brought to the emergency department after a painful fall against a rocky ledge. His temperature is 37.5°C (99.5°F), pulse is 95/min, respirations are 18/min, and blood pressure is 118/70 mm Hg. He has dull pain in the lateral shoulder with

radiation to the proximal arm. An x-ray of the arm shows a hairline fracture of the surgical neck of the humerus. Which of the following tests is best for assessing the status of the nerve associated with this injury?

A. Have the patient abduct the limb while holding a 4.5 kg (10-lb) weight

B. Have the patient shrug the shoulders

C. Test for presence of skin sensation over the lateral side of the shoulder

D. Test for normal sensation over the medial skin of the axilla

E. Have the patient push against an immovable object like a wall and assess the position of the scapula

77. A 27-year-old man is brought to the emergency department after a motorcycle collision. Vitals are within normal limits. Physical examination shows bruising on the upper body and loss of the soft tissue on the dorsum of his left hand. The functions of the left extensor carpi radialis longus and brevis tendons are lost. An x-ray of the upper limbs shows no other abnormalities. A decision to replace those tendons with the palmaris longus tendons of both forearms is made. Postoperatively, sensation is absent on the lateral palm and palmar surfaces of the first three digits bilaterally. There is also paralysis of thumb opposition. What is the most likely cause of the sensory and motor deficits?

A. Bilateral loss of spinal nerve T1 with fractures of first rib bilaterally

B. Lower plexus (lower trunk) trauma

C. Dupuytren contracture

D. Left radial nerve injury in the posterior compartment of the forearm

E. The palmaris longus was absent bilaterally; the nerve normally deep to it looked like a tendon and was cut

78. A 15-year-old boy is brought to the emergency department 30 minutes after sustaining a gunshot wound to the ventral surface of the upper limb. Three months after the injury, the patient comes to the physician for a follow-up examination. Physical examination shows a complete clawing of the digits of his left hand, but the patient is able to extend his wrist. He has severe paresthesia of all five digits of the affected hand. Which of the following mechanisms is most likely responsible for these findings?

A. The ulnar nerve has been severed at the wrist.

B. The median nerve has been injured in the carpal tunnel.

C. The median and ulnar nerves are damaged at the wrist.

D. The median and ulnar nerves have been injured at the elbow region.

E. The median, ulnar, and radial nerves have been injured at mid-humerus.

79. A 68-year-old woman is brought to the emergency department after falling on a flexed wrist in an attempt to break her fall when she missed the last step of her motorhome. Her temperature is 37°C (98.6°F), pulse is 80/min, respirations are 16/min, and blood pressure is 138/75 mm Hg. Physical examination shows a deformity of the distal wrist. An x-ray of the wrist shows a fracture of the distal radius with volar angulation of the distal fragment. Which of the following is the most likely type of fracture in this patient?

A. Colles fracture

B. Scaphoid fracture

C. Bennett fracture

D. Smith fracture

E. Boxer's fracture

80. A 27-year-old-man is brought to the emergency department after he was hit on a fingertip while attempting to catch a ball bare-handed. Physical examination shows that the ballplayer cannot straighten the DIP joint of the middle finger of his right hand. Which of the following is the most likely diagnosis?

A. Claw hand deformity

B. Boutonnière deformity

C. Swan-neck deformity

D. Dupuytren contracture

E. Mallet finger

81. A 31-year-old-woman is brought to the emergency department following an injury that forced her to withdraw from a figure skating competition. Her partner missed catching her from an overhead position and instead grasped her forearm powerfully. Physical examination shows bruising of the forearm. She is unable to flex the DIP joint of the index finger on clasping the hands and is unable to flex the terminal phalanx of the thumb. There is loss of sensation over the thenar aspect of the hand. What is the most likely mechanism of her injury?

A. Median nerve injured within the cubital fossa

B. Anterior interosseous nerve injury at the pronator teres

C. Radial nerve injury at its entrance into the posterior forearm compartment

D. Median nerve injury at the proximal skin crease of the wrist

E. Ulnar nerve trauma halfway along the forearm

82. A 19-year-old man is brought to the emergency department after he fell from a cliff while hiking in the mountains. He broke his fall by grasping a tree branch. His vital signs are within normal limits. Physical examination shows hyperextension of the MCP joint and flexion at the IP joints of the fourth and fifth digits. Which of the following nerves is responsible for sensory deficits in the affected limb?

A. Inferior lateral brachial cutaneous nerve

B. Musculocutaneous nerve

C. Intercostobrachial nerve

D. Medial antebrachial cutaneous nerve

E. Median nerve

83. A 52-year-old woman underwent mastectomy for invasive ductal carcinoma of the left breast. During the procedure the tumor and the pectoral, central axillary, and apical axillary lymph node groups were excised. Six months later she comes to the physician for a follow-up examination. Physical examination shows a deep, hollow area inferior to the medial half of the clavicle. The patient has no motor or sensory deficits. Which of the following is the most likely cause of the findings on physical examination?

A. Part of the pectoralis major muscle was cut and removed in the mastectomy

B. The pectoralis minor muscle was removed entirely in the surgery

C. The lateral pectoral nerve was cut

D. The medial pectoral nerve was cut

E. The lateral cord of the brachial plexus was injured

84. A 54-year-old woman was brought to the emergency department after being found unconscious at the scene of a motor vehicle collision. Spine injury was suspected, and her neck was immobilized in a cervical collar. On arrival, her temperature is 37°C (98.6°F), pulse is 120/min, respirations are 16/min, and blood pressure is 142/84 mm Hg. Physical examination shows unilateral absence of her brachioradialis reflex. Injury to which of the following spinal nerves is most likely responsible for the absence of this reflex?

A. C5

B. C6

C. C7

D. C8

E. T1

85. A 43-year-old man is brought to the emergency department after a motor vehicle collision in which he sustained a whiplash injury. On arrival, his temperature is 37°C (98.6°F), pulse is 110/min, respirations are 18/min, and blood pressure is 140/82 mm Hg. Physical examination shows loss of elbow extension, loss of extension of the MCP joints, and absence of ipsilateral triceps reflex. An MRI shows an intervertebral disc herniation in the cervical region. Which of the following spinal nerves is most likely affected?

A. C5

B. C6

C. C7

D. C8

E. T1

86. A 29-year-old man comes to the physician because of 2-day history of worsening pain of his right elbow. The patient fell off a ladder 2 days ago at work and applied an ice pack to the site. Physical examination shows a swollen and discolored right elbow with tenderness to palpation. An x-ray of the left upper limb shows a dislocated elbow with separation of the ulna and the medial aspect of the distal humerus. Which of the following joint classifications best describes the articulation formed between the two bones involved in this patient injury?

A. Trochoid

B. Ginglymus

C. Enarthrodial

D. Synarthrosis

E. Sellar

87. A 45-year-old woman is brought to the emergency department after sustaining injuries from a motorbike collision. She was propelled over the handlebars of her bike, landing on the point of her left shoulder. Her temperature is 37°C (98.6°F), pulse is 100/min, respirations are 15/min, and blood pressure is 145/87 mm Hg. Physical examination shows a swollen, pale, and cool proximal arm. Any movement of the arm causes severe pain. An x-ray of the arm shows a fracture of the humerus and the formation of a large hematoma. A diagnosis of Volkmann ischemic contracture is made. At which of the following locations has the fracture most likely occurred?

A. Surgical neck of humerus

B. Radial groove of humerus

C. Supracondylar line of humerus

D. Olecranon

E. Lateral epicondyle

88. A 55-year-old-woman comes to the emergency department because of a painful, swollen wrist after she fell from the stage into the orchestra pit while conducting during rehearsal. Physical examination shows tenderness in the medial wrist. An x-ray of the wrist shows a fracture of the styloid process of the ulna as well as a distal radial fracture. Disruption of the triangular fibrocartilage complex is suspected. The ulna articulates at the wrist with which of the following bones?

A. Triquetrum

B. Hamate

C. Radius and lunate

D. Radius

E. Pisiform and triquetrum

89. A 67-year-old woman comes to the emergency department after falling on an outstretched hand while walking her dog the evening before. Neurologic examination finds weakness of flexion of the wrist in a medial direction, a loss of sensation on the medial side of the hand, and clawing of the fingers. An x-ray of her elbow shows no abnormalities. At which of the following locations has the nerve injury most likely occurred?

A. Behind the medial epicondyle

B. Between the pisiform bone and the flexor retinaculum

C. Within the carpal tunnel

D. At the cubital fossa, between the ulnar and radial heads of origin of flexor digitorum superficialis

E. At the radial neck, 1 cm distal to the humerocapitellar (HCA) joint

90. An 18-year-old man comes to the emergency department after he sustained a wrist laceration. His temperature is 37.5°C (99.5°F), pulse is 82/min, respirations are 14/min, and blood pressure is 120/72 mm Hg. Physical examination shows a 2.5-cm laceration at the distal crease of the medial wrist with underlying tissues exposed. Which of the following signs is most likely found on physical examination?
   A. The patient could not touch the tip of the thumb to the tips of the other digits
   B. There would be loss of sensation on the dorsum of the medial side of the hand
   C. The patient would be unable to flex the IP joints
   D. There would be decreased ability to extend the IP joints
   E. There would be no serious functional problem at all to the patient

91. A 45-year-old man comes to the office after a digit of his left hand was injured when a door was slammed on his hand. A superficial cut on his middle finger was sutured. Physical examination shows functional deficits of the finger. The PIP joint is pulled into constant flexion, whereas the DIP joint is held in a position of hyperextension. What is the most likely diagnosis?
   A. Mallet finger
   B. Boutonnière deformity
   C. Dupuytren contracture
   D. Swan-neck deformity
   E. Dinner fork wrist deformity

92. A 67-year-old man comes to the office because of a 6-month history of progressively worsening pain in his hands associated with a gradual loss of function which is more prominent while he is painting. Physical examination of the hands shows flexion of the MCP joints, extension of the PIP joints, and slight flexion of the DIP joints. What is the most likely diagnosis?
   A. Mallet finger
   B. Boutonnière deformity
   C. Dupuytren contracture
   D. Swan-neck deformity
   E. Dinner fork wrist deformity

93. A 32-year-old woman comes to the physician for a follow-up examination. One month ago, she underwent surgical dissection of her right axilla for the removal of lymph nodes for staging and treatment of her breast cancer. She has weakness and pain of her right shoulder and has difficulty raising her left arm above her head when combing her hair. Physical examination shows medial scapular winging accentuated when the patient is asked to push against a wall. In a subsequent consult visit with her surgeon, she was told that a nerve was injured during the surgical procedure. What is the origin of the injured nerve?
   A. The upper trunk of her brachial plexus
   B. The posterior division of the middle trunk
   C. Ventral rami of the brachial plexus

   D. The posterior cord of the brachial plexus
   E. The lateral cord of the brachial plexus

94. A 72-year-old man comes to the physician because of an abnormal thickening of the skin at the base of his ring fingers over the past year. He has no pain in his hand but has a gradual decrease in the range of motion of his fingers. Physical examination of both hands shows localized and firm ridges in the palmar skin that extend to the base of the ring finger. He is unable to fully flex and extend the ring fingers. What is the most likely diagnosis?
   A. Ape hand
   B. Dupuytren contracture
   C. Claw hand
   D. Wrist drop
   E. Mallet finger

95. A 24-year-old woman is brought to the emergency department after sustaining an injury to her shoulder during a basketball game. The right shoulder is externally rotated and abducted. Physical examination shows loss of the lateral contour of the shoulder. An x-ray shows anterior shoulder dislocation. What nerve is most commonly injured in this type of injury?
   A. Axillary
   B. Radial
   C. Median
   D. Ulnar
   E. Musculocutaneous

96. An 85-year-old man is brought to the emergency department with a painful left arm after lifting a case of wine. Physical examination shows swelling and bruising at the anterior of the elbow and loss of the biceps brachii reflex (Fig. 6.5). Which of the following is the most likely location of the rupture?
   A. Intertubercular groove
   B. Midportion of the biceps brachii muscle
   C. Junction with the short head of the biceps brachii muscle
   D. Proximal end of the combined biceps brachii muscle
   E. Bony insertion of the muscle

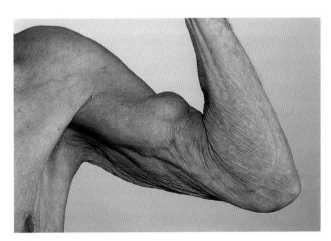

• **Fig. 6.5**

97. A 55-year old man comes to the physician because of a 2-week history of weakness and pain in his left shoulder that disturbs his sleep at night. Physical examination shows point-tenderness below the acromion. Tenderness is elicited when the patient abducts and internally rotates his arm against resistance. An MRI of the shoulder shows injury to the tendon of the supraspinatus muscle. Which of the following is true about the supraspinatus muscle?
  A. It inserts onto the lesser tubercle of the humerus.
  B. It initiates adduction of the shoulder.
  C. It is innervated chiefly by the C5 spinal nerve.
  D. It is supplied by the upper subscapular nerve.
  E. It originates from the lateral border of the scapula.

98. A 5-year-old boy is brought to the emergency department after falling from a tree. The patient cradles his injured arm. Neurovascular examination finds no abnormalities. An x-ray shows a non-displaced fracture. The child's parents are informed that their son's fracture is the most commonly occurring fracture in children and can be treated nonoperatively. Which of the following bones was most likely fractured?
  A. Humerus
  B. Radius
  C. Ulna
  D. Scaphoid
  E. Clavicle

99. A 22-year-old woman comes to the physician because of a long history of pain in her left upper limb. She has difficulty with fine motor tasks of the hand and paresthesia along the medial surface of the forearm and palm. Physical examination shows weakness and atrophy of gripping muscles ("long flexors") and the intrinsic muscles of the hand. The radial pulse is diminished when her neck is rotated to the ipsilateral side (positive Adson test). What is the most likely diagnosis?
  A. Erb-Duchenne paralysis
  B. Aneurysm of the brachiocephalic trunk, with plexus compression
  C. Thoracic outlet syndrome
  D. Carpal tunnel syndrome
  E. Injury to the medial cord of the brachial plexus

100. A 25-year-old man comes to the physician with numbness and tingling of the hand after playing a game on his phone while leaning his elbows against a desk for 6 hours. Physical examination shows weakness of wrist adduction, loss of sensation on the medial aspect of the hand, and clawing of the digits. Which of the following mechanisms is most likely responsible for this patient's presentation?
  A. Compression of a nerve passing between the humeral and ulnar heads of origin of flexor carpi ulnaris
  B. Compression of a nerve passing at Guyon canal between the pisiform bone and flexor retinaculum
  C. Compression of a nerve passing through the carpal tunnel

D. Compression of a nerve passing between the ulnar and radial heads of origin of flexor digitorum superficialis
  E. Compression of a nerve passing deep to brachioradialis muscle

Questions 101–125

101. A 22-year-old G1P0, at 32 weeks of gestation was admitted urgently to the hospital in preterm labor. Physical examination shows a breech footling presentation. The baby is delivered vaginally with considerable amounts of traction. The newborn is shown in Fig. 6.6. Which of the following structures was most likely injured during the childbirth?
  A. Radial nerve
  B. Upper trunk of the brachial plexus
  C. Lower trunk of the brachial plexus
  D. Median, ulnar, and radial nerves
  E. Upper and lower trunks of the brachial plexus

102. A 17-year-old girl comes to the physician because of pain in her right hand for the past 6 months which worsened after taking a martial arts class. The patient says that she had been breaking concrete blocks with her right hand. Physical examination shows a flattened hypothenar eminence of the right hand and weakness of abduction and adduction of her fingers.

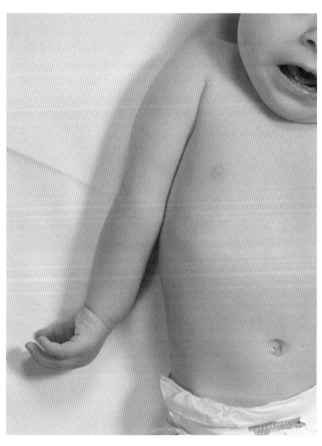

• **Fig. 6.6**

She is able to flex the digits normally. There is also decreased sensation over the palmar surfaces of the fourth and fifth digits. Which of the following best describes the nature of her injury?

A. Compression of the median nerve in the carpal tunnel

B. Fracture of the triquetrum, with injury to the dorsal branch of thc ulnar nerve

C. Dislocation of a bone in the proximal row of the carpus

D. Fracture of the body of the fifth metacarpal

E. Injury of the ulnar nerve in Guyon canal

103. A 10-year-old boy is brought to the emergency department after a dog bite that entered the common flexor synovial sheath (also known as the ulnar bursa) of his forearm. The wound was cleaned and dressed, and he was further treated with rabies antiserum. Two days later, the patient returns to the hospital with a temperature of 38°C (100.4°F) and swelling of his palm. Following the anatomy of the typical common flexor sheath, which of the following digits is most susceptible to the spread of the infection?

A. First

B. Second

C. Third

D. Fourth

E. Fifth

104. A 23-year-old man comes to the emergency department 2 days after sustaining a knife wound to his left hand. He develops a temperature of 38°C (100.4°F). Physical examination shows a red and swollen wound on the palmar aspect of the fifth digit at the base of the distal phalanx. The infection spreads to the sheath of the flexor digitorum profundus tendons. If left untreated, which of the following spaces could the infection most likely spread to?

A. Central compartment

B. Hypothenar compartment

C. Midpalmar space

D. Thenar compartment

E. Thenar space

105. A 36-year-old man comes to the emergency department because of a dull ache in his shoulder and axilla (Fig. 6.7). Vital signs are within normal limits. The pain is exacerbated with activity and is relieved by rest. Four days ago, he was hospitalized and a central venous line was placed. Physical examination shows a swollen right arm. What is the most likely cause of the patient's current presentation?

A. Axillary-subclavian vein thrombosis

B. Compression of C5–C8 spinal nerve

C. Disc herniation of C4–C8

D. Impingement syndrome

E. Injury to radial, ulnar, and median nerves

106. A 22-year-old woman is brought to the emergency department 1 hour after sustaining a severe knife

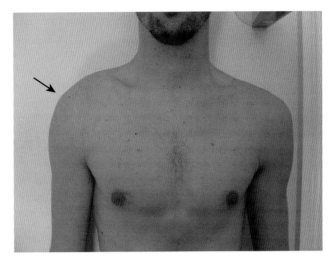

• Fig. 6.7

wound to the upper chest. Her temperature is 36.9°C (98.4°F), pulse is 82/min, respirations are 16/min, and blood pressure is 115/72 mm Hg. Physical examination shows a 3-cm deep entry wound at the deltopectoral groove. Vascular clamps are applied proximal and distal to the site of injury between the second and third parts of the axillary artery to control the bleeding. Which of the following arteries most likely provides collateral circulation to the scapula?

A. Transverse cervical and suprascapular

B. Posterior circumflex humeral and deep brachial

C. Suprascapular and circumflex scapular

D. Supreme (superior) thoracic and thoracoacromial

E. Lateral thoracic and suprascapular

107. A 24-year-old man is brought to the emergency department 2 hours after sustaining a knife wound to the arm during a fight. Physical examination shows a penetrating wound on the proximal forearm. There is weakness of pronation of the forearm and the patient is unable to oppose the thumb. Sensation is decreased in the lateral 3½ digits on the palmar surface of the hand. Which of the following is most likely seen on physical examination when the patient is asked to make a fist?

A. The MCP and IP joints of the second and third digits of the hand will be in a condition of extension.

B. The third and fourth digits will be held in a slightly flexed position.

C. The thumb will be flexed and slightly abducted.

D. The first, second, and third digits will be held in a slightly flexed position.

E. The MCP and IP joints of the second and third digits of the hand will be in a condition of flexion.

108. A 55-year-old man is brought to the emergency department after sustaining blunt trauma to his right axilla. Physical examination shows pronounced medial winging of the scapula and partial paralysis of the right side of the diaphragm. Which of the

following parts of the brachial plexus has most likely been injured?

A. Cords

B. Divisions

C. Ventral rami

D. Terminal branches

E. Trunks

109. A 69-year-old man comes to the physician because of a 3-month history of numbness and pain of the first 3½ digits of his right hand which interrupts his sleep at night. He retired 9 years ago after working as a carpenter for 30 years. Physical examination shows atrophy of the thenar eminence and weakness of thumb opposition (see Fig. 6.2). What is the most likely cause of this patient's atrophy?

A. Compression of the median nerve in the carpal tunnel

B. Formation of the osteophytes that compress the ulnar nerve at the ulnar condyle

C. Hypertrophy of the triceps brachii muscle compressing the brachial plexus

D. Osteoarthritis of the cervical spine

E. Repeated trauma to the ulnar nerve

110. A 54-year-old woman comes to the physician because of pain and numbness in her right wrist after a fall. Two hours ago, the patient slipped on wet bathroom tiles and fell forcefully on her outstretched hand. Neurologic examination finds decreased sensation in the palmar aspect of the lateral 3½ digits. An x-ray of the hand shows anterior dislocation of a carpal bone that articulates with the radius (see Fig. 6.3). Which of the following bones is most commonly dislocated?

A. Capitate

B. Lunate

C. Scaphoid

D. Pisiform

E. Triquetrum

111. A 32-year-old man comes to the physician with a 3-month history of intermittent pain, paresthesia, and numbness of the digits of his right hand. The symptoms are more severe in the fourth and fifth digits and occur when he raises his arm over his shoulder. Physical examination shows weakness of the right arm. An x-ray of the right shoulder shows the presence of a cervical rib and accessory scalene musculature. Which of the following structures is most likely compressed?

A. Axillary nerve

B. Upper trunk of brachial plexus

C. Subclavian artery

D. Lower trunk of brachial plexus

E. Brachiocephalic artery and lower trunk of brachial plexus

112. A 23-year-old woman comes to the emergency department because of severe pain in her left forearm. Two days ago, she was involved in a motor vehicle collision and sustained a contusion of the forearm. Physical examination shows a swollen and tender forearm with loss of two-point discrimination. Passive dorsiflexion of the wrist causes severe pain. An MRI of the forearm shows a compartment syndrome originating at the interosseous membrane between the radius and ulna. Which of the type of joint is most likely affected?

A. Synarthrosis

B. Symphysis

C. Synchondrosis

D. Trochoid

E. Ginglymus

113. A 28-year-old woman is brought to the emergency department after experiencing severe pain in her chest while lifting weights. The pain was substernal and radiated to the mandible and her left arm. The woman felt dizzy and after 10 minutes she collapsed and became unconscious. A physician attempted to locate her radial pulse. The radial artery lies between two tendons near the wrists. Which of the following is the correct pair of tendons?

A. Flexor carpi radialis and palmaris longus

B. Flexor carpi radialis and brachioradialis

C. Brachioradialis and flexor pollicis longus

D. Flexor pollicis longus and flexor digitorum superficialis

E. Flexor pollicis longus and flexor digitorum profundus

114. A 59-year-old woman is brought to the emergency department after a motor vehicle collision. She is unconscious and appears markedly pale. Physical examination shows several lacerations on her body. Her respirations are 18/min, and blood pressure is 80/60 mm Hg. Her radial pulse is absent. After crossing the radiocarpal joint, where can the radial artery most likely be identified?

A. Between the two heads of the first dorsal interosseous muscle

B. In the anatomical snuffbox

C. Below the tendon of the flexor pollicis longus

D. Between the first and second dorsal interossei muscles

E. Between the first dorsal interosseous muscle and the adductor pollicis longus

115. A 69-year-old woman comes to the physician because of numbness and tingling of her hand for the past 3 months. Physical examination shows weakness of the abductor pollicis brevis, opponens pollicis, and the first two lumbrical muscles. Sensation was decreased over the lateral palm and the palmar aspect of the first 3½ digits of her right hand. Which of the following nerves is most likely compressed?

A. Ulnar

B. Radial

C. Recurrent branch of median

D. Median

E. Posterior interosseous

116. A 32-year-old man comes to the physician for a postoperative follow up 5 months after being involved a motor vehicle collision. Previous x-rays showed multiple right upper limb fractures that required surgical intervention. Physical examination shows normal abduction of the arm and extension of the forearm and normal sensation of the forearm and hand. He is unable to extend his wrist against gravity and has weakness in handgrip and supination. Which of the following nerves were most likely injured during the surgical procedure?
A. Posterior cord of the brachial plexus
B. Radial nerve at the distal third of the humerus
C. Radial and ulnar
D. Radial, ulnar, and median
E. Radial and musculocutaneous

117. A 52-year-old man is brought to the emergency department after falling on wet pavement. Physical examination shows weakened abduction of the thumb and extension of the MCP joints of the digits. Dorsal and radial deviation is noted on extension of the wrist. An x-ray of the forearm shows a fracture of the radius and an MRI shows an expanding hematoma between the fractured radius and supinator muscle. Which of the following nerves is most likely injured?
A. Anterior interosseous
B. Deep branch of radial nerve
C. Radial nerve
D. Deep branch of ulnar nerve
E. Median nerve

118. A 34-year-old woman is brought to the emergency department after being involved in a motor vehicle collision. She has dull pain in the left shoulder. Vital signs are within normal limits. Physical examination shows that the patient is unable to flex the elbow and shoulder and is also unable to initiate abduction of her arm without first establishing lateral momentum of the limb. An x-ray of the arm shows marked edema, hematoma of the proximal arm, and no fractures. Which portion of the brachial plexus is most likely injured?
A. Superior trunk
B. Middle trunk
C. Inferior trunk
D. Lateral cord
E. Medial cord

119. A 22-year-old man is brought to the emergency department 1 hour after being involved in a motor vehicle collision. He has severe pain in the right arm. Physical examination shows bruising of the right upper limb with no open wounds. The patient is unable to extend his hand and fingers. There is loss of sensation over the posterior forearm and dorsolateral hand. An x-ray of the arm shows an oblique fracture of the humerus. The damaged nerve is most likely composed of fibers from which of the following spinal levels?
A. C5, C6
B. C5, C6, C7

C. C5, C6, C7, C8, T1
D. C6, C7, C8, T1
E. C7, C8, T1

120. A 56-year-old woman is brought to the emergency department after being involved in a motor vehicle collision. A large area of her chest wall needed to be surgically removed and replaced with a musculo-osseous scapular graft involving the medial border of the scapula. Which of the following arteries will most likely compensate for the blood supply to the entire scapula?
A. Suprascapular
B. Dorsal scapular artery
C. Posterior circumflex humeral artery
D. Lateral thoracic
E. Superior thoracic artery

121. A 56-year-old woman is brought to the emergency department after falling on her left hand. She has a history of osteoporosis diagnosed 2 years ago. She is alert, awake, and oriented. Physical examination shows limited movement, tenderness, and swelling of the left wrist. An x-ray of the left hand shows a Colles fracture. Which of the following carpal bones are most likely fractured or dislocated in this type of fracture?
A. Triquetrum and scaphoid
B. Triquetrum and lunate
C. Scaphoid and lunate
D. Triquetrum, lunate, and scaphoid
E. Triquetrum and pisiform

122. A 3-year-old girl is brought to the emergency department because of severe pain in her left upper extremity. Her mother recalls that she violently lifted the girl by her raised arm to prevent her from walking in front of a moving car. Physical examination shows that the patient's forearm is pronated and extended at the elbow and she resists any movement due to pain. Which of the following is the most likely cause of the child's pain?
A. Compression of the median nerve
B. Separation of the head of the radius from its articulation with the trochlea of the humerus
C. Separation of the head of the radius from its articulation with the ulna and the capitulum of the humerus
D. Separation of the ulna from its articulation with the trochlea of the humerus
E. Stretching of the radial nerve as it passes behind the medial epicondyle of the humerus

123. A 61-year-old man is brought to the emergency department after being hit by a bat on the left arm. Physical examination shows weakness of extension at the wrist and MCP joints, and loss of sensation on the dorsum of the hand proximal to the first two digits. An x-ray of the left arm shows a hairline fracture of the body of the humerus just distal to its midpoint. Which of the following nerves is most likely injured?
A. Median
B. Ulnar

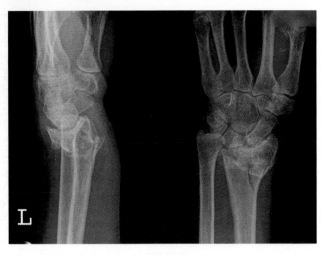

• **Fig. 6.8**

C. Radial

D. Musculocutaneous

E. Axillary

124. A 34-year-old man is brought to the emergency department 30 minutes after he was involved in a motor vehicle collision. Vital signs are within normal limits and he is awake, alert, and oriented. Physical examination shows numerous lacerations over his left forearm, wrist, and hand. Paralysis of the muscles that act to extend the IP joints is noted (Fig. 6.8). Which of the following nerves is most likely injured?

A. Ulnar

B. Recurrent branch of median

C. Radial

D. Musculocutaneous

E. Anterior interosseous

125. A 45-year-old woman is brought to the emergency department by her husband because of a 2-week history of progressively increasing neck pain. Her pulse is 80/min, respirations are 20/min, and blood pressure is 128/32 mm Hg. Physical examination shows pain with mobilization, restricted range of motion of the neck, and weakness on extension of the forearm at the elbow. An MRI examination finds a herniated disc in the cervical region. Which of the following spinal nerves is most likely compressed?

A. C5

B. C6

C. C7

D. C8

E. T1

Questions 126–150

126. A 34-year-old woman is brought to the emergency department after being involved in a motor vehicle collision. Vital signs are within normal limits. She has severe pain and limited mobility of the finger. Physical examination shows a mallet finger. Which of

the following is expected to be present during radiographic examination?

A. A lesion of the ulnar nerve at the distal flexor crease of the wrist

B. A separation of the extension expansion over the middle IP joint

C. Compression of the deep ulnar nerve by dislocation of the lunate bone

D. Avulsion fracture of the dorsum of the distal phalanx

E. Fracture of the fourth or fifth metacarpal bone

127. A 42-year-old woman comes to the physician for a follow-up after injuring her left shoulder. Two months ago, she was hit on the left shoulder by a falling tree branch and was diagnosed with Erb-Duchenne palsy. She has progressively worsening pain and limited movement. Previous x-rays showed no fracture of the bones of the shoulder girdle. Which of the following conditions is also expected to be present during physical examination?

A. Winged scapula

B. Inability to laterally rotate the arm

C. Paralysis of intrinsic muscles of the hand

D. Paresthesia in the medial aspect of the arm

E. Loss of sensation in the dorsum of the hand

128. A 41-year-old woman is brought to the emergency department after being involved in a motor vehicle collision. Vital signs are within normal limits. Physical examination shows a laterally deviated proximal portion of the radius. An x-ray of the forearm shows a transverse fracture of the radius proximal to the attachment of the pronator teres muscle. Which of the following muscles is most likely responsible for this deviation?

A. Pronator teres

B. Pronator quadratus

C. Brachialis

D. Supinator

E. Brachioradialis

129. A 45-year-old woman comes to the emergency department after being bitten by a dog on the lateral side of her hand 2 days ago. Her temperature is 39.4°C (102.9°F); other vital signs are within normal limits. Physical examination shows an open wound on the lateral side of her left hand and swollen lymph nodes. Which group of lymph nodes is most likely the first to be involved?

A. Central axillary

B. Humeral

C. Pectoral

D. Subscapular

E. Parasternal

130. A 25-year-old woman is brought to the emergency department after being involved in a motor vehicle collision. Physical examination shows that the right arm appears swollen, pale, and cool. Radial pulse is absent and any movement of the arm causes severe

pain. An x-ray of the right arm shows a fracture at the radial groove of the humerus and a cast is placed. Three days later she has severe pain over the length of her arm. Which of the following conditions will most likely explain the findings on physical examination?

A. Venous thrombosis
B. Thoracic outlet syndrome
C. Compartment syndrome
D. Raynaud disease
E. Injury of the radial nerve

131. A 22-year-old woman is brought to the emergency department after falling from a tree. She has pain and limited mobility of her left wrist. Vital signs are within normal limits. Physical examination shows tenderness and swelling of the left wrist. An x-ray of the hand shows fractured pisiform and hamate bones. Which of the following nerves will most likely be injured?

A. Median
B. Recurrent branch of median
C. Radial
D. Anterior interosseous
E. Deep ulnar

132. A 43-year-old man comes to the physician because of a 2-week history of a painful right shoulder. He has pain when reaching over his head and difficulty sleeping on his right side. Physical examination shows tenderness to palpation below the acromion. The empty can test is positive. Which of the following is most likely present when the patient abducts his arm?

A. Painful abduction 0 to 15 degrees
B. Painful abduction 0 to 140 degrees
C. Painful abduction 70 to 140 degrees
D. Painful abduction 15 to 140 degrees
E. Painful abduction 40 to 140 degrees

133. A 54-year-old woman is brought to the emergency department after falling on an outstretched hand. She has severe pain in her right wrist. Physical examination shows tenderness over the anatomical snuffbox. An x-ray of the hand shows dislocation of the carpal bones. Which of the following carpal bones will most likely be involved?

A. Scaphoid-lunate
B. Trapezoid-trapezium
C. Hamate-lunate
D. Pisiform-triquetrum
E. Hamate-capitate

134. A 62-year-old man is brought to the emergency department after falling on wet pavement. He has pain in the left hand. Vital signs are within normal limits. Physical examination shows a dislocation of the carpometacarpal (CMC) joint of the left hand. An x-ray of the hand shows a fracture at the base of the first metacarpal bone that extends into the CMC joint. Which of the following is most likely diagnosis?

A. Colles fracture
B. Scaphoid fracture
C. Bennett fracture

D. Smith fracture
E. Boxer's fracture

135. A 23-year-old woman is brought to the emergency department after injuring her thumb from a fall while skiing. Vital signs are within normal limits. Physical examination shows a severely tender and swollen first digit of the right hand, and weakness of thumb abduction. MRI of the right hand shows rupture of the ulnar collateral ligament of the MCP joint of the thumb. What is the most likely diagnosis?

A. Gamekeeper's thumb
B. Scaphoid fracture
C. Bennett fracture
D. Smith fracture
E. Boxer's fracture

136. A 54-year-old woman is brought to the emergency department after being found unconscious. The Glasgow coma scale score is 6, her temperature is 37°C (98.6°F), pulse is 97/min, respirations are 19/min, and blood pressure is 129/79 mm Hg. Physical examination shows an absent biceps brachii reflex. What is the spinal level of the afferent component of this reflex?

A. C5
B. C6
C. C7
D. C8
E. T1

137. A 54-year-old woman is brought to the emergency department after a fall. She has pain along the left arm and limited mobility of the left upper limb. Vital signs are within normal limits. Physical examination shows absence of the brachioradialis reflex. The ventral ramus of which spinal nerve is responsible for this reflex?

A. C5
B. C6
C. C7
D. C8
E. T1

138. A 55-year-old woman is brought to the emergency department after being involved in a motor vehicle collision. She is awake, alert, and oriented. Vital signs are within normal limits. Physical examination shows exquisite tenderness of the flexor muscles of the forearm on palpation and fixed flexion of the digits. Swelling, cyanosis, and decreased sensation of the hand is also noted. Which of the following is the most likely diagnosis?

A. Colles fracture
B. Scaphoid fracture
C. Bennett fracture
D. Volkmann ischemic contracture
E. Boxer's fracture

139. A 62-year-old man comes to the emergency department because of a 3-hour history of pain and swelling of the right hand after a fall. Vital signs are within

normal limits. Physical examination shows tenderness to palpation and significant swelling of the right hand. An x-ray of the right hand shows a fracture of the pisiform bone and a hematoma of the surrounding area. Which of the following nerves is most likely affected?

A. Ulnar
B. Radial
C. Median
D. Deep ulnar
E. Deep radial

140. A 32-year-old woman comes to the emergency department 1 hour after injuring her elbow when she fell from her bicycle. Vital signs are within normal limits. Physical examination shows a Benediction sign of the hand with the first three digits in the extended position and the fourth and fifth fingers in the flexed position. Which of the following nerves are most likely injured?

A. Injury to median and radial nerves
B. Injury to median nerve
C. Injury to radial and ulnar nerves
D. Injury to ulnar nerve
E. Injury to median, ulnar, and radial nerves

141. A 54-year-old man is brought to the emergency department because of constant severe substernal chest pain and sweating for 2 hours. An ECG shows ST-segment elevation in leads V1–V3 and the patient is diagnosed with an anterior wall myocardial infarction. Angiography is performed and coronary artery bypass surgery using a radial artery graft is proposed. Which of the following tests should be performed during physical examination before the bypass graft operation?

A. Allen test
B. Triceps reflex
C. Tinel test
D. Brachioradialis reflex
E. Biceps reflex

142. A 34-year-old man comes the emergency department with pain in the arm after a fall onto a concrete floor. The patient denies head trauma or loss of consciousness. Physical examination shows weakness in abduction and adduction of his fingers. Flexion of the digits is normal. Sensation over the palmar surface of the fourth and fifth fingers is decreased. Which of the following is the most likely diagnosis?

A. Compression of the median nerve in the carpal tunnel
B. Injury of the radial nerve from fractured humerus
C. Compression of the median nerve as it passes between the two heads of the pronator teres
D. Compression of the radial nerve by the supinator
E. Injury of the ulnar nerve by a fractured pisiform

143. A 65-year-old man is brought to the emergency department after falling on his outstretched hand. The patient complains of severe right shoulder pain.

Physical examination shows an externally rotated and slightly abducted right arm. Flattening of the deltoid muscle is noted and sensation is also absent over the right deltoid muscle. Which of the following is the most likely diagnosis?

A. Anterior dislocation of the humerus
B. AC joint subluxation
C. Clavicular fracture
D. Spiral fracture of the humeral mid-body
E. Rotator cuff tear

144. A 4-year-old boy is brought to the emergency department because of left arm pain after being lifted by his parents. Movement of his right upper extremity is restricted due to pain. He holds his arm at his side with his elbow extended and forearm pronated. There are no visible hematomas or swelling. Which of the following structures is most likely injured in this patient?

A. Annular ligament
B. Biceps brachii tendon
C. Interosseous membrane
D. Radial collateral ligament
E. Ulnar collateral ligament

145. A 35-year-old man is brought to the emergency department after falling from a motorcycle and injuring his shoulder. The patient is alert and responsive. Vital signs are within normal limits. Physical examination shows the loss of the normal contour of the shoulder and an abnormal appearing depression below the acromion. Which of the following injuries did the patient most likely sustain?

A. Avulsion of the coronoid process
B. Dislocated shoulder joint
C. Fracture of the mid-body of the humerus
D. Fracture of the surgical neck of the humerus
E. Laceration of the posterior cord

146. A 22-year-old woman comes to the physician for a routine examination. During venipuncture, the phlebotomist is unable to withdraw blood and quickly realizes that she passed the needle completely through the vein. Which of the following structures located deep to the median cubital vein has acted as a barrier and has prevented her from puncturing an artery?

A. Flexor retinaculum
B. Pronator teres muscle
C. Bicipital aponeurosis
D. Brachioradialis muscle
E. Biceps brachii tendon

147. A 21-year-old man is brought to the emergency department after sustaining a laceration on the anterior surface of his left wrist distal to the skin fold crease. Physical examination shows a broad, glistening white structure deep to the superficial fascia on extension of the wrist. The patient has no numbness or tingling and no loss of motion of any of the fingers or the hand. Sensation to pinprick is normal in all of

the fingers and the palm of the hand. Which structure has the physician located?

A. Flexor retinaculum
B. Flexor carpi ulnaris tendon
C. Palmar skin
D. Flexor digitorum superficialis tendons
E. Flexor digitorum profundus tendons

148. A 34-year-old woman is brought to the emergency department after injuring her hand while she was carving wood. Physical examination shows a laceration on the proximal aspect of her palm from the base of the thumb to the pisiform bones, and weakness in opposition of the thumb. Sensation in the hand is normal. Which of the following injuries best accounts for her findings?

A. Injury of the median nerve in the carpal tunnel
B. Injury of the palmar branch of the median nerve
C. Injury of the recurrent and palmar branch of the median nerve
D. Injury of the recurrent branch of median nerve at the wrist
E. Injury of the radial and ulnar nerves

149. A 22-year-old football player is brought to the emergency department because of a wrist injury after falling on his outstretched hand. During surgery, the anatomical snuffbox is exposed and an artery is visualized crossing the fractured bone that forms the floor for this space. Which of the following arteries was most likely visualized?

A. Ulnar
B. Radial
C. Anterior interosseous
D. Posterior interosseous
E. Deep palmar arch

150. A 36-year-old man is brought to the emergency department because of a deep knife wound on the medial side of his distal forearm. Vital signs are within normal limits. Physical examination shows weakness on abduction and adduction of the digits. He is unable to hold a piece of paper between his fingers. Sensation of the fifth digit and the medial side of the fourth digit is absent. Which of the following nerves is most likely injured?

A. Axillary
B. Median
C. Musculocutaneous
D. Radial
E. Ulnar

Questions 151–175

151. A 28-year-old man is brought to the emergency department after falling off a street pole and landing directly on his right shoulder. His temperature is 37°C (98.6°F), pulse is 68/min, respirations are 12/min, and blood pressure is 109/79 mm Hg. Physical examination shows tenderness on movement of the shoulder. An x-ray of the right shoulder shows a

fracture through the entire length of the floor of the intertubercular sulcus of the right humerus. The muscle most likely affected by the fracture is innervated by a nerve composed of which of the following nerve roots?

A. C3 and C4
B. C6–C8
C. C4 and C5
D. C2–C4
E. C5–C7

152. A 21-year-old woman comes to the physician for a follow-up appointment. One week ago, she sustained a dislocated glenohumeral joint of her shoulder while playing soccer and the shoulder was reduced in the emergency department. Physical examination shows decreased strength on medial rotation of her arm at the shoulder during today's visit. This finding was most likely caused by a tear in which of the following muscles?

A. Infraspinatus
B. Pectoralis major
C. Subscapularis
D. Supraspinatus
E. Teres minor

153. A 29-year-old man comes to the physician because of weakness of his right hand. A few weeks ago, he grabbed a branch as he was falling from a tree. Physical examination shows weakness in abduction and adduction of his digits. He is unable to oppose the thumb of his right hand. Which of the following structures was most likely injured?

A. Lower trunk of the brachial plexus
B. Median nerve
C. Musculocutaneous nerve
D. Ulnar nerve
E. Upper trunk of the brachial plexus

154. A 28-year-old man is brought to the emergency department after injuring his right hand in a knife fight. Physical examination shows loss of extension of the fourth and fifth digits at the IP joints, and loss of abduction of the fingers of the right hand. Which of the following muscles is most likely responsible for the loss of IP extension of the medial two fingers?

A. Dorsal interosseous muscles
B. Extensor digitorum
C. Lumbrical muscles
D. Palmar interosseous muscles
E. Extensor digiti minimi

155. A 72-year-old woman is brought to the emergency department after a fall on her outstretched left arm. She has significant elbow pain. Physical examination shows a palpable defect over her biceps brachii tendon, and pain during elbow flexion without any restriction on movement. An x-ray of the left arm does not show fractures or dislocations. She is diagnosed with rupture of the biceps brachii tendon. Which of

the following muscles most likely allow the patient to continue to flex her elbow?

A. Brachialis and brachioradialis

B. Flexor carpi ulnaris and flexor carpi radialis

C. Flexor digitorum superficialis and flexor digitorum profundus

D. Pronator teres and supinator

E. Triceps brachii and coracobrachialis

156. A 16-year-old girl is brought to the emergency department after attempting suicide by cutting her wrist. She has a history of depression. Physical examination shows the deepest part of the wound between the tendons of the flexor carpi radialis and the flexor digitorum superficialis. This patient will be most likely to have a deficit of which of the following?

A. Adduction and abduction of the fingers

B. Extension of the index finger

C. Flexion of the ring and little finger

D. Sensation over the base of the little finger

E. Opposition of the thumb and slightly weakened flexion of the second and third digits

157. A 36-year-old man is brought to the emergency department by his wife because of worsening pain in his right wrist. He has not been able to perform his work duties or drive a car due to the pain. 2 days ago he fell off a ladder with his hand outstretched. Physical examination shows tenderness on the lateral side of the wrist at the base of the first metacarpal. What is the most likely diagnosis?

A. Fracture of the first metacarpal

B. Fracture of the trapezium

C. Tenosynovitis of thumb extensors

D. Fracture of the scaphoid

E. First CMC joint arthritis

158. A 55-year-old man is brought to the emergency department after sustaining a blow from a baseball bat at the junction of his neck and shoulder on the right. Physical examination shows asymmetry of the right scapula on pushing forward with the arm. There is also asymmetry during diaphragmatic excursion. Which part of the brachial plexus is most likely injured?

A. Cords

B. Divisions

C. Ventral rami

D. Terminal branches

E. Trunks

159. A 55-year-old woman comes to the clinic because of a 1-week history of right elbow pain. The pain started after a game of tennis. The pain begins at the elbow and extends into the dorsum of the forearm. Physical examination shows mild swelling and tenderness over the lateral epicondyle. Which one of the following wrist movements will most likely exacerbate the pain?

A. Radial deviation

B. Ulnar deviation

C. Flexion

D. Extension

E. Flexion and ulnar deviation

160. A newborn girl is brought to the physician because of limited movement of the right arm following a complicated delivery. Her mother has a history of diabetes. Vital signs are within normal limits. Physical examination shows an adducted and medially rotated right arm. Her right forearm is extended and pronated and the wrist is flexed. Which of the following ventral rami is most likely injured?

A. C5 and C6

B. C6 and C7

C. C7 and C8

D. C8 and T1

E. C5–T1

161. A 48-year-old woman comes to the physician because of pain and numbness in the right wrist. She works as a secretary in a large law firm. Physical examination shows that maximal flexion of the wrist with the elbows in a flexed and abducted position reproduces the pain in the right hand. Tinel sign is positive. Which of the following muscles will most likely be weakened by this condition?

A. Dorsal and palmar interossei

B. Lumbricals III and IV

C. Thenar and lumbricals I and II

D. Flexor digitorum superficialis and profundus

E. Hypothenar

162. A 24-year-old man comes to the physician because he has difficulty with buttoning his shirts. Vital signs are within normal limits. Physical examination shows that he is able to grip a sheet of paper between his second and third fingers and there are no sensory deficits in the hand. Signs of tenderness and inflammation are absent. Which of the following nerves is mostly likely affected?

A. Deep branch of ulnar

B. Anterior interosseous

C. Median

D. Recurrent branch of median

E. Deep branch of radial

163. A 22-year-old man comes to the emergency department because of a hand injury from broken glass. Physical examination shows a deep laceration across the entire length of the distal transverse crease on the anterior surface of the wrist. There is no injury to the flexor retinaculum. During physical examination which neuromuscular deficits will most likely be found on physical examination?

A. Weakened pronation of the forearm

B. Inability to abduct the thumb

C. Weakened flexion of the thumb

D. Weakened opposition of the thumb

E. Inability to adduct the thumb

164. A 23-year-old man comes to the physician because of pain in the right upper extremity for several weeks. The pain is sharp, exacerbated by movement, and is

progressively worsening since he increased his training for the upcoming basketball season. Examination of the right upper extremity shows no deformity. The pain is reproduced during the initial phase of abduction of the right arm, and when the arm is abducted against resistance. There is weakness in lateral rotation of the right shoulder. Which nerve was most likely injured?

A. Lower subscapular
B. Axillary
C. Radial
D. Suprascapular
E. Upper subscapular

165. A 35-year-old man comes to the physician for a follow-up examination. Three days ago, he sustained a laceration to the tip of his thumb. He had a low-grade fever and redness and swelling localized to the injured part of the thumb on physical examination. During this visit, the entire thumb and thenar eminence is also erythematous and swollen. Which of the following lymph nodes will most likely be the first to receive lymphatic drainage from this injury?

A. Posterior axillary
B. Subclavian
C. Lateral axillary
D. Anterior axillary
E. Central axillary

166. A 4-year-old boy is brought to the emergency department by his mother because of left arm pain. His mother explains the pain started after she tugged his left arm when crossing the road to pull him out of the way of an oncoming car. Over the next few hours, his mother became worried as her son was not moving his left arm while playing with his toys. On physical examination, the child's arm is slightly flexed and pronated. An x-ray of the left upper extremity is performed and shown below. The laxity of which of the following structures resulted in this finding?

A. Annular
B. Joint capsule
C. Interosseous membrane
D. Radial collateral
E. Ulnar collateral

167. A 62-year-old woman is brought to the physician by her daughter because of worsening deformity of her hand. A photograph of her hand is shown in Fig. 6.9. Physical examination shows pain and numbness over her fifth digit and decreased pinch strength. An x-ray of the wrist shows a hairline fracture of the hamate at the ulnar or Guyon canal. Which of the following will most likely be present during physical examination?

A. Numbness and weakness of the fourth and fifth digits
B. Wrist drop
C. Atrophy of the thenar muscles
D. Positive Tinel test
E. Weakness in wrist adduction

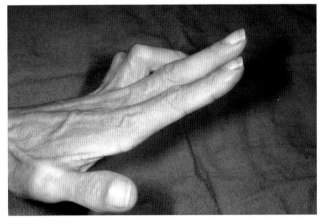

• Fig. 6.9

168. A 25-year-old woman comes to the physician because of numbness and tingling in her right hand. Her first episode was four weeks ago while carrying a piece of luggage. Physical examination shows no motor or sensory deficits in the upper limb. When asked to abduct her upper limb to 90 degrees and to maintain this position, while repeatedly closing and opening her hands, the symptoms are reproduced along the medial border of the limb, from the axilla to the hand. Which nerve structure(s) is/are most likely compressed?

A. Ulnar nerve at the medial epicondyle
B. Radial nerve at the neck of the radius
C. Median nerve in the carpal tunnel
D. Inferior trunk of the brachial plexus
E. Posterior divisions of the brachial plexus

169. A 50-year-old woman comes to the physician because of sudden "locking" of her index finger when playing her viola. Physical examination shows the index finger "stuck" in the flexed position when asked to extend her index finger. During passive extension and flexion of the finger a snapping sound can be heard. She has pain on the distal palmar aspect of the finger. There is no erythema or atrophy. What is the most likely diagnosis?

A. Tenosynovitis stenosans (trigger finger)
B. Dupuytren contracture
C. Mallet finger
D. Boutonniere deformity
E. Boxer's fracture

170. A 25-year-old woman comes to the physician because of an unsightly lump on her wrist that is causing her great distress. She has a tingling sensation on the lateral three and a half digits of the palmar aspect of her hand. During physical examination a pen torch is used to illuminate the lump. The contents of the lump are drained, which cause immediate relief of her symptoms. Which of the following is the most likely diagnosis?

A. Neurofibroma
B. Ganglion cyst

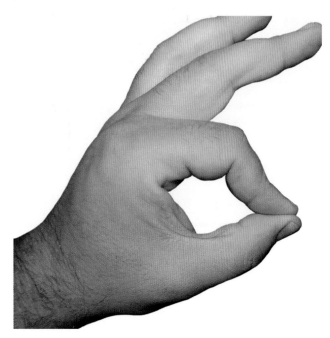

• Fig. 6.10

C. Chondroma

D. Osteoma

E. Osteophyte

171. A 19-year-old man comes to the physician because of numbness and pain in his fingers. He is a professional cyclist and has been training long distances on rough terrain. Physical examination shows sensory loss to the medial two and a half digits on the dorsal aspect of his hand. A diagnosis of handlebar neuropathy is made. What other signs may be elicited during physical examination?

A. Sensory loss of the medial one and a half digits on the palmar aspect of the hand

B. Weakness in abduction of the thumb

C. Weakness in extension of the thumb

D. Thenar muscle atrophy

E. Tinel sign at the scaphoid

172. A 20-year-old man comes to the physician because of an inability to grip his racquet during racquetball practice. He denies any recent trauma. Physical examination shows atrophy of the thenar eminence, inability to oppose the thumb, and difficulty in flexing the middle IP joints of the digits. What is the most likely diagnosis?

A. Hypertrophy of the supinator

B. Pronator syndrome

C. Medial supracondylar fracture

D. Tennis elbow

E. Golfer's elbow

173. A 54-year-old man comes to the physician because of weakness in his fingers. He attempts to make a ring between his thumb and index finger by bringing the tips together as shown in Fig. 6.10. He is able to successfully hold a piece of paper between his thumb and index finger. Physical examination shows weakness in pronation of the forearm and wrist flexion. Which of the following nerves is most likely affected?

A. Ulnar nerve at Guyon canal

B. Median nerve in the carpal tunnel

C. Anterior interosseous nerve beneath the ulnar head of pronator teres

D. Deep branch of the radial nerve beneath the supinator

E. Median nerve beneath the bicipital aponeurosis

174. A 24-year-old man is brought to the emergency department after being involved in a motor vehicle collision. He sustained multiple injuries including complex fractures of the right wrist. Her temperature is 7°C (98.6°F), pulse is 115/min, respirations are 19/min, and blood pressure is 110/78 mm Hg. His injuries are stabilized and surgical repair is planned. Physical examination shows weakness of thumb adduction and finger adduction and abduction. There is decreased sensation along the medial border of the hand and the fourth and fifth digits. Flexion of the DIP joints of the fourth and fifth digits is normal. If the nerve injury is not repaired, which of the following will most likely become apparent in the affected hand over the next few months?

A. Flattening of the thenar eminence

B. Wrist drop

C. Radial deviation at the wrist

D. Ulnar deviation at the MCP joints

E. Prominent metacarpal bones with "guttering" between adjacent metacarpals

175. A 30-year-old man is brought into the emergency department 3 hours after stumbling down the stairs and falling on his outstretched hand. He has constant pain in his wrist, and a tingling and burning pain over the past 30 minutes. Vital signs are within normal limits. An x-ray of the forearm shows fractures of both the radial and ulnar styloid processes and dislocation of a carpal bone. Which of the following abnormal sensory and motor findings are most likely to be found on examination?

A. Dysesthesia (tingling in response to light touch) along the medial border of the hand and little finger and weakness in adduction of the thumb

B. Dysesthesia over the palm and palmar aspect of the thumb, index, and middle fingers and weakness in thumb opposition

C. Numbness along the medial border of the hand and little finger and weakness in wrist extension

D. Numbness over the dorsum of the hand laterally including the dorsal aspect of the thumb, index, and middle fingers and weakness in grip strength

E. Numbness over the palm and palmar aspect of the thumb, index, and middle fingers and weakness in adduction of the thumb

Questions 176–186

176. A 25-year-old man comes to the emergency department after falling on a slippery trail and injuring his elbow and hand. Physical examination shows abrasions over the olecranon, medial epicondyle, and palm of the hand. Sensation is decreased with "pins and needles" (paresthesia) along the ulnar border of the hand and medial one and a half digits. There is also weakness of finger abduction and adduction, thumb adduction, and flexion at the DIP of the ring and little fingers. Which structure was most likely injured?
A. Ulnar nerve at the medial epicondyle
B. Ulnar nerve at Guyon (ulnar) canal
C. Median nerve in the cubital fossa
D. Median nerve in the carpal tunnel
E. Medial cord of brachial plexus in the axillary inlet

177. A 29-year-old woman comes to the emergency department after falling on an outstretched hand. Physical examination shows pain on movement of the wrist associated with numbness and tingling on the radial side of the palm and palmar aspect of the thumb, index, and middle fingers. X-ray of the wrist shows anterior dislocation of a carpal bone. Which of the following carpal bones is most likely dislocated?
A. Pisiform compressing ulnar nerve
B. Hook of the hamate compressing ulnar artery
C. Scaphoid compressing the radial artery
D. Lunate compressing the median nerve
E. Trapezoid bone compressing the superficial radial nerve

178. A 54-year-old woman is brought to the emergency department after being involved in a motor vehicle collision. Vital signs are within normal limits. Physical examination shows soft tissue edema and bruising around the neck. An x-ray of the left arm shows a mid-body humeral fracture. Which of the following areas will most likely have impaired or absent sensation?
A. Lateral aspect of the forearm
B. Medial aspect of the arm
C. Medial aspect of the arm and forearm
D. Posterior aspect of the forearm
E. Lateral and posterior aspect of the forearm

179. A 52-year-old man is brought to the emergency department after a fall. Vital signs are within normal limits. Physical examination shows weakness of wrist extension, abduction and extension of the thumb, and extension of the MCP and IP joints of the fingers. There are no sensory deficits. An x-ray of the right arm shows a fracture at the neck of the radius and a hematoma at the fracture site. Which nerve is most likely affected?
A. Anterior interosseous
B. Deep radial
C. Radial
D. Ulnar
E. Superficial radial

180. A 42-year-old woman is brought to the emergency department after a fall. She has tingling and numbness along the medial border of her left hand. Vital signs are within normal limits. Physical examination shows several abnormalities including Froment sign. Weakness of which of the following muscles most likely explains the presence of Froment sign?
A. First dorsal interosseous muscle
B. Opponens pollicis
C. Adductor pollicis
D. Flexor pollicis longus
E. Flexor pollicis brevis

181. A 43-year-old woman comes to the physician because of 2-week history of pain and numbness in the right hand. There is no history of trauma. Physical examination shows tenderness of the lateral three and a half digits with percussion over the flexor retinaculum. Which of the following conditions is most likely associated with this sign?
A. Carpal tunnel syndrome
B. De Quervain tenosynovitis
C. Thoracic outlet syndrome
D. Mallet finger
E. Radial nerve damage

182. A 25-year-old woman comes to the physician because of numbness and tingling in her right arm and hand while carrying a piece of luggage. Physical examination shows no motor or sensory deficits in the upper limb. When asked to abduct her upper limb to 90 degrees and to maintain this position while repeatedly flexing and extending the digits of the hand, the symptoms are reproduced along the medial border of the limb, from the axilla to the hand. Which nerve structure(s) is/are most likely compressed?
A. Ulnar nerve at the medial epicondyle
B. Radial nerve at the neck of the radius
C. Median nerve in the carpal tunnel
D. Inferior trunk of the brachial plexus
E. Divisions of the brachial plexus

183. A 55-year-old woman is brought to the emergency department after being involved in a motor vehicle collision. She has pain in the left hand. Physical examination shows swelling and tenderness to palpation of the dorsal wrist. Her temperature is 37°C (98.6°F), pulse is 97/min, respirations are 19/min, and blood pressure is 129/79 mm Hg. X-ray of the left hand shows a fractured carpal bone in the floor of the anatomical snuffbox. Which of the following carpal bones is most likely fractured?
A. Triquetrum
B. Scaphoid
C. Capitate
D. Hamate
E. Trapezoid

184. A 21-year-old man comes to the emergency department because of a pain in the right shoulder after a fall. Vital signs are within normal limits. Physical

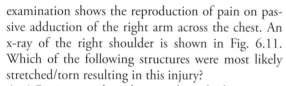

• **Fig. 6.11**

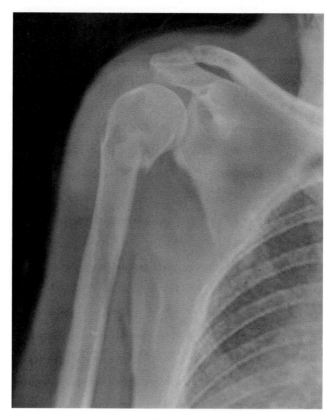

• **Fig. 6.12**

examination shows the reproduction of pain on passive adduction of the right arm across the chest. An x-ray of the right shoulder is shown in Fig. 6.11. Which of the following structures were most likely stretched/torn resulting in this injury?

A. AC joint capsule and coracoclavicular ligament
B. AC joint capsule and coracoacromial ligament
C. Sternoclavicular joint capsule and coracoacromial ligament
D. Coracoclavicular and transverse scapular ligaments
E. Coracoclavicular and coracoacromial ligaments

185. A 67-year-old woman is brought to the emergency department after injuring her left shoulder from a fall. She has a history of osteoporosis. Physical examination shows bruising and dimpling of the upper part of the arm with exquisite tenderness over the affected area. An x-ray of the left shoulder is shown in Fig. 6.12. Which of the following nerves is most likely injured?

A. Radial
B. Axillary

C. Ulnar
D. Median
E. Musculocutaneous

186. A 14-year-old boy is brought to the emergency department after falling on his outstretched hand. Physical examination shows point tenderness above the humeral epicondyles and a pulsatile mass just above the cubital fossa. There is weakness on pronation, wrist flexion, and grip strength. Thumb flexion and opposition are also impaired. Flexion at the DIP joints of the fourth and fifth digits is normal. An x-ray shows a supracondylar fracture of the humerus. Which of the following structures are most likely injured?

A. Axillary nerve and posterior circumflex humeral artery
B. Radial nerve and deep brachial artery
C. Median nerve and brachial artery
D. Superficial radial nerve and radial artery
E. Ulnar nerve and ulnar artery

Answers

Answers 1–25

1. D. The suspensory ligaments of the breast, also known as Cooper ligaments, are fibrous bands that run from the dermis of the skin to the deep fascia covering the pectoralis major muscle and are primary supports for the breasts against gravity. Ptosis of the breast is usually due to the stretching of these ligaments and can be repaired with plastic surgery.

A. Scarpa fascia is the membranous layer of the superficial fascia of the anterior abdominal wall.

B and C. The pectoralis major and pectoralis minor are muscles that move the upper limb and lie deep to the breast but do not provide direct support to the structure of the breast, although the suspensory ligaments of the breast attach to the pectoral fascia covering the pectoralis major muscle.

E. The serratus anterior muscle is involved in the movements of the scapula, for example, protraction.
GAS 133, 140–142; N 188; ABR/McM 185

2. **A.** The lower subscapular nerve arises from the C5 and C6 spinal nerves. It innervates the lower border of subscapularis and the teres major muscles. The subscapularis and teres major muscles are both responsible for adducting and medially rotating the arm. A lesion of this nerve would result in weakness in these motions.

B. The axillary nerve also arises from cervical spinal nerves 5 and 6 and innervates the deltoid and teres minor muscles. The deltoid muscle is large and covers the entire surface of the shoulder, and contributes to arm movement in any plane. The teres minor muscle is a lateral rotator of the arm and a member of the rotator cuff group of muscles.

C. The radial nerve arises from the posterior cord of the brachial plexus. It is the largest branch, and it innervates the triceps brachii and anconeus muscles in the arm and the extensors of the forearm.

D. The accessory nerve is cranial nerve XI, and innervates the trapezius muscle, which elevates and depresses the scapula.

E. The supraspinatus and infraspinatus muscles originate from the supraspinous and the infraspinous fossae, respectively, and attach to the greater tubercle of the humerus. Both muscles are innervated by the suprascapular nerve. The supraspinatus is responsible for initiation of arm abduction, and the infraspinatus allows for lateral rotation of the shoulder.
GAS 703–706; N 417; ABR/McM 150

3. **C.** The thenar muscles (and lumbricals I and II) are innervated by the median nerve which runs through the carpal tunnel. The carpal tunnel is formed anteriorly by the flexor retinaculum and posteriorly by the carpal bones. Carpal tunnel syndrome is caused by a compression of the median nerve due to reduced space in the carpal tunnel. The carpal tunnel contains the tendons of flexor pollicis longus, flexor digitorum profundus, and flexor digitorum superficialis muscles and their synovial sheaths.

A, B, D, E. The interossei, lumbricals III and IV, and hypothenar muscles are all innervated by the ulnar nerve.
GAS 788–789, 799; N 455; ABR/McM 168

4. **D.** Fracture of the medial epicondyle can cause damage to the ulnar nerve due to its position in the groove behind the epicondyle. The ulnar nerve innervates one and a half muscles in the forearm, the flexor carpi ulnaris and the medial half of the flexor digitorum profundus muscles. The nerve continues on to innervate most of the intrinsic muscles in the hand.

A. The flexor digitorum superficialis is innervated by the median nerve.

B. The biceps brachii muscle is innervated by the musculocutaneous nerve.

C and E. The radial nerve innervates both the brachioradialis and supinator muscles.
GAS 741, 753–758; N 437; ABR/McM 153

5. **C.** A mid-body humeral fracture can result in injury to the radial nerve and deep brachial artery because they lie in the radial or spiral groove located on the posterior surface of the mid-body of the humerus.

A. Injury to the median nerve and brachial artery can be caused by a supracondylar fracture that occurs by falling on an outstretched hand and partially flexed elbow.

B. A fracture of the surgical neck of the humerus can injure the axillary nerve and posterior circumflex humeral artery.

D. The suprascapular artery and nerve can be injured in a shoulder dislocation.

E. The long thoracic nerve and lateral thoracic artery may be damaged during a mastectomy procedure.
GAS 752; N 422; ABR/McM 152

6. **B.** A supracondylar fracture often results in injury to the median nerve. The course of the median nerve is anterolateral, and at the elbow it lies medial to the brachial artery on the brachialis muscle.

A. The axillary nerve passes posteriorly through the quadrangular space, accompanied by the posterior circumflex humeral artery, and winds around the surgical neck of the humerus. Injury to the surgical neck may damage the axillary nerve.

C. The musculocutaneous nerve pierces the coracobrachialis muscle and descends between the biceps brachii and brachialis muscle. It continues into the forearm as the lateral antebrachial cutaneous nerve.

D. The radial nerve courses anterior to the lateral epicondyle of the humerus, through the cubital fossa.

E. The ulnar nerve descends behind the medial epicondyle in its groove and is easily injured and produces "funny bone" symptoms.
GAS 750, 752; N 438; ABR/McM 151

7. **C.** The radial nerve descends posteriorly between the long and lateral heads of the triceps brachii muscle and passes inferolaterally on the back of the humerus between the medial and lateral heads of the triceps brachii muscle. It eventually enters the anterior compartment and descends to enter the cubital fossa, where it divides into superficial and deep branches. The deep branch of the radial nerve winds laterally around the radius and runs between the two heads of the supinator muscle and innervates the extensor muscles of the forearm. Some refer to the deep radial nerve distal to the supinator muscle as the posterior interosseous nerve.

A. Ulnar: The ulnar nerve passes down the medial aspect of the forearm and works to flex and adduct the hand at the wrist as well as flex the 4th and 5th metacarpals at the distal interphalangeal joint.

B. The anterior interosseous nerve arises from the median nerve and supplies the radial half of flexor digitorum profundus, flexor pollicis longus, and pronator quadratus muscles, none of which seem to be injured in this example.

D. Injury to the median nerve causes a characteristic flattening (atrophy) of the thenar eminence.

E. Because this injury does not result in loss of sensation over the skin of the upper limb, it is likely that the superficial branch of the radial nerve is not injured. If the radial nerve were injured very proximally, the woman would not be able to extend her elbow. The branches of the radial nerve to the triceps brachii muscle arise proximal to where the nerve runs in the radial groove.
GAS 733–745, 750, 752, 777, 792; N 435; ABR/McM 161

8. **B.** The musculocutaneous nerve supplies the biceps brachii and brachialis muscles, which are the flexors of the elbow. The musculocutaneous nerve continues as the lateral antebrachial cutaneous nerve, which supplies sensation to the lateral side of the forearm (with the forearm in the anatomical position). The biceps brachii muscle is the most powerful supinator muscle. Injury to this nerve would result in weakness of supination and forearm flexion and lateral forearm sensory loss.

A. Injury to the radial nerve would result in weakened extension and a characteristic wrist drop.

C. Injury to the median nerve causes paralysis of flexor digitorum superficialis muscle and other flexors in the forearm and results in a characteristic flattening of the thenar eminence.

D. The lateral cord of the brachial plexus gives origin both to the musculocutaneous and lateral pectoral nerves. There is no indication of pectoral paralysis or weakness. Injury to the lateral cord can result in weakened flexion and supination in the forearm, and weakened adduction and medial rotation of the arm.

E. The lateral antebrachial cutaneous nerve is a branch of the musculocutaneous nerve and does not supply any motor innervation. Injury to the musculocutaneous nerve alone is unusual but can follow penetrating injuries.
GAS 749; N 465; ABR/McM 150

9. **C.** Tenosynovitis can be due to an infection of the synovial sheaths of the digits. Tenosynovitis in the thumb may spread through the synovial sheath of the flexor pollicis longus tendon, also known as the radial bursa.

A and B. The tendons of the flexor digitorum superficialis and profundus muscles are enveloped in the common synovial flexor sheath or ulnar bursa.

D and E. Neither the flexor carpi radialis nor flexor pollicis brevis tendons are contained in synovial flexor sheaths.

GAS 792–793; N 451; ABR/McM 145

10. **A.** The three chief contents of the cubital fossa are the biceps brachii tendon, brachial artery, and median nerve (lateral to medial).

B and D. The common and anterior interosseous arteries arise distal to the cubital fossa.

C and E. The ulnar and radial arteries are the result of the bifurcation of the brachial artery deep within the cubital fossa. Venipuncture involves superficial veins.
GAS 758–760; N 438; ABR/McM 160

11. **D.** Lymph from the skin of the anterior chest wall primarily drains to the axillary lymph nodes.

A and E. The deep inguinal nodes receive efferents from the deep lymphatics of the lower limb, some efferents from the superficial inguinal nodes, and lymphatic drainage from the glans penis or clitoris.

B, C, E. The horizontal group of superficial inguinal lymph nodes drains structures in the perineum whereas the vertical group of superficial lymph nodes receive lymph from most of the superficial tissues of the lower limb.
GAS 737–738; N 416; ABR/McM 185

12. **C.** The anterior intercostal arteries are twelve small arteries, two in each of the upper six intercostal spaces at the upper and lower borders. The upper artery lying in each space forms an anastomosis with the posterior intercostal arteries, whereas the lower one usually joins the collateral branch of the posterior intercostal artery.

A. The musculophrenic artery is a terminal branch of the internal thoracic artery (also known as the internal mammary artery), and it supplies the pericardium, diaphragm, and muscles of the lower intercostal spaces and the abdominal wall. It anastomoses with the deep circumflex iliac artery.

B. The superior epigastric artery is the other terminal branch of the internal thoracic artery, and it supplies the diaphragm, peritoneum, and the anterior abdominal wall and anastomoses with the inferior epigastric artery.

D. The lateral thoracic artery runs along the lateral chest wall and supplies the pectoralis major, pectoralis minor, and serratus anterior.

E. The thoracodorsal artery accompanies the thoracodorsal nerve in supplying the latissimus dorsi muscle and lateral thoracic wall.
GAS 156; N 197; ABR/McM 189

13. **D.** The location for palpation of the radial pulse is lateral to the tendon of the flexor carpi radialis, where the radial artery can be compressed against the distal radius. The radial pulse can also be felt in the anatomical snuffbox between the tendons of the extensor pollicis brevis and extensor pollicis longus muscles, where the radial artery can be compressed against the scaphoid.

A, B, C, E. Palmaris longus, flexor pollicis longus, flexor digitorum profundus, and flexor digitorum superficialis tendons are not used to localize the radial pulse.
GAS 772, 818; N 437; ABR/McM 169

14. A. The flexor digitorum profundus muscle is dually innervated by the ulnar nerve to the medial two fingers and the median nerve for the middle and index fingers. Because of the superficial course of the ulnar nerve, it is vulnerable to laceration. Such an injury would result in an inability to flex the DIP joints of the fourth and fifth digits because the flexor digitorum profundus muscle is the only muscle that flexes this joint.

  B. The flexor digitorum superficialis muscle flexes the proximal, not distal, IP joints of the fingers.

  C. The lumbricals function to flex the MPtop joints and assist in extending the IP joints.

  D. The flexor carpi ulnaris acts to flex and medially deviate the hand at the wrist.

  E. The interossei adduct and abduct the fingers and can also flex the MP while extending the IP joints of the fingers.

  GAS 771; N 437; ABR/McM 169

15. D. The recurrent branch of the median nerve is motor to the muscles of the thenar eminence, which is an elevation caused by the abductor pollicis brevis, flexor pollicis brevis, and opponens pollicis muscles. If the opponens pollicis is paralyzed, one cannot oppose the pad of the thumb to the pads of the other digits because this is the only muscle that can oppose the thumb by moving the first metacarpal on the trapezium. The recurrent branch of the median nerve does not have a cutaneous distribution.

  A. Holding a piece of paper between the fingers is a simple test of adduction of the fingers. These movements are controlled by the deep branch of the ulnar nerve, which is not injured in this patient.

  B. The anterior interosseous nerve does not travel distal to the wrist.

  C. Median nerve damage would involve loss of cutaneous sensation on the radial 3½ digits.

  E. The deep branch of the radial nerve does not usually travel distal to the wrist.

  GAS 808; N 463; ABR/McM 168

16. B. The condition described in this patient is called "winging" of the scapula. "Winging" of the scapula occurs when the medial border of the scapula lifts off the chest wall when the patient pushes against resistance, such as a vertical wall. The serratus anterior muscle holds the medial border of the scapula against the posterior chest wall and is innervated by the long thoracic nerve. The serratus anterior assists in rotation of the scapula above the horizontal plane so that the glenoid fossa is directed more superiorly.

  A. The posterior cord of the brachial plexus gives rise to the upper and lower subscapular nerves, thoracodorsal nerve, axillary nerve, and radial nerve. The long thoracic nerve does not arise from the posterior cord but from C5 to C7 ventral spinal nerve roots.

  C. The upper trunk of the brachial plexus is comprised of the C5 and C6 nerve roots and gives rise to the suprascapular nerve. The upper trunk of the brachial plexus does not supply fibers to the long thoracic nerve.

  D. The middle subscapular nerve branches from the posterior division of the brachial plexus. It is also known as the thoracodorsal nerve and innervates the latissimus dorsi muscle. The lower subscapular nerve originates from C5 to C6 spinal nerves, branches from the posterior cord of the brachial plexus, and innervates the lower aspect of the subscapularis muscle and the teres major.

  E. The long thoracic nerve is formed from the ventral rami of C5–C7. C8–T1 will not contribute to the formation of the long thoracic nerve.

  GAS 716; N 417; ABR/McM 149

17. A. The annular ligament is a fibrous band that encircles the head of the radius, forming a collar that attaches to the ulna and fuses with the radial collateral ligament and articular capsule of the elbow. The annular ligament functions to prevent displacement of the head of the radius from the humeroradial joint. In a child of this age, the head of the radius is almost the same diameter as the body of the bone, so the head is relatively easy to dislocate.

  B. The joint capsule functions to allow free rotation of the joint and does not function in its stabilization.

  C. The interosseous membrane is a fibrous layer between the radius and ulnar that assists in holding these two bones together.

  D. The radial collateral ligament extends from the lateral epicondyle to the annular ligament of the radius.

  E. The ulnar collateral ligament is a triangular ligament that extends from the medial epicondyle to the olecranon of the ulna (*GAS* Figs. 7.73A and 7.72).

  GAS 753–755; N 428; ABR/McM 154

18. E. The injury being described is also known as Erb-Duchenne paralysis or "waiter's tip hand" and is relatively common in children after a difficult delivery. This usually results from an injury to the upper trunk of the brachial plexus, presenting with loss of abduction, flexion, and lateral rotation of the arm. The superior trunk of the brachial plexus consists of spinal nerve ventral rami C5–C6.

  A, B, C, D. Injury to any of these structures would not result in the classic presentation of Erb-Duchenne palsy.

  GAS 727–736; N 420; ABR/McM 145

19. C. The superficial branch of the ulnar nerve supplies the skin of the little finger and the medial side of the ring finger.

  A. The superficial branch of the radial nerve provides cutaneous innervation to the radial (lateral) dorsum of the hand and the radial two and a half digits over the proximal and middle phalanges.

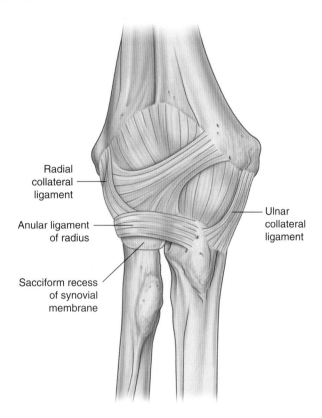

Radial collateral ligament

Anular ligament of radius

Sacciform recess of synovial membrane

Ulnar collateral ligament

• *GAS* Fig. 7.73A

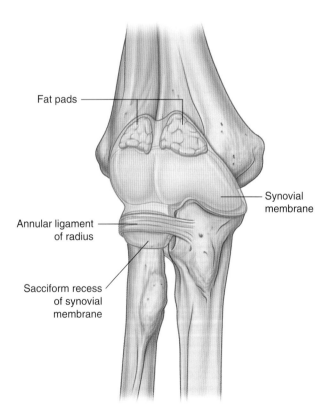

Fat pads

Annular ligament of radius

Sacciform recess of synovial membrane

Synovial membrane

• *GAS* Fig. 7.72

B. The common palmar digital branches of the median nerve innervate the lateral aspect of the palmar hand, the palmar surface of the radial 3½

digits, and the dorsal aspect of distal phalanges of the second and third finger as well as the lateral part of the fourth digit.

D. The deep radial nerve supplies the extensor carpi radialis brevis and supinator muscles and all of the distal extensor muscles before continuing as the posterior interosseous nerve, which is sensory to the wrist joint (note: some consider the posterior interosseous nerve as synonymous with the deep radial nerve).

E. The recurrent branch of the median nerve supplies the abductor pollicis brevis, flexor pollicis brevis, and opponens pollicis muscles.

GAS 683–687; N 463; ABR/McM 169

20. B. The anatomical snuffbox is formed by the tendons of the extensor pollicis brevis accompanying the abductor pollicis longus, and the extensor pollicis longus. The floor is formed by the scaphoid bone, and it is here that one can palpate for a possible fractured scaphoid. Within the first 2 to 6 weeks after injury, plain radiographs are limited in the detection of scaphoid fractures. Patients with a scaphoid fracture are at greatest risk of developing avascular necrosis of the proximal part of the scaphoid bone due to an interruption to its retrograde vasculature.

A. The lunate is the most commonly dislocated bone in the wrist.

C, D, E. The capitate, hamate, and trapezoid are not as commonly fractured as the scaphoid.

GAS 791–792; N 434; ABR/McM 174

21. E. The ulnar nerve innervates the palmar interossei, which adduct the fingers. This is the movement that would maintain the paper between the fingers.

A. The axillary nerve does not innervate muscles of the hand.

B. The median nerve supplies the first and second lumbricals, the opponens pollicis, abductor pollicis brevis, and the flexor pollicis brevis muscles. None of these muscles would affect the ability to hold a piece of paper between the fingers.

C and D. The musculocutaneous and radial nerves do not supply muscles of the hand.

GAS 799; N 455; ABR/McM 171

22. D. The supraspinatus muscle is one of the four rotator cuff muscles—the other three being the infraspinatus, teres minor, and subscapularis muscles. The tendon of the supraspinatus muscle is relatively avascular and is often injured when the shoulder is dislocated. This muscle initiates abduction of the arm, and damage would impair this movement.

A. The coracobrachialis muscle, which runs from the coracoid process to the humerus near its midbody, functions in adduction and flexion of the arm.

B. The main function of the triceps brachii muscle is to extend the forearm at the elbow, although its long head can also help in arm extension and adduction. Damage to its long head would not affect abduction.

C. The pectoralis minor muscle functions as an accessory respiratory muscle and to stabilize the scapula and is not involved in abduction.

E. The teres major muscle functions to adduct and medially rotate the arm.

GAS 706; N 415; ABR/McM 143

23. **E.** The coracoacromial ligament contributes to the coracoacromial arch, preventing superior displacement of the head of the humerus. Because this ligament is very strong, it will rarely be damaged; instead, the ligament can cause inflammation or erosion of the tendon of the supraspinatus muscle as the tendon moves back and forth under the ligament.

A. The AC ligament, connecting the acromion with the lateral end of the clavicle, is not in contact with the supraspinatus tendon.

B. The coracohumeral ligament is located too far anteriorly to impinge upon the supraspinatus tendon.

C. The glenohumeral ligaments or bands are located in the anterior glenohumeral capsule, deep to the subscapularis muscle primarily, and would not contribute to injury of the supraspinatus muscle.

D. The transverse scapular ligament crosses the scapular notch and is not in contact with the supraspinatus tendon.

GAS 693–694; N 415; ABR/McM 142

24. **A.** The median nerve supplies sensory innervation to the thumb, index, and middle fingers and also to the lateral half of the ring finger. The median nerve also provides motor innervation to muscles of the thenar eminence. Compression of the median nerve in the carpal tunnel explains these deficits in conjunction with normal functioning of the flexor compartment of the forearm because these muscles are innervated by the median nerve proximal to the carpal tunnel. Also, sensory innervation in the proximal palm will be normal because the palmar branch of the radial nerve usually branches off proximal to the flexor retinaculum which forms the roof of the carpal tunnel.

B and E. The ulnar nerve is not implicated in these symptoms. It does not provide sensation to digits 1 to 3.

C. Compression of the brachial plexus could not be attributed to pressure from the triceps brachii because this muscle is located posterior and distal to the plexus. In addition, brachial plexus symptoms would include other upper limb deficits, rather than the focal symptoms described in this case.

D. Osteoarthritis of the cervical spine would also lead to increasing complexity of symptoms.

GAS 788; N 452; ABR/McM 169

25. **C.** The radial nerve innervates the extensor compartments of the arm and the forearm. It supplies the triceps brachii proximal to the radial groove, so elbow

extension is intact here. It also provides sensory innervation to much of the posterior arm and forearm as well as the dorsal thumb, index, and middle fingers up to the level of the fingernails. Symptoms are described only in the distal limb due to the midhumeral location of the lesion.

A and B. The median nerve innervates flexors of the forearm and thenar muscles and provides sensory innervation to the lateral 3½ digits and palmar hand.

D. Upon exiting the cubital fossa the radial nerve terminates by dividing into the superficial and deep branch. Because both motor and sensory function of the radial nerve is impaired, this patient most likely has injured the radial nerve proximal to its division into deep (motor) and superficial sensory branches.

E. The ulnar nerve supplies only the flexor carpi ulnaris and the medial half of the flexor digitorum profundus in the forearm. Additionally, its sensory distribution is to the medial 1½ digits on the palmar aspect and 2½ digits on the dorsal aspect of the medial hand. It does not supply extensor muscles of the wrist.

GAS 735, 750; N 422; ABR/McM 152

Answers 26–50

26. **D.** The musculocutaneous nerve innervates the brachialis and biceps brachii muscles, which are the main flexors at the elbow. The biceps brachii inserts on the radius and is an important supinator. Because the musculocutaneous nerve is damaged in this case, it leads to loss of sensory perception to the lateral forearm, which is supplied by the distal continuation of the musculocutaneous nerve (known as the lateral antebrachial cutaneous nerve). The name "musculocutaneous" indicates it is "muscular" in the arm and "cutaneous" in the forearm.

A. Adduction and abduction of the fingers are mediated by the ulnar nerve and would not be affected in this instance.

C. The flexor pollicis brevis muscle flexes the thumb and is mainly innervated by the recurrent branch of the median nerve.

B. Flexion of the fingers is performed by the long flexors of the fingers, innervated by the median and ulnar nerves.

E. Sensory innervation of the medial forearm is provided by the medial antebrachial cutaneous nerve, usually a direct branch of the medial cord of the brachial plexus.

GAS 735; N 421; ABR/McM 151

27. **E.** The deep branch of the radial nerve courses between the two parts of the supinator muscle and is located just medial and distal to the lateral epicondyle. After the nerve emerges from the supinator it is called the posterior interosseous nerve. It can be irritated by hypertrophy of the supinator, which compresses the nerve, causing pain and weakness.

A. The ulnar nerve courses laterally behind the medial epicondyle and continues anterior to the flexor carpi ulnaris muscle.

B and C. The median nerve passes into the forearm flexor compartment.

D. The superficial radial nerve courses down the lateral aspect of the posterior forearm and would not cause pain due to pressure applied to the posterior forearm.

GAS 782; N 469; ABR/McM 161

28. **B.** The lunate is the most commonly dislocated carpal bone because of its shape and relatively weak ligaments anteriorly. This dislocation may result in an entrapment neuropathy involving the median nerve within the carpal tunnel.

C and E. Dislocations of the scaphoid and triquetrum are relatively rare.

A and D. The trapezoid and capitate bones are located in the distal row of the carpal bones.

GAS 783; N 442; ABR/McM 173

29. **A.** The medial antebrachial cutaneous nerve carries sensory fibers derived from the C8 and T1 levels.

B. The long thoracic nerve characteristically arises from the anterior rami of the nerve roots C5–C7.

C. The lateral antebrachial cutaneous nerve is the distal continuation of the musculocutaneous nerve, carrying fibers from the C5, C6, and C7 levels.

D, E. The deep branch of the ulnar nerve and the anterior interosseous nerve carry predominantly motor fibers. The sensory fibers coursing in the radial nerve are derived from the C5–C8 levels.

GAS 683–687, 731; N 463; ABR/McM 157

30. **C.** The contraction of the extensor mechanism produces extension of the DIP joint. When the tendon of the extensor digitorum is torn from the distal phalanx, the digit is pulled into flexion by the flexor digitorum profundus muscle. If a piece of the distal phalanx is attached to the torn tendon, it is an avulsion fracture.

A. The palmar digital branches of the median nerve supply lumbrical muscles and carry sensation from their respective digits.

B. Vincula longa are slender, bandlike connections from the deep flexor tendons to the phalanx that can carry blood supply to the tendons.

D and E. The insertions of the flexor digitorum superficialis and profundus are on the flexor surface of the middle and distal phalanges, respectively, and act to flex the IP joints.

GAS 777–778, 799; N 454; ABR/McM 175

31. **E.** A fracture of the distal radius with deviation toward the palm of the distal segment often displaces the lunate bone.

A, B, C. D. The other listed bones are unlikely to be displaced in a palmar direction by Smith fracture.

GAS 761–764; N 442; ABR/McM 173

32. **B.** The abductor pollicis longus and extensor pollicis brevis muscles occupy the first dorsal compartment of the wrist.

A. The extensor carpi radialis longus and brevis are in the second compartment.

C and D. The extensor digitorum is in the third compartment, as is the extensor indicis.

E. The extensor carpi ulnaris is located in the sixth dorsal compartment.

GAS 775–780; N 435; ABR/McM 175

33. **E.** The medial cord has been injured by traction on the lower trunk of the brachial plexus. The medial cord is the continuation of the inferior (lower) trunk of the brachial lexus, which is formed by C8 and T1.

A. C5 and C6 are typically associated with the superior (upper) trunk level and thus the lateral cord.

B, C, D. C7 forms the middle trunk. An injury to the posterior cord would usually involve the C7 spinal nerve. This is a typical Klumpke palsy.

GAS 729–736; N 420; ABR/McM 145

34. **A.** A mid-body fracture of the humerus in the radial groove results in injury to the radial nerve. The flexor carpi ulnaris muscle is not innervated by the radial nerve but rather by the ulnar nerve.

B, C, D, E. The brachioradialis, extensor carpi radialis longus and brevis, and supinator muscles are all innervated by the radial nerve distal to the radial groove.

GAS 767, 777; N 422; ABR/McM 158

35. **A.** Injury to the radial nerve in the radial groove will paralyze the abductor pollicis longus muscle and both extensors of the thumb. This injury will also lead to wrist drop (inability to extend the wrist). Weakness of grip would also occur, although this is not mentioned in the question. If the wrist is flexed, finger flexion and grip strength are weakened because the long flexor tendons are not under tension. Note how much your strength of grip is increased when your wrist is extended versus when it is flexed.

GAS 752, 809; N 431; ABR/McM 152

36. **A.** The deep brachial artery passes down the arm with the radial nerve.

B. The radial collateral artery arises from the deep brachial artery and anastomoses with the radial recurrent branch of the radial artery proximal to the elbow laterally.

C. The superior ulnar collateral artery: The superior ulnar collateral artery travels along the posterior side of the medial epicondyle, along with the ulnar nerve, and anastomoses with the posterior ulnar recurrent artery.

D. The inferior ulnar collateral artery arises from the brachial artery and accompanies the median nerve into the forearm.

E. The anterior ulnar recurrent artery arises from the ulnar artery and anastomoses with the inferior ulnar collateral artery anterior to the elbow.

GAS 745–747; N 438; ABR/McM 158

37. C. Adduction of the fifth digit is produced by contraction of the third palmar interosseous muscle. All of the interossei are innervated by the deep branch of the ulnar nerve.
    A. Flexion of the PIP joint of the fifth digit (little finger): Flexion of the PIP joint of the fifth digit is a function of the flexor digitorum superficialis, which is supplied by the median nerve.
    B. Complete extension of the thumb is a function of the extensor pollicis longus. It is supplied by the deep branch of the radial nerve.
    D. Abduction of the thumb is a function of the abductor pollicis longus and abductor pollicis brevis. The abductor pollicis longus is innervated by the deep branch of the radial nerve and the abductor pollicis brevis is innervated by the recurrent branch of the median nerve.
    E. Opposition of the thumb is a function of the opponens pollicis, supplied by the recurrent branch of the median nerve.
    GAS 799; N 455; ABR/McM 171

38. C. The radial nerve is the most likely nerve compressed to cause these symptoms. This type of nerve palsy is often called "Saturday night palsy." One reason for this nickname is that people would supposedly fall asleep after being intoxicated on a Saturday night with their arm over the back of a chair or bench, thereby compressing the nerve in the radial groove. The radial nerve innervates all of the extensors of the elbow, wrist, and fingers. It innervates the triceps brachii muscle but the motor branch typically comes off proximal to the site of compression, so the patient can still extend the elbow.
    A. Paralysis of the lateral cord of the brachial plexus would result in loss of the musculocutaneous nerve and the lateral pectoral nerve, which do not mediate extension of the forearm or hand.
    B. The medial cord of the brachial plexus branches into the median nerve and ulnar nerve. Neither of these nerves innervates muscles that control extension.
    D. The median nerve innervates flexors of the forearm and the thenar muscles.
    E. The lateral and median pectoral nerves innervate the pectoralis major and minor muscles and do not extend into the arm.
    GAS 750–752; N 419; ABR/McM 145

39. A. The basilic vein can be used for dialysis, especially when the cephalic vein is judged to be too small, as in this case. The basilic vein can be elevated from its position as it passes through the fascia on the medial side of the arm (brachium).
    C. The cephalic vein passes more laterally up the limb.
    B. The lateral cubital vein is a tributary to the cephalic vein.

C. The median cubital vein joins the basilic and cephalic veins at the level of the cubital fossa.
D. The median antebrachial vein courses up the midline of the forearm (antebrachium) ventrally.
GAS 688, 748, 758–760; N 405; ABR/McM 157

40. A. The patient exhibits the classic "benediction attitude" of the thumb and lateral fingers from injury to the median nerve proximally in the forearm. The thumb is somewhat extended (radial supplied abductor and extensors unopposed); digits 2 and 3 are extended (by extensor digitorum and indicis unopposed); digits 4 and 5 are partially flexed (by their intact flexor digitorum profundus). A lesion of the median nerve would result in weakened flexion of the PIP joints of all digits (flexor digitorum superficialis muscle), loss of flexion of the IP joint of the thumb, the DIP joints of digits 2 and 3 (flexor digitorum profundus muscle), and weakened flexion of the MCP joints of the second and third digits (first and second lumbricals).
    B. A lesion of both the ulnar and median nerves would cause weakness or paralysis of flexion of all of the digits.
    C and D. A lesion of the ulnar nerve would mostly cause weakness in flexion of the DIP of the fourth and fifth digits and would affect all of the interosseous muscles and the lumbricals of the fourth and fifth digits.
    D and E. A lesion of the radial nerve would cause weakness in extension of the wrist, thumb, and MCP joints.
    GAS 774, 808; N 438; ABR/McM 158

41. C. The head of the humerus is displaced inferiorly because in that location it is not supported by rotator cuff muscle tendons or the coracoacromial arch. It is also pulled anteriorly (relative to the tendon of the triceps brachii) beneath the coracoid process by pectoralis and subscapularis muscles.
    A. The head of the humerus is displaced laterally: It would not be displaced laterally because it is supported by the deltoid muscle.
    B. It would not be displaced posteriorly because it is supported by the teres minor and infraspinatus muscle tendons.
    D. It would not be displaced superiorly because the coracoacromial ligament and supraspinatus reinforce in that direction.
    E. A medial dislocation is resisted by the subscapularis tendon.
    GAS 701; N 410; ABR/McM 142

42. A. The anterior axillary (or anterior pectoral) nodes are the first lymph nodes to receive most of the lymph from the breast parenchyma, areola, and nipple. From there, lymph flows through central axillary, apical axillary, and supraclavicular nodes in sequence.
    B. The interpectoral or Rotter nodes lie between the pectoral muscles and are, unfortunately, an

alternate route in some patients, speeding the rate of metastasis.

C. The parasternal nodes lie along the internal thoracic artery and vein and receive lymph from the medial part of the breast.

D. The central axillary lymph nodes receive lymph from the anterior, posterior, and lateral group of axillary lymph nodes.

E. The apical axillary group of lymph nodes receive the efferent lymph vessels from all the other axillary nodes.

GAS 737; N 407; ABR/McM 185

43. D. The left accessory nerve (CN XI) has been injured posterior to the sternocleidomastoid muscle, resulting in paralysis of the trapezius, allowing the shoulder to droop and the superior angle of the scapula to protrude posteriorly. The sternocleidomastoid muscles are intact, as demonstrated by symmetry in strength in turning the head to the right and left.

A and C. There is no indication of paralysis of the lateral rotators of the shoulder or elbow flexors (suprascapular nerve or upper trunk).

B. Injury to the dorsal scapular nerve results in the lateral deviation of the ipsilateral scapula and a weakness in retracting the shoulder.

E. Thoracodorsal nerve injury would result in paralysis of the latissimus dorsi muscle, an extensor and medial rotator of the humerus.

GAS 703; N 417; ABR/McM 138

44. C. Inability to extend the MCP joints. The tendons of the extensor digitorum, extensor indicis, and extensor digiti minimi muscles, innervated by the radial nerve, are responsible for extension of the MCP and, to a much lesser degree, the proximal (PIP) and distal (DIP) interphalangeal joints.

A and B. Abduction and adduction of the MCP joints are functions of the interossei, all of which are innervated by the deep ulnar nerve.

D and E. Extension of the PIP and DIP joints is performed by the lumbricals and interossei. The first two lumbricals are supplied by the median nerve; the other lumbricals and the interossei, by the deep branch of the ulnar nerve.

GAS 782, 805–809; N 454; ABR/McM 164

45. C. Fracture of the surgical neck of the humerus often injures the axillary nerve, which innervates the deltoid and teres minor muscles. Abduction of the humerus between 15 degrees and horizontal is performed by the deltoid muscle. Lateral rotation of the humerus is mainly performed by the deltoid muscle, teres minor, and the infraspinatus. The deltoid and teres minor are both lost in this case.

A. The ulnar nerve would be potentially compromised in a fracture of the medial epicondyle of the humerus.

B. Fracture of the glenoid fossa would lead to drooping of the shoulder.

D. Fracture of the anatomical neck of the humerus will similarly lead to a drooping of the shoulder but would not necessarily affect abduction of the humerus. It is also quite unusual.

E. Fracture of the middle third of the humerus would most likely injure the radial nerve.

GAS 693; N 409; ABR/McM 146

46. B. When cutaneous lymphatics of the breast are blocked by tumor emboli, the skin becomes edematous, except where hair follicles cause small indentations of the skin. This gives the skin an overall resemblance to an orange peel, hence the term peau d'orange.

A. Shortening of the suspensory ligaments (of Cooper) or retinacula cutis leads to pitting of the overlying skin, pitting that is intensified if the patient raises her arm above her head.

C. Inversion of areolar skin with involvement of the ducts would also be due to involvement of the retinacula cutis.

D and E. Peau d' orange of breast cancer is not caused by the invasion of the cancer into the pectoralis major. Invasion of the pectoralis major by cancer can result in fixation of the breast, seen upon elevation of the ipsilateral limb.

GAS 737; N 190; ABR/McM 185

47. D. The subclavian vein lies anteriorly between the clavicle and first rib and is the most superficial structure to be damaged following a fracture of the clavicle.

A. The subclavian artery runs posterior to the subclavian vein, and though it is in the appropriate location, it would likely not be damaged because of its deeper anatomical position.

B. The cephalic vein is a tributary to the axillary vein after ascending on the lateral side of the arm. Its location within the body is too superficial and lateral to the site of injury.

C. The lateral thoracic artery is a branch from the axillary artery that runs lateral to the pectoralis minor. It courses inferior and medial from its point of origin from the axillary artery, and it does not maintain a position near the clavicle during its descent.

E. The internal thoracic artery arises from the first part of the subclavian artery before descending deep to the costal cartilages. Its point of origin from the subclavian artery is lateral to clavicular injury. Furthermore, its course behind the costal cartilages is quite medial to the clavicular fracture.

GAS 682, 725–736; N 419; ABR/McM 135

48. A. A Colles fracture is a fracture of the distal end of the radius. The proximal portion of the radius is displaced anteriorly, with the distal bone fragment projecting posteriorly. The displacement of the radius from the wrist often gives the appearance of a dinner fork, thus a Colles fracture is often referred to as a "dinner fork" deformity.

B. A scaphoid fracture results from a fracture of the scaphoid bone and would thus not cause displacement of the radius. This fracture usually occurs at the narrow aspect ("waist") of the scaphoid bone.

C and E. Bennett and boxer's fractures both result from fractures of the metacarpals (first and fifth, respectively).

D. Volkmann ischemic contracture is a muscular deformity that can follow a supracondylar fracture of the humerus, with arterial laceration into the flexor compartment of the forearm. Ischemia and muscle contracture, with extreme pain, accompany this fracture.

GAS 761–764; N 442; ABR/McM 130

49. B. In shoulder separation, either or both the AC and coracoclavicular ligaments can be partially or completely torn through. The AC joint can be interrupted and the distal end of the clavicle may deviate upward in a complete separation, while the upper limb droops away inferiorly, causing a "step off" that can be palpated and sometimes observed.

A. Displacement of the head of the humerus is shoulder dislocation, not separation.

C. The coracoacromial ligament is not torn in separation (but it is sometimes used in the repair of the torn coracoclavicular ligament).

D. The transverse scapular ligament is not involved in shoulder separation.

E. Disruption of the glenoid labrum often accompanies shoulder dislocation.

GAS 699; N 415; ABR/McM 142

50. A. The nail was fired explosively from the nail gun and then pierced the ulnar nerve near the coronoid process of the ulna and the trochlea of the humerus. Paralysis of the medial half of the flexor digitorum profundus muscle would result (among other significant deficits), with loss of flexion of the DIP joints of fourth and fifth digits.

B. Trauma of the ulnar nerve at the wrist would not affect the IP joints, although it would cause paralysis of the hypothenar, medial 2 lumbrical, interossei, and adductor pollicis muscles.

C. Median nerve damage proximal to the pronator teres would affect PIP joint flexion and DIP joint flexion of digits 2 and 3 as well as thumb flexion and opposition.

D. Median nerve injury at the wrist would cause loss of thenar muscles but not long flexors of the fingers.

E. Trauma to spinal nerve ventral ramus C8 would affect all long finger flexors.

GAS 774, 805; N 438; ABR/McM 158

Answers 51–75

51. C. The injury has occurred just beyond the third part of the axillary artery. The only collateral arterial channel between the third part of the axillary artery and the brachial artery is between the posterior circumflex humeral and the ascending branch of the deep

brachial. This anastomotic path is often inadequate to supply the arterial needs of the limb.

A. The suprascapular artery anastomoses with the circumflex scapular deep to the infraspinatus.

B. The dorsal scapular artery (passing beneath the medial border of the scapula) has no anastomosis with thoracodorsal within the scope of the injury.

D. The lateral thoracic artery has no anastomoses with the brachial artery.

E. The superior thoracic artery (first part of axillary artery) has no helpful anastomoses with the thoracoacromial (second part of axillary) (*GAS* Figs. 7.39 and 7.50).

GAS 708–710; N 424; ABR/McM 145

52. E. The scaphoid (or the older term, navicular) bone is the most commonly fractured carpal bone.

A. The trapezium is located just distal to the scaphoid bone, however it is not the most commonly fractured carpal bone.

B. The lunate is the most commonly dislocated carpal bone.

C. The pisiform is a sesamoid bone that is located most medially in the proximal row of carpal bones. It is not the most commonly fractured carpal bone.

D. The hamate is located most medially in the distal row of carpal bones. It is not the most commonly fractured carpal bone.

GAS 787; N 442; ABR/McM 173

53. E. The anterior interosseous nerve is a branch of the median nerve that supplies the flexor pollicis longus, the lateral half of the flexor digitorum profundus, and the pronator quadratus muscles. If it is injured, flexion of the IP joint of the thumb will be compromised.

A. The median nerve gives rise to the anterior interosseous nerve. However, injury to this nerve would result in more widespread deficits.

B. The deep branch of the radial nerve supplies extensors in the forearm, not flexors.

C. The radial nerve gives rise to superficial and deep branches and the continuation of the deep branch, the posterior interosseous nerve and is not associated with the anterior interosseous nerve; therefore, it would not have any effect on the flexors of the forearm.

D. The recurrent median nerve is also a branch of the median nerve but supplies the thenar eminence muscles, and its injury would result in problems with opposable motion of the thumb (*GAS* Fig. 7.89.

GAS 774; N 466; ABR/McM 160

54. C. The tendon of the long head of the biceps brachii muscle passes through the glenohumeral joint, surrounded by synovial membrane.

A. The glenohumeral ligaments or bands are thickenings of the glenohumeral joint capsule anteriorly.

B. The long head of the triceps brachii arises from the infraglenoid tubercle, beneath the glenoid fossa.

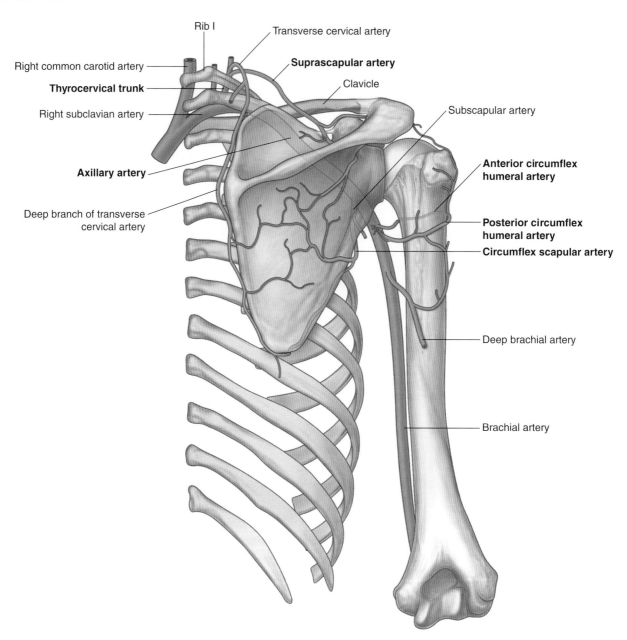

Rib I

Transverse cervical artery

Right common carotid artery

Suprascapular artery

Thyrocervical trunk

Clavicle

Right subclavian artery

Subscapular artery

Axillary artery

Anterior circumflex humeral artery

Deep branch of transverse cervical artery

Posterior circumflex humeral artery

Circumflex scapular artery

Deep brachial artery

Brachial artery

• *GAS* **Fig. 7.39**

D. The infraspinatus tendon passes posterior to the head of the humerus to insert on the greater tubercle.

E. The coracobrachialis arises from the coracoid process and inserts on the humerus.

GAS 695; N 421; ABR/McM 143

55. E. The suprascapular artery passes over, and the suprascapular nerve passes under, the superior transverse scapular ligament. This ligament bridges the superior scapular notch in the upper border of the scapula, converting the notch to foramen. The artery and nerve then pass deep to the supraspinatus muscle thereafter, supplying it and then passing through the inferior scapular (spinoglenoid) notch to supply the infraspinatus.

A. The subscapular artery is a branch of the third part of the axillary artery; it divides into circumflex scapular and thoracodorsal branches.

B. The transverse cervical artery courses anterior to this site.

C. The dorsal scapular artery and nerve pass along the medial border of the scapula.

D. The posterior circumflex humeral branch of the axillary artery passes through the quadrangular space with the axillary nerve.

GAS 708–709; N 418; ABR/McM 139

56. A. The patient has suffered injury to the radial nerve in the mid-humeral region. The nerve that provides sensation to the dorsum of the hand proximal to the thumb and index finger is the superficial branch of the radial nerve.

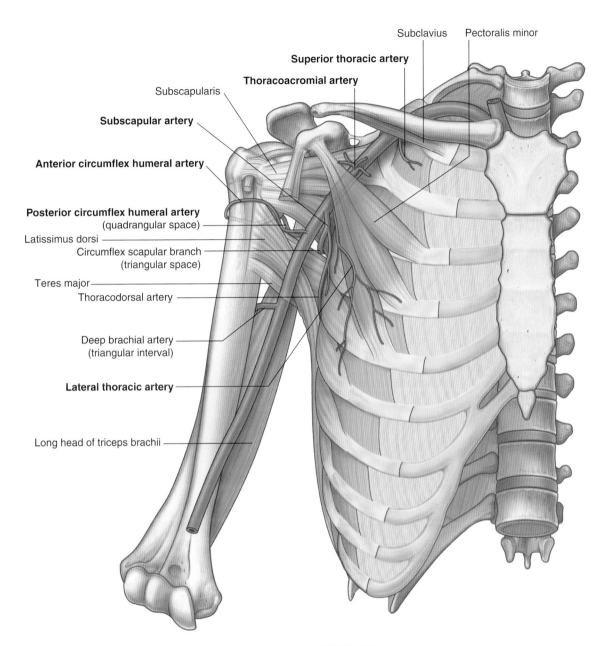

Subclavius   Pectoralis minor

Superior thoracic artery

Thoracoacromial artery

Subscapularis

Subscapular artery

Anterior circumflex humeral artery

Posterior circumflex humeral artery
(quadrangular space)

Latissimus dorsi

Circumflex scapular branch
(triangular space)

Teres major

Thoracodorsal artery

Deep brachial artery
(triangular interval)

Lateral thoracic artery

Long head of triceps brachii

• *GAS* **Fig. 7.50**

B. The posterior interosseous nerve supplies proprioceptive sensory information from the wrist joint.

C. The lateral antebrachial cutaneous nerve is a continuation of the musculocutaneous nerve and supplies the lateral side of the forearm.

D. The medial antebrachial cutaneous is a direct branch of the medial cord and supplies skin of the medial side of the forearm.

E. The dorsal cutaneous branch of the ulnar nerve supplies the medial half of the dorsum of the hand.
GAS 750, 782; N 422; ABR/McM 152

57. C. The seventh cervical nerve makes a major contribution to the radial nerve, and this nerve is the prime mover in wrist extension. The dermatome of C7 is in the region described, which runs down the posterior arm, forearm, and hand and over digits 2 and 3.

A. Loss of C5 would affect shoulder movement and skin over the deltoid.

B. C6 loss would affect arm flexion and skin on the lateral side of the upper limb.

D. C8 loss would affect forearm muscles primarily and skin on the medial side of the upper limb.

E. T1 loss would affect hand muscles and skin of the arm medially.
GAS 734, 777, 780; N 420; ABR/McM 162

58. B. As the radial artery passes from the ventral surface to the dorsum of the wrist, it crosses through the anatomical snuffbox and passes over the scaphoid bone.

A. The ulnar artery is located on the medial side of the wrist, passing from beneath the flexor carpi ulnaris to reach Guyon canal between the pisiform bone and the flexor retinaculum. Guyon canal is adjacent to but not in communication with the carpal tunnel.

C and D. The anterior interosseous and posterior interosseous arteries arise from the common interosse-

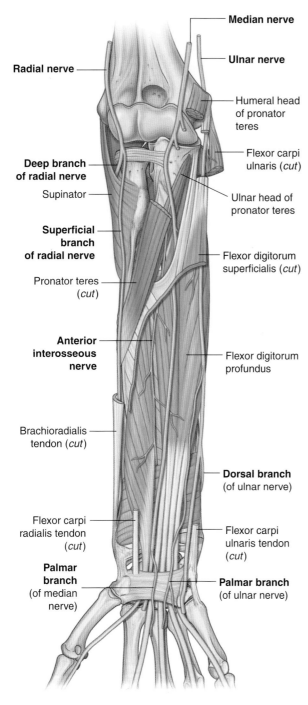

• GAS Fig. 7.89

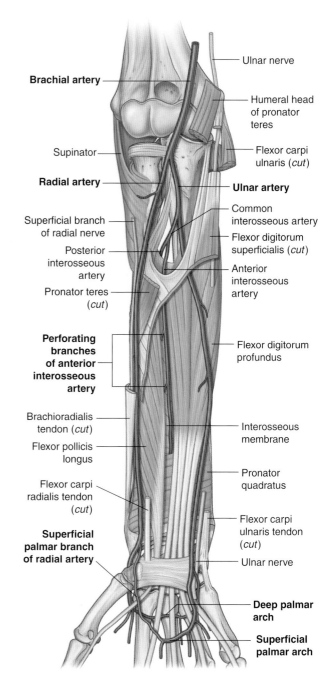

• GAS Fig. 7.88

ous branch of the ulnar artery and pass proximal to distal in the forearm between the radius and ulna, in the flexor and extensor compartments, respectively.

E. The deep palmar branch of the ulnar artery passes between the two heads of the adductor pollicis to anastomose with the radial artery in the palm (*GAS* Fig. 7.88).

GAS 801–805; N 457; ABR/McM 176

59. D. The patient is suffering from subacromial or subdeltoid bursitis. (If the pain on palpation is less when the arm has been elevated to the horizontal, the bursitis may be thought of as being more subacromial, that is, associated more with the supraspinatus tendon

perhaps, for such a bursa may be drawn back under the acromion when the limb is abducted.)

A. The subscapular bursa, beneath the subscapularis muscle, would not present as superficial pain. It can communicate with the glenohumeral joint cavity.

B. The main function of the infraspinatus muscle is lateral rotation of the shoulder. The infraspinatus muscle is not involved in overhead shoulder movements.

C. Inflammation or arthritic changes within the glenohumeral joint present as more generalized shoulder pain than that present here.

E. The teres minor muscle and tendon are located inferior to the point of marked discomfort.
GAS 696, 713; N 424; ABR/McM 142

60. E. The axillary sheath is a fascial continuation of the prevertebral layer of the deep cervical fascia extending into the axilla. It encloses the nerves of the neurovascular bundle of the upper limb.

A and B. Superficial fascia is loose connective tissue between the dermis and the deep investing fascia and contains fat, cutaneous vessels, nerves, lymphatics, and glands. C. The buccopharyngeal fascia covers the buccinator muscles and the pharynx is continuous anteriorly with the pretracheal fascia.

D. The clavipectoral fascia invests the clavicle and pectoralis minor muscle. The axillary fascia is continuous with the pectoral and latissimus dorsi fascia and forms the hollow of the armpit.
GAS 710, 730; N 416; ABR/McM 367

61. C. The accessory nerve (CN XI) arises from the ventral rootlets of C1–C4 that ascend through the foramen magnum to then exit the cranial cavity through the jugular foramen. It innervates the sternocleidomastoid and trapezius muscles, which function in head rotation and elevating the shoulders.

A. The suprascapular nerve receives fibers from C5 to C6 (occasionally from C4 if the plexus is "prefixed") and innervates the supraspinatus muscle, which is responsible for the first 15 degrees of arm abduction. Erb point of the brachial plexus is at the union of C5–C6 spinal nerves.

B. The long thoracic nerve arises from plexus routes C5, C6, and C7, and supplies the serratus anterior.

D. The accessory nerve (CN XI) arises from the ventral rootlets of C1–C4.

E. Radial nerve is not involved in rotation of the neck.
GAS 703; N 422; ABR/McM 138

62. D. The AC ligament connects the clavicle and the acromion of the scapula. Separation of the shoulder, also known as AC joint separation, is associated with damage to the AC joint and the AC ligament which reinforces it. In more severe forms, the coracoclavicular ligament may also be damaged. The glenohumeral ligaments or bands may be injured by an anterior dislocation of the humerus but are not likely to be injured by a separated shoulder. The coracoacromial ligament, superior transverse scapular ligament, and tendon of the long head of triceps brachii are not likely to be injured by separation of the shoulder.

A. Glenohumeral ligament: The glenohumeral ligaments or bands may be injured by an anterior dislocation of the humerus but are not likely to be injured by a separated shoulder.

B. Coracoacromial ligament: This ligament attaches the coracoid process to the acromion. It protects the head of the humerus. This ligament is not likely to be injured by separation of the shoulder.

C. Tendon of long head of biceps brachii: This tendon arises from the supraglenoid tubercle above the glenoid cavity of the scapula, then runs through the intertubercular sulcus of the humerus and attaches to the radial tuberosity of the radius. This ligament is not likely to be injured by separation of the shoulder.

D. Transverse scapular ligament: This ligament connects two borders of the scapular notch on the upper border of the scapula. The suprascapular nerve passes below this ligament. It is not likely to be injure by separation of the shoulder.
GAS 694; N 410; ABR/McM 142

63. A. The quadrangular space is bordered medially by the long head of the triceps brachii muscle, laterally by the surgical neck of the humerus, superiorly by the teres minor muscle, and inferiorly by the teres major muscle. Both the axillary nerve and posterior circumflex humeral vessels traverse this space.

B, C, D, E. The other structures listed are not contained within the quadrangular space. The cephalic vein is located in the deltopectoral triangle, and the radial nerve is located in the triangular interval between the lateral and long heads of the triceps brachii.
GAS 718–720, 730; N 417; ABR/McM 144

64. B. Froment sign is positive for ulnar nerve palsy. More specifically it tests the action of the adductor pollicis muscle. The patient is asked to hold a sheet of paper between the thumb and a flat palm.

A. The flexor pollicis longus is innervated by the anterior interosseous branch of the median nerve.

C. The flexor digiti minimi is innervated by the deep branch of the ulnar nerve and would not be used to hold a sheet of paper between the thumb and palm.

D. The flexor carpi radialis is innervated by the median nerve.

E. The extensor indicis is innervated by the deep radial nerve (Fig. 6.13).
GAS 814–816, 826; N 467; ABR/McM 166

65. C. The recurrent branch of the median nerve innervates the thenar muscles (opponens pollicis, abductor pollicis brevis, and flexor pollicis brevis) and is not responsible for any cutaneous innervation. Damage to the palmar cutaneous branches of the median or ulnar nerve would not cause weakness of opposition of the thumb for they are principally sensory in function.

A. The first common palmar digital branch of the median nerve is not responsible for movement of the thenar muscles.

B. The second common palmar digital branch of the median nerve is not responsible for movement of the thenar muscles.

D. The deep branch of the ulnar nerve supplies the hypothenar muscles, adductor and abductor muscles of digits 2 to 5, and adductor pollicis and does not innervate the abductor pollicis brevis.

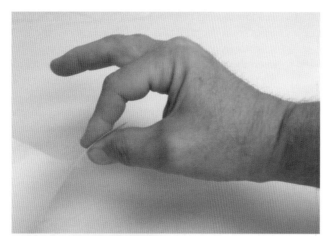

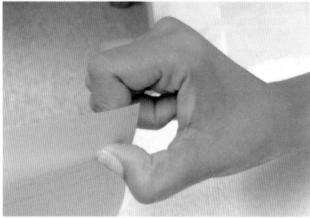

• Fig. 6.13

E. Anterior interosseous nerve supplies the deep muscles of the flexor forearm. It is not responsible for movement of the thenar muscles.
GAS 817; N 466; ABR/McM 168

66. D. Injury to the deep branch of the ulnar nerve results in paralysis of all interosseous muscles and the lumbrical muscles of the fourth and fifth digits. Extension of the MCP joints is intact, which is a function of the radial nerve. IP extension of the fourth and fifth digits is absent, due to the loss of their respective lumbricals and the loss of all interosseous muscles. Some weak IP joint extension is still present in the second and third digits because the lumbricals of these two fingers are innervated by the median nerve.
A and B. The radial nerve and the median nerve appear to be intact in this case.
C. If the ulnar nerve were injured in the mid-forearm region, there would be sensory loss in the palm and digits 4 and 5 and on the dorsum of the hand.
E. The recurrent branch of the median nerve supplies the thenar muscles; it does not supply lumbricals. Moreover, paralysis of this nerve would have no effect on the IP joints.
GAS 805–807; N 467; ABR/McM 168

67. A. The thoracodorsal artery arises from the subscapular artery. It provides the latissimus dorsi.
B. The dorsal scapular artery passes between the ventral rami of the brachial plexus and then deep rhomboid muscles along the medial border of the scapula.
C. The transverse cervical artery arises from the thyrocervical trunk at the root of the neck and can provide origin for a dorsal scapular branch (in 30%).
D and E. The lateral thoracic and thoracoacromial arteries are branches of the second part of the axillary artery and provide no supply to the latissimus dorsi.
GAS 709–710; N 418; ABR/McM 149

68. C. The surgical neck of the humerus is a typical site of fractures. The fracture line lies above the insertions of the pectoralis major, teres major, and latissimus dorsi muscles. The supraspinatus muscle abducts the proximal fragment, whereas the distal fragment is elevated and adducted. The elevation results from contraction of the deltoid, biceps brachii, and coracobrachialis muscles. The adduction is due to the action of pectoralis major, teres major, and latissimus dorsi.
A, B, D, E. These answer choices will not result in adduction of the distal aspect of the fragmented humerus.
GAS 693; N 417; ABR/McM 148

69. B. The fracture line of the upper third of the radius lies between the bony attachments of the supinator and the pronator teres muscles. The distal radial fragment and hand are pronated due to unopposed contraction of pronator teres (A) and pronator quadratus (C) muscles. The proximal fragment deviates laterally by the unopposed contraction of the supinator muscle.
D. The brachioradialis inserts distally on the radius.
E. The brachialis inserts on the coronoid process of the ulna and would not be involved in the lateral deviation of the radius.
GAS 762–764; N 435; ABR/McM 161

70. A. The palmaris longus passes along the midline of the flexor surface of the forearm and passes distally superficial to the flexor retinaculum.
B. The flexor carpi radialis is seen in the lateral portion of the forearm superficially, passing over the trapezium to insert at the base of the second metacarpal.
C. The abductor pollicis longus tendon is laterally located in the wrist, where it helps form the lateral border of the anatomical snuffbox.
D. The flexor carpi ulnaris tendon can be seen and palpated on the medial side of the wrist ventrally.
E. The flexor pollicis longus tendon passes deep through the carpal tunnel.
GAS 767; N 437; ABR/McM 167

71. B. The patient has fractured the neck of the 5th metacarpal when hitting the machine with his fist. This type of fracture is known as a "boxer's fracture."
A, C, D. Neither a fracture of the ulnar styloid nor a Colles fracture nor Smith fracture of the distal radius

would present with the absence of a knuckle as observed here.

    E. Bennett fracture involves dislocation of the CMC joint of the thumb. Indications are that the injury is on the medial side of the hand, not the wrist, nor the lateral side of the hand or wrist.
GAS 783–784; N 443; ABR/McM 173

72. **E.** Scoliosis (severe lateral curvature of the spine) in the patient is causing compression or stretching of the T1 spinal nerve ramus by the first rib as the nerve ascends to join C8 and form the lower trunk of the brachial plexus. T1 provides sensation for the medial side of the forearm, via the medial antebrachial cutaneous nerve from the medial cord of the brachial plexus. T1 is the principal source of motor supply to all of the intrinsic muscles in the palm. Its dysfunction affects all fine motor movements of the digits. Long flexors of the fingers are intact; therefore, the median nerve (A) and ulnar nerve are not injured. The extensors of the wrist are functional; therefore, the radial nerve (C) is not paralyzed. The only sensory disturbance is that of the T1 dermatome.

    B and D. The compression of middle and lower trunk of the brachial plexus would not give rise to the symptoms observed in this patient.
GAS 683–687, 744–745; N 170; ABR/McM 98

73. **D.** "Gamekeeper's thumb" was a term coined because this injury was most commonly associated with Scottish gamekeepers who killed small animals such as rabbits by breaking their necks between the ground, the thumb, and the index finger. The resulting valgus force on the abducted MCP joint caused injury to the ulnar collateral ligament. These days this injury is more commonly seen in skiers who land awkwardly with their hand braced on a ski pole, causing the valgus force on the thumb.

    A. De Quervain syndrome (tenosynovitis) affects the tendons of the lateral aspect of the wrist. It presents with wrist pain upon turning the wrist, grasping, or making a fist.

    B. A navicular fracture is also known as a scaphoid fracture. The scaphoid is the carpal bone which is most likely to be fractured.

    C. A boxer's thumb is a fracture dislocation at the base of the thumb.

    E. Bennett thumb refers to fracture of the base of the first metacarpal bone. It continues to the CMC joint.
GAS 785–786; N 443; ABR/McM 172

74. **A.** The long head of the biceps brachii muscle assists in shoulder flexion and during a tendinopathy would cause pain in the anterior compartment of the shoulder, where it originates at the supraglenoid tubercle. Forced contraction would cause a greater tension force on the tendon that will result in more pain.

    B. Pain will not be felt in the lateral shoulder during forced contraction of the biceps brachii muscle as

the heads of the biceps originates from the supraglenoid tubercle and the coracoid process of the scapula.

    C. Pain will not be felt during abduction and flexion of the shoulder joint as this movement is not a function of the biceps brachii muscle.

    D. Contraction of the biceps brachii muscle will result in flexion of the arm; extension and adduction of the arm is not a function of this muscle.

    E. The patient will not experience pain in the lateral shoulder during flexion of the shoulder joint.
GAS 721; N 423; ABR/McM 142

75. **C.** The common extensor tendon originates from the lateral epicondyle, and inflammation of this tendon is lateral epicondylitis, nicknamed "tennis elbow" because the tendon is often irritated during the backhand stroke in tennis. Because the extensors of the wrist originate as part of the common extensor tendon, resisted extension of the wrist will exacerbate the pain of lateral epicondylitis.

    A. Nerve conduction studies are used to confirm signs and symptoms that are consistent with neuropathies (e.g., numbness and paresthesia) such as in carpal tunnel syndrome.

    B. In tennis elbow, there would be no pain on flexion or passive extension of the elbow as the extensor carpi radialis brevis only abduct and extend the wrist.

    D. The numbness and tingling in the fourth and fifth digit will not present in tennis elbow. These signs are consistent with medial epicondylitis (golfer's elbow).

    E. Tenderness will not be felt over the distal styloid process of the radius in tennis elbow. The origin of the forearm common extensor tendon is located at the proximal forearm. The brachioradialis is a forearm extensor muscle and will contribute to symptoms of lateral epicondylitis.
GAS 757, 775; N 431; ABR/McM 161

Answers 76–100

76. **C.** The axillary nerve passes dorsally beside the surgical neck of the humerus (accompanied by the posterior circumflex humeral artery) and can be injured when the humerus is fractured at that location. The axillary nerve provides sensation to the skin over the upper, lateral aspect of the shoulder. Although the patient might not be able to abduct the arm from 15 to 90 degrees because of the injury (A), a simple test of skin sensation can indicate whether there is associated nerve injury of the axillary nerve.

    B. Shrugging the shoulders can help assess trapezius function, thereby testing the performance of the accessory nerve (CN XI).

    D. Intact sensation of the skin on the medial aspect of the axilla and arm is an indication that the medial brachial cutaneous and intercostobrachial nerves are functional.

E. Pushing against an immovable object tests the serratus anterior muscle and the long thoracic nerve.

GAS 707–709; N 468; ABR/McM 145

77. E. The surgeon took the distal segments of the median nerves from both forearms, instead of the palmaris longus tendons. Both of the structures lie in the midline of the ventral surface of the distal forearm and often have similar appearance in color and diameter. The nerve is located deep to the tendon, when the tendon is present. When the tendon of the palmaris longus is absent, the median nerve appears to be in the anatomical position of the tendon.

A. There is no evidence of rib fractures. Additionally, a fractured rib would not explain loss of sensation on the lateral portion of the palm.

B. Lower plexus trauma (C8, T1) would result in paralysis of forearm flexor muscles and all intrinsic hand muscles and sensory loss over the medial dorsum and palmar surfaces of the hand.

C. Dupuytren contracture is a flexion contracture of (usually) digits 4 and 5 from connective tissue disease in the palm.

D. Radial nerve injury in the posterior forearm would affect MCP joint extension, thumb extension, and so on, not palmar disturbances.

GAS 774–775; N 437; ABR/McM 159

78. C. Trauma both to the median and ulnar nerves at the wrist results in total clawing of the fingers. The MCP joints of all digits are extended by the unopposed extensors because the radial nerve is intact. All interossei and lumbricals are paralyzed because the deep branch of the ulnar nerve supplies all of the interossei; lumbricals I and II are paralyzed, as they are innervated by the median nerve; lumbricals III and IV are paralyzed, since the deep ulnar nerve provides their motor innervation. The interossei and lumbricals are responsible for extension of the IP joints. When they are paralyzed, the long flexor tendons pull the fingers into a position of flexion, completing the "claw" appearance.

A. If ulnar nerve was only damaged and median nerve spared, the clawing of the hand would be less prominent in the index and middle fingers. This is because the lumbricals of those digits would still be capable of some degree of extension of those IP joints.

B. If the median nerve alone is injured in the carpal tunnel, there would be loss of thenar opposition but not clawing.

D. If the median and ulnar nerves are both transected at the elbow, the hand appears totally flat because of the loss of long flexors, in addition to paralysis of the intrinsic muscle of the hand. E. Radial nerve at mid-humerus would be intact in this patient.

GAS 774, 805–809; N 438; ABR/McM 166

79. D. Smith fracture is a fracture of the distal radius with the distal fragment displaced in a volar direction. Smith fracture is sometimes referred to as a reverse Colles fracture.

A. Colles fracture is a fracture of the distal radius with the distal fragment displaced dorsally.

B. The scaphoid is the most commonly fractured bone in the wrist and does not involve the radius.

C. Bennett thumb (boxer's thumb) refers to fracture of the base of the first metacarpal bone. It continues to the CMC joint.

E. A boxer's fracture is a fracture of the 5th metacarpal neck.

GAS 761–764; N 443; ABR/McM 162

80. E. The extensor tendons of the fingers insert distally on the distal phalanx of each digit. If the tendon is avulsed, or the proximal part of the distal phalanx is detached, the DIP joint is pulled into total flexion by the unopposed flexor digitorum profundus muscle. This result gives the digit the appearance of a mallet.

A. Claw hand occurs with lesions to the median and ulnar nerves at the wrist. In this clinical problem all intrinsic muscles are paralyzed, including the extensors of the IP joints. The MCP joint extensors, supplied by the radial nerve, and the long flexors of the fingers, supplied more proximally in the forearm by the median and ulnar nerves, are intact and are unopposed, pulling the fingers into the "claw" appearance.

B. In boutonnière deformity, the central portion of the extensor tendon expansion is torn over the PIP joint, allowing the tendon to move toward the palmar, causing the tendon to act as a flexor of the PIP joint. This causes the DIP joint to be hyperextended.

C. Swan-neck deformity involves slight flexion of the MCP joints, hyperextension of PIP joints, and slight flexion of DIP joints. This condition results most often from shortening of the tendons of intrinsic muscles, as in rheumatoid arthritis.

D. Dupuytren contracture results from connective tissue disorder in the palm, usually causing irreversible flexion of digits 4 and 5.

GAS 777–780, 802; N 454; ABR/McM 162

81. A. Because the median nerve is injured within the cubital fossa, the long flexors are paralyzed, including the flexor pollicis longus muscle. Loss of lateral palmar sensation also confirms median nerve injury.

B. If only the anterior interosseous nerve were damaged, there would be no cutaneous sensory deficits.

C. The radial nerve supplies wrist extensors, long thumb abductor, and MCP joint extensors. The radial nerve also supplies cutaneous innervation to the dorsum of the hand. D. The flexor pollicis longus would not be paralyzed if the median nerve were injured at the wrist.

E. The ulnar nerve does not supply sensation to the lateral palm.
GAS 757, 795; N 438; ABR/McM 158

82. D. The physical examination findings of this patient are consistent with Klumpke palsy. Most cases of Klumpke palsy are associated with birth injuries. However, the injury can occur in older children and adults if they injure the C8 and T1 nerves, as in this case where the patient fell from a tree and reached for a tree branch to break a fall. In a lesion of the lower trunk of the brachial plexus, or the C8 and T1 ventral rami, there is sensory loss on the medial arm and forearm and the medial side of the hand (dorsal and ventral). The medial cord is an extension of the lower trunk. The medial cord gives origin to the medial brachial and medial antebrachial cutaneous nerve, which supplies the T1 dermatome of the medial side of the brachium and antebrachium.

A. The inferior lateral brachial cutaneous nerve arises from the radial nerve, C5 and C6 which itself arises from the upper trunk of the brachial plexus.

B. The musculocutaneous nerve arises from the lateral cord, ending in the lateral antebrachial cutaneous nerve, with C5 and C6 dermatome fibers.

C. The intercostobrachial nerve is the lateral cutaneous branch of the T2 ventral primary ramus and supplies skin on the medial side of the arm.

E. The median nerve distributes C6 and C7 sensory fibers to the lateral part of the palm, thumb, index, middle finger, and half of the ring finger.
GAS 729–734; N 420; ABR/McM 144

83. C. The lateral pectoral nerve is typically the only source of motor supply to the clavicular head of the pectoralis major muscle. If it is injured (as in this case of an iatrogenic injury when the apical axillary lymph nodes were removed), this part of the muscle undergoes atrophy, leaving an infraclavicular cosmetic deficit.

A and B. The medial pectoral nerve provides motor supply to the sternocostal part of the pectoralis major and all of the pectoralis minor. Physical examination reveals no obvious motor or sensory deficits.

D. Loss of the medial pectoral nerve would have no effect on the clavicular head of pectoralis major.

E. Injury to the lateral cord would lead to loss not only of all of the lateral pectoral nerve but also the musculocutaneous nerve, resulting in biceps brachii and brachialis paralysis and lateral antebrachial sensory loss, and loss of the proximal distribution of the median nerve.
GAS 713, 731; N 419; ABR/McM 149

84. B. The C6 spinal nerve is primarily responsible for the brachioradialis reflex.

A and B. C5 and C6 are both involved in the biceps brachii reflex; C5 for motor, C6 for the sensory part of the reflex arc; C7 is the key spinal nerve in the triceps reflex.

D. C8 is responsible for the finger jerk reflex.
E. T1 is not responsible for deep tendon reflexes.
GAS 744; N 437; ABR/McM 151

85. C. The main spinal nerve that contributes to the radial nerve and innervates the triceps brachii is C7. Absence of the triceps reflex is usually indicative of a C7 radiculopathy or injury.

A and B. The C5 and C6 spinal nerves are involved in the biceps brachii reflex pathway.

D and E. The C8 and T1 spinal nerves are not involved in reflexes of the upper limb.
GAS 734–735, 756; N 420; ABR/McM 152

86. B. Ginglymus joint is the correct technical term to describe a hinge joint. It allows motion in one axis (flexion and extension in the case of the humeroulnar joint) and is therefore a uniaxial joint.

A, C, D, E. The other types of joints listed allow motion in more than one axis.
GAS 19, 753; N 445; ABR/McM 126

87. C. A fracture of the humerus just proximal to the epicondyles is called a supracondylar fracture. This is the most common cause of a Volkmann ischemic fracture. The sharp bony fragment often lacerates the brachial (or other) artery, with bleeding into the flexor compartment. Diminution of arterial supply to the distal limb results in the ischemia. Bleeding into the compartment causes greatly increased pressure, first blocking venous outflow from the compartment, then reducing the arterial flow into and through the compartment as the pressure rises to arterial levels. The ischemic muscles then undergo unrelieved contracture. A humeral fracture is sometimes placed in a cast from shoulder to wrist, often concealing the ischemia until major tissue loss occurs. Cold, insensate digits, and great pain are warnings of this compartment syndrome, demanding that the cast be removed and the compartment opened ("released") for pressure reduction and vascular repair.

A. Fracture of the surgical neck endangers the axillary nerve and posterior circumflex humeral artery, although not ischemic contracture.

B. Fracture of the humerus in the radial groove can injure the radial nerve and deep brachial artery.

D. Fracture of the olecranon does not result in Volkmann contracture, although the triceps brachii can displace the distal fracture fragment of the ulna.

E. Fracture of the lateral epicondyle is quite rare. This type of fracture usually occurs as a result of sudden traction on the common extensor origin by the extensor muscles or due to direct trauma.
GAS 755; N 424; ABR/McM 158

88. D. Normally the distal part of the ulna articulates only with the radius at the distal radioulnar joint at the wrist, a joint that participates in pronation and supination.

A, B, C. The head of the ulna does not articulate with any of the carpal bones; instead, it is separated from the triquetrum and lunate bones by the triangular fibrocartilage complex between it and the radius.

E. The pisiform articulates with the triquetrum. The carpal articulation of the radius is primarily that of the scaphoid (the old name is navicular) bone.

GAS 753–754; N 442; ABR/McM 129

89. **A.** The force of the woman's fall on the outstretched hand was transmitted up through the forearm, in this case resulting in dislocation of the olecranon at the elbow, putting traction on the ulnar nerve as it passes around the medial epicondyle of the humerus. Ulnar trauma at the elbow can cause weakness in medial flexion (adduction) at the wrist, from loss of the flexor carpi ulnaris. Ulnar nerve injury also results in sensory loss in the medial hand and paralysis of the interossei and medial two lumbricals, with clawing especially of fourth and fifth digits.

B. Injury of the ulnar nerve at the pisiform bone would not affect the flexor carpi ulnaris, nor would it produce sensory loss on the dorsum of the hand because the dorsal cutaneous branch of the ulnar branches off proximal to the wrist.

C. Carpal tunnel problems affect median nerve function, which is not indicated in this patient's case.

D. The ulnar nerve passes medial to the cubital fossa between the heads of the flexor carpi ulnaris, not between the heads of the flexor digitorum superficialis.

E. Injuries at the radial neck affect the site of division of the radial nerve, and its paralysis would not result in the clinical problems seen in this patient.

GAS 757, 784; N 467; ABR/McM 153

90. **D.** The interossei are the most important muscles in extension of the IP joints because of the manner of their insertion into the extensor expansion of the fingers, which passes dorsal to the transverse axes of these joints. The lumbrical muscles assist in IP extension, in addition to flexing the MCP joints. Ulnar nerve injury at the wrist results in paralysis of all the interossei and the medial two lumbricals as well as the adductor pollicis.

A. Impairment of thumb opposition is a manifestation of median nerve injury or injury to the opponens pollicis. The median nerve lies in the midline of the wrist deep to the flexor retinaculum. The patient's injury and physical examination findings are inconsistent with median nerve injury.

B. The ulnar nerve supplies cutaneous innervation to the palmar surface and dorsum of the fifth and medial half of the fourth digit. However, the cutaneous branch of the ulnar nerve (dorsal branch of the ulnar nerve) originates from the ulnar nerve at the distal ⅓ of the forearm which is proximal to the wrist. An injury of the ulnar nerve at the wrist would not result in sensory deficits in the hands.

C. Extensors of the MCP joints are innervated by the deep radial nerve. Unopposed extension of the MCP joints causes them to be held in extension

whereas unopposed long flexors of the fingers (supplied by median and ulnar nerves proximally in the forearm) cause them to be flexed into the "claw" position. The lumbricals of digits 2 and 3 are still intact because they are supplied by the median nerve, so clawing is not seen as much on these digits. Loss of opposition would result from median or recurrent nerve paralysis.

E. This statement is false.

GAS 799–800; N 454; ABR/McM 168

91. **B.** In boutonnière deformity, the central portion of the extensor tendon expansion is torn over the PIP joint, allowing the tendon to move toward the palm, causing the tendon to act as a flexor of the PIP joint. This causes the DIP joint to be hyperextended. The tear in the extensor tendon is said to resemble a buttonhole (boutonnière in French), and the head of the proximal phalanx may stick through the hole.

A, C, D, E. None of the other answer choices would cause this distinctive appearance.

GAS 784–786; N 454; ABR/McM 176

92. **D.** Swan-neck deformity involves slight flexion of the MCP joints, hyperextension of the PIP joints, and slight flexion of the DIP joints. This condition results most often from shortening of the tendons of intrinsic muscles, as in rheumatoid arthritis. When asked to straighten the injured finger, the patient is unable to do so and the curvature of the finger somewhat resembles the neck of a swan.

A, B, C, E. None of the other answer choices would cause this appearance.

GAS 784–786; N 454; ABR/McM 168

93. **C.** The long thoracic nerve was injured during the axillary dissection, resulting in paralysis of the serratus anterior muscle. The serratus anterior is important in upward rotation of the scapula in raising the arm above the level of the shoulder. Its loss results in protrusion of the medial border ("winging" of the scapula), which is more obvious when one pushes against resistance. The long thoracic nerve arises from the ventral rami of C5, C6, and C7.

A. The upper trunk (C5, C6) supplies rotator and abductor muscles of the shoulder and elbow flexors.

B. The posterior division of the middle trunk contains C7 fibers for distribution to extensor muscles; likewise, the posterior cord supplies extensors of the arm, forearm, and hand.

D. The axillary nerve and radial nerve originate from the posterior cord of the brachial plexus. These nerves provide motor innervation to the deltoid and arm extensor respectively. Thus an injury to these nerves will not result in wing scapula.

E. The lateral cord (C5, C6, and C7) gives origin to the lateral pectoral nerve, the musculocutaneous nerve, and the lateral root of the median nerve. There is no sensory loss in the limb in this patient;

injury to any of the other nerve elements listed here would be associated with specific dermatome losses. *GAS 715–716; N 417; ABR/McM 144*

94. B. Dupuytren contracture or deformity is a result of fibromatosis of the palmar aponeurosis, resulting in irregular thickening of the fascial attachments to the skin, which causes gradual contraction of the digits, especially the fourth and fifth digits. In 50% of cases, it is bilateral in occurrence.

   A. Ape hand, or flat hand, is a result of loss of the median and ulnar nerves at the elbow, with paralysis of all long flexors of the fingers and all intrinsic hand muscles. The term can also be specific for just median nerve injury and a flattened thenar eminence.

   C. Claw hand results from paralysis of IP joint extension by interossei and lumbricals, innervated primarily by the ulnar nerve.

   D. Wrist drop occurs with radial nerve paralysis and loss of the extensors carpi radialis longus and brevis.

   E. Mallet finger results from detachment of the extensor mechanism from the distal phalanx of a finger and unopposed flexion of that DIP joint.

   GAS 791; N 449; ABR/McM 166

95. A. The axillary nerve is a direct branch of the posterior cord and wraps around the surgical neck of the humerus to innervate the teres minor and the deltoid muscles. With this anatomical arrangement, the axillary nerve is tightly "tethered" to the proximal humerus. When the head of the humerus is dislocated anteriorly, it often puts traction on the axillary nerve.

   B, C, D, E. These nerves are not injured in an anterior shoulder dislocation.

   GAS 707–708; N 417; ABR/McM 150

96. A. The tendon of the long head of the biceps brachii muscle runs in the intertubercular groove on the proximal humerus as it changes direction and turns medially to attach to the supraglenoid tubercle of the scapula. This change in direction within an osseous structure predisposes the tendon to wear and tear, particularly in people who overuse the biceps brachii muscle. This type of injury presents with a characteristic sign called the "Popeye sign" after the cartoon character.

   B. Midportion of the biceps brachii muscle is an unlikely area for rupture of the muscle and loss of the biceps brachii reflex.

   C. Junction with the short head of the biceps brachii muscle is an unlikely area for rupture of the muscle and loss of the biceps brachii reflex.

   D. The combined tendon that travels through the intertubercular groove is more vulnerable to injury.

   E. The tendon is more vulnerable to injury due to its course through the intertubercular groove.

   GAS 720–721; N 421; ABR/McM 120

97. C. The supraspinatus muscle inserts on the greater tubercle of the humerus and is said to initiate abduction of the arm at the shoulder. It is supplied principally by spinal nerve C5.

   A. The subscapularis muscle is the only muscle that inserts on the lesser tubercle.

   B. The supraspinatus muscle does not initiate adduction of the arm but rather abduction.

   D. The subscapularis muscle is innervated by the upper and lower subscapular nerves.

   E. The teres minor muscle takes origin from the lateral border of the scapula; the teres major muscle takes origin from the region of the inferior angle and the lateral border of the scapula.

   GAS 706; N 415; ABR/McM 121

98. E. During a fall on an outstretched upper limb, the forces are conducted through the hand on up through the bones of the limb in succession. Often these bones do not fracture but rather pass the compressive forces proximally. The appendicular skeleton joins with the axial skeleton at the sternoclavicular joint. The forces are not sufficiently transferred to the sternum, causing the clavicle to absorb the force, resulting in the common pediatric fracture of this sigmoidal-shaped bone.

   A, B, C, D. The clavicle is the most common fractured bone in this scenario.

   GAS 699; N 465; ABR/McM 118

99. C. The patient is suffering from thoracic outlet syndrome, involving neural and vascular elements. This results from any condition that decreases the dimensions of the superior thoracic aperture (the formal name of the thoracic outlet). It could be a result of a cervical rib, accessory muscles, and/or atypical connective tissue bands at the root of the neck. In this case, symptoms involve the arm, forearm, and hand. Paresthesia along the medial forearm and hand and atrophy of long flexors and intrinsic muscles point to a possible compression or traction problem of the lower trunk (C8, T1) rather than a lesion of either the median or ulnar nerve. The lateral palm has no sensory problem, which tends to rule out median nerve involvement. Changes in the radial artery pulse point to vascular compression.

   A. Erb-Duchenne paralysis of the upper trunk would affect proximal limb functions, such as arm rotation and abduction.

   B. This lesion is on the left side, so the brachiocephalic trunk could not be involved because it arises from the right side of the aortic arch; moreover, it would not compress the brachial plexus.

   D. Carpal tunnel syndrome would not explain the problems of the forearm and medial hand, or the long flexor atrophy.

   E. An isolated medial cord lesion would not explain the atrophy of all long flexors and intrinsic muscles and does not explain the radial pulse characteristics. The ischemic pain in the arm is due to vascular compression.

GAS 151; N 192; ABR/McM 144

100. A. The ulnar nerve enters the forearm by passing between the two heads of the flexor carpi ulnaris and descends between and innervates the flexor carpi ulnaris (for medial wrist deviation) and flexor digitorum profundus (medial half) muscles. Injuring the ulnar nerve results in claw hand. It enters the hand superficial to the flexor retinaculum and lateral to the pisiform bone, where it is vulnerable to damage.

B. The ulnar nerve also enters Guyon canal, the passage between the pisiform and hook of the hamate at the wrist, but damage to it here would not present with the aforementioned symptoms.

C. The median nerve enters the carpal tunnel and the radial nerve passes deep to the brachioradialis.

D. The median nerve passes between the ulnar and radial heads of origin of flexor digitorum superficialis and does not give rise to the symptoms observed.

E. The radial nerve passes deep to brachioradialis muscle and has nothing to do with the patient's presentation.

GAS 767, 774; N 467; ABR/McM 153

Answers 101–125

101. B. During a breech delivery as described here, downward traction is applied to the shoulders and upper limbs as the baby is forcibly extracted from the birth canal. This exerts traction on the upper trunk of the brachial plexus, often causing a traction injury from which the baby can often recover. If the ventral rami of C5 and C6 are avulsed from the spinal cord, the injury is permanent.

A, C, D, E. These nerves are not commonly injured by this mechanism.

GAS 729, 736; N 420; ABR/McM 35

102. E. Striking the concrete blocks with the medial side of her hand has injured the ulnar nerve in Guyon canal. This is the triangular tunnel formed by the pisiform bone medially, the flexor retinaculum attaching to the hook of the hamate laterally, and the palmar carpal ligament anteriorly. This injury would result in loss of sensation to the medial palm and the palmar surface of the medial one and a half digits and motor loss of the hypothenar muscles, the interossei, and the medial two lumbricals.

A. The median nerve is not involved because the thenar muscles and lateral palmar sensations are intact.

B. The dorsal branch of the ulnar nerve arises proximal to the wrist, thus it would not be lost.

C. If the lunate bone (the most frequently dislocated carpal bone) were dislocated, it would not cause compression of the ulnar nerve at the wrist.

D. There is no indication of fifth metacarpal fracture, the so-called boxer's fracture.

GAS 774, 805–806; N 452; ABR/McM 168

103. E. The common flexor sheath or ulnar bursa encloses the long flexor tendons of the fingers in the carpal tunnel and proximal palm. This sheath is usually continuous with the flexor sheath of the little (fifth) finger, which continues within the palm, having no connection with sheaths of the other digits (A, B, C, D), which do not extend into the digits.

GAS 791–793; N 451; ABR/McM 167

104. C. The infectious agent was introduced into the synovial sheath of the long tendons of the little (fifth) finger. Proximally, this sheath runs through the midpalmar space (or central compartment), and inflammatory processes typically rupture into this space unless aggressively treated with the appropriate antibiotics

A, B, D. These compartments do not correlate with the long tendons of the fifth finger.

E. The thenar space contains the flexor pollicis longus within its synovial sheath, the tendons of the index finger, first lumbrical muscle, and the palmar digital vessels and nerves of the thumb and lateral portion of the index finger.

GAS 800–801; N 451; ABR/McM 167

105. A. Axillary-subclavian vein thrombosis is becoming much more common in recent years because of the extensive use of catheters in cancer patients and other chronic medical conditions. Effort-induced thrombosis is seen with strenuous use of the dominant arm with hyperabduction and lateral rotation of the arm, or backward and downward rotation of the shoulder as in playing cricket, volleyball, baseball, or chopping wood. The symptoms of subclavian stenosis are fairly dramatic; most patients present promptly, usually within 24 hours. They complain of a dull ache in the shoulder and axilla, with worsening pain upon activity. Conversely, rest and elevation often relieve the pain. Patients with catheter-associated axillary-subclavian deep vein thrombosis have similar symptoms at the arm or shoulder on the side with the indwelling catheter.

B, C, D, E. These conditions are not complications of central venous line placement.

GAS 748; N 419; ABR/McM 218

106. C. The injury is at the second part of the axillary artery. The suprascapular artery is a branch of the thyrocervical trunk off the subclavian artery, proximal to the axillary artery. The subscapular artery is the major branch of the third part of the axillary artery, giving off the thoracodorsal and the circumflex scapular arteries. In this case blood from the suprascapular artery would be flowing into the circumflex scapular artery and then in a retrograde direction into the axillary artery, supplying blood distal to the injury.

A, B, D, E These arteries do not provide collateral circulation around the scapula.
GAS 709–710; N 424; ABR/McM 140

107. A. This proximal injury to the median nerve would paralyze all of the long flexors of the digits, except for the medial half of the flexor digitorum profundus muscle that flexes the DIP joints of digits 4 and 5, thereby swinging the "balance of power" to the muscles that extend the digits, all of which are innervated by the radial nerve. The intrinsic hand muscles can aid in flexion of the MCP joints and are innervated by the ulnar nerve. However, they are of insufficient size to compensate for the extensor forces exerted on fingers.
B. The third digit will be extended following injury to the median nerve.
C. With paralysis of the median nerve, there will be weakness in thumb abduction and opposition.
D. The second and third digit will be extended following median nerve injury.
E. The MCP and DIP joints of the second and third digit will be extended due to unopposed action of the radial nerve.
GAS 731–735; N 466; ABR/McM 157

108. C. The winged scapula results from a lesion of the long thoracic nerve, which supplies the serratus anterior muscle. This muscle is responsible for rotating the scapula upward, which occurs during abduction of the arm above the horizontal. The long thoracic nerve arises from the ventral rami of C5–C7 of the brachial plexus. The diaphragm is supplied by the phrenic nerve, which comes from the ventral rami of C3–C5 (mnemonic: C3, 4 and 5 keep the diaphragm alive).
A, B, D, E. These sites are distal to the origin of the long thoracic nerve.
GAS 716; N 417; ABR/McM 135

109. A. The median nerve supplies sensory innervation to the thumb, index, and middle fingers as well as to the lateral half of the ring finger. The median nerve also provides motor innervation to muscles of the thenar eminence. Compression of the median nerve in the carpal tunnel explains these deficits in conjunction with normal functioning of the flexor compartment of the forearm.
B and E. The ulnar nerve is not implicated in these symptoms.
C. Compression of the brachial plexus could not be attributed to pressure from hypertrophy of the triceps brachii muscle because it is located distal to the plexus. In addition, symptoms would include several upper limb deficits rather than the focal symptoms described in this instance.
D. Osteoarthritis of the cervical spine would also lead to increasing complexity of symptoms.
GAS 734, 817; N 466; ABR/McM 168

110. B. The lunate bone is the most commonly dislocated carpal bone. Displacement is anterior in the majority of the cases. Dislocation of the lunate bone can precipitate the signs typically associated with carpal tunnel syndrome.
A, D, E. These bones are not commonly dislocated and do not articulate with the radius.
C. The scaphoid articulates with the radius but is more commonly fractured than dislocated.
GAS 783–785; N 446; ABR/McM 128

111. D. A cervical rib (usually found at C7) may cause thoracic outlet syndrome, a condition characterized by weak muscle tone in the hand and loss of radial pulse when the upper limb is abducted above the shoulder. The symptoms suggest a lower trunk injury to the brachial plexus.
A. The axillary nerve supplies the shoulder muscles, which show no loss of function.
B. The upper trunk of the brachial plexus supplies innervation to the shoulder muscles, which are unaffected based on the patient's presenting abnormalities.
C. The subclavian artery is located anterior to the brachial plexus until the plexus separates into cords as it passes under the clavicle.
E. The brachiocephalic artery and (D) the lower trunk of the brachial plexus is only partially correct; the brachiocephalic artery is not directly associated with the brachial plexus due to its location near the midline of the body behind the sternum.
GAS 151; N 192, 420; ABR/McM 135

112. A. A synarthrosis joint is a fibrous connection that allows limited movement. In this case, pronation/supination movement is allowed by the interosseous membrane joint between the radius and ulna.
B. Symphysis joints are permanent fibrocartilaginous fusions between two bones; pubic symphysis is an example.
C. Synchondrosis is a temporary joint made of cartilage that transitions to bone typically after growth completes (i.e., epiphyseal plate).
D. Trochoid joints are pivot joints, and the humeroradial portion of the elbow joint is an example.
E. Ginglymus joints are hinge joints such as those located at the IP junctions in the hand and foot (PIPs and DIPs).
GAS 17–19, 774–775; N 429; ABR/McM 154

113. B. The radial pulse is best located on the forearm (antebrachium) just proximal to the wrist joint. At this point, the radial artery travels on the distal radius between the flexor carpi radialis and brachioradialis tendons.
A. The palmaris longus tendon travels more medially to the radial artery and above the flexor retinaculum.

C, D, E. The flexor pollicis longus tendon is a deeper structure in the antebrachium and is also located medially to the radial artery.
GAS 818; N 437; ABR/McM 170

114. **B.** The radial artery enters the hand through the anatomical snuffbox.
    A. The artery then moves on to pierce through the two heads of the first dorsal interosseous muscle and enter the deep aspect of the palm.
    C. The flexor pollicis longus tendon runs on the palmar aspect of the hand and the radial artery runs on the dorsal aspect of the hand before entering the deep aspect of the palm, and therefore the radial artery does not run below this tendon.
    D. The radial artery does not run between the first and second interosseous muscle and therefore cannot be used as a landmark to identify the artery.
    E. The radial artery does not run between the first dorsal interosseous muscle and the adductor pollicis longus.
    GAS 791, 812; N 457; ABR/McM 170

115. **D.** The median nerve provides innervation to most of the muscles in the flexor compartment of the forearm; cutaneous innervation of the palmar aspect of the second, third, and fourth digits and the lateral palm; and innervation of five intrinsic hand muscles: first and second lumbricals, abductor pollicis brevis, opponens pollicis, and flexor pollicis brevis. The thenar compartment contains the abductor pollicis brevis, opponens pollicis, and flexor pollicis brevis muscles, and these muscles are innervated by the recurrent branch of the median nerve. The patient has weakening of the first two lumbricals and not simply the thenar muscles, so the median nerve is most likely to be compressed. Another indication that the median nerve is compressed is the vigorous shaking of the wrist. Because the median nerve traverses the carpal tunnel, carpal tunnel compression could lead to this action on the part of the patient.
    A. The ulnar nerve provides innervation for part of the flexor digitorum profundus and flexor carpi ulnaris muscles. These muscles are not weakened in this patient.
    B. The radial nerve provides cutaneous supply to the dorsum of the hand and forearm as well as extensor muscles of the forearm.
    C. Recurrent branch of median: The recurrent branch of the median nerve innervates the thenar muscles, opponens pollicis, abductor pollicis brevis, and flexor pollicis brevis, however since sensation over the palmar surface is also decreased, it is unlikely due to compression of this nerve.
    E. The posterior interosseous nerve is a branch of the radial nerve and provides sensory innervation of the wrist joint.
    GAS 734, 784; N 466; ABR/McM 166

116. **B.** The patient can extend his forearm, which suggests that the triceps brachii muscle is not weakened. Supination appears to be weak along with hand grasp and wrist drop. This would indicate that part of the radial nerve has been lost below the innervation of the triceps brachii and above the branches to the supinator and extensors in the forearm. However, sensation on the forearm and hand is intact, indicating that the superficial branch of the radial nerve is intact. The superficial branch of the radial nerve separates from the deep radial nerve at the distal third of the humerus.
    A. The posterior cord of the brachial plexus is responsible for providing innervation of the axillary and radial nerves. This patient does have some radial nerve innervation and no loss of axillary nerve function.
    C and D. The patient does not have weakened adduction of the wrist, indicating that the ulnar nerve is not injured.
    E. If both the radial and musculocutaneous nerves are injured, supination would not be possible as the supinator and biceps brachii muscles provide supination of the forearm.
    GAS 750–752, 785; N 468; ABR/McM 151

117. **B.** The deep branch of the radial nerve, after it emerges distal to the supinator, is responsible for innervation of several muscles in the extensor compartment of the posterior aspect of the forearm, including extension of the MCP joints. The deep radial nerve courses laterally around the radius and passes between the two heads of the supinator muscle and is thus likely to be compressed by a hematoma between the fractured radius and the supinator muscle.
    A. The anterior interosseous nerve is a branch of the median nerve and supplies the flexor digitorum profundus, flexor pollicis longus, and the pronator quadratus muscles.
    C. Though the radial nerve gives rise to its deep branch, this answer choice is too general and would not indicate the precise injured branch of the radial nerve.
    D and E. Both the deep branch of the ulnar nerve and the median nerve traverse the medial and anteromedial aspect of the arm, respectively. These nerves primarily supply the flexor compartment of the arm (GAS Fig. 7.92).
    GAS 775, 782; N 469; ABR/McM 161

118. **A.** The superior trunk of the brachial plexus includes C5 and C6, which give rise to the suprascapular nerve, which innervates the supraspinatus muscle. The supraspinatus muscle is the primary muscle involved in abduction of the arm from 0 to 15 degrees. The deltoid muscle, supplied primarily by C5, abducts the arm from 15 to 90 degrees.
    B. The middle trunk is just C7 and has nothing to do with the muscle involved in initial abduction of the arm.

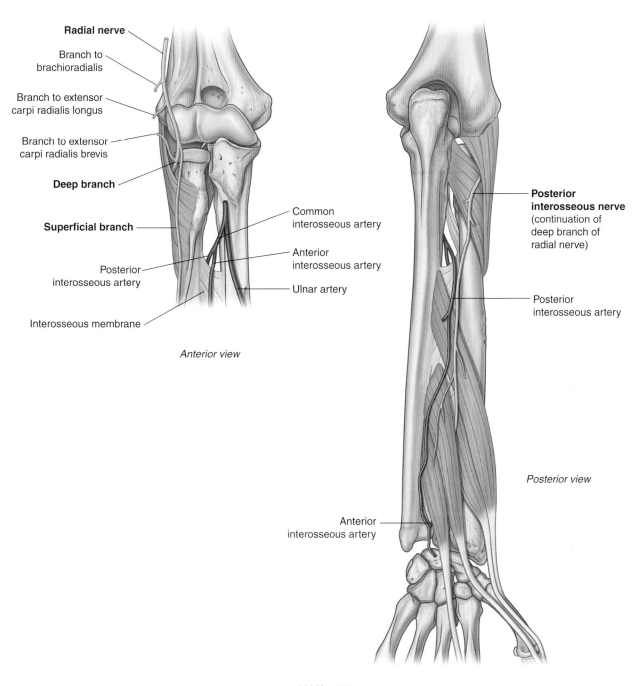

Radial nerve

Branch to brachioradialis

Branch to extensor carpi radialis longus

Branch to extensor carpi radialis brevis

Deep branch

Superficial branch

Posterior interosseous artery

Interosseous membrane

Common interosseous artery

Anterior interosseous artery

Ulnar artery

Anterior view

Posterior interosseous nerve (continuation of deep branch of radial nerve)

Posterior interosseous artery

Anterior interosseous artery

Posterior view

• *GAS* **Fig. 7.92**

C. The inferior trunk is composed of C8–T1 and does not supply the supraspinatus muscle; therefore, it is not the right answer.

D and E. The cords are distal to the branching of the supraspinatus muscle; therefore, neither lateral cord nor medial cord is the correct answer.
GAS 729, 736; N 420; ABR/McM 28

119. C. The radial nerve is responsible for extension of the hand and fingers. This nerve is derived from all the ventral rami of C5–T1.

A, B, D, E. None of the other answers include all the ventral rami.
GAS 734–735; N 420; ABR/McM 100

120. A. The suprascapular artery arises as a major branch of the thyrocervical trunk from the subclavian artery. It has rich anastomoses with the circumflex scapular artery and could provide essential blood supply to the scapula. The dorsal scapular artery would be lost with the graft. None of the other vessels listed is in position to provide adequate supply to the scapula.
GAS 709; N 418; ABR/McM 31

121. C. The scaphoid and lunate carpal bones have a direct articulation with the radius, which is fractured in a Colles fracture; therefore, they would most likely be disrupted or fractured.

A, B, D, E The other carpal bones listed do not have direct contact with the radius and have a more distal location; therefore, they would not be as likely to be injured with a Colles fracture.

GAS 764; N 442; ABR/McM 129

122. C. This type of dislocation is common in children and results when the radius is dislocated and slips out from the annular ligament, which holds it in place, articulating with the ulna and the capitulum of the humerus. In adults the annular ligament has a good "grip" at the radial neck, but in young children the radial head is not fully developed, leading to an indistinct neck.

A. Compression of the median nerve is not likely due to its medial position in the cubital fossa.

B. The radius does not articulate with the trochlea of the humerus; the ulna articulates at this position.

D. The ulna is not likely to be dislocated because it is more stable than the radius, which has only the annular ligament for its support.

E. The radial nerve does not pass behind the medial epicondyle; rather, the ulnar nerve does this, so this is not the correct answer.

GAS 755–757, 775; N 428; ABR/McM 154

123. C. Injury to the radial nerve can be caused by a blow to the midhumeral region because the nerve winds around the body of the humerus. The symptoms described include the loss of wrist and finger extension and a loss of sensation in an area of skin supplied by the radial nerve.

A. The median nerve provides sensory innervation to the lateral 3½ digits on the palmar aspect of the hand. The median nerve is not responsible for wrist extension.

B. Ulnar nerves provide sensory innervation to the medial 1½ digits on the palmar aspect of the hand and the medial 2½ digits on the dorsal aspect of the hand. The ulnar nerve is not responsible for wrist extension.

D. The musculocutaneous nerve provides sensory innervation to the lateral forearm.

E. The axillary nerve provides sensory innervation to the deltoid region of the shoulder.

GAS 752; N 468; ABR/McM 152

124. A. The ulnar nerve innervates the dorsal and palmar interossei, which act to abduct and adduct the fingers and assist the lumbricals in their actions of flexing the MCP joints and extending the IP joints.

B. The recurrent branch of the median nerve innervates the thenar muscle group that functions in the movement of the thumb.

C. The radial nerve is responsible for wrist extension.

D. The musculocutaneous nerve does not innervate any muscles in the forearm or hand.

E. The anterior interosseous innervates the flexor pollicis longus and the pronator quadratus as well as the radial half of the flexor digitorum profundus.

GAS 799–800; N 467; ABR/McM 168

125. C. The triceps brachii muscle is innervated by the radial nerve (primarily C7), which comes off C5–T1 spinal nerves.

A and B. As the patient's only motor deficit involves the triceps brachii muscles, one can rule out C5 and C6, which supply fibers to the axillary, musculocutaneous, and upper subscapular nerves. Damage to either of these ventral rami would result in additional motor deficits of the shoulder and flexor compartment of the arm.

D and E. One can also rule out C8–T1 because these ventral rami form the medial pectoral nerve and the medial brachial and antebrachial cutaneous nerves, as well as the ulnar and the distal distribution of the median nerve. Damage to these ventral rami would result in loss of pectoral muscle function and cutaneous sensation over the medial surface of the upper limb, and loss of hand function.

GAS 734, 750; N 420; ABR/McM 100

Answers 126–150

126. D. Mallet finger, also known as baseball finger, is a deformity in which the finger is permanently flexed at the DIP joint due to avulsion of the insertion of the extensor tendon at the distal phalanx.

A. A lesion of the ulnar nerve at the distal flexor crease of the wrist: This injury would lead to decreased sensation over the medial palm and 4th and 5th metacarpals. In addition, weakness of various muscles in the hand would be expected as well.

B. A separation of the extension expansion over the middle IP joint: Mallet finger is an avulsion injury of the tendon at the DIP. The PIP joint is not involved.

D. Compression of the deep ulnar nerve by dislocation of the lunate bone: Weakness of various muscles in the hand would be expected, such as the hypothenar muscles, interosseous muscles, 3rd and 4th lumbricals, and adductor pollicis.

E. Fracture of the fourth or fifth metacarpal bone: This injury would not lead to the formation of mallet finger, which is specifically an avulsion injury of the tendon at the DIP.

GAS 793; N 446; ABR/McM 175

127. B. Injury to the superior trunk of the brachial plexus can damage nerve fibers going to the suprascapular, axillary, and musculocutaneous nerves. Damage to the suprascapular and axillary nerves causes impaired abduction and lateral rotation of the arm. Damage to the musculocutaneous nerve causes impaired flexion of the forearm.

A. A winged scapula would be caused by damage to the long thoracic nerve. The long thoracic nerve is formed from spinal cord levels C5, C6, and C7, so the serratus anterior muscle would be weakened from the damage to C5 and C6, but the muscle would not be completely paralyzed. C. Most of the intrinsic muscles of the hand are innervated by the ulnar nerve, which would most likely remain intact.

D. Paresthesia in the medial aspect of the arm would be caused by damage to the medial brachial cutaneous nerve (C8–T1; inferior trunk).

E. Loss of sensation on the dorsum of the hand would be caused by damage to either the ulnar or radial nerves (C6–T1).

GAS 729, 747; N 420; ABR/McM 31

128. **D.** The supinator muscle attaches to the radius proximally and when fractured would cause a lateral deviation.

A. The pronator teres muscle originates on the medial epicondyle and coronoid process of the ulna and inserts onto the middle of the lateral side of the radius, pulling the radius medially below the fracture.

B. The pronator quadratus muscle originates on the anterior surface of the distal ulna and inserts on the anterior surface of the distal radius, pulling the radius medially.

C. The brachialis muscle originates in the lower anterior surface of the humerus and inserts in the coronoid process and ulnar tuberosity, hence not causing an action on the radius.

E. The brachioradialis muscle originates on the lateral supracondylar ridge of the humerus and inserts at the base of the radial styloid process, far below the fracture.

GAS 767, 777–778; N 430; ABR/McM 127

129. **B.** Lymph from the lateral side of the hand drains directly into epitrochlear, then lateral axillary, and then to the central axillary nodes (A).

C. Pectoral nodes receive lymph mainly from the anterior thoracic wall, including most of the breast.

D. Subscapular nodes receive lymph from the posterior aspect of the thoracic wall and scapular region.

E. Parasternal nodes receive lymph from the lower medial quadrant of the breast (GAS Fig. 7.57).

GAS 737–738; N 407; ABR/McM 371

130. **C.** Compartment syndrome is characterized by increased pressure within the confined space of a fascial compartment, which impairs blood supply, resulting in paleness and loss of pulses distal to the compartment.

A. Venous thrombosis would not result in loss of the radial pulse and it is not associated with trauma or injury to a muscle compartment.

B. Thoracic outlet syndrome affects nerves in the brachial plexus and the subclavian artery and blood vessels between the neck and the axilla, far above the cast.

D. Raynaud disease affects blood flow to the limbs when they are exposed to temperature changes or stress.

E. The fracture at the radial groove probably resulted in a radial nerve injury but would not be responsible for these symptoms.

GAS 582, 763; N 437; ABR/McM 151

131. **E.** The deep branch of the ulnar nerve arises at the level of the pisiform bone and passes between the pisiform and the hook of the hamate; hence the deep branch of the ulnar nerve is most likely to be injured in this patient.

A. The median nerve enters the palm in the midline through the carpal tunnel.

B. The recurrent branch of the median nerve branches off after the median nerve enters the palm through the carpal tunnel.

C. The radial nerve divides into superficial and deep branches when it enters the cubital fossa.

D. The anterior interosseous arises from the median nerve as the latter courses between the two head of the pronator teres muscle. It continues on to the anterior aspect of the interosseous membrane between the flexor digitorum profundus and flexor pollicis longus muscles.

GAS 805; N 455; ABR/McM 171

132. **A.** The empty can test assesses the function of the supraspinatus muscle, which initiates the first 15 degrees of abduction of the arm; palpation of the tendon during this phase would result in pain from a tendinopathy of the supraspinatus.

B, C, D, E The deltoid muscle is responsible for abduction of the arm beyond the first 15 degrees and is not assessed during the empty can test.

GAS 706; N 415; ABR/McM 138

133. **A.** The hallmark fracture caused by a fall on an outstretched hand is a scaphoid-lunate fracture; the scaphoid and lunate are the two wrist bones most proximal to the styloid process of the radius.

B, C, D, E. All the other wrist bones are less likely to be affected by this injury.

GAS 783–784, 797; N 442; ABR/McM 128

134. **C.** Bennett fracture is a CMC fracture at the base of the thumb.

A. Colles fracture is also called "dinner fork deformity" because the distal fragment is displaced posteriorly.

B. Scaphoid fracture would be indicated by pain in the anatomical snuffbox.

D. Smith fracture is also called a reverse Colles fracture and is caused when the distal fragment of the radius angles forward.

E. Boxer's fracture refers to a fracture of the neck of a metacarpal bone, usually the fifth or fourth metacarpal bone.

GAS 783–786; N 442; ABR/McM 128

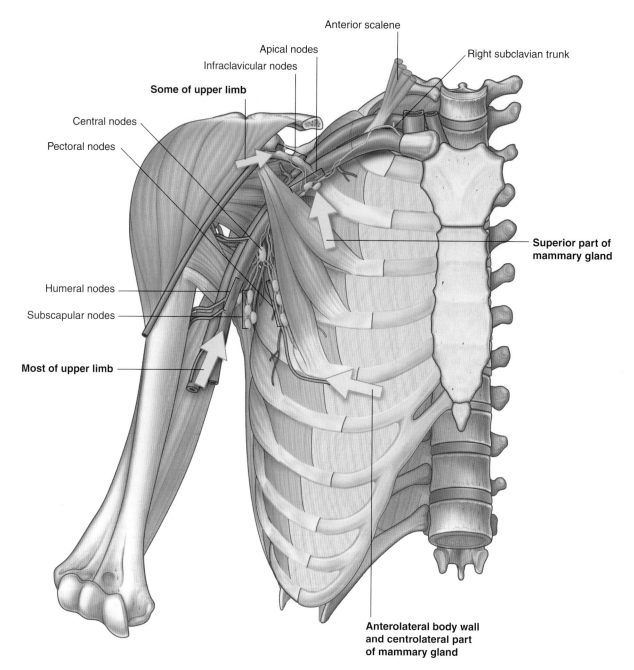

Anterior scalene

Apical nodes

Infraclavicular nodes

Right subclavian trunk

Some of upper limb

Central nodes

Pectoral nodes

Superior part of mammary gland

Humeral nodes

Subscapular nodes

Most of upper limb

Anterolateral body wall and centrolateral part of mammary gland

• *GAS* Fig. 7.57

135. A. Interestingly, "gamekeeper's thumb" was a term coined to describe an injury common among Scottish gamekeepers who, it is said, killed small animals such as rabbits by breaking their necks between the ground and the gamekeeper's thumb and index finger. The resulting valgus force on the abducted MCP joint caused injury to the ulnar collateral ligament. Today this injury is more commonly seen in skiers who land awkwardly with their hand braced on a ski pole, causing the valgus force on the thumb, as seen in this patient. Whereas the term "skier's thumb" is sometimes used, "gamekeeper's thumb" is still in common usage.

B. Scaphoid fracture occurs after a fall on an outstretched hand, involving the scaphoid and lunate bones.

C. Bennett fracture is a fracture at the base of the first metacarpal.

D. Smith fracture is also called a reverse Colles fracture and is caused when the distal radius is fractured and the distal radial fragment is angled forward. Colles fracture is also called dinner fork deformity because the distal fragment of the radius is displaced posteriorly.

E. Boxer's fracture is a fracture of the necks of the second and third (and sometimes the fifth) metacarpals.

GAS 783–786; N 445; ABR/McM 173

136. B. The biceps brachii reflex is elicited by tapping on the tendon of the biceps near its insertion on the radius. The biceps brachii reflex involves C5 and C6 spinal nerves. C5 provides the motor component; C6 the afferent side of the reflex arc.

A. C5 provides the efferent component of the biceps brachii reflex.

C, D, E These nerves are not involved in the biceps brachii reflex.

GAS 720–721; N 421; ABR/McM 157

137. B. The brachioradialis reflex is elicited by tapping the tendon of the brachioradialis muscle. The reflex involves spinal nerves C5, C6, and C7. The major contribution is from C6.

A, C, D, E These nerves are not involved in the brachioradialis reflex.

GAS 775–777; N 437; ABR/McM 159

138. D. Volkmann contracture is a flexion deformity of the fingers and sometimes the wrist from an ischemic necrosis of the forearm flexor muscles.

A. Colles fracture is also called dinner fork deformity because the distal fragment of the radius is displaced posteriorly. Smith fracture is also called a reverse Colles fracture and is caused when the distal radius is fractured, with the radial fragment angled forward.

B. Scaphoid fractures occur after a fall on an outstretched hand and involve the scaphoid and lunate bones.

C. Bennett fracture is a fracture at the base of the first metacarpal. E. Boxer's fracture is a fracture of the necks of the second and third (and sometimes the fifth) metacarpal.

GAS 764; N 437; ABR/McM 159

139. D. The ulnar nerve enters the forearm by passing between the two heads of the flexor carpi ulnaris and descends between and innervates the flexor carpi ulnaris and flexor digitorum profundus (medial half) muscles. It enters the hand superficial to the flexor retinaculum and lateral to the pisiform bone, where it is vulnerable to damage and provides the deep ulnar branch.

A. The deep ulnar branch is more likely injured than the ulnar nerve.

B. The radial nerve is not located lateral to the pisiform bone.

C. The median nerve is not located lateral to the pisiform bone.

E. The deep branch of the radial nerve arises proximally in the forearm.

GAS 774; N 467; ABR/McM 158

140. B. Benediction sign of the hand with the index and middle fingers extended and the ring and little fingers flexed is caused by an injury to the median nerve. The long flexors of the digits are supplied by the median nerve; the unopposed radial nerve and deep ulnar nerve supply the extensors of the digits 1 to 3, causing them to be in the extended position. Digits 4 and 5 are slightly flexed because the flexors of the PIP joints are supplied by the ulnar nerve.

A, C, D, E. The radial nerve is spared due to the unopposed extension of digits 1 to 3, while the ulnar nerve is spared due to flexion of digits 4 and 5.

GAS 774, 807; N 466; ABR/McM 166

141. A. The Allen test involves compression of the radial and ulnar arteries at the wrist with the fingers flexed tightly to move the blood out the palm. Pressure is then released on the radial and ulnar arteries successively to determine the degree of supply to the hand by either vessel and the patency of the anastomoses between them. The usefulness of the radial artery for bypass can thereby be assessed. If the palm does not flush with blood when the radial artery is released, then the ulnar artery is not sufficient to supply the hand if the radial artery is harvested for a graft. The other tests have nothing to do with the patency of the radial artery.

B, C, E. These are neurological tests and do not assess integrity of the vasculature. D. Tinel test is a clinical test to assess carpal tunnel syndrome due to compression of the median nerve.

GAS 805; N 438; ABR/McM 169

142. E. The ulnar nerve enters the hand superficial to the flexor retinaculum and lateral to the pisiform bone and innervates all the interossei and adductor pollicis via the deep branch. These muscles are responsible for adduction and abduction of the fingers. Flexion of the fingers is spared because the flexor digitorum superficialis and the radial half of the flexor digitorum profundus are innervated by the median nerve, which is unaffected by this injury.

A. Had the median nerve been compressed in the carpal tunnel, one would have difficulty with motion of the thumb as a result of a lack of innervation of the thenar muscles.

B and D. An injury of the radial nerve in the arm results in extension deficit in the forearm and hand.

C. The median nerve does not innervate muscles of abduction and adduction of the fingers. It only provides sensory innervation to the palmar surface of the first three digits.

GAS 805; N 455; ABR/McM 167

143. A. The glenohumeral joint is an extremely mobile joint with a wide range of movement. Anterior dislocation is the most common. Anterior dislocations of the humerus usually follow injuries where abnormal force is applied to the shoulder while the arm is extended, abducted, and externally rotated. When the head of the humerus is displaced anteriorly and

inferiorly, there is flattening of the deltoid prominence (due to the increased weight of the humerus pulling on the muscle), protrusion of the acromion, and anterior axillary fullness (due to the movement of the humeral head into this location). The most commonly injured nerve is the axillary nerve, which innervates the teres minor and deltoid and also provides cutaneous supply to the skin overlying the deltoid muscle.

B. AC joint subluxation typically results from a blow to the tip of the shoulder when the arm is at the side and slightly adducted. It produces swelling and superior displacement of the clavicle. It is not associated with specific major nerve injuries or sensory deficits.

C. The clavicle is a commonly fractured bone typically after direct trauma. Most fractures occur in the middle third of the clavicle. There is local swelling and tenderness but rarely any neurovascular damage.

D. A spiral humerus mid-body fracture may result from a fall on an outstretched hand. The radial nerve is commonly fractured as it runs in the radial groove.

E. Rotator cuff tears usually occur when there is some degenerative injury to the tendons. The rotator cuff is made up of the subscapularis, supraspinatus, infraspinatus, and teres minor and tendons.

GAS 695; N 422, 428; ABR/McM 142

144. **A.** The patient is experiencing radial head subluxation ("nursemaid's elbow"), the most common elbow injury in children. The injury often results from a sharp pull on the hand while the forearm is pronated and the elbow is extended. The underdevelopment of the radial head and the laxity of the annular ligament allows for the radial head to sublux (partially dislocate) from this cuff of tissue. This condition is extremely painful but can be easily treated with supination and compression of the elbow joint.

B. Although it is uncommon for muscle tendons to rupture, the most common is the tendon of the long head of the biceps brachii. It produces a characteristic deformity when flexing the elbow: an extremely prominent bulge of unattached muscle belly called the "Popeye sign."

C. The interosseous membrane is an expansive sheet of connective tissue that connects the radius and ulna at their bodies. It serves as an attachment site for the muscles of the forearm.

D. The radial collateral ligament lies on the lateral side of the elbow joint reinforcing the radiohumeral joint.

E. The ulnar collateral ligament lies on the medial side of the elbow joint reinforcing the ulnohumeral joint.

GAS 753–755; N 428; ABR/McM 154

145. **B.** The glenohumeral joint is an extremely mobile joint with a wide range of motion. Anterior dislocation of the humerus is most common and usually associated with an isolated traumatic incident. When the head of the humerus is displaced anteriorly and inferiorly, flattening of the deltoid prominence occurs, leading to loss of the normal contour of the humerus. There is protrusion of the acromion, and the slope of the shoulder lateral to the acromion is depressed and has a "dented" appearance.

A. Avulsion of the coronoid process of the ulna can occur with elbow hyperextension, which affects the elbow joint.

C. A fracture of the mid-body of the humerus damages the radial nerve.

D and E. Although a fracture to the surgical neck of the humerus and a laceration of the posterior cord affect the axillary nerve, which innervates the deltoid muscle, there will not be any depression beneath the acromion in either case.

GAS 695; N 428; ABR/McM 142

146. **C.** The median cubital vein is a superficial vein that lies on the bicipital aponeurosis. The bicipital aponeurosis or lacertus fibrosus is a flat sheet of connective tissue that fans out from the medial side of the biceps brachii tendon to blend with the antebrachial fascia of the forearm flexor muscles. It reinforces the cubital fossa and protects the brachial artery, which runs deep to it.

A. The flexor retinaculum covers the carpal bones on the palmar side of the hand and thus forms the carpal tunnel.

B. The pronator teres muscle has two attachments: to the medial epicondyle of the humerus and the ulnar head arising from the medial coronoid process of the ulna. The brachial artery runs lateral to the pronator teres muscle.

D. The brachioradialis muscle flexes the elbow and pronates and supinates depending on the position of the forearm. It lies on the lateral side of the forearm forming the lateral limit of the cubital fossa.

E. The biceps brachii tendon inserts on the radial tuberosity. The bicipital aponeurosis originates from the medial side of the biceps brachii tendon, and the brachial artery lies underneath the aponeurosis.

GAS 757–758; N 407; ABR/McM 157

147. **A.** The flexor retinaculum is a thick connective tissue band that spans the space between the medial and lateral sides of the carpal tunnel. It protects and stabilizes the tendons that run beneath it.

B, D and E. Damage to the flexor carpi ulnaris tendon, flexor digitorum superficialis tendons, and flexor digitorum profundus tendons result in functional losses in the hand.

C. The palmar skin is made of loose connective tissue and does not have a shiny, glistening appearance (GAS Fig. 7.107).

GAS 788–790; N 452; ABR/McM 167

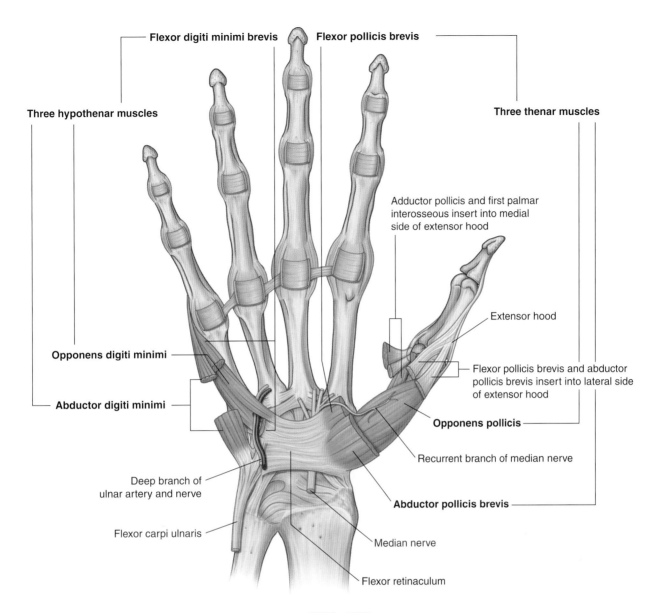

Flexor digiti minimi brevis

Flexor pollicis brevis

Three hypothenar muscles

Three thenar muscles

Adductor pollicis and first palmar
interosseous insert into medial
side of extensor hood

Extensor hood

Opponens digiti minimi

Flexor pollicis brevis and abductor
pollicis brevis insert into lateral side
of extensor hood

Abductor digiti minimi

Opponens pollicis

Recurrent branch of median nerve

Deep branch of
ulnar artery and nerve

Abductor pollicis brevis

Flexor carpi ulnaris

Median nerve

Flexor retinaculum

• *GAS* **Fig. 7.107**

148. D. The recurrent branch of the median nerve usually originates from the lateral side of the median nerve at the distal margin of the flexor retinaculum. It innervates the three thenar muscles: the opponens pollicis, flexor pollicis brevis, and abductor pollicis brevis.

A and C. Injury of the median nerve in the carpal tunnel, as well as injury of the recurrent and palmar branch of the median nerve, causes both sensory and motor deficits. B. Injury of the palmar branch of the median nerve results in loss of sensation only of the palm.

E. Injury to the radial and ulnar nerves results in sensory and motor deficits in the distribution of theses nerves (GAS Fig. 7.107).
GAS 808; N 466; ABR/McM 166

149. B. The radial artery enters the anatomical snuffbox as it passes to the posterior aspect of the hand between the two heads of the first dorsal interosseous muscle.

A. The ulnar artery courses in the anterior forearm and enters the hand on the palmar surface.

C and D. The anterior and posterior interosseous arteries are found anteriorly and posteriorly, respectively, on or near the interosseous membrane, which is located between the radius and ulna.

E. The deep palmar arch is an anastomosis on the palmar surface of the hand that is formed by the terminal part of the radial artery and the deep branch of the ulnar artery.
GAS 772, 791, 801–806; N 457; ABR/McM 170

150. E. The ulnar nerve is responsible for cutaneous innervation to the medial one and a half digits and motor innervation to most of the intrinsic muscles of the hand including the interossei. The interossei muscles are responsible for adduction of the digits, which is the action that would be used to hold a piece of paper between the finger

A. The axillary nerve innervates the deltoid and teres minor muscles in the arm. This nerve also carries sensory information from the shoulder joint and the skin over the inferior part of the deltoid muscle.

B. The median nerve is responsible for cutaneous innervation of the lateral three and a half fingers, and the lateral palm including the thenar eminence. It innervates the thenar muscles and the lateral two lumbricals. These muscles function to oppose the thumb and flex the MCP joints, respectively.

C. The musculocutaneous nerve is responsible for innervation of the anterior compartment of the arm, ending as the lateral antebrachial cutaneous nerve below the elbow.

D. The radial nerve innervates the extensors of the hand. It also carries sensory information from the dorsum of the hand. Therefore, damage to this nerve will not lead to this array of symptoms (GAS Fig. 7.113).

GAS 805–806; N 467; ABR/McM 168

Answers 151–175

151. B. The latissimus dorsi attaches into the intertubercular sulcus of the humerus. This muscle is innervated by the thoracodorsal nerve, which is a branch of the posterior cord and is made up of roots C7–C8 with some C6 involvement possible.

A and D. Nerve roots C2, C3, and C4 are part of the cervical plexus and supply the "strap" muscles.

C. The C4 and C5 nerve roots are the main contributions to the phrenic nerve. The C5 nerve root does not usually contribute to the thoracodorsal nerve.

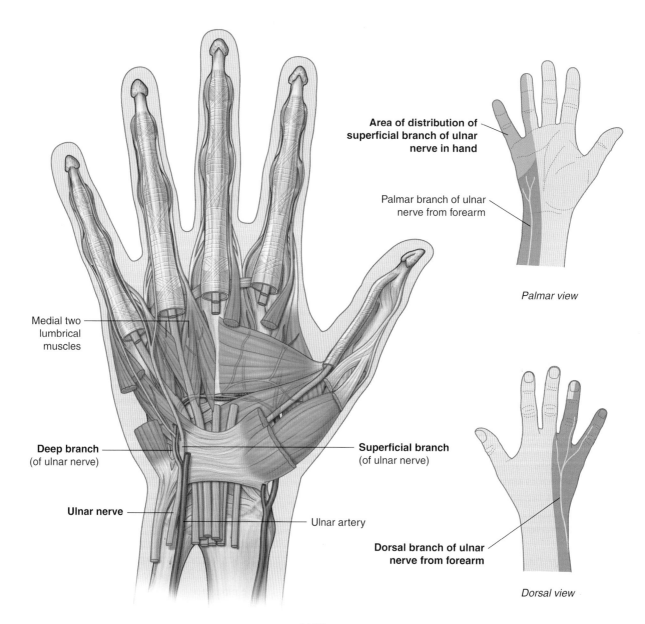

Area of distribution of superficial branch of ulnar nerve in hand

Palmar branch of ulnar nerve from forearm

Palmar view

Medial two lumbrical muscles

Deep branch (of ulnar nerve)

Superficial branch (of ulnar nerve)

Ulnar nerve

Ulnar artery

Dorsal branch of ulnar nerve from forearm

Dorsal view

• *GAS* **Fig. 7.113**

E. The C5 nerve root contributes to the phrenic nerve, while C7 and C8 together with C6 form the thoracodorsal nerve.
GAS 717; N 420; ABR/McM 121

152. **C.** Anterior dislocation of the shoulder can damage the nerves located in the axilla or cause tears in the rotator cuff muscles. Internal or medial rotation of the arm is the primary function of subscapularis muscle, and this is the only action impaired in this patient.
A and E. The infraspinatus and teres minor muscles function as lateral rotators.
B. The pectoralis major is responsible for flexion, adduction, and medial rotation and would not likely be damaged during a shoulder dislocation.
D. The supraspinatus muscle is responsible for the first 15 degrees of arm abduction.
GAS 700; N 415; ABR/McM 142

153. **A.** The nerve responsible for innervation of the interosseous muscles that are weakened is the deep branch of the ulnar nerve. Innervation of the muscles responsible for opposition of the thumb is via the recurrent branch of the median nerve. Both of these nerves are formed by the C8 and T1 ventral rami, which combine to form the inferior trunk of the brachial plexus.
B and D. Damage to either the median or ulnar nerves alone will not produce all of these symptoms. Median nerve damage would involve all of the flexors of the wrist, except the flexor carpi ulnaris, and most digits, except for the IP joints of the fourth and fifth fingers. It will also result in loss of function of the entire thumb. Ulnar nerve damage will result in weakness of the medial half of flexor digitorum profundus (fourth and fifth IP joint flexion), as well as the intrinsic muscles (interossei and medial two lumbricals) of the hand, except for the lateral two lumbricals.
C. The musculocutaneous nerve innervates muscles of the anterior arm, namely the coracobrachialis, biceps brachii, and most of the brachialis. Additionally, it carries sensory information from the lateral forearm. Therefore, injury to this nerve will result in loss of flexion at the elbow joint, supination, pronation, and loss of sensation in the lateral forearm.
E. The upper trunk receives contributions from the C5 and C6 ventral rami and divides into the musculocutaneous, median, and suprascapular nerves. Injury to the upper trunk will lead to deficits in the distribution of these nerves, for example loss of flexion at the elbow joint.
GAS 805; N 420; ABR/McM 166

154. **C.** The patient likely has damage to the ulnar nerve, which affected both the interossei and medial two lumbricals. The lumbricals extend the IP joints of the ring and little fingers, while the interossei are responsible for abduction and adduction of the digits as well as assisting in MCP flexion and IP extension.

A and D. The dorsal interossei are responsible for abduction, while the palmar interossei are responsible for adduction of the digits. Interossei also assist in MCP flexion and IP extension.
B. Injury to the extensor digitorum would lead to loss of extension of the four digits.
E. The extensor digiti minimi is responsible for extension of the fifth digit, and if damaged will not affect the fourth digit.
GAS 805; N BP105; ABR/McM 168

155. **A.** Flexion of the elbow is achieved by contraction of the biceps brachii, brachialis, and brachioradialis muscles. The brachialis muscle is the major flexor of the elbow joint and together with the brachioradialis will continue to flex the elbow if the biceps brachii is damaged.
B. The flexor carpi ulnaris and radialis are primarily responsible for flexion of the wrist.
C. The flexor digitorum superficialis and profundus are responsible for flexion of the digits at the MCP and IP joints, respectively.
D. The pronator teres and supinator are responsible for pronation and supination, respectively.
E. The coracobrachialis does not cross the elbow joint while the triceps brachii is the elbow extensor.
GAS 744; N 421; ABR/McM 159

156. **E.** Opposition is a complex movement that begins with the thumb in the extended position and initially involves abduction and medial rotation of the first metacarpal. This is produced by the action of the opponens pollicis muscle at the CMC joint, by the flexor pollicis brevis muscle, and then by flexion at the MCP joint. The opponens pollicis and flexor pollicis brevis muscles are supplied by the recurrent branch of the median nerve (C8, T1). The median nerve is the principal nerve of the anterior compartment of the forearm and the thenar muscles of the hand. It passes through the carpal tunnel with the tendons of the flexor digitorum profundus, flexor digitorum superficialis, and flexor pollicis longus to supply the thenar muscles of the hand.
A. Adduction and abduction of the fingers: The interosseous muscles adduct and abduct the fingers.
B. The extensor indicis extends the index finger.
C. The fourth and fifth fingers are flexed by the medial two tendons of the flexor digitorum superficialis (supplied by the median nerve) and the medial two tendons of the flexor digitorum profundus (supplied by the ulnar nerve).
D. The ulnar nerve carries sensory information from the base of the fifth digit.
GAS 808; N 455; ABR/McM 168

157. **D.** The scaphoid is the most frequently fractured carpal bone. Fracture often results from a fall on the palm when the hand is abducted, the fracture occurring across the narrow part ("waist") of the scaphoid. Pain occurs primarily on the lateral side of the wrist, especially during dorsiflexion and abduction of the hand. If the only blood supply to the scaphoid enters the bone distally, avascular necrosis (pathological death of bone resulting from inadequate blood supply) of the proximal fragment of the scaphoid may occur and produce degenerative joint disease of the wrist.

A. First metacarpal fractures are usually caused by an axial blow directed against the partially flexed metacarpal.

B. An isolated fracture of the trapezium is an uncommon injury. A fracture of the trapezium can occur alongside other carpal injuries. Clinical presentation is highly variable and depends on fracture displacement and involvement of the CMC joint. Patients may have pain at the base of the thumb or restricted movement of the thumb. The injury occurs with a fall on the hand with the wrist extended and radially deviated.

C. Tenosynovitis is an infection of the digital synovial sheaths. Symptoms of tenosynovitis include pain, swelling, and difficulty moving the particular joint where the inflammation occurs.

E. CMC joint arthritis is a degenerative joint disease affecting the first CMC joint.
GAS 787; N 447; ABR/McM 168

158. C. The long thoracic nerve arises from the upper three ventral rami of the brachial plexus (C5–C7). The long thoracic nerve innervates the serratus anterior, which protracts the scapula. An injury to the long thoracic nerve will result in winging of the scapula. Additionally, the phrenic nerve, which innervates the diaphragm, arises from ventral rami (C3–C5). Thus an injury involving ventral rami of C3, C4, or C5 can impair the diaphragm, reducing excursion of the ipsilateral part of the diaphragm.

A. Cords of the brachial plexus do not contribute to the innervation of the diaphragm. The nerves arising from the cords of the brachial plexus provide innervation to muscles that stabilize the shoulder girdle.

B. There are no nerves arising from the divisions of the brachial plexus.

D. Terminal branches of the brachial plexus provide motor innervation to the upper extremity and shoulder girdle. An injury to any of the terminal branches of the brachial plexus will not impair function of the diaphragm.

E. Nerves arising from the upper trunk of the brachial plexus are the suprascapular nerve and the nerve to the subclavius. Thus, trauma to these nerves will not affect the function of the serratus anterior muscle or the diaphragm.
GAS 716, 730; N 417; ABR/McM 149

159. D. The lateral epicondyle is the common extensor origin. Most of the extensor muscles of the forearm originate from this area. Putting those muscles in

action will exacerbate pain on the lateral epicondyle, a condition nicknamed "tennis elbow."

A. Radial deviation of the wrist will not exacerbate the pain of lateral epicondylitis.

B. Ulnar deviation of the wrist will not exacerbate the pain of lateral epicondylitis.

C. Flexion exacerbates the pain of medial epicondylitis (also known as golfer's elbow).

E. Asking the patient to flex and medially deviate the wrist will worsen the pain of medial epicondylitis.
GAS 741, 757; N 431; ABR/McM 153

160. A. Erb palsy in newborns commonly occurs following a difficult delivery during which the angle between the neck and shoulder is increased extensively for the baby to transit the birth canal. Stretching of the neck can shear the nerve fibers of the superior roots of the brachial plexus (C5 -C6). Infants will have the affected upper limb resting at their side, medially rotated, with the forearm extended and the wrist pronated. This posturing of the limb is similar to a waiter grasping a tip and hence the alternative name of waiter's tip sign. Injuries to the lower trunk of the brachial plexus (Klumpke paralysis) are much less common. Injury of the inferior trunk (C8 and T1) may avulse the roots of the spinal nerves from the spinal cord. The small muscles of the hand are affected, and patients will present with a claw hand deformity (GAS Fig. 7.52 A).

B. In a C6-C7 injury, flexion of the arm may be affected due to decrease in innervation of musculocutaneous nerve to coracobrachialis, brachialis, and biceps brachii muscles. The pectoral muscles would also be affected leading to decreased adduction and medial rotation of arm. In addition, extension of the arm may be affected due to involvement of the radial nerve.

C. In a C7-C8 injury, extension of the arm would be affected due to decrease in sensation of triceps brachii muscles by the radial nerve. In addition, weakness to the muscles of the hand may be affected, due to involvement of the ulnar nerve.

D. Injury of the inferior trunk (C8 and T1) may avulse the roots of the spinal nerves from the spinal cord. The small muscles of the hand are affected, and patients will present with a claw hand deformity (Klumpke paralysis).

E. A C5 -T1 injury of the brachial plexus will result in paralysis to most of the entire upper limb.
GAS 729; N 455; ABR/McM 168

161. C. Carpal tunnel syndrome is a relatively common condition that causes pain, numbness, and a tingling sensation in the hand and fingers. Carpal tunnel syndrome is caused by compression of the median nerve, which supplies the thenar muscles and the first and second lumbricals.

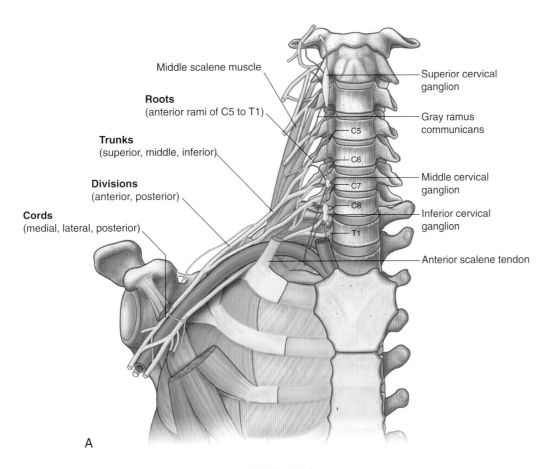

Middle scalene muscle

Roots
(anterior rami of C5 to T1)

Trunks
(superior, middle, inferior)

Divisions
(anterior, posterior)

Cords
(medial, lateral, posterior)

Superior cervical ganglion

Gray ramus communicans

C5

C6

Middle cervical ganglion

C7

C8

Inferior cervical ganglion

T1

Anterior scalene tendon

A

• *GAS* **Fig. 7.52A**

A. Dorsal and palmar interossei are innervated by the deep branch of the ulnar nerve.

B. Lumbricals III and IV are innervated by ulnar nerve.

D. The flexor muscles of the forearm are supplied by the median nerve before it travels through the carpal tunnel.

E. The hypothenar muscles are innervated by the ulnar nerve.

GAS 788–789; N 452; ABR/McM 168

162. D. Recurrent branch of the median nerve is the correct answer. This branch, which supplies the thenar muscles, is given off after the median nerve passes through the carpal tunnel. The opponens pollicis muscle, which is part of the thenar muscle group, is used while buttoning a shirt, an action that requires thumb opposition (GAS Fig. 7.52A).

A. The deep branch of the ulnar nerve supplies motor innervations to all the intrinsic muscles of the hand except the thenar muscles the lateral two lumbricals. It also supplies sensation to the medial one and a half fingers on the palmar side and two and a half fingers on the dorsal side.

B. The patient can still grip a piece of paper between the second and third digits, a function largely performed by the interossei muscles, which are innervated by the deep branch of the ulnar nerve.

C. The median nerve supplies sensation to the lateral palm as well as the first 3.5 digits. In addition, it supplies motor innervations to the thenar muscles and the 1st and 2nd lumbricals.

E. The deep branch of the radial nerve provides motor innervation to the long extensors of the wrist.

163. E. Inability to adduct the thumb is the correct answer because the ulnar nerve travels superficial to the flexor retinaculum and innervates the adductor pollicis muscle, which adducts the thumb.

A. Pronation of the forearm is carried out by muscles innervated by the median nerve.

B. Abduction of the thumb is performed by muscles innervated by the median and radial nerves.

C. The flexor pollicis longus flexes the thumb. This muscle is innervated by a branch of the median nerve called the anterior interosseous nerve. The median nerve courses deep to the flexor retinaculum and would not be injured with a laceration sparing the integrity of the flexor retinaculum.

D. Opposition of the thumb is also performed by muscles innervated by the median nerve. Since the median nerve travels deep to the flexor retinaculum, the nerve would not be injured with a laceration sparing the integrity of the flexor retinaculum.

GAS 805–806; N 455; ABR/McM 166

164. D. The supraspinatus is innervated by the suprascapular nerve (C5, C6) and the nerve continues through the inferior scapular notch and innervates the infraspinatus. The supraspinatus initiates abduction of the arm up to the first 15 to 20 degrees.

    A. The subscapular nerves, superior and inferior, supply the subscapularis and the inferior subscapular nerve innervates the teres major. Both muscles medially rotate the arm.

    B. The axillary nerve supplies the deltoid and teres minor muscles and also a patch of skin on the lateral side of the shoulder. The deltoid abducts the arm beyond 20 degrees, and the teres minor muscle, although a lateral rotator, does not abduct the arm.

    C. The radial nerve supplies muscles in the posterior compartments of the arm and forearm, which are extensors of the elbow, wrist, and fingers in that order.

    E. The upper subscapular nerve supplies the subscapularis, a medial rotator of the arm.

    GAS 706, 731; N 417; ABR/McM 144

165. C. With the involvement of the thenar muscles, lymph drains initially to the epitrochlear nodes and then to the lateral axillary (humeral) nodes.

    A. The posterior axillary nodes receive lymph from the upper back and shoulder.

    B. The subclavian or apical axillary nodes receive lymph from all the axillary nodes.

    D. The anterior axillary (pectoral) nodes receive lymph from most of the breast and the upper side of the anterolateral chest wall.

    E. All anterior, lateral, and posterior axillary nodes drain to the central axillary nodes.

    GAS 737; N 407; ABR/McM 371

166. A. "Nursemaid's elbow," a condition commonly found in children below 5 years of age, is caused by a sharp pull of the child's hand. In children, the annular ligament, which holds the head of the radius in place, is lax and allows the radial head to sublux (dislocate) when the hand is pulled distally. The radial head in children is small and has not fully ossified to the adult size, thus the annular ligament is unable to provide its full capacity of support to the radial head adding to the increased risk of radial subluxation.

    B. The joint capsule of the radioulnar joint is not attached to the radius; rather it passes around the neck of the radius inferiorly to attach to the coronoid process of the ulna.

    C. The interosseous membrane binds the radius and ulna together along their bodies and does not maintain stability of the joint.

    D. The radial collateral ligament attaches the lateral side of the head of the radius to the lateral condyle of the humerus.

    E. The ulnar collateral ligament attaches the medial side of the ulnar head to the medial condyle of the humerus.

    GAS 755; N 428; ABR/McM 154

167. A. This patient has a classic claw hand due to the damage of the deep branch of the ulnar nerve caused by a fractured hamate at the ulnar or Guyon canal. The ulnar nerve supplies the intrinsic muscles of the hand except for the lateral two lumbricals and the thenar muscles. The lumbricals and interossei insert at the back of the fingers via the dorsal (extensor) hood. This hood extends from the MCP joint to the distal phalanx. Through this mechanism, the muscles flex the MCP joint and extend the IP joint. This function is lost with damage to the deep branch of the ulnar nerve resulting in flexion of the IP joints and extension of the MCP joint, giving the appearance as shown in the photograph. The superficial branch of the ulnar nerve also supplies cutaneous innervation to the medial one and a half fingers (ring and little fingers) on the palmar side.

    B. Injury to the radial nerve produces the clinical sign of wrist drop. The radial nerve provides motor innervation to the extensor compartment of the arm and forearm and sensory innervation to the C5–C8 dermatomes. Depending on the level of injury of the radial nerve, either motor or sensory deficits, or both, may be impaired. The radial nerve is often injured with mid-body humeral fractures or from compression in the axilla that may occur from sleeping with the arm hanging over a chair.

    C. Atrophy of the thenar muscles occurs with chronic compression of the median nerve, as it courses through the carpal tunnel. Thenar compartment atrophy is a common finding in patients with carpal tunnel syndrome.

    D. A positive Tinel test is a clinical sign that also indicates compression of the median nerve at the carpal tunnel. Like thenar muscle atrophy, a positive Tinel test is a clinical sign of carpal tunnel syndrome.

    E. The flexor carpi ulnaris muscle is innervated by the ulnar nerve. Contractions of this muscle allows adduction (ulnar deviation) of the wrist. Proximal damage to the ulnar nerve (e.g., at the region of the elbow) can result in the inability to adduct the wrist. A proximal injury may also cause sensory deficit in the forearm and the hand. However, this patient has a fractured hamate which is a distal injury, thus adduction of the wrist will not be impaired.

    GAS 807; N 467; ABR/McM 168

168. D. In thoracic outlet syndrome—sometimes caused by a cervical rib or a cervical fibrous/muscular band—ventral rami or trunks of the brachial plexus can be compressed as they travel from the neck to the axilla. In this case, the inferior trunk of the brachial plexus is being compressed by a cervical rib. The anterior division of the inferior trunk continues as the medial cord of the brachial plexus. The medial brachial cutaneous nerve (medial cutaneous nerve of the arm) and medial antebrachial cutaneous nerve (medial cutaneous nerve of the forearm) are branches of the medial cord of the plexus, with the ulnar nerve as its terminal branch. Additionally, there is a medial cord contribution to the median nerve. Compression of the inferior cord of the brachial plexus, therefore, presents with numbness and paresthesia on the medial part of the arm, forearm, and hand.

A. Ulnar nerve compression at the medial epicondyle, also known as cubital tunnel syndrome, present as tingling and numbness in the ring and little fingers. Symptoms worsen with elbow flexion.

B. Compression of the radial nerve at the neck of the radius will cause decreased sensation at the dorsoradial aspect of the forearm. Symptoms are exacerbated by wrist flexion and pronation of the forearm.

C. Median nerve compression at the wrist will lead to symptoms such as pain and paresthesias in the first three digits and radial half of the fourth digit. Physical examination will show positive Tinel and Phalen signs. Risk factors include hypothyroidism, obesity, and rheumatoid arthritis.

E. The trunks of the brachial plexus give rise to six divisions: anterior and posterior divisions of the upper, middle, and lower trunks. The posterior divisions unite to form the posterior cord which does not provide contributions to the ulnar nerve.
GAS 151; N 419; ABR/McM 149

169. **A.** Tenosynovitis stenosans or trigger finger occurs after swelling or nodular growth of the flexor tendon, which interferes with it gliding through the pulley and produces a snap or click on active extension or flexion.

B. Dupuytren contracture is a progressive fibrotic deformity that occurs as a result of thickening and contractures of the fascia on the palmar surface of the hand eventually leading to permanent partial flexion of the MCP and PIP joints. It mostly affects the ring and little fingers. Risk factors include tobacco and alcohol use and diabetes mellitus.

C. Mallet finger is caused by damage of the terminal extensor tendon distal to the DIP joint. Patient presents with painful and swollen DIP joint most often after a traumatic impaction injury to the finger. Physical examination shows fingertip resting at approximately 45 degrees and lack of active extension of the DIP joint.

D. Boutonnière deformity occurs due to disruption of the central slip over the PIP joint. This can be secondary to trauma or laceration. The patient presents with PIP flexion and DIP extension.

E. Boxer's fracture is a fracture of the fifth metacarpal neck caused by direct trauma to a closed fist. Physical examination shows tenderness to palpation over the fifth metacarpal neck and dorsal angulation proximal to the fracture.
GAS 793; N 451; ABR/McM 166

170. **B.** Ganglion cysts are outpouchings of the joint capsule or sheath of the tendons and may occur anywhere in the hand or feet. They contain synovial-like fluid and can be transilluminated when light is shined through them. On palpation, they are firm and well circumscribed. They commonly occur on the dorsum of the hand and may be surgically treated. The others are all solid tumors and cannot be drained.

A. Neurofibroma is a benign tumor of neuroepithelial origin. It is a solid tumor that cannot be drained.

C. Chondromas are benign tumors of cartilaginous origin. They are also solid tumors.

D. Osteomas are benign pieces of bony outgrowths mostly found in the head.

E. Osteophytes are bony projections at the joints and are associated with cartilaginous degeneration.
GAS 791–792, 807; N 443; ABR/McM 167

171. **A.** The term handlebar neuropathy is a condition that commonly affects long-distance cyclists. The ulnar nerve in the wrist becomes compressed due to the direct pressure of the upper body weight resting on the handlebars. The symptoms correspond to the loss of ulnar nerve function at the wrist, thus handlebar or ulnar neuropathy causes sensory loss of the palmar aspects of the medial one and a half digits and the dorsal aspect of the medial two and a half digits.

B. Abduction of the thumb is by the abductor pollicis longus supplied by the radial nerve and the abductor pollicis brevis supplied by the median nerve.

C. Extensors of the thumb are supplied by the radial nerve.

D. Median nerve palsy can result in thenar muscle atrophy.

E. A Tinel sign might be observed near the hamate at Guyon canal but not laterally at the scaphoid.
GAS 805–807; N 467; ABR/McM 168

172. **B.** Pronator syndrome is due to damage of the median nerve as it passes between the two heads of a hypertrophied pronator teres muscle. It will present with loss of opposition, atrophy of the thenar muscles, and flexion difficulty of the digits and sensory loss of the lateral three and a half digits.

A. Hypertrophy of the supinator muscle will affect the deep branch of the radial nerve that continues distally as the posterior interosseous nerve and also provides sensation from the wrist joint.

C. A medial supracondylar fracture might affect the ulnar nerve.

D. Tennis elbow affects only the common extensor muscle origin and will not cause flexor or opposition difficulties of the digits and thumb, respectively (GAS Fig. 7.85).

E. Medial epicondylitis, also known as golfer's elbow, is an overuse injury that causes pain in the myotendinous junction between the medial epicondyle and the wrist flexors. It presents as tenderness at the medical epicondyle and pain is elicited with elbow extension.
GAS 767; N 466; ABR/McM 160

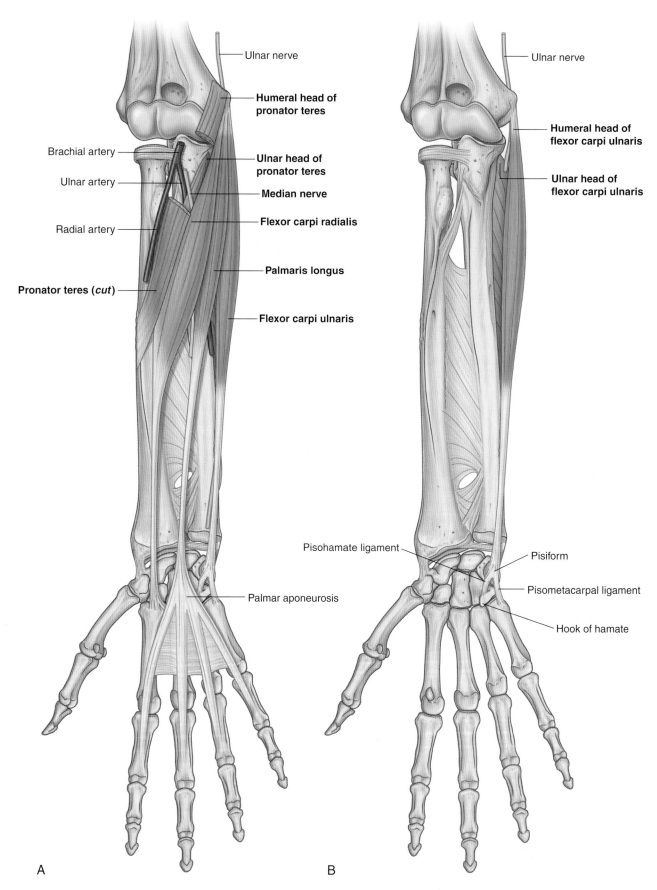

Ulnar nerve

**Humeral head of
pronator teres**

Brachial artery

**Ulnar head of
pronator teres**

Ulnar artery

Median nerve

Flexor carpi radialis

Radial artery

Palmaris longus

Pronator teres (*cut*)

Flexor carpi ulnaris

Palmar aponeurosis

Ulnar nerve

**Humeral head of
flexor carpi ulnaris**

**Ulnar head of
flexor carpi ulnaris**

Pisohamate ligament

Pisiform

Pisometacarpal ligament

Hook of hamate

A

B

• *GAS* **Fig. 7.85**

173. C. The anterior interosseous nerve runs distally and anterior to the interosseous membrane supplying the radial half of the flexor digitorum profundus muscle, which sends nerves to the fourth and fifth fingers), flexor pollicis longus, and the pronator quadratus muscle, hence the weakness in pronation and wrist flexion (GAS Fig. 7.89).

A. The ulnar nerve supplies the medial aspect of the hand.

B. The median nerve at the carpal tunnel will present as tingling and numbness in the areas supplied by the median nerve in the hand.

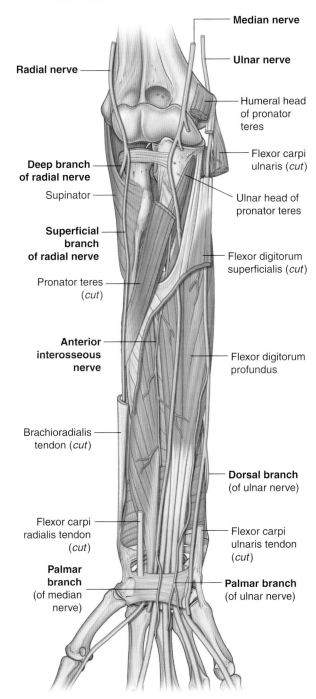

Median nerve
Ulnar nerve
Radial nerve
Humeral head of pronator teres
Flexor carpi ulnaris (*cut*)
Deep branch of radial nerve
Supinator
Ulnar head of pronator teres
Superficial branch of radial nerve
Pronator teres (*cut*)
Flexor digitorum superficialis (*cut*)
Anterior interosseous nerve
Flexor digitorum profundus
Brachioradialis tendon (*cut*)
Dorsal branch (of ulnar nerve)
Flexor carpi radialis tendon (*cut*)
Flexor carpi ulnaris tendon (*cut*)
Palmar branch (of median nerve)
Palmar branch (of ulnar nerve)

• *GAS Fig. 7.89*

D. The deep branch of the radial nerve innervates the wrist extensors. Wrist extension will be weakened, not flexion.

E. Compression of the median nerve at the elbow by the pronator teres causes pronator syndrome characterized by pain and/or numbness in the areas supplied by the distal median nerve as well as the weakness of the muscles innervated by the anterior interosseous nerve.

GAS 774; N 466; ABR/McM 160

174. A. Since the median nerve is intact there will be no thenar atrophy.

B. If the wrist extensors, which are supplied by radial nerve, are intact, no wrist drop will be observed.

C. Radial deviation is not seen due to action of the extensor carpi ulnaris which contributes to wrist extension and pulls the hand toward the medial (ulnar) side. Extensor carpi ulnaris is supplied by the radial nerve.

D. Ulnar deviation at the MCP joint is a characteristic of rheumatoid arthritis and not as a result of damage to the ulnar nerve.

E. Injury to the ulnar nerve would cause wasting to many of the intrinsic muscles of the end, leading to atrophy and the appearance of prominent metacarpal bones with "guttering" in the web spaces between metacarpals.

GAS 805–807; N 467; ABR/McM 153

175. B. The lunate is the most commonly dislocated carpal bone. It helps to form the floor of the carpal tunnel. When it is dislocated, it displaces into the carpal tunnel, potentially compressing the median nerve. The patient will then present with dysesthesia over the palm and palmar aspect of the thumb, index, and middle fingers, and weakness in thumb opposition.

A. Dysesthesia along the medial border of the hand is a result of damage to the ulnar nerve.

C. Numbness along the medial border of the hand and weakness of wrist extension are characteristics of ulnar and radial nerves, respectively.

D. Weakened grip strength is due to damage to the ulnar nerve. Numbness over the dorsum of the hand laterally is a result of compromise to the median nerve and radial nerve.

E. Sensory innervation of the palmar aspect of the first three and half digits is by the median nerve. Adductor pollicis adducts the thumb and is innervated by the deep branch of the ulnar nerve.

GAS 782–785; N 442; ABR/McM 128

Answers 176–186

176. A. The deficits describe ulnar nerve damage close to its entry into the forearm. The ulnar nerve passes behind the medial epicondyle and is relatively unprotected, making this area prone to nerve injury. In the forearm, via its muscular branches, it innervates the flexor carpi ulnaris muscle and the medial half of the flexor digitorum profundus muscle. In the hand, the deep branch of the ulnar nerve innervates the hypothenar muscles, adductor pollicis, abductor digiti minimi, flexor digiti minimi brevis, third and fourth lumbricals, and opponens digiti minimi. The sensory innervation is to the fifth and medial half of the fourth digits and corresponding part of the hand, which can explain the deficits experienced by the patient.

B. Entrapment of the ulnar nerve in the ulnar or Guyon canal leads to tingling and numbness in the ring and little fingers without the other symptoms.

C. Compression of the median nerve in the cubital fossa causes the symptoms of pronator syndrome in addition to deficits in the muscles supplied by the anterior interosseous nerve which branches from the median nerve before the latter enters the carpal tunnel.

D. Median nerve compression in the carpal tunnel causes the symptoms of carpal tunnel syndrome and affects sensation of the lateral border of the hand.

E. The medial cord gives rise to the medial brachial and antebrachial cutaneous nerves, ulnar nerve, and also contributes to the median nerve. This patient has no sensory loss in the arm or forearm.
GAS 774; N 466; ABR/McM 160

177. D. The lunate is compressing the median nerve.

A. The pisiform compressing the ulnar nerve is incorrect as the ulnar nerve innervates the skin on the medial one and a half digits.

B. The hook of hamate compressing the ulnar artery is also incorrect. The hook of the hamate forms part of the ulnar or Guyon canal; compression of the ulnar artery will not produce the deficits described because of the collateral circulation and anastomoses that exist with the radial artery.

C. The scaphoid compressing the radial artery is incorrect because there is collateral circulation from the palmar arches to compensate for radial artery occlusion.

E. The trapezoid is not compressing the superficial radial nerve because the superficial branch of the radial nerve supplies the radial aspect of the thumb and radial side of the index finger via its lateral and medial branches.
GAS 782, 808; N 455; ABR/McM 177

178. D. In the mid-body region of the humerus the radial nerve runs in the radial groove; fracture of the humerus at this point will likely impinge directly on the radial nerve, producing a sensory deficit along the posterior aspect of the forearm.

A. The lateral aspect of the forearm is innervated by the lateral antebrachial cutaneous nerve, which is derived from the musculocutaneous nerve. These nerves may not be affected by a mid-body fracture of the humerus because they are well separated from the bone by muscle.

B. The medial aspect of the arm and (C) forearm is supplied by the intercostobrachial nerve and the medial antebrachial cutaneous nerve that takes its origin from the medial cord of the brachial plexus where it runs superficially, making it extremely difficult to injure both nerves during a mid-body fracture of the humerus.

E. The lateral and posterior aspects of the forearm are unlikely choices because the displaced bone not only has to impinge on the radial nerve but must also affect the very superficially located lateral antebrachial cutaneous nerve.
GAS 752; N 468; ABR/McM 152

179. B. The deep branch of the radial nerve innervates the extensors of the wrist, abductor pollicis longus, extensor indicis, extensor digiti minimi, and extensor pollicis longus muscles. It does not have any cutaneous branches, making it the best answer.

A. The anterior interosseous nerve innervates flexors of the lateral three digits.

C. Although the radial nerve does give rise to the deep branch, there are no cutaneous sensory deficits mentioned, so the radial nerve proper was not affected.

D. The ulnar nerve also innervates flexors in the hand but since no sensory deficits were noted ulnar nerve injury can be ruled out.

E. The superficial radial nerve is a cutaneous nerve.
GAS 775–777; N 469; ABR/McM 161

180. C. Froment test is a special test to aid in the diagnosis of ulnar nerve palsy. The test evaluates the function of adductor pollicis muscle.

A. The first dorsal interosseous is tested by abducting the index finger against resistance.

B. The opponens pollicis muscle is evaluated using pulp-to-pulp opposition and the squeeze test.

C. The flexor pollicis longus muscle is a flexor of the thumb and is tested by instructing the patient to flex the tip of the thumb against resistance while the proximal phalanx is held in extension.

D. The flexor pollicis brevis muscle flexes the thumb at the MCP joint and is tested by asking the individual to flex the proximal phalanx of the thumb against resistance.
GAS 805–807; N 455; ABR/McM 168

181. A. Tinel sign is used to aid in the diagnosis of carpal tunnel syndrome. It is performed by lightly percussing above the carpal tunnel where the median nerve is located.

B. De Quervain tenosynovitis is inflammation of the sheath or tunnel that surrounds tendons that control the thumb, for example, extensor pollicis brevis. It is tested using Finkelstein test, where the examiner grips the thumb of the individual being tested and ulnarly deviates the hand sharply.

C. Thoracic outlet syndrome is tested using Adson test.

D. Mallet finger describes a finger deformity due to extensor digitorum tendon injury.

E. Radial nerve damage is tested by evaluating the cutaneous distribution of the radial nerve or by testing the extensor muscles of the hand.
GAS 788–789; N 452; ABR/McM 166

182. D. A 45-year-old man comes to the emergency department because of difficulty breathing through his nose. Physical examination shows signs of an obstruction of the nasal airway in both nostrils. A CT scan of the head shows bilateral nasal obstruction with left maxillary sinus involvement. (Fig. 7.14). Drainage from which of the following structures will most likely be impaired from the obstruction?

A, B, C. Compression of the ulnar nerve at the medial epicondyle, radial nerve at the neck of the radius, or median nerve in the carpal tunnel would not cause the motor deficits present in this patient.

E. There are no nerves originating directly from the divisions of the brachial plexus.
GAS 729, 736; N 420; ABR/McM 135

183. B. The scaphoid is the most commonly fractured carpal bone as a result of the relationship with the styloid process of the radius in the distal forearm. When a person falls as described in this question, the scaphoid gets pushed against the styloid process, usually at the narrowest ("waist") part of the scaphoid and fractures as a result of the forces transmitted through the bones.

A. The triquetrum articulates with the lunate laterally, the ulnar proximally, and the hamate distally. This bone has no association with the anatomical snuff box.

C. The capitate is the largest of the carpal bones. The capitate articulates proximally with the lunate and scaphoid and distally with the bases of the second, third, and fourth metacarpals. The capitate has no associations with the anatomical snuff box.

D. The hamate is also a medially oriented carpal bone and does not form the floor of the anatomical snuff box.

E. The trapezoid is a laterally oriented carpal bone with proximal articulation with the second metacarpal and distal articulation with the scaphoid. The trapezoid is not associated with the floor of the anatomical snuff box.
GAS 787; N 457; ABR/McM 128

184. A. The AC and coracoclavicular ligaments are critical to the stability of the shoulder. In particular, the coracoclavicular ligament provides much of the weight-bearing support for the upper limb on the clavicle. The AC joint capsule attaches the acromion (of the scapula) to the clavicle and the coracoclavicular ligament attaches the coracoid process to the clavicle. Interruption of these ligaments would cause dislocation of the AC joint as seen on the x-ray.

B. The coracoacromial ligament extends between the acromion and the coracoid process of the scapula.

C. The sternoclavicular joint exists between the manubrium and the proximal end of the clavicle and is unrelated to either the injury or the x-ray.

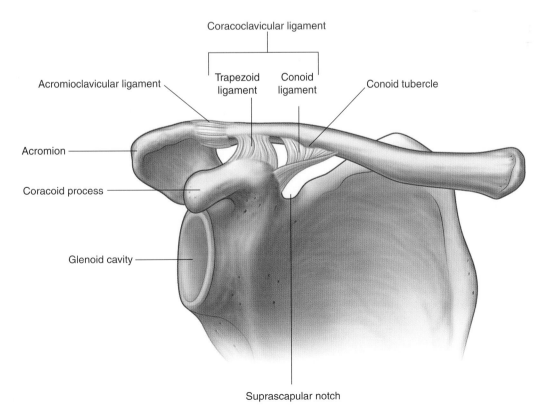

Coracoclavicular ligament

Acromioclavicular ligament

Trapezoid ligament

Conoid ligament

Conoid tubercle

Acromion

Coracoid process

Glenoid cavity

Suprascapular notch

• *GAS* **Fig. 7.24**

D. The transverse scapular ligament lies above the superior scapular notch and converts it into a foramen through which the suprascapular nerve runs (GAS Fig. 7.24).

E. See explanation for A and B.

GAS 694; N 410; ABR/McM 142

185. B. The x-ray shows a fracture of the humerus at the surgical neck. The bruising and dimpling of the upper arm would result from this injury. The axillary nerve leaves the brachial plexus as a terminal branch of the posterior cord. It passes through the quadrangular space and wraps around the surgical neck of the humerus on its way to provide innervation to the teres minor, the deltoid, and the portion of skin over the lower aspect of the deltoid that is known as the "sergeant's patch."

A. The radial nerve travels in the radial groove along the body of the humerus and would be injured in a fracture of the body of the humerus.

C. The ulnar nerve could be injured in a fracture of the medial epicondyle.

D. The median nerve travels too deep to be injured here and could be compressed at the carpal tunnel or at the cubital fossa.

E. The musculocutaneous nerve is likewise within the tissue and will not be affected by this injury.

GAS 692–693; N 422; ABR/McM 142

186. C. The median nerve and brachial artery were injured. Injury to the median nerve is indicated by the weakness of pronation, wrist flexion, and grip strength. The median nerve innervates the muscles that govern or carry out these movements. The brachial artery is near the median nerve and can also be injured. Flexion at the DIP joints of the ring and little fingers indicates that the ulnar nerve is intact. The x-ray indicates a supracondylar fracture of the humerus, which is the region in which the median nerve passes.

A. A fracture at the surgical neck would injure the axillary nerve and posterior circumflex humeral artery.

B. A fracture of the body of the humerus would injure the radial nerve and deep brachial artery.

D. The superficial radial nerve and radial artery would be damaged by injury over or in the anatomical snuffbox.

E. Ulnar nerve palsy would present with a clawed hand deformity. A supracondylar fracture will not disrupt the integrity of the ulnar nerve. The ulnar artery is a distal branch of the brachial artery. Supracondylar fracture will not cause direct injury to the ulnar nerve.

GAS 745, 750, 757; N 438; ABR/McM 158

7

Head and Neck

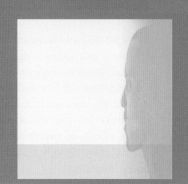

Questions

Questions 1–25

1. A 2-month-old boy is brought to the physician for a routine examination. Physical examination shows a small pit at the anterior border of his left sternocleidomastoid muscle with mucus dripping intermittently from the opening. The area appears slightly tender to palpation. A CT scan of the head and neck shows the pit extending to the tonsillar fossa as a branchial fistula. Which of the following embryologic structures is most likely involved in this anomaly?
   A. Second pharyngeal arch
   B. Second pharyngeal pouch and groove
   C. Third pharyngeal pouch
   D. Thyroglossal duct
   E. Second pharyngeal pouch and cervical sinus

2. A 6-month-old girl is brought to the physician by her parents for follow up examination for her cleft palate. The parents say the child is developing and feeding well despite the defect. Physical examination shows a cleft palate and an otherwise healthy child with no other abnormalities. The major portion of the palate develops from which of the following embryonic structures?
   A. Lateral palatine process
   B. Median palatine process
   C. Intermaxillary segment
   D. Median nasal prominences
   E. Frontonasal eminence

3. A 3-month-old boy is brought to the office by his mother because she noticed a small area of his right iris is missing. Physical examination shows age-appropriate eye movements, a normal ciliary body, and macular sparing of the left and right eye. Examination of the right eye shows a defect consistent with a coloboma. Which of the following is the most likely embryological cause of this condition?
   A. Failure of the retinal/choroid fissure to close
   B. Abnormal neural crest formation
   C. Abnormal interactions between the optic vesicle and ectoderm
   D. Posterior chamber cavitation
   E. Weak adhesion between the inner and outer layers of the optic vesicle

4. A 28-year-old woman delivers a boy by spontaneous vaginal delivery without any complications. Physical examination of the boy shows a depression of the skull. The physician reassures the mother that the depression in the boy's skull is normal and will close at a certain age. Which of the following fontanelles is located at the junction of the sagittal and coronal sutures and at what age does this fontanelle typically close?
   A. Posterior fontanelle, which closes at about 2 years
   B. Mastoid fontanelle, which closes at about 16 months
   C. Lambdoid fontanelle, which closes at 8 months to 1 year
   D. Sphenoidal fontanelle, which closes at about 3 years
   E. Anterior fontanelle, which closes at about 18 months

5. A 3-year-old boy is brought to the physician by his mother after she noticed a lump in his neck. The child had recently recovered from an upper respiratory tract infection. Physical examination shows a soft, anterior, midline cervical mass which is tender to palpation. When he is asked to protrude his tongue, the mass in the neck is observed to move upward. Which of the following is the most likely diagnosis?
   A. Thyroglossal duct cyst
   B. Defect in sixth pharyngeal arch
   C. Branchial cyst
   D. Cystic fistula of the third pharyngeal arch
   E. Defect in first pharyngeal arch

6. A 25-year-old woman delivers a girl by cesarean section. The pregnancy and delivery were uncomplicated. Physical examination shows a gap in her upper lip, and no other malformations or deficits are observed. A diagnosis of cleft lip was made. Failure of fusion of which of the following structures is the most likely the cause of this condition?
   A. Lateral nasal and maxillary prominences/processes
   B. Medial nasal prominences/processes
   C. Lateral nasal and medial nasal prominences/processes
   D. Lateral prominences/processes
   E. Maxillary prominences/processes and the intermaxillary segment

7. A 30-year-old woman delivers a boy by an uncomplicated spontaneous vaginal delivery. Physical examination shows hypoplasia of the mandible, cleft palate, and defects of the eye and ear. All defects were found unilaterally on the right side. The rest of the examination shows no other abnormalities. Abnormal development of which of the following pharyngeal arches would most likely produce such symptoms?
   A. First arch
   B. Second arch
   C. Third arch
   D. Fourth arch
   E. Sixth arch

8. A 28-year-old woman delivers a boy at preterm who was brought to the neonatal intensive care unit for observation. Physical examination of the boy shows a tuft of hair over the sacrum. Ultrasonography of his head shows a dilation of the lateral and third ventricles, with a normal-sized fourth ventricle. Stenosis of the cerebral aqueduct (of Sylvius) is also seen. Which of the following conditions is the most likely diagnosis?
   A. Nonobstructive hydrocephalus
   B. Anencephaly
   C. Obstructive hydrocephalus
   D. Meroanencephaly
   E. Holoprosencephaly

9. A 5-year-old girl is brought to the physician by her mother because she noticed a mass in the neck. The child has no difficulty in swallowing. Physical examination shows a midline neck mass. Lung sounds are clear to auscultation bilaterally. A biopsy of the mass shows thymic tissue. Based on embryonic origin of the thymus, which of the following additional structures is most likely to have an ectopic location?
   A. Jugulodigastric lymph node
   B. Lingual tonsil
   C. Parathyroid gland
   D. Submandibular gland
   E. Thyroid gland

10. A 3-month-old boy with a history of low birth weight is brought to the physician for a follow up. Physical examination shows no abnormalities. Laboratory results show hypocalcemia and ultrasound shows thyroid hypoplasia, and absence of the thymus. Abnormal development of which of the following pharyngeal pouches or arches will most likely produce these defects?
    A. First and second
    B. Second and third
    C. Third and fourth
    D. Fourth
    E. Fourth and sixth

11. A 31-year-old woman delivers a term girl by an uncomplicated vaginal delivery. Physical examination of the neonate shows a gap in her upper lip, no other malformations or deficits are observed. A diagnosis of a cleft lip was made. Which of the following is considered to be the most important causative factor in the production of this anomaly?
    A. Riboflavin deficiency
    B. Infectious disease
    C. Mutant genes
    D. Cortisone administration during pregnancy
    E. Irradiation

12. A 5-month-old boy is brought to the physician after his parents witnessed unusual muscle-jerking and twitching on a few occasions. Physical examination shows no abnormalities. Laboratory studies show hypocalcemia. An ultrasound examination of the neck shows absence of the thymus and inferior parathyroid glands. Which of the following pharyngeal pouches is most likely involved?
    A. First
    B. Second
    C. Third
    D. Fourth
    E. Fifth

13. A 1-month-old girl was brought to the physician by her mother because of harsh sounds during breathing. The mother says the breathing is less noisy when the infant is laying on her stomach. Physical examination shows a stridor. An x-ray of the neck shows the greater cornua and the inferior part of the hyoid bone were absent at birth. A defect in an associated muscle has the potential to compromise the act of swallowing. The girl appears to respire and feed well. The failure of development of which of the following embryonic structures most likely led to these defects?
    A. Maxillary prominence
    B. Mandibular prominence
    C. Second pharyngeal arch
    D. Third pharyngeal arch
    E. Fourth pharyngeal arch

14. A 22-year-old woman comes to the emergency department because of 1-week history of a swelling on the right side of her neck. She says the swelling was bigger and tender. Physical examination shows a small area of swelling that is painless on palpation. An ultrasound examination of the neck shows a well-defined cystic mass at the angle of the mandible anterior to the sternocleidomastoid muscle. What is the most likely diagnosis?
    A. Dermoid cyst
    B. Inflamed lymph node
    C. Accessory thyroid gland tissue
    D. Thyroglossal duct cyst
    E. Lateral cervical cyst

15. A preterm 5-day-old boy is kept for observation after birth because an enlarged head. The prenatal course and delivery were uncomplicated. Physical examination shows a small infant with an enlarged head and no other abnormalities. An MRI of the head confirms the diagnosis of noncommunicating hydrocephalus (Fig. 7.1). Which of the following is the most likely cause of such a condition?

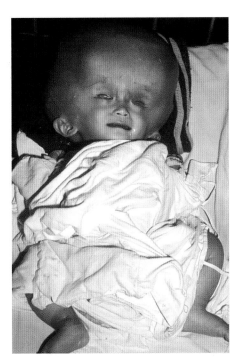

• Fig. 7.1

A. Obstruction in the circulation of the cerebrospinal fluid (CSF)
B. Excess production of CSF
C. Increased size of the head
D. Disturbances in the resorption of CSF
E. Failure of the neural tube to close

16. A 1-month-old boy is brought to the physician for routine examination. The prenatal course and delivery were uncomplicated. His Appearance, Pulse, Grimace, Activity, and Respiration (APGAR) scores were 8 and 9 at 1 and 5 minutes, respectively. He is at the 90th percentile for weight and height. Physical examination shows an atretic external acoustic meatus on the right side. Which of the following conditions is most likely the cause of this defect?
A. Otic pit did not form
B. Development of the first pharyngeal pouch was affected
C. Meatal plug did not canalize
D. Auricular hillocks did not develop
E. The tubotympanic recess degenerated

17. A 65-year-old woman comes to the physician because of a burning pain in the area of her chin and lower lip. Physical examination shows no abnormalities, and she was sent home with over-the-counter analgesics. A few days later, the woman returns with small vesicles over the same area, some of which have erupted. She is diagnosed with a dermatomal herpes zoster inflammation (shingles). Which of the following nerves is most likely to contain the virus?
A. Auriculotemporal
B. Buccal
C. Lesser petrosal
D. Mental
E. Infraorbital

18. A 68-year-old woman is brought to the emergency department because of sudden, excruciating bouts of pain over the area of her midface. The patient has a history of trigeminal neuralgia (tic douloureax). Three months ago, she ran out of medication while her primary care physician was on holiday. In this condition, which ganglion is most likely responsible for mediating the pain?
A. Geniculate
B. Trigeminal (semilunar or Gasserian)
C. Inferior glossopharyngeal
D. Otic
E. Pterygopalatine

19. A 17-year-old girl is brought to the emergency department because of an intense headache and a "bulging" sensation in her eyes. Physical examination shows photophobia with difficulty of lateral gaze in both eyes. An MRI of the head confirms the diagnosis of cavernous sinus thrombosis. Thrombophlebitis in the "danger area" of the face can easily spread to the cavernous sinus and involve the ophthalmic branch of the trigeminal nerve. If this occurs, which of the following symptoms will most likely be present during physical examination?
A. Pain in the hard palate
B. Anesthesia of the upper lip
C. Pain from the eyeball
D. Pain over the lower eyelid
E. Tingling sensation over the buccal region of the face

20. A 40-year-old man is brought to the emergency department because of a severe headache, dizziness, and vomiting. The patient has a history of chronic headaches for 6 months. Physical examination shows weakness in protrusion of the tongue and no other deficits or abnormalities. An MRI of the head shows a mass at the hypoglossal canal. Which of the following muscles will most likely be affected by this mass?
A. Geniohyoid
B. Mylohyoid
C. Palatoglossus
D. Genioglossus
E. Thyrohyoid

21. A 45-year-old woman is brought to the emergency department because of a severe headache, dizziness, and vomiting. Physical examination shows that the patient has dryness of the nasal and paranasal sinuses, loss of lacrimation, and loss of taste from the anterior two-thirds of the tongue. An MRI of the brain shows an intracranial tumor. Which of the following structures has most likely been affected by the tumor to cause these symptoms?
A. Auriculotemporal nerve
B. Lesser petrosal nerve
C. Facial nerve
D. Inferior salivatory nucleus
E. Pterygopalatine ganglion

22. A 17-year-old girl comes to the physician because of symptoms of pain and discoloration of her right hand for the past month. She first noticed the symptoms while she was brushing her hair or talking on the phone. An MRI of the neck confirms the diagnosis of thoracic outlet syndrome. Which symptom would most likely be present in this syndrome?
    A. Problems with respiration because of pressure on the phrenic nerve
    B. Reduced blood flow to the thoracic wall
    C. Reduced venous return from the head and neck
    D. Numbness in the upper limb
    E. Distention of the internal jugular vein

23. A 31-year-old woman is brought to the emergency department after being involved in a motor vehicle collision. She has a Glasgow Coma Scale (GCS) of 12. Physical examination shows right pupillary miosis, ptosis of the eyelid, and anhidrosis of the right side of face. A CT scan of the head shows a fracture and large hematoma inferior to the right jugular foramen. Which of the following ganglia is most likely affected by the hematoma?
    A. Submandibular
    B. Trigeminal (semilunar or Gasserian)
    C. Superior cervical
    D. Geniculate
    E. Ciliary

24. A 35-year-old man is brought to the emergency department because of sudden bouts of severe headaches. He describes the pain to be on the right side and involving his right eye at times. Physical examination shows a loss of general sensation from the anterior two-thirds of his tongue, but taste and salivation are intact. An MRI of the head shows a tumor within the infratemporal fossa. Which of the following nerves is most likely affected by the tumor?
    A. Lingual proximal to its junction with the chorda tympani
    B. Chorda tympani
    C. Inferior alveolar
    D. Lesser petrosal
    E. Glossopharyngeal

25. A 60-year-old woman is brought to the emergency department with chronic episodic headaches and enlarged lymph nodes. The patient says she has been having sudden bouts of dizziness causing her to have to sit or lie down and close her eyes. She also mentions a feeling of fullness in her right ear. A CT scan of the head shows a tumor at the jugular foramen. Which of the following would be the most likely neurologic deficit?
    A. Loss of tongue movements
    B. Loss of facial expression
    C. Loss of sensation from the face and the scalp
    D. Loss of hearing
    E. Loss of gag reflex

Questions 26–50

26. A 34-year-old man is brought to the emergency department after being hit on the head with a baseball bat. He is unconscious and unresponsive. Physical exam shows a large hematoma on the right temporal region of the patient's head. A CT scan of the head shows a fractured pterion and an epidural hematoma. Branches of which of the following arteries are most likely to be injured?
    A. External carotid
    B. Superficial temporal
    C. Maxillary
    D. Deep temporal
    E. Middle meningeal

27. A 48-year-old woman is brought to the emergency department by her family after being found unconscious. The patient has a history of chronic headaches and her daughter says they seem to be getting worse lately. Physical examination shows no abnormalities. A CT scan shows a tumor in her brain. When the woman regains consciousness, her right eye is directed laterally and downward, with complete ptosis of her upper eyelid, and her pupil is dilated. Which of the following structures was most likely affected by the tumor to result in these symptoms?
    A. Oculomotor nerve
    B. Optic nerve
    C. Facial nerve
    D. Ciliary ganglion
    E. Superior cervical ganglion (SCG)

28. A 55-year-old man is brought to the emergency department after sustaining an injury to the head during work. The patient is distraught, but conscious and oriented to person, place, and time. Physical examination shows severe scalp lacerations and profuse bleeding. The wounds were quickly cleaned and sutured. After 3 days, the wound is inflamed, swollen, and painful. Between which tissue layers is the infection most likely located?
    A. The periosteum and bone
    B. The aponeurosis and the periosteum
    C. The dense connective tissue and the aponeurosis
    D. The dense connective tissue and the skin
    E. The dermis and the epidermis

29. A 36-year-old woman is brought to the emergency department after being involved in a motor vehicle collision. The patient is conscious, oriented to person, place, and time, and says she has significant pain in her neck. Physical examination shows tenderness over her neck without any lacerations. The uvula is found to be deviated to the right. No other abnormalities were found. A CT scan of the head shows no fractures. Which nerve is most likely affected to result in this deviation?
    A. Left vagus
    B. Right vagus
    C. Right hypoglossal
    D. Left glossopharyngeal
    E. Right glossopharyngeal

30. A 22-year-old man is brought to the emergency department after being found unconscious on the street. The man is not responsive and breathing very slowly. His oxygen saturation is dangerously low and intubation is initiated by passing an endotracheal tube through an opening between the vocal folds. What is the name of this opening?
    A. Piriform recess
    B. Vestibule
    C. Ventricle
    D. Vallecula
    E. Rima glottidis

31. A 55-year-old man is brought to the emergency department with left-sided tooth pain in his upper jaw. Physical examination shows tenderness on the left side of his face and ipsilateral maxillary teeth when tapping on his left maxilla. The patient has no allergies. Which of the following conditions will be the most likely diagnosis?
    A. Sphenoid sinusitis
    B. Anterior ethmoidal sinusitis
    C. Posterior ethmoidal sinusitis
    D. Maxillary sinusitis
    E. Frontal sinusitis

32. A 70-year-old man is brought to the emergency department because of severe headaches that have gotten progressively worse in the past few weeks. He describes the pain as severe and has no history of trauma or changes to his vision. The patient also has difficulty coughing and swallowing. An MRI of the head shows a tumor affecting a cranial nerve. Which nerve is most likely affected?
    A. Mandibular
    B. Maxillary
    C. Glossopharyngeal
    D. Vagus
    E. Hypoglossal

33. A 7-year-old boy is brought to the emergency department because of 2-day history of high fever. The boy says he has pain in his right ear and throat. Physical examination shows a red and inflamed pharynx. The tympanic membranes are intact and translucent without any exudate. A diagnosis of viral pharyngitis is made. Which of the following structures most likely provided a pathway for the infection to spread to the tympanic cavity (middle ear)?
    A. Choanae
    B. Internal acoustic meatus
    C. External acoustic meatus
    D. Auditory tube
    E. Pharyngeal recess

34. A 33-year-old woman is brought to the emergency department after falling and hitting her head. The patient is unresponsive but breathing. There is no obvious sign of bleeding. Physical examination shows responsive pupillary light test reflex bilaterally. The integrity of which of the following nerves is being checked during this reflex?
    A. Optic and facial
    B. Optic and oculomotor

C. Maxillary and facial
D. Ophthalmic and oculomotor
E. Ophthalmic and facial

35. A 48-year-old man comes to the physician because of a 2-week history of double vision. The patient has not experienced any recent trauma. Physical examination shows that he is unable to adduct his left eye and lacks a corneal reflex on the left side. An MRI of the head confirms an intracranial lesion. Where is the most likely location of the lesion causing these symptoms?
    A. Inferior orbital fissure
    B. Optic canal
    C. Superior orbital fissure
    D. Foramen rotundum
    E. Foramen ovale

36. A 34-year-old man comes to the physician because of recent sensitivity to sound. He works as security personnel during concerts and festivals. Physical examination shows no abnormalities with the tympanic membrane or external acoustic meatus. The patient says he does not have trouble hearing, but he has some ringing in his ears. A diagnosis of hyperacusis is made. Which of the following cranial nerve's injury is most likely responsible for these symptoms?
    A. Hypoglossal
    B. Facial
    C. Accessory
    D. Vagus
    E. Glossopharyngeal

37. A 34-year-old man comes to the physician because of 1-week history of pain in his right ear. When the patient is asked about events preceding his condition, he mentions swimming regularly in the lake nearby. Physical examination shows an external acoustic meatus infection (otitis externa) and the patient coughs while the external acoustic meatus is inspected with a speculum. The cough results from irritation to which nerve innervating an area of the external acoustic meatus?
    A. Vestibulocochlear
    B. Vagus
    C. Trigeminal
    D. Facial
    E. Accessory

38. A 29-year-old woman comes to the physician for a follow-up examination, two weeks after undergoing a thyroidectomy. She was diagnosed with intractable Graves disease. She says her wound has healed well and she has noticed a significant improvement in her symptoms, but her voice has become hoarse and has not improved. Which of the following nerves was most likely injured during the operation?
    A. Internal laryngeal
    B. External laryngeal
    C. Recurrent laryngeal
    D. Superior laryngeal
    E. Glossopharyngeal

39. A 48-year-old man comes to the physician because his wife recently noticed something strange with his right eye. Physical examination under normal lighting shows that the patient's right and left pupil are 2 mm and 4 mm, respectively; when the lights are off, they are 2 mm and 6 mm, respectively. His vision in both eyes is normal. These findings are most likely because of a lesion involving which of the following right-sided structures?
    A. Oculomotor nerve
    B. SCG
    C. Nervus intermedius
    D. Edinger-Westphal nucleus
    E. Trigeminal (semilunar, Gasserian) ganglion

40. A 55-year-old woman comes to the physician for worsening chronic headaches from a right-sided tumor at the base of the skull. She has recently noticed her right eye and right nostril constantly feel dry. Which of the following nerves is most likely compressed by a tumor to result in a decreased secretion from the lacrimal gland and mucous membrane of her nasal passage?
    A. Chorda tympani
    B. Deep petrosal
    C. Greater petrosal
    D. Lesser petrosal
    E. Nasociliary

41. A 24-year-old man is brought to the emergency department after a street fight. The patient was punched in the eye and is having difficulty seeing out of his left eye. He says that he did not fall or lose consciousness during or after the fight. Physical examination shows a sunken left orbit surrounded by edematous soft tissue. A CT scan of the head shows an inferior (blow-out) fracture of the orbit with the left globe ectopically positioned. Orbital structures would most likely be found in which of the following spaces?
    A. Ethmoidal cells
    B. Frontal sinus
    C. Maxillary sinus
    D. Nasal cavity
    E. Sphenoidal sinus

42. A 35-year-old woman is brought to the emergency department by her family because of worsening fever. Her family says that she has had a severe case of sinusitis for the past week that has not gotten better and this morning she seemed confused. Physical examination shows a lethargic woman with fever, tachycardia, and tachypnea. Laboratory studies show leukocytosis and a negative urine dip. A CT scan of the head shows a thrombus within the cavernous sinus. A diagnosis of sepsis secondary to cavernous sinus thrombosis is made. Which of the following is the most direct route for spread of infection from the face to the cavernous sinus?
    A. Pterygoid venous plexus
    B. Superior ophthalmic vein
    C. Frontal venous plexus

D. Basilar venous plexus
E. Parietal emissary vein

43. A 7-year-old boy was brought to the emergency department by his parents for a complication of otitis media which became a mastoiditis. A mastoidectomy with myringotomy was performed to treat the infection. Five days postoperatively, the boy develops several facial deficits. Physical examination shows that the right corner of his mouth was drooping, he was unable to close his right eye, and there was food collection in his right oral vestibule. Which of the following nerves was most likely injured during the surgery?
    A. Glossopharyngeal
    B. Vagus
    C. Facial
    D. Maxillary division of the trigeminal nerve
    E. Mandibular division of the trigeminal nerve

44. A 55-year-old man comes to the emergency department because of a severe headache. The patient has a history of smoking and hypertension. A CT scan of the head shows an aneurysm in the cerebral arterial circle (of Willis). Which of the following vessels does not contribute to the circle?
    A. Anterior communicating
    B. Posterior communicating
    C. Middle cerebral
    D. Internal carotid
    E. Posterior cerebral

45. A 45-year-old woman comes to the physician with severe ear pain for the past 3 days. She says that the pain was initially mild then progressively got worse, and yesterday she developed a fever. A CT scan of the head shows an infection of the mastoid cells. In mastoiditis, the infection can erode the thin layer of the bone between the mastoid cells and the posterior cranial fossa. If this occurs, the infection can spread into the skull through the venous system. Which of the following venous structures is most likely the route of infection?
    A. Superior sagittal sinus
    B. Inferior sagittal sinus
    C. Straight sinus
    D. Cavernous sinus
    E. Sigmoid sinus

46. A 63-year-old man comes to the physician because he has been having trouble hearing from his left ear. He says that food doesn't seem to taste the same and at times he catches himself drooling from the left side of his mouth. A CT scan of the head shows a tumor compressing a nerve within the skull. Through which of the following openings is the nerve most likely passing?
    A. Foramen ovale
    B. Foramen rotundum
    C. Internal acoustic meatus
    D. Jugular foramen
    E. Superior orbital fissure

47. A 70-year-old man comes to the physician for a scheduled biopsy of a growth he has had on his lower lip for the past 6 months. The patient has smoked 1 pack of cigarettes daily for 40 years and lost 9 kg (20 lb) over the last 3 months. A biopsy of his lower lip shows a squamous cell carcinoma. The patient is evaluated for surgical excision with lip reconstruction. If the cancer was to metastasize, which lymph nodes will most likely be involved the first?

A. Occipital
B. Parotid
C. Retropharyngeal
D. Jugulodigastric
E. Submental

48. A 54-year-old man comes to the physician because of 5-month history of headaches. He says that the pain is throbbing in nature with intermittent episodes of double vision. He does not have a history of migraines and he has been healthy otherwise. Physical examination shows no abnormalities. A CT scan of the head shows an internal carotid artery aneurysm inside the cavernous sinus. Which of the following nerves would most likely be affected first?

A. Abducens nerve
B. Oculomotor nerve
C. Ophthalmic nerve
D. Maxillary nerve
E. Trochlear nerve

49. A 24-year-old man comes to the physician 2 weeks after he had his wisdom teeth extracted from both sides of his lower jaw. Right after the procedure when the local anesthetic wore off, the patient noticed that he did not have any sensation in the front of his tongue. Physical examination shows that he has lost his sense of taste from the anterior two-thirds of his tongue. Which of the following nerves was most likely injured during the procedure?

A. Auriculotemporal
B. Chorda tympani
C. Lingual
D. Mental
E. Inferior alveolar

50. A 56-year-old woman is brought to the emergency department because of a 3-month history of ear pain. She has a history of rheumatoid arthritis that affects her temporomandibular joint. The patient has no other symptoms. An MRI scan is shown in Fig. 7.2. Which of the following nerves is most likely responsible for the pain sensation?

A. Facial
B. Auriculotemporal
C. Lesser petrosal
D. Vestibulocochlear
E. Chorda tympani

Questions 51–75

51. A 56-year-old man is admitted to the hospital for a tumor resection below the base of his skull. After healing, the patient notices that his mouth is somewhat drier during eating than before his surgery. An MRI

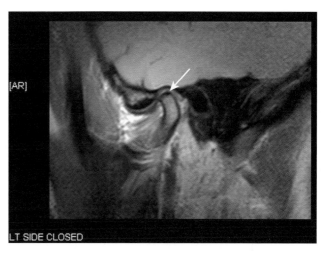

• Fig. 7.2

examination shows that the mandibular division of the trigeminal nerve is damaged, most likely during the procedure because of its involvement with the tumor. Which of the following ganglia is most likely damaged?

A. Trigeminal (semilunar, Gasserian)
B. Geniculate
C. Superior cervical
D. Otic
E. Submandibular

52. In the case of overproduction of CSF, drainage of CSF through the arachnoid villi may not be able to keep pace with the amount of CSF being produced, and hydrocephaly may result. The arachnoid villi allow CSF to pass between which two of the following spaces?

A. Choroid plexus and subdural space
B. Subarachnoid space and superior sagittal sinus
C. Subdural space and cavernous sinus
D. Superior sagittal sinus and jugular vein
E. Epidural and subdural space

53. A 22-year-old woman is brought to the emergency department after she was hit by a soccer ball in her right eye. She did not lose consciousness and her vital signs are within normal limits. Physical examination shows that her vision and extraocular eye movements are all intact and unchanged. The corneal reflex is tested and found to be normal. Which of the following nerves is responsible for the afferent limb of this reflex?

A. Frontal
B. Lacrimal
C. Nasociliary
D. Oculomotor
E. Optic

54. A 21-year-old man was brought to the emergency department because of a severe nosebleed. The bleeding has stopped, and the patient is otherwise stable. The area known as Kiesselbach (or Little) plexus is the most common area where epistaxis originates from. This area is exposed to environmental changes and trauma. Which of the following arteries most likely provide anastomoses to this area?

A. Ascending palatine and ascending pharyngeal

B. Posterior superior alveolar and accessory meningeal

C. Lateral branches of posterior ethmoidal and middle meningeal

D. Septal branches of the sphenopalatine and superior labial

E. Descending palatine and tonsillar branches of the pharyngeal

55. A 12-year-old boy is brought to the emergency department because of trouble swallowing for the past few days. Physical examination shows fever and swollen palatine tonsils. As this was his third case of tonsillitis within 6 months, a tonsillectomy is recommended. The palatine tonsils are located between the anterior and posterior tonsillar pillars. Which of the following muscles form these pillars?

A. Levator veli palatini and tensor veli palatini

B. Palatoglossus and palatopharyngeus

C. Styloglossus and stylopharyngeus

D. Palatopharyngeus and salpingopharyngeus

E. Superior and middle pharyngeal constrictors

56. A 35-year-old woman comes to the physician for a scheduled laparoscopic cholecystectomy. In the operating room, a laryngeal mask airway has been placed to deliver continuous anesthesia and ensure proper oxygenation during the surgery. This mask is composed of an air tube with an inflatable or self-sealing cuff. It is inserted through the mouth until the cuff rests against the top of the glottis and helps keep the airway open. Under normal conditions, the rima glottidis is opened by which pair of muscles?

A. Posterior cricoarytenoids

B. Lateral cricoarytenoids

C. Thyroarytenoids

D. Transverse arytenoids

E. Cricothyroids

57. A 32-year-old man comes to the physician because of a 3-day history of a painful swelling of his right cheek. The swelling is localized at the right lower jaw and is worse during meals. The patient says that he can also feel a soft, thin ridge of tissue along the inside of his cheek, running forward from his right lower jaw toward his right upper molars. He is concerned because he has never felt that structure before. The physician reassures him that the structure is normal and it has just become inflamed because of the infection. Which of the following is the most likely structure she is feeling?

A. Facial artery

B. Maxillary artery

C. Parotid duct

D. Marginal mandibular branch of the facial nerve

E. Facial vein

58. A 43-year-old man comes to the physician for a persistent sore throat and worsening hoarseness for the past year. The patient is found to have a laryngeal carcinoma. A surgical procedure is performed, and the tumor is successfully removed from the larynx. During the surgery, the right ansa cervicalis is anastomosed with the right recurrent laryngeal nerve in order to reinnervate the muscles of the larynx and restore phonation. Which of the following muscles will most likely be paralyzed after the surgery?

A. Sternocleidomastoid

B. Platysma

C. Sternohyoid

D. Trapezius

E. Cricothyroid

59. A 67-year-old woman is brought to the emergency department with a painful, erythematous swelling on the right side of her neck. An ultrasound examination shows a fluid-filled structure with hyperechoic debris that is consistent with an abscess. The abscess, located in the middle of the posterior cervical triangle, is drained surgically. During recovery, physical examination shows right shoulder droop and inability to raise her right hand above her head. Which of the following nerves has most likely been injured?

A. Accessory

B. Ansa cervicalis

C. Facial

D. Hypoglossal

E. Suprascapular

60. A 20-year-old man was brought to the emergency department with a stab wound in the superior region of his neck during a bar fight. Vital signs are within normal limits. A CT scan of the neck shows that the wound has not affected any major structures. Following surgical repair of the wound, physical examination shows that the patient has lost sensation from the skin over the angle of the jaw. Which of the following nerves is most likely injured?

A. Supraclavicular

B. Transverse cervical

C. Great auricular

D. Greater occipital

E. Lesser occipital

61. A 2-year-old boy is brought to the physician for a routine examination. He was born via spontaneous vaginal delivery which was complicated causing his head posture to be continuously tilted. Physical examination shows his right ear is held close to his right shoulder and his face is turned superiorly to the left. No neck masses are visible. A diagnosis of congenital torticollis is made, and the child is started on a trial of physical therapy before considering medical management. Which of the following muscles was most likely damaged during birth?

A. Anterior scalene

B. Omohyoid

C. Sternocleidomastoid

D. Trapezius

E. Platysma

62. A 35-year-old woman is brought to the emergency department after being involved in a motor vehicle collision. On arrival, the patient is unconscious with an

upper airway obstructed by blood and mucus. After vacuum suctioning, a midline tracheostomy inferior to the thyroid gland isthmus is performed to secure her airway. Which of the following vessels are most likely to be present at the site of incision and will need to be cauterized?

A. Middle thyroid vein and inferior thyroid artery
B. Inferior thyroid artery and inferior thyroid vein
C. Inferior thyroid vein and thyroidea ima artery
D. Cricothyroid artery and inferior thyroid vein
E. Left brachiocephalic vein and inferior thyroid artery

63. A 34-year-old woman comes to the emergency department because of a large mass at the center of her neck. Physical examination and subsequent ultrasound show a tumor of the thyroid gland. Biopsy suggests a benign tumor but because of its large size a partial thyroidectomy is performed. Twenty-four hours following the surgery, in which the inferior thyroid artery was ligated, the patient develops hoarseness and has difficulty breathing on exertion. Which of the following nerves was most likely injured during the surgical procedure?

A. Internal branch of superior laryngeal
B. Ansa cervicalis
C. Ansa subclavia
D. Recurrent laryngeal
E. External branch of superior laryngeal

64. A 65-year-old woman is brought to the emergency department because of fatigue and weight loss. She also has been having recurring headaches and difficulty swallowing. Recently, the patient's fluid intake has decreased because of frequently aspirating fluids when attempting to drink. She has lost 9 kg (20 lb) over 3 months. Physical exam shows loss of skin turgor and dysphagia. A CT scan of the head shows a skull base tumor occupying the space behind the jugular foramen. Involvement of which of the following structures is most likely responsible for these findings in the patient?

A. Ansa cervicalis
B. Cervical sympathetic trunk
C. External laryngeal nerve
D. Hypoglossal nerve
E. Vagus nerve

65. A 55-year-old woman is brought to the emergency department after feeling dizzy and falling. Recently, she has been having frequent episodes of headaches and dizziness. Her pulse is 100/min, blood pressure is 190/110 mm Hg, and respirations are 18/min. Physical examination shows carotid bruits bilaterally. The patient is undergoing an arteriogram that shows 90% occlusion in both common carotid arteries. A carotid endarterectomy is performed, and large atherosclerotic plaques are removed. Postoperatively, physical examination shows that her tongue deviated toward the right when she was asked to protrude it. Which of the following nerves was most likely injured during the procedure?

A. Right glossopharyngeal
B. Right hypoglossal
C. Left hypoglossal
D. Left lingual
E. Left vagus

66. A 34-year-old woman comes to the physician for a scheduled partial thyroidectomy. In the recovery room, she has been having difficulties drinking fluid and is noted to aspirate into her lungs. The patient failed her swallow evaluation. Physical examination shows that the area of the piriform recess above the vocal fold of the larynx was anesthetized. Which of the following nerves was most likely injured?

A. External branch of the superior pharyngeal
B. Hypoglossal
C. Internal branch of the superior laryngeal
D. Lingual
E. Recurrent laryngeal

67. A 38-year-old man comes to the physician because of a large mass in his lower anterior neck. The patient works at a nuclear power plant. He says that the lump does not cause any pain, but he has some difficulty swallowing. An ultrasound examination confirms a benign tumor of the thyroid gland and a partial thyroidectomy is performed. Twenty-four hours following the surgery, physical examination shows the patient could not abduct the true vocal cords. Which of the following muscles was most likely denervated during the operation?

A. Posterior cricoarytenoid
B. Lateral cricoarytenoid
C. Thyroarytenoid
D. Arytenoid
E. Cricothyroid

68. A 46-year-old woman is brought to the hospital for a scheduled thyroidectomy to remove a thyroid gland tumor. During the procedure, the superior thyroid artery is identified and used as a landmark in order to not damage its small companion nerve. Which of the following nerves is most likely to accompany this artery?

A. Cervical sympathetic trunk
B. External branch of the superior laryngeal
C. Inferior root of the ansa cervicalis
D. Internal branch of the superior laryngeal
E. Recurrent laryngeal

69. A 3-year-old girl is brought to the emergency department after accidentally inserting a pencil into her ear. The child is crying in pain. Physical examination shows a ruptured tympanic membrane with a few drops of blood in the external acoustic meatus. There is concern that there might have been injury to the nerve that principally innervates the external surface of the tympanic membrane. Which of the following clinical tests can be performed to check for injury to this nerve?

A. Check the taste in the anterior two-thirds of the tongue
B. Check the sensation to the pharynx and palate

C. Check if there is paresthesia at the temporomandibular joint

D. Check for sensation in the larynx

E. Check for sensation in the nasal cavity

70. A 27-year-old woman is brought to the emergency department after she was thrown from a motorcycle without wearing a helmet. An MRI of the head and neck shows a type I LeFort fracture and comminuted fracture of the mandible and temporomandibular joint. The patient underwent extensive reconstructive surgery and is recovering well. During the subsequent follow-up examination, the patient experiences high sensitivity to loud sounds. Which of the following muscles is most likely paralyzed?

A. Posterior belly of digastric

B. Stapedius

C. Tensor veli palatini

D. Stylohyoid

E. Cricothyroid

71. A 43-year-old man is brought to the emergency department after being hit in the head with a bat. Physical examination shows a deep skull laceration, facial bruising, and a hematoma. A CT scan of the head shows a fracture at the base of his skull. An MRI of the head shows that the right greater petrosal nerve has also been injured. Which of the following signs and/or symptoms need to be identified during physical examination in order to confirm the diagnosis of this nerve injury?

A. Partial dryness of the mouth because of lack of salivary secretions from the submandibular and sublingual glands

B. Partial dryness of the mouth because of lack of salivary secretions from the parotid gland

C. Dryness of the right cornea because of lack of lacrimal gland secretion

D. Loss of taste sensation from the right anterior two-thirds of the tongue

E. Loss of general sensation from the right anterior two-thirds of the tongue

72. A 12-year-old girl is brought to emergency department because of a fever and right ear pain. She has a history of recurrent middle ear infections. Her temperature is 38.9°C (102°F), pulse is 101/min, blood pressure 125/80 mm Hg. Physical examination shows a lesion in the tympanic plexus in the middle ear cavity. Since the preganglionic parasympathetic fibers that pass through the plexus have been lost, which of the following conditions will be found during physical examination?

A. Diminished mucus in the nasal cavity

B. Diminished mucus on the soft palate

C. Diminished saliva production by the parotid gland

D. Diminished saliva production by the submandibular and sublingual glands

E. Diminished tear production by the lacrimal gland

73. A 38-year-old woman comes to the dental clinic with acute tooth pain. The woman admits to eating a lot of sweets and rarely seeing a dentist. The dentist found several dental caries, with the worst being a penetrating cavity affecting one of the mandibular molar teeth. Which of the following nerves would the dentist need to anesthetize to treat the caries in that tooth?

A. Lingual

B. Inferior alveolar

C. Buccal

D. Mental

E. Mylohyoid

74. A 59-year-old man comes to the physician because of 3-month history of mandibular pain that has been getting worse. The pain has increased to the point where he cannot eat properly and is getting constant headaches. He always had trouble with his jaw as he used to be a boxer. Physical examination shows he has a grinding and clicking sensation when he moves his jaw. An MRI of the head shows an acute inflammation of the temporomandibular joint because of arthritis. Which of the following muscles will most likely be affected by the inflammatory process of this joint?

A. Temporalis

B. Medial pterygoid

C. Masseter

D. Lateral pterygoid

E. Buccinator

75. A 62-year-old woman is brought to the emergency department after a fall down a flight of stairs. The patient says she is feeling fine and she just fell because of double vision. Physical examination shows worsening diplopia when she attempts to look downward. A CT scan of the head shows no intracranial process or fracture. A lesion of which of the following nerves is most likely responsible for this patient's complaint?

A. Optic

B. Oculomotor

C. Abducens

D. Trochlear

E. Frontal

Questions 76–100

76. A 65-year-old man comes to the physician because of experiencing episodes of double vision. He says that double vision is intermittent and has been going on for 3 months. The patient is wondering if he has to change his prescription glasses. The patient has not had any headaches or dizziness. Physical examination shows that the patient experiences diplopia, and when he is asked to turn his right eye inward toward his nose and look down, he is able to look inward but not down. Which nerve is most likely involved?

A. Abducens

B. Nasociliary

C. Oculomotor, inferior division

D. Oculomotor, superior division

E. Trochlear

77. A 44-year-old woman comes to the physician for follow-up examination. She is being treated for Raynaud

disease and systemic lupus erythematosus. Her medication regimen contains a sympathetic blocking drug that is administered in high doses. Which of the following conditions will most likely be expected to occur as an adverse effect of the drug?

A. Exophthalmos and dilated pupil
B. Enophthalmos and dry eye
C. Dry eye and inability to accommodate for reading
D. Wide open eyelids and loss of depth perception
E. Ptosis and miosis

78. A 47-year-old woman is brought to the emergency department with signs of cavernous sinus thrombosis. An MRI of the head shows a pituitary gland tumor involving the cavernous sinus, confirming the initial diagnosis (Fig. 7.3). The right abducens nerve appears to be compressed by the tumor. A complete eye examination is conducted to identify potential nerve damage. In which direction will the physician most likely ask the patient to turn her right eye to assess for damage of the abducens nerve?

A. Inward
B. Outward
C. Downward
D. Down and out
E. Down and in

79. A 9-year-old boy is brought to the emergency department because of a drooping right eyelid (ptosis) (Fig. 7.4). Physical examination shows classical signs of Horner syndrome. The mother is very anxious as their family has a significant family history of strokes occurring at a young age. The patient is admitted to the hospital for further evaluation. Which of the following additional signs on the right side would be found in the patient?

A. Constricted pupil
B. Dry eye
C. Exophthalmos
D. Pale, blanched face
E. Sweaty face

80. A 32-year-old woman is brought to the emergency department because of sudden onset of headaches and dizziness. Physical examination shows that the patient has partial ptosis, miosis, and anhidrosis on the right side of her face. She says this has never happened before. It was her sister that noticed her eyelid was drooping. Which of the following muscles is most likely paralyzed to cause her ptosis?

A. Orbicularis oculi, orbital part
B. Orbicularis oculi, palpebral part
C. Levator palpebrae superioris
D. Superior oblique
E. Superior tarsal (of Müller)

81. A 16-year-old boy is brought to the emergency department because of fever, drowsiness, and altered mental state. The patient is awake but not oriented to person, place, or time. He has a history of severe acne for the past 2 years. Physical examination shows papules, pustules, and nodules predominantly around his nose and periorbital edema on the right side. A CT scan of the head shows cavernous sinus thrombosis. Which of the following routes of entry to the cavernous sinus would most likely be responsible for the infection and thrombosis?

A. Carotid artery
B. Mastoid emissary vein
C. Middle meningeal artery
D. Superior ophthalmic vein
E. Parietal emissary vein

82. A 68-year-old man is brought to the emergency department after a sudden onset of one-sided weakness. The patient has difficulty speaking and is unable to walk on his own. A CT scan of the head shows an acute cerebral vascular accident in the anterior inferior

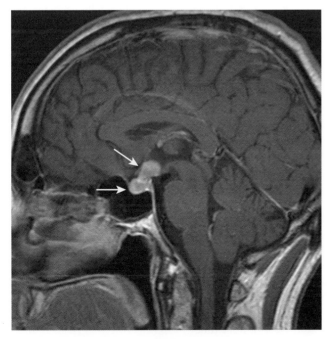

• Fig. 7.3

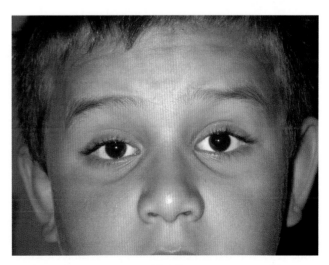

• Fig. 7.4

cerebellar artery, resulting in a small hemorrhage of the artery at its origin from the main trunk. Which of the following nerves will most likely be immediately affected by the hemorrhage?

A. Optic nerve
B. Oculomotor nerve
C. Trochlear nerve
D. Trigeminal nerve
E. Abducens nerve

83. A 5-year-old boy is brought to the emergency department by his parents because of left ear pain. The patient had a history of recurrent otitis media and this is his fourth episode in 6 months. Otoscopic examination shows a bulging and inflamed tympanic membrane. It is decided to incise the tympanic membrane to relieve the pressure and drain the fluid. Which of the following is the best location to make an opening (myringotomy) for drainage?

A. The anterior superior quadrant of the tympanic membrane
B. The posterior superior quadrant of the tympanic membrane
C. Directly through the site of the umbo
D. The anterior inferior quadrant of the tympanic membrane
E. A vertical incision should be made in the tympanic membrane, from the 12 o'clock position of the rim of the tympanic membrane to the 6 o'clock position of the rim

84. A 56-year-old man comes to the physician because of recent diagnosis of an extradural tumor in the posterior cranial fossa. During physical examination, when the patient is asked to protrude his tongue straight out, his tongue deviates to the right. Which of the following pairs of muscles and/or nerves are most likely injured?

A. Right hypoglossal nerve and right genioglossus
B. Left hypoglossal nerve and left genioglossus
C. Right hyoglossus and left styloglossus
D. Right geniohyoid and first cervical nerve
E. Contralateral vagus and hypoglossal nerves

85. A 62-year-old man comes to the physician for the first time for gradually worsening vision for the past 6 months. He says he has difficulty driving because of poor vision. Physical examination shows limited peripheral visual field. Tonometry shows a high intraocular pressure, and a diagnosis of glaucoma is made. Which of the following spaces first receives the aqueous humor secreted by the epithelium of the ciliary body?

A. Anterior chamber
B. Posterior chamber
C. Pupil
D. Vitreous
E. Lacrimal sac

86. A 17-year-old girl comes to the physician for a scheduled tonsillectomy because of recurrent infections.

The procedure was done without complication. The patient returns to the clinic a week later for a follow-up appointment. The patient has not had any issues with her tonsils, however, since the surgery, she has been experiencing pain in her ear. Which of the following nerves was most likely injured during the surgical procedure?

A. Auriculotemporal
B. Lesser petrosal
C. Vagus
D. Glossopharyngeal
E. Chorda tympani

87. A 49-year-old woman is brought to the emergency department because of sudden bout of dizziness and vomiting. The patient says she has been having recurrent headaches and dizziness for the past year. However, this was the first time it lasted for hours which caused her to vomit. Physical examination shows that when the right side of the pharyngeal wall is touched with a tongue depressor, the uvula deviates to the left and the left pharyngeal wall contracts upward. When the left pharyngeal wall is touched, the response is similar. A CT scan of the head shows a tumor in the jugular canal. Given the findings from her physical examination, which of the following nerves have most likely been affected by the tumor?

A. Right glossopharyngeal
B. Left glossopharyngeal
C. Right mandibular
D. Left hypoglossal
E. Right vagus

88. A 45-year-old man is brought to the emergency department with severe dyspnea. Physical examination shows a significant swelling in the floor of his mouth and pharynx with nearly totally occluded airway. A swelling in his lower jaw and upper neck is also noted. His wife says that he just had one of his lower molars extracted a week ago and he had been feeling progressively worse since that day. Which of the following will be the most likely diagnosis?

A. Quinsy
B. Torus palatinus
C. Ankyloglossia
D. Ranula
E. Ludwig angina

89. A 5-year-old girl is brought to the physician by her parents because of fever and cough for the last 2 days. Her mother is concerned she may be having trouble breathing and says that the patient may have decreased hearing. Physical examination shows a tender right ear with a golden-brown fluid that can be observed through the tympanic membrane. Which is the most likely direct route for the spread of an infection from the upper respiratory tract to the middle ear cavity?

A. Auditory tube
B. Choanae

C. Nostrils
D. Facial canal
E. Internal acoustic meatus

90. A 54-year-old man is brought to the emergency department for severe pain in his nasal cavity. He says that he has been having recurring nosebleeds and pain within his nasal cavity for the past year. When they first started, they were occasional and went away without treatment, but lately they have become more intense and frequent. Patient has no trauma or history of picking his nose. A CT scan of the head shows a mass in his nasal cavity. In which of the following locations would the carcinoma block the hiatus of the maxillary sinus?
A. Inferior meatus
B. Middle meatus
C. Superior meatus
D. Nasopharynx
E. Sphenoethmoidal recess

91. A 54-year-old man comes to the physician for a recent diagnosis of an aneurysm in the basilar artery, close to the cavernous sinus. Because of the risk of rupture, the vascular surgery team has recommended an endovascular aneurysm repair. An anterior approach to the sella turcica through the nasal cavity is chosen. Through which of the following routes is the surgeon most likely to gain access to the cranial cavity?
A. Cribriform plate
B. Cavernous sinus
C. Frontal sinus
D. Maxillary sinus
E. Sphenoidal sinus

92. A 10-year-old girl is brought to the physician for a follow-up visit 1 week after a scheduled tonsillectomy. The surgery was performed without any complications. Physical examination shows absence of the gag reflex on the left when the posterior part of the tongue is depressed. The sensory portion of which of the following nerves was most likely injured?
A. Facial
B. Glossopharyngeal
C. Mandibular
D. Maxillary
E. Hypoglossal

93. A 56-year-old woman comes to the physician for a scheduled total thyroidectomy because of a large thyroid gland tumor. After she recovered from the anesthesia, she started to experience hoarseness that lasted for 3 weeks. Subsequent examination shows a permanently adducted vocal fold on the right side. Surgical trauma to which of the following muscles is most likely to be responsible for the adducted right vocal fold?
A. Aryepiglottic
B. Posterior cricoarytenoid
C. Thyroarytenoid
D. Transverse arytenoids
E. Vocalis

94. A 45-year-old man comes to the physician because of headache, ear pain, difficulty hearing in one ear, and recurring nosebleeds. The patient says that he has been having difficulty breathing through his nose and he had unexplained weight loss for the last 3 months. Physical examination shows fluid in the middle ear cavity. CT scan of the head shows a postnasal tumor. Hypertrophy of which of the following structures would be most likely to compromise the drainage of the auditory tube?
A. Lingual tonsil
B. Palatine tonsil
C. Pharyngeal tonsil
D. Superior constrictor muscle
E. Uvula

95. A 10-year-old boy is brought to the emergency department because of fever and swollen tonsils. The boy is fatigued and is having difficulty swallowing because of pain. A rapid strep test was positive and the patient is subsequently diagnosed with severe pharyngitis. Infection in the nasopharynx may spread to the middle ear cavity along the derivative of which embryonic pharyngeal pouch?
A. First
B. Second
C. Third
D. Fourth
E. Sixth

96. A 25-year-old man comes to the physician with a stinging sensation in his mouth for 1 day. The patient ate burnt toast yesterday in a rush when he was late for his class. He believes that the burnt parts of the toast scratched the roof of his mouth which caused the stinging sensation. Which of the following nerves is responsible for the sensory innervation of that area?
A. Posterior superior alveolar
B. Inferior alveolar
C. Lingual
D. Greater palatine
E. Lesser palatine

97. A 32-year-old woman comes to the physician for a scheduled partial thyroidectomy because of thyroid gland cancer. Two months postoperatively, the patient says that she often chokes when she is eating or drinking. Physical examination shows that the patient has lost the ability to detect the presence of foreign objects in the laryngeal vestibule. Which of the following nerves was most likely injured?
A. Internal branch of superior laryngeal nerve
B. External branch of superior laryngeal nerve
C. Glossopharyngeal nerve
D. Hypoglossal nerve
E. Recurrent laryngeal nerve

98. A 1-year-old boy is brought to the physician because he was found to have an ankyloglossia at birth. The boy did not have any problems with feeding. The physician referred him for possible surgery because his congenital abnormality may affect his speech. Which of the following surgical procedures would be most appropriate for this condition?

A. Removal of pterygomandibular raphe

B. Resection of the pterygoid hamulus bilaterally

C. Cutting the lingual frenulum

D. Repair of the palate

E. Removal of the central segment of the hyoid bone

99. An 8-year-old boy is brought to the emergency department because of a severe infection of the right middle ear. Within the antibiotic course of a week, the infection had spread to the mastoid antrum and the mastoid air cells. The patient did not respond to antibiotics, and a radical mastoid operation was performed. Following the operation, it was noticed that the boy's face is distorted. His mouth is drawn upward to the left, and he is unable to close his right eye. Saliva tends to accumulate in his right cheek and dribble from the corner of his mouth. What structure was most likely damaged during the operation?

A. Mandibular nerve

B. Parotid duct

C. Vagus nerve

D. Facial nerve

E. Glossopharyngeal nerve

100. An 8-year-old boy is brought to the emergency department because of an ear infection. The patient was started on antibiotics, but his symptoms persistently got worse for the next 7 days. The patient underwent mastoidectomy. Postoperatively, physical examination shows accumulation of saliva in the vestibule of his oral cavity and dribble from the corner of his mouth. He is diagnosed with Bell palsy. Which of the following muscles was most likely paralyzed?

A. Zygomaticus major

B. Orbicularis oculi

C. Buccinator

D. Levator palpebrae superioris

E. Orbicularis oris

Questions 101–125

101. A 32-year-old man is brought to the emergency department because of difficulties with his vision. Physical examination shows a loss of the lateral halves of the fields of vision in both eyes (bitemporal hemianopia). An MRI of the head shows a tumor of the adenohypophysis. Which of the following structures was most likely compressed by the tumor?

A. Optic nerve

B. Optic chiasm

C. Optic tract

D. Oculomotor

E. Abducens nerve

102. A 45-year-old woman is brought to the emergency department after falling down a flight of concrete stairs. The patient has a contusion on her head with bruising of her arms and legs. Physical examination shows weakness of patient's downward medial gaze. The patient admits she's been having headaches and vision problems recently. A CT scan of the head shows no intracranial bleeding or fractures. A cerebral arteriography and an MRI show a nerve being compressed by an arterial aneurysm inferior to the tentorium cerebelli. Which of the following arteries is most likely compressing the associated nerve?

A. Internal carotid artery/abducens nerve

B. Middle cerebral artery/oculomotor nerve

C. Posterior cerebral artery (PCA)/ophthalmic nerve

D. Basilar artery/ophthalmic nerve

E. Superior cerebellar artery/trochlear nerve

103. A 72-year-old woman is brought to the emergency department by her family because she has been excessively tired and unresponsive at times. The family says the patient has been losing weight. Physical examination shows ptosis and miosis of the right eye. Cardiac examination shows no murmurs, and lungs are clear to auscultation bilaterally. There is tenderness to palpation of the chest in the upper right thorax. Which of the following is the most likely diagnosis?

A. Raynaud disease

B. Frey syndrome

C. Bell palsy

D. Quinsy

E. Pancoast tumor

104. A 32-year-old man comes to the clinic because of a headache and difficulties with vision. The dilator pupillae muscle, the smooth muscle cell fibers of the superior tarsal muscle (of Müller, part of the levator palpebrae superioris), and the smooth muscle cells of the blood vessels of the ciliary body are supplied by efferent nerve fibers. Which of the following structures contains the nerve cell bodies of these fibers?

A. Pterygopalatine ganglion

B. Intermediolateral nucleus (lateral horn) C1 to C4

C. Geniculate ganglion

D. Nucleus solitarius

E. SCG

105. A 22-year-old man is brought to the emergency department after being hit in the right eye with a ball during baseball practice. Physical examination shows considerable swelling and discoloration of the right eyelid. The patient could not turn his pupil laterally from forward gaze, indicating possible muscle entrapment. Which of the following bones was most likely fractured?

A. Orbital plate of the frontal bone

B. Lamina papyracea of the ethmoid bone

C. Orbital surface of the maxilla

D. Cribriform plate of the ethmoid bone

E. Greater wing of the sphenoid bone

106. A 57-year-old man is brought to the emergency department because of dizziness and a severe headache. Physical examination shows the patient's eyeball is fixed in an abducted position, slightly depressed,

the pupil is dilated and the upper lid is droopy. When the patient is asked to move the pupil toward the nose, the pupil rotates medially. Consensual corneal reflexes are normal. A CT scan of the head shows a tumor in the superior orbital fissure. Which of the following nerves is most likely affected?

A. Trochlear nerve

B. Oculomotor nerve

C. Abducens nerve and sympathetic nerve plexus accompanying the ophthalmic artery

D. Ophthalmic nerve and short ciliary nerve

E. Superior division of oculomotor nerve and the nasociliary nerve

107. A 57-year-old man is brought to the emergency department after falling from a tree. The patient says he hit his face on a branch as he was falling but has no loss of consciousness. A CT scan of the head shows a fracture of the cribriform plate (Fig. 7.5). Which of the following conditions will most likely be present during the physical examination?

A. Entrapment of the eyeball

B. Anosmia

C. Hyperacusis

D. Tinnitus

E. Deafness

108. A 45-year-old woman came to the clinic because of swelling on the side of her face for 2 months. Ultrasound-guided needle biopsy confirmed a parotid gland tumor. The patient undergoes tumor resection without complications. Three months postoperatively, the patient comes to the physician because her face sweats profusely when she tastes or smells food. A diagnosis of Frey syndrome (gustatory sweating) is

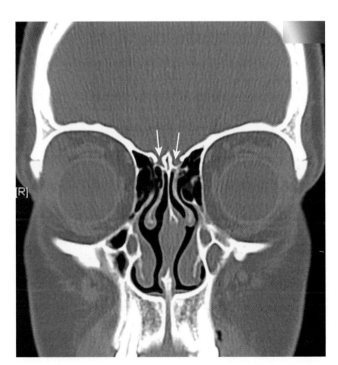

• **Fig. 7.5**

made. Which of the following nerves was most likely injured during the procedure?

A. Buccal

B. Inferior alveolar

C. Auriculotemporal

D. Facial

E. Lingual

109. A 54-year-old man is scheduled to undergo a bilateral thyroidectomy. During the consenting process, he is informed that during surgery there is a risk of losing the airway if a particular nerve is injured bilaterally. This nerve controls a pair of muscles that open the airway. The patient is informed that in the event that both nerves are lesioned, there may be a need to intubate or surgically open the airway in order to prevent asphyxiation. Which of the following pairs of muscle opens the airway?

A. Cricothyroids

B. Posterior cricoarytenoids

C. Arytenoids

D. Thyroarytenoids

E. Lateral cricoarytenoids

110. An 11-year-old boy is brought to the office because of a fever and sore throat. Physical examination shows enlarged tonsils with exudate. This is the patient's seventh bout of tonsillitis in 1 year and the physician recommends a tonsillectomy. The physician discusses the benefits and risks of the surgery with his parents. The patient's mother asks if there is a significant risk of bleeding during the procedure. Which of the following arteries supplies most of the blood to the tonsils?

A. Ascending pharyngeal

B. Facial

C. Lingual

D. Descending palatine

E. Superior thyroid

111. A 55-year-old man is brought to the emergency department because of severe ear pain. He accidentally punctured his tympanic membrane with an ear pick when he was suddenly startled by a loud noise. Physical examination shows the ear pick still in his ear as the patient was afraid to pull it out himself. Which of the following nerves is responsible for the sensory innervation of the inner surface of the tympanic membrane?

A. Glossopharyngeal

B. Auricular branch of facial

C. Auricular branch of vagus

D. Great auricular

E. Lingual

112. A 45-year-old man comes to the emergency department because of excruciating facial pain. He was diagnosed with trigeminal neuralgia (tic douloureux) 10 years ago. Physical examination shows tenderness to light touch of the skin between the lower eyelid and the upper lip. A treatment option is to lesion the nerve involved by injecting alcohol into it. To reach

the nerve, the needle will most likely need to be inserted through which of the following openings?

A. Foramen ovale

B. Foramen spinosum

C. Infraorbital foramen

D. Mandibular foramen

E. Foramen magnum

113. A 32-year-old woman comes to the physician because of weight loss, diarrhea, and heat intolerance. She is diagnosed with hyperthyroidism and is scheduled to have a thyroidectomy. Following surgery, the patient is unable to pass her swallow test. The patient has most likely lost sensation of the larynx from the vocal folds to the entrance into the larynx, causing aspiration of liquids into the airway. Which of the following nerves is most likely injured?

A. Internal branch of superior laryngeal nerve

B. External branch of superior laryngeal nerve

C. Glossopharyngeal nerve

D. Hypoglossal nerve

E. Recurrent laryngeal nerve

114. A 55-year-old man is brought to the emergency department after hitting his head when he slipped and fell on wet pavement. He has no loss of consciousness or drowsiness. His vital signs are within normal limits. Physical examination shows a hematoma that formed in the "danger zone" of the scalp, spreading to the area of the eyelids. Which of the following layers is regarded as the "danger zone"?

A. Loose, areolar layer

B. Skin

C. Galea aponeurotica

D. Pericranium

E. Subcutaneous layer

115. A 45-year-old woman comes to the emergency department because of a severe headache. Her blood pressure is 190/100 mm Hg, pulse is 115/min, and respirations are 20/min. An ECG shows atrial fibrillation and a chest x-ray shows no acute cardiopulmonary events. To reduce the patient's blood pressure, a pressure point located deep to the anterior border of the sternocleidomastoid muscle at the level of the superior border of the thyroid cartilage is massaged. Which of the following structures is targeted by the massage?

A. Carotid sinus

B. Carotid body

C. Thyroid gland

D. Parathyroid gland

E. Inferior cervical ganglion

116. A 59-year-old man was brought to the emergency department after falling from a three-story scaffolding. On arrival, the patient is unconscious with a fractured jaw, broken teeth, facial lacerations, and an open tibial fracture. To secure an airway, an emergency tracheotomy is performed where brisk arterial bleeding suddenly occurred from the midline incision over the trachea. Which of the following vessels was most likely cut?

A. Inferior thyroid branch of thyrocervical trunk

B. Cricothyroid branch of the superior thyroid artery

C. Thyroidea ima artery

D. Middle thyroid vein

E. Jugular arch connecting the anterior jugular veins

117. A 21-year-old man is brought to the emergency department after collapsing on the basketball court because of severe dizziness. Physical examination shows the patient demonstrates lack of equilibrium and memory impairment. A 3-cm wound is noted on his scalp from an injury in a game several weeks earlier. A CT scan of the head shows an intracranial hematoma. A lumbar puncture was also performed that showed no signs of infection or blood in the CSF. Which of the following is the most likely diagnosis?

A. The middle meningeal artery was torn, resulting in epidural hematoma

B. There is a fracture in the pterion with injury to the adjacent vasculature

C. The injury resulted in the bursting of a pre-existing aneurysm of the anterior communicating artery of the cerebral circle

D. A cerebral vein is torn

E. The cavernous sinus has a thrombus

118. A 63-year-old man is brought to the hospital because of back pain and headaches. He has a history of removal of a prostate gland tumor 2 years ago following a diagnosis of prostate cancer. CT and MRI examinations show the cancer has spread from the pelvis to the posterior cranial fossa by way of the internal vertebral venous plexus (of Batson). Physical examination shows that the right shoulder droops lower than the left, there is considerable weakness when the patient turns his head to the left. The patient's tongue points to the right when he attempts to protrude it from his mouth. There are no other significant findings. Which of the following nerves are most likely affected?

A. Right vagus, right accessory, and right hypoglossal nerves

B. Left accessory, right glossopharyngeal, right vagus, and left hypoglossal nerves

C. Left hypoglossal, right trigeminal, and left glossopharyngeal nerves

D. Right accessory and right hypoglossal nerves

E. Left facial, left accessory, right accessory, and vagus nerves

119. A 3-month-old boy is brought to the emergency department for irritability and inconsolable crying. Physical examination shows the infant has a dry right eye and an ophthalmologist consult is called for further evaluation. An MRI shows a lesion at the neural cell bodies of the preganglionic axons of the fibers that terminate in the pterygopalatine ganglion. Which of the following structures contains the neural cell bodies of the preganglionic axons?

A. SCG
B. Edinger-Westphal nucleus
C. Superior salivatory nucleus
D. Inferior salivatory nucleus
E. Nucleus ambiguus

120. A 22-year-old woman comes to the physician because of progressively worsening throat pain. The pain started as a dull ache but intensified and localized to the right side over the past 2 days. Her temperature is 38°C (100.4°F), pulse is 80/min, respirations are 16/min, and blood pressure is 110/84 mm Hg. She says she has pain on swallowing and is unable to eat because of the pain. Physical examination shows a peritonsillar abscess (quinsy) on the right side, which was subsequently confirmed with ultrasound. The patient is sent to the hospital for incision and drainage of the lesion. During this procedure, which of the following arteries is at greatest risk of injury?
A. Lingual artery
B. A branch of facial artery
C. Superior laryngeal artery
D. Ascending pharyngeal artery
E. Descending palatine artery

121. A 17-year-old girl comes to the physician because of severe facial acne. Physical examination shows a prominent and painful lesion on the side of her nose. The patient was given antibiotics and warned not to press or pick at the large, inflamed swelling as this may result in an infection which can spread to the brain. Which of the following pathways will most likely result in the spread of infection?
A. Nasal venous tributary to angular vein, to superior ophthalmic vein, then to cavernous sinus
B. Retromandibular vein to supraorbital vein, then to inferior ophthalmic vein, then to cavernous sinus
C. Dorsal nasal vein to superior petrosal vein, then inferior ophthalmic vein to cavernous sinus
D. Facial vein to maxillary vein, then middle meningeal vein to cavernous sinus
E. Transverse facial vein to superficial temporal vein to emissary vein to cavernous sinus

122. A 73-year-old man comes to the emergency department because of a progressive loss of vision in his right eye. The patient says he has swelling and difficulty looking to the right side with his right eye. Physical examination of the right eye shows periorbital edema, limited lateral movement, and macular edema through the ophthalmoscope. An MRI of the head shows thrombophlebitis of the cavernous sinus. Which of the following structures will most likely contain a thrombus to cause these symptoms in this patient?
A. Subarachnoid space
B. Central artery of the retina
C. Central vein of the retina
D. Optic chiasm
E. Ciliary ganglion

123. A 67-year-old man comes to the physician because of difficulty with his vision. The patient has no pain and says that he actually didn't notice the vision loss until he started bumping into furniture repeatedly. A visual field test shows significant loss of peripheral vision. The patient is referred to an ophthalmologist where he is diagnosed with open angle glaucoma, where the aqueous humor does not drain properly into the scleral venous sinus at the iridoscleral angle of the eyeball. In a normal eye, the aqueous fluid is secreted by the epithelium of the ciliary body, directly into which of the following spaces?
A. Iridoscleral angle
B. Posterior chamber
C. Pupil
D. Vitreous body
E. Lacrimal sac

124. A 2-month-old girl is brought to the physician because of an enlarged head. The patient is quickly sent to the hospital for an MRI and admitted for further evaluation. The MRI of the head shows a complete dilation of the entire ventricular system. The treatment team is currently evaluating whether to place a shunt or consider surgery. Which of the following conditions most likely led to this type of clinical picture?
A. Lack of absorption through arachnoid granulations into venous system
B. Occlusion of cerebral aqueduct (of Sylvius)
C. Blockage of the lateral aperture (of Luschka) of the fourth ventricle
D. Congenital absence of the cisterna magna
E. Closure of the interventricular foramina (of Monro)

125. A 54-year-old man is brought to the emergency department after being struck by a moving vehicle. On arrival, the patient has a GCS of 10 and stable vital signs. The patient has no obvious signs of bleeding and a Facial drooping, Arm weakness, Speech difficulties and Time (FAST) examination is also negative. A CT scan of the head shows a fracture through the crista galli of the anterior cranial fossa, resulting in slow, local bleeding. Which of the following is the most likely source of bleeding?
A. Middle meningeal artery
B. Great cerebral vein (of Galen)
C. Superior sagittal sinus
D. Straight sinus
E. Superior ophthalmic vein

Questions 126–150

126. A 55-year-old woman comes to the physician because of deteriorating vision. Ophthalmologic examination tests the globe, the retina, and the cornea of each eye and all extraocular eye movements are observed to ensure full range of motion, smoothness of movements, and synchronicity bilaterally. Which of the following nerves must be functioning properly if the patient is able to abduct the eye without difficulty and without upward or downward deviation?

A. Superior division of oculomotor, ophthalmic nerve, abducens nerve
B. Trochlear nerve, abducens nerve, nasociliary nerve
C. Inferior division of oculomotor, trochlear, abducens
D. Oculomotor and ophthalmic nerves
E. Superior division of oculomotor, trochlear, and abducens nerves

127. A 45-year-old man comes to the emergency department because of hoarseness for the past 3 months. The patient has a long history of smoking. A CT scan shows a cancerous growth in his larynx with no evidence of metastasis. In addition, the area in which the tumor is growing is characterized by very limited lymphatic drainage. Which of the following locations is most likely to contain a tumor with these characteristics?
    A. Anterior commissure of the vocal ligaments
    B. Interarytenoid fold
    C. Laryngeal ventricle
    D. Cricothyroid ligament
    E. Middle segment of the vocal cord

128. A 55-year-old man comes to the emergency department because of progressively severe headaches. His temperature is 38°C (100.4°F), otherwise his vital signs are within normal limits. Physical examination shows neck stiffness and pain on passive movement of the neck. A lumbar puncture is performed and shows traces of blood in the CSF. Which of the following conditions has most likely occurred in this patient?
    A. Fracture of the pterion with vascular injury
    B. A ruptured "berry" aneurysm
    C. Leakage of branches of the middle meningeal vein within the temporal bone
    D. A tear of a superior cerebral vein at its entrance to the superior sagittal sinus
    E. Occlusion of the internal carotid artery by a clot generated in the left atrium

129. A 55-year-old man comes to physician for a scheduled resection of a tumor in the left jugular canal. Postoperatively, the patient has no gag reflex when the ipsilateral pharyngeal wall is stimulated, although the pharynx moved upward and a gag reflex resulted when the right pharyngeal wall was stimulated. The uvula deviated to the right and the left vocal cord drifted toward the midline. Which of the following structures will contain the neural cell bodies for the motor supply of the paralyzed muscles?
    A. Nucleus solitarius
    B. Trigeminal motor nucleus
    C. Dorsal motor nucleus
    D. Nucleus ambiguus
    E. Superior or inferior ganglia of vagus

130. A 65-year-old man is brought to the emergency department after sustaining facial injuries during a motor vehicle collision. Physical examination shows several lacerations and abrasions in the lower jaw and face.

A CT scan shows that the inferior alveolar nerve is injured at its origin. Which of the following muscles would most likely be paralyzed as a result of this injury?
    A. Geniohyoid
    B. Hyoglossus
    C. Mylohyoid
    D. Stylohyoid
    E. Palatoglossus

131. A 64-year-old man is brought to the emergency department by his son after being found unconscious at home. The patient has a history of diabetes mellitus and hypertension. A CT scan of the head shows that the patient had a cerebral vascular accident, with a small hematoma produced by the superior cerebellar artery. Which of the following nerves will most likely be affected by the hematoma?
    A. Trochlear nerve
    B. Abducens nerve
    C. Facial nerve
    D. Vestibulocochlear nerve
    E. Glossopharyngeal nerve

132. A 65-year-old man comes to the emergency department 3 weeks after hitting his head. He had the accidental head bump while moving furniture and did not have any significant pain at that time. Currently, the pain has been progressively worsening. Physical examination shows mental confusion and poor physical coordination. A CT scan of the head shows an intracranial thrombus probably due to leakage from a cerebral vein over the right cerebral hemisphere. Which of the following is the most likely diagnosis?
    A. Subarachnoid bleeding
    B. Epidural bleeding
    C. Intracerebral bleeding into the brain parenchyma
    D. Subdural bleeding
    E. Bleeding into the cerebral ventricular system

133. A 27-year-old man comes to the physician because of jaw pain after a boxing match. He says he feels pain during jaw movement. Physical examination shows decreased strength and asymmetry in opening of the jaws. Strength and symmetry of strength in opening the jaws are tested. Which of the following muscles is the most important in jaw protrusion and depressing the mandible?
    A. Anterior portion of temporalis
    B. Lateral pterygoid
    C. Medial pterygoid
    D. Masseter
    E. Platysma

134. A 6-month-old girl is brought to the physician by her mother because of slow growth and no tooth development. The mother had an uncomplicated pregnancy and an uneventful delivery. There is no history of developmental delays. The physician reassures the mother and informs her about the expected age for teeth development. Which of the following teeth are expected to appear first?

A. Superior medial incisor teeth at 8 to 12 months of age

B. Inferior medial incisor teeth at 6 to 10 months of age

C. Superior lateral incisor teeth at 8 to 10 months of age

D. Inferior lateral incisor teeth at 12 to 14 months of age

E. First molar tooth at 6 to 8 months of age

135. A 56-year-old man comes to the physician because of severe headaches and ear pain. The patient also has ringing in his ears (tinnitus). He is otherwise healthy and his vital signs are within normal limits. The patient has no family history of cancer. A CT scan of the head shows a tumor in the middle ear cavity, invading through the bony floor. Which of the following structures will most likely be affected?

A. The cochlea and lateral semicircular canal

B. The internal carotid artery

C. The sigmoid venous sinus

D. The superior jugular bulb

E. The aditus ad antrum of the mastoid region and the facial nerve

136. A 52-year-old man is brought to the emergency department after sustaining a bullet wound in the lower jaw. Physical examination shows a bullet wound in the infratemporal fossa. There is unilateral loss of temperature, pressure, and pain sensation in the anterior ⅔ of the tongue. Taste and salivary function are intact. Which of the following is the most likely diagnosis?

A. The facial nerve was transected distal to the origin of the chorda tympani

B. Receptors for hot, cold, pain, and pressure are absent in the patient's tongue

C. The glossopharyngeal nerve has been injured in the pharynx

D. The superior laryngeal nerve was obviously severed by the bullet

E. The lingual nerve was injured at its origin near the foramen ovale

137. A 12-year-old boy is brought to the emergency department because of fever and fatigue. Physical examination shows neck stiffness and neck tenderness with passive movement. The patient was diagnosed with meningitis and a lumbar puncture is performed to determine the etiology of infection. However, lumbar puncture should not be performed when CSF pressure is elevated. Which of the following conditions would most likely indicate an elevated CSF pressure?

A. Papilledema

B. Separation of the pars optica retinae anterior to the ora serrata

C. The fovea centralis exhibits hemorrhage from medial retinal branches

D. Obvious opacity of the lens

E. Pitting or compression of the optic disc

138. A 65-year-old woman is brought to the emergency department after being diagnosed with cavernous sinus thrombosis. The patient has headaches but is otherwise stable. A CT scan of the head shows an aneurysm of the internal carotid artery within the cavernous sinus. Which of the following will most likely be present during physical examination if nerve compression was suspected within the cavernous sinus?

A. Inability to gaze downward and laterally on the affected side

B. Complete ptosis of the superior palpebra (upper eyelid)

C. Bilateral loss of accommodation and loss of direct pupillary reflex

D. Ipsilateral loss of the consensual corneal reflex

E. Ipsilateral paralysis of abduction of the pupil

139. A 54-year-old man is brought to the emergency department after being involved in a motor vehicle collision. Physical examination shows multiple lacerations in the upper eyelid and the sclera contains small fragments of broken glass. A CT scan of the face shows a fracture at the frontozygomatic suture. What is the preferred site for needle insertion to anesthetize the orbital contents and then the area of the eyelid injury?

A. Into the sclera in the limbic region and also into the infraorbital foramen

B. Into the fossa for the lacrimal sac and also beneath the lateral bulbar conjunctiva

C. Into the supraorbital foramen and also into the lacrimal caruncle

D. Through the upper eyelid deeply toward the orbital apex and also between the orbital septum and the palpebral musculature laterally

E. Directly posteriorly through the anulus tendineus and superior orbital fissure

140. A 45-year-old man comes to the emergency department after falling on his chin on a protruding nail. The patient says he feels moderate pain. Vital signs are within normal limits. Physical examination shows a nail penetrating the skin overlying the submental triangle lateral to the midline. The wound is inflamed and swollen, but the bleeding has stopped. Which of the following muscles would most likely be the last to be penetrated by the nail?

A. Platysma

B. Mylohyoid

C. Anterior belly of the digastric

D. Geniohyoid

E. Genioglossus

141. A 55-year-old woman comes to the physician because of swelling on the side of her face for the past 2 months. An ultrasound-guided needle biopsy confirms a malignant parotid tumor. The patient is scheduled for tumor resection. Following surgery, physical examination shows marked weakness in the musculature of the patient's lower lip. Which of the following

nerves was most likely injured during the procedure to cause this symptom?

A. Marginal mandibular branch of facial
B. Zygomatic branch of facial
C. Mandibular division of the trigeminal nerve
D. Buccal branch of facial
E. Buccal nerve

142. A 15-year-old boy is brought to the emergency department because of a daily dull headache for the past 4 months. Physical examination shows that the patient's visual field is limited bitemporally. An MRI of the head shows a craniopharyngioma occupying the sella turcica, primarily involving the suprasellar space. Which of the following is the most likely cause of this tumor?

A. Persistence of a small portion of Rathke pouch
B. Abnormal development of pars tuberalis
C. Abnormal development of the interventricular foramina (of Monro)
D. Abnormal development of the alar plates that form the lateral wall of diencephalon
E. Abnormal development of diencephalon

143. A 1-day-old girl is brought to the physician for neonatal examination. Vital signs are within normal limits. Physical examination shows a telencephalic vesicle; the eyes are fused, and a single nasal chamber is present in the midline. An MRI of the head shows that the olfactory bulbs, olfactory tracts, and the corpus callosum are hypoplastic. Which of the following is the most likely diagnosis?

A. Holoprosencephaly
B. Smith-Lemli-Opitz syndrome
C. Schizencephaly
D. Exencephaly
E. Meningoencephalocele

144. A 1-day-old boy is brought to the neonatal care unit after being diagnosed with meningohydroencephalocele. The patient was born at term by normal vaginal delivery with no complications. Physical examination shows an enlarged head. A CT scan of the head shows protrusion of the brain and ventricular system. Which of the following bones is most commonly affected?

A. Squamous part of temporal bone
B. Petrous part of temporal bone
C. Squamous part of occipital bone
D. Sphenoid bone
E. Ethmoid bone

145. A 28-year-old woman delivers a stillborn boy. The prenatal course was complicated with polyhydramnios. Physical examination shows the absence of a nasal bone, and the vault of the boy's skull is undeveloped leaving the malformed brain exposed. A diagnosis of exencephaly is made. What is the most common embryological cause of this condition?

A. Toxoplasmosis infection
B. Failure of closure of the cephalic part of the neural tube

C. Ossification defect in the bones of the skull
D. Caudal displacement of cerebellar structures
E. Maternal alcohol abuse

146. A 6-month-old girl is brought to the emergency department because of poor feeding, irritability, and sleepiness. Physical examination shows an enlarged head and a small sac extending through the spine identifying as a spina bifida cystica. An MRI of the head and neck shows a caudal displacement of the cerebellar vermis through the foramen magnum. Which of the following is the most likely diagnosis?

A. Chiari II malformation
B. Holoprosencephaly
C. Smith-Lemli-Opitz syndrome
D. Schizencephaly
E. Exencephaly

147. A 1-year-old boy is brought to the emergency department because the parents noticed he does not respond to auditory stimuli. An MRI of the head shows abnormal development of the membranous and bony labyrinths. The patient was diagnosed with congenital deafness. Which of the following can lead to this condition?

A. Infection with rubella virus
B. Failure of the second pharyngeal arch to form
C. Failure of the dorsal portion of first pharyngeal cleft
D. Abnormal development of the auricular hillocks
E. Failure of the dorsal portion of first pharyngeal cleft and second pharyngeal arch

148. A 3-month-old boy is brought to the emergency department by his parents' because they found white patches in his eyes. The patient was not vaccinated because of the parent's religion. The patient has not been hospitalized since birth. An ophthalmoscopic examination shows a congenital cataract. Which of the following is responsible for this condition?

A. Infection with rubella virus
B. Choroid fissure fails to close
C. Persistent hyaloid artery
D. Toxoplasmosis infection
E. Cytomegalovirus (CMV) infection

149. A newborn infant is transferred to the pediatric intensive care unit because the ocular lens failed to develop. The patient's parents are both adopted and they are not aware of their family history. Genetic study of the newborn shows a mutation in the *PAX6* gene. Which of the following conditions can explain the physical examination findings of the newborn?

A. Cyclopia
B. Coloboma
C. Anophthalmia
D. Aphakia and aniridia
E. Microphthalmia

150. A 2-month-old girl is brought to the physician because of facial asymmetry. Physical examination shows a small and flat maxillary, temporal, and zygomatic

bones, anotia, and a dermoid tumor in the eyeball on the right side. Which of the following is the most likely diagnosis?

A. Hemifacial microsomia
B. Treacher Collins syndrome
C. Robin sequence
D. DiGeorge syndrome
E. Velocardiofacial syndrome

Questions 151–175

151. A 3-month-old girl is brought to the physician because of abnormal facial features. The patient was born in Ghana and immigrated to the United States 1 month ago. Physical examination shows small, low-set ears, short width of eye openings, a long face, cleft palate, and an enlarged nose tip. An x-ray of the head shows a thymic hypoplasia and a basic metabolic panel showed hypocalcemia. An echocardiogram of the heart shows a ventricular septal defect. Which of the following genes is defective?

A. 22q11
B. Sonic Hedgehog (SHH)
C. PAX 2
D. PAX 6
E. 47XXY

152. A 3-day-old boy has a noticeably small mandible. Physical examination shows hypoplasia of the mandible, underdevelopment of the bones of the face, downward-slanting palpebral fissures, defects of the lower eyelids, and deformed external ears. Abnormal development of which of the pharyngeal arches most likely caused these symptoms?

A. First arch
B. Second arch
C. Third arch
D. Fourth arch
E. Sixth arch

153. A 1-year-old boy is brought to the emergency department with fever. His vaccination history is up to date. His parents say that the boy fell several times in the playground the day before. Physical examination shows stiff neck and Kernig sign. Meningitis is suspected. A CT scan of the head shows a sinus infection. Which of the following sinuses is present at this age?

A. Frontal sinus
B. Maxillary sinus
C. Sphenoid sinus
D. Middle ethmoidal cells
E. Posterior ethmoidal cells

154. A newborn infant is found to have severe brain abnormalities. Physical examination shows that the calvaria is defective and the brain is protruding from the cranium. A rudimentary brainstem and some functioning neural tissue are present. A diagnosis is made of meroencephaly. Which of the following is the most likely cause of this condition?

A. Failure of the rostral neuropore to close in the fourth week
B. CMV infection
C. Failure of the hypophyseal diverticulum to develop
D. Failure of the neural arch to develop
E. Abnormal neural crest formation

155. A 55-year-old man is brought to the emergency department because of fever for 4 days accompanied by throat pain and difficulty swallowing. His temperature is 40°C (104°F), pulse is 102/min, respirations are 25/min, and blood pressure is 140/79 mm Hg. Physical examination shows excessive drooling, an enlarged right palatine tonsil and swelling of the right posterior pharynx. A CT scan of the neck shows fluid collection in the retropharyngeal space extending to the posterior mediastinum. The infection is most likely located between which of the following fascial layers?

A. Between alar and prevertebral
B. Between alar and pretracheal
C. Between pretracheal and prevertebral
D. Between buccopharyngeal and alar
E. Between buccopharyngeal and prevertebral

156. A 24-year-old man is brought to the emergency department after a street fight. His temperature is 37°C (98.6°F), pulse is 56/min, respirations are 25/min, and blood pressure is 128/79 mm Hg. Physical examination shows limited movement of the right eye with enophthalmos. An x-ray of the head shows an inferior blow-out fracture of the right orbit. Which of the following nerves is particularly vulnerable with this type of injury?

A. Infraorbital
B. Supratrochlear
C. Frontal
D. Inferior alveolar
E. Optic

157. A 67-year-old man comes to the physician because of progressive difficulty hearing in his right ear when there is background noise. The patient says that he has "heart problems" and his current medication includes low-dose aspirin. During physical examination the Rinne test is performed. Which of the following is the most likely location for the tuning fork to be placed to test bone conduction?

A. Temporal bone
B. Frontal bone
C. Mastoid process
D. External occipital protuberance
E. Vertex of the head

158. A 55-year-old man comes to the office because of pain while chewing for the past 3 months. Physical examination shows hoarseness of voice and pain on swallowing. A lateral x-ray of the neck shows a mass at the tracheoesophageal groove. Which of the following nerves is most likely affected by the mass?

A. Recurrent laryngeal
B. Internal laryngeal
C. Vagus
D. External laryngeal
E. Phrenic

159. A 34-year-old man is brought to the emergency department because of head injury after falling off his motorbike. The patient was not wearing a helmet. His temperature is 37.1°C (98.78°F), pulse is 97/min, respirations are 25/min, and blood pressure is 100/70 mm Hg. Physical examination shows multiple lacerations over the frontal bone. If his wounds become infected, which of the following veins could most likely provide a pathway of infection transmission from the veins of the scalp to the underlying dural venous sinuses?
A. Supratrochlear vein
B. Diploic veins
C. Anterior cerebral veins
D. Superior sagittal sinus
E. Supraorbital vein

160. A 65-year-old man is brought to the emergency department after an episode of a transient ischemic attack. His temperature is 37.4°C (99.32°F), pulse is 97/min, respirations are 25/min, and blood pressure is 170/100 mm Hg. An MRI of the head shows an aneurysm in the region between the PCA and superior cerebellar artery. Which of the following nerves will most likely be compressed by the aneurysm?
A. Trochlear
B. Abducens
C. Oculomotor
D. Vagus
E. Optic

161. A 36-year-old woman is brought to the emergency department after being struck in the left orbital region by a ball. Physical examination of the left eye shows the eye is unable to abduct. An x-ray of the head shows a blow-out fracture of the medial wall of the orbit. Which of the following muscles is most likely injured or trapped?
A. Lateral rectus
B. Medial and inferior recti
C. Medial rectus
D. Medial rectus and superior oblique
E. Inferior rectus

162. A 16-year-old girl is brought to the emergency department after being hit in the eye with a tennis ball during her tennis practice. She has vertical and torsional diplopia. Physical examination shows that the pupil of her eye cannot be turned upward. An x-ray of the head shows a blow-out fracture of the inferior wall of the orbit. Which of the following muscle(s) is (are) most likely injured?
A. Inferior rectus and inferior oblique
B. Medial and inferior recti
C. Inferior oblique

D. Medial rectus, inferior rectus, and inferior oblique
E. Inferior rectus

163. A 36-year-old man is brought to the emergency department with a painful rash of the nose. Physical examination shows herpetic lesions over the dorsum of the nose and on the right eye. Which of the following nerves is most likely to be responsible for the transmission of the virus to the eye?
A. Nasociliary
B. Supratrochlear
C. Infraorbital
D. Posterior ethmoidal
E. Anterior ethmoidal

164. A 22-year-old man is brought to the emergency department after he was injured in a street fight (Fig. 7.6). His vital signs are within normal limits. Physical examination shows a discolored and swollen right eye. An x-ray of the head shows a fracture of a facial bone. Because of the patient's severe pain, an anesthetic solution is injected into his orbit. Which of the following nerves is most likely to be anesthetized?
A. Ophthalmic
B. Infraorbital
C. Anterior ethmoidal
D. Frontal
E. Optic

165. A 34-year-old woman is brought to the emergency department after being involved in a motor vehicle collision. The patient says that she was the passenger in the vehicle and during the collision she hit her right cheekbone and eye against the dashboard. Physical examination shows that she is unable to depress the right eye when the pupil is in the adducted position. An MRI of the head shows a severed nerve. What is the most common location at which this nerve will be injured?
A. As it pierces the dura of the tentorium cerebelli in the tentorial notch
B. At the cavernous sinus
C. At the sella turcica

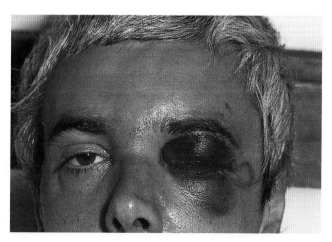

• **Fig. 7.6**

D. At the inferior orbital fissure
E. At the superior orbital fissure

166. A 56-year-old woman comes to the emergency department because of right eye pain. Her vital signs are within normal limits. Physical examination shows redness of the right eye. She also experiences pain in the right eye while the H-test is conducted. An MRI of the head shows an inflammation of the right optic nerve. Which of the following is the most likely explanation for the patient's symptoms?
A. The annular tendon (of Zinn) is inflamed
B. The inflammation has affected the nerves innervating the eye muscles
C. The muscles are contracting because of generalized inflammation
D. The nasociliary nerve is affected
E. The ophthalmic artery is constricted

167. A newborn preterm boy is brought to the neonatal intensive care unit after an uncomplicated vaginal delivery. The neonate's mother did not receive prenatal care throughout the pregnancy. His vital signs are within normal limits. Physical examination shows smaller than usual eyes bilaterally. Ultrasound of the head shows enlarged ventricles with multiple bright echogenic foci within the surrounding brain matter. Which of the following is the most likely cause of this condition?
A. Infection with rubella virus
B. Choroid fissure failed to close
C. Persistent hyaloid artery
D. Toxoplasmosis infection
E. Epstein-Barr virus (EBV) infection

168. A 2-month-old boy is brought to the emergency department by his parents after falling from his stroller. His vital signs are within normal limits. Physical examination shows bruises on the head and face. There is loss of the nasolabial fold on the left side of the infant's face, drooping of the left side of the patient's mouth, and the absence of forehead creases. Where is the most likely place for nerve injury in the infant?
A. At the stylomastoid foramen
B. Inferior to the parotid gland
C. Anterior to the parotid gland
D. Proximal to the stylomastoid foramen
E. At the location in which the mandibular and buccal branches are distributed

169. A 6-year-old boy is brought to the emergency department with a fever and pain over the parotid gland (Fig. 7.7). His development is normal, however he is behind with his scheduled vaccines. His temperature is 38.3°C (101.0°F), pulse is 100/min, respirations are 18/min, and blood pressure is 120/90 mm Hg. Physical examination shows bilaterally enlarged and tender parotid glands. A diagnosis of mumps parotitis is made. Which of the following nerves is responsible for painful sensations from the region of the parotid gland?

A. Facial
B. Auriculotemporal
C. Lesser petrosal
D. Lingual
E. Chorda tympani

170. A 55-year-old woman comes to the physician because of episodes of hearing loss, ringing of the right ear, and feeling of fullness or pressure in her right ear for the past 4 months. Physical examination shows decreased hearing in the right ear. A diagnosis of Ménière disease is made. Which of the following structures is most likely affected by the edema associated with Ménière disease?
A. Middle ear
B. Endolymphatic sac
C. Semicircular canals
D. Cochlea
E. Helicotrema

171. A 55-year-old woman comes to the physician because of swelling in her neck. Her vital signs are within normal limits. Physical examination shows a non-tender mass on the right side of the patient's neck. An ultrasound examination of the neck shows a thyroid gland mass. A biopsy of the lesion shows a thyroid gland cancer. She subsequently undergoes a thyroidectomy. Three days after the thyroidectomy, a CT-scan of the head shows air bubbles. Which of the following is the most likely cause of the air bubbles?
A. Injury to inferior thyroid artery
B. Injury to inferior and superior thyroid arteries
C. Injury to superior thyroid artery and vein
D. Injury to superior and middle thyroid veins
E. Injury to superior, middle, and inferior thyroid veins

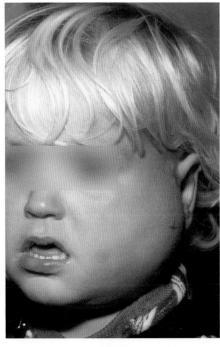

• **Fig. 7.7**

172. A 32-year-old man is brought to the emergency department after being involved in a motor vehicle collision. His temperature is 37.4°C (99.32°F), pulse is 105/min, respirations are 25/min, and blood pressure is 90/70 mm Hg. Physical examination shows an unconscious man with multiple lacerations on his face and blood within the oral cavity. An emergency airway is established with a cricothyrotomy. An artery is injured during the cricothyrotomy procedure. Two days later the patient shows signs of aspiration pneumonia. Which of the following arteries was most likely injured?

A. Superior thyroid
B. Inferior thyroid
C. Cricothyroid
D. Superior laryngeal
E. Suprahyoid

173. A 22-year-old woman is brought to the emergency department by ambulance after falling from her bicycle. The patient lost consciousness in the field. Her temperature is 37.5°C (99.5°F), pulse is 70/min, respirations are 26/min, and blood pressure is 140/90 mm Hg. Physical examination shows a laceration on the right side of her head. An emergency tracheotomy is performed. What is the most common tracheal cartilage level at which a tracheotomy incision should be performed?

A. First to second
B. Second to third
C. Third to fourth
D. Fourth to fifth
E. Fifth to sixth

174. A 36-year-old woman is brought to the emergency department after being involved in a motor vehicle collision. Her temperature is 37.4°C (99.32°F), pulse is 105/min, respirations are 22/min, and blood pressure is 130/70 mm Hg. Physical examination shows several lacerations on her head and face, and her palate elevates asymmetrically toward the right. Which of the following muscles is paralyzed?

A. Left levator veli palatini
B. Left tensor veli palatini
C. Right levator veli palatini
D. Right tensor veli palatini
E. Right tensor veli palatini and left levator veli palatini

175. A 45-year-old man is brought to the emergency department after stumbling and hitting his head on a table in a restaurant. His vital signs are within normal limits. Photographs were taken of the patient's eyes during neurologic examination (Fig. 7.8). Which of the following nerves to the left eye was most likely injured?

A. Trochlear
B. Abducens
C. Oculomotor
D. Optic
E. Oculomotor and abducens

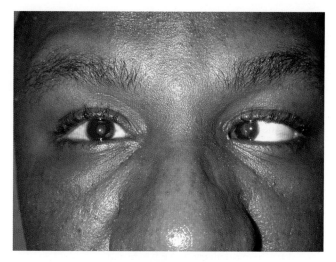

• **Fig. 7.8**

Questions 176–200

176. A 32-year-old woman is brought to the emergency department after losing consciousness and collapsing in the middle of the street. Her vital signs are within normal limits. Physical examination shows bruises on the face and head on the right side. There is an absence of the accommodation reflex of the right eye. Which of the following structures is most likely involved in the pathology of this patient?

A. Superior salivatory nucleus
B. SCG
C. Nervus intermedius
D. Edinger-Westphal nucleus
E. Trigeminal ganglion

177. A 32-year-old man comes to the emergency department because of nausea, vomiting, and a severe headache for 3 days. His vital signs are within normal limits. Physical examination shows nystagmus. An MRI of the head shows an acoustic neuroma (Fig. 7.9). Which of the following nerves is most likely compressed by the tumor?

A. Facial
B. Oculomotor
C. Vagus
D. Hypoglossal
E. Abducens

178. A 3-year-old boy is brought to the physician by his parents because of swelling of the side of his neck. Physical examination shows a mass of tissue anterior to the superior one-third of the sternocleidomastoid muscle (Fig. 7.10). The swelling is fluctuant and nontender to palpation. Which of the following is the most likely diagnosis?

A. Branchial cleft cyst
B. Ruptured sternocleidomastoid muscle
C. Lymph node inflammation
D. Torticollis
E. External carotid artery aneurysm

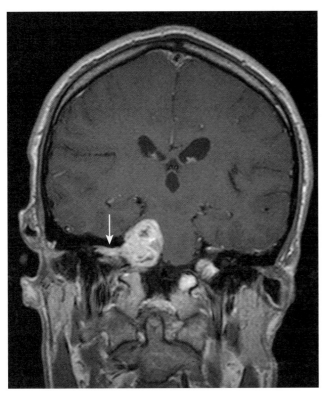

• Fig. 7.9

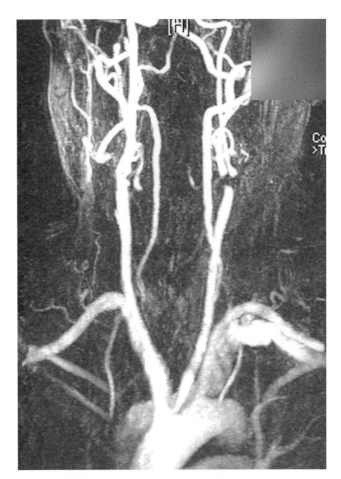

• Fig. 7.11

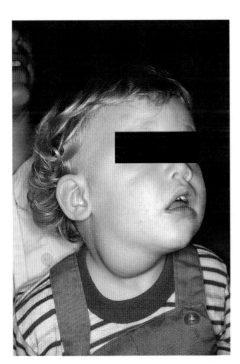

• Fig. 7.10

179. A 68-year-old woman comes to the physician because of chronic dizziness and headaches. She has a history of multiple transient ischemic attacks, hypertension, and diabetes mellitus. Her temperature is 37.0°C (98.6°F), pulse is 80/min, respirations are 15/min, and blood pressure is 145/90 mm Hg. Cranial and cervical angiography (Fig. 7.11) shows an occluded vessel. Which of the following vessels is most likely involved?
   A. External carotid
   B. Internal carotid
   C. Common carotid
   D. Vertebral
   E. Superior thyroid

180. A 9-year-old girl comes to the emergency department with painful swelling behind her right ear. Her temperature is 38.3°C (101.0°F), pulse is 110/min, respirations are 15/min, and blood pressure is 120/90 mm Hg. Physical examination shows erythema, swelling, and tenderness behind the right ear. An MRI of the head shows mastoiditis (Fig. 7.12). Which of the following structures is most likely to be affected by the inflammation?
   A. Sigmoid sinus
   B. Petrous part of the temporal bone
   C. Inner ear
   D. Occipital sinus
   E. Internal carotid artery

181. A 34-year-old woman comes to the emergency department with a painful left eye. Her vital signs are within normal limits. Physical examination shows a lump on the lower eyelid of the left eye (Fig. 7.13). A diagnosis of a chalazion is made. An obstruction of which of the

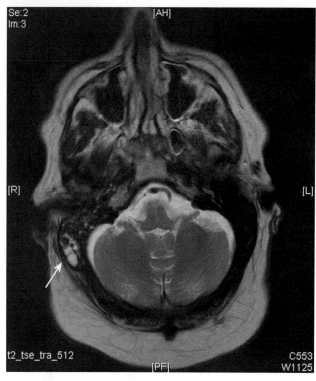

• **Fig. 7.12**

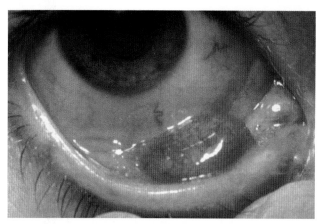

• **Fig. 7.13**

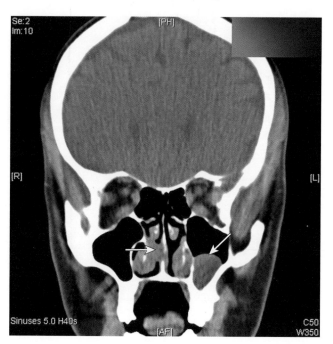

• **Fig. 7.14**

A. Sphenoid sinus
B. Maxillary sinus and nasolacrimal duct
C. Ethmoidal cells
D. Frontal sinus
E. Nasolacrimal duct

183. A 58-year-old man comes to the physician because of progressive unilateral hearing loss and ringing in the affected ear (tinnitus) of 4 months duration. His vital signs are within normal limits. Physical examination shows hearing loss in the right ear. An MRI of the head shows a tumor at the cerebellopontine angle. Which of the following nerves is most likely affected?
A. Vagus
B. Hypoglossal
C. Vestibulocochlear
D. Glossopharyngeal
E. Trigeminal

184. A newborn boy is brought to the neonatal intensive care unit after a difficult delivery requiring forceps. The pregnancy was complicated by maternal diabetes. His vital signs are within normal limits. Physical examination shows a cephalohematoma on the right side of his head because of rupture of small periosteal arteries. The blood from the lesion will most likely accumulate between which of the following tissues?
A. Between skin and dense connective tissue layer
B. Between loose connective tissue layer and galea aponeurotica
C. Between galea aponeurotica and pericranium
D. Between pericranium and calvaria
E. In the subcutaneous layer

following structures is most likely responsible for the patient's ocular pathology?
A. Lacrimal ducts
B. Tarsal glands
C. Sclera
D. Pupil
E. Nasolacrimal duct

182. A 45-year-old man comes to the emergency department because of difficulty breathing through his nose. Physical examination shows signs of an obstruction of the nasal airway in both nostrils. A CT scan of the head shows bilateral nasal obstruction with left maxillary sinus involvement. (Fig. 7.14). Drainage from which of the following structures will most likely be impaired from the obstruction?

185. A 54-year-old woman is brought to the emergency department because of a severe headache, nausea, and vomiting. Physical examination shows that she

is unconscious. When she regains consciousness, her right eye is directed laterally and inferiorly. There is also complete ptosis of her upper eyelid and pupillary dilation of the affected eye. An MRI of the head shows a tumor in her brain producing a transtentorial herniation. Which of the following lobes of the brain is most likely affected by the tumor?

A. Parietal
B. Temporal
C. Occipital
D. Frontal
E. Parietal and temporal

186. A 54-year-old man comes to the emergency department because of a severe headache and vomiting. His vital signs are within normal limits. Physical examination of the eye shows bilateral papilledema. An MRI of the brain shows a tumor occupying a portion of the anterior cranial fossa. Which of the following is responsible for the sensation of pain in this case?

A. Meningeal branches of the maxillary nerve
B. Meningeal branches of the mandibular nerve
C. Meningeal branches of the ethmoidal nerves
D. Tentorial nerve
E. C2 and C3 fibers

187. A 55-year-old woman is brought to the emergency department because of chest pain. Physical examination shows a diaphoretic woman with no tenderness of the anterior chest wall. An ECG shows an acute myocardial infarction. A series of medications is administered to the patient, including sublingual nitroglycerin. Which of the following structures is most likely to be the route of absorption of this drug?

A. Deep lingual vein
B. Submandibular duct
C. Sublingual duct
D. Lingual vein
E. Sublingual vein

188. A 35-year-old man comes to the emergency department because of a lump on the right side of his face. Physical examination shows a hard, non-tender mass in the right submandibular region. A biopsy of the mass shows a malignancy of the submandibular gland. The submandibular gland and its duct are removed. Which of the following nerves is most prone to injury in this type of procedure?

A. Buccal
B. Lingual
C. Inferior alveolar
D. Nerve to mylohyoid
E. Glossopharyngeal

189. A 22-year-old man comes to the physician because of a runny nose, fever, and progressive vision loss. Physical examination shows loss of transillumination of the maxillary sinuses bilaterally and swelling of the nasal mucosa bilaterally. A diagnosis of acute sinusitis is made. Injury to which of the following structures is most likely to result in the loss of vision in this patient?

A. Ophthalmic artery
B. Nasociliary nerve
C. Anterior ethmoidal nerve
D. Trochlear nerve
E. Optic nerve

190. A 55-year-old man is brought to the emergency department after falling from the roof of his one-story home. Physical examination shows a laceration of the scalp. An x-ray of the head shows a small, depressed fracture of the vertex of the skull. A non-contrast CT scan of the head shows thrombosis of the superior sagittal sinus. A day later the patient becomes unconscious. What is the most likely cause of his loss of consciousness?

A. Obstruction of CSF resorption
B. Obstruction of the cerebral aqueduct (of Sylvius)
C. Laceration of the middle meningeal artery
D. Fracture of the cribriform plate with CSF rhinorrhea
E. Aneurysm of the middle cerebral artery

191. An 11-year-old boy is brought to the physician by his parents because of fever and a sore throat for 2 days. He has a history of a genetic immunodeficiency with recurrent tonsillitis. Physical examination shows enlarged erythematous palatine tonsils with petechiae and pus. Which of the following lymph nodes is most likely first to become visibly enlarged during tonsillitis?

A. Submandibular
B. Parotid
C. Jugulodigastric
D. Submental
E. Retropharyngeal

192. A 45-year-old man comes to the physician because of a red and painful left eye. His 3-year-old daughter was diagnosed with viral conjunctivitis 3 days ago. Physical examination of the left eye shows an injected conjunctiva. Which of the following groups of lymph nodes is first to become involved if the infection were to spread?

A. Submandibular
B. Preauricular
C. Jugulodigastric
D. Submental
E. Superficial parotid

193. A 45-year-old woman comes to the physician because of difficulty swallowing and night-time coughing fits. The patient says that she regurgitated stale food items from a meal she had 2 days ago. She has a history of repeated chest infections. Physical examination shows a palpable swelling in her neck. Barium swallow of the esophagus shows an outpouching of the esophagus collecting contrast in the cervical region. Between which muscles is this pouch most likely located?

A. Between styloglossus and stylopharyngeus
B. Between palatoglossal arch and median glossoepiglottic fold
C. Between upper and middle pharyngeal constrictors
D. Between the cricopharyngeal and thyropharyngeal portions of inferior pharyngeal constrictor
E. Between the middle and inferior pharyngeal constrictors

194. A 5-year-old boy is brought to the emergency department unconscious after falling from a tree. An emergency tracheostomy is performed to establish an airway. During the procedure, profuse dark venous bleeding suddenly occurs from the midline incision over the trachea. Which of the following vessels was most likely cut?
A. Superior thyroid vein
B. Middle thyroid vein
C. Left brachiocephalic vein
D. Inferior thyroid vein
E. Jugular venous arch connecting the anterior jugular veins

195. A 55-year-old woman comes to the physician because of a sore throat and ear pain. Her vital signs are within normal limits. A CT scan of the head and neck shows Eagle syndrome in which the styloid process and stylohyoid ligament are elongated and calcified. Which of the following nerves is most likely affected by this syndrome in this patient?
A. Vagus
B. Facial
C. Glossopharyngeal
D. Hypoglossal
E. Vestibulocochlear

196. A 62-year-old man comes to the physician because of spontaneous lacrimation of the right eye that occurs while eating. Three weeks ago, the patient was diagnosed with Bell palsy. His vital signs are within normal limits. Physical examination shows no neurologic deficits. Which of the following nerves has developed a lesion to cause this condition?
A. Facial nerve proximal to the geniculate ganglion
B. Greater petrosal nerve
C. Lesser petrosal nerve
D. Lacrimal nerve
E. Chorda tympani

197. A 54-year-old woman comes to the emergency department because of difficulty with her vision over the past 5 days. Physical examination shows loss of vision in the temporal visual fields bilaterally. An MRI of the head shows an aneurysm of one of the arteries at the base of the brain compressing the optic chiasm. Which of the following arteries is most likely be involved?
A. Middle cerebral
B. Anterior communicating
C. Anterior cerebral
D. Superior cerebellar
E. Posterior inferior cerebellar

198. A 22-year-old woman comes to the physician because of a sinus infection that has lasted 2 weeks. Her temperature is 38.3°C (101.0°F), pulse is 96/min, respirations are 15/min, and blood pressure is 120/90 mm Hg. Physical examination shows focal inflammation with mucosal edema in the inferior nasal meatus. Drainage from which of the following structures is most likely to be obstructed by this inflammation and edema?
A. Anterior ethmoidal cells
B. Frontonasal duct
C. Maxillary sinus
D. Middle ethmoidal cells
E. Nasolacrimal duct

199. A 40-year-old woman is brought to the emergency department after being involved in a motor vehicle collision. Her temperature is 37.5°C (99.5°F), pulse is 96/min, respirations are 16/min, and blood pressure is 130/90 mm Hg. Physical examination shows bruises on the face, chest, and upper limbs. An x-ray of the head shows a fracture of the temporal bone resulting in a lesion of the facial nerve proximal to the origin of the chorda tympani in the posterior wall of the tympanic cavity. Which of the following functions would most likely remain intact in this patient?
A. Control of muscles in lower half of face
B. Control of secretions by submandibular gland
C. Taste sensation from anterior two-thirds of tongue
D. Tear production by the lacrimal gland
E. Voluntary closure of the eyelid

200. A 17-year-old boy is brought to the emergency department after cutting himself while trying to shave. Physical examination shows a 2 cm laceration over the angle of the mandible. The area of the laceration is anesthetized and the wound is sutured. Cutaneous sensation over this area is normally supplied by which of the following nerves?
A. Cervical branch of facial
B. Great auricular nerve
C. Mandibular branch of trigeminal nerve
D. Marginal mandibular branch of facial nerve
E. Transverse cervical nerve

Questions 201–225

201. A 72-year-old man comes to the physician with abdominal pain and changes in his bowel habits. Physical examination shows a cachectic man and a mass is palpated in the right lower quadrant. A CT-scan shows findings that are consistent with malignant tumor of the cecum. Which of the following cervical lymph nodes is most frequently associated with malignant tumors as seen in this patient?
A. Left inferior deep cervical
B. Left supraclavicular
C. Right inferior deep cervical
D. Right supraclavicular
E. Jugulodigastric

202. A 60-year-old man comes to the physician with worsening hoarseness and difficulty swallowing. He has smoked two packs of cigarettes for the past 30 years. Physical examination shows a mass on the right side of the neck and firm fixed regional lymph nodes are palpated. Direct laryngoscopy shows a mass protruding into the piriform recess of the larynx. The mucosa of the piriform recess must be anesthetized for removal of the tumor. Which of the following nerves is responsible for general sensation to the mucosa where the tumor is located?
    A. External branch of superior laryngeal
    B. Inferior laryngeal
    C. Glossopharyngeal
    D. Hypoglossal
    E. Internal branch of superior laryngeal

203. A 25-year-old man is brought to the emergency department after he was found unconscious on the floor of his apartment. He was pronounced dead on arrival. At autopsy, examination shows crepitus over the midline of the neck. An x-ray shows a fractured hyoid bone, but the calvaria and other bones appear to be intact. Which of the following is the most likely cause of death?
    A. Myocardial infarction
    B. A fall from a height that resulted in fatal internal bleeding
    C. Subdural hematoma
    D. Strangulation
    E. Ingestion of a poisonous substance

204. A 40-year-old woman comes to the emergency department with severe headaches, vomiting, and dizziness. Physical examination shows gait instability and left-sided hemineglect. An MRI of the head shows necrotic lesions in the cerebellum and a solitary lesion in the right cerebral hemisphere. A biopsy of the right cerebral hemisphere lesion shows an advanced melanoma. She dies 2 months later. At autopsy, examination shows no pigmented lesions of her skin or scalp. Which of the following is the most likely source of the malignant melanoma cells?
    A. Superior sagittal sinus
    B. Sphenoidal sinus
    C. Retina of the eye
    D. Pituitary gland
    E. Thymus

205. A 3-month-old girl is brought to the physician by her parents because of mucus dripping from the side of her neck. Her vital signs are within normal limits. Physical examination shows a small pit on the anterior border of sternocleidomastoid with mucus dripping intermittently from its opening. Which of the following embryologic structures is involved in this anomaly?
    A. Persistence of the second pharyngeal arch
    B. Persistence of the proximal part of the second pharyngeal groove

C. Persistence of the third pharyngeal pouch
    D. Thyroglossal duct
    E. Persistence of the fourth pharyngeal pouch

206. A 3-year-old boy is brought to the emergency department after having a seizure. He was born at term with no complications. Medical history includes a repaired cleft palate and a heart murmur. Physical examination shows low-set ears and a small mandible. Laboratory studies show hypocalcemia. A chromosome analysis shows a deletion in the long arm of chromosome 22. Failure of neural crest cells to migrate into which area(s) best explains the patient's condition?
    A. First pharyngeal arch
    B. Third and fourth pharyngeal pouches
    C. The developing heart
    D. Second pharyngeal pouch
    E. First, second, and third pharyngeal arches

207. A 2-month-old girl is brought to the physician for a cleft lip surgery consultation. The infant was born at term with no complications. She has normal development. Physical examination shows a unilateral upper cleft lip on the right side. Failure of fusion of which of the following structures is the most likely cause of this congenital defect?
    A. Lateral nasal and maxillary prominences/processes
    B. Right and left medial nasal prominences/processes
    C. Lateral nasal and medial nasal prominences/processes
    D. Lateral nasal prominences/processes
    E. Maxillary prominence/process and the intermaxillary segment

208. A primigravid woman comes to the physician at 18 weeks of gestation for a routine prenatal examination. Vital signs are within normal limits. Physical examination shows a uterine fundus height above the umbilicus. Ultrasound examination shows polyhydramnios and spina bifida. Which of the following conditions is expected to be found during the ultrasound examination of the fetus?
    A. Anencephaly
    B. Bilateral renal agenesis
    C. Agenesis of the vagina
    D. Hydrocephalus
    E. Omphalocele

209. A 4-month-old girl is brought to the physician for a neonatal wellness follow-up. She was born at 38 weeks' gestation via a spontaneous vaginal delivery with no complications. She received all scheduled vaccinations and her development has been normal. Physical examination shows a small defect in the 6 o'clock position of the right iris. She is referred to an ophthalmologist. A detailed ophthalmologic examination shows a defect in the inferior sector of the iris, the pupillary margin, the ciliary body, and the retina. What is the etiology of the infant's condition?
    A. Failure of the retinal/optic fissure to close
    B. Abnormal neural crest formation

C. Abnormal interactions between the optic vesicle and ectoderm

D. Posterior chamber cavitation

E. Weak adhesion between the inner and outer layers of the optic cup

210. A 26-year-old man is brought to the emergency department with face pain after being knocked out during a boxing match. His vital signs are within normal limits. Physical examination shows swelling and bruising over the left jaw. He is unable to fully open his mouth. A CT scan of the head shows severe trauma to the articular disc and fracture of the neck of the mandible. This could result in injury to a muscle that developed from which of the following embryonic structures?

A. First pharyngeal pouch

B. Second pharyngeal pouch

C. First pharyngeal arch

D. First pharyngeal cleft

E. Second pharyngeal arch

211. A 2-day-old boy is admitted to the hospital for correction of a large defect in the occipital bone (cranium bifidum). An MRI of the head shows that the defect contains meninges and part of the brain including the ventricular system protruding through the bony defect. What is the most likely diagnosis?

A. Cranial meningocele

B. Encephalocele

C. Meroencephaly

D. Meningohydroencephalocele

E. Microcephaly

212. A 30-year-old man comes to the physician because of a mass in his neck that he ignored for several years. Physical examination shows a soft, midline mass about 2 cm in diameter in the neck. A CT scan of the neck shows a well-defined, fluid-filled mass (Fig. 7.15). Persistence of which embryological structure most likely accounts for this mass?

A. Second pharyngeal cleft

B. Foramen cecum

C. Thyroglossal duct

D. Third pharyngeal pouch

E. Cervical sinus

213. A newborn boy is brought to the pediatric intensive care unit after a spontaneous vaginal delivery. The pregnancy and delivery were uncomplicated. Physical examination shows down-slanting palpebral fissures, defects of the lower eyelids, and deformed external ears. He is diagnosed with Treacher Collins syndrome (mandibulofacial dysostosis). Abnormal development of which pharyngeal arch will most likely produce this syndrome?

A. First

B. Second

C. Third

D. Fourth

E. Sixth

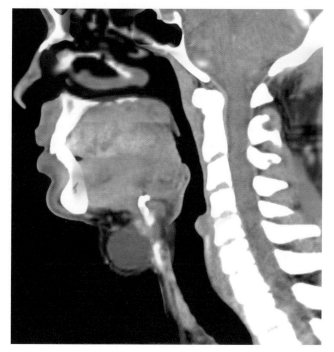

• **Fig. 7.15**

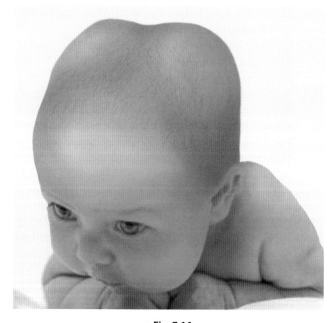

• **Fig. 7.16**

214. A 28-year-old woman gives birth to a boy. A vacuum device was used to assist in the delivery. Physical examination of the infant after birth shows bilateral swellings on the infant's head that do not cross suture lines (Fig. 7.16). Transillumination of the skull appears to be normal and neurologic examination is normal. Which of the following is most likely responsible for this patient's symptoms?

A. Intracranial bleeding

B. Blockage of the interventricular foramen

C. Failure of cleavage of the prosencephalon

D. Collection of blood beneath the periosteum of the bone

E. Collection of edema fluid above the periosteum of the bone

215. A 2-month-old girl is brought to the emergency department because of a seizure. Her vital signs are within normal limits. Physical examination shows severe chorioretinitis bilaterally. A CT scan of the head shows hydrocephalus and several areas of intracranial calcifications. What is the most likely cause of these symptoms?

A. The mother was treated with tetracyclines during pregnancy

B. The mother was infected with rubella during the first trimester of pregnancy

C. The mother was infected with CMV during the first trimester of pregnancy

D. The mother was infected with *Treponema pallidum* during pregnancy exhibiting congenital syphilis

E. The mother was infected with *Toxoplasma gondii* during the first trimester of pregnancy

216. A 3-month-old boy is brought to the physician because of a lump in his neck. His vital signs are within normal limits. Physical examination shows a soft mass of tissue on the neck and a biopsy of the mass shows ectopic thymus tissue. Which other developmentally related structure could also have an ectopic location?

A. Jugulodigastric lymph node

B. Lingual tonsil

C. Inferior parathyroid gland

D. Submandibular gland

E. Palatine tonsil

217. A 6-year-old girl was brought to the physician by her mother who was concerned about her daughter's teeth. The child is developing normally and has no problems in school. Her vital signs are within normal limits. Physical examination shows a yellowish-brown discoloration of the child's deciduous teeth. What is the most likely cause of this discoloration?

A. The mother continued to smoke during the pregnancy

B. The mother was treated with tetracycline during the pregnancy

C. Poor calcification of dentin because of calcium deficiency during the pregnancy

D. The mother was infected with rubella during the pregnancy

E. The mother continued to use alcohol during the pregnancy

218. A 23-year-old woman gives birth to a preterm boy. The mother did not seek prenatal care throughout the pregnancy. The boy is transferred to the neonatal intensive care unit for evaluation of low birth weight. His vital signs are within normal limits. Physical examination shows a small head circumference and bilateral cataracts. Cardiac auscultation shows a

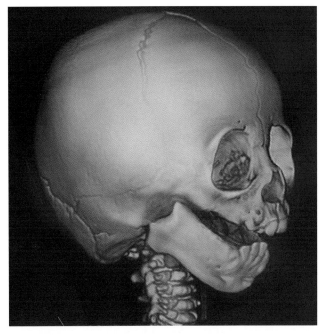

• Fig. 7.17

continuous machine-like murmur. Which of the following is the most likely cause of these findings?

A. The mother was taking thalidomide during pregnancy

B. The mother was infected with rubella during the first trimester of pregnancy

C. The mother was infected with CMV during the first trimester of pregnancy

D. The mother used cocaine during pregnancy

E. The mother was infected with *T. gondii* during the first trimester of pregnancy

219. A 1-year-old boy is brought to the physician for a follow-up visit. He was born at term via an uncomplicated spontaneous vaginal delivery. Physical examination shows multiple craniofacial abnormalities and a cleft palate. CT scans, including the 3D reconstruction shown in Fig. 7.17 are obtained to guide surgical planning. Which other abnormalities are likely to be found with appropriate investigation?

A. Hyperthyroidism

B. Hypoplasia of the hyoid bone

C. Malformation of laryngeal cartilages

D. Hypoplasia of the thymus

E. Hearing loss

220. A 14-year-old boy is brought to the physician because of a mass on the left side of his neck. He had an upper respiratory infection 3 weeks ago that resolved uneventfully. Physical examination shows a soft fluid-filled mass on the left side of the neck at the level of the laryngeal prominence. A CT scan of the neck shows a well-defined, 4-cm diameter, fluid-filled mass with a thin outer rim (Fig. 7.18). A diagnosis of a branchial cyst is made. Which embryological structure most likely contributes to this mass?

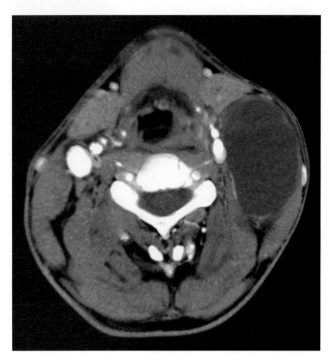

• **Fig. 7.18**

   A. First pharyngeal pouch
   B. Second pharyngeal arch
   C. Third pharyngeal pouch
   D. Cervical sinus
   E. Ectopic thyroid gland

221. A newborn boy was delivered via spontaneous vaginal delivery with no complications. Physical examination of the neonate shows hypoplasia of the mandible and zygomatic bones, slanted palpebral fissures, and malformed external ears. No cardiac murmurs are detected on auscultation. There is a family history of similar findings in his father. What is the most likely diagnosis?
   A. Pierre Robin syndrome
   B. DiGeorge syndrome
   C. Fetal alcohol syndrome (FAS)
   D. Chiari I malformation
   E. Treacher Collins syndrome

222. A 22-year-old woman is brought to the emergency department after falling from the 9th floor of an apartment complex. Her temperature is 37.5°C (99.5°F), pulse is 103/min, respirations are 20/min, and blood pressure is 140/90 mm Hg. Physical examination shows multiple fractures of the mandible. She undergoes surgical reconstruction of the mandible. Postoperatively, she has numbness of the lower lip and chin. Which nerve was most likely injured?
   A. Auriculotemporal
   B. Buccal
   C. Lesser petrosal
   D. Mental
   E. Infraorbital

223. A 22-year-old man is brought to the emergency department after being involved in a motor vehicle collision. His temperature is 37.5°C (99.5°F), pulse is 105/min, respirations are 22/min, and blood pressure is 100/90 mm Hg. Physical examination shows severe facial trauma. A CT scan of the head shows multiple fractures of the facial bones. He is taken to the operating room for surgical repair. Following surgery, taste sensation at the tip of the tongue is lost. Which ganglion contains the neuron cell bodies of the taste fibers from this part of the tongue?
   A. Trigeminal
   B. Geniculate
   C. Inferior glossopharyngeal
   D. Submandibular ganglion
   E. Pterygopalatine

224. A 21-year-old man comes to the emergency department because of fever and a severe headache. His temperature is 38.5°C (102.02°F), pulse is 106/min, respirations are 16/min, and blood pressure is 130/90 mm Hg. A CT scan of the head shows a ring enhancing lesion compressing the ophthalmic branch of the trigeminal nerve. Which of the following additional symptoms would the patient most likely experience?
   A. Pain in the hard palate
   B. Anesthesia of the upper lip
   C. Painful eyeball
   D. Pain over the lower eyelid
   E. Tingling sensation over the buccal region of the face

225. A 72-year-old man comes to the physician because of difficulty when eating for the past few weeks. His vital signs are within normal limits. Physical examination shows a cachexic man. An MRI of the head shows a tumor of the brainstem affecting the contents of the hypoglossal canal. Which of the following muscles would be affected by such a tumor?
   A. Geniohyoid
   B. Mylohyoid
   C. Palatoglossus
   D. Genioglossus
   E. Stylohyoid

Questions 226–250

226. A 71-year-old man comes to the physician with a dry itchy right eye and nose. He often uses eye drops to relieve the dryness. He was diagnosed with a nonresectable brain tumor 4 months ago. Physical examination shows a red dry eye with no visual impairment. Which cranial nerve nucleus will the tumor most likely involve?
   A. Inferior salivatory nucleus
   B. Dorsal vagal nucleus
   C. Superior salivatory nucleus
   D. Edinger-Westphal nucleus
   E. Nucleus ambiguus

227. A 23-year-old man comes to the physician with right arm pain and weakness. His vital signs are within normal limits. Physical examination shows a pale appearing right hand that is cooler than the left hand. A CT scan of his neck shows hypertrophied scalene muscles on the right. The patient is diagnosed with thoracic outlet syndrome. Which of the following symptoms is also consistent with this diagnosis?
  A. Problems with respiration because of pressure on the phrenic nerve
  B. Reduced blood flow to the thoracic wall
  C. Reduced venous return from the head and neck
  D. Numbness in the upper extremity
  E. Distension of the internal jugular vein

228. A 29-year-old woman comes to the physician because of a lump on her neck. After thorough investigation, she undergoes a thyroidectomy to remove the tumor. In the postoperative period the patient develops swelling of her neck. Physical examination shows partial ptosis of the right eyelid, with pupillary constriction of the ipsilateral eye. The symptoms of this patient are most likely caused by compression of which of the following ganglions?
  A. Submandibular
  B. Trigeminal
  C. Superior cervical
  D. Geniculate
  E. Ciliary

229. A 26-year-old man is brought to the emergency department after sustaining a traumatic injury to the midface during a street fight. His vital signs are within normal limits. Physical examination shows intact taste and salivation, but there is loss of general sensation from the anterior tongue. Which of the following nerves was most likely injured?
  A. Lingual nerve proximal to its junction with the chorda tympani
  B. Chorda tympani
  C. Inferior alveolar
  D. Lingual distal to its junction with the chorda tympani
  E. Glossopharyngeal

230. An 82-year-old man comes to the physician for a follow-up examination after being diagnosed with a tumor of the posterior cranial fossa. An MRI of the head shows perineural spread of the tumor along nervous tissue at the jugular foramen. Which deficit would be expected to be found on physical examination of this patient?
  A. Loss of tongue movements
  B. Loss of facial expression
  C. Loss of sensation from the face and the scalp
  D. Loss of hearing
  E. Loss of gag reflex

231. A 25-year-old man is brought to the emergency department after injuring himself during a soccer game. His coach says that the patient hit his head against the

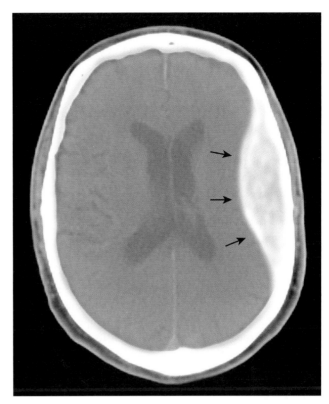

• **Fig. 7.19**

goal post while trying to reach for the oncoming ball. The patient did not lose consciousness but was confused for several minutes. He later resumed playing. Four hours later, he was found unconscious in the locker room. A CT scan of his head shows a hemorrhage (Fig. 7.19, *arrows*). The vessel that was ruptured to produce this hemorrhage enters the skull through which of the following openings?
  A. Foramen spinosum
  B. Foramen ovale
  C. Jugular foramen
  D. Hypoglossal canal
  E. Foramen lacerum

232. A 55-year-old woman is brought to the emergency department by her husband after she was found unconscious in their home. She has a history of poorly controlled hypertension. Her temperature is 37.5°C (99.5°F), pulse is 90/min, respirations are 16/min, and blood pressure is 175/100 mm Hg. Physical examination shows ptosis of the right eye and right pupillary mydriasis. The right eye is also deviated inferolaterally. A non-contrast CT scan shows a subarachnoid hemorrhage. Angiography is most likely to show a hematoma compressing which of the following structure structures?
  A. Oculomotor nerve
  B. Optic nerve
  C. Facial nerve
  D. Ciliary ganglion
  E. SCG

233. A 20-year-old man comes to the emergency department with a wound on the back of his head. Physical examination shows a laceration in the occipital region of the scalp. The wound was sutured. Three days later, the patient returns to the emergency department because of a tender, erythematous wound that has become infected and has spread anteriorly on the scalp. Between which layers of the scalp has the infection spread?
    A. The periosteum and bone
    B. The aponeurosis and the periosteum
    C. The dense connective tissue and the aponeurosis
    D. The dense connective tissue and the skin
    E. The dermis and the epidermis

234. A 73-year-old patient comes to the physician because of a 6-month history of neck pain, hoarseness, and weight loss. Physical examination shows tenderness on deep palpation of the anterior neck. Laryngoscopy is performed and a large tumor is identified on one of the true vocal folds. The laryngoscope is unable to pass through the opening between the folds. What is the name of this opening?
    A. Piriform recess
    B. Vestibule
    C. Ventricle
    D. Vallecula
    E. Rima glottidis

235. An 82-year-old man comes to the physician because of a neck mass. Physical examination shows an enlarged, hard, non-tender cervical lymph node on the right side of the neck. Visualization with a flexible laryngoscope shows a mass located in the piriform recess. Performing a biopsy of the mass, care must be shown to avoid injuring which of the following nerves?
    A. Mandibular
    B. Maxillary
    C. Glossopharyngeal
    D. Internal branch of superior laryngeal
    E. Hypoglossal

236. A 3-year-old girl was brought to the physician because of a severe throat infection. Her temperature is 38.3°C (101.0°F), pulse is 100/min, respirations are 26/min, and blood pressure is 102/60 mm Hg. Physical examination shows a bulging and erythematous tympanic membrane. What is the embryologic origin of the structure that allowed the infection to spread from the pharynx to the middle ear cavity?
    A. Second pouch
    B. First groove
    C. Second groove
    D. First pouch
    E. Third pouch

237. A 35-year-old man was brought to the emergency department after being involved in a motor vehicle collision. His temperature is 37.5°C (99.5°F), pulse is 110/min, respirations are 27/min, and blood pressure is 90/60 mm Hg. Physical examination shows

a comatose patient unresponsive to tactile or verbal feedback. A laceration was observed on the left side of his head. During neurologic examination the light is directed into the right eye and the pupil constricts. Which of the following two cranial nerves are being tested?
    A. Optic and facial
    B. Optic and oculomotor
    C. Maxillary and facial
    D. Ophthalmic and oculomotor
    E. Ophthalmic and facial

238. A 27-year-old woman comes to the physician because of vision problems. Physical examination shows that the right pupil is dilated and unresponsive to light. A CT angiography of the head shows a large aneurysm of the superior cerebellar artery just after it branches off from the basilar artery, compressing the nerve responsible for the symptoms. Which cranial nerve is being compressed by the aneurysm?
    A. Oculomotor
    B. Trigeminal
    C. Facial
    D. Vagus
    E. Abducens

239. An 88-year-old man comes to the physician because of blurry vision and headache for the past 6 months. Physical examination shows an inability to abduct his right eye and ipsilateral absence of the corneal reflex. A CT scan of the head shows a dural mass. A growth located in which of the following structures of the skull is most likely responsible for the symptoms of this patient?
    A. Inferior orbital fissure
    B. Optic canal
    C. Superior orbital fissure
    D. Foramen rotundum
    E. Foramen ovale

240. A 72-year-old woman comes to the physician because of pain in her left ear. She says that this pain started suddenly 2 days ago and is so severe that she must hold the phone away from her ear because it sounds too loud. Physical examination shows a hyperacusis of the left ear and Bell palsy of the left side of the face. Which cranial nerve is most likely to be affected by the infection to result in hyperacusis?
    A. Hypoglossal
    B. Facial
    C. Spinal accessory
    D. Vagus
    E. Glossopharyngeal

241. A 70-year-old man comes to the physician for evaluation of sudden hearing loss in his right ear. Physical examination shows a large amount of cerumen (earwax) in the right external acoustic meatus which is removed to fully evaluate the tympanic membrane. During this process the patient begins to cough. The cough results from stimulation of an area of the

meatus that is innervated by which of the following nerves?

A. Vestibulocochlear
B. Vagus
C. Trigeminal
D. Facial
E. Accessory

242. A 30-year-old woman comes to the physician because of hoarseness of her voice after undergoing a total thyroidectomy for a cancerous thyroid nodule 3 weeks ago. Physical examination shows a well-healing surgical scar. She is able to swallow sips of water without difficulty. Which nerve was most likely injured during the operation?

A. Internal branch of superior laryngeal
B. External branch of superior laryngeal
C. Recurrent laryngeal
D. Superior laryngeal
E. Glossopharyngeal

243. An 82-year-old man is brought to the physician by his daughter for a follow-up visit. His vital signs are within normal limits. Physical examination shows anisocoria. The extraocular muscles are intact. Which of the following tests should be used to differentiate a sympathetic nerve lesion from an oculomotor nerve lesion?

A. Startle reflex
B. Blink reflex
C. Pupillary light reflex
D. H-test
E. Vision test (reading chart)

244. A 22-year-old man comes to the emergency department after being hit in the eye by a baseball bat. Physical examination shows inability to move his eye normally and to focus on close objects. Injury to which of the following nerve structures would most likely be the cause of his condition?

A. Trochlear nerve and abducens nerve
B. Oculomotor nerve and abducens nerve
C. SCG and long ciliary nerves
D. Short ciliary nerves and ciliary ganglion
E. Infratrochlear nerve and ciliary ganglion

245. A 75-year-old man comes to the physician because of a painful rash on his forehead. Physical examination shows a vesicular rash and a diagnosis of orofacial herpes is made. Herpetic lesions of the forehead require expeditious treatment because the infection can spread to the cavernous sinus, leading to intracranial complications. Which venous structure is the most likely route of transmission of this infectious process to the cavernous sinus?

A. Pterygoid venous plexus
B. Superior ophthalmic vein
C. Superior petrosal sinus
D. Basilar venous plexus
E. Parietal emissary vein

246. An 87-year-old woman underwent surgery to remove a vestibular schwannoma (tumor at the internal

acoustic meatus). Physical examination postoperatively shows drooping of the right corner of the mouth and food collection in the right oral vestibule. She is unable to close the right eye. Which of the following cranial nerves was injured during the surgery?

A. IX
B. X
C. VII
D. V2
E. V3

247. A 51-year-old man comes to the office because of hearing loss in his left ear, poor balance, a loss of taste sensation, and drooling from the left side of his mouth. A CT scan of the head shows a tumor on the left side of the posterior cranial fossa. Which of the following locations of the tumor would result in the symptoms observed by this patient?

A. Foramen ovale
B. Foramen rotundum
C. Internal acoustic meatus
D. Jugular foramen
E. Superior orbital fissure

248. A 50-year-old man comes to the physician because of a lower lip lesion. He has a 30 pack-year smoking history and a long history of alcohol abuse. Physical examination shows an ulcerated lesion with raised margins on the left side of the lower lip. Biopsy of the lesion shows nests of large, squamous epithelial cells with abundant eosinophilic cytoplasm and keratin pearls. The patient is diagnosed with squamous cell carcinoma. Which lymph nodes are first to be affected by the spread of the tumor cells?

A. Occipital
B. Parotid
C. Retropharyngeal
D. Jugulodigastric
E. Submental

249. An 84-year-old man comes to the emergency department because of double vision. Physical examination shows inability to abduct his right eye. In which of the locations indicated in the arteriogram (Fig. 7.20) will an aneurysm most likely be located to cause the nerve compression resulting in these symptoms/signs?

A. A
B. B
C. C
D. D
E. E

250. A 3-year-old boy is brought to the physician because of a painful swelling on the right side of his face. Imaging (Fig. 7.21) shows an obstructed and enlarged structure (arrows) with inflammation of the associated salivary gland. Which of the following nerves is most likely responsible for the pain?

A. Facial
B. Auriculotemporal
C. Lingual

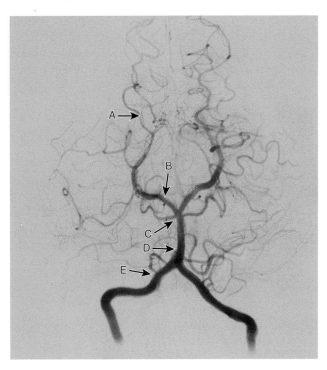

• Fig. 7.20

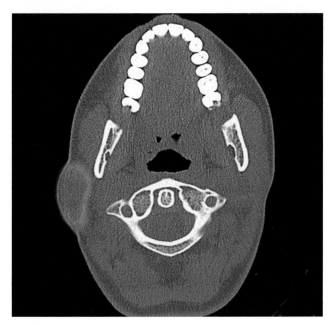

• Fig. 7.22

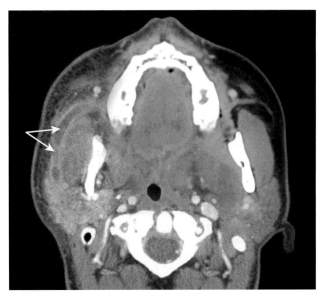

• Fig. 7.21

D. Vagus

E. Chorda tympani

Questions 251–275

251. A 44-year-old woman comes to the physician because of persistent difficulty with her speech. She underwent a thyroidectomy 4 days ago. Physical examination shows a well-healing scar on the anterior neck. Fiberoptic laryngoscopy shows normal-appearing vocal folds that meet in the midline. The patient is diagnosed with surgical injury of the left superior laryngeal nerve. Which of the following additional abnormal findings would be expected with injury to this nerve?

A. Decreased/absent sensation above the vocal folds

B. Decreased/absent sensation below the vocal folds

C. Poorly coordinated swallowing reflex

D. Bilateral weakness/paralysis of the posterior crico-arytenoid muscles

E. Weakness/paralysis of the left posterior cricoarytenoid muscle

252. A 59-year-old man comes to the office 2 weeks after undergoing resection of a brainstem tumor. Physical examination shows a well-healing scar on the posterior aspect of his head. A postoperative CT scan of the head shows a nonobstructive (communicating) hydrocephalus. Between which structures is malabsorption most likely to occur?

A. Choroid plexus and subdural space

B. Subarachnoid space and superior sagittal sinus

C. Subdural space and cavernous sinus

D. Superior sagittal sinus and jugular vein

E. Epidural and subdural space

253. A 52-year-old man comes to the physician because of a growing lump on the left side of his face and neck for the past several months. The lump has become painful in the past 2 weeks. Based on the mass in the CT image (Fig. 7.22), which of the following neurologic abnormalities will most likely be shown on physical examination as a direct result of the growing mass?

A. Contralateral deviation of the uvula during elevation of the soft palate

B. Ipsilateral deviation on protraction of the tongue

C. Ipsilateral pupillary constriction and partial ptosis

D. Ipsilateral weakness in elevation of the mandible

E. Ipsilateral weakness in tight closure of the eyelids

254. A 55-year-old man with a history of cocaine abuse is brought to the emergency department because of severe uncontrolled bleeding from his nose. Physical examination shows bright red blood dripping from his left nasal cavity. Flexible nasal endoscopy shows the bleeding originates in Kiesselbach area. Anastomotic connections between which arteries are involved in this condition?

A. Descending palatine and ascending pharyngeal

B. Posterior superior alveolar and accessory meningeal

C. Lateral branches of posterior ethmoidal and middle meningeal

D. Branches of sphenopalatine, superior labial, and anterior ethmoidal

E. Descending palatine and tonsillar branches of the ascending pharyngeal

255. A 49-year-old woman is brought to the emergency department because of fever, sore throat, and difficulty swallowing for the past week. Her temperature is 38°C (100.4°F), pulse is 100/min, respirations are 19/min, and blood pressure is 139/80 mm Hg. Physical examination shows swollen palatine tonsils bilaterally and a tonsillectomy is performed. Which nerve coursing within the tonsillar fossa needs to be spared during the surgery?

A. Vagus

B. Hypoglossal

C. Glossopharyngeal

D. Internal laryngeal

E. External laryngeal

256. A 39-year-old man comes to the physician because of a 1-month history of hoarseness. Physical examination shows no obvious findings. A laryngoscopy shows nodules on the vocal cords with normal movement. Which of the following muscles functions to open the rima glottidis?

A. Posterior cricoarytenoids

B. Lateral cricoarytenoids

C. Thyroarytenoids

D. Transverse arytenoids

E. Cricothyroids

257. A 61-year-old man is brought to the emergency department because he was found unconscious by his daughter. Shortly after arriving, he regains consciousness. Physical examination shows that he is unable to shrug his shoulder on the right side and turn his head to the left. A CT scan of the head and neck shows a large aneurysm of an artery compressing the nerve responsible for his symptoms. In which of the following arteries is the aneurysm located?

A. Superior cerebellar

B. Posterior cerebral

C. Anterior inferior cerebellar

D. Posterior inferior cerebellar

E. Basilar

258. A 64-year-old woman is brought to the emergency department because of an acute onset of uncoordinated swallowing and difficulty with phonation. She has a long history of type II diabetes. A CT scan of the head shows a brainstem stroke. The cranial nerve responsible for the dysfunction in this patient will most likely also produce which of the following symptoms?

A. Weakness/paralysis of muscles of mastication on one side

B. Weakness/paralysis of muscles of facial expression on one side

C. Hearing loss and balance problems

D. Decreased/absent sensation in the oropharynx

E. Decreased/absent cough reflex

259. A 44-year-old woman comes to the physician 2 weeks after undergoing a thyroidectomy for multiple benign thyroid nodules. Physical examination shows injury to the left external laryngeal nerve. An injury to this nerve may result in which of the following symptoms?

A. Inability to abduct the vocal fold

B. Monotone, easily fatigued voice with poor pitch control

C. Decreased/absent sensation above the vocal folds

D. Decreased/absent sensation below the vocal folds

E. Decreased/absent cough reflex

260. A 49-year-old woman comes to the physician because of difficulty swallowing. Physical examination shows that the patient's uvula deviates to the right. Physical examination shows that when the left side of the pharyngeal mucosa is touched, the gag reflex is weaker than when the mucosa on the right side is touched. Which nerve is most likely injured to cause these symptoms?

A. Left vagus

B. Left glossopharyngeal

C. Right vagus

D. Left V3

E. Right glossopharyngeal

261. A 40-year-old woman comes to the physician because of 3-day history of headache and pain in the region of her left jaw and left ear. The patient says that she often grinds her teeth (bruxism). She is concerned because she is a singer, and it is painful when she opens her mouth wide to sing. Physical examination shows the left side of the jaw deviates slightly to the left on elevation. A clicking sound is noted when she opens her mouth. Physical examination shows a painful area around the left mandibular condyle on palpation. Mandibular depression is difficult to perform because of pain. There is tightness indicative of a muscle spasm along the left mandibular ramus. Palpation shows no other area of tightness. Spasms of which of the following muscles are most likely associated with this condition?

A. Buccinator

B. Masseter

C. Mylohyoid

D. Posterior belly of the digastric

E. Lateral pterygoid

262. A 62-year-old woman comes to the physician for a routine examination. During a test of the cough reflex, she inhales air containing different amounts of particles that will adhere to mucus primarily in the trachea. Blockade of afferent neurons in which cranial nerve will most likely suppress this woman's cough reflex?
    A. Glossopharyngeal
    B. Hypoglossal
    C. External laryngeal
    D. Trigeminal
    E. Vagus

263. During neurological examination of a 27-year-old woman, the physician strokes a wisp of cotton across a patient's left cornea without a response. The physician then strokes the cotton across the patient's right cornea and both eyes blink. The most likely explanation of these findings is damage to which of the following cranial nerves on the left?
    A. Optic
    B. Oculomotor
    C. Trigeminal
    D. Abducens
    E. Facial

264. A 12-year-old girl is brought to the physician by her parents because of a sore neck for the past 4 days. Her temperature is 37.7°C (99.9°F), pulse is 95/min, respirations are 20/min, and blood pressure is 120/80 mm Hg. Physical examination shows a tender swelling anterior to, and just above, the thyroid notch of the neck. An ultrasound examination shows a cyst in the tract along which the thyroid gland descended. All of the tract tissue must be removed between which of the following two structures to treat this patient's condition?
    A. Left lobe of thyroid gland and tonsillar fossa
    B. Right lobe of thyroid gland and epiglottis
    C. Right lobe of thyroid gland and hyoid bone
    D. Thyroid isthmus and foramen cecum
    E. Thyroid isthmus and piriform recess

265. A 34-year-old man comes to the physician because of 2-week history of double vision that becomes worse when reading a newspaper or walking down the stairs. Physical examination shows weakness of downward movement of the left eye. A CT scan of the head shows a large aneurysm in one of the arteries of the posterior cerebral circulation that compresses the nerve resulting in the symptoms. In which artery in the diagram (Fig. 7.23) is the aneurysm located?
    A. A
    B. B
    C. C
    D. D
    E. E

266. A 63-year-old woman comes to the emergency department because of drooping of the left eye. Physical examination shows the left eye is abducted and depressed with an absent light reflex. Angiography shows an aneurysm (*arrow*, Fig. 7.24) of an artery

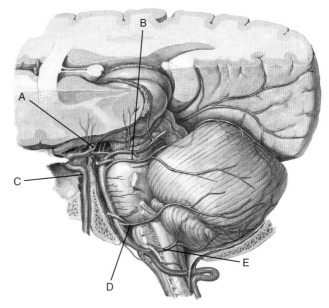

• **Fig. 7.23**

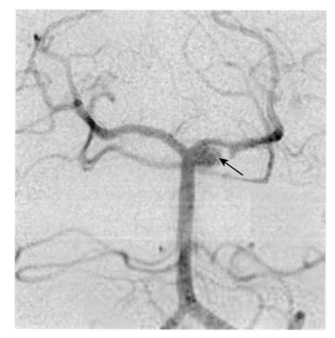

• **Fig. 7.24**

compressing the nerve responsible for the symptoms. Which of the following describes the location of the aneurysm?
    A. Internal carotid artery in the cavernous sinus
    B. Division of the internal carotid artery into middle and anterior cerebral arteries
    C. Left vertebral artery at the junction with the basilar artery
    D. Union of left and right vertebral arteries forming basilar artery
    E. Basilar artery between the left superior cerebellar and posterior cerebral arteries

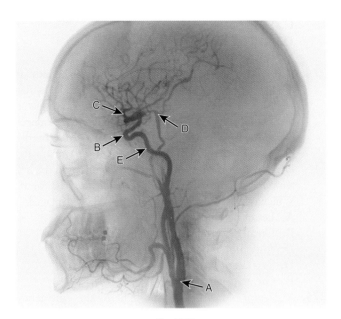

• Fig. 7.25

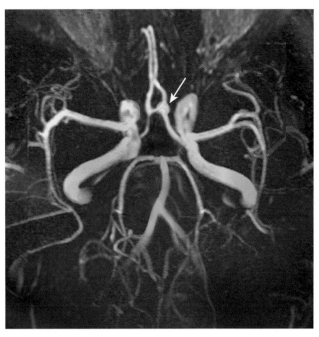

• Fig. 7.26

267. A 75-year-old woman comes to the emergency department because of double vision. Physical examination shows inability to abduct her right eye. In which of the locations indicated in the arteriogram (Fig. 7.25) would an aneurysm most likely be located to cause the nerve compression resulting in these symptoms?
A. PCA
B. Internal carotid artery
C. External carotid artery
D. Anterior cerebral artery
E. Posterior communicating artery

268. A 49-year-old man is brought to the emergency department by his wife because of headaches and dizziness for the past 2 months. A CT scan of the head shows a saccular (berry) aneurysm (Fig. 7.26, *arrow*). An aneurysm at this location would most likely cause nerve compression resulting in which of the following additional findings on neurologic examination?
A. Inability to abduct the eye
B. Inability to depress the adducted eye
C. Loss of corneal sensation
D. Ptosis
E. Visual field deficits

269. A 16-year-old boy is brought to the emergency department because of pain and blurred vision after he was hit by a baseball bat to his left eye during practice. Physical examination shows his eyes move as seen in the photograph (Fig. 7.27B) when asked to gaze upward. A CT scan of the head shows a fracture, as indicated by the arrow in the image (Fig. 7.27A). Which of the following muscles is most likely affected?
A. Levator palpebrae superioris
B. Inferior oblique
C. Inferior rectus
D. Medial rectus
E. Superior rectus

270. A 10-year-old boy is brought to the emergency department because of severe ear pain, headache, and fever for the past 5 days. His temperature is 39.16°C (102.5°F), pulse is 98/min, and respirations are 18/min. Physical examination shows an ill appearing boy with a red and bulging tympanic membrane with purulent effusion. There is tenderness over the area indicated by the arrow in the coronal CT (Fig. 7.28). Assuming that this area is now infected, which of the following venous channels is most at risk for thrombosis as a direct result of the proximity to the infected/inflamed bone?
A. Cavernous sinus
B. Pterygoid venous plexus
C. Sigmoid sinus
D. Straight sinus
E. Superior petrosal sinus

271. A 12-year-old boy is brought into the office because of headaches, runny nose, and a fever. His temperature is 37.2°C (99°F), pulse is 90/min, and respirations are 18/min. Physical examination shows tenderness when the physician taps the area slightly superior to the midportion of the patient's eyebrows. Which of the following anatomic areas is the physician most likely examining?
A. Maxillary sinus
B. Transverse sinus
C. Frontal sinus
D. Sphenoid sinus
E. Ethmoid sinus

272. A 12-year-old boy was brought to the physician by his mother because of pain behind his ear. His vital signs are within normal limits. During physical examination, the physician palpates the mastoid process of the adolescent with tenderness elicited upon

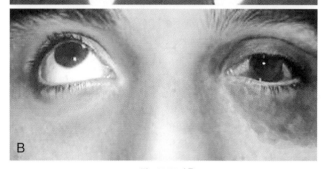

• Fig. 7.27 AB

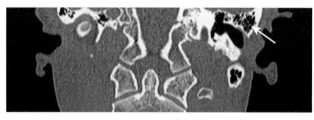

• Fig. 7.28

palpation. Which of the following bones is the physician palpating?

A. Occipital
B. Zygomatic
C. Temporal
D. Parietal
E. Sphenoid

273. A 45-year-old man comes to the physician for a routine examination. An ophthalmoscopic examination shows clear macula lutea, optic disc, and several branching arteries emanating from the optic disc. These arteries are most likely derived from which of the following?

A. Central retinal artery
B. Long posterior ciliary artery

C. Short posterior ciliary artery
D. Ophthalmic artery
E. Anterior ciliary artery

274. A 16-year-old girl is brought to the physician because of loss of sensation on the left side of her head. She says that while at a party last night, she asked her friend to pierce the tragus of her left ear. While attempting to pass a needle through the tragus, the friend slips and the needle deeply punctures the skin directly anterior to the tragus. Physical examination shows loss of sensation on the left temporal side of her scalp up to the vertex of her head. Which of the following nerves is most likely damaged?

A. Lesser occipital
B. Greater occipital
C. Auriculotemporal
D. Zygomaticotemporal
E. Great auricular

275. A 27-year-old woman is brought to the emergency department because of ringing in his ear and a drooping smile. Physical examination shows loss of left nasolabial fold and asymmetry of the patients smile. An MRI of her head shows a small tumor located at the internal acoustic meatus. Which of the following cranial nerves is most likely being compressed by the tumor?

A. V
B. VI
C. VII
D. IX
E. X

Questions 276–300

276. A 62-year-old man is brought to the physician by his wife because of difficulty walking and behavioral changes. His vital signs are within normal limits. Physical examination shows inattentiveness, memory impairment, and broad-based gait. An MRI of the head shows a brain tumor near the crista galli and cribriform plate of the ethmoid bone. Which of the following will most likely be an additional symptom this patient experiences?

A. Paralysis of facial muscles
B. Loss of vision
C. Difficulty swallowing
D. Loss of smell
E. Loss of hearing

277. A 20-year-old man is brought to the emergency department after his motorcycle slammed into a guardrail. His temperature is 37.5°C (99.5°F), pulse is 110/min, respirations are 27/min, and blood pressure is 100/80 mm Hg. Physical examination shows multiple lacerations and bruises on the face. A CT scan of his head shows a fracture of the sella turcica. Which of the following bones was most likely damaged in this patient?

A. Sphenoid
B. Temporal
C. Occipital

D. Ethmoid

E. Frontal

278. A 21-year-old man comes to the emergency department because of severe headache and nausea. Five days ago, he sustained a deep cut on his scalp while shaving his head with a razor blade. The man did not seek medical attention for this injury. His temperature is 39.5°C (103.1°F), pulse is 110/min, respirations are 27/min, and blood pressure is 90/60 mm Hg. Physical examination shows a lethargic man. A CT scan of his head shows an infection of the superior sagittal sinus. Which of the following veins was most likely responsible for this patient's current infection?

A. Intercavernous sinus

B. Inferior sagittal sinus

C. Diploic vein

D. Basal vein

E. Emissary vein

279. A 20-year-old man is brought to the emergency department after being cut in the face with a broken glass bottle. His vital signs are within normal limits. Physical examination shows a deep, 10-cm laceration running obliquely across his right cheek. He is unable to close his right eye and cannot smile on the right side. Which of the following structures was most likely damaged in this patient?

A. Vertebral artery

B. Common carotid artery

C. Parotid gland

D. Lateral pterygoid muscle

E. Temporalis muscle

280. A 25-year-old man is brought to the emergency department after sustaining a blow to the back of the head. He is unconscious on arrival. His temperature is 39.5°C (103.1°F), pulse is 80/min, respirations are 15/min, and blood pressure is 130/60 mm Hg. Physical examination shows a 5-cm scalp hematoma. A CT scan of the head shows a fracture in the occipital bone extending superiorly from the foramen magnum. Which of the following structures is transmitted through this foramen?

A. Cranial nerve I

B. Cranial nerve IX

C. Cranial nerve X

D. Cranial nerve XI

E. Cranial nerve XII

281. An 11-year-old girl is brought to the physician for a follow-up examination. She has a history of repeated upper respiratory tract infections and tonsillitis since she was 7 years old. She subsequently undergoes bilateral tonsillectomy. While performing the procedure, the nerve that lies in the tonsillar fossa deep and inferior to the palatine tonsil is damaged. Which of the following is most likely to result from this injury?

A. Loss of sensation on the posterior one third of the tongue

B. Loss of taste on the anterior two-thirds of the tongue

C. Paralysis of the constrictor muscles of the pharynx

D. Paralysis of the muscles of the soft palate

E. Paralysis of the muscles of the tongue

282. A 70-year-old man comes to the physician because of 2-month history of progressive hoarseness. He has smoked 12 cigarettes per day for the past 45 years. His vital signs are within normal limits. Physical examination shows firm lymph nodes in the neck. Laryngoscopy shows a polyp overlying the mucosa of the right vocalis muscle. Which of the following is most likely located immediately lateral to this muscle?

A. Lateral cricoarytenoid muscle

B. Aryepiglottic muscle

C. Posterior cricoarytenoid muscle

D. Oblique arytenoid muscle

E. Thyroarytenoid muscle

283. A 34-year-old woman is brought to the emergency department with difficulty breathing. She was trying out food at a new restaurant in town 30 minutes ago. Her temperature is 37.6°C (99.68°F), pulse is 105/min, respirations are 28/min, blood pressure is 120/80 mm Hg, and oxygen saturation is approximately 80%. Physical examination shows a swollen tongue protruding from her mouth. The patient oxygen saturation does not improve with bag-mask ventilation. Intubation is unsuccessful because of massive soft tissue edema of her pharynx. A decision is made to perform a cricothyrotomy. After palpation of the neck to identify the appropriate landmarks, an incision should most likely be made at which of the following locations?

A. The cricothyroid membrane, which is located at the junction of the clavicle and the sternum

B. The cricothyroid membrane, which is located between the thyroid cartilage and the cricoid cartilage below

C. The thyrohyoid membrane, which is located between the thyroid cartilage (Adam's apple) and the hyoid bone above

D. The sternal notch, which is located at the junction of the clavicle and the sternum

E. The trachea, which is located below the cricoid cartilage

284. A 26-year-old man is brought to the emergency department after being involved in a motor vehicle collision. His temperature is 37.6°C (99.68°F), pulse is 110/min, respirations are 28/min, blood pressure is 90/60 mm Hg, and oxygen saturation is 82%. Physical examination shows a patient in acute distress and an intubation procedure is initiated. The tube is inserted immediately without anesthesia and the tube touches the epiglottis causing pain and discomfort to the patient. Which of the following cranial nerves most likely allows the patient to sense pain and discomfort from the procedure?

A. Vagus

B. Glossopharyngeal

C. Vestibulocochlear

D. Hypoglossal

E. Facial

285. A 55-year-old man comes to the physician because of a 3-month history of hearing loss and a continuous strange buzzing noise in his right ear. Physical examination shows right-sided hearing loss, asymmetric smile, and decreased corneal reflex in his right eye. A CT scan of the head shows a large intracranial tumor. Which of the following will most likely be the location of the tumor?

A. Between the medulla and the cerebellar hemisphere

B. Above the diaphragma sellae

C. Over the lateral hemispheric fissure

D. Between the cerebellum and the lateral pons

E. Between the cerebellar peduncles

286. A 28-year-old woman comes to the physician because of pain in her ear. Her vital signs are within normal limits. Physical examination shows erythema at the external acoustic meatus. As the speculum is introduced into the external acoustic meatus in close contact with its posterior wall, the patient starts coughing and is feeling dizzy. Irritation of which of the following nerves was most likely stimulated by the speculum?

A. Vestibulocochlear

B. Vagus

C. Trigeminal

D. Facial

E. Accessory

287. A 60-year-old man comes to the physician for a follow-up examination of his thyroid cancer. Three weeks later he undergoes a total thyroidectomy procedure. During the procedure, the superior thyroid artery is ligated. There is a concern about injury to an adjacent nerve. Which of the following muscles is innervated by this nerve?

A. Thyroarytenoid

B. Lateral cricoarytenoid

C. Posterior cricoarytenoid

D. Cricothyroid

E. Vocalis

288. A 55-year-old woman comes to the emergency department because of a 2-week history of severe headaches. She has no fever, neck stiffness, or photophobia. Her temperature is 37.4°C (99.32°F), blood pressure is 155/95 mm Hg, pulse is 99/min, and respirations are 20/min. Physical examination shows a woman who is in pain and distress. Range of movement of the neck is normal, and fundoscopy shows no abnormalities on the retina. A CT angiography of the brain shows a dilated branch of the basilar artery at the junction of the pons and medulla on the right side. She is referred to the neurosurgeon for assessment and further management. Which of the following best describes the clinical features with which this patient might show?

A. Weak abduction and depression of the right eye

B. Weak adduction of the left eye

C. Weak adduction and elevation of the right eye

D. Weak abduction of the right eye

E. Weak abduction of the left eye

289. A 65-year-old woman comes to the emergency department because of a 2-week history of severe headaches. Her temperature is 36°C (96.8°F), blood pressure 160/89 mm Hg, pulse 110/min, and respirations are 16/min. Physical examination shows normal range of neck movements. Fundoscopy shows no abnormalities of the retina. A CT angiography of the brain shows a dilated branch of the basilar artery at the junction of the pons and midbrain on the right side. Which of the following best describes the clinical features with which this patient might show?

A. Weak abduction of the right eye

B. Blurred vision from the right eye and full ptosis of the right upper eyelid

C. Loss of vision from lateral fields of right eye and medial fields of left eye

D. Inability to detect odors through the right nostril

E. Loss of sensation of the skin over the right forehead, cheek, and mandible

290. A 60-year-old man comes to the physician with numbness to the right side of the lower jaw and the inside of the right cheek. Physical examination shows loss of sensation over the scalp in the posterior temporal region and skin over the auricle anteriorly. There is weak lateral deviation of the mandible to the right. A CT scan of the brain shows a mass in the infratemporal fossa. What other functions are most likely affected in this patient?

A. Weak elevation of the corner of the right side of the mouth

B. Loss of sensation over the upper lip and to the upper teeth

C. Inability to sense a foreign body in the right eye

D. Decreased secretion from the parotid gland

E. Inability to abduct the right eye

291. A 40-year-old woman comes to the emergency department because of swelling and pain over the left side of her face. Physical examination shows a tender, warm swelling over the left mandible anterior to the ear. An ultrasound shows a hyperechoic mass within the lumen of the parotid duct, which was distended proximally. What other clinical features are most likely present in this patient?

A. Weak deviation of the mandible to the right

B. Complete ptosis of the left eyelid

C. Numbness of the skin over the left lower mandible

D. Excessive tearing

E. Pain over the anterior auricle, tragus, and anterior helix

292. A 40-year-old man is brought to the emergency department after falling through a glass window to the ground 5 feet below. His vital signs are within normal limits. Physical examination shows multiple

superficial lacerations on the limbs, but no deformities of bones or joints were evident. There was a 5-cm longitudinal laceration over the left jaw. Exploration of the wound shows the presence of a foreign body. A CT scan of the head shows a 3 × 2 cm foreign body lodged between the two heads of the lateral pterygoid muscle. Which of the following clinical findings are most likely to be found in this patient?

A. Weak elevation of the jaw
B. Weak deviation of the jaw to the right side
C. Numbness over the skin of the tragus and helix of the left ear
D. Numbness over the skin and mucosa of the anterior cheek
E. Decreased volume of saliva

293. A 30-year-old man is brought to the emergency department after being involved in a head-on motor vehicle collision. He was not wearing a seatbelt and was found unconscious in the driver's seat. He has low blood pressure and tachycardia. Physical examination shows several lacerations about his face and body. A "step-off" is palpated over the root of the nose and the glabella. There is also clear fluid draining from the nasal cavity. Once the patient was stabilized, a CT of the head was performed and shows a fracture in the middle region of the anterior cranial fossa. Which of the following signs will the patient most likely describe once he regains consciousness?

A. Blurred vision
B. Diplopia
C. Anosmia
D. Blindness
E. Dry left eye

294. A 30-year-old man is brought to the emergency department after falling from a building scaffold. His temperature is 36°C (96.8°F), blood pressure is 90/83 mm Hg, pulse 110/min, and respirations are 23/min. Physical examination shows a poorly responsive patient and several lacerations on his face and body. Once the patient is stabilized, a CT scan of the head shows a fracture near the apex of the orbit with narrowing of the opening to the orbit in the area. Which of the following functions will most likely be maintained or spared in this patient?

A. Secretions from the right lacrimal gland
B. Ability to detect a foreign body on the cornea
C. Sensation over the anterior scalp
D. Sensation to the upper eyelid
E. Ability to abduct the eye

295. A 30-year-old man is brought to the emergency department after being involved in a motor vehicle collision. He has low blood pressure and tachycardia. Physical examination shows a poorly responsive patient with several lacerations on his face and body. There is a bony deformity of the right mandible where abnormal mobility of the bone is noted when the bone is palpated along the ramus. A CT scan of the head shows a displaced, transverse fracture of the ramus proximal to the angle of the mandible. Which of the following will most likely be affected?

A. Elevation of the jaw
B. Lateral deviation of the jaw to the left side
C. Salivation; sensation and taste from the anterior tongue
D. Sensation from skin over anterior cheek and tongue
E. Salivation; sensation from posterior temporal skin and tragus of the ear

296. A 20-year-old man is brought to the emergency department after his motorcycle collided with a light pole. He was unable to recall all events of the incident and he feels pain on the right side of the head and face, lower back, right elbow, and right knee. His vital signs are within normal limits. Physical examination shows an alert and oriented man with multiple abrasions to his upper and lower limbs. There is a tender 6 × 6 cm swelling over the right temporal bone and a laceration to the superior aspect of the helix of the right ear. A CT scan of the head shows a minimally displaced fracture of the floor of the middle cranial fossa involving the pterygoid canal. Which of the following describes all fiber types that are most likely affected in this injury?

A. Presynaptic parasympathetic
B. Postsynaptic sympathetic; presynaptic parasympathetic
C. Postsynaptic sympathetic; postsynaptic parasympathetic
D. Special sensory; postsynaptic parasympathetic
E. General sensory; postsynaptic parasympathetic

297. A 20-year-old man is brought to the emergency department because of 5-day history of fever, swelling over the right temple of his head, and headache. One week ago he was involved in a motorcycle collision and had a minimally displaced open fracture of right temporal bone. The wound was irrigated and debrided and after 24 hours he was discharged. The man appears to be in painful distress. Physical examination shows a tender erythematous swelling over the right temporal bone where the patient received sutures. Neurologic examination shows findings consistent with neuritis of the nerve passing through the distal part of the facial canal. Which of the following functions is likely to be spared by this lesion?

A. Taste from the anterior two-thirds of the tongue
B. Movements of the right side of the face
C. Secretions from the submandibular gland
D. Secretions from the sublingual gland
E. Secretions from the lacrimal gland

298. A 20-year-old woman is brought to the emergency department with pain on the left side of her face, hand, and elbow, as well as double vision after falling from her horse. She says she had no loss of consciousness. Physical examination shows periorbital

edema and bruising of the inferior skin of the eye. There is a swelling over the superolateral aspect of the left eye with a bony defect that is tender to palpation. Pupillary light reflexes are normal, and fundoscopy shows no abnormalities of the retina. A CT scan of the head shows a comminuted, depressed fracture of the frontal process of the left zygomatic bone involving the orbit. Which of the following describes the most likely consequence of her injury?

A. Weak abduction of the eye
B. Diplopia
C. Blurred vision
D. Decreased secretions from the left lacrimal gland
E. Partial ptosis

299. A 30-year-old man is brought to the emergency department because of severe pain to the right eye and double vision. Physical examination shows right periorbital edema and bruising of the skin and tenderness over the inferior orbital margin. A defect of the bone along the inferior orbital margin is also palpated. A CT scan of the head and face shows a displaced fracture of the inferior margin and floor of the orbit along the suture line between the zygomatic and maxillary bones. Which of the following is an additional physical examination of this patient?

A. Partial ptosis of the upper eyelid
B. Complete ptosis of the upper eyelid
C. Inability to elevate the adducted eyeball
D. Inability to depress the adducted eyeball
E. Inability to produce tears

300. A 40-year-old woman comes to the physician with vertigo, nausea, and reduced hearing in her left ear for 3 months. She also complains of dry mouth and dryness of the left eye. Her vital signs are within normal limits. Physical examination shows findings consistent with Paget disease. A CT scan of the head shows thickening of the bones of the skull. Which of the following areas was most likely affected to produce this patient's symptoms?

A. Petrous temporal bone
B. Infratemporal fossa
C. Facial canal
D. Middle ear
E. Inner ear

Questions 301–308

301. A 15-year-old boy is brought to the emergency department with right ear pain. While attempting to clean his ear with a cotton swab, his little brother bumped into his elbow, causing the swab to penetrate deeply into the ear. Physical examination with the otoscope shows clotted blood in the right external acoustic meatus. A pearly-white right tympanic membrane with no cone of light is visualized. On Rinne test, bone conduction was greater than air conduction in the right ear. Weber test shows that sound lateralizes to the right ear. Which of the following best describes

the nerves responsible for the perception of pain from the injured area?

A. Auriculotemporal and great auricular
B. Facial, glossopharyngeal, and vagus
C. Lesser occipital and great auricular
D. Chorda tympani and glossopharyngeal
E. Tympanic plexus and lesser petrosal

302. A 20-year-old woman delivered a girl at term via a spontaneous vaginal delivery after an uneventful pregnancy. Newborn physical examination shows that the iris of the left eye had a defect inferolaterally. The mother is reassured that the physical examination would not likely cause any significant visual impairment, as the defect is very small. Which of the following is the best explanation of the defect observed?

A. Failed induction of surface ectoderm by the neuroectoderm
B. Failed obliteration of the intraretinal space
C. Failed closure of the choroid fissure
D. Optic cup does not overlap the developing lens
E. Lens vesicle remains connected to surface ectoderm

303. A 30-year-old woman comes to the physician with nasal congestion, runny nose, and headache for 2 days. Her temperature is 38.5°C (101.5°F), blood pressure is 136/87 mm Hg, pulse 99/min, and respirations are 18/min. Physical examination shows an erythematous nasal mucosa with swelling of the conchae. There is tenderness over the forehead above the root of the nose and at the areas on either side of the glabella. She was diagnosed with an upper respiratory tract infection. Which of the following is the most likely structure that allowed passage for the spread of the infection in this patient?

A. Auditory tube
B. Ethmoidal infundibulum
C. Nasolacrimal duct
D. Sphenoethmoidal recess
E. Superior nasal meatus

304. A 20-year-old woman delivered a girl at term after an uneventful pregnancy. The mother says she used alcohol and tobacco throughout the pregnancy. Physical examination shows a groove connecting the medial canthus of the right eye to the right corner of the upper lip. There was a clear, watery discharge from the groove. A defect in which of the following developmental processes most likely resulted in the deformity seen in this infant?

A. Fusion of maxillary processes to each other
B. Fusion of medial nasal prominences to each other
C. Migration of ectoderm between maxillary and lateral nasal prominences
D. Fusion of the maxillary and lateral nasal processes
E. Fusion of the intermaxillary segment with the maxillary processes

305. A 20-year-old woman delivered a boy at term by spontaneous vaginal delivery. Newborn physical examination

shows the corners of the eyes are downward slanting and the pinnae and mandible were underdeveloped. As the mother attempts breast feeding, she notes that the boy has difficulty sucking. When bottle feeding the milk often refluxed through his nose. The mother says that the child's father had similar facial abnormalities. Which of the following is the most likely cause of the deformities seen in this infant?

A. Failed fusion of lateral nasal prominences and maxillary processes

B. Lack of fusion of medial nasal prominences

C. Failed migration of neural crest cells to the first pharyngeal arch

D. Failed migration of neural crest cells to the third and fourth pharyngeal pouches

E. Failed migration of ectoderm between maxillary and lateral nasal prominences

306. A 40-year-old woman comes to the physician because of a 4-month history of constant, worsening headaches. She says that the pain is worse on the right side. She is not having fever, neck stiffness, or aversion to light. Vital signs are within normal limits. Physical examination shows no motor weakness of the upper or lower limbs. A CT scan angiography of the brain shows a berry aneurysm of the right superior cerebellar artery. Which of the following will most likely be identified during physical examination on this patient?

A. Lack of accommodation, adduction of the right eye

B. Blurred vision, complete ptosis, abduction of the right eye

C. Partial ptosis, adduction, and downward rotation of the right eye

D. Complete ptosis, abduction, and upward rotation of the right eye

E. Complete ptosis, abduction, and downward rotation of the right eye

307. A 20-year-old woman delivered a boy at term by cesarean section. The second trimester ultrasound showed enlarged ventricles of the fetal brain. Neonatal physical examination shows a head circumference of 40 cm (normal range, 34 to 36 cm). There is decreased movement of the limbs. A CT scan of the head shows dilatation of all the ventricles. Which of the following is likely to be the cause of the infant's condition?

A. Narrowing of the median aperture

B. Narrowing of the lateral aperture

C. Abnormality of arachnoid granulations

D. Lack of choroid plexus in the lateral ventricles

E. Increased blood flow in the cerebral arteries

308. A 64-year-old man comes to the physician because of excessive facial sweating on the right side of his face. His medical history includes a parotidectomy over a year ago for a malignant tumor of the right parotid gland. He says that when he sees appetizing food, he sweats excessively on the right side of his face where the tumor was removed. Physical examination shows a well healed surgical scar. There are no cranial nerve deficits observed. Where are the nerve cell bodies for the nerve fibers that are now innervating his sweat glands located?

A. Ciliary ganglion

B. Pterygopalatine ganglion

C. Otic ganglion

D. Submandibular ganglion

E. Superior salivatory nucleus

Answers

Answers 1–25

1. E. The child in this case suffers from a fistula that indicates an open malformation. This implies that the defect must be because of the failure of closure of both an internal and an external structure. A branchial fistula results from the failure of closure of both the second pharyngeal pouch and the cervical sinus, the cervical sinus being the consolidation of the second through fourth pharyngeal clefts, all being external structures.

A and C. This excludes the second pharyngeal arch and third pharyngeal pouch from being the answers alone.

B. The second pharyngeal groove merges with the third and fourth pharyngeal grooves to form the cervical sinus. Failure of closure of the second groove alone would not present with an open fistula.

D. The thyroglossal duct extends from the thyroid to the tongue and failure of its closure would not result in an external defect.

GAS 995; N 77; ABR/McM 28–35

2. A. The largest part of the palate is formed by the secondary palate which is embryologically derived from the lateral palatine processes.

B. The median palatine process gives rise to the smaller primary palate located anteriorly.

C. The intermaxillary segment gives rise to the middle upper lip, premaxillary part of the maxilla, and the primary palate.

D. The median nasal prominences merge with each other and with the maxillary prominences to give rise to the intermaxillary segment.

E. The frontonasal eminence gives rise to parts of the forehead, nose, and eyes.

GAS 1059–1060; N 73, 77; ABR/McM 1, 9

3. A. A coloboma of the iris is caused by the failure of the retinal fissure to close during the sixth embryonic week.

B. Abnormal neural crest formation would lead to abnormal development of choroid, sclera, and cornea.

C. Abnormal interaction between the optic vesicle and ectoderm would lead to abnormal development of the entire eye because a lens placode may fail to develop or develop abnormally.

  D. The iris would not be affected by abnormal development of the posterior chamber.

  E. Weak adhesion between the layers of the optic vesicle leads to congenital retinal detachment.

  GAS 925–926; N 94; ABR/McM 51

4. E. The anterior fontanelle is located at the junction of the sagittal and coronal sutures and closes at around 18 months of age.

  A. The posterior fontanelle is located at the junction of the sagittal suture and lambdoid suture, and it closes at around 2 to 3 months.

  B and C. The mastoid fontanelle is located at the junction of the squamous suture and the lambdoid suture, and it closes at the end of the first year. There is a lambdoid suture but not a lambdoid fontanelle.

  D. The sphenoidal fontanelle is located at the junction of the squamous suture and the coronal suture and closes at around 2 to 3 months.

  GAS 852; N 13, 16; ABR/McM 14

5. A. Thyroglossal duct cysts occur because of retention of a remnant of the thyroglossal duct along the path followed by the descending thyroid gland during development. The path begins at the foramen cecum of the tongue and descends in the midline to the final position of the thyroid.

  B. The sixth pharyngeal arch provides origin to muscles and cartilage of the neck and would produce a midline mass connected to the tongue.

  C. A branchial cyst would not be present in the midline, it would be present on the lateral neck.

  D. The third pharyngeal arch provides origin to the stylopharyngeus muscle and hyoid bone.

  E. The first pharyngeal arch gives rise to muscles of mastication and the malleus and incus.

  GAS 998; N 77; ABR/McM 33

6. E. The most common cause of cleft lip is failure of fusion of the maxillary process and the intermaxillary segment.

  A. Defects located between the lateral nasal prominences and the maxillary processes would affect the development of the nasolacrimal duct.

  B. Failure of fusion of the medial nasal prominences would produce a median cleft lip, a rare congenital anomaly.

  C. The lateral and median nasal processes both arise from the nasal placodes and do not undergo subsequent fusion.

  D. The lateral nasal prominences do not fuse with each other.

  GAS 1066; N 53; ABR/McM 14

7. A. The listed symptoms are typical of first pharyngeal (branchial) arch syndrome as the first arch gives rise to muscles of mastication, mylohyoid, anterior belly of the digastric, tensor tympani, tensor veli palatini, malleus, and the incus.

  B. Abnormal development of the second arch would affect the muscles of facial expression, the stapes, and parts of the hyoid bone.

  C. Abnormal development of the third pharyngeal arch would affect only the stylopharyngeus muscle and parts of the hyoid bone.

  D and E. Abnormal development of the fourth and sixth arch would affect various muscles and cartilages of the larynx and pharynx and would not produce the hypoplastic mandible characteristic of first arch syndrome.

  GAS 950, 966, 998; N 55–56, 105; ABR/McM 35, 39, 57

8. C. Obstructive hydrocephalus refers to a condition in which flow of CSF is obstructed within the ventricular system. In this case the obstruction results from the stenosis of the cerebral aqueduct (of Sylvius). This leads to pressure increasing in the CSF upstream from the obstruction expanding the lateral and third ventricles while the fourth ventricle is unaffected.

  A. Nonobstructive hydrocephalus is because of either excessive CSF production or ineffective CSF reabsorption. This would lead to enlargement of all ventricular chambers.

  B and D. Anencephaly, also known as meroanencephaly, is a partial absence of the brain and is because of defective closure of the anterior neuropore.

  E. Holoprosencephaly is a failure of cleavage of the forebrain and would result in a single fused ventricle.

  GAS 865–866; N 157; ABR/McM 72, 81

9. C. Both the inferior parathyroid glands and the thymus are derived from the third pharyngeal (branchial) pouch. Therefore, an ectopic thymus is likely to be associated with ectopic parathyroid tissue, indicating an abnormal development of the third pharyngeal pouch.

  A. Development of jugulodigastric lymph nodes are not associated with development of the thymus.

  B. The lingual tonsil develops from an aggregation of lymph nodules on the tongue and is not associated with development of the thymus.

  D. The submandibular gland develops from endodermal buds in the floor of the stomodeum and is not associated with development of the thymus.

  E. The thyroid gland arises from an out pocketing of the floor of the primitive oral cavity, descending along the route of the thyroglossal duct, and it is not associated with development of the thymus.

  GAS 1011; N 89; ABR/McM 30

10. C. The defect is likely in the development of third and fourth pharyngeal pouches because the superior parathyroid glands are derived from the fourth pouch, whereas the inferior parathyroid glands are derived from the third pouch. In addition, the third pouch gives rise to the thymus, and the parafollicular cells of the thyroid gland are derived from the fourth pharyngeal pouch.

  A and B. The first pouch gives rise to the tympanic membrane and cavity. The second pouch gives rise to the palatine tonsils and tonsillar sinus.

D and E. Abnormal development of the fourth and sixth arch would affect various muscles and cartilages of the larynx and pharynx and would not produce the hypoplastic mandible characteristic of first arch syndrome.
GAS 1011; N 89; ABR/McM 30

11. C. Whereas all forms of clefts are considered to have a multifactorial etiology, cleft lip in particular seems to have a **strong genetic factor.** This has been determined using studies of twins.
A, B, D, and E. The other listed factors may or may not play a role in the development of a cleft lip, but genetics remains the most important determining factor.
GAS 1066; N 53; ABR/McM 14

12. C. Absence of the thymus and inferior parathyroid glands would be because of defective development of the third pharyngeal pouch, their normal site of origin.
A. The first pouch gives rise to the tympanic membrane and cavity.
B. The second pouch gives rise to the palatine tonsils and tonsillar sinus.
D. The fourth pharyngeal pouch gives rise to the superior parathyroid glands and the parafollicular cells of the thyroid gland.
E. The fifth pharyngeal pouch contributes to the formation of the parafollicular cells of the thyroid gland.
GAS 1011; N 89; ABR/McM 30

13. D. The third pharyngeal arch gives rise to the greater cornua and lower part of the hyoid bone, in addition to the stylopharyngeus muscle.
A. The maxillary prominence is important in the development of the cheeks and upper lip.
B. The mandibular prominence is important in development of the mandible.
C. The second pharyngeal arch gives rise to the lesser cornu and upper part of the hyoid body.
E. The fourth pharyngeal arches, while extensively involved in development of the cartilage and muscles of the larynx, play no part in the development of the hyoid bone.
GAS 1080; N 22; ABR/McM 48

14. E. A lateral cervical cyst is caused by remnants of the cervical sinus and would present anterior to the sternocleidomastoid.
A. A dermoid cyst is a cystic teratoma that often occurs near the lateral aspect of the eyebrow.
B. A swollen lymph node is likely to present with pain.
C. Accessory thyroid tissue is normally situated along the route of descent of the thyroglossal duct, either in the posterior tongue or along the midline of the neck.
D. A cyst of the thyroglossal duct would be found in locations similar to where accessory thyroid tissue is found.
GAS 1005; N 77; ABR/McM 28–35

15. A. Noncommunicating hydrocephalus, also known as obstructive hydrocephalus, is because of an obstruction to flow of CSF within the ventricular system.

B. Excess production of CSF or disturbed resorption of CSF gives rise to communicating or nonobstructive hydrocephalus.
C. An increased size of the head can occur as a result of hydrocephalus but would not be a causative factor for hydrocephalus.
D. Disturbances in the resorption of CSF may occur in cases of subarachnoid hemorrhage where absorption of CSF from arachnoid granulations may be affected. This causes communicating hydrocephalus and not non-communicating hydrocephalus since the communication between the ventricles are still fine.
E. Failure of the neural tube to close may lead to anencephaly or spina bifida, depending on the portion of the tube affected, but would not result in hydrocephalus.
GAS 865–866; N 157; ABR/McM 72, 81

16. C. A normal APGAR score indicates that the child appeared normal and healthy at birth, based on skin color, pulse, reflexes, muscle tone, and breathing (Appearance, Pulse, Grimace, Activity, and Respiration). An atretic external acoustic canal occurs because of failure of the meatal plug to canalize, an event that normally occurs in late fetal life.
A. Failure of the otic pit to form results in an absent otic vesicle and the membranous labyrinth.
B. The first pharyngeal pouch gives rise to the tympanic membrane and cavity, and an abnormal development would not affect the external acoustic meatus.
D. Failure of the auricular hillocks to develop results in failure of the external ear to develop.
E. A degenerated tubotympanic recess would not lead to an atretic external acoustic meatus.
GAS 945; N 106; ABR/McM 57

17. D. The chin and lower lip area are supplied by the mental nerve, a branch of the inferior alveolar nerve, which in turn is a branch of the mandibular division of the trigeminal nerve (CN V₃).
A. The auriculotemporal nerve supplies the temporomandibular joint, the temporal region, the parotid gland, and the ear anteriorly.
B. The buccal nerve is sensory to the external and internal surface of the cheek.
C. The lesser petrosal nerve is a parasympathetic nerve and would not be affected by herpes zoster, a disease of the dorsal root ganglia.
E. The infraorbital nerve provides sensory innervation to the lower eyelid, side of the nose, and upper lip.
GAS 975; N 59; ABR/McM 38

18. B. The trigeminal ganglion, also known as the semilunar or Gasserian ganglion, is the location of the sensory neuron cell bodies of the trigeminal nerve (CN V). Trigeminal neuralgia (also know as tic douloureux) is a condition in which pain occurs over the area of distribution of trigeminal nerve branches.
A. The geniculate ganglion is found on the facial nerve (CN VII) and receives sensory fibers for

taste and transmits preganglionic parasympathetic fibers.

C. The inferior glossopharyngeal ganglion is part of the glossopharyngeal nerve (CN IX), not the trigeminal nerve, and is not the site of the cell bodies mediating the pain.

D. The otic ganglion, located on the mandibular division of the trigeminal nerve, contains postganglionic parasympathetic cell bodies for parotid gland secretion.

E. The pterygopalatine ganglion, located in the pterygopalatine fossa, also contains postganglionic parasympathetic cell bodies for lacrimation and mucosal secretion.

GAS 910; N 133; ABR/McM 81

19. C. The ophthalmic branch of the trigeminal nerve (CN V1) supplies sensory innervation to the eyeball, leading to pain when damaged.

A. B, and D. Pain in the hard palate and lower eyelid, and anesthesia of the upper lip would be carried by the maxillary branch of the trigeminal nerve (CN V$_2$).

E. Paresthesia over the buccal portion of the face would be mediated by the mandibular division of the trigeminal nerve (CN V$_3$).

GAS 903; N 61; ABR/McM 81

20. D. A tumor at the hypoglossal canal would compress the hypoglossal nerve (CN XII) and affect the genioglossus, a muscle it supplies.

A. The geniohyoid is supplied by C1, which runs with the hypoglossal nerve after it passes through the hypoglossal canal, and would therefore be unaffected.

B. The mylohyoid is supplied by the nerve to mylohyoid, a branch of the mandibular division of the trigeminal nerve (CN V$_3$).

C. The palatoglossus is innervated by the vagus nerve (CN X).

E. The thyrohyoid is innervated by fibers from C1 to C2 carried by hypoglossal nerve.

GAS 1086–1087; N 70; ABR/McM 48

21. C. The superior salivatory nucleus is the autonomic nucleus for the facial nerve (CN VII). Parasympathetic fibers carried by the greater petrosal branch of the facial nerve are responsible for supply of the lacrimal gland and sinuses, via the pterygopalatine ganglion. The geniculate ganglion contains the cell bodies for taste from the anterior two-thirds of the tongue carried by the chorda tympani branch of the facial nerve. This branch also carries the parasympathetic supply for the submandibular and sublingual salivary glands.

A. The auriculotemporal nerve provides sensory innervation to the skin of the temporal region of the head, the temporomandibular joint, and general sensation from the anterior-most portion of the external ear.

B and D. The inferior salivatory nucleus and lesser petrosal nerve provide preganglionic parasympathetic fibers carried by the glossopharyngeal nerve (CN IX) that synapse in the otic ganglion, providing parotid gland stimulation.

E. The pterygopalatine ganglion includes fibers that innervate only lacrimation and the paranasal sinuses, but not taste on the anterior two-thirds of the tongue (*GAS* Fig. 8.87).

GAS 900; N 134; ABR/McM 39

22. D. Thoracic outlet syndrome is characterized by the presence of a cervical rib, accessory muscles, or connective tissue bands that constrict the limited dimensions of the thoracic outlet. The cervical rib is usually located on the C7 vertebra and can impinge on the brachial plexus, resulting in loss of some feeling to the upper limb.

A. There would be no impingement on the phrenic nerve because it leaves the ventral rami of C3 to C5 directly parallel with the vertebral column.

B. The syndrome does not include reduction of blood flow to the thoracic wall because of extensive anastomoses between the vessels that supply blood to the anterior thoracic wall.

C and E. Venous return from the head and neck is mainly through the internal jugular vein and would not be affected because of thoracic outlet syndrome. This is because the location of the vein is near the midline of the body and would not be occluded or distended.

GAS 151; N 191, 195; ABR/McM 218

23. C. The superior cervical ganglion, which is the uppermost part of the sympathetic trunk, supplies sympathetic innervation to the head and neck. The usual symptoms for SCG injury, commonly known as Horner syndrome, are miosis, ptosis, and anhidrosis in the head and neck region. Postganglionic sympathetic nerves usually run on the arteries leading into the head and neck region.

A. The submandibular ganglion does not carry sympathetic nerves to areas of the head and neck.

B. The trigeminal ganglion includes only cell bodies from afferent sensory nerves from the head.

D. The geniculate ganglion includes cell bodies for taste sensation from the anterior two-thirds of the tongue, carried by the facial nerve; it also transmits parasympathetic innervation to many sections of the head and face.

E. The ciliary ganglion provides parasympathetic innervation to the eye, and also has some sympathetic fibers coursing through but not synapsing; thus, it would not account for the symptoms of the face.

GAS 1025; N 142; ABR/McM 47

24. A. The chorda tympani joins the lingual nerve in the infratemporal fossa, and a lesion to the lingual nerve before it is joined by the chorda tympani would

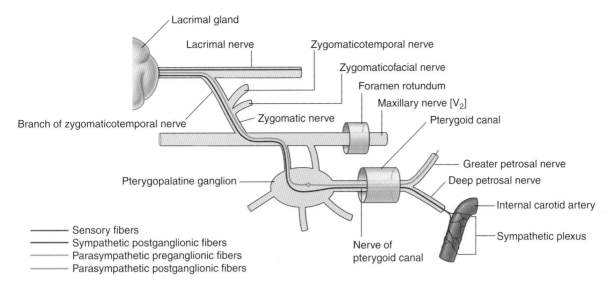

Lacrimal gland
Lacrimal nerve
Zygomaticotemporal nerve
Zygomaticofacial nerve
Foramen rotundum
Maxillary nerve [V₂]
Pterygoid canal
Branch of zygomaticotemporal nerve
Zygomatic nerve
Greater petrosal nerve
Deep petrosal nerve
Internal carotid artery
Pterygopalatine ganglion
Sympathetic plexus
Nerve of pterygoid canal

Sensory fibers
Sympathetic postganglionic fibers
Parasympathetic preganglionic fibers
Parasympathetic postganglionic fibers

• *GAS* Fig. 8.87

account for the loss of general sensation, with no loss to the special sense of taste and saliva production.

B. If the chorda tympani were injured, the patient would present with a loss of taste (from the anterior two-thirds of tongue) and a decrease in saliva production because the submandibular and sublingual salivary glands would be denervated.

C. The inferior alveolar nerve provides sensory innervation to the mandibular teeth, but no such loss is present.

D. The lesser petrosal nerve innervates postganglionic neurons supplying the parotid gland, but no loss of salivation is present.

E. The glossopharyngeal nerve provides taste innervation to the posterior third of the tongue and sensation related to the gag reflex, but there is no deficit present in this patient.
GAS 1090; N 53; ABR/McM 82

25. E. The jugular foramen is the route of exit for three nerves (glossopharyngeal [CN IX], vagus [CN X], and accessory [CN XI] nerves) and one vein (internal jugular vein) from the cranial cavity. The glossopharyngeal nerve provides the sensory input for the gag reflex, whereas the vagus nerve provides the motor output. Nerve compression within this foramen would lead to a loss of both systems and thus no gag reflex.

A. Tongue movements are almost entirely supplied by the hypoglossal nerve (CN XII), which exits the skull through the hypoglossal canal.

B. The facial nerve (CN VII) innervates the muscles of the face and would not be affected by this injury.

C. Loss of sensation from the face and scalp would be present only if there was involvement of the trigeminal nerve.

D. Loss of hearing would be present with any compression of the vestibulocochlear nerve (CN VIII).

The vestibulocochlear nerve was formally called the *auditory nerve* but *vestibulocochlear* clearly refers to its dual function.
GAS 858; N 20; ABR/McM 11

Answers 26–50

26. E. The middle meningeal artery is a branch of the maxillary artery and courses between the dura mater and skull close to the area of the pterion. Any fracture or impact trauma to this location typically results in a laceration of the middle meningeal artery resulting in an epidural hematoma.

A. B, and C. The external carotid artery ends behind the mandible by dividing into the maxillary and the superficial temporal arteries, and neither of these arteries directly affects the meninges of the brain.

D. The deep temporal arteries do not penetrate the bony skull and thus would not contribute to an epidural hematoma (*GAS* Fig. 8.33).
GAS 979; N 112; ABR/McM 42

27. A. An injury to the oculomotor nerve (CN III) would cause the eye to point downward and laterally because of the unopposed contractions of the muscles innervated by the trochlear (CN IV) and abducens (CN VI) nerves (superior oblique and lateral rectus muscles, respectively). The oculomotor nerve also provides innervation to the levator palpebrae superioris; thus, any injury will cause complete ptosis or inability to raise the eyelid. The constriction of the pupil is provided by parasympathetic nerves via the oculomotor nerve.

B. The optic nerve is responsible only for the sensory aspect of light via the retina in the eye.

C. The facial nerve innervates the facial muscles, including the orbicularis oculi, which closes the eyelid for the blink reflex.

Position of pterion

Middle meningeal artery

Anterior meningeal arteries
(from ethmoidal arteries)

Middle
meningeal artery

Maxillary artery

Posterior meningeal artery
(from ascending
pharyngeal artery)

Meningeal branch
(from ascending
pharyngeal artery)

Meningeal branch
(from occipital artery)

Meningeal branch
(from vertebral artery)

Ascending pharyngeal artery

Occipital artery

External carotid artery

• *GAS* **Fig. 8.33**

D. The ciliary ganglion could be damaged in this patient, but the loss of parasympathetic supply will not adequately explain the ptosis of the eyelid.

E. The SCG provides sympathetic innervation to the head and neck including the smooth muscle in the upper lid (superior tarsal muscle of Müller), but no loss of sympathetics is evident in this patient.

GAS 889–890; N 64; ABR/McM 52–54

28. B. The scalp is divided into five layers: skin, dense connective tissue, aponeurosis, loose connective tissue, and periosteum. A handy mnemonic is SCALP (skin, connective tissue, aponeurosis, loose connective tissue, and periosteum). Typically, infections will be located between the aponeurosis and periosteum, within the loose connective tissue, because of the ease with which infectious agents spread via the many veins located in this region. This area is usually referred to as the "danger zone" of the scalp mainly because scalp infections here can be transmitted into the skull via emissary veins, then via diploic veins of the bone to the cranial cavity.

A. The periosteum and bone are tightly bound together; thus, it is not likely to find infections between these layers.

C and D. The areas between the dense connective tissue and aponeurosis, and between the connective tissue and the skin layers, do not include connecting veins but mainly superficial veins of the head.

E. The skin provides a very strong barrier against infections; the epidermis and dermis layers are rarely seen separated, and thus the likelihood of an infection between these areas would be rare.

GAS 911; N 10, 31; ABR/McM 5, 4

29. A. An injury to the left vagus nerve (CN X) would cause the uvula to become deviated to the right. This is because the vagus nerve innervates the musculus uvulae that makes up the core of the uvula. If only one side is effectively innervated, contraction of the active muscle will deviate the uvula to the contralateral side of the injury (ipsilateral side of the uninjured vagus nerve). In addition, the intact levator veli palatini will pull the uvula to the intact side.

B. Injury to the right vagus nerve would pull the uvula to the left side.

C. The right and left hypoglossal nerves innervate the tongue muscles and would not affect the uvula.

D and E. The glossopharyngeal nerve supplies sensory innervation to the oropharynx and nasopharynx, but not motor innervation to these areas.

GAS 889; N 82, 137; ABR/McM 47

30. E. The rima glottidis is the opening between the vocal folds and the arytenoid cartilages on the right and left sides.

   A. The piriform recess is the recess in the laryngopharynx lateral to the laryngeal opening.

   B. The vestibule is the region between the epiglottis and rima glottidis.

   C. The ventricle is the area between the true and false vocal cords.

   D. The vallecula is a bilateral recess in the laryngopharynx anterior to the epiglottis just posterior to the tongue (*GAS* Fig. 8.221).

   GAS 1049; N 91; ABR/McM 49

31. D. Maxillary sinusitis is an infection of the maxillary sinus, which is located in the body of the maxillary bone. Sharp pain can be a major symptom of maxillary sinusitis. The difference between the remaining answer choices is the location of the sinus.

   A. The sphenoidal sinus is located posterosuperior to the nasopharynx.

   B and C. The ethmoidal sinuses are located laterosuperiorly to the nasal septum.

   E. The frontal sinus is located in the frontal bone in the anterior part of the face.

   GAS 1063–1064; N 49–51; ABR/McM 43, 82

32. D. The vagus nerve is responsible for sensation in the mucosa of the larynx, and also motor innervation of the muscles that initiate a cough reflex and swallowing (motor).

   A. The mandibular division of the trigeminal nerve provides sensory innervation to the mouth and lower and lateral face and motor innervation to the muscles of mastication.

   B. The maxillary division of the trigeminal nerve provides only sensory innervation to the midfacial region surrounding the maxillary bone.

   C. The glossopharyngeal nerve provides sensory innervation to the oropharynx (gag reflex) and motor innervation to the stylopharyngeus muscle.

   E. The hypoglossal nerve innervates most of the muscles of the tongue and is not associated with the cough reflex.

   GAS 892, 1041–1042; N 82; ABR/McM 45

33. D. The auditory (eustachian) tube connects the middle ear and the nasopharynx and is the conduit for spreading infections.

   A. The choanae are the openings between the nasal cavity and the nasopharynx, but they are not involved in spreading infection.

   B and C. The internal and external acoustic meatuses are not directly associated with the middle ear but are associated with the inner and outer ear, respectively.

   E. The pharyngeal recess is a slit-like opening located behind the entrance to the auditory tube in the nasopharynx. Adenoids, enlarged masses of lymphoid tissue, can develop there.

   GAS 945, 947, 949; N BP29, 115; ABR/McM 57–58

34. B. The optic and oculomotor nerves are responsible for the sensory and motor portions, respectively, of the pupillary light reflex.

   A. The optic nerve would include the sensory portion, but the facial nerve only closes the eyelid and does not affect the pupil.

   C. The maxillary division of the trigeminal nerve only provides sensory innervation to the skin surrounding the maxillary bone.

   D. The ophthalmic division of the trigeminal nerve provides sensory innervation to the cornea for the corneal reflex, but not the light reflex.

   GAS 889; N 97; ABR/McM 51

35. C. The superior orbital fissure is the opening that allows the passage of the oculomotor nerve and the trochlear nerve; the lacrimal, frontal, and nasociliary branches of ophthalmic division of the trigeminal nerve; the abducens nerve; the superior and inferior divisions of the ophthalmic vein; and the sympathetic fibers from the cavernous plexus. The sensory and motor components of the corneal reflex are the ophthalmic division of the trigeminal nerve and the oculomotor nerve, whereas the eye impairment is because of a lesion to the oculomotor nerve, all of which are transmitted through the superior orbital fissure.

   A. The inferior orbital fissure contains the maxillary division of the trigeminal nerve, infraorbital vessels, and branches of the pterygopalatine ganglion.

   B. The optic canal contains the ophthalmic artery and optic nerve, in addition to sympathetic fibers.

   D. The foramen rotundum contains the maxillary nerve.

   E. The foramen ovale contains the lesser petrosal nerve, the mandibular division of the trigeminal nerve, the accessory middle meningeal artery, and an emissary vein.

   GAS 889, 923; N BP26; ABR/McM 23, 25

36. B. The facial nerve innervates the stapedius muscle, which is responsible for limiting movement of the stapes, thereby reducing the intensity of the sound entering the inner ear.

   A. The hypoglossal nerve innervates tongue muscles.

   C. The accessory nerve supplies the trapezius and sternocleidomastoid muscles.

   D. The vagus nerve does not provide any innervation for sound in the ear.

   E. The glossopharyngeal nerve only supplies sensation to the posterior third of the tongue, the oropharynx (gag reflex), middle ear cavity, and tympanic membrane, and muscle innervation to the stylopharyngeus muscle.

   GAS 884, 887–888; N 107; ABR/McM 57–58

37. B. The vagus nerve innervates a part of the external acoustic meatus and, when stimulated, can trigger a cough reflex in about 20% of people. This is thought to be because of "referred sensation" from the vestibule of the larynx, which is innervated by the vagus nerve.

   A. The vestibulocochlear nerve is associated only with the inner ear.

   C. The trigeminal nerve does provide some innervation to the external acoustic meatus but does not affect the cough reflex as does the vagus nerve.

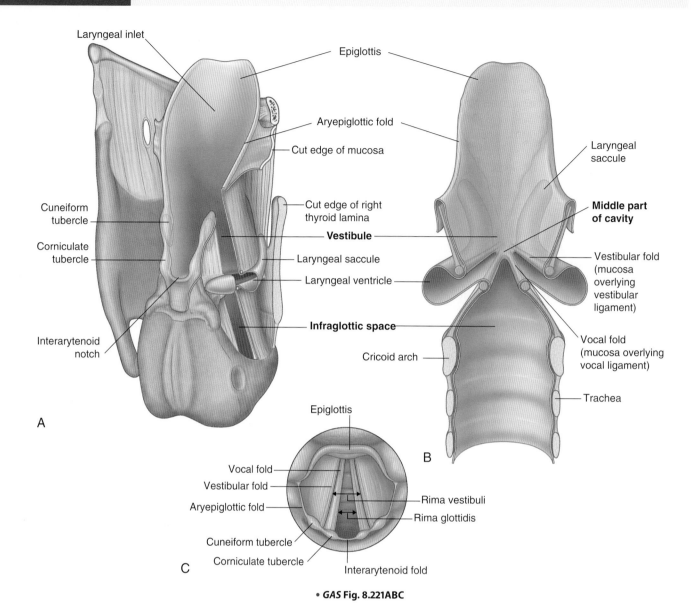

Laryngeal inlet

Epiglottis

Aryepiglottic fold

Cut edge of mucosa

Laryngeal saccule

Middle part of cavity

Cuneiform tubercle

Cut edge of right thyroid lamina

Vestibule

Corniculate tubercle

Laryngeal saccule

Laryngeal ventricle

Vestibular fold (mucosa overlying vestibular ligament)

Interarytenoid notch

Infraglottic space

Cricoid arch

Vocal fold (mucosa overlying vocal ligament)

Trachea

A

Epiglottis

B

Vocal fold

Vestibular fold

Rima vestibuli

Aryepiglottic fold

Rima glottidis

Cuneiform tubercle

Corniculate tubercle

Interarytenoid fold

C

• *GAS* **Fig. 8.221ABC**

D. The auricular branch of the facial nerve only provides a small amount of general sensory supply to the external ear; it is not associated with the cough reflex.

E. The accessory nerve does not provide innervation to the external ear.

GAS 945; N 106; ABR/McM 57–58

38. C. The recurrent laryngeal nerve supplies most of the motor innervation to the larynx and sensation below the true vocal folds. The thyroid gland and the recurrent laryngeal nerve are in close proximity and thus the nerve is the most likely to be injured with a thyroidectomy. Injury to the recurrent laryngeal nerve can result in speech defects, including hoarseness.

A, B, and D. The superior laryngeal nerve has two branches: the internal laryngeal nerve innervates the mucous membranes of the larynx above the vocal folds, and the external laryngeal nerve innervates the cricothyroid muscle, which tenses the vocal folds.

E. The glossopharyngeal nerve is located superiorly to the true vocal folds and would not be affected by this procedure.

GAS 1010; N 89; ABR/McM 49

39. B. The SCG provides sympathetic innervation to the face and neck regions. Sympathetics travel along the branches of the internal carotid artery, and one result of stimulation of these nerves is to dilate the pupil during a sympathetic response ("flight or fight").

A. The oculomotor nerve would not affect the dilation of the pupil; rather, its stimulation results in the constriction (parasympathetic nerves).

C. The nervus intermedius is the parasympathetic component to the facial nerve and affects only lacrimation of the eye.

D. The Edinger-Westphal nucleus is the location of the cell bodies of the preganglionic parasympathetic neurons that are carried by the oculomotor nerve (not sympathetics).

E. The trigeminal ganglion only provides sensory innervation to the face and eye but has no motor effect on the pupil.
GAS 920, 1025; N 142; ABR/McM 44

40. C. The greater petrosal nerve, a parasympathetic branch of the facial nerve, provides innervation to the lacrimal gland in the orbit.

A. The chorda tympani provides innervation to the submandibular and sublingual glands and also taste to the anterior two-thirds of the tongue.

B. The deep petrosal nerve carries sympathetic innervation to the blood vessels and mucous glands of the head and neck.

D. The lesser petrosal nerve provides parasympathetic innervation to the parotid gland.

E. The nasociliary nerve provides sensory innervation to the ethmoidal sinuses and the cornea as well as innervation to the skin of the upper eyelid medially as well as the superior nose regions laterally.
GAS 921–922; N 134; ABR/McM 51–54

41. C. The maxillary sinus is located directly inferior to the orbit. Any trauma to the inferior bony wall of the orbit will likely displace the orbital structures in the compartment to the space below the orbit (maxillary sinus). In most people the sclera of the eyeball is stronger than in the orbital floor, so a blow-out fracture is more likely than rupture of the eyeball.

A. The ethmoidal cells are located medial to the orbit.

B. The frontal sinus is located superiorly to the orbit.

D. The nasal cavity is toward the midline and is not inferior to the orbit.

E. The sphenoidal sinus is deeper into the facial region but is not inferior to the orbit.
GAS 1063, 1065; N 49–51; ABR/McM 18

42. B. The superior ophthalmic vein drains directly into the cavernous sinus. The "danger area" of the face is located in the triangular region from the lateral angle of the eye to the middle of the upper lip, near the nose, and is drained by the facial vein. The facial vein communicates directly with the cavernous sinus through the superior ophthalmic vein.

A. The pterygoid venous plexus communicates with the cavernous sinus through the inferior ophthalmic vein, but it is not directly connected to the cavernous sinus.

C and E. The frontal venous plexus and parietal emissary veins do not communicate directly with the cavernous sinus.

D. The basilar venous plexus connects the inferior petrosal sinuses and communicates with the internal vertebral venous plexus.
GAS 876; N 84; ABR/McM 59

43. C. A lesion of the facial nerve is likely to lead to the symptoms described (drooping mouth, unable to close right eye, and food collection in the oral vestibule) because the muscles of facial expression are paralyzed. There is a bony prominence over the facial nerve located on the medial wall of the middle ear. Because of its close proximity, the facial nerve can be very rarely damaged because of otitis media.

A, B, D, and E. The other nerves listed are not located in close proximity to the middle ear and, if injured, would not present with the symptoms described.
GAS 875; N 110; ABR/McM 61

44. C. The middle cerebral artery is the lateral continuation of the internal carotid artery and therefore not part of the arterial circle. Although it receives its blood supply from the cerebral arterial circle (of Willis), it does not actually form any part of the circle.

A, B, D, and E. The cerebral arterial circle (of Willis) receives its blood supply from the internal carotid and vertebral arteries. The actual circle is formed by the bifurcation of the basilar, posterior cerebral, posterior communicating, internal carotid, anterior cerebral, and anterior communicating arteries. (*GAS* Fig. 8.38A).
GAS 871; N 151; ABR/McM 67

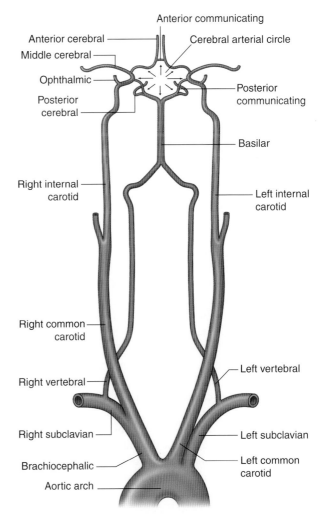

• *GAS* **Fig. 8.38A**

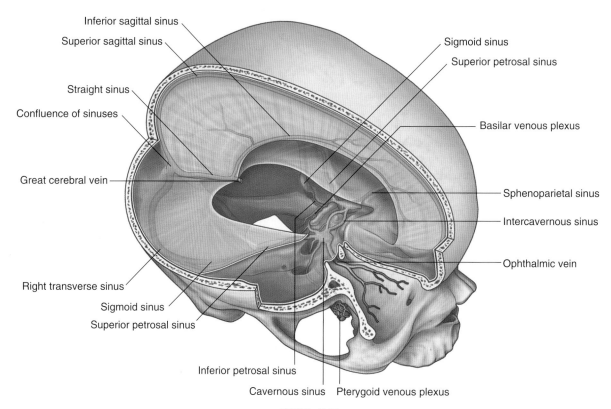

Inferior sagittal sinus

Superior sagittal sinus

Straight sinus

Confluence of sinuses

Great cerebral vein

Right transverse sinus

Sigmoid sinus

Superior petrosal sinus

Inferior petrosal sinus

Cavernous sinus   Pterygoid venous plexus

Sigmoid sinus

Superior petrosal sinus

Basilar venous plexus

Sphenoparietal sinus

Intercavernous sinus

Ophthalmic vein

• *GAS* **Fig. 8.44**

45. E. The sigmoid venous sinus empties into the internal jugular vein and drains the brain and skull. It runs along the posterior cranial fossa near the suture between the temporal and occipital bones just lateral to the mastoid cells.

A. The superior sagittal sinus lies within the superior aspect of the longitudinal fissure, between the two cerebral hemispheres.

B. The inferior sagittal sinus runs inferior to the superior sagittal sinus within the falx cerebri and joins the great cerebral vein (of Galen) to form the straight sinus.

C. The straight sinus drains the great cerebral vein (of Galen) into the confluence of sinuses.

D. The cavernous sinus is located within the middle cranial fossa and receives the superior ophthalmic vein, the sphenoparietal sinus, and other venous vessels (*GAS* Fig. 8.44).

GAS 875; N 110; ABR/McM 61

46. C. The tumor is compressing the facial nerve, which runs through the internal acoustic meatus along with the vestibulocochlear nerve. The facial nerve provides the sensation of taste to the anterior two-thirds of the tongue via the chorda tympani and also mediates all of the facial muscles, except the muscles of mastication.

A. The mandibular branch of the trigeminal nerve courses through the foramen ovale and mediates motor to the muscles of mastication, tensor tympani, tensor veli palatini, mylohyoid, and the

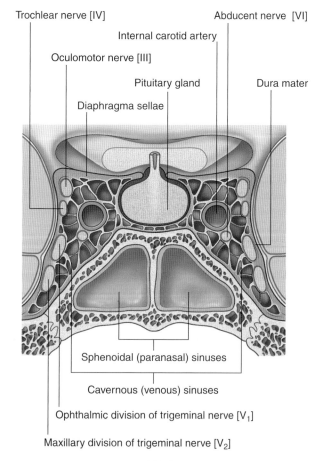

Trochlear nerve [IV]

Abducent nerve [VI]

Internal carotid artery

Oculomotor nerve [III]

Pituitary gland

Dura mater

Diaphragma sellae

Sphenoidal (paranasal) sinuses

Cavernous (venous) sinuses

Ophthalmic division of trigeminal nerve [V₁]

Maxillary division of trigeminal nerve [V₂]

• *GAS* **Fig. 8.45**

anterior belly of digastric as well as sensation to the lower third of the face.

B. The maxillary branch of the trigeminal branch passes through the foramen rotundum and is sensory to the middle third of the face.

D. The jugular foramen has the glossopharyngeal, vagus, and accessory nerves coursing through it.

E. The superior orbital fissure has the ophthalmic branch of the trigeminal nerve coursing through it, along with the oculomotor, trochlear, and abducens nerves.
GAS 887–888; N 105; ABR/McM 58

47. E. The submental lymph nodes drain approximately the anterior two-thirds of the mouth and tongue, including the lower lips.

A. The occipital nodes serve the inferoposterior aspect of the head.

B. The parotid nodes lie anterior to the ear and serve the region of the lateral aspect of the eye, the parotid gland, and anterior ear.

C. The retropharyngeal nodes lie posterior to the pharynx and drain the posterior aspect of the throat and pharynx.

D. The jugulodigastric node is a large node posterior to the parotid gland and just below the angle of the mandible. It receives lymph from much of the face, scalp, and oropharynx and is commonly enlarged in tonsillitis.
GAS 909; N 86; ABR/McM 13

48. A. The abducens nerve would be affected first in a case of aneurysmal dilation of the internal carotid artery because the nerve runs in closest proximity to the artery within the cavernous sinus.

B, C, D, and E. The other nerves running in the wall of the cavernous sinus are the oculomotor nerve, trochlear nerve, and both the maxillary and ophthalmic branches of the trigeminal nerve. Each of these nerves, however, courses along, or within, the lateral walls of the cavernous sinus and may not be immediately affected by an aneurysm of the internal carotid artery (*GAS Fig. 8.45*).
GAS 876; N 115; ABR/McM 59

49. C. The lingual nerve is the most likely nerve damaged because there is loss both of taste and general sensory supply to the anterior two-thirds of the tongue, which is innervated by the lingual nerve, which at this point has been joined by the chorda tympani.

A. The auriculotemporal nerve is a posterior branch of the mandibular division of the trigeminal nerve and innervates skin of the ear anteriorly as well as the temporal region.

B. The chorda tympani would be a likely choice; however, it carries only taste and does not mediate other general sensation to the tongue.

D and E. The mental nerve is the terminal branch of the inferior alveolar nerve and innervates the skin of the chin.
GAS 1090; N 133; ABR/McM 35

50. B. The auriculotemporal nerve is a posterior branch of the mandibular division of the trigeminal nerve. It encircles the middle meningeal artery and courses medially to the temporomandibular joint and then ascends up near the auricle. Because this nerve supplies the temporomandibular joint and skin of the external acoustic meatus and ear, pain from the joint can be referred to the ear as in this case.

A. The facial nerve courses over the ramus of the mandible, passing superficial to the masseter muscle and below the temporomandibular joint through the parotid gland, and would not be involved in this problem.

C. The lesser petrosal nerve courses through the middle cranial fossa and exits through the foramen ovale, where it joins the otic ganglion.

D. The vestibulocochlear nerve exits the cranial cavity through the internal acoustic meatus and innervates structures in the inner ear.

E. The chorda tympani is a branch of the facial nerve and joins the lingual nerve from the mandibular division of the trigeminal nerve anterior to the temporomandibular joint.
GAS 974–975; N 133; ABR/McM 29

Answers 51–75

51. D. The otic ganglion is the location of the postganglionic parasympathetic neural cell bodies innervating the parotid gland. The ganglion lies on the medial surface of the mandibular division of the trigeminal nerve near the foramen ovale.

A. The trigeminal ganglion contains cell bodies for neurons innervating sensory aspects of the face.

B. The geniculate ganglion contains the nerve cell bodies for taste from the anterior two-thirds of the tongue, primarily.

C. The SCG has the cell bodies of postganglionic sympathetic fibers traveling into the head and upper neck.

E. The submandibular ganglia contain the cell bodies of postganglionic parasympathetic fibers innervating the sublingual and submandibular salivary glands.
GAS 877–892; N 145; ABR/McM 33

52. B. The arachnoid villi are extensions of the arachnoid mater into dural venous sinuses such as the superior sagittal sinus. The villi allow for proper drainage of the CSF into the venous bloodstream from the subarachnoid space in which the CSF circulates. These villi are a crucial element in maintaining proper intracranial pressure and circulation of the CSF.

A, C, D, and E. Though the choroid plexus primarily produces CSF, the CSF flows within the subarachnoid space. CSF does not flow within the other spaces listed.
GAS 864; N 113; ABR/McM 62

53. C. The afferent/sensory limb of the corneal (blink) reflex is carried by the nasociliary nerve. It is a branch of the ophthalmic division of the trigeminal nerve.

A and B. The frontal and lacrimal nerves provide cutaneous supply to parts of the upper eyelid and forehead, but they do not innervate the cornea. The facial nerve is the efferent limb of the corneal reflex and mediates the closing of both eyes in response to irritation of the cornea.

D. The oculomotor nerve mediates the reopening of the eyes by contraction of the levator palpebrae superioris.

E. The optic nerve also innervates the eye for the sense of vision and is the afferent limb of the pupillary light reflex.

GAS 889; N 97; ABR/McM 44, 51–52

54. D. Kiesselbach plexus (also called Little area) is an anastomosis of four arteries on the anterior nasal septum. The four arteries are the anterior ethmoidal artery, sphenopalatine artery, superior labial artery, and greater palatine artery. The two largest contributors, however, are the septal branches of the sphenopalatine (from the maxillary artery) and superior labial arteries (branches of the facial artery, which in turn is a branch of the external carotid artery).

A, B, C, and E. These pairs of arteries do not contribute to Kiesselbach plexus. (*GAS* Fig. 8.243AB).

GAS 987–988; N 47; ABR/McM 42

55. B. The palatine tonsils lie in the tonsillar fossae with muscular anterior and posterior pillars (covered with mucosa) forming the boundaries of the fossa. These pillars are formed by the palatoglossal arch, anteriorly, and the palatopharyngeal arch, posteriorly. The anterior pillar, part of the palatoglossal arch, contains the palatoglossus muscle; the posterior pillar, provided by the palatopharyngeal arch, is formed by the palatopharyngeus muscle.

A, C, D, and E. These pairs of muscles do not form the tonsillar arches.

GAS 1033; N 67; ABR/McM 49

56. A. The posterior cricoarytenoid muscles lie on the posterior aspect of the lamina of the cricoid cartilage. When these muscles contract, they cause lateral rotation (abduction) of the vocal processes of the arytenoid cartilages, thereby opening the space between the vocal folds, the rima glottidis.

B. The lateral cricoarytenoid is involved with adducting the arytenoid cartilage and closing the rima glottidis.

C. The thyroarytenoid muscles lie alongside either vocal ligament and are also involved in adducting the vocal folds.

D. The transverse arytenoid muscle connects both arytenoid cartilages and also aids in closing the rima glottidis.

E. The cricothyroid muscle is located on the anterior aspect of the cricoid cartilage and aids in elongation and tensing of the vocal folds, thus preparing the vocal cords to vibrate or raising the pitch of the voice.

GAS 1048–1050; N 65; ABR/McM 47

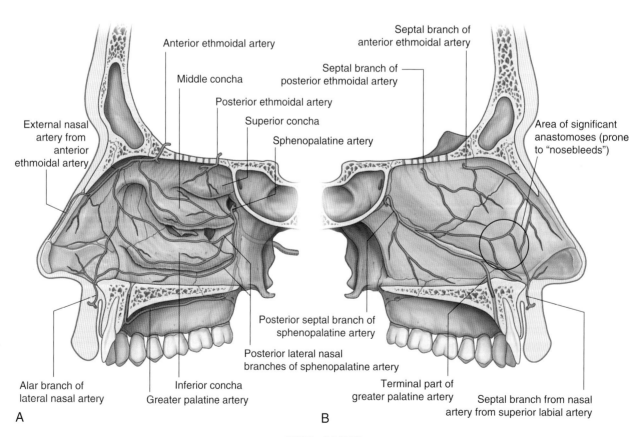

Anterior ethmoidal artery

Middle concha

Posterior ethmoidal artery

Superior concha

Sphenopalatine artery

External nasal artery from anterior ethmoidal artery

Septal branch of anterior ethmoidal artery

Septal branch of posterior ethmoidal artery

Area of significant anastomoses (prone to "nosebleeds")

Alar branch of lateral nasal artery

Inferior concha
Greater palatine artery

Posterior septal branch of sphenopalatine artery

Posterior lateral nasal branches of sphenopalatine artery

Terminal part of greater palatine artery

Septal branch from nasal artery from superior labial artery

A

B

• *GAS* **Fig. 8.243AB**

57. C. The parotid duct, also known as the Stensen duct, crosses the masseter muscle transversely and extends to the oral cavity where it opens into the oral vestibule opposite the upper second molar. This structure is typically not palpable but can become enlarged because of blockage or parotid gland infection.

    A. The facial artery can be palpated in the groove anterior to the mandibular angle. The facial vein lies anterior to the artery, passing toward the angle of the lips, but does not ascend in close proximity to the masseter.

    B, D, and E. All of the other vessels are located more deeply and cannot be palpated.

    GAS 900; N 65; ABR/McM 40

58. C. Because of the surgical division of the ansa cervicalis, the sternohyoid muscle will most likely be paralyzed following this tumor resection. The ansa cervicalis innervates the strap muscles, including the sternohyoid, sternothyroid, and omohyoid muscles.

    A. The sternocleidomastoid is innervated by the accessory nerve and will not be involved with this surgery.

    B. The platysma is located most superficially on the neck and is innervated by the cervical branch of the facial nerve.

    D. The trapezius muscle is also innervated by the accessory nerve and plays no role in ansa cervicalis functions.

    E. The cricothyroid muscle is innervated by the external branch of the superior laryngeal nerve, from vagus, and would not be affected by the surgery.

    GAS 1005; N 38; ABR/McM 31, 33

59. A. The accessory nerve passes across the posterior triangle of the neck after innervating the sternocleidomastoid muscle and then innervates the trapezius muscle on the respective side of the body. Upon surgical division of the nerve, the patient will lose the ability to raise the ipsilateral shoulder. The trapezius will also lose tone and the shoulder will droop.

    B. The ansa cervicalis innervates strap muscles of the neck and, if cut, would not produce drooping of the shoulder.

    C. The facial nerve does not pass through any of the triangles of the neck; however, if it were divided, paralysis would result in the muscles of facial expression.

    D. The hypoglossal nerve innervates the intrinsic muscles of the tongue, plus the genioglossus, hyoglossus, and styloglossus and, if injured, would not result in any of the patient's symptoms.

    E. The suprascapular nerve innervates the supraspinatus and infraspinatus muscles, which mainly contributes to abduction of the arm well below shoulder level and external rotation of the humerus.

    GAS 89; N 39; ABR/McM 29, 30, 32

60. C. Four nerves participate in providing cutaneous supply to the neck. The area over the angle of the jaw is innervated by the great auricular nerve. It ascends from spinal segments from C2 and C3 and innervates the skin over the angle of the jaw, posteroinferior to the auricle of the ear, as well as most of the auricle. The other nerves include the supraclavicular, transverse cervical, and the lesser occipital.

    A. The supraclavicular nerves originate from C3 to C4 and innervate the more inferior aspects of the neck, the upper deltoid region, and skin inferior to the clavicles.

    B. The transverse cervical also originates from the C2 to C3 spinal segments but passes anteriorly to innervate the anterior and lateral aspects of the neck.

    D. The greater occipital nerve does not provide cutaneous sensation to the neck.

    E. The lesser occipital nerve innervates skin in the area of the back of the neck and posterior occiput.

    GAS 973–974; N 9; ABR/McM 29, 30, 31, 33

61. C. Because of its size and vulnerable position during birth, the sternocleidomastoid muscle is injured more often than other muscles of the head and neck during birth especially if the delivery is difficult. When acting alone, the action of this muscle is to turn the head to the opposite side and bend it toward the ipsilateral shoulder. When using both muscles, the head will flex toward the chest. Therefore, the most likely muscle to have been injured here is the left sternocleidomastoid muscle.

    A, B, D, and E. While injury to these muscles could contribute to this presentation, it is unlikely for it to be the sole contributor. The most fitting and most common injury causing this presentation is the sternocleidomastoid muscle.

    GAS 1013; N 36; ABR/McM 31, 32

62. C. The most likely structures one would encounter while performing a midline incision below the isthmus of the thyroid gland would be the inferior thyroid vein and the thyroidea ima artery. The inferior thyroid vein drains typically to the left brachiocephalic vein, which crosses superficially, just inferior to the isthmus. The thyroidea ima artery arises from the aortic arch, vertebral artery, or other source but is present in less than 10% of people.

    A. The middle thyroid veins drain the thyroid gland to the internal jugular vein and are superior to the incision site.

    B. The inferior thyroid arteries branch from either subclavian artery and meet the thyroid gland at an oblique angle. They would not be ligated with a midline incision.

    D. The cricothyroid artery courses superior to the isthmus of the thyroid gland.

    E. The brachiocephalic veins are inferior to the site of incision.

GAS 1008; N 38, 84, 87–89, 204, 215, 241; ABR/ McM 30, 32, 37, 218

63. D. The recurrent laryngeal nerve is the most likely nerve damaged during the surgery because it runs in close proximity to the inferior thyroid artery and is easily injured or transected with the artery if extreme care is not exercised during operative procedures. The recurrent laryngeal nerve innervates the majority of the vocal muscles that open and close the rima glottidis, in addition to providing sensory supply to the larynx below the vocal folds. Even relatively mild trauma to the nerve can result in hoarseness and difficulty in opening the glottis.

A. The internal branch of the superior laryngeal nerve is not in close proximity to the inferior thyroid artery and pierces the thyrohyoid membrane to enter the laryngopharynx.

B. The ansa cervicalis lies lateral to the site of surgery and does not innervate any structures that, if paralyzed, would cause hoarseness.

C. The ansa subclavia is part of the cervical sympathetic trunk that forms a loop around the subclavian artery; it does not contribute to vocal cord movement, and thus would not cause hoarseness if injured.

E. The external branch of superior laryngeal innervates the cricothyroid muscle, tensing the vocal cords. Damage to this nerve would cause hoarseness but would not cause difficulty in breathing.

GAS 1009–1010, 1023, 1058; N 30, 39, 80, 82, 87–89, 92, 137, 141, 213–216, 230, 235–236, 243, 245–246; ABR/McM 35–36, 47, 49–50, 84

64. E. The vagus nerve exits the skull at the jugular foramen and is responsible for motor innervation to the smooth muscles of the trachea, bronchi, and digestive tract, in addition to the muscles of the palate, pharynx, larynx, and superior two-thirds of the esophagus.

A. The ansa cervicalis innervates the strap muscles of the neck, with the exception of the thyrohyoid muscle.

B. The cervical sympathetic trunk does not enter into the jugular foramen; it runs behind the carotid sheath, parallel with the internal carotid artery; its internal carotid branch accompanies the artery into the carotid canal and carries sympathetic fibers to deep areas of the head.

C. Damage to the external laryngeal nerve would result in paralysis of the cricothyroid muscle, presenting as an easily fatigued voice with hoarseness.

D. Injury to the hypoglossal nerve would result in protrusion of the tongue toward the affected side and moderate dysarthria.

GAS 883–884, 890, 892, 1023; N 19, 33, 39–41, 49, 64, 66, 82–83, 87–89, 115, 124, 127–128, 136–138, 141–142, 146, 173, 210, 213–215, 231, 236, 243, 304–307, 321; ABR/McM 29–30, 34–35, 47, 66, 71, 84, 219

Sensory

Anterior two thirds (oral)
- General sensation mandibular nerve [V$_3$] via lingual nerve
- Special sensation (taste) facial nerve [VII] via chorda tympani

Posterior one third (pharyngeal)
- General and special (taste) sensation via glossopharyngeal nerve [IX]

Motor

Hypoglossal nerve [XII]
- Intrinsic muscle
- Genioglossus
- Hyoglossus
- Styloglossus

Palatoglossus – vagus nerve [X]

• *GAS* **Fig. 8.261**

65. B. The hypoglossal nerve provides motor innervation to the muscles of the tongue, with the exception of the palatoglossus. Injury to the hypoglossal nerve would result in deviation of the tongue toward the affected side when the tongue is protruded (in this case the right side), mainly because of the unilateral contraction of left genioglossus, and moderate dysarthria.

A. Injury to the glossopharyngeal nerve would result in loss of taste in the posterior third of the tongue, loss of oropharyngeal sensation, and loss of gag reflex on the affected side. The inferior alveolar nerve supplies the tissues of the chin and lower teeth.

C. Injury to the left hypoglossal would cause the tongue to deviate to the left when the tongue is protruded.

D. The lingual nerve conveys parasympathetic preganglionic fibers to the submandibular ganglion and general sensation and taste fibers for the anterior two-thirds of the tongue.

E. Injury to the vagus nerve would cause sagging of the soft palate, deviation of the uvula to the unaffected side, hoarseness, and difficulty in swallowing and speaking (*GAS* Fig. 8.261).

GAS 883–884, 890–892; N 19, 40–41, 49, 68, 59, 64, 70, 82–84, 86, 115, 124, 128–129, 139–140; ABR/ McM 44, 66, 70, 85

66. C. During removal of the tumor, the internal branch of the superior laryngeal nerve was injured. Injury to this nerve results in loss of sensation above the vocal cords, at the entrance to the larynx, and loss of taste on the epiglottis. Loss of sensation in the laryngeal vestibule can precipitate aspiration of fluid into the larynx, trachea, and lungs. The pharyngeal nerve from the vagus nerve supplies motor innervation to the muscles of the pharynx, except the stylopharyngeus (glossopharyngeal nerve).

A. Injury to the external branch of the superior pharyngeal would cause an inability to change the pitch of the voice, leading to a monotone voice, as well as hoarseness.

B. Injury to the hypoglossal nerve would result in protrusion of the tongue toward the affected side and moderate dysarthria.

D. The lingual nerve conveys parasympathetic preganglionic fibers to the submandibular ganglion and general sensation and taste fibers for the anterior two-thirds of the tongue.

E. The recurrent laryngeal provides sensory fibers to the larynx below the vocal cords and motor fibers to all of the muscles of the larynx except for the cricothyroid.

GAS 1057; N BP25, 78, 75, 80, 82, 87–89, 91, 92, 137; ABR/McM 47, 84

67. A. The posterior cricoarytenoids are the only muscles of the larynx that abduct the vocal cords.

B, C, D, and E. The remaining answer choices are muscles that act in adduction of the vocal cords.

GAS 1050–1051; N 75, 80, 91, 93, 92, 160; ABR/McM 47–49

68. B. The external branch of the superior laryngeal nerve courses together with the superior thyroid artery for much of its route.

A. The cervical sympathetic trunk is located quite posteriorly to this location.

C. The inferior root of the ansa cervicalis is located more laterally in the anterior neck.

D. The internal branch of the superior laryngeal nerve takes a route superior to that of the external branch and the superior thyroid artery and would be unlikely to be injured in this case.

E. The recurrent laryngeal nerve terminates inferiorly, passing into the larynx in relation to the inferior thyroid artery or its branches.

GAS 1057; N 82, 87–89, 92, 137; ABR/McM 47, 84

69. C. The external surface of the tympanic membrane is innervated primarily by the auriculotemporal nerve, a branch of the mandibular division of the trigeminal nerve. Damage to this nerve would additionally result in painful movements of the temporomandibular joint because this joint receives innervation from the same nerve.

A. Taste in the anterior two-thirds of the tongue is supplied by the facial nerve and would be unaffected in this injury. (The chorda tympani could be injured,

but its superior location on the medial side of the tympanic membrane would make this unlikely.)

B. The oro- and laryngopharynx receive their sensory fibers from the glossopharyngeal and vagus nerves. The nasopharynx and palate are supplied by the maxillary division of the trigeminal nerve and would be unaffected by this injury.

D. Sensory innervation to the larynx is provided by the vagus nerve.

E. The sensory innervation of the nasal cavity is supplied by the ophthalmic and maxillary divisions of the trigeminal nerve and would be unaffected by injury to the tympanic membrane.

GAS 901, 904, 974–975, 1093; N 9, 25, 53, 56–57, 59, 82–83, 133, 136, 145; ABR/McM 29, 39–40, 56, 82–81

70. B. Both the stapedius and tensor tympani normally function to dampen movements of the middle ear ossicles, thereby muting sound and preventing hyperacusis. A stapedius would be the source of hyperacusis in this problem because it receives its innervation from the facial nerve.

A and D. The posterior belly of the digastric and the stylohyoid receive innervation from the facial nerve, but their paralysis would not cause hyperacusis.

C. The tensor veli palatini receives motor innervation from the mandibular division of the trigeminal nerve but does not dampen movements of the ear ossicles.

E. Damaged innervation of the cricothyroid, which is supplied by the external branch of the superior laryngeal nerve, would not result in hyperacusis.

GAS 952, 958–960; N 64, 107, 129, 134, 160; ABR/McM 57–58

71. C. The greater petrosal nerve carries parasympathetic fibers that are involved in the innervation of the lacrimal gland, as well as the mucosal glands of the nose, palate, and pharynx. As a result, an injury to the right greater petrosal nerve would be expected to result in decreased lacrimal secretions for the right eye.

A. The sublingual and submandibular glands receive their parasympathetic fibers from the facial nerve via the chorda tympani and the lingual nerve. They would be unaffected by this lesion.

B. The parotid gland receives its parasympathetic secretory innervation from the glossopharyngeal nerve via the lesser petrosal and auriculotemporal nerves and would be unaffected.

D and E. Taste to the anterior tongue is provided by the facial nerve via the chorda tympani, and general sensation to the anterior tongue is provided by the mandibular division of the trigeminal nerve via the lingual nerve.

GAS 958, 977, 986, 1094–1095; N 20, 46, 62, 64, 66, 97, 107, 134–136, 142, 144, 146; ABR/McM 44, 58, 85

72. C. Parasympathetic innervation of the parotid gland is provided by axons carried by the glossopharyngeal nerve that emerge from the tympanic plexus of the middle ear as the lesser petrosal nerve. These preganglionic parasympathetic fibers terminate at synapses in the otic ganglion, which supplies the secretory parasympathetic innervation to the parotid gland.

A, B and E. Glandular secretions of the nasal cavity, soft palate, and lacrimal gland all receive parasympathetic innervation from the fibers of the greater petrosal nerve and would remain intact following a tympanic plexus lesion.

D. Axons for secretory innervation to the sublingual and submandibular glands are carried by the facial nerve, then course through the chorda tympani, before synapsing in the submandibular ganglion, with postganglionic fibers eventually reaching the glands via the lingual nerve (*GAS* Figs. 8.120 and 8.125).

GAS 953, 978; N 19–20, 59, 97, 106–107, 133–134, 136, 145; ABR/McM 44, 84–85

73. **B.** The inferior alveolar branch of the mandibular division of the trigeminal nerve provides sensory innervation to the mandibular teeth and would require anesthesia to abolish painful sensation.

A. The lingual nerve provides taste and sensation to the anterior two-thirds of the tongue and carries general sensory fibers, taste fibers, and parasympathetic fibers. It does not provide sensory innervation to the teeth.

C. The buccal nerve provides sensory innervation to the inner and outer surface of the cheek.

D. The mental nerve is the distal continuation of the inferior alveolar nerve as it exits the mental foramen of the mandible and does not affect the teeth.

E. The nerve to the mylohyoid is a motor branch of the inferior alveolar nerve that supplies the mylohyoid and the anterior belly of the digastric.

GAS 883, 885, 886–887, 889–890, 978; N 25, 68, 56–57, 59, 69, 66, 82, 133, 142, 145; ABR/McM 42, 59, 81–82

74. **D.** Part of the lateral pterygoid muscle has its insertion on the articular disc within the temporomandibular joint and would be most affected by the inflammation of this joint.

A. The temporalis muscle inserts on the coronoid process and anterior margin of the mandibular ramus and retracts the jaw.

B. The medial pterygoid muscle extends from the medial surface of the lateral pterygoid plate to the mandible and functions in elevation of the jaw.

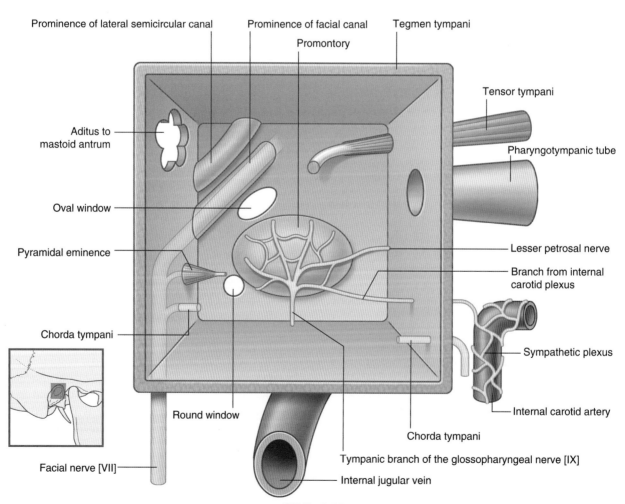

Prominence of lateral semicircular canal

Prominence of facial canal

Tegmen tympani

Promontory

Tensor tympani

Aditus to mastoid antrum

Pharyngotympanic tube

Oval window

Pyramidal eminence

Lesser petrosal nerve

Branch from internal carotid plexus

Chorda tympani

Sympathetic plexus

Internal carotid artery

Round window

Chorda tympani

Tympanic branch of the glossopharyngeal nerve [IX]

Facial nerve [VII]

Internal jugular vein

• *GAS* **Fig. 8.120**

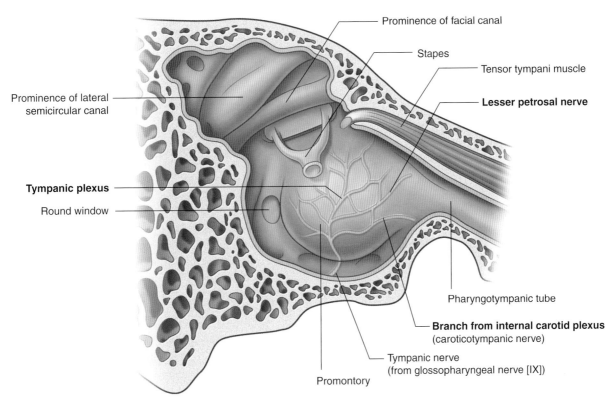

Prominence of facial canal

Stapes

Tensor tympani muscle

Lesser petrosal nerve

Prominence of lateral semicircular canal

Tympanic plexus

Round window

Pharyngotympanic tube

Branch from internal carotid plexus
(caroticotympanic nerve)

Tympanic nerve
(from glossopharyngeal nerve [IX])

Promontory

• *GAS* **Fig. 8.125**

C. The masseter extends from the zygomatic arch to the lateral surface of the ramus of the mandible and elevates the jaw.

E. The buccinator pulls back the angle of the mouth and flattens the cheek.

GAS 966, 972, 974; N 13, 49, 56–57, 59, 160; ABR/ McM 10, 19, 42–44

75. D. The trochlear nerve innervates the superior oblique muscle, which acts to move the pupil downward and laterally. It is the only muscle that can depress the pupil when the eye is adducted. When an individual walks downstairs, this eye motion is initiated, and diplopia results if it is not functioning properly.

A. The optic nerve provides vision, and a lesion of this nerve would not result in diplopia when an affected individual walks down the stairs, but rather diminished vision or blindness.

B. The oculomotor nerve supplies the superior, inferior, and medial rectus as well as the inferior oblique. Overall, innervation from the oculomotor nerve results in upward and inward movements of the eye, and a lesion of this nerve would not induce diplopia in an individual walking downstairs.

C. The abducens nerve innervates the lateral rectus muscle, which abducts the eye, and damage would not induce the diplopia presented in this problem.

E. The frontal nerve is a branch of the ophthalmic division of the trigeminal nerve and provides sensory innervation to the forehead.

GAS 883–884, 886, 889–890, 932–933; N 64, 96, 97, 115, 124–125, 127–129, 132, 155; ABR/McM 60, 56, 80

Answers 76–100

76. E. The superior oblique muscle turns the pupil downward from the adducted position. Inability to perform this motion, in conjunction with diplopia when walking downstairs, indicates damage to the trochlear nerve.

A. The abducens innervates the lateral rectus, resulting in abduction of the eye.

B. The nasociliary nerve is a sensory nerve originating from the ophthalmic branch of the trigeminal nerve.

C and D. The oculomotor nerve supplies the superior, inferior, and medial rectus as well as the inferior oblique muscles. Overall, innervation from the oculomotor nerve results in upward and downward movements of the eye. Damage to this nerve would not induce diplopia when an affected individual walks downstairs. In addition, inability to gaze downward in the adducted position does not indicate oculomotor nerve damage. In this position the oculomotor nerve would be responsible for upward movement.

GAS 883–884, 886, 889–890, 932–933; N 64, 96, 97, 115, 124–125, 127–129, 132, 156; ABR/ McM 61, 56, 80

77. E. Ptosis and miosis occur in response to blocking of sympathetic innervation. Ptosis (drooping of the eyelid) results from lack of innervation of the superior tarsal muscle (of Müller), and miosis (pupillary constriction) results from unopposed parasympathetic innervation of the pupil.

A. A dilated pupil would not occur because this requires the action of the sympathetically innervated dilator pupillae.

B and C. Dry eye would occur because of lacrimal gland insufficiency, but because this is mediated by parasympathetic fibers, it would remain unaffected in this case. The same holds true for the parasympathetically mediated accommodation pathway.

D. Depth perception involves the visual pathway and is not mediated by the sympathetic system.
GAS 918–920; N 94, 142; ABR/McM 37, 53

78. B. The right abducens nerve innervates the right lateral rectus, which mediates outward movement (abduction) of the right eye.

    A. Inward movement is accomplished by the medial rectus, supplied by the oculomotor nerve.

    C. Downward movement in the midline is accomplished by joint activation of the superior oblique and inferior rectus muscle, supplied by oculomotor and trochlear nerves, respectively.

    D. Down and out motion is mediated by the combined actions of the lateral rectus, inferior rectus, and superior oblique muscles, which are innervated by the abducens, oculomotor, and trochlear nerves respectively.

    E. Down and inward movement of the pupil is a function of the inferior and medial rectus muscles, which are innervated by the inferior division of oculomotor nerve.
    GAS 883–884, 887, 889–890, 933; N 20, 64, 96, 97, 124, 128, 132; ABR/McM 66, 80, 83, 80

79. A. Horner syndrome involves interruption of sympathetic supply to the face. This results in ptosis (drooping eyelid), miosis (constricted pupil), and anhidrosis (lack of sweating) of the face.

    B. The eye is lubricated by the lacrimal gland, which secretes in response to parasympathetic stimulation, and would be unaffected.

    C. Exophthalmos (protrusion of the globe) is frequently caused by hyperthyroidism and is not present in Horner syndrome.

    D. Loss of sympathetic innervation leads to unopposed vasodilatation of the vessels to the face, leading to flushing rather than paleness.

    E. Horner syndrome results in lack of sweating of the face.
    GAS 917–920; N 94, 142; ABR/McM 37

80. E. The superior tarsal muscle (of Müller), innervated by sympathetics, is smooth muscle that assists in elevating the eyelids and maintaining this position. Loss of sympathetic innervation will result in partial ptosis of the eyelid.

    A and B. The orbicularis oculi, innervated by the facial nerve, is responsible for closure of the eye. The palpebral part closes the eyelids ordinarily; the orbital part contracts when the eye is closed more forcibly, resulting in increased tear movement across the globe (perhaps to flow down the cheeks).

    C. Damage to the levator palpebrae superioris, innervated by the oculomotor nerve, would result in complete, rather than partial, ptosis.

    D. The superior oblique, innervated by the trochlear nerve, moves the pupil downward from the adducted position (for example, as when the right eye gazes down toward the left foot). To test the trochlear nerve, ask the patient to look with each eye toward the tip of the nose.
    GAS 917–920; N 94; ABR/McM 37, 80

81. D. Cavernous sinus thrombosis can often result from squeezing pimples or other infectious processes located around the danger area of the face, which includes the area of the face directly surrounding the nose. This physical pressure has the potential to move infectious agents from the pimple into the superior ophthalmic vein, which then carries it to the cavernous sinus. The pterygoid venous plexus and ophthalmic vein both communicate with the cavernous sinus and therefore offer a route of travel for the spread of infection, but the path provided by the superior ophthalmic vein is a more direct route. The superior ophthalmic vein receives blood supply from the supraorbital, supratrochlear, and angular veins that supply the area around the nose and lower forehead. (Venous blood in the head can flow in either direction because these veins do not possess valves.)

    A. The carotid artery would not offer a route of communication between the area of infection and the cavernous sinus.

    B and E. The emissary veins communicate between the venous sinuses and the veins of the scalp and would therefore not be involved in the spread of infection between the nose and cavernous sinus.

    C. The middle meningeal artery courses between the dura and periosteum, (often called the preicranium in this loacation) whereas the carotid artery, specifically the internal carotid artery, traverses through the cavernous sinus and provides origin to the ophthalmic artery. (*GAS* Fig. 8.68).
    GAS 875–876, 909, 916; N 20, 84, 99, 104, 115; ABR/McM 47, 59

82. E. The anterior inferior cerebellar artery is a major supplier of the anterior inferior portion of the cerebellum. Nerves located in close proximity would likely be affected by hemorrhage of this artery. The abducens nerve is situated at the pontomedullary junction and is therefore most likely to be damaged following hemorrhage of the anterior inferior cerebellar artery A, B, and C. The optic, oculomotor, and trochlear nerves are all associated with the midbrain region and would likely not suffer any damage with a possible hemorrhage.

    D. The trigeminal nerve is situated in the pons and is thus located too far rostrally to be affected.
    GAS 870; N 147, 149–152, 154, 176; ABR/McM 67

83. D. The anterior inferior quadrant of the tympanic membrane is the only portion of the tympanic membrane

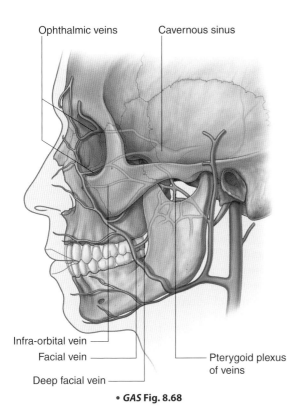

Ophthalmic veins   Cavernous sinus

Infra-orbital vein
Facial vein
Deep facial vein
Pterygoid plexus
of veins

• *GAS* Fig. 8.68

that would allow for an incision with minimal or no damage to adjacent important structures.

A and B. Incision in the anterior and posterior superior quadrants of the tympanic membrane would likely damage the malleus, which is situated immediately superior and medially to the tympanic membrane.

C. The umbo is situated in close proximity to the handle of the malleus and might be damaged during incision.

E. A vertical incision through the tympanic membrane would almost certainly damage the malleus of the middle ear. Damage to the malleus from surgical incision would interfere with the auditory conduction through the middle ear cavity, and this should be avoided to prevent conductive hearing loss.
GAS 945–947, 960; N 105–107, 109; ABR/McM 44, 57–58

84. A. The hypoglossal nerve innervates the muscles of the tongue and is therefore directly involved in alteration of shape and movement of the tongue. A lesion in this nerve would cause deviation of the tongue toward the injured side, which could be observed upon protrusion of the tongue. The genioglossus is the major muscle involved in protrusion of the tongue. The genioglossus muscles arise from the inside of the mandible and pass posteriorly to insert into the deep aspect of the tongue. When the genioglossus muscles contract, they pull the tongue forward, and out of the mouth, in protrusion. If one genioglossus is paralyzed, it acts as a restraint on one side of the tongue when the tongue is pulled forward, causing the tip of the tongue to point to the nonmoving side.

B. Damage to the left hypoglossal nerve and left genioglossus muscle would cause the tongue to deviate to the left on protrusion.

C. The styloglossus muscle is responsible for retraction and elevation of the tongue. D. Neither the geniohyoid muscle nor the first cervical nerve contribute to tongue movement.

E. Vagus nerve does not contribute to tongue movements. Damage to a hypoglossal nerve would cause the tongue to deviate to the ipsilateral side.
GAS 883–884, 892, 889–890; N 19, 40–41, 49, 68, 59, 64, 70, 82–84, 86, 115, 124, 128–129, 139–140; ABR/McM 44, 66, 85

85. B. The posterior chamber receives ciliary body secretions first. The ciliary body produces aqueous humor and is located in the posterior chamber. Increased production of fluid from this site would cause an increase in intraocular pressure if drainage is inadequate.

A. The iridoscleral angle of the anterior chamber is the location of drainage of the aqueous humor; therefore, a blockage of drainage in this location can cause increased intraocular pressure.

C. The pupil is the connection between the anterior and posterior chamber; a collection of fluid does not occur here, for this is simply an aperture to allow light onto the retina.

D. The vitreous body is not directly connected to the production of aqueous humor.

E. The lacrimal sac is the upper dilated end of the nasolacrimal duct and opens up into the inferior nasal meatus of the nasal cavity. The nasolacrimal duct has nothing to do with increased intraocular pressure.
GAS 936–937, 939; N 100–101; ABR/McM 51

86. D. The glossopharyngeal nerve mediates general somatic sensation from the pharynx, the auditory tube, and from the middle ear. Painful sensations from the pharynx, including the auditory tube, can be referred to the ear by this nerve, as in this case of tonsillectomy.

A. The auriculotemporal nerve supplies skin of the auricle and tympanic membrane and scalp anterosuperior to the auricle. This nerve would not be involved directly or indirectly in the operation.

B. The lesser petrosal nerve contains preganglionic parasympathetic fibers that run in the glossopharyngeal and tympanic nerves before synapsing in the otic ganglion.

C. The vagus nerve mediates general somatic afferent supply to the auricle and external acoustic meatus; stimulation of the meatus can trigger a gag reflex or coughing reflex.

E. The chorda tympani mediates taste for the anterior two-thirds of the tongue.
GAS 883–884, 886, 888, 889–890, 932–933; N 41, 49, 64, 66, 82–83, 124, 127–128, 134, 136–137, 141–142, 144–146, 214; ABR/McM 44, 66, 84

87. E. In this case, the uvula deviates to the left, indicating that the left palatal muscles are unaffected, and the **right** muscles are not working properly. The uvula deviates toward the unaffected side of the pharyngeal muscles because of the pull of the unopposed levator veli palatini. The pharyngeal constrictor muscles, as well as muscles of the palate, are all innervated by the **vagus nerve** (except tensor veli palatini—mandibular division of the trigeminal nerve).

    A. Even though a tumor of the jugular canal could potentially affect the glossopharyngeal, vagus, and accessory nerves, the patient's presentation indicates a lesion on the vagus nerve. A lesion on the glossopharyngeal nerve would produce symptoms such as loss of taste from the posterior $\frac{1}{3}$ of the tongue, loss of gag reflex, impairment of swallow or cough—the patient does not present these symptoms.

    B. The pharyngeal wall on the left side is also drawn upward by the non-paralyzed stylopharyngeus, supplied by the left glossopharyngeal nerve; thus, it is intact.

    C. The right mandibular nerve (or the mandibular division of trigeminal nerve) provides sensory innervation to the face and motor supply to the masticatory muscles and does not innervate the muscles of the pharynx.

    D. The left hypoglossal nerve innervates the intrinsic and extrinsic muscles of the left side of the tongue. Compression or injury of this nerve would not lead to uvula deviation.

    GAS 883–884, 890, 892, 1023; N 19, 33, 39–41, 49, 64, 66, 82–83, 87–89, 115, 124, 127–128, 136–138, 141–142, 146, 173, 210, 213–215, 231, 236, 243, 306–307, 321; ABR/McM 47, 61, 66–71, 84, 219

88. E. An infection of the submandibular space is usually the result of a dental infection in the mandibular molar area in the floor of the mouth (Ludwig angina). If the patient is not treated with antibiotics promptly, the pharyngeal and submandibular swelling can lead to asphyxiation.

    A. Quinsy, also known as peritonsillar abscess, is a pus-filled inflammation of the tonsils that can occur because of tonsillitis.

    B. Torus palatinus is a benign bony growth on the hard palate; a torus mandibularis is a similar growth on the inside of the mandible. Such growths are usually benign and would not typically cause pain.

    C. Ankyloglossia, which is also known as tongue-tie, is a congenital defect that results in a shortened lingual frenulum that restricts movement of the tongue. The affected person will usually have a speech impediment.

    D. A ranula is a mucocele found on the floor of the mouth, often resulting from dehydration in older individuals, with coagulation (inspissation) of salivary secretions. It can be caused by acute local trauma; however, they are usually asymptomatic.

    GAS 977, 1092; N 31–32, 35; ABR/McM 18, 30, 32–33, 40

89. A. The auditory (eustachian or pharyngotympanic) tube is a mucosal-lined tube that provides a direct connection from the nasopharynx to the middle ear cavity. A respiratory infection can travel from the upper respiratory tract to the oropharynx or nasopharynx and then on into the middle ear via the auditory tube.

    B. The choanae are paired openings from the nasal cavity into the nasopharynx and do not connect with the auditory tube or the middle ear.

    C. The nostrils do not connect with the auditory tube or middle ear.

    D and E. The facial canal and the internal acoustic meatus are passages for facial and vestibulocochlear nerves, respectively. Neither of these is a likely site for the spread of infection from the upper respiratory tract to the middle ear.

    GAS 943, 950, 955, 1035–1037, 1079; N 43, 49, 56, 67, 72, 75, 77–80, 105–107, 109, BP29, 136; ABR/McM 60, 55, 57–58

90. B. The maxillary sinus drains via the middle nasal meatus, specifically into the semilunar hiatus. The middle nasal meatus and semilunar hiatus are located under the middle nasal concha.

    A. The inferior nasal meatus drains the lacrimal secretions carried by the nasolacrimal duc.

    C. The superior nasal meatus drains the posterior ethmoidal cells.

    D and E. The nasopharynx and sphenoethmoidal recess are not situated in close proximity to the maxillary sinus and are therefore not involved in its drainage. The sphenoidal sinuses drain into the sphenoethmoidal recesses (*GAS Fig. 8.235*).

    GAS 1058–1060; N 43–44, 50–51; ABR/McM 3, 12, 16, 44, 55

91. E. The sphenoidal sinus provides the most direct access to the pituitary gland, which is situated directly above this sinus.

    A. The cribriform plate could offer a point of entry into the cranium; entry at that site would lead to damage of the olfactory cells and nerve, but it would also lead to entry into the subarachnoid space, with leakage of CSF and potential meningitis. The cribriform plates are also located too far anteriorly from the pituitary gland.

    B. The cavernous sinus is situated within the cranial cavity lateral to the pituitary gland; it is not a site for surgical entrance to the cranial cavity.

    C and D. Neither the frontal sinus nor maxillary sinus has any direct communication with the interior of the cranial cavity and would therefore not allow the surgeon a potential access point to the pituitary gland.

    GAS 1064–1065; N 45–46; ABR/McM 12, 17, 25, 43, 47, 55, 79

92. B. The gag reflex is composed of both an afferent and an efferent limb. These reflexes are mediated by the glosso-pharyngeal and vagus nerves, respectively. Together, the glossopharyngeal and vagus nerves are responsible for the contraction of the muscles of the pharynx involved in the gag reflex. In this case the glossopharyngeal nerve was injured when the tonsils were excised, resulting in the loss of the sensory side of the reflex.

A. The facial nerve is involved with taste of the anterior two-thirds of the tongue; however, it does not mediate the gag reflex.

C and D. The mandibular and maxillary nerves are part of the trigeminal nerve and are thus largely associated with the sensory supply of the face, sinuses, and oral cavity.

E. The hypoglossal nerve innervates most of the muscles of the tongue.

GAS 1089; N 66; ABR/McM 29, 35, 36, 44, 66, 84

93. B. The recurrent laryngeal nerve is often at risk of being damaged during a thyroidectomy. Patients who have a transected or damaged recurrent laryngeal will often present with a characteristic hoarseness following surgery. The posterior cricoarytenoid is supplied by the recurrent laryngeal nerve and would thus be impaired following damage to the nerve. The posterior cricoarytenoid is the only muscle responsible for abduction of the vocal cords, and paralysis of this muscle would result in a permanently adducted position of the involved vocal cord.

A, C, D, and E. The other muscles listed are all adductors of the vocal cords, and paralysis of these would not lead to closure of the airway.

GAS 1051; N 91–93; ABR/McM 47–49

94. C. The pharyngeal tonsil is situated in a slit-like space, the pharyngeal recess, in the nasopharynx behind the opening of the auditory (eustachian) tube, and a pharyngeal tonsil in this location can lead to blockage of the drainage of the auditory tube.

A and B. The lingual tonsil is located in the posterior aspect of the tongue, whereas the palatine tonsil is contained within the tonsillar fossa between the palatoglossal and palatopharyngeal arches. An enlargement of the lingual tonsil or the palatine tonsil will not occlude the auditory tube because of their location in the oropharynx.

D. The superior pharyngeal constrictor would not be involved in occlusion of the auditory tube because it is located more posteriorly.

E. The uvula is drawn upward during deglutition and prevents food from entering the nasopharynx; it does not block the auditory tube.

GAS 1036; N 43; ABR/McM 60, 366

95. A. Infection can spread from the nasopharynx to the middle ear by way of the auditory tube, which opens to both spaces. The first pharyngeal pouch is responsible for formation both of the auditory tube and middle ear (tympanic) cavity.

B. The second pharyngeal pouch persists as the tonsillar sinus and tonsillar crypts.

C. The third pharyngeal pouch develops into the inferior parathyroid gland and thymus,

D. The fourth pharyngeal pouch forms the superior parathyroid gland and the ultimobranchial body.

E. The sixth pharyngeal pouch is not well defined and would therefore not contribute to the development of the auditory tube.

GAS 950; N 105; ABR/McM 45–47, 49

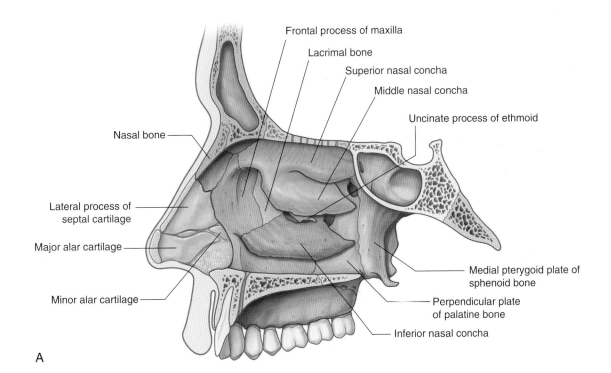

Frontal process of maxilla
Lacrimal bone
Superior nasal concha
Middle nasal concha
Uncinate process of ethmoid
Nasal bone
Lateral process of septal cartilage
Major alar cartilage
Minor alar cartilage
Medial pterygoid plate of sphenoid bone
Perpendicular plate of palatine bone
Inferior nasal concha

A

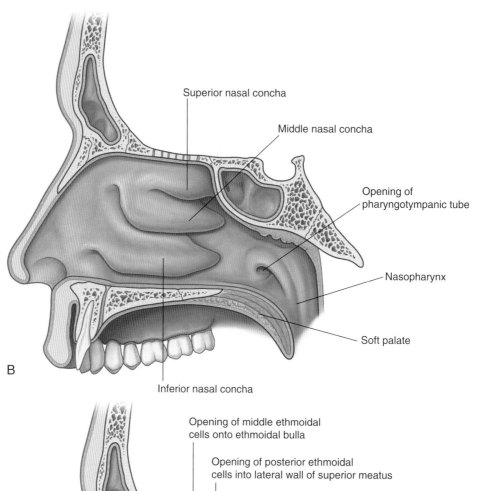

Superior nasal concha

Middle nasal concha

Opening of
pharyngotympanic tube

Nasopharynx

Soft palate

Inferior nasal concha

B

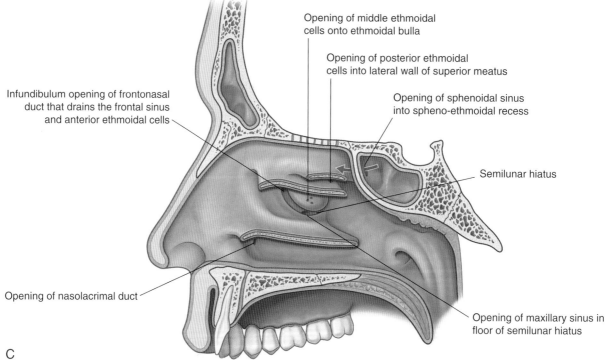

Opening of middle ethmoidal
cells onto ethmoidal bulla

Opening of posterior ethmoidal
cells into lateral wall of superior meatus

Opening of sphenoidal sinus
into spheno-ethmoidal recess

Infundibulum opening of frontonasal
duct that drains the frontal sinus
and anterior ethmoidal cells

Semilunar hiatus

Opening of nasolacrimal duct

Opening of maxillary sinus in
floor of semilunar hiatus

C

• *GAS* Fig. 8.235

96. D. The greater palatine nerve is responsible for the sensory innervation of the hard palate, or the hard part of the roof of the mouth.

  A. The posterior superior alveolar nerve supplies multiple structures, including posterior portions of the gums, cheeks, and the upper posterior teeth. However, it is not involved in nerve supply to the hard palate.

  B. The inferior alveolar nerve has several branches, including the mental nerve, incisive branch, nerve to the mylohyoid, and inferior dental branch. These nerves do not supply the roof of the mouth and thus are not involved.

  C. The lingual nerve supplies taste and general sensation to the anterior two-thirds of the tongue.

  E. The lesser palatine nerve supplies the soft palate and upper portion of the palatine tonsil but is not involved in supply to the hard palate.

  GAS 984, 1112–1113; N 46, 48, 62–64, 67, 66, 82, 133, 142; ABR/McM 44, 55

97. A. Damage to the internal branch of superior laryngeal nerve would result in a general loss of sensation to the larynx above the vocal cords, leaving the patient with an inability to detect food or foreign objects in the laryngeal vestibule.

  B and E. The external branch of superior laryngeal nerve and recurrent laryngeal nerve are both at risk during thyroidectomy. Damage to the recurrent laryngeal nerve would result in paralysis of all the laryngeal muscles except the cricothyroid; it would render the patient hoarse, with a loss of sensation below the vocal cords. Loss of the external branch of superior laryngeal nerve would lead to paralysis of the cricothyroid muscle and hoarseness.

  C. Damage to the glossopharyngeal nerve would result in loss of sensation in the tonsils, pharynx, middle ear, and posterior $\frac{1}{3}$ of the tongue (taste and sensation).

  D. Injury to the hypoglossal nerve would result in weakness or paralysis of muscle movement of the tongue.

  GAS 1057; N 66, 75, 78, 80, 82, 87–88, 91–92, 137; ABR/McM 49–50, 84

98. C. Ankyloglossia (tongue-tie) is characterized by a lingual frenulum that extends all the way to the tip of the tongue. This condition can cause problems with speech, feeding, and oral hygiene as a result of the low range of motion of the tongue. Ankyloglossia can be treated surgically by cutting the lingual frenulum.

  A, B, D, and E. None of the other procedures described would treat this condition.

  GAS 1057; N 53, 65; ABR/McM 43, 47, 49, 56

99. D. Of the answer choices listed, the left facial nerve of the patient is the most likely to be damaged during the mastoidectomy. The facial nerve exits the skull via the stylomastoid foramen, just anterior to the mastoid process. A lesion of the facial nerve is likely to cause the symptoms described as a result of paralysis of the facial muscles. Depending upon the site of injury, the patient could also lose the chorda tympani branch of the facial nerve, leading to loss of taste from the anterior two-thirds of the tongue ipsilaterally as well as loss of functions of the submandibular and sublingual salivary glands.

  A, B, C, and E. The other nerves listed are not likely to be damaged during a mastoidectomy.

  GAS 959; N 107; ABR/McM 58, 39, 40, 83

100. C. Normally, the tonus of the buccinator muscle prevents the accumulation of saliva and foodstuffs in the oral vestibule.

  A, B, D, and E. Although a lesion of the facial nerve would paralyze the other muscles listed, the buccinator is the predominant muscle of the cheek.

  G GAS 893, 898, 900, 1081; N 31, 53–55, 59, 57, 78; ABR/McM 39–40, 4

Answers 101–125

101. B. Compression of the optic chiasm can cause bitemporal hemianopia because of compression of nerve fibers coming from the nasal (medial) hemiretinas of both eyes. The optic chiasm is located in very close proximity above the pituitary gland.

  A. Compression of an optic nerve would cause complete blindness in the affected eye.

  C. Compression of an optic tract would cause homonymous hemianopia.

  D. Compression of the oculomotor nerve would cause the eye to deviate "out and down" (paralysis of the four extraocular muscles innervated by this nerve), ptosis (paralysis of levator palpebrae), and mydriasis (paralysis of constrictor pupillae).

  E. Compression of the abducens nerve would cause paralysis of the lateral rectus muscle, leading to medial deviation (adduction) of the eye.

  GAS 878; N 115, 117, 118; ABR/McM 59, 66

102. E. A lesion of the trochlear nerve causes weakness of downward medial gaze. As a result, patients with trochlear nerve lesions commonly have difficulty walking down a flight of stairs. The superior cerebellar artery branches from the basilar artery just before it bifurcates into the posterior cerebral arteries. The trochlear nerve emerges from the dorsal aspect of the midbrain and can easily be compressed by an aneurysm of the superior cerebellar artery as it wraps around the midbrain.

  A, B, C, and D. Aneurysms of the other arteries mentioned are not likely to compress the trochlear nerve, and lesions of the nerves listed are not likely to cause problems walking down stairs.

  GAS 870; N 154; ABR/McM 59, 66, 66–67

103. E. A Pancoast tumor is located in the pulmonary apex, usually in the right lung. (This is because inhaled gases tend to collect preferentially in the upper right lung, in part because of the manner of branching of the tertiary bronchi.) These tumors can involve the upper thoracic sympathetic ganglia and cause Horner syndrome (ptosis, miosis, and anhidrosis). The other conditions listed are not likely to cause symptoms of Horner syndrome.

A. Raynaud disease, a vascular disorder that affects the extremities, is caused by excessive tone of sympathetic vasoconstriction.

B. Frey syndrome, a rare malady resulting from parotidectomy, is characterized by excessive facial sweating in the presence of food or when thinking about it.

C. Bell palsy is characterized by a lesion of the facial nerve, with weakness or paralysis of mimetic muscles.

D. Quinsy is characterized by painful, pus-filled inflammation of the tonsils.

ABR/McM 218

104. E. The dilator pupillae, levator palpebrae superioris, and smooth muscle cells of blood vessels in the ciliary body all receive sympathetic innervation. The postsynaptic cell bodies of the sympathetic neurons that innervate these structures are located in the SCG.

A, C, and D. These structures do not contain sympathetic cell bodies.

B. The intermediolateral cell column contains presynaptic sympathetic neurons, but it is located only at spinal cord levels T1 to L2.

GAS 1024–1025; N 143; ABR/McM 36

105. B. A fracture of the lamina papyracea of the ethmoid bone is likely to entrap the medial rectus muscle, causing an inability to gaze laterally.

A. A fracture of the orbital plate of the frontal bone could perhaps entrap the superior oblique or superior rectus muscle, but this would be very unusual.

C. A fracture of the orbital surface of the maxilla can entrap the inferior rectus or inferior oblique muscles, limiting upward gaze.

D. A fracture of the cribriform plate could damage olfactory nerves and result in leakage of CSF through the nose (CSF rhinorrhea), with associated meningeal infection.

E. A fracture of the greater wing of the sphenoid is not likely to entrap any extraocular muscles.

GAS 1061, 1062; N 11, 13, 15; ABR/McM 12, 17, 26

106. B. A lesion of the oculomotor nerve will cause the eye to remain in a "down and out" position. This is because of the actions of the unopposed lateral rectus (supplied by the abducens nerve) and the superior oblique (supplied by the trochlear nerve). The tertiary function of the superior oblique is to cause intorsion (internal rotation) of the eyeball, a function that is not usually seen unless the oculomotor nerve is paralyzed. The patient is also likely to present with a full or partial ptosis because of paralysis of the levator palpebrae muscle. The pupil will remain dilated because of loss of stimulation by parasympathetic fibers that innervate the constrictor pupillae muscle.

A, C, D, and E. Damage to the other nerves listed will not lead to the conditions described.

GAS 990; N 96–97; ABR/McM 44, 59, 61, 52, 56, 80

107. B. The axons of olfactory nerves run directly through the cribriform plate to synapse in the olfactory bulb. Damage to this plate can damage the nerve axons, causing anosmia (loss of the sense of smell).

A. A fracture of the cribriform plate is not likely to entrap the eyeball.

C. Hyperacusis can occur following paralysis of the stapedius muscle.

D and E. A lesion of the vestibulocochlear nerve can cause tinnitus and/or deafness.

GAS 1061–1062; N 15; ABR/McM 11–12, 26, 59

108. C. Frey syndrome occurs when parasympathetic axons in the auriculotemporal nerve are cut during a parotidectomy. When these postganglionic cholinergic axons grow peripherally after parotid gland surgery, they establish synapses upon the cholinergic sweat glands, which are innervated normally only by sympathetic fibers. As the peripheral nerves make new connections, aberrant connections can be formed between the auriculotemporal nerve and sweat glands (not usually innervated by the auriculotemporal nerve). This results in flushing and sweating in response to the thought, smell, or taste of food, instead of the previous, normal salivary secretion by the parotid gland.

A, B, D, and E. The other nerves listed do not correlate with Frey syndrome.

GAS 838, 979; N 9; ABR/McM 39–40, 42, 56, 81–82

109. B. The posterior cricoarytenoid muscle is the only abductor of the larynx that opens the rima glottidis by rotating the vocal processes of the arytenoid cartilages laterally.

A, C, D, and E. All of the other listed muscles have adduction as part of their function and thus are not required to maintain the airway.

GAS 1051; N 91, 93, 92; ABR/McM 47–49

110. B. The palatine tonsils are highly vascular and are primarily supplied by the tonsillar branch of the facial artery; therefore, care is taken to identify and ligate or cauterize this artery while performing a tonsillectomy.

A, C, D, and E. The palatine tonsil also receives arterial supply from the ascending pharyngeal, the dorsal lingual, and the lesser palatine, but the supply from the facial artery is by far the most significant.

GAS 1001–1002, 906–907; N 72; ABR/McM 28–32, 39–40

111. A. The inner surface of the tympanic membrane is supplied by the glossopharyngeal nerve.

B and C. The auricular branches of the facial and vagus nerves and the auriculotemporal branch of the trigeminal nerve innervate the external surface of the tympanic membrane.

D. The great auricular nerve arises from C2 and C3 and supplies the posterior auricle and skin over the parotid gland.

E. The lingual nerve does not have anything to do with sensory supply of the tympanic membrane.
GAS 946, 948; N 107, 129; ABR/McM 23, 57

112. C. The infraorbital branch of the maxillary division of the trigeminal nerve exits the front of the skull below the orbit through the infraorbital foramen. A needle inserted into the infraorbital foramen and directed posteriorly will pass into the maxillary division of the trigeminal nerve.
    A. The mandibular division of the trigeminal nerve exits the skull through the foramen ovale.
    B. The middle meningeal artery exits the infratemporal fossa through the foramen spinosum to enter the cranial cavity.
    D. The inferior alveolar branch of the mandibular division passes into the mandibular foramen to then descend in the jaw to supply the mandibular teeth.
    E. The foramen magnum is where the spinal cord exits the skull and where the accessory nerve ascends into the skull after arising from the cervical spinal cord and brainstem.
    GAS 923; N 11, 13, 21, 42; ABR/McM 1, 12, 21, 38

113. A. If there is an injury to the internal branch of superior laryngeal nerve, there is a loss of sensation above the vocal cords. In this case, for internal laryngeal injury to occur, one must conclude that the operative field extended above the position of the thyroid gland to the level of the thyrohyoid membrane.
    B. The external branch of superior laryngeal nerve can be injured during a thyroidectomy, but its injury would result in paralysis of the cricothyroid muscle and weakened voice/hoarseness.
    C. Injury of the glossopharyngeal nerve would result in more widespread symptoms, including loss of sensation from the oropharynx, posterior tongue, and middle ear.
    D. Injury to the hypoglossal nerve would cause deficits in motor activity of the tongue.
    E. Damage to the recurrent laryngeal nerve would result in paralysis of most laryngeal muscles, with possible respiratory obstruction, hoarseness, and loss of sensation below the vocal cords.
    GAS 1057; N 66, 78, 75, 80, 82, 87–89, 91–92, 137; ABR/McM 49–50, 8

114. A. The loose areolar connective tissue layer is known as the "danger zone" because infections can spread easily from this layer into the skull by means of emissary veins that pass into and through the bones of the skull.
    B, C, D, and E. None of the other scalp layers listed is referred to as the "danger zone."
    GAS 911–912; N 10; ABR/McM 5

115. A. The carotid sinus is a baroreceptor that can be targeted for carotid massage to decrease blood pressure. The carotid sinus receptors are sensitive to changes in pressure. For this reason, sustained compression of the carotid sinuses can lead to unconsciousness or death as the pulse is reflexively reduced.
    B. The carotid body is a chemoreceptor, responsive to the balance of oxygen and carbon dioxide.
    C and D. Neither the thyroid gland nor the parathyroid gland has anything to do with acute control of blood pressure because of mechanical stimuli.
    E. The inferior cervical ganglion fuses with the first thoracic ganglion to form the stellate ganglion. It gives rise to the inferior cervical cardiac nerve and provides postganglionic sympathetic supply to the upper limb.
    N 136, 141–142, 147, 214; ABR/McM 35, 45

116. C. The thyroidea ima artery is present in about 10% of people; when present it supplies the thyroid gland and ascends in front of the trachea; therefore, it would be easily injured in an emergency tracheostomy with a midline incision over the trachea.
    A. The inferior thyroid branch of the thyrocervical trunk does not run along the front of the trachea in such a position that a midline incision could damage it.
    B. The cricothyroid branch of the superior thyroid artery passes across the cricothyroid ligament, well above the site of incision.
    D and E. Arterial bleeding would not result from damage to either the middle thyroid vein or the jugular venous arch.
    GAS 1008; N 41, 83, 87, 89; ABR/McM 29–32

117. D. A torn cerebral vein often results in a relatively slow-bleeding subdural hematoma. Such a hematoma can be involved in gradual compression of the brain, resulting in confusion, dizziness, clumsiness, and memory loss. There would be no sign of blood in the CSF because the bleeding is into the subdural space, not the subarachnoid space. This would fit the description of symptoms in this case.
    A. Middle meningeal artery rupture results in an epidural hematoma, which is much more acute and often includes a brief period of unconsciousness followed by a lucid interval and can proceed to death if the bleeding is left untreated.
    B. Fracture of the pterion also can result in an epidural hematoma because the middle meningeal artery is the adjacent vasculature mentioned.
    C. Rupture of the anterior communicating artery would result in a subarachnoid hematoma, and there would be blood in the CSF upon lumbar puncture.
    E. In a cavernous sinus thrombosis there would be cranial nerve involvement because of compression of those nerves that run through or in the wall of the cavernous sinus, including the oculomotor, trochlear, trigeminal (maxillary and mandibular divisions), and abducens nerves.
    GAS 874; N 111; ABR/McM 62

118. D. Paralysis of the right accessory and hypoglossal nerves is present in this patient. Drooping of the right

shoulder occurs as a result of paralysis of the trapezius because of injury to the right accessory nerve. Loss of the right accessory nerve would also result in weakness in turning the head to the left, a function of the right sternocleidomastoid muscle, which is also supplied by this nerve. The tongue deviation to the right is because of the unopposed activity of the left tongue muscles since the right hypoglossal nerve (which innervates the right tongue muscles) is affected.

A, B, C, and E. The other combinations of affected cranial nerves would not produce the specific symptoms described here.
GAS 883–884, 889–892; N 138–139; ABR/McM 29, 32–33, 44, 66–67, 84–85

119. C. The neural cell bodies whose axons synapse in the pterygopalatine ganglion are located in the superior salivatory nucleus, which is in the pons; this nucleus provides the general visceral efferent (GVE) fibers of the facial nerve for lacrimal and salivary secretion.
    A. The SCG is a sympathetic ganglion containing postganglionic neurons and is not concerned with the pterygopalatine ganglion, which is a parasympathetic ganglion.
    B. The Edinger-Westphal nucleus is located in the midbrain and contains the cell bodies of the GVE fibers of the oculomotor nerve, which are responsible for constriction of the pupil via synapse in the ciliary ganglion and supply to the sphincter pupillae muscle and accommodation via the ciliary muscle.
    D. The inferior salivatory nucleus is located in the medulla and gives origin to GVE fibers of the glossopharyngeal nerve to the otic ganglion for secretion of saliva from the parotid gland.
    E. The nucleus ambiguus contains the cell bodies of nerves innervating muscles of the soft palate, pharynx, and larynx—largely associated with speech and swallowing.
    GAS 883–884, 887–890; N 62, 127–128, 134, 144; ABR/McM 85

120. B. A branch of the facial artery would be of primary concern because its branches supply the oropharynx and it is the primary source of arterial supply to the palatine tonsil.
    A. The location of the lingual artery is inferior to the oropharynx and it would be less likely to be injured in the event of a surgical procedure.
    C. The superior laryngeal artery is also located lower and would not be subject to injury by surgery in the area of the oropharynx.
    D. The ascending pharyngeal artery arises in the carotid triangle from the external carotid artery and gives rise to pharyngeal, palatine, inferior tympanic, and meningeal branches. This vessel is located inferiorly to the site of surgery.
    E. Terminal branches of the descending palatine artery could be encountered at the upper pole of

the palatine tonsil, but the main stem of the vessel would not be endangered in the surgical treatment here.
GAS 1034–1037; N 68, 65, 67, 71–72, 77, 79; ABR/McM 28, 39–40, 43

121. A. Infection in the "danger area of the face" can lead to cavernous sinus thrombosis because infection spreads from the nasal venous tributary to the angular vein, then to the superior ophthalmic vein, which passes into the cavernous sinus.
    B, C, D, and E. None of the other routes listed would be correct for drainage from the danger area of the face.
    GAS 907–908; N 99, 115, 147, 151; ABR/McM 47, 51, 59

122. C. The thrombus may pass through the central vein of the retina to reach the cavernous sinus. The patient would suffer blindness because the central vein is the only vein draining the retina and if it is occluded, blindness will ensue.
    A. The subarachnoid space would not be associated with the blindness experienced.
    B. Thrombus of the central artery would not cause cavernous sinus thrombophlebitis.
    D. The optic chiasm is a neural structure that does not transmit thrombi.
    E. The ciliary ganglion is a parasympathetic ganglion; a thrombus in the cavernous sinus would not pass through it.
    GAS 937; N 100, 103–104; ABR/McM 59, 79

123. B. Aqueous humor is secreted by the ciliary body into the posterior chamber of the eye, just behind the iris. The humor flows through the pupil into the anterior chamber and then is filtered by a trabecular meshwork, then drained by the scleral venous sinus (also called the canal of Schlemm).
    A. The iridoscleral angle is the angle formed between the iris and the sclera, where the scleral venous sinus or canal of Schlemm resides.
    C. The pupil is the opening in the iris, which leads from the posterior chamber to the anterior chamber.
    D. Vitreous humor, not aqueous humor, is found in the vitreous body.
    E. The lacrimal sac is involved with tears, not the secretion of aqueous humor.
    GAS 936; N 89; ABR/McM 51–54, 80

124. A. With all of the ventricles enlarged and no obvious single site of complete ventricular obstruction, the problem must be a condition of communicating hydrocephalus, with inadequate absorption through the arachnoid granulations into the superior sagittal sinus. There is no evidence of obstruction of CSF flow somewhere in the ventricular system.
    B, C, D, and E. The other choices listed are all examples of noncommunicating hydrocephalus that result from obstruction, not just overproduction or filtration problems (*GAS Fig. 8.35*).

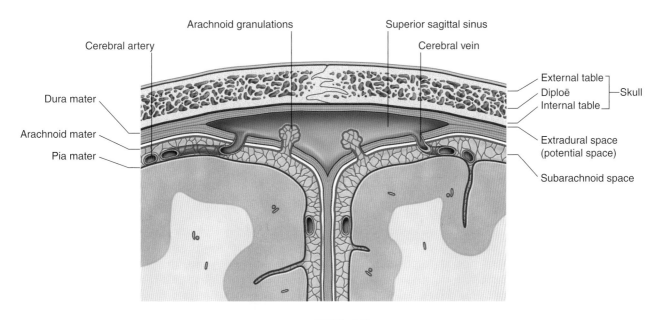

Arachnoid granulations

Superior sagittal sinus

Cerebral artery

Cerebral vein

External table
Diploë — Skull
Internal table

Dura mater

Arachnoid mater

Pia mater

Extradural space
(potential space)

Subarachnoid space

• *GAS* Fig. 8.35

GAS 865–866; N 157; ABR/McM 72

125. C. The superior sagittal sinus would most likely be the source of the bleeding because it attaches anteriorly to the crista galli and because of the slow nature of the bleed.

A. The middle meningeal artery would not be a good answer because its location is near the pterion on the temporal aspect of the skull but its bleeding would be profuse, not slow.

B. The great cerebral vein (of Galen) is located posteriorly in the cranial cavity and is not in the right location for an injury of this type to disrupt it.

D. The straight dural venous sinus is also posterior, receiving blood from the inferior sagittal sinus and the great cerebral vein (of Galen). It drains posteriorly to the confluence of sinuses (eponym: torcular Herophilus).

E. The superior ophthalmic vein drains from the orbit to the cavernous sinus; further, it is located inferiorly to the crista galli and is not directly related to the superior sagittal sinus.

GAS 852, 875–876, 1072–1073; N 111–112, 114; ABR/McM 47, 60–62

Answers 126–150

126. C. For proper movements of the eye to occur, all the cranial nerves that innervate the extraocular eye muscles are required (oculomotor, trochlear, and abducens nerves). The inferior division of the oculomotor innervates the inferior rectus, the medial rectus, and the inferior oblique. Lateral movement of the eye is initiated by the lateral rectus (abducens nerve), assisted thereafter by the superior oblique (trochlear nerve) and the inferior oblique (inferior division of oculomotor nerve). The inferior rectus (inferior division of the oculomotor nerve) balances the

upward deviation exerted by the superior rectus (superior division of the oculomotor nerve). The medial rectus (superior division of the oculomotor nerve) must relax to facilitate the lateral excursion.

A. B, and D. Include branches of the trigeminal nerve, which have no role in motor movement of the eye. E. The superior division of oculomotor nerve innervates the superior rectus and the levator palpebrae superioris and these muscles are not required for abduction of the eye.

GAS 926–929; N 96, 103; ABR/McM 51–54

127. E. The middle of the vocal cord would be the most likely location of the tumor because there is poor lymph drainage from this region.

A, B, C, and D. All other locations mentioned are drained by lymphatics. Areas above the vocal cords are drained by the superior deep cervical nodes, and areas below the vocal cords drain to pretracheal nodes before draining into the inferior deep cervical nodes.

GAS 1038–1039; N 85–86; ABR/McM 365, 367

128. B. When a berry aneurysm ruptures, the blood flows into the subarachnoid space and therefore mixes with CSF; thus, blood would be present in the CSF when a lumbar puncture is performed.

A. The pterion overlies the anterior branch of the middle meningeal vessels, and damage to these vessels would result in an epidural hematoma, with compression of the brain.

C. Leakage of branches of the middle meningeal vein within the temporal bone would cause blood vessels within the bone to leak, without direct connection to the CSF fluid.

D. A tear of a superior cerebral vein as it joins the superior sagittal sinus would lead to a subdural hematoma, in which the blood collects in the subdural space, without entry to CSF.

E. The occlusion of the internal carotid artery by way of clot would not lead to leakage of blood into the CSF.

GAS 873–874; N 147–154; ABR/McM 67

129. D. The nucleus ambiguus gives rise to efferent motor fibers of the vagus nerve, which supply the laryngeal and pharyngeal muscles. If supply to this region is interrupted, an individual loses the swallowing, cough, and gag reflexes.

A. The nucleus solitarius is located in the brainstem and is responsible for receiving general visceral sensation and taste from the facial, glossopharyngeal, and vagus nerves.

B. The trigeminal motor nucleus contains motor neurons that innervate the muscles of mastication, the tensor tympani, tensor veli palatini, mylohyoid, and anterior belly of the digastric.

C. The dorsal motor nucleus contains the cell bodies of preganglionic parasympathetic fibers of the vagus nerve innervating the heart muscle and smooth musculature and glands of the respiratory and intestinal tract.

E. The superior ganglion of the vagus contains cell bodies of general somatic afferent fibers, and the inferior ganglion of the vagus is chiefly visceral afferent in function concerning sensations (with the exclusion of painful sensation) from the heart, lungs, larynx, and alimentary tract.

GAS 826, 884–886; N137; ABR/McM 84

130. C. Just before it passes into the mandible to supply the lower teeth and chin, the inferior alveolar nerve gives rise to the mylohyoid nerve, a motor nerve supplying the **mylohyoid** and anterior belly of the digastric.

A. The geniohyoid muscle is innervated by motor fibers from spinal nerve C1 that run with the hypoglossal nerve.

B. The hyoglossus muscle is innervated by the hypoglossal nerve.

D. The stylohyoid muscle is innervated by the facial nerve.

E. The palatoglossus muscle is innervated by the vagus nerve.

GAS 975–978; N 133–134, 136–137, 139, 144, 146; ABR/McM 81–85

131. A. The superior cerebellar artery arises near the termination of the basilar artery, passes immediately below the oculomotor nerve, and eventually winds around the cerebral peduncle, close to the trochlear nerve, as it continues on toward the upper surface of the cerebellum where it will divide into branches that anastomose with the inferior cerebellar arteries. The trochlear nerve passes between the PCA and the superior cerebellar artery, and therefore a hematoma of the superior cerebellar artery can easily injure the trochlear nerve.

B. The abducens nerve originates from the anterior surface of the pons, thus is not within the vicinity of the superior cerebellar artery.

C and D. The facial and vestibulocochlear nerves both enter the skull via the internal acoustic meatus in the temporal bone and do not have an intimate relationship with the superior cerebellar artery.

E. The glossopharyngeal nerve passes through the jugular foramen, and as it exits from the skull it passes forward between the internal jugular vein and internal carotid artery.

GAS 868–871; N 147, 149–152, 154, 176; ABR/McM 59, 66–67

132. D. Subdural bleeding usually results from tears in veins that cross the subdural space, between the dura and the arachnoid. This bleeding may cause a gradual increase in intracranial pressure and may result in leakage of venous blood over the right cerebral hemisphere with a variable rate of progression.

A. A subarachnoid bleed is because of rupture of an artery into the subarachnoid space surrounding the brain, between the arachnoid membrane and the pia mater. Hydrocephalus may result if the subarachnoid bleeding or subsequent fibrosis creates obstructions to CSF flow through the subarachnoid space or drainage of the CSF.

B. Epidural bleeding results in most cases from tearing of the middle meningeal artery, and this rapidly expanding, space-occupying lesion can cause death within 12 hours.

C. Intracerebral bleeding into the brain parenchyma is focal bleeding from a blood vessel into the brain parenchyma, most likely caused by hypertension and/or atherosclerosis. Typical symptoms include focal neurologic deficits, with abrupt onset of headache, nausea, and impairment of consciousness.

E. Bleeding into the cerebral ventricular system may be because of trauma or hemorrhage of blood from nearby arteries, especially those related to the supply of the choroid plexus.

GAS 891–893; N 150–154; ABR/McM 66

133. B. The lateral pterygoid muscle is a muscle of mastication innervated by the lateral pterygoid nerve of the mandibular division of the trigeminal nerve. The lateral pterygoid acts to protrude the mandible and open the jaw.

A. The anterior portion of temporalis is a muscle of mastication innervated by the deep temporal nerves from the mandibular division of the trigeminal nerve that elevates the mandible when contracted.

C. The medial pterygoid muscle is a muscle of mastication innervated by the nerve to medial pterygoid from the mandibular division of the trigeminal nerve. This muscle closes the jaw and works with the contralateral medial pterygoid in side-to-side (grinding) jaw movements.

D. The masseter muscle is a muscle of mastication innervated by the masseteric branch of the mandibular division of the trigeminal nerve that specifically assists in chewing.

E. The platysma is a thin muscle of facial expression that lies within the superficial fascia of the neck and lower face. It is innervated by the cervical branch of the facial nerve. The platysma produces a slight wrinkling of the surface of the skin of the neck in an oblique direction, depresses the lower jaw, and draws down the lower lip and angle of the mouth. *GAS 977–978, 983; N 13, 49, 56–57, 59, 82, 133, 160; ABR/McM 42–44*

134. B. The inferior medial incisor teeth erupt first at 6 to 10 months. Teeth tend to erupt earlier in girls than in boys, and quite a range exists in the normal distribution curve.

A and C. The superior medial incisor teeth erupt at 8 to 12 months and superior lateral incisor teeth erupt at 9 to 13 months.

D. The inferior lateral incisor teeth erupt at 10 to 16 months.

E. The first molar teeth erupt at 13 to 19 months. *GAS 1114–1119; N 12, 52, 73–74; ABR/McM 13*

135. D. The sigmoid sinus collects venous blood from the transverse sinuses and empties it into a small cavity known as the superior jugular bulb, the inferior portion of which is located beneath the bony floor of the middle ear. A paraganglioma is a tumor that may originate from paraganglia cells found in the middle ear and on the superior jugular bulb. Tumors that originate from the superior jugular bulb can grow to fill the entire bulb and may effectively block blood returning to the heart from that side of the brain. Blood flow from the brain is gradually diverted toward the opposite sigmoid sinus and superior jugular bulb, causing the opposite venous system to expand and accommodate increased blood flow.

A. The cochlea and lateral semicircular canals are located in the inner ear and are not directly affected by such a tumor.

B. The internal carotid artery is related to the anterior wall of the middle ear cavity and is not likely to be affected by a tumor penetrating the middle ear.

C. The sigmoid venous sinus collects venous blood beneath the temporal bone and follows a tortuous (S-shaped) course to the jugular foramen where it becomes continuous with the internal jugular vein at the superior jugular bulb.

E. The aditus ad antrum is the entrance to the mastoid antrum, which is the common cavity in the mastoid process into which mastoid cells open. Below the aditus ad antrum is an elevation of bone, the pyramid of the stapes, which is occupied by the stapedius muscle.

GAS 874–876; N 64, 110, 114–115; ABR/McM 71

136. E. The lingual nerve supplies sensory innervation to the mucous membrane of the anterior two-thirds of the tongue and via chorda tympani fibers that join it in the infratemporal fossa, taste sensation to the anterior part of the tongue, and parasympathetic fibers to the submandibular and sublingual glands.

A. The chorda tympani branch of the facial nerve is responsible for carrying taste fibers from the anterior two-thirds of the tongue and preganglionic parasympathetic fibers for the submandibular ganglion. Injury to the chorda tympani branch of the facial nerve will result in loss of taste and salivary function.

B. This patient's loss of tongue sensation is likely because of nerve damage rather than lack of receptors.

C. Injury to the glossopharyngeal nerve would result in loss of general sensory and taste fibers from the posterior third of the tongue and parasympathetic supply for the parotid gland.

D. Injury to the superior laryngeal nerve, a branch of the vagus nerve, will result in loss of sensation from the laryngopharynx and the larynx above the vocal folds (*GAS Fig. 8.150A*).

GAS 1098, 1101, 1103; N 53, 68, 56–57, 59, 65, 69–70, 66, 82, 133–134, 142, 144–146; ABR/McM 29, 35, 81–82

137. A. Papilledema is optic disc swelling ("edema of the papilla") that is caused by increased intracranial or CSF pressure. If a lumbar puncture is performed in a patient with elevated CSF pressure and fluid is withdrawn from the lumbar cistern, the brain can become displaced caudally and the brainstem may be compressed by the herniated cerebellar tonsils.

B. Separation of the pars optica retinae anterior to the ora serrata, or retinal detachment, may result in vision loss or blindness.

C. A hemorrhage from medial retinal branches may result in damage to the fovea centralis and can result in macular degeneration.

D. Opacity of the lens (cataracts) will cause gradual yellowing and may reduce the perception of blue colors. Cataracts typically progress slowly to cause vision loss and are potentially blinding if untreated.

E. Compression of the optic disc, resulting from increased intrabulbar pressure, will lead to an excessive accumulation of serous fluid in the tissue space.

GAS 931; N 103; ABR/McM 43–44, 79

138. E. Within the cavernous sinus, the abducens nerve is in intimate contact with the internal carotid artery. Therefore, an aneurysm of the internal carotid artery could quickly cause tension or compression on the abducens nerve. This would result in ipsilateral paralysis of abduction of the pupil.

Otic ganglion (medial to [V₃]) Lesser petrosal nerve [IX]

Auriculotemporal nerve

Top of parotid gland

Petrotympanic fissure

Lingual nerve

Auriculotemporal nerve

Chorda tympani from [VII]

Lingual nerve

Tongue

Submandibular ganglion

Sublingual gland

——	Preganglionic parasympathetic fibers from glossopharyngeal nerve [IX]
··········	Postganglionic parasympathetic fibers from otic ganglion
——	Preganglionic parasympathetic fibers from facial nerve [VII]
··········	Postganglionic parasympathetic fibers from submandibular ganglion

Mylohyoid Submandibular gland

• *GAS* **Fig. 8.150A**

A. Inability to gaze downward and laterally would be because of the trochlear nerve, which is not in the cavernous sinus.

B. Complete ptosis would be a result of a complete lesion in the oculomotor nerve, which is not apparent here.

C. Bilateral loss of accommodation and loss of pupillary reflex would be the result of bilateral loss of the oculomotor nerve, which is not likely in this situation.

D. Ipsilateral loss of the consensual corneal reflex is a result of loss of both the ophthalmic division of the trigeminal nerve and the facial nerve, supplying the afferent and efferent limbs of the reflex, respectively.

GAS 876; N 115; ABR/McM 47, 59, 80

139. D. It is necessary to anesthetize the conjunctival covering of the sclera, which is supplied by the nasociliary branch of the ophthalmic division of the trigeminal nerve. To do that, the needle should be placed through the upper eyelid deeply toward the orbital apex to infiltrate the nasociliary nerve, and also between the orbital septum and the palpebral musculature laterally to anesthetize lateral sensory supply from the lacrimal nerve and (perhaps) twigs from the maxillary division of the trigeminal nerve.

A and E. Both these answers result in puncturing of the sclera and would most likely cause further damage to the eye.

B and C. The fossa for the lacrimal sac, which is occupied by the lacrimal sac portion of the nasolacrimal duct, is too medial, whereas the supraorbital foramen is above the eye. Injections into either location would not result in anesthetizing of the sclera. *GAS 931–935; N 20, 61, 97, 132–133, 142–143; ABR/McM 44, 51, 80–81*

140. E. During a puncture wound as described in this case, passing up from below the chin, the nail would pierce the genioglossus last.

A, B, C, and D. The nail would first pierce the platysma, then the anterior belly of the digastric, then the mylohyoid, then the geniohyoid, and finally the genioglossus. *GAS 896, 899, 995–997; N 32, 36, 38; ABR/McM 28, 205*

141. A. The facial nerve passes through the parotid gland and is therefore at risk during surgery of the parotid gland. Since this patient's symptoms involved paralysis of the muscles of the lower lip, the branch of the facial nerve that supplies these muscles, the marginal mandibular branch, is the one that has suffered the iatrogenic injury. The muscles controlling the lower lip include depressor labii inferioris, depressor anguli oris, and mentalis.

B. Zygomatic branch of facial nerve runs across the zygomatic bone to supply the orbicularis oculi muscle. Damage to this nerve would cause weakness in closing one's eye tightly.

C. Mandibular division of trigeminal nerve is the largest division of the trigeminal nerve, consisting of both motor and sensory innervation. The motor component consists of the muscles of mastication, the mylohyoid, the anterior belly of the digastric muscle, and tensor tympani and tensor veli palatini muscles. The sensory component includes branches for the auriculotemporal, lingual, inferior alveolar, and buccal nerves.

D. The buccal branch the facial nerve is a motor nerve that controls several muscles used in facial expressions, but none of which directly control the lower lip.

E. The buccal nerve is a branch of the mandibular division, which provides sensory to the skin of the cheek and the mucosa of the oral vestibule.

GAS 900–901; N 54; ABR/McM 40

142. A. During embryologic development of the pituitary gland, an outgrowth from the roof of the pharynx (Rathke pouch) grows cephalad and forms the anterior lobe (pars tuberalis) of the pituitary gland. A craniopharyngioma is a tumor derived from the epithelium of the Rathke pouch. It is slow growing, found in the suprasellar location, and more common supratentorial tumor in children.

B. Pars tuberalis is a sheath that wraps the anterior lobe of the pituitary gland; it is not associated with craniopharyngiomas.

C. The interventricular foramen (of Monro) is a bilateral connection between the lateral ventricles and the third ventricle that is not involved in formation of craniopharyngiomas.

D. The alar plate is part of the dorsal neural tube and a caudal portion will eventually form sensory axons of the spinal cord. It is involved in general somatic and visceral sensory impulses and not associated with craniopharyngiomas.

E. Diencephalon is the portion of the embryonic neural tube that gives rise to the thalamus, hypothalamus, pineal gland, and posterior lobe of the pituitary gland. It is not associated with craniopharyngiomas.

GAS 854–855; N 52; ABR/McM 47

143. A. In holoprosencephaly, loss of midline structures results in malformations of the brain and face. There is a single telencephalic vesicle, fused eyes, and a single nasal chamber. Also, there is often hypoplasia of the olfactory bulbs, olfactory tracts, and corpus callosum.

B. Children with Smith-Lemli-Opitz syndrome have craniofacial and limb defects and 5% have holoprosencephaly.

C. Schizencephaly is rare and is characterized by large clefts in the cerebral hemispheres, which in some cases cause a loss in brain tissue.

D. Exencephaly is caused by failure of the cephalic part of the neural tube to close; therefore, the skull does not close, leaving the brain exposed.

E. Meningoencephalocele is a deficit of the cranium involving the squamous part of the occipital bone and, in some cases, the posterior aspect of the foramen magnum. It can include the meninges if the herniation or protruding brain includes part of the ventricular system.

N 117; ABR/McM 46

144. C. Usually, deficits of the cranium involve the squamous part of the occipital bone and, in some cases, the posterior aspect of the foramen magnum. If the herniation or protruding brain includes part of the ventricular system (most likely the posterior horn of the lateral ventricles), then it is referred to as meningohydroencephalocele. The deficit in the squamous part of the occipital bone usually occurs at the posterior fontanelle of the skull.

A. B, D, and E. These portions of the skull are not typically involved in cranial defects.

GAS 856–857; N 15; ABR/McM 27

145. B. The rostral neuropore closes during the fourth week of development. If this does not occur, the forebrain primordium is abnormal and the calvaria or vault fails to develop.

A. Toxoplasmosis infection during embryologic development leads to microcephaly, in which the brain and calvaria are small in size. These patients usually have mental retardation because of an undeveloped brain.

C. An ossification defect in the bones of the skull is often a result of hydrocephalus.

D. Caudal displacement of the cerebellar structures would not lead to an undeveloped calvaria or vault.

E. Maternal alcohol abuse leads to intrauterine growth restriction (IUGR), causing microcephaly and mental retardation.

N 120; ABR/McM 60

146. B. Holoprosencephaly is caused by failure of the prosencephalon to properly divide into two cerebral hemispheres. In severe cases, this is incompatible with life, but in less severe cases, such as the one presented here, babies have normal or near-normal brain development, sometimes with facial abnormalities. In this case, the child has a myelomeningocele. Almost all of these patients with this condition have a concomitant Chiari II malformation.

A. Chiari II malformation is where the cerebellar vermis, fourth ventricle, and associated brainstem are herniated through the foramen magnum and into the upper cervical spinal canal.

C. Smith-Lemli-Opitz syndrome is characterized by craniofacial and limb defects; 5% of whom have holoprosencephaly. D. Schizencephaly is characterized by large clefts in the cerebral hemispheres.

E. Exencephaly is a condition where the brain is exposed because of failure of the skull to close. It is typically because of failure of cephalic portion of neural tube to close.

N 116; ABR/McM 66

147. A. Congenital deafness is because of a maldevelopment of the conducting system of the middle and external ear or neurosensory structures of the inner

ear. **Rubella infection** during a critical time of ear development can lead to a malformed spiral organ (neurosensory hearing loss) or congenital fixation of the stapes, resulting in conducting hearing loss.

  B. Failure of the second pharyngeal arch to form would lead to a middle ear without a stapes bone. However, in congenital deafness, there is a fixation of the stapes.

  C. Failure of the dorsal portion of the first pharyngeal cleft would lead to undeveloped malleus and incus. These are not affected in congenital deafness, however.

  D. Abnormal development of the auricular hillocks does not lead to deafness but is a marker for other potential congenital anomalies.

  E. (As explained in B and C)

  N 105; ABR/McM 57

148. **A.** With congenital cataracts, the lens appears opaque and grayish white and blindness will result. Infection by teratogenic agents such as **rubella virus** (German measles) can cause congenital cataracts. This infection can affect the development of the lens, which has a critical period of development between the fourth and seventh week.

  B. Choroid fissure failure would lead to coloboma, a condition that can lead to a cleft and eye abnormalities but not congenital cataracts.

  C. A persistent hyaloid artery would not lead to a cataract but rather a freely moving, wormlike structure (as interpreted by the patient) projecting on the optic disc.

  D. Toxoplasmosis infection would lead to microcephaly and eventually mental retardation because of an undeveloped brain.

  E. CMV would cause microcephaly and mental retardation.

  N 102; ABR/McM 51

149. **D.** A mutation of the *PAX6* gene usually results in congenital aphakia (absence of the lens) and aniridia (absence of the iris).

  A. Cyclopia is a condition in which there is a single eye and is usually caused by a mutation of the *SHH* gene, leading to a loss of midline tissue and underdevelopment of the forebrain and frontonasal prominence.

  B. Coloboma occurs if the choroid fissure fails to fuse, which is usually caused by a mutation of the *PAX2* gene.

  C. Anophthalmia is a disorder in which there is a complete absence of the eye.

  E. In microphthalmia, the eye is small in its development, typically less than two-thirds its normal size. This condition usually results from an infection such as CMV and toxoplasmosis.

  GAS 1063–1064; N 102; ABR/McM 51

150. **A.** In hemifacial microsomia the craniofacial anomalies that usually occur unilaterally and involve small and flat maxillary, temporal, and zygomatic bones.

Ear and eye anomalies also occur with this syndrome. Ear abnormalities include tumors and dermoids of the eyeball.

  B. Treacher Collins syndrome is normally characterized by malar hypoplasia (caused by undeveloped zygomatic bones), mandibular hypoplasia, downslanted palpebral fissures, lower eyelid colobomas, and malformed ears.

  C. Robin Sequence is caused by an altered first arch structure, with the development of the mandible most affected. Infants with Robin Sequence normally have micrognathia, cleft palate, and glossoptosis.

  D and E. DiGeorge syndrome is a severe craniofacial defect that includes velocardiofacial syndrome and conotruncal anomalies face syndrome. It is characterized by cleft palate, cardiac defects, abnormal face, thymic hypoplasia, and hypocalcemia.

  N 11, 43, 215; ABR/McM 30

Answers 151–175

151. **A.** Abnormal face, cardiac defects, thymic hypoplasia, cleft palate, and hypocalcemia are characteristics of DiGeorge syndrome. A deletion of the long arm of chromosome 22 (**22q11**) causes this developmental defect.

  B. A defect of the *SHH* gene can lead to cyclopia. *PAX2* and *PAX6* gene mutations lead to malformations of the eye.

  C and D. Specifically, PAX2 mutations are responsible for coloboma, and PAX6 mutations characterize congenital aphakia and aniridia. E. Turner syndrome (47XXY) is characterized by a webbed neck and small stature.

  N 11, 43, 215; ABR/McM 30

152. **A.** The first pharyngeal arch, which is often associated with the mandible, is responsible for development of Meckel cartilage, malleus, incus, and mandible. Additionally, it is innervated by the trigeminal nerve, specifically the mandibular division that innervates the muscles of mastication. This patient presents with features characteristic of developmental defects in the first arch.

  B. The second pharyngeal arch gives rise to the stapes, styloid process, lesser cornu, Reichert cartilage, and the upper half of the hyoid bone. It is innervated by the facial nerve.

  C. The third pharyngeal arch is responsible for formation of the greater cornu and the lower half of the hyoid bone and is innervated by the glossopharyngeal nerve.

  D and E. The fourth and sixth pharyngeal arches give rise to the laryngeal cartilages, in addition to being innervated by the vagus nerve.

  N 11, 105; ABR/McM 21

153. **B.** The maxillary sinus arises late in fetal development and is the only sinus present at birth.

  A. The frontal sinus develops at approximately 7 years of age.

C. The sphenoidal sinus develops during adolescence.
D and E. The ethmoid cells develop at approximately 2 years of age.
GAS 1063–1064; N 87; ABR/McM 47

154. A. Meroencephaly often results from a failure of the rostral neuropore to close during the fourth week of development. The calvaria (i.e., skullcap) is absent, with a resultant extrusion of the brain from the cranium. Defects are often found along the vertebral column as well.

    B. CMV infection can cause microcephaly, in which both the brain and cranium are drastically reduced in size. However, there is no extrusion of the brain from the cranium.

    C. The hypophyseal diverticulum is associated with the pituitary gland and usually regresses to leave only a remnant stalk. Failure of this diverticulum to develop would not be associated with meroencephaly.

    D. Failure of neural arch development would affect the vertebral column, not the cranium.

    E. Neural crest cells give rise to a variety of cell types, and abnormal formation would likewise not be associated with meroencephaly.

    N 113; ABR/McM 62

155. D. The retropharyngeal space extends from the inferior aspect of the skull to the posterior mediastinum behind the esophagus. An infection or abscess in this space could thus travel toward the posterior mediastinum. The retropharyngeal space is enclosed between the buccopharyngeal layer of visceral fascia covering the posterior wall of the pharynx and the alar fascia. The buccopharyngeal fascia begins superiorly at the base of the skull and merges with the fascia of the esophagus before continuing into the thoracic cavity. The buccopharyngeal fascia also invests the superior pharyngeal constrictor and buccinator muscles. The alar fascia is formed from bilateral anterior extensions of the prevertebral fascia. The alar fascia is continuous with the carotid sheath and provides the posterior and inferior boundary for what is referred to as the true retropharyngeal space. Attachments of the alar fascia to the buccopharyngeal fascia result in separation of the danger space from the true retropharyngeal space.

    B. The pretracheal fascia is the anterior layer of the visceral fascia that encloses the trachea, esophagus, and thyroid gland.

    C. The prevertebral fascia invests the vertebral column and the intrinsic muscles of the neck and back. The prevertebral fascia is separated from the visceral fascia by the alar fascia, therefore there is no potential spaces between these fascial layers.

    A. Between the alar fascia and the more posterior prevertebral fascia covering the skeletal musculature is the inferior portion of the retropharyngeal space referred to as the so-called danger space of the neck. This space is continuous superiorly to the base of the skull and continues inferiorly through the posterior mediastinum to the level of the respiratory diaphragm.

    E. The alar fascia separates the buccopharyngeal and prevertebral fasciae (*GAS* Fig. 8.163).

    GAS 991–992; N 87; ABR/McM 47

156. A. An inferior fracture of the orbit would likely damage the infraorbital nerve. A blow-out fracture often results in a displaced orbital wall, and in this case, the floor or inferior wall. The infraorbital nerve leaves the skull immediately inferior to the inferior aspect of the orbital margin, via the infraorbital foramen, after traveling through the floor of the orbit within the infraorbital groove and canal. Thus, this nerve is the most likely to be damaged.

    B and C. The frontal nerve courses superiorly over the orbital contents before dividing into the supratrochlear and supraorbital nerves.

    D. The inferior alveolar nerve originates from the mandibular division of trigeminal nerve and is not close to the orbit therefore not likely to be damaged.

    E. The optic nerve is located behind the eyeball and travels posteriorly away from the orbit to enter the cranium. These nerves are therefore unlikely to be damaged.

    GAS 904; N 63; ABR/McM 80–82

157. C. Rinne test is often employed during physical examination to determine possible conduction hearing loss. A tuning fork is struck and placed on the mastoid process for maximum bone conduction to the inner ear structures. It is then placed near the external ear until the patient can no longer detect vibrations. In a normal healthy patient the air conduction will be better than the bone conduction. Rinne test is often used in conjunction with the Weber test to rule out sensorineural hearing loss.

    A, B, D, and E. The tuning fork is not placed on any of these areas during the Rinne test.

    GAS827, 1110; N 49; ABR/McM 4, 7, 9, 16

158. A. The right and left recurrent laryngeal nerves loop around the right subclavian artery and the arch of the aorta, respectively. These nerves then travel superiorly in the tracheoesophageal groove to the larynx. Damage to the recurrent laryngeal nerve as a result of surgical intervention or the presence of a tumor in the tracheoesophageal groove would render the patient hoarse. This hoarseness is because of a lack of innervation by the recurrent laryngeal nerve to most of the muscles of the larynx.

    B. Damage to the internal laryngeal nerve would cause a loss of sensation above the vocal cords, in addition to a loss of taste on the epiglottis.

    C. The vagus nerve gives rise to the recurrent laryngeal nerves; damage to this nerve, however,

Buccopharyngeal fascia
(posterior portion of
pretracheal layer)

Investing layer

Infrahyoid muscles

Pretracheal fascia

Pretracheal space

Manubrium of sternum

Prevertebral layer

Retropharyngeal space

Fascial space within prevertebral layer

• *GAS* Fig. 8.163

would result in numerous symptoms beyond just hoarseness.

D. Damage to the external laryngeal nerve, which can occur during thyroidectomy, will result in a loss of innervation to the cricothyroid muscle, with resultant vocal weakness. Patients with this lesion will often present with a fatigued voice.

E. Irritation or compression of the phrenic nerve can cause problems with breathing and triggered hiccup reflex not painful swallowing or hoarseness

GAS 999, 1000, 1023, 1058; N 234–235; ABR/McM 47, 49, 50, 84

159. B. Diploic veins are responsible for communication between the veins of the scalp and the venous sinuses of the brain. Diploic veins are situated within the layers of bone of the skull and connect the emissary veins of the scalp to the venous sinuses located between two layers of dura. The diploe is of clinical significance in that the diploic veins within this layer provide a pathway of communication between the veins of the scalp and underlying venous sinuses of the brain, by means of emissary veins. The emissary veins and diploe provide a potential vascular pathway of infection.

A and E. The supratrochlear and supraorbital veins are located superficially on the scalp, immediately superior to the upper eyelid, and do not communicate directly with the venous sinuses of the brain.

C. The anterior cerebral vein is an intracranial vein and, as such, does not maintain a direct communication with the external veins of the scalp.

D. The superior sagittal sinus receives blood from the superior cerebral, diploic, and emissary veins; however, it does not provide a pathway of communication to the veins of the scalp.

GAS 874; N 32–33; ABR/McM 11

160. C. The oculomotor nerve passes between the posterior cerebral artery (PCA) and the superior cerebellar artery near the junction of the midbrain and pons. A. Although the trochlear nerve could be compressed by the superior cerebellar artery, it would not likely be damaged by an aneurysm of the PCA.

B and D. The abducens nerve is located in the pons, and the vagus is situated near the postolivary sulcus in the medulla. Neither of these nerves is likely to be compressed by the arteries mentioned here because of their more distal location.

E. The optic nerve arises near the arterial circle of Willis close to the internal carotid artery. Its location would thus prevent compression following an aneurysm at the PCA and superior cerebellar artery.

GAS 838, 883, 884, 886, 889–890, 932; N 9, 42, 61–64, 84; ABR/McM 80

161. C. A blow-out fracture of the medial wall of the orbit would likely render the medial rectus muscle nonfunctional by entrapment of the muscle between the fracture fragments of the cracked medial wall formed by the fragile ethmoid bone. The medial rectus is responsible for adduction of the eye, but in this case the muscle acts as a tether or anchor on the eyeball, preventing lateral excursion (abduction) of the eye. There is no nerve damage here, and the muscle is not paralyzed.

A. The lateral rectus is responsible for abduction of the eye, and the inferior rectus rotates the eyeball downward. Damage to these muscles or their nerve supply would result in an inability to move the eye laterally and inferiorly, respectively.

B and E. Inferior rectus muscle is located at the floor of the orbit and will be responsible for the eye movement deficits seen in this patient.

D. The superior oblique muscle located at the roof of the orbit. This muscle abducts, depresses, and internally rotates the eye.
GAS 927–929; N 13; ABR/McM 52–53, 80

162. **A.** The inferior rectus and inferior oblique muscles are entrapped in the fissure between the parts of the fractured orbital floor. Normally, the superior rectus and the inferior oblique are responsible for an upward movement of the eyeball. In this case, however, the broken orbital plate of the maxilla has snared or entrapped the inferior rectus and inferior oblique muscles, causing them to act as anchors on the eyeball, preventing upward movement of the eye. The muscles are not necessarily damaged and there is no apparent nerve injury in this patient. Freeing the muscles from the bone will allow free movement of the eye again, barring any other injury.
B. Damage to the medial and inferior recti would result in a laterally and superiorly deviated eye.
C. D, and E. The inferior oblique rotates the eye upward and laterally. Damage to this muscle would therefore cause the pupil to be directed somewhat downward. Damage to the medial rectus would result in lateral deviation of the eyeball. The inferior rectus is responsible for downward movement of the eye, and damage to this muscle would result in a superiorly deviated eyeball or an inability to gaze upward symmetrically with both eyes.
GAS 927–929; N 33, 40, 58, 82, 92, 141, 236, 243

163. **A.** A herpes rash on the dorsum of the nose is known as Hutchinson sign. This indicates that the virus is located in cell bodies of the ophthalmic division of the trigeminal nerve. This nerve branches into nasociliary, frontal, and lacrimal branches. The nasociliary nerve has direct branches that carry sensory innervation from the eye. The nasociliary nerve also gives off the ethmoidal nerves that innervate the superior nasal mucosa, in addition to providing the origin of the dorsal nasal nerve.
B. The supratrochlear nerve is a branch of the frontal nerve and carries sensory innervation from the skin superior to the orbit.
C. The infraorbital nerve is a branch from the maxillary division of the trigeminal nerve and carries sensory innervation from the skin of the face between the orbit and the upper lips.
D. Posterior ethmoidal nerve is a branch from the nasociliary nerve that provides sensory innervation to the sphenoidal sinus and posterior ethmoidal cells.
E. Anterior ethmoidal nerve provides sensory innervation to the nasal cavity and the dorsum of the nose. The anterior ethmoidal nerve is also a branch from the nasociliary nerve.
GAS 935–936, 1075; N 111, 113; ABR/McM 44, 51, 80–81

164. **A.** Anesthetics are injected into the submuscular layer of delicate (areolar) connective tissue, the layer that contains nerves of the eyelid. This space is continuous with the "danger zone" of the scalp. A blow to the forehead can result in a hematoma known as a "black eye," with the passage of blood into the submuscular space. Infections can, likewise, pass within this space. One can insert a needle through the upper eyelid, near the orbital margin, and then direct it deeply toward the orbital apex. The anesthetic can then infiltrate the branches of the ophthalmic division of the trigeminal nerve, including its nasociliary branch, resulting in anesthesia of the area.
B. The infraorbital nerve branches from the maxillary branch of the trigeminal nerve after the later exits the infraorbital canal. Injection of anesthesia near the orbital margin is less likely to affect this nerve.
C. The anterior ethmoidal nerve provides sensory innervation to the nasal cavity and dorsum of the nose. It is a continuation of the nasociliary nerve after it enters the anterior ethmoidal foramen. The anterior ethmoidal nerve would not be anesthetized by an orbital margin injection.
D. The frontal nerve is a branch of the ophthalmic nerve that gives rise to the supraorbital and supratrochlear nerve.
E. The optic nerve is the second cranial nerve and is located at the back of the eye. It plays a role in the transmission of visual information from the retina to the brain. The optic nerve would not be affected by an orbital margin injection at the upper eyelid.
GAS 838, 887, 902, 904, 933–936, 1074, 1075; N 96–97; ABR/McM 44, 56, 81

165. **A.** Paralysis of the trochlear nerve results in loss of ability for the affected eye to be directed downward when the pupil is in the adducted position (the primary action of the superior oblique muscle). The patient must tilt her head toward the opposite side to allow the two pupils to converge on an object on the floor. Paralysis of the trochlear nerve is not unusual when a patient's head has hit the dashboard in an automobile crash—the delicate nerve is easily torn where it pierces the dura of the tentorium cerebelli at the tentorial notch because the brain and brainstem move forward and backward with the force of impact (a "coup-contrecoup" injury).
B, C, D, and E. The most common site of injury to the trochlear nerve after a traumatic injury is at the point where it pierces the dura of the tentorium cerebelli as explained above.
GAS 862; N 95, 132, 160; ABR/McM 44, 59–61

166. **A.** The dural covering of the optic nerve is connected to the annular tendon which serves as the origin of the rectus muscles; therefore, when there is an

inflammation of the optic nerve, contractions of the rectus muscles can evoke severe pain.

B. Inflammation affecting all nerves innervating the muscles of the eye is highly unlikely.

C. Generalized inflammation causing ocular muscle contraction is unlikely.

D. The nasociliary nerve is a branch of the ophthalmic nerve. It gives off a number of branches such as the long ciliary, posterior and anterior ethmoidal, and infratrochlear nerves and does not play a role in eye movement.

E. Constriction or occlusion of the ophthalmic artery can cause loss of vision which is not observed in this patient

N 96, 132, 160; ABR/McM 54

167. D. Toxoplasmosis infection is caused by the parasite *Toxoplasma gondii*, which is associated with undercooked meat and the feces of cats. Once a person is exposed to toxoplasmosis, immunity is developed. However, the biggest concern is when exposure occurs in a pregnant woman who has no previous exposure. Congenital malformations such as microphthalmia can occur if the infection is passed on to the fetus.

A. Congenital rubella infection is likely to occur when a pregnant woman lacks immunization with the Measles, Mumps, and Rubella (MMR) vaccine prior to pregnancy. The MMR vaccine is a live vaccine and should not be given in pregnancy. Neonates exposed to the virus in-utero are more likely to have symptoms such as sensorineural deafness, eye abnormalities, and patent ductus arteriosus.

B. Failure of the choroid fissure to close will result in the formation of a coloboma.

C. The hyaloid artery is a branch of the ophthalmic artery which usually regresses prior to birth. Sometimes pieces of the hyaloid artery may persist as "floaters."

E. EBV is associated with ocular malformations, however infection or reactivation of the virus during pregnancy does not yield any specific patterns of congenital malformations

N 20, 61, 97, 132, 133, 142, 143; ABR/McM 54

168. A. At the point where the facial nerve exits the stylomastoid foramen it is most susceptible to shearing forces. In the absence of a skull fracture whereby the facial nerve can be damaged within the facial canal, the nerve is most commonly injured as it exits the stylomastoid foramen. In infants, in whom the mastoid process has not yet developed, the facial nerve lies unprotected, just beneath the skin.

B. Injury to the facial nerve inferior to the parotid gland would only affect platysma and perhaps the muscles of the lower lip.

C. There are several branches of the facial nerve anterior to the parotid gland. Given the mechanism of the infant's injury, it would be unlikely for injury

to an individual branch of the facial nerve anterior to the parotid gland to have occurred.

D. An injury of the facial nerve proximal to the stylomastoid foramen will also impair the function of the chorda tympani. Given the mechanism of the patient's injury, this type of facial nerve injury is unlikely to occur.

E. Injury to specific terminal branches of the facial nerve such as the mandibular and buccal branches is not likely to occur with mechanism of injury presented in this patient, because the location of these nerves are far from the site of injury.

GAS 858, 910, 959; N 9, 59, 61, 64, 97, 115, 132–133, 142–146; ABR/McM 9, 14, 23, 57

169. B. The auriculotemporal nerve, a branch of the mandibular division of the trigeminal nerve (CV V3) leads into the parotid gland, and its compression in mumps can be associated with severe pain. The compressive effects are due in large part to the continuity of the fascial capsule of the parotid gland with the tough layer of superficial investing fascia of the neck, a layer that is almost nondistensible. When the gland swells, sensory fibers for pain are triggered rapidly, and can be referred to the ear. None of the other nerves listed supply the parotid gland.

A. The facial nerve is a motor nerve, not sensory, as it passes through the parotid gland, hence no painful sensation will be experienced by the patient secondary to compression of this nerve.

C. The lesser petrosal nerve carries secretory fibers from the tympanic plexus to the parotid gland. It does not provide any generalized sensory innervation to the region of the parotid gland.

D and E. The chorda tympani originates from the facial nerve as it passes inferiorly in its facial canal and it provides sensory innervation to the anterior two-thirds portion of the tongue via the lingual nerve. Painful sensations over the parotid gland would not be observed because of compression of these nerves.

GAS 901, 904, 974, 975, 1093; N 97, 114–115, 155–156; ABR/McM 29, 38–40, 42, 56–57, 81–82

170. B. Hydrops (edema) results from accumulation of excessive fluid in the endolymphatic sac. Labyrinthine hydrops or endolymphatic hydrops is known as Ménière disease. This disease can result in hearing loss, roaring noises in the ear, and episodic dizziness (vertigo) associated with nausea and vomiting. About 10% of patients require surgical intervention for persistent, incapacitating vertigo; others are treated with diuretics, low salt intake, and reduction of stimulants like caffeine to lower the volume of body fluids and alleviate the symptoms of Ménière disease.

A, C, D, and E. As stated above, Ménière disease is a result of excessive endolymph accumulation in the endolymphatic sac. None of these other structures are involved in endolymph accumulation.

GAS 957; N 96–97, 132; ABR/McM 57–58

171. D. The superior thyroid vein is a tributary to the internal jugular vein; it accompanies the superior thyroid artery. The middle thyroid vein is typically a short, direct tributary to the internal jugular vein. The inferior thyroid vein usually drains vertically downward to one or both of the brachiocephalic veins. The superior and middle thyroid veins can be torn in thyroid surgery, perhaps admitting an air bubble (because of negative pressure in the veins) that can ascend in the internal jugular vein into the skull, with deleterious or lethal results.

A, B, and C. The most likely cause of air bubbles in this patient is an injury to the superior or middle thyroid vein.

E. The inferior thyroid vein usually drains into the left brachiocephalic vein. An injury to this structure is less likely to be a cause of air bubbles on CT scan.
GAS 1008, 1009; N 87; ABR/McM 28–30, 32–33

172. C. The cricothyroid artery is a small branch of the superior thyroid artery. It anastomoses with the cricothyroid artery of the opposite side at the upper end of the median cricothyroid ligament, a common site for establishing an emergency airway. The cricothyroid artery can be pushed into the airway during a cricothyrotomy. The vessel(s) can bleed directly into the trachea which can go unnoticed by medical personnel, with potentially fatal aspiration of blood by the patient.

A. The superior thyroid artery branches off the external carotid artery typically at the level of the hyoid bone. It provides the majority of the blood supply to the thyroid gland and is located laterally to the incision point of the cricothyrotomy procedure. Hence, it is less likely to be injured.

B. The inferior thyroid artery typically arises from the thyrocervical trunk and ascends into the posterior surface of the thyroid gland. It is less likely to be injured because of its location.

D. The superior laryngeal artery originates from the superior thyroid artery and courses beneath the thyrohyoid to pierce the thyrohyoid membrane laterally. It is less likely to be injured by a midline cricothyrotomy.

E. The suprahyoid artery is a branch of the lingual artery and runs superficially to the hyoglossus muscle. It is not in the vicinity of the cricothyrotomy procedure.
GAS 837, 1046; N 17, 19, 54, BP29, 134, 136; ABR/McM 34

173. C. An incision at the level of the third and fourth tracheal cartilages usually results in the fewest complications *during a tracheotomy*. The isthmus of the thyroid gland (a richly vascular structure) is usually at the level of the second tracheal cartilage and this incision is just inferior to that. However, other vascular structures such as a thyroidea ima artery or tributaries of the external jugular veins make a tracheostomy a surgical procedure to be performed with care.

A, B, D, and E. Because of the highly vascularized nature of the thyroid gland, incision at the any other level might cause injury to important neurovascular structures.
GAS 1054; N 9, 25, 53, 56–57, 59, 82–83, 133, 136, 145; ABR/McM 36, 37, 209

174. A. The uvula would move toward the intact right side. This is because the intact levator veli palatini would be unopposed by the opposite, paralyzed left levator veli palatini.

B, D, and E. The tensor veli palatini are one of the 5 paired muscles of the soft palate. They act to tense the palatine aponeurosis which helps to open the auditory tube during swallowing. This allows for pressure equalization between the pharynx and middle ear. They do not play a role in palatal elevation.

C. A paralyzed right levator veli palatini will cause elevation of the soft palate on the left.
GAS 834, 971, 1033, 1096, 1098; N 109; ABR/McM 10, 47

175. B. If the left abducens nerve is injured, there will be a loss of function of the left lateral rectus muscle so the patient will be unable to abduct his left eye to the same degree as the unaffected right eye.

A. The trochlear nerve supplies the superior oblique muscle, which if injured would cause the patient to lose the ability to turn the pupil downward when it is in the adducted position. As an example, the affected patient could not turn the pupil to look downward to the left if the right trochlear nerve were paralyzed. This deficiency can make it difficult for individuals to descend stairs if they have trochlear nerve palsy.

C and E. If the oculomotor nerve were injured, the pupil would be directed "down and out" because of unopposed actions of the lateral rectus and superior oblique, which are innervated by the abducens and trochlear nerves, respectively.

D. If the optic nerve were injured, the patient would have blindness in the affected eye. If the oculomotor and abducens nerves were injured, the patient would have only the actions of the superior oblique muscle, and the eye would be directed downward and outward from the position of forward gaze.
GAS 883–884, 887, 889–890, 933; N 38, 84, 87–89, 92, 204, 215, 241; ABR/McM 59, 61, 52–54, 66–67, 80, 83, 86

Answers 176–200

176. D. The accommodation reflex is performed by constriction of the pupil when trying to focus on a near object. This function is controlled by the parasympathetic nerve fibers carried in the oculomotor nerve from the Edinger-Westphal nucleus of the midbrain that synapse in the ciliary ganglion. Postganglionic axons act on the sphincter pupillae muscle to cause reduction in pupil diameter and on the ciliary muscle to cause relaxation of the suspensory ligament of the lens, allowing the lens to adopt a more spherical shape for near focusing. If there is a lack of accommodation, it means the action of the ciliary muscle is compromised. The ciliary muscle also gets parasympathetic innervation by postganglionic neurons evoked from the ciliary ganglion by GVE fibers of oculomotor nerve whose cell bodies are located in the Edinger-Westphal nucleus.

A. The superior salivatory nucleus is involved with lacrimation and salivation, not the ciliary muscle and accommodation.

B. The SCG is a sympathetic ganglion; its postganglionic axons innervate the dilator pupillae muscle, which causes mydriasis, but not the miosis of accommodation.

C. The nervus intermedius is a part of the facial nerve that contains special sensory, somatic sensory, and secretomotor fibers. It innervates the sublingual, submandibular, and lacrimal ducts and plays no role in the accommodation reflex.

E. The trigeminal ganglion is a sensory ganglion and does not have parasympathetic fibers and does not innervate the ciliary muscle for accommodation (*GAS* Fig. 8.107).
N 83, 87; ABR/McM 79

177. **A.** An acoustic neuroma (vestibular schwannoma or neurolemmoma) is a benign tumor of the vestibulocochlear nerve (CN VIII), which causes compression of the facial nerve (CN VII). The vestibulocochlear nerve leads from the inner ear to the brain. Although many such tumors will not grow or grow very slowly, growth can in some cases result ultimately in brainstem compression (as in this example), hydrocephalus, brainstem herniation, and death. It is diagnosed on MRI with gadolinium contrast as shown. Extension of the neuroma into the right internal acoustic meatus can be seen on the coronal MRI (see arrow in Fig. 7.9). The exact cause of the tumor is unknown; most people with acoustic neuromas (vestibular schwannoma) are diagnosed between the ages of 30 and 60. Because of advances in microsurgery, including intraoperative monitoring of facial and cochlear function, the risks of facial paralysis and hearing loss have been greatly reduced. Many acoustic neuromas can now be treated effectively with both surgery and targeted radiation therapy (e.g., gamma knife). The outcomes for those with small acoustic neuromas are better, whereas those with neuromas larger than 2.5 cm are likely to experience significant hearing loss postsurgery.
B. C, D, and E. Acoustic neuroma does not cause compression of any of these other cranial nerves
GAS 838, 883, 884, 887–892, 901, 905–906, 910, 958–960, 1002; N 208

178. **A.** Pharyngeal (branchial) cleft cysts are the most common congenital cause of a neck mass. They are epithelial cysts that arise anterior to the superior third of the sternocleidomastoid muscle from a

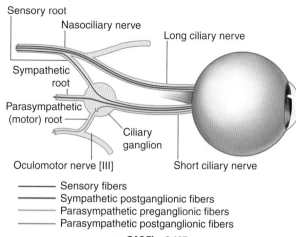

• *GAS* Fig. 8.107

failure of obliteration of the second branchial cleft in embryonic development. The second pharyngeal arch grows caudally and, ultimately, covers the third and fourth arches. The buried clefts become ectoderm-lined cavities that normally involute. Occasionally this process is arrested and the entrapped remnant forms an epithelium-lined cyst, in some cases with a sinus tract to the overlying skin. Many branchial cleft cysts are asymptomatic; others may become tender, enlarged, or inflamed, or they may develop abscesses that rupture, resulting in a purulent draining sinus to the skin or pharynx. Surgery is indicated in these cases.

B. A ruptured sternocleidomastoid muscle will present as difficulty with pointing the chin contralaterally. There will be no mass present.

C. A mass secondary to lymph node inflammation will be tender to palpation which is not observed in this patient.

D. Torticollis is an abnormal contracture of the sternocleidomastoid muscle. This causes the head tilting to the affected side and head rotation to the opposite side.

E. An external carotid artery aneurysm is highly unlikely in this case presentation.
N 49, 56, 67, 78, 72, 75, 81, 137, 160; ABR/McM 32

179. **C.** The angiograph provided clearly shows that the radiopaque medium injected into the patient did not completely fill the common carotid artery. Portions of the internal and external carotid arteries are filled above the common carotid because of "back fill" provided by the collateral circulation. However, vascular supply to the brain is still compromised in this patient, leading to her symptoms.
A, B, D, and E. These vessels are not the cause of the occlusion seen in the angiography.
GAS 136, 860, 999–1000; N 20, 64, 96–97, 115, 124, 128, 132; ABR/McM 224

180. **A.** Mastoiditis is an infection of the cells within the mastoid process of the temporal bone, often caused by untreated acute otitis media.

A known complication of mastoiditis is inflammation of the sigmoid sinus. Necrosis of the bone because of untreated infection will often affect the sigmoid sinus.

B. The petrous part of the temporal bone is unlikely to experience inflammation.

C. Infection in the middle ear is usually the preceding event to mastoiditis rather than occurring as a result of it.

D. The occipital sinus is located far posteromedial to the mastoid process and is unlikely to be affected.

E. Because of its position, the internal carotid artery will not be affected by this inflammation.
GAS 947–953; N 127, 128, 132, 143; ABR/McM 57–58, 16

181. **B.** A chalazion is caused by an obstructed tarsal gland of the eyelid.

A. Swellings of the lacrimal gland usually present on the upper lateral eyelid and are not indicative of a chalazion.

C and D. A chalazion is not an infection within the eye, so this excludes sclera and pupil from being the correct answers.

E. The nasolacrimal duct runs from the medially located lacrimal sac to the inferior nasal meatus of the nose and would be unaffected in the case of a chalazion.
GAS 921; N 20, 41, 49, 57, 59, 62, 64, 68, 82, 105, 107, 110, 115, 124, 128, 133–134, 142, 145–146; ABR/McM 52–54

182. **B.** The nasal polyp also involved the maxillary sinus, located immediately lateral to the nasal cavity.

A. The sphenoidal sinus, located superior to the nasopharynx, is unlikely to be affected by a nasal polyp.

C. The ethmoidal cells, located medially to the orbit and lateral to the nasal cavity, are also unlikely to be affected by a nasal polyp, although this possibility cannot be ruled out.

D. The frontonasal ducts draining the frontal sinuses are located superomedially to the eyes and are unlikely to be affected by the nasal polyp.

E. The nasolacrimal ducts are located between the lacrimal and maxillary bones of the bony orbit. They are unlikely to be obstructed by a nasal polyp.
GAS 1063–1065; N 63; ABR/McM 3, 12, 16

183. **C.** A tumor at the cerebellopontine angle, such as an acoustic schwannoma, is most likely to affect first the vestibulocochlear nerve and then the facial nerve. This excludes the vagus (A), hypoglossal (B), glossopharyngeal (D), and trigeminal (E) nerves from being the correct answers.
GAS 942, 959; N 10, 33, 37–38, 40–41, 64, 82–84, 87–89, 136, 139, 141–142, 144–145, 147, 149, 196, 204, 214, 236, 240; ABR/McM 11, 17, 23

184. **D.** Rupture of the periosteal arteries resulting in a cephalohematoma is defined as a collection of blood underneath the periosteum. On the head, it is located between the pericranium (periosteum of the skull) and the calvaria (skull).

A, B, and C. The galea aponeurotica, skin, and areolar connective tissue are all located superficial to the site of bleeding and hematoma.

E. Bleeding from a cephalohematoma does not involve the subcutaneous tissues
GAS 911–914; N 105–111; ABR/McM 5

185. **B.** The tentorial/uncal herniation described in this case is most likely to occur as a result of a temporal lobe tumor. The uncus is part of the temporal lobe, and when enlarged, it will be compressed against the foramen magnum. This results in the symptoms manifested by damage to the nearby oculomotor nerve.

A and E. Herniation of the parietal lobe is highly unlikely to produce the symptoms observed in this patient which are secondary to the compression of the oculomotor nerve.

C. Occipital lobe tumors would not cause oculomotor nerve compression.

D. Frontal lobe tumors can present as behavioral changes, impaired judgment, and memory loss. These symptoms are not seen in this patient.
GAS 850, 856; N 117–118; ABR/McM 9

186. **C.** A tumor involving the meningeal branches of the ethmoidal nerves that originate from the ophthalmic division of the trigeminal nerve is likely to cause pain from pressure and nerve injury in the anterior cranial fossa.

A and B. The maxillary and mandibular divisions of the trigeminal nerve provide sensory innervation to the middle and posterior aspects of the meninges, respectively.

D. The tentorial nerve, a branch of the ophthalmic division of the trigeminal nerve, supplies the tentorium cerebelli and the falx cerebri.

E. Spinal nerves C2 and C3 fibers do not provide meningeal innervation.
GAS 913, 838, 883; N 9, 132–133; ABR/McM 44, 61

187. **A.** The deep lingual vein is located most superficially on the underside of the tongue. It is therefore the most direct route for absorption of the administered nitroglycerin.

B and C. The submandibular and sublingual ducts are excretory in function and do not function to absorb a drug, such as nitroglycerin.

D and E. The lingual and sublingual vein are located more deeply within the floor of the mouth and do not provide the most direct route for absorption.
GAS 1089 N 70; ABR/McM 29, 35

188. **B.** The lingual nerve initially courses directly underneath the mucosa of the floor of the mouth and superior to the deep portion of the submandibular gland, and specifically passes lateral to and beneath the submandibular duct to reach the tongue. This nerve is therefore at risk for ligation, division, or trauma during excision of the gland and duct. The lingual nerve

is part of the mandibular division of the trigeminal nerve and carries fibers from the chorda tympani, a branch of the facial nerve (CN VII). These latter fibers supply taste to the anterior two-thirds of the tongue and preganglionic parasympathetic axons involved in salivary gland secretion. Fibers of the mandibular division of the trigeminal nerve (CN V3) give rise to the lingual nerve and supply general sensation to the anterior two-thirds of the tongue. The lingual nerve passes deep both to the lateral pterygoid muscle and the ramus of the mandible and subsequently travels deep to the submandibular gland itself

A. The buccal nerve, also a branch of the mandibular division of the trigeminal nerve, supplies the skin and mucosa of the cheek and is not in close proximity to the gland or duct.

C. The inferior alveolar nerve, though close in proximity to the submandibular gland, travels deep to the lateral pterygoid muscle and later enters the mandibular canal to supply the lower teeth.

D. The nerve to the mylohyoid, a branch of the inferior alveolar nerve, supplies the mylohyoid muscle and the anterior belly of the digastric. While it is somewhat at risk for damage during excision of the submandibular gland and duct as it passes forward on the undersurface of the mylohyoid muscle in the submandibular triangle, the submandibular gland usually hangs below the nerve to mylohyoid within the triangle.

E. The glossopharyngeal nerve is a mixed nerve carrying sensory and motor fibers. It is responsible for sensory innervation to the oropharynx and posterior one-third of the tongue and motor innervation to the stylopharyngeus muscle.
GAS 1089–1090; N 70; ABR/McM 29, 35

189. A. The ophthalmic artery is a branch of the internal carotid artery and provides origin to the ocular and orbital vessels, including the central artery of the retina, which supplies the retina. The central artery of the retina is an end artery that has no anastomoses with other arterial sources; therefore, occlusion of this artery will result in loss of vision.

B. The nasociliary nerve is a branch of the ophthalmic division of the trigeminal nerve. It is the general sensory nerve for the eye and is the afferent limb of the corneal blink reflex; it has no direct effect on vision.

C. The anterior ethmoidal nerve is a branch of the nasociliary nerve and supplies the anterior ethmoid cells, the nasal septum, and the lateral walls of the nasal cavity anterosuperiorly; it also supplies the skin on the bridge of the nose.

D. The trochlear nerve is the fourth of the 12 cranial nerves and innervates the superior oblique muscle, one of the six extraocular muscles. The extraocular muscles function in the movement of the eyeball and not the perception of light.

E. The optic nerve is the second of the 12 cranial nerves and is responsible for vision. A lesion of the optic nerve would lead to blindness; however, based on the location of the patient's infection, the optic nerve was not affected directly by the infection but indirectly by the loss of arterial supply.
GAS 923; N 147–149; ABR/McM 53–54

190. A. CSF is mostly secreted from the choroid plexuses of the lateral, third, and fourth ventricles of the brain. The CSF enters the subarachnoid space from the fourth ventricle, via the lateral and median apertures (foramina of Luschka and Magendie). The CSF then circulates in the subarachnoid space until it is finally resorbed back into the venous side of the circulation through the arachnoid granulations into the superior sagittal sinus. A thrombus of the superior sagittal sinus can lead to an obstruction of CSF absorption (communicating hydrocephalus) in which all of the ventricles of the brain are enlarged and the intracranial pressure is increased.

B. Obstruction of the cerebral aqueduct (of Sylvius) will result in a non-communicating hydrocephalus.

C. Laceration of the middle meningeal artery will not result in hydrocephalus. Injury to the middle meningeal artery will most likely cause an epidural hematoma.

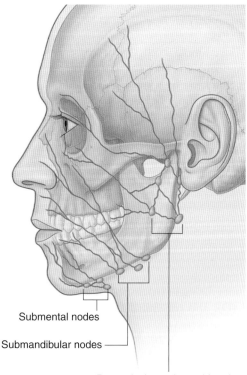

Submental nodes

Submandibular nodes

Pre-auricular and parotid nodes

• *GAS* **Fig. 8.69**

D. Fracture of the cribriform plate can cause CSF rhinorrhea; however this injury will not result in hydrocephalus.

E. Aneurysm of the middle cerebral artery can compress the oculomotor nerve. If an aneurysm of the middle cerebral artery ruptures, a subarachnoid hematoma will form. An aneurysm of the middle cerebral artery will not cause hydrocephalus.
GAS 875; N 119–121; ABR/McM 72–76

191. C. The jugulodigastric node, also known as the tonsillar lymph node, receives drainage from the palatine tonsils, tongue, and pharynx. It is often enlarged during tonsillitis.

A. The submandibular lymph nodes drain the back of the tongue, gums, upper lip, parts of the lower lip, and sides of the face. They drain into the deep cervical group of nodes.

B. The parotid nodes are located superficially and deep to the parotid gland and drain aspects of the cheek, external acoustic meatus, the lateral aspects of the eyelids, and posterior orbit.

D. The submental nodes drain the tip of the tongue bilaterally, the lower lip, and floor of the mouth.

E. The retropharyngeal lymph nodes drain the nasopharynx, nasal cavities, and auditory tubes (*GAS* Fig. 8.69).

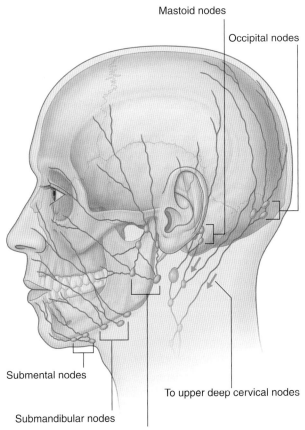

Mastoid nodes

Occipital nodes

Submental nodes

To upper deep cervical nodes

Submandibular nodes

Pre-auricular and parotid nodes

• *GAS* **Fig. 8.75**

GAS 1027–1028; N 85–86; ABR/McM 32

192. B. The preauricular lymph nodes are also known as the deep parotid nodes. They are located deep to the parotid gland and drain lymph from the posterior orbit.

A. The submandibular nodes drain the side of the cheek and lateral aspects of the nose and lips.

C. The jugulodigastric nodes receive drainage from all of the superior nodes of the face and also drain the tonsils.

D. The submental lymph nodes drain the tip of the tongue, floor of the oral cavity anteriorly, and the chin (*GAS* Fig. 8.75).

E. The superficial parotid lymph nodes lie superficial to the parotid gland and drain the lateral angles of the eyelids, aspects of the nose, and the external acoustic meatus.
GAS 909, 1027–1028; N 85; ABR/McM 39–41

193. D. The pharyngeal (Zenker) diverticulum is usually located between the cricopharyngeal and thyropharyngeal portions of the inferior pharyngeal constrictor. This is the most common site for development of a pharyngeal diverticulum because of the inherent weakness between the pharyngeal muscles in this location. Stasis of materials within this diverticulum can lead to inflammation, infection, and abscess. This site is also known as Killian triangle.

A, B, C, and E. A Zenker diverticulum is most likely to occur at Killian triangle.
GAS 1031–1034; N 88; ABR/McM 49, 60

194. D. The inferior thyroid veins drain the inferior aspects of the thyroid gland and often unite to form a midline vein that descends anterior to the trachea to join the left brachiocephalic vein, although the right inferior thyroid vein may join the right brachiocephalic vein separately.

A. The superior thyroid veins drain the superior aspects of the thyroid glands and join the internal jugular veins bilaterally and superiorly to the site of incision.

B. The middle thyroid veins drain the middle portions of the thyroid glands and also terminate in the internal jugular veins laterally, superior to the incision site.

C. The left brachiocephalic vein lies within the superior mediastinum, joining the right brachiocephalic vein to form the superior vena cava, which is located just to the right of the midline.

E. The jugular venous arch connecting the anterior jugular veins is quite variable and lies just superior to the suprasternal notch of the manubrium and is not typically a source of concern if encountered surgically.
GAS 135, 158, 172; N 215–216; ABR/McM 36–37

195. C. The glossopharyngeal nerve (CN IX) enters the posterior oropharynx by coursing between the stylohyoid ligament and the stylopharyngeus muscle. Calcification of the stylohyoid ligament can readily affect this nerve by irritation or compression. The glossopharyngeal nerve carries sensory nerve fibers from the posterior third of the tongue and the oropharynx. A lesion of this nerve could cause loss of both general sensation and taste sensation from the posterior third of the tongue and general sensation from the oropharynx.

A. The vagus nerve carries sensory, motor, and parasympathetic fibers and is not close to the styloid process.

B. The facial nerve carries motor and sensory fibers and is not close to the styloid process.

D. The hypoglossal nerve provides motor innervation to the intrinsic and extrinsic muscles of the tongue.

E. The vestibulocochlear nerve carries information about hearing and balance.

GAS 887–888; N 127–128; ABR/McM 35–36

196. A. There is a lesion of the facial nerve (CN VII) proximal to the geniculate ganglion. At the geniculate ganglion, the greater petrosal nerve branches from the facial nerve and ultimately runs to the pterygopalatine ganglion where preganglionic fibers synapse on postganglionic neurons that innervate the lacrimal gland. There is a disruption of the facial nerve proximal to this branch that allows the greater petrosal nerve to be stimulated by factors that would normally stimulate the submandibular and sublingual glands. These glands are innervated via the chorda tympani that arises from the facial nerve distal to the geniculate ganglion.

B. The greater petrosal nerve originates from the facial nerve at the geniculate ganglion and provides preganglionic parasympathetic fibers to the pterygopalatine ganglion, which serves the lacrimal gland as well as mucous glands of the nasal cavity and paranasal sinuses.

C. The lesser petrosal nerve carries secretory fibers from the tympanic plexus to the otic ganglion, which serves the parotid gland. It is not involved in lacrimation.

D. The lacrimal nerve is a derivative of the ophthalmic branch of the trigeminal nerve. It provides sensory innervation to the conjunctiva and skin of the lateral upper eyelid as well as the lateral forehead and lateral canthus.

E. The chorda tympani originates from the mastoid segment of the facial nerve just prior to the latter's exit from the stylomastoid foramen. It carries afferent sensory fibers to the anterior two-thirds of the tongue via the lingual nerve but also provides secretomotor innervation to the sublingual and submandibular glands.

GAS 910, 958–959; N 134–136; ABR/McM 44, 58

197. B. The anterior communicating artery, a portion of the cerebral arterial circle (of Willis), is the most common site of intracranial aneurysm. It lies directly superior to the optic chiasm, and an aneurysm of this artery would likely compress the chiasm, as in this patient.

A. The middle cerebral artery branches off the internal carotid and is not close to the optic chiasm.

C. The anterior cerebral artery arises from the internal carotid and supplies the frontal and parietal lobes.

D. The superior cerebellar artery branches off the basilar artery and is not close to the optic chiasm.

E. The posterior inferior cerebellar artery branches off the vertebral artery.

GAS 869; N 151; ABR/McM 67

198. E. The nasolacrimal duct is the only duct that normally drains into the inferior nasal meatus and therefore would be affected by a focal inflammation in this region.

A, B, and D: The ethmoidal cells are collectively known as the ethmoid sinus. The ethmoidal sinus consists of three paired sets of small chambers, which are the anterior, middle, and posterior ethmoid cells. The anterior ethmoid cells open into the ethmoidal infundibulum. The middle ethmoidal cells drain onto the ethmoidal bulla and the posterior ethmoidal cells into the superior nasal meatus.

C. The maxillary sinus is a paired structure. The maxillary sinus drains into the middle nasal meatus via the semilunar hiatus.

GAS 1066–1068; N 95; ABR/McM 51, 55

199. D. The greater petrosal nerve is a branch of the facial nerve that ultimately supplies the lacrimal gland. This branch comes off the facial nerve (CN VII) at the geniculate ganglion proximal to the chorda tympani. The greater petrosal nerve is unlikely to be involved in a lesion of the facial nerve as described.

A. The facial nerve branches supplying the muscles of facial expression arise after the facial nerve has emerged from the stylomastoid foramen, below the temporal bone.

B. Lesion of the facial nerve proximal to the origin of the chorda tympani would denervate the submandibular and sublingual salivary glands.

C. Lesion of the facial nerve proximal to the origin of the chorda tympani would cause a loss of taste from the anterior two-thirds of the tongue on the affected side.

E. Branches of the facial nerve arising below the temporal bone supply the orbicularis oculi that closes the eyelid.

GAS 1095; N 135; ABR/McM 44, 58, 85

200. B. The great auricular nerve is derived from the ventral rami of the second and third cervical nerves and supplies the skin over the angle of the mandible and auricle up to the level of the temporomandibular joint.

A. The cervical branch of the facial nerve innervates the platysma muscle.

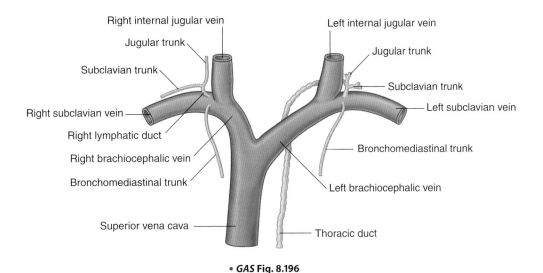

• **GAS Fig. 8.196**

C. The mandibular branch is the largest division of the trigeminal nerve. It provides sensory innervation to the cheek skin and oral mucosa via the buccal nerve as well as the teeth, the skin over the mandible, and skin anterosuperior to the ear on the ipsilateral side.

D. The marginal mandibular branch of the facial nerve supplies motor innervation to the lower lip. It innervates the depressor anguli oris, depressor labii inferioris, and the mentalis muscles.

E. The transverse cervical nerve is a cutaneous branch of the cervical plexus and provides sensory innervation to the skin of the anterior cervical region.

GAS 943–944; N 9; ABR/McM 29–32

Answers 201–225

201. B. The supraclavicular lymph node on the left side is associated with the thoracic duct. The thoracic duct receives lymph from below the diaphragm, including the gastrointestinal tract. Malignant cells that travel up the thoracic duct are known to involve the left supraclavicular lymph node. Historically this is called Virchow node or Troisier sign when enlargement is found on palpation (*GAS* Fig. 8.196).

A and C. The deep cervical lymph nodes receive all the lymph drainage from the head and neck either directly or indirectly via the superficial lymph nodes. Their efferent vessels converge to form the jugular lymphatic trunk together with vessels from the superior deep cervical lymph nodes.

D. The right supraclavicular lymph node drains the esophagus, lungs, and the chest on the right side.

E. The jugulodigastric lymph nodes receive lymph from the tongue, palatine tonsils, and pharynx.

GAS 136–137; N 85; ABR/McM 30

202. E. The internal branch of the superior laryngeal nerve, often called the internal laryngeal nerve, supplies the

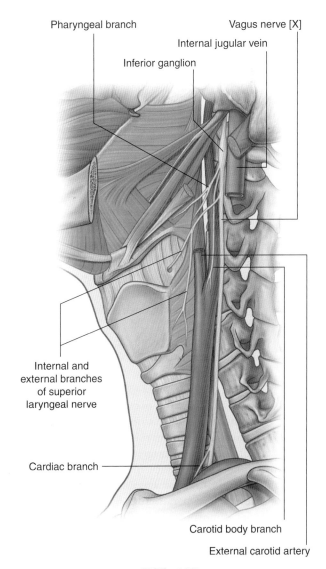

• **GAS Fig. 8.173**

mucosa of the larynx above the vocal folds (which includes the vestibule of the larynx) and the piriform recess.

- **A.** The external branch of the superior laryngeal nerve (external laryngeal nerve) provides motor innervation to the cricothyroid and inferior pharyngeal constrictor muscles.
- **B.** The inferior laryngeal nerve supplies the mucosa of the larynx below the vocal folds.
- **C.** The glossopharyngeal nerve (CN IX) supplies sensation to the posterior third of the tongue and to the oropharynx.
- **D.** The hypoglossal nerve (CN XII) is a motor nerve and innervates all tongue musculature except for the palatoglossus which is innervated by the vagus nerve. (GAS Fig. 8.173).

GAS 1057; N 141–142; ABR/McM 48, 84

203. D. A fractured hyoid bone suggests strangulation. B and C. A fall from a height and subdural hematoma would likely be accompanied by fractured bones.
    A and E. Whereas myocardial infarction or poison remain possibilities, the medical examiner would have a high index of suspicion for strangulation because of the fractured hyoid bone.
    GAS 833, 837; N 53, 68; ABR/McM 31, 33

204. C. Melanocytes in the pigmented layer of the retina are a potential source of malignant melanoma cells. The tumor spreads hematogenously directly to the brain and has a very poor prognosis.
    A, B, D, and E. None of the other listed structures contains melanocytes.
    GAS 936; N 103; ABR/McM 79

205. B. A branchial sinus results from the failure of the second pharyngeal groove and the cervical sinus to obliterate. It typically opens anywhere along the inferior third of the anterior border of sternocleidomastoid.
    D. Thyroglossal duct cysts or sinuses are usually found in the median plane of the neck and found just below the hyoid or open anterior to the laryngeal cartilages.
    A, C and E. A branchial sinus results from retention of a portion of pharyngeal or branchial clefts 2–4, not pharyngeal pouches or arches.
    N 32–33, 91; ABR/McM 32–33

206. B. DiGeorge syndrome occurs because of failure of differentiation of the third and fourth pouches into thymus and parathyroid glands as a result of failure of neural crest migration into the third and fourth pouches. Absence of normal T-cell development leads to poor immunity and hypocalcemia from lack of parathyroid hormone. However, the facial dimorphism is because of lack of neural crest cell involvement in first pharyngeal arch development.
    A. First pharyngeal arch develops into the maxillary and mandibular processes.

- **C.** The heart derives from the mesodermal germ layer cells.
- **D.** The second pharyngeal pouch forms the palatine tonsil.
- **E.** The first, second, and third arches are not involved in the formation of the thymus and parathyroid glands.

N 234–235; ABR/McM 14

207. E. Cleft lip is a result of failure of the mesenchyme in the medial nasal and maxillary prominences to fuse. Unilateral cleft occurs if the maxillary prominence on the affected side fails to fuse with the intermaxillary segment, whereas bilateral cleft occurs if there is failure of fusion on both sides. Median cleft occurs from failure of formation of the intermaxillary segment from the medial nasal processes. A and D. The lateral nasal processes form the ala of the nose.
    B and C. The medial nasal prominences form the intermaxillary segment.
    GAS 844; N 21, 52; ABR/McM 26, 14

208. A. Severe cases of spina bifida are often associated with anencephaly because of the fact that they all occur from different types of nonfusion defects in the neural tube. Anencephaly is usually seen in conjunction with polyhydramnios because of lack of neurologic control to initiate and complete swallowing of amniotic fluid for absorption in the gastrointestinal tract. These conditions lead to high alpha-fetoprotein levels in the amniotic fluid.
    B, C, D, and E. These do not occur from nonfusion defects in the neural tube.
    GAS 72; N 307; ABR/McM 93

209. A. Coloboma of the iris and retina is because of defective closure of the retinal fissure during the sixth week of life and may involve the ciliary body.
    B. Neural crest cells in the eye form the choroid, sclera, and corneal endothelium.
    C and D. These are not processes involved in the pathogenesis of a coloboma.
    E. Weak adhesion between the layers of the optic cup leads to congenital retinal detachment.
    GAS 936; N 102–103; ABR/McM 79

210. C. The lateral pterygoid muscle attaches to the articular disc, capsule of the temporomandibular joint, and neck of the mandibular condyle and as such any damage here will injure the muscle. The muscles of mastication including the lateral pterygoid muscle are derived from the first pharyngeal arch.
    A. The first pouch gives rise to the tubotympanic recess.
    B. The second pouch forms the tonsillar sinus.
    D. The first cleft gives rise to the external acoustic meatus.

E. The second arch gives rise to the muscles of facial expression.
GAS 966; N56–57, 59; ABR/McM 42–44

211. D. In cranium bifidum, if the protruding brain contains part of the ventricular system the condition is known as meningohydroencephalocele.
   A. It is a cranial meningocele if only the meninges herniate.
   B. It is encephalocele if it contains brain matter and meninges.
   C. Meroencephaly is a neural tube defect in which only a rudimentary brain or minor functioning neural tissue is present instead of a whole brain.
   E. Microcephaly is an abnormally small head, which is a result of an abnormally small brain.
   GAS 72; N 307; ABR/McM 93

212. C. Thyroglossal duct cysts are because of the failure of obliteration of the thyroglossal duct. The thyroglossal duct is formed as the thyroid gland primordium descends from the posterior aspect of the tongue to its usual location. The thyroglossal duct may persist and form cysts, which are usually found in the median plane of the neck and just below the hyoid bone.
   A. The second pharyngeal cleft is usually obliterated.
   B. The only other midline structure is the foramen cecum, which is a persistence of the proximal part of the thyroglossal duct and is above the hyoid bone.
   D. The third pharyngeal pouch forms the inferior parathyroid glands and the thymus.
   E. The cervical sinus is formed by the merging of the 2nd, 3rd, and 4th pharyngeal grooves.
   GAS 1009; N 71, 77; ABR/McM 60

213. A. The first pharyngeal arch gives rise to the maxillary and mandibular prominences. Failure or insufficient migration of neural crest cells here leads to mandibulofacial dysostosis (Treacher Collins syndrome) in which there is malar hypoplasia, down-slanting palpebral fissures, defects of the lower eyelids, and external ear deformities.
   B, C, D, and E. These arches are not involved in the formation of the maxillary and mandibular prominences.
   N 71, 77; ABR/McM 49

214. D. Cephalohematoma is hemorrhage between the cranium and the periosteum of the cranial bones by rupture of vessels crossing the periosteum. In contrast, subgaleal (subaponeurotic) hemorrhage is hemorrhage between the periosteum and the aponeurotic layer and is more extensive with more complications. The swelling does not cross suture lines in cephalohematoma but does in subgaleal hemorrhage.
   A, B, and C. These are not involved in the formation of a cephalohematoma.
   E. Caput succedaneum is a collection of edema fluid above the periosteum of the cranial bones.
   GAS 911–914; N 111; ABR/McM 5

215. E. The *T. gondii* organism crosses the placental membrane and infects the fetus, causing destructive changes in the brain (intracranial calcifications) and eyes (chorioretinitis) that result in mental deficiency, microcephaly, microphthalmia, and hydrocephaly. Fetal death may follow infection, especially during the early stages of pregnancy.
   A. Administration of tetracycline to a pregnant woman is associated with stained teeth and hypoplasia of enamel in her baby.
   B. Rubella virus is associated with various anomalies such as IUGR, postnatal growth retardation, cardiac and great vessel abnormalities, microcephaly, sensorineural deafness, cataract, microphthalmos, glaucoma, pigmented retinopathy, mental deficiency, neonatal bleeding, hepatosplenomegaly, osteopathy, and tooth defects.
   C. Infection with CMV is the most common viral infection of the fetus, occurring in approximately 1% of neonates. Most pregnancies end in spontaneous abortion (miscarriage) when the infection occurs during the first trimester. CMV infection later in pregnancy may result in severe birth defects, including IUGR, microphthalmia, chorioretinitis, blindness, microcephaly, cerebral calcification, mental deficiency, deafness, cerebral palsy, and hepatosplenomegaly. Primary maternal infections (acquired during pregnancy) nearly always cause serious fetal infection and birth defects.
   D. Early fetal manifestations of untreated maternal syphilis are congenital deafness, abnormal teeth and bones, hydrocephalus, and mental deficiency.
   N 111; ABR/McM 34

216. C. In the fifth week, epithelium of the dorsal region of the third pouch differentiates into the inferior parathyroid gland while the ventral region forms the thymus.
   A. Lymph nodules develop in the mucosa of the respiratory and alimentary systems and are derived from mesenchymal cells.
   B. The lingual tonsil develops from an aggregation of lymph nodules in the root of the tongue.
   D. The submandibular glands appear late in the sixth week. They develop from endodermal buds in the floor of the stomodeum.
   E. The palatine tonsil is derived from the second pharyngeal pouch.
   N 88; ABR/McM 46

217. B. Tetracycline crosses the placental membrane and is deposited in the embryo's bones and teeth at sites of active calcification. Tetracycline therapy during the fourth to ninth months of pregnancy may also cause tooth defects (e.g., enamel hypoplasia), yellow to brown discoloration of the teeth, and diminished growth of long bones. Calcification of the permanent teeth begins at birth and, except for the third molars,

is complete by 7 to 8 years of age; hence, long-term tetracycline therapy during childhood can affect the permanent teeth.

A, C, and E. These are not associated with the symptoms seen in this case.

D. Rubella virus is associated with various anomalies such as IUGR, postnatal growth retardation, cardiac and great vessel abnormalities, microcephaly, sensorineural deafness, cataract, microphthalmos, glaucoma, pigmented retinopathy, mental deficiency, neonate bleeding, hepatosplenomegaly, osteopathy, and tooth defects.

N 13; ABR/McM 62

218. **B.** Rubella virus (German measles) is associated with various anomalies such as IUGR, postnatal growth retardation, cardiac and great vessel abnormalities, microcephaly, sensorineural deafness, cataract, microphthalmos, glaucoma, pigmented retinopathy, mental deficiency, neonatal bleeding, hepatosplenomegaly, osteopathy, and tooth defects.

A. Thalidomide is a potent teratogen. The characteristic presenting feature is meromelia, but the defects range from amelia (absence of limbs) through intermediate stages of development (rudimentary limbs) to micromelia (abnormally small and/or short limbs).

C. CMV infection later in pregnancy may result in severe birth defects such as IUGR, microphthalmia, chorioretinitis, blindness, microcephaly, cerebral calcification, mental deficiency, deafness, cerebral palsy, and hepatosplenomegaly.

D. The effects of cocaine include spontaneous abortion, prematurity, IUGR, microcephaly, cerebral infarction, urogenital anomalies, neurobehavioral disturbances, and neurologic abnormalities.

E. The *T. gondii* organism crosses the placental membrane and infects the fetus causing destructive changes in the brain (intracranial calcifications) and eyes (chorioretinitis) that result in mental deficiency, microcephaly, microphthalmia, and hydrocephaly.

N 103; ABR/McM 52–55

219. **E.** In Treacher Collins syndrome (mandibulofacial dysostosis), which is caused by an autosomal dominant gene, there is malar hypoplasia (underdevelopment of the zygomatic bones of the face) with down-slanting palpebral fissures, defects of the lower eyelids, deformed external ears, and sometimes abnormalities of the middle and internal ears. From the CT it is clear that there is no external acoustic meatus.

A, B, C, and D. These are not associated with Treacher Collins syndrome.

GAS 1063–1065; N 22; ABR/McM 3, 12, 17

220. **D.** Cervical cysts, sinuses, and fistulas may develop from parts of the second pharyngeal groove, the cervical sinus, or the second pharyngeal pouch that fail to obliterate.

A. The first pharyngeal pouch gives rise to the tympanic cavity, mastoid antrum, and auditory tube.

B. The second pharyngeal pouch is associated with the development of the palatine tonsil.

C. The thymus is derived from the third pair of pharyngeal pouches. The parathyroid glands are formed from the third and fourth pairs of pharyngeal pouches.

E. An ectopic thyroid gland results when the thyroid gland fails to descend completely from its site of origin in the tongue.

GAS 942, 960; N 87–89; ABR/McM 11, 17, 24

221. **E.** In Treacher Collins syndrome (mandibulofacial dysostosis), which is caused by an autosomal dominant gene, there is malar hypoplasia (underdevelopment of the zygomatic bones of the face) with down-slanting palpebral fissures, defects of the lower eyelids, deformed external ears, and sometimes abnormalities of the middle and internal ears.

A. Pierre Robin sequence, an autosomal recessive disorder, is associated with hypoplasia of the mandible, cleft palate, and defects of the eye and ear.

B. Patients with DiGeorge syndrome are born without a thymus and parathyroid glands and have defects in cardiac outflow tracts. In some cases, ectopic glandular tissue has been found.

C. Symptoms of FAS are IUGR, mental deficiency, microcephaly, ocular anomalies, joint abnormalities, and short palpebral fissure.

D. Chiari I malformation is inferior displacement of the cerebellar tonsils more than 5 mm through the foramen magnum into the cervical vertebral canal.

N 22; ABR/McM 13

222. **D.** The mental nerve and vessels pass through the mental foramen in the mandible. The mental nerve supplies the skin and mucous membrane of the lower lip from the mental foramen to the midline, including the skin of the chin. It is a branch of the inferior alveolar nerve, which comes off the posterior division of the mandibular division of the trigeminal nerve.

A. The auriculotemporal nerve, from mandibular division of trigeminal nerve, and the great auricular nerve, a branch of the cervical plexus composed of fibers from C2 and C3 spinal nerves, innervate the parotid sheath as well as the overlying skin.

B. The buccal nerve is a branch of the anterior division of the mandibular nerve, which supplies the skin over the cheek and the mucosa lining the oral vestibule.

C. The lesser petrosal nerve is the visceral motor component of the glossopharyngeal nerve (CN IX), carrying parasympathetic fibers from the tympanic plexus to the parotid gland.

E. The infraorbital nerve innervates (sensory) the lower eyelid, upper lip, and part of the nasal vestibule and exits the infraorbital foramen of the maxilla.

GAS 904; N 117–119; ABR/McM 17

223. B. The taste sensation is via chorda tympani, from the facial nerve, which have their cell bodies in the geniculate ganglion. The general sensory supply of the mucous membrane of the oral part (anterior two-thirds), but not the region of the vallate papillae, is by the lingual nerve.

    A. General sensation is via the mandibular division of the trigeminal nerve (with cell bodies in the trigeminal ganglion).

    C. This ganglion is not responsible for the taste sensation described in this case.

    D and E. The submandibular and pterygopalatine ganglia are where the presynaptic parasympathetic fibers from chorda tympani and greater petrosal nerves synapse, respectively.

    GAS 958; N 9, 132–134; ABR/McM 44, 51

224. C. The Ophthalmic nerve (ophthalmic division of the trigeminal nerve, CN V1) carries sensory branches from the eye, conjunctiva, and orbital contents, including the lacrimal gland. It also receives sensory branches from the nasal cavity, frontal sinus, ethmoidal cells, falx cerebri, dura in the anterior cranial fossa and superior part of the tentorium cerebelli, upper lid, dorsum of the nose, and anterior part of the scalp. Branches of ophthalmic nerve are the lacrimal, frontal, and nasociliary nerves.

    A, B, D, and E. Maxillary nerve (CN V2) and mandibular nerve (CN V3) carry sensory information from other regions of the face.

    GAS 904; N 70; ABR/McM 29, 35

225. D. The hypoglossal nerve (CN XII) passes through hypoglossal canal. All the muscles of the tongue, intrinsic and extrinsic, are supplied by the hypoglossal nerve (except palatoglossus). Extrinsic tongue muscles supplied by hypoglossal nerve include the genioglossus, hyoglossus, and styloglossus.

    A, B, C, and E. These muscles will not be affected.

    GAS 1089–1091; N 70; ABR/McM 29, 35

Answers 226–250

226. C. Superior salivatory nucleus (or superior salivary nucleus) of the facial nerve is a visceromotor cranial nerve nucleus located in the pontine tegmentum. Preganglionic parasympathetic fibers arise from the nucleus and pass laterally to exit the pons with motor VII axons. Then some of the preganglionic fibers pass to the pterygopalatine ganglion via the greater petrosal nerve (via the pterygoid canal, also known as the Vidian canal) and synapse in the pterygopalatine ganglion. Postganglionic efferent fibers travel to innervate the lacrimal gland and the mucosal glands of the nose, palate, and pharynx, whereas the other preganglionic parasympathetic fibers are also distributed partly via the chorda tympani and lingual nerves to the submandibular ganglion, and postsynaptic fibers to the submandibular gland and sublingual gland. Therefore, other symptoms in this patient will be reduced salivary secretion from submandibular and sublingual glands.

    A. The inferior salivatory nucleus is responsible for parasympathetic input to the parotid gland via the glossopharyngeal nerve.

    B. The dorsal nucleus of the vagus is responsible for parasympathetic input to the abdomen and thorax.

    D. The Edinger-Westphal nucleus is responsible for parasympathetic input to the iris sphincter muscle and the ciliary muscle.

    E. The nucleus ambiguus contains motor neurons that innervate muscles in the larynx, pharynx, and the soft palate. It also contains preganglionic parasympathetic neurons that innervate the heart.

    GAS 923; N 147–150; ABR/McM 54–56

227. D. The superior thoracic aperture is variably referred to as the thoracic inlet as well as the thoracic outlet. Obstruction actually occurs outside the aperture in the root of the neck, and the manifestations of thoracic outlet syndrome involve the upper limb through this aperture. A supernumerary (extra cervical) rib or a fibrous connection extending from its tip to the first thoracic rib may elevate structures normally lying above the first rib and place pressure on these structures, notably the subclavian artery or inferior trunk of the brachial plexus, and may cause symptoms. Other etiologies could include an elongated transverse process of the C7 vertebra and muscular abnormalities (e.g., in the scalenus anterior muscle, a sickle-shaped scalenus medius). Most common symptoms include discoloration of the hands, one hand colder than the other hand, weakness of the hand and arm muscles, and tingling.

    A, B, C, and E. These symptoms are not associated with this condition.

    GAS 29–31; N 119–122; ABR/McM 71

228. C. The SCG lies at the base of the cranium. It lies deep to the sheath of the internal carotid artery and internal jugular vein (carotid sheath), and anterior to the longus capitis muscle. It contains neurons that supply sympathetic innervation to a number of target organs within the head and also contributes gray rami communicantes to the cervical plexus. The postsynaptic sympathetic fibers stimulate contraction of the blood vessels (vasomotor) and erector muscles associated with hairs (pilomotor), and cause sweating (sudomotor). Postsynaptic sympathetic fibers in the cranium also innervate the dilator muscle of the iris (dilator pupillae); therefore compression causes complete pupillary constriction. It also innervates the muscle that maintains elevation of the upper lid (holding the eye open); therefore compression causes partial ptosis (drooping of the upper lid). Paralysis of the CN III causes complete ptosis. (*GAS* Fig. 8.194).

• **GAS Fig. 8.194**

A. The submandibular ganglion is responsible for parasympathetic innervation to the oral mucosa, submandibular, and the sublingual gland.

B. The trigeminal ganglion is a sensory ganglion of the trigeminal nerve.

D. The geniculate ganglion contains fibers for somatic sensation and taste.

E. The ciliary ganglion is a parasympathetic ganglion responsible for constriction of the pupil and accommodation.

GAS 1027–1029; N 85–87; ABR/McM 33

229. A. The lingual nerve is joined by the chorda tympani about 2 cm below the base of the skull, deep to the lower border of the lateral pterygoid muscle. It supplies the anterior two-thirds of the tongue with general sensation and taste, the latter mediated by fibers in the chorda tympani. The secretomotor fibers of the chorda tympani are given off to the submandibular ganglion, which is suspended from the lingual nerve. They relay in the ganglion for the submandibular gland, and some postganglionic fibers rejoin the lingual nerve for transport to the sublingual salivary glands in the floor of the mouth. The lingual nerve also supplies all the mucous membrane of the floor of the mouth and the lingual gingiva (gums).

B, C, D, and E. These nerves are not involved.

GAS 909, GAS 1027–1029; N 91; ABR/McM 39–42

230. E. Perineural spread of a tumor (or spread of tumor along a nerve) is one of the more insidious forms of tumor metastasis. This form of spread is more commonly found in malignant rather than benign lesions. In this case the tumor spreads along tissue at the jugular foramen, thus involving the glossopharyngeal (CN IX), vagus (CN X), and accessory nerves (CN XI). The pharyngeal reflex (gag reflex) would be affected because the sensory limb is mediated predominantly by CN IX (glossopharyngeal nerve) and motor limb by CN X (vagus nerve).

A, B, C, and D. Tongue movements, facial expression, sensation, and hearing are mediated by cranial nerves XII, VII, V, and VIII respectively.

GAS 1031–1034; N 94; ABR/McM 49, 61

231. A. Extradural (epidural) hemorrhage is arterial in origin. Blood from torn branches of a middle meningeal artery which passes through foramen spinosum collects between the periosteal layer of the dura and the calvaria. The extravasated blood strips the dura from the cranium. Usually this follows a hard blow to the head; an extradural (epidural) hematoma then forms. Typically, a brief concussion (loss of consciousness) occurs, followed by a lucid interval of some hours. Later, drowsiness and coma (profound unconsciousness) occur, and if the pressure is not relieved the patient will die (*GAS* Fig. 8.47).

B. The foramen ovale is located on the greater wing of the sphenoid bone. The accessory meningeal artery and an emissary vein pass through this foramen.

C. The internal jugular vein and the cranial nerves IX, X, and XI pass through this foramen.

D. The hypoglossal nerve passes through the hypoglossal canal.

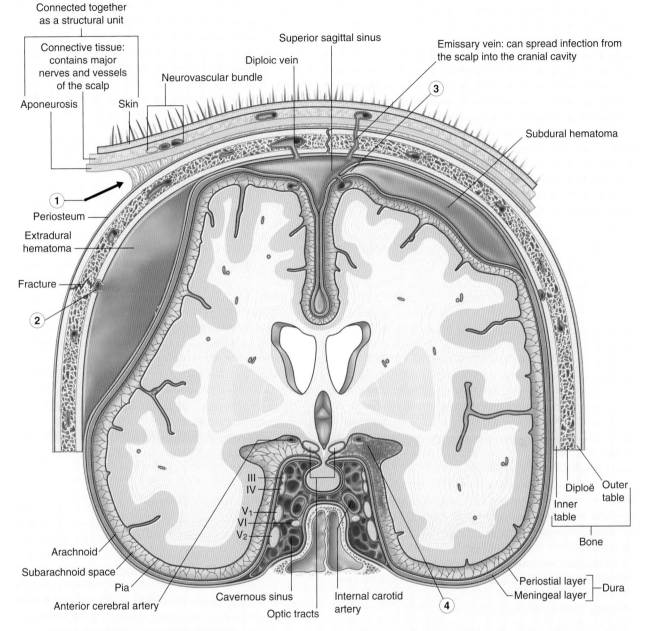

1 **Loose connective tissue (danger area)**
  - In scalping injuries, this is the layer in which separation occurs.
  - Infection can easily spread in this layer.
  - Blunt trauma can result in hemorrhage in this layer (blood can spread forward into the face, resulting in "black eyes").

2 Rupture of the middle meningeal artery (branches) by fracture of the inner table of bone results in extradural hematoma. Under pressure, the blood progressively separates dura from the bone.

3 Tear to cerebral vein where it crosses dura to enter cranial venous sinus can result in subdural hematoma. The tear separates a thin layer of meningeal dura from that which remains attached to the periosteal layer. As a result, the hematoma is covered by an inner limiting membrane derived from part of the meningeal dura.

4 **Aneurysm**
  - Ruptured aneurysms of vessels of the cerebral arterial circle hemorrhage directly into the subarachnoid space and CSF.

• **GAS Fig. 8.47**

E. The nerve and artery of the pterygoid canal pass through the foramen lacerum.
GAS 135, 158, 175; N 215–217; ABR/McM 36–37

232. A. The oculomotor nerve (CN III) supplies the majority of the muscles controlling eye movements. Thus, damage to this nerve results in the eye displaced outward and downward as a result of unopposed lateral rectus (innervated by the abducens nerve, CN VI) and superior oblique (innervated by the trochlear nerve, CN IV). The ciliary muscle within the ciliary body changes the shape of the lens. In the absence of nerve stimulation, the diameter of the relaxed muscular ring is larger, making the lens flatter for far vision. Parasympathetic stimulation via the oculomotor nerve (CN III) causes sphincter-like contraction of the ciliary muscle and the lens gets thicker for near vision. These fibers also innervate the sphincter pupillae. Thus, interruption of these fibers causes dilation of the pupil because of the unopposed action of the sympathetically innervated dilator pupillae muscle. Because the oculomotor nerve supplies the levator palpebrae superioris, a lesion there causes paralysis of the muscle; the patient cannot raise the superior eyelid (cannot open the eye). Partial ptosis is related more to paralysis of the superior tarsal muscle, which is sympathetically innervated.
  B. The optic nerve carries sensory fibers from the retina.
  C. The facial nerve is responsible for controlling the muscles of facial expression and taste sensation from the anterior two-thirds of the tongue.
  D. The ciliary ganglion is responsible for parasympathetics to the muscles of the eye.
  E. The SCG is a sympathetic ganglion near the second and third vertebrae.
  GAS 888–889; N 127–129; ABR/McM 52–53

233. B. Scalp lacerations are the most common type of head injury requiring surgical care. These wounds bleed profusely because the arteries entering the periphery of the scalp bleed from both ends owing to abundant anastomoses. The arteries do not retract when lacerated because they are held open by the dense connective tissue in the second layer of the scalp. The scalp is composed of five layers, the first three of which are connected intimately and move as a unit. Each letter in the word SCALP serves as a mnemonic for one of its five layers, skin, connective tissue, aponeurosis, loose areolar tissue, and pericranium. The loose connective tissue layer (fourth layer) of the scalp is the danger area of the scalp because pus or blood spreads easily in it. Infection in this layer can also pass into the cranial cavity through small emissary veins, which pass through parietal foramina in the calvaria and reach intracranial structures such as the meninges.
  A, C, D, and E. The infection is less likely to spread to these layers.

GAS 910, 957–960; N 134–137; ABR/McM 44, 62
234. E. The rima glottidis is the opening between the true vocal cords. The diameter of this opening is regulated by the laryngeal muscles to modulate pitch of sound.
  A. The piriform fossa is a shallow space found on the lateral side of the laryngeal orifice bounded laterally by the thyroid cartilage and medially by the aryepiglottic fold.
  B. The laryngeal vestibule is the upper portion of the laryngeal airway, between the laryngeal inlet and the false vocal folds. It is much wider than the rima glottidis or the space between the true vocal folds.
  C. The ventricle is the space between the true and false vocal folds in the larynx.
  D. The vallecula is a depression behind the root of the tongue that serves to hold saliva for lubrication and prevention of premature initiation of deglutition reflex.
  GAS 869; N 27; ABR/McM 49–50

235. D. The mucosa of the piriform fossa receives sensory innervation from the internal branch of the superior laryngeal nerve. This nerve also supplies somatic sensory fibers to the larynx above the vocal cords, epiglottis, and vallecula. Owing to its superficial location in the mucosa of the piriform fossa, it could be damaged during procedures involving the piriform fossa with loss of sensation in the areas it innervates and loss of protective reflex of the larynx.
  A. The mandibular division of the trigeminal nerve (CN V3) supplies somatic sensation from the lower face and motor innervation to muscles of mastication. It also sends sensory fibers to the meninges including the external acoustic meatus.
  B. The maxillary division of the trigeminal nerve (CN V2), although a sensory component of the trigeminal, does not innervate the piriform fossa.
  C. The glossopharyngeal nerve (CN IX) supplies special visceral efferent to the stylopharyngeus muscle, parasympathetic to the parotid gland, general visceral afferent to the carotid sinus and body, special sensory to the posterior one third of the tongue, and general somatic efferent to the external ear, internal part of the tympanic membrane, posterior third of the tongue, and the oropharynx.
  E. The hypoglossal nerve (CN XII) innervates the intrinsic and extrinsic muscles of the tongue.
  GAS 1067–1070; N 136, 139, 237; ABR/McM 49–45

236. D. The first pharyngeal pouch gives rise to the tympanic recess, with its membrane giving rise to the tympanic membrane. The tympanic recess itself gives rise to the tympanic cavity and the mastoid antrum. The auditory tube (eustachian), a part of the tympanic cavity, connects the tympanic cavity to the pharynx. Infections of the pharynx (pharyngitis) can spread from the pharynx to the middle ear through the auditory tube.

A. The second pharyngeal pouch usually obliterates with its tiny remains forming the tonsillar sinus with the remaining mesenchyme forming the lymphoid nodules of the palatine tonsil.

B, C, and E. These structures do not form the auditory tube.

GAS 1093–1096; N BP29, 43; ABR/McM 57–58, 46

237. **B.** The pupillary light reflex is mediated by an afferent limb carried by the optic nerve (CN II) and the efferent limb carried by the oculomotor nerve (CN III). The pupil constricts when the light is shone because the optic nerve was able to pick up the light sensation while the oculomotor nerve mediates the contraction of the sphincter pupillae muscle of the iris that results in pupillary constriction. This muscle is specifically innervated by the parasympathetic component of the oculomotor nerve, which has its preganglionic cell bodies at the Edinger-Westphal nucleus and postganglionic fibers at the ciliary ganglion.

A, C, D, and E. The pupillary light reflex is not mediated by the combination of the other nerves.

GAS 943–945; N 132; ABR/McM 54

238. **A.** The oculomotor nerve (CN III) is the efferent limb of the pupillary reflex. It carries parasympathetic nerve fibers with preganglionic cell bodies in the Edinger-Westphal nucleus and postganglionic cell bodies in the ciliary ganglion and supplies the sphincter pupillae of the iris. The oculomotor nerve is found between the superior cerebellar artery and the PCA. Aneurysm of the superior cerebellar artery can therefore compress on the oculomotor nerve resulting in pupillary dilatation (because of unopposed sympathetic innervation of the dilator pupillae) and unresponsiveness of the affected eye.

B, C, D, and E. The trigeminal, facial, vagus, and abducens nerves do not participate in the pupillary light reflex.

GAS 136–138; N 132; ABR/McM 67

239. **C.** The superior orbital fissure is an opening in the skull found between the lesser and greater wings of the sphenoid bone and communicates with the orbit and maxillary sinus. Among other structures, it transmits the oculomotor nerve (CN III), branches of the ophthalmic division of trigeminal nerve (CN V1), abducens nerve (CN VI), and ophthalmic vein. Tumors around the superior orbital fissure can compress these structures. Abduction of the eye is done by the abducens nerve, and the ophthalmic nerve supplies sensation to the cornea and serves as the afferent limb of the corneal reflex. These functions were lost because of compression of these nerves.

A. The inferior orbital fissure is located inside of the orbit, transmitting the zygomatic and infraorbital branches of the maxillary nerve and branches of the pterygopalatine ganglion.

B. The optic canal is found in the anterior cranial fossa and transmits the optic nerve and ophthalmic artery.

D and E. The foramen rotundum and ovale are located in the middle cranial fossa.

N 141–143; ABR/McM 11, 80

240. **B.** Herpes zoster can affect spinal and cranial nerves. It usually follows reactivation of a dormant varicella infection, which resides in a sensory ganglion. Illness, stress, or immunosuppression can reactivate the dormant virus, which may result in both motor and sensory dysfunction. In this case, a dominant herpes infection in the geniculate ganglion of the facial nerve has been reactivated, resulting in dysfunction of the facial nerve branch that supplies the stapedius muscle (nerve to the stapedius). The stapedius muscle inserts in the neck of the stapes bone in the middle ear and functions to dampen the vibrations of the stapes by way of putting tension on the neck of the stapes. Denervation of this muscle results in the perception of loudness of sound in the ear (hyperacusis) (*GAS* Fig. 8.124).

A, C, D, and E. These nerves are not responsible for the hyperacusis.

N 53, 55, 58; ABR/McM 83

241. **B.** The vagus nerve (CN X) makes a small sensory contribution to the external acoustic meatus (via its auricular branch, also called the nerve of Arnold) and the vagus is the afferent limb of the cough reflex since it innervates the interior of the larynx.

A. The vestibulocochlear nerves mediate hearing and balance.

C. Although the auriculotemporal branch of the trigeminal contributes to the innervations of the external acoustic meatus, it does not participate in the cough reflex.

D. The facial nerve, which also contributes to the innervations of the external acoustic meatus, has no role in the cough reflex.

E. The accessory nerve is motor to the sternocleidomastoid and trapezius muscles.

GAS 885–886, 892; N 137; ABR/McM 84

242. **C.** The recurrent laryngeal nerve, a branch of the vagus nerve (CN X), supplies motor innervation to all the intrinsic muscles of the larynx excluding the cricothyroid muscle and also supplies sensory fibers to the larynx below the vocal cord. Being paired (right and left), the left recurrent laryngeal nerve upon emerging from the vagus nerve in the neck hooks (recurs) under the ligamentum arteriosum at the arch of aorta and then travels within the tracheoesophageal groove to the larynx. The right nerve hooks under the right subclavian artery. In the course of their recurrent path into the neck, these nerves are posterior to the middle part of the thyroid gland. Therefore, the recurrent laryngeal nerve may be inadvertently damaged during thyroidectomy.

A. The internal branch of the superior laryngeal nerve supplies sensory fibers to the laryngeal mucosa above the vocal cord. Injury to this nerve causes anesthesia in the larynx above the vocal cord.

Malleus   Incus

Tensor tympani muscle

Tendon of
stapedius muscle

Pyramidal eminence

Footplate of stapes

Pharyngotympanic tube

Tympanic membrane

• *GAS* Fig. 8.124

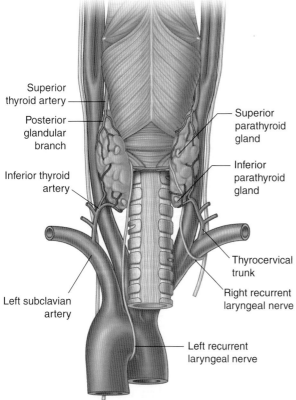

Superior
thyroid artery

Posterior
glandular
branch

Inferior thyroid
artery

Left subclavian
artery

Superior
parathyroid
gland

Inferior
parathyroid
gland

Thyrocervical
trunk

Right recurrent
laryngeal nerve

Left recurrent
laryngeal nerve

• *GAS* Fig. 8.180

B. The external branch of the superior laryngeal nerve supplies the cricothyroid muscle. This muscle serves to tense the vocal cord. Paralysis of the external laryngeal nerve results in a monotonous voice because of inability to tense the vocal cord.

D. Paralysis of the superior laryngeal nerve will also result in anesthesia above the vocal cord and loss of the protective reflex of the larynx (*GAS* Fig. 8.180). E. The glossopharyngeal nerve carries sensory and motor fibers.

GAS 1008–1009; N 87–89; ABR/McM 84

243. C. The pupillary light reflex is used to test the ability of the eyes to perceive light sensation. The afferent limb of this reflex arc is the optic nerve while the oculomotor is the efferent limb. By shining light into the eye from a penlight, each eye is tested individually for a direct constriction of the pupil on the ipsilateral side and then for a consensual reflex on the contralateral side.

A. The startle reflex is a kind of acoustic reflex that occurs in reaction to sudden auditory stimulation.

B. The blink or corneal reflex is a reflex that is produced in reaction to stimulation of the cornea of the eye. This reflex is mediated by the ophthalmic branch of the trigeminal (afferent limb) and the facial nerve (efferent limb).

D. The H-test is a maneuver used to test the extra-ocular muscles, which are innervated by the oculomotor, trochlear, and abducens nerves.

E. The vision test, also known as visual acuity test, is used to assess the ability of the eye to read or identify letters from different distances.

GAS 883–886; N 97, 132; ABR/McM 80

244. D. The short ciliary nerves and ciliary ganglion is the correct answer option. It is clear from the vignette that the problem lies with accommodation, which involves pupil accommodation, lens accommodation, and convergence. Eye movements were not compromised and as such parasympathetic deficit is the likely cause of his condition. Preganglionic axons from the Edinger-Westphal nucleus are carried by the oculomotor nerve. These parasympathetics travel to the ciliary ganglion located in the posterior orbit and from here postganglionic axons, carried by the short ciliary nerves, go on to innervate the sphincter pupillae muscle, which constricts the pupil and innervates the ciliary muscle. Contraction of the ciliary muscle relieves tension on the zonular fibers, allowing the lens to be more convex. Absence of action of the ciliary muscles and sphincter pupillae results in loss of the ability to focus on near objects.

A, B, C, and E. The trochlear nerve and abducens nerves innervate the superior oblique and lateral rectus muscles, respectively. Since eye movements were unaffected, this combination can be eliminated as an answer option immediately. Other combinations are also incorrect.

GAS 864; N 111–113; ABR/McM 61, 72

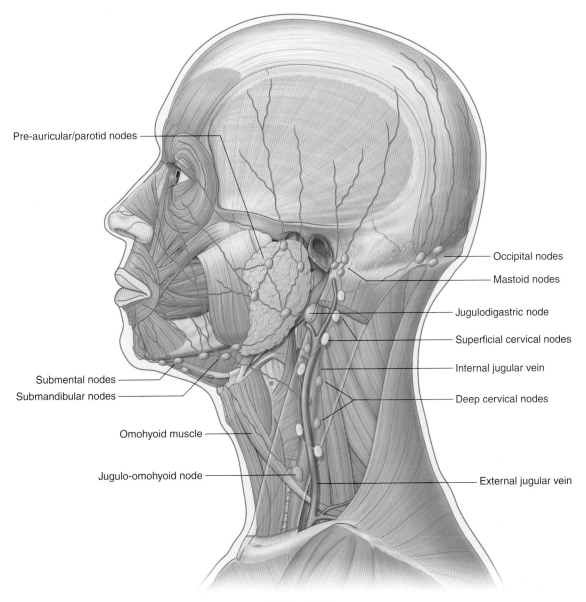

Pre-auricular/parotid nodes

Occipital nodes

Mastoid nodes

Jugulodigastric node

Superficial cervical nodes

Internal jugular vein

Deep cervical nodes

Submental nodes

Submandibular nodes

Omohyoid muscle

Jugulo-omohyoid node

External jugular vein

• *GAS* **Fig. 8.197**

245. B. The herpetic infection of the forehead likely spread to supratrochlear veins, which join to form a single trunk that runs down near the middle line of the forehead parallel with the vein of the opposite side. The two veins are joined, at the root of the nose, by a transverse branch, called the nasal arch. At the medial angle of the orbit, it joins the supraorbital vein to form the angular vein and drains into the superior ophthalmic vein, which communicates with the cavernous sinus. The infection can also make its way to the inferior ophthalmic vein via facial and deep facial veins to spread to the cavernous sinus.
  A. The pterygoid venous plexus has communication with the anterior facial vein and communicates with the cavernous sinus but is not the danger area of the face since it does not drain directly into the pterygoid plexus.
  C. The superior petrosal sinus is located in the superior petrosal sulcus of the petrous part of the temporal bone. It drains the cavernous sinus and travels posterolaterally to drain into the transverse sinus.
  D. The basilar venous plexus is made up of multiple venous channels between the layers of the dura mater above the clivus, where it interconnects the two inferior petrosal sinuses.
  E. The parietal emissary vein connects the superior sagittal sinus with tributaries of the superficial temporal vein.
  GAS 875–876; N 64, 85–86, 99; ABR/McM 47

246. C. The facial nerve is a mixed cranial nerve, which carries both motor and (special) sensory fibers. The motor component of the facial nerve arises from the facial nerve nucleus and forms the facial nerve proper, while the sensory and parasympathetic parts of the facial nerve emerge from the brain as nervus intermedius. The motor and sensory parts of the facial nerve enter the petrous part of the temporal bone via the internal acoustic meatus, which is very close to the inner ear; it then courses through the facial canal, after which it emerges from the stylomastoid foramen and passes through the parotid gland, where it divides into five major branches. The facial nerve provides special sensory fibers to the anterior two-thirds of the tongue, motor to the muscles of facial expression and the stylohyoid and posterior belly of the digastric muscles.
  A, B, D, and E. These cranial nerves are not responsible for the control of muscles of facial expression.
  GAS 883–887; N 110, 135; ABR/McM 83

247. C. The internal acoustic meatus is a canal in the petrous part of the temporal bone. The facial nerve (CN VII) and vestibulocochlear nerve (CN VIII) course through this canal. The vestibulocochlear nerve consists of the cochlear nerve, carrying special sensory hearing, and the vestibular nerve, carrying signals for balance and equilibrium. The facial nerve carries special sensory taste to the anterior two-thirds of the tongue and motor fibers that control the muscles of facial expression.
  A, B, D, and E. These do not involve the cranial nerves VII and VIII.
  GAS 958–960; N 18, 20; ABR/McM 83

248. E. The submental nodes are located between the anterior bellies of the digastric muscles. The central portions of the lower lip and anterior floor of the mouth and the apex of the tongue drain into these nodes. Efferent lymphatic from these nodes go to the submandibular lymph nodes and partly to the juguloomohyoid node of the deep cervical group of nodes.
  A. The occipital nodes drain the occipital region of the scalp.
  B. The parotid nodes drain the root of the nose, the eyelids, the frontotemporal region, and the external acoustic meatus, and a deep group drains the nasal part of the pharynx and the posterior parts of the nasal cavities.
  C. The retropharyngeal nodes are found in the buccopharyngeal fascia and drain the nasal cavities, the nasal part of the pharynx, and the auditory tubes.
  D. The jugulodigastric nodes drain the tonsils primarily (*GAS* Fig. 8.197).
  GAS 909, 915; N 85–86

249. D. Aneurysms of the anterior inferior cerebellar artery cause direct impingement on the abducens nerve as it emerges from the brainstem at the pontomedullary junction between the labyrinthine artery above and the anterior inferior cerebellar artery below. Impingement of this nerve leads to loss of function to the lateral rectus muscle ipsilaterally, resulting in the inability to abduct the eye.
  A. The anterior communicating artery does not relate to the abducens nerve.
  B and C. Aneurysms affecting the PCA will likely affect the oculomotor nerve.
  E. Vertebral artery aneurysm will likely affect the hypoglossal nerve.
  GAS 869–870; N 149–154; ABR/McM 67

250. B. The parotid gland receives visceromotor postganglionic parasympathetic and somatosensory fibers (to the parotid capsule) from the auriculotemporal nerve. As the nerve passes between the neck of the mandible and the sphenomandibular ligament, it gives off parotid branches and then turns superiorly, posterior to the mandibular condyle, and gives off branches to the skin of the anterior portion of the auricle as well as anterosuperior to the auricle.
  A, C, D, and E. These nerves do not provide somatosensory innervation to the parotid gland.
  GAS 906–908; N 134, 145; ABR/McM 33, 39, 40

Answers 251–275

251. A. Sensory innervation to the area of the larynx superior to the vocal folds is supplied by the superior laryngeal nerve.

B. The recurrent laryngeal nerve supplies sensation to the area inferior to the vocal cords.

C. The vagus (CN X) and glossopharyngeal (CN IX) nerves bring about the swallowing reflex.

D, E. Weakness to the posterior cricoarytenoid muscles would be because of recurrent laryngeal nerve damage.

GAS 1057; N 87–89; ABR/McM 47

252. B. A nonobstructive hydrocephalus occurs as a result of decreased reabsorption of CSF via the arachnoid villi.

A, C, D, E. The subdural and epidural spaces are potential spaces, and these do not contain CSF. The choroid plexus produces the CSF, which flows into the subarachnoid space and is reabsorbed into the superior sagittal sinus via the arachnoid villi.

GAS 874–876; N 111–115; ABR/McM 60–61

253. E. The location of the growing lump is close to the external acoustic meatus and is likely compressing on the facial nerve as it exits the stylomastoid foramen. The facial nerve is responsible for tight closure of the eyelids.

B, D. Protraction of the tongue is because of innervation of the hypoglossal nerve and elevation of the mandible by the mandibular nerve.

C. Pupillary constriction and partial ptosis result from damage to the oculomotor nerve.

A. Vagus nerve innervates levator veli palatini muscle.

GAS 889–890; N 17, 110, 135; ABR/McM 58

254. D. Branches of the sphenopalatine, superior labial, and anterior ethmoidal anastomose anteriorly on the nasal septum and are prone to bleeding.

A, E. The descending palatine and ascending pharyngeal arteries are located posteriorly in the pharynx.

B. The posterior superior alveolar artery travels within the maxilla and the accessory meningeal artery is found within the cranial cavity.

C. Posterior ethmoidal and middle meningeal arteries do not supply the nasal septum.

GAS 1072; N 47; ABR/McM 55

255. C. The glossopharyngeal nerve is located in the lower part of the tonsillar fossa after it passes behind and then lateral to the stylopharyngeus muscle, which it innervates.

A. The vagus nerve forms part of the pharyngeal plexus for supply of the pharynx and continues in the carotid sheath.

B. The hypoglossal nerve is found inferior to the tongue.

D, E. The external and internal laryngeal nerves, or the external and internal branches of the superior laryngeal nerve, are found in the neck.

GAS 877, 890–891; N 72, 80, 82, 136; ABR/McM 84

256. A. The function of the posterior cricoarytenoid muscle is to abduct the vocal cords.

B, D. The transverse arytenoid and lateral cricoarytenoid muscle adducts the vocal cords, bringing them into apposition for phonation.

C, E. Cricothyroid stretches the vocal cords taut for phonation and thyroarytenoid muscles reduce this tension on the vocal cords to adjust the pitch of the voice. *GAS 1050–1051; N 91–93; ABR/McM 49*

257. D. Sternocleidomastoid and trapezius muscles are supplied by the accessory nerve, which enters the skull via the foramen magnum. The posterior inferior cerebellar artery is the artery nearest the accessory nerve.

A, B, C, E. The other arteries listed are not close to the accessory nerve.

GAS 870, 888–890; N 150, 152, 154; ABR/McM 32

258. E. The nerve responsible for innervating the muscles of the larynx and pharynx is the vagus nerve, which also initiates the cough reflex.

A, B. The muscles of mastication and facial expression are supplied by trigeminal and facial nerves, respectively.

C. The vestibulocochlear nerve mediates hearing and balance.

D. The oropharyngeal mucosa is supplied by the glossopharyngeal nerve.

GAS 885–886, 888; N 137; ABR/McM 84

259. B. The external laryngeal nerve, the external branch of the superior laryngeal nerve, supplies the cricothyroid muscle responsible for tensing the vocal cords.

C, D, E. Loss of sensation would not result from injury to a motor nerve.

A. Inability to abduct the vocal folds would result from damage to the recurrent laryngeal nerve.

GAS 1008–1009; N 87–89; ABR/McM 49

260. A. The vagus nerve is responsible for motor innervation to the soft palate (except tensor veli palatini).

C. if damaged, the uvula would deviate from the side of the lesion.

B and E. Glossopharyngeal nerve damage could reduce the gag reflex because it is the afferent limb but would not produce the other symptoms.

D. Damage to the trigeminal nerve would not produce any of these symptoms.

GAS 834, 840–841; N 66, 136–137; ABR/McM 84

261. B. The masseter muscle originates on the zygomatic bone and inserts on the lateral surface of the ramus of the mandible. It is a powerful elevator of the mandible. Grinding of the teeth can lead to hypertrophy of the muscles of mastication, especially the masseter. Patients will have difficulty in depressing the mandible because of spasms of this enlarged muscle.

A. The buccinator muscle is located between the maxilla and the mandible. Its main action is to compress the cheek against the teeth. It is also involved in whistling, smiling, and speech production.

C. The mylohyoid muscle runs from the mandible to the hyoid bone and forms part of the floor of the oral cavity.

D. The posterior belly of the digastric muscle originates from the mastoid process and connects to the hyoid bone via the intermediate tendon. It plays a role in the opening of the jaw when the masseter and temporalis are relaxed.

E. The lateral pterygoid plays a role in mouth opening and jaw protrusion.
GAS 966–967; N 55–56; ABR/McM 39–41

262. E. The vagus nerve mediates both the afferent and efferent limbs of the cough reflex: afferent to the mucus membranes and efferent to the muscles of the larynx.

A. The glossopharyngeal nerve is involved in the gag reflex as the afferent limb.

B. The hypoglossal nerve innervates most of the tongue musculature except for the palatoglossus which is innervated by the vagus nerve.

C. The external laryngeal nerve is a branch of superior laryngeal nerve, from vagus nerve, that provides only motor innervation to the cricothyroid and cricopharyngeus muscles.

D. The trigeminal nerve provides sensory innervation to the face.
GAS 889, 1003; N 137; ABR/McM 84

263. C. The trigeminal nerve is the major sensory nerve of the face. It has three branches: ophthalmic, maxillary, and mandibular. The neurologist was trying to elicit the corneal reflex where the afferent limb (sensation on the eyeball) is via the trigeminal nerve and the efferent limb is the facial nerve (closing the eye).

A. The optic nerve is responsible for vision.

B and D. The oculomotor and abducens nerves innervate extraocular muscles.

E. The facial nerve plays a role in the efferent limb of the corneal reflex, but since both eyes blink when the right cornea is stroked, both facial nerves appear to be intact.
GAS 838, 887, 890; N 97, 132–134, 142; ABR/McM 81

264. D. The thyroid gland develops as a diverticulum from the floor of the primitive pharynx. It is temporarily connected to the tongue at the foramen cecum by the thyroglossal duct, which then degenerates. It descends in the neck, passing anterior to the hyoid bone. Incomplete degeneration of the thyroglossal duct can lead to a cystic mass in the path of the descent of the thyroid gland.

A, B, C, E. The thyroglossal duct passes from foramen cecum of the tongue to the isthmus of the thyroid gland.
GAS 1007–1008; N 71, 77; ABR/McM 36

265. B. The paired superior cerebellar arteries are the penultimate branches of the basilar artery. Each artery originates from the basilar artery and runs laterally to supply the superior and medial parts of the cerebellum. In its course, it travels very close to the trochlear nerve. This nerve innervates the superior oblique muscle, which is responsible for depression of the eyeball when it is in the adducted state. This allows for proper vision when reading a newspaper or walking downstairs.

A. Damage to the middle cerebral arteries may cause facial motor deficits but it would not be

specific to the trochlear nerve which supplies the superior oblique muscle.

C. Internal carotid artery occlusion would not lead to focalized deficits of the trochlear nerve but may cause generalized motor deficits on one side of the body or monocular blindness.

D and E. Aneurysms of the anterior inferior cerebellar artery and the posterior inferior cerebellar artery are extremely rare. Symptoms caused may be vertigo, tinnitus, nausea and hearing loss.
GAS 869–870; N 149–154; ABR/McM 67

266. E. The aneurysm is located near the basilar artery between the left superior cerebellar and posterior cerebral arteries. This location is the origin of the oculomotor nerve, which innervates the extraocular eye muscles with the exception of the lateral rectus (innervated by the abducens nerve) and the superior oblique (done by the trochlear nerve). Compression of this nerve by an aneurysm will result in the eye being abducted (lateral rectus) and depressed (superior oblique).

A, B, C, and D. None of these other locations describe the origin of the oculomotor nerve and therefore would not be implicated in its deficit.
GAS 869–870; N 149–154; ABR/McM 67

267. B. The internal carotid is the artery that supplies the majority of the blood supply to the brain. It has several parts including the cervical, petrous, lacerum, cavernous, clinoid, ophthalmic, and communicating segments. The cavernous sinuses are paired dural sinuses that are located on the lateral wall of the sphenoid bone on either side of the sella turcica. The internal carotid artery and the abducens nerve run through it. Damage to this part of the internal carotid would affect the abducens nerve and the patient's ability to abduct the eye.

A, C, D, and E. Aneurysms of the other arteries would not result in a compression of the abducens nerve as they are not situated in the cavernous sinus.
GAS 869, 875; N 115; ABR/McM 67

268. E. The patient is suffering from an aneurysm of the anterior communicating artery. This artery connects the two anterior cerebral arteries across the beginning of the longitudinal fissure superior to the optic chiasm. An aneurysm in this area compresses the optic chiasm, resulting in blindness in the outer half of both right and left visual fields (bitemporal hemianopsia).

A. An aneurysm of the anterior inferior cerebellar artery compresses the abducens nerve, which results in an inability to abduct the eye.

B. An aneurysm of the superior cerebellar artery can also cause compression of the trochlear nerve and an inability to depress the adducted eye.

C. Ptosis is as a result of compression to the oculomotor nerve, which can be compressed by an aneurysm in the superior cerebellar or the posterior cerebral arteries.

D. Loss of corneal sensation is because of damage to the trigeminal nerve.

GAS 876; N 150–152; ABR/McM 67

269. C. The CT scan shows an orbital (blow-out) fracture. The inferior rectus muscle originates from the inferior part of the common tendinous ring and inserts on the inferior anterior part of the eyeball. With an orbital fracture, an injury to the floor of the orbit may result in entrapment of the inferior rectus muscle by a fragment of bone. This tethers the inferior rectus muscle to bone, resulting in loss of function of the muscle. Patients experience diplopia when attempting upward gaze.

A, B, D, and E. These muscles would not be affected with the resulting fracture or cause the symptoms this patient is experiencing.

GAS 927; N 96; ABR/McM 51

270. C. The area indicated by the *arrow* is the mastoid cells of the mastoid process. The infection likely spread via mastoid emissary veins, which passed through the mastoid foramen of the temporal bone to the sigmoid sinus. The sigmoid sinus begins beneath the temporal bone and travels to the jugular foramen, at which point it joins the inferior petrosal sinus to form the jugular vein.

A. The cavernous sinus does not have any direct relations to the mastoid process or mastoid cells.

B. The pterygoid venous plexus is located in the infratemporal fossa and communicates with the anterior facial vein and the cavernous sinus, by branches through the sphenoidal emissary foramen (of Vesalius), foramen ovale, and foramen lacerum. It has no relation to the mastoid process or mastoid emissary veins.

D. The straight sinus is located within the dura mater, where the falx cerebri meets the midline of tentorium cerebelli.

E. The superior petrosal sinus is located in the petrosal sulcus on the petrous part of the temporal bone. It receives blood from the cavernous sinus and passes backward and laterally to drain into the transverse sinus.

GAS 876, 953; N 110, 114, 115; ABR/McM 36

271. C. The frontal sinuses are located in the frontal bone above the orbital margin.

A. The maxillary sinus is located on the sides of the nose below the cheeks and above the teeth, within the maxillary bone.

B. The transverse sinus is a dural venous sinus that drains the confluence of sinuses and runs along the inner aspect of the occipital bone surface.

D. The sphenoidal sinus is within the sphenoid bone and cannot be palpated externally.

E. The ethmoid sinus is a collection of small air cells located within the ethmoid bone between the nose and the eye.

GAS 1063–1068; N 49, 51; ABR/McM 11, 16, 17

272. C. The temporal bone parts include mastoid, petrous, squamous, and tympanic portions. The mastoid process is part of the mastoid portion of the temporal bone.

A. The occipital bone is located at the back of the skull and lower part of the skull.

B. The zygomatic bone is located at the upper and lateral aspect of the face. It is also referred to as the "cheekbone" and forms most of the prominence of the cheek.

D. The parietal bone forms the upper central part of the cranium.

E. The sphenoid bone is located in the middle of the skull between the frontal, ethmoid, and maxillary bones anteriorly and the occipital and temporal bones posteriorly.

GAS 961–962; N 13, 17; ABR/McM 4, 7, 6

273. A. The central retinal artery is the major blood supply to the intima of the eye. It is a branch of the ophthalmic artery and travels within the optic nerve close to the eyeball to get to the intima or retina of the eye.

B. C, and E. The ciliary arteries arise from the ophthalmic artery and supply the sclera, choroid, conjunctiva, ciliary processes, and rectus muscles. The central retinal artery only rarely arises from the posterior ciliary arteries.

D. The ophthalmic artery branches off the internal carotid artery as the latter exits the cavernous sinus. It gives rise to several other smaller arteries including the ciliary arteries as described above.

GAS 931; N 103; ABR/McM 53

274. C. The auriculotemporal nerve, a branch of the mandibular division of the trigeminal nerve, passes posteriorly, deep to the ramus of the mandible and superior to the deep part of the parotid gland, emerging posterior to the temporomandibular joint to supply the skin anterior to the auricle and anteriorly on the auricle, as well as skin of the temporal region posteriorly. The nerve distributes to the skin of the tragus and adjacent helix of the auricle and therefore of the external acoustic meatus and skin of the superior portion of the tympanic membrane. The lesser occipital nerve, a branch of the cervical plexus, supplies the skin posterior to the auricle. The great auricular nerve, also a cervical plexus branch, supplies the skin overlying the mandible and the capsule of the parotid gland, as well as the majority of the lateral surface of the auricle. The zygomaticotemporal nerve supplies the hairless patch of skin over the anterior part of the temporal fossa. The greater occipital nerve supplies the occipital part of the scalp.

A, B, D, E. The arteries indicated are not related to cranial nerves that are responsible for depression of the gaze.

GAS 974–975; N 53, 57, 59, 82, 133; ABR/McM 83

275. C. The two nerves found in the internal acoustic meatus are the facial nerve and vestibulocochlear nerve. Of the two, the facial nerve supplies facial muscles and can cause unilateral facial paralysis.

A, B, D, and E. The remainder of the cranial nerves do not share spatial orientations with the internal acoustic meatus.

GAS 958–960; N 18, 20; ABR/McM 58

276. D. The olfactory nerves arise from cells in the superior part of the lateral and septal walls of the nasal cavity. The processes of these cells (forming the olfactory nerve) pass through the cribriform plate and end in the olfactory bulbs, which lie on either side of the crista galli. Therefore, a tumor here compresses these nerves, and the sense of smell will be affected. The optic tract and chiasm are not likely to be affected. Similarly, the vagus, vestibulocochlear, and facial nerves are not in close proximity.

A. B, C, and E. The remainder of the cranial nerves mentioned do not share spatial orientations with the crista galli

GAS 897, 1074; N 46, 130; ABR/McM 55

277. A. The butterfly-shaped middle cranial fossa has a central part composed of the sella turcica on the body of the sphenoid and large, depressed lateral parts on each side.

B. The temporal bones are situated at the sides and base of the skull and consist of the squama temporalis, mastoid portion, petrous portion, tympanic part, zygomatic process, and styloid process.

C. The occipital bone is situated at the back and lower part of the skull and is pierced by a large oval opening, the foramen magnum.

D and E. The ethmoid and frontal bones are found in the anterior cranial fossa.

GAS 855; N 18; ABR/McM 4, 11, 12

278. E. The loose connective tissue layer (layer four) of the scalp is the danger area of the scalp because purulence or blood spreads easily in it. Infection in this layer can also pass into the cranial cavity through small emissary veins, which pass through foramina in the calvaria, and reach intracranial structures such as the meninges.

A and B. The intercavernous sinus and the inferior sagittal sinus are venous sinuses formed in the dura mater.

C. The diploic veins are found within the bones of the cranial vault and drain the diploic space. This is found in the marrow-containing area of cancellous bone between the inner and outer layers of compact bone.

D. The basal veins of Rosenthal are paired veins that drain into the great vein of Galen.

GAS 874, 878; N 10, 111, 113; ABR/McM 5

279. C. The muscles of facial expression are supplied by the facial nerve, which emerges from the stylomastoid foramen and passes through the parotid gland. The nerve gives off five major branches within the parotid gland from superior to inferior: temporal, zygomatic, buccal, marginal mandibular, and cervical. A fun mnemonic for these five branches is To Zanzibar By Motor Car.

A and B. The common carotid artery provides branches to supply the neck and the face while the vertebral artery supplies the spinal cord and the posterior part of the brain and brainstem.

D and E. The lateral pterygoid and temporalis muscles are muscles of mastication and are supplied by the mandibular division of the trigeminal nerve (CN V3).

GAS 913–915; N 145; ABR/McM 34, 39, 40

280. D. The area behind the foramen magnum consists of the squamous part of the occipital bone. The foramen magnum is in the basilar part of the occipital bone (basiocciput). The dura mater is attached to the margins of the foramen as it sweeps down from the posterior cranial fossa. Within the tube of dura mater, the lower medulla, with the vertebral and spinal arteries and the spinal roots of the accessory nerves, traverse the foramen in the subarachnoid space.

A. CN I passes through the cribriform plate of the ethmoid bone.

B, C, and E. The glossopharyngeal, vagus, and accessory nerves arise from the side of the medulla oblongata. The three nerves run laterally across the occipital bone and pass through the jugular foramen.

GAS 890–892; N 20, 154; ABR/McM 11, 61

281. A. The glossopharyngeal nerve emerges from the surface of the medulla and travels laterally in the pontine cistern to enter the anterior compartment of the jugular foramen. It gives off the tympanic nerve, which supplies the middle ear and forms the lesser petrosal nerve, a carotid branch to innervate the carotid body, the nerve to the stylopharyngeus, pharyngeal branches, a lingual branch, and a tonsillar branch. The tonsillar branch provides afferent fibers for the tonsillar mucosa and the lingual branch conveys common sensation and taste from the posterior third of the tongue, as well as secretomotor fibers for lingual glands.

B and E. Taste of the anterior two-thirds of the tongue is innervated by the chorda tympani, a branch of the facial nerve (CN VII).

C and D. The vagus nerve (CN X) innervates the muscles of the soft palate (except for tensor veli palatini) and the constrictor muscles of the pharynx.

GAS 834, 840–841; N 66, 136, 137; ABR/McM 44, 84

282. E. The vocalis muscles lie medial to the thyroarytenoid muscles and lateral to the vocal ligaments within the vocal folds. The vocalis muscles produce minute adjustments of the vocal ligaments, selectively relaxing the anterior and posterior parts, respectively, of the vocal folds during animated speech and singing.

A, B, C, D. The other muscles listed are not closely related to the vocalis muscle

GAS 1050–1051; N 91–93; ABR/McM 49

283. B. Cricothyrotomy is an emergency airway procedure performed to ensure immediate airway ventilation in cases of laryngeal obstruction. It is performed by making an incision at the cricothyroid membrane, which is located between the thyroid cartilage and the cricoid cartilage.

A, C, D, and E. All the other options are incorrect because the cricothyroid membrane is located between the thyroid cartilage and the cricoid cartilage and this is where the incision is made.
GAS 1041, 1046; N 90; ABR/McM 48, 49

284. A. The larynx receives sensory innervation from the vagus nerve via the internal branch of superior laryngeal nerve.
  B. The glossopharyngeal nerve does not innervate the epiglottis.
  C. The vestibulocochlear nerve mediates hearing and balance.
  D. The hypoglossal nerve supplies motor fibers to the tongue muscles.
  E. The facial nerve, while performing many functions including motor supply to muscles of facial expression and taste in the anterior two-thirds of the tongue, does not supply sensory nerves to the epiglottis.
  GAS 1057; N 92, 137; ABR/McM 49, 84

285. D. An acoustic neuroma is an intracranial tumor that arises from the Schwann cell sheath investing the vestibulocochlear nerve. As this tumor grows, it eventually occupies a large portion of the cerebellopontine angle. Since cranial nerves VII and VIII are in close proximity to this location, these nerves are also usually affected, with subsequent manifestation of symptoms of impaired hearing, vertigo, loss of balance and nystagmus, paralysis of muscles of facial expression, hyperacusis, loss of taste sensation on the anterior two-thirds of the tongue, loss of corneal reflex and sensation around the mouth and nose, and paralysis of muscles of mastication.
  A, B, C, E. The other locations listed are not related to the facial and vestibulocochlear nerves.
  GAS 954; N 150, 154; ABR/McM 61

286. B. The patient described in the question has experienced vasovagal syncope after stimulation of the posterior wall of her external acoustic meatus by an otoscope speculum. In this form of syncope, parasympathetic outflow via the vagus nerve (CN X) leads to decreased pulse and blood pressure. The posterior part of the external acoustic meatus is innervated by the small auricular branch of the vagus nerve.
  A. The vestibulocochlear nerve has dual innervations. The vestibular portion innervates the vestibular system in the middle ear which is responsible for detecting balance. The vestibular nerve also detects head movement and works with the oculomotor and abducens nerve to stabilize the eyes on an image while the head moves. The cochlear nerve traverses the cochlear in the middle ear and forms the spiral ganglia which serves the sense of hearing.
  C. Most of the remainder of the external acoustic meatus, including the external portion of the

tympanic membrane, is innervated by the mandibular division of the trigeminal nerve via its auriculotemporal branch. The inner surface of the tympanic membrane is innervated by the glossopharyngeal nerve (CN IX) via its tympanic branch.
  D. The facial nerve acts as the motor component of the corneal reflex.
  E. The accessory nerve supplies the sternocleidomastoid and trapezius muscle.
  GAS 838, 945; N 137; ABR/McM 84

287. D. The superior thyroid artery, a branch of the external carotid artery, and the inferior thyroid artery, a branch of the thyrocervical trunk, provide the blood supply to the thyroid and parathyroid glands. The superior thyroid artery, superior thyroid vein, and external branch of the superior laryngeal nerve course together in a neurovascular triad that originates superior to the thyroid gland and lateral to the thyroid cartilage. Because the external branch of the superior laryngeal nerve courses close to the superior thyroid artery, it is at risk of injury during thyroidectomy.
  A, B, C and E. Thyroarytenoid, lateral cricoarytenoid, posterior cricoarytenoid and vocalis muscles are all innervated by the recurrent laryngeal nerve which may course more close with the inferior thyroid artery and not the superior thyroid artery.
  GAS 1050–1051; N 87, 92; ABR/McM 48, 49

288. D. The basilar artery is formed by the two vertebral arteries at the inferior part of the brainstem. At the pontomedullary junction, the basilar artery gives rise to two branches: the anterior inferior cerebellar artery first and then the labyrinthine artery. The abducens nerve (cranial nerve VI) emerges at the pontomedullary junction and is usually found between the anterior inferior cerebellar and the labyrinthine arteries. The abducens nerve supplies the lateral rectus muscle, which abducts the eyes. This function of the nerve can be impaired if the nerve is compressed by a nearby aneurysm. If this condition occurs on the right side, it can result in weak abduction of the right eye.
  A. Weak abduction and depression of the right eye would occur if the inferior rectus muscle innervation by the oculomotor nerve was affected.
  B. Weak adduction of the left eye would occur if the aneurysm affected the oculomotor innervation of the medial rectus.
  C. Weak adduction and elevation of the right eye would occur if the right inferior oblique's muscle innervation by the oculomotor nerve was affected
  E. Weak abduction of the left eye would occur if the abducens nerve (CN VI) was affected as this nerve supplies the lateral rectus muscle responsible for this movement.
  GAS 869–870; N 150, 152, 154; ABR/McM 67, 68

289. B. The cranial nerve emerging anterolaterally at the junction of the pons and midbrain is the oculomotor

(CN III). It passes between the superior cerebellar and posterior cerebral arteries (above). Both arteries are branches of the basilar artery. An aneurysm of the PCA could result in compression of the nerve and lead to oculomotor nerve palsy. This will result in the individual being unable to move the eye normally. The affected eye will be in a down and out position. The outward location of the eye is because of the lateral rectus (innervated by the sixth cranial nerve), which maintains muscle tone in comparison to the paralyzed medial rectus. The downward location is because the superior oblique muscle (innervated by the fourth cranial or trochlear nerve) is not antagonized by the paralyzed superior rectus, inferior rectus, and inferior oblique muscles.

A. The abducens nerve (cranial nerve VI) emerges at the pontomedullary junction and is usually found between the anterior inferior cerebellar and the labyrinthine arteries. The abducens nerve supplies the lateral rectus muscle, which abducts the eyes.

C. Contralateral homonymous hemianopia occurs due to lesions affecting the optic track leading to one side of the brain. Loss of vision from lateral fields of right eye and medial fields of left eye can occur due to lesions affecting the right optic track and would lead to visual disturbances in the left visual fields causing a left homonymous hemianopia.

D. Inability to detect odors through the right nostril. Unilateral anosmia may be caused by several things affecting the olfactory nerve including head trauma (most common), tumors of the floor of the anterior fossa, or subarachnoid hemorrhage.

E. Loss of sensation of the skin over the right forehead, cheek, and mandible may occur due to damage of the 3 separate branches of the trigeminal nerve (ophthalmic, mandibular, maxillary).
GAS 869–870; N 150, 152, 154; ABR/McM 67, 68

290. D. The infratemporal fossa is a wedge-shaped region. It is located inferior to the temporal fossa and between the ramus of the mandible laterally and the wall of the pharynx medially. The contents of the fossa include the temporalis, masseter, and lateral and medial pterygoid muscles. The pterygoid venous plexus and branches of the maxillary artery are also found in this fossa. Nerves passing through the fossa include the mandibular, auriculotemporal, inferior alveolar, lingual, buccal, and chorda tympani nerves. Tumors involving the infratemporal fossa present with a variety of symptoms depending on the structures involved. The auriculotemporal nerve carries the postsynaptic parasympathetic fibers for parotid gland innervation, so secretions of this gland will be affected by compression to the nerves in the infratemporal fossa.

A. Weak elevation of the corner of the right side of the mouth would be cause by damage to the right facial nerve.

B. Loss of sensation over the upper lip and to the upper teeth would be caused by damage to the maxillary branch of the trigeminal nerve which can be compressed in the pterygopalatine fossa through which it traverses just posterior to the upper jaw.

C. Inability to sense a foreign body in the right eye would occur due to damage of the ophthalmic branch of the trigeminal nerve which passes through the superior orbital fissure.

E. Inability to abduct the right eye would occur due to damage of the abducens nerve which can occur due to aneurysms of blood vessels near the pontomedullary junction.
GAS 961; N 82–85; ABR/McM 9

291. E. Because of the mass in the lumen of the parotid duct and distended parotid gland, nerves passing through the gland can be affected. Pain sensation over the anterior auricle, tragus, and anterior helix is because of compression of the auriculotemporal nerve, which passes through the parotid gland and ascends just anterior to the ear, supplying the external acoustic meatus, surface of the tympanic membrane, and large area of the temple.

A. The trunk of the facial nerve divides into temporofacial and cervicofacial divisions, which then further divide into temporal (supplies temple, forehead, and supraorbital muscles), zygomatic (orbital and upper lip muscles), buccal (upper lip and muscles at the corner of mouth), marginal mandibular (lower lip and chin muscles), and cervical branches (platysma muscle). Compression of any or all of the branches affects corresponding muscles and their functions.

B. Complete ptosis of the left eyelid would occur due to damage of the oculomotor nerve (CN III).

C. Numbness of the skin over the left lower mandible would occur due to damage of the mandibular division of the trigeminal nerve.

D. Excessive tearing may be caused by loss of innervation to the orbicularis oculi from the facial nerve which may cause an inability to close the eyes tightly resulting in a spillage of tears.
GAS 913–915; N 54, 53, 145; ABR/McM 39, 40

292. D. The nerves involved are the lingual and buccal nerves, which are branches of the mandibular branch of the trigeminal nerve. These branches provide sensation to mucosa of the anterior two-thirds of the tongue (general sensation), adjacent gums, cheek mucosa, and overlying skin.

A and B. Weak movement of the jaw would be caused by damage to the mandibular branch of the trigeminal nerve but more specifically the masseteric branch which supplies the masseter muscle responsible for jaw movement.

C. Numbness over the skin of the tragus and helix of the left ear would occur due to damage of the auriculotemporal nerve.

E. The lingual and buccal nerves have no role in salivation.
GAS 974–977; N 59; ABR/McM 44

293. C. If the orbital rim is involved in the fracture, the patient may demonstrate a palpable bony "step-off" and complain of pain with palpation of the rim. Presentations of anterior cranial fossa fractures often include CSF rhinorrhea and bruising around the eyes. A fracture of the cribriform plate may cause anosmia, or lack of the sense of smell, due to damage to the olfactory nerves that pass up through the cribriform plate.

A and B. Blurred vision and diplopia may be due to damage of the cranial nerves supplying the ocular muscles including the trochlear, oculomotor and abducens nerve which may occur due to aneurysms occurring in vessels around the brainstem.

D. Blindness may occur due to damage of the optic tracts or the optic nerve nerve itself or injury to the occipital lobe.

E. Dry left eye would occur due to damage of the lacrimal nerve which is a nerve coming off of the ophthalmic branch of the trigeminal nerve.

GAS 885, 1061, 1074; N 18, 46, 130; ABR/McM 12

294. A. The nerves that control lacrimal secretion pass within the zygomatic nerve, from the maxillary nerve and the pterygopalatine ganglion, through the inferior orbital fissure, which is found in the orbit between the greater wing of the sphenoid and the orbital surface of the maxilla. The zygomatic nerve would not be affected by a fracture near the apex of the orbit. The abducens nerve, the nasociliary nerve, and divisions of the oculomotor nerve all pass through the middle part of the fissure, which results in options B, C, D, and E being likely consequences of the injury as they are closer to the apex of the orbit.

GAS 923; N 20, 63, BP 26, 133; ABR/McM 11, 12

295. A. Fracture of the mandibular ramus would weaken elevation of the jaw, since the most powerful jaw elevator, the temporalis muscle, attaches to the coronoid process above the fracture. Masseter and medial pterygoid muscles, the other two elevators of the mandible, could still function to elevate the jaw.

B. Unopposed action of the lateral pterygoid on the left would cause deviation of the jaw to the right.

C, D, E. Salivation and sensation would not be affected by the fracture of the ramus.

GAS 975–977; N 82; ABR/McM 55

296. B. Coursing through the pterygoid canal are the artery, vein, and nerve of the pterygoid canal (Vidian canal).

A, C, D, E. The nerve of the pterygoid canal (Vidian nerve) contains presynaptic parasympathetic fibers from the facial nerve via the greater petrosal nerve, which eventually go on to synapse in the pterygopalatine ganglion, and postsynaptic sympathetic fibers from the deep petrosal nerve, which do not synapse in pterygopalatine ganglion (*GAS Fig. 8.157A*).

GAS 982, 984; N 46, 61, 62, 63; ABR/McM 25

297. E. The nerves that control lacrimal secretion pass through the inferior orbital fissure, which is found in the orbit between the orbital surface of the maxilla and greater wing of the sphenoid bone.

A, C, D. Taste from the anterior two-thirds of the tongue and secretions from the submandibular and sublingual glands were likely affected because their nerve signals are carried by the chorda tympani, which joins the facial nerve in the facial canal located in the petrous part of the temporal bone.

B. Movements of the right side of the face are also likely compromised or deficient because these muscles are innervated by branches of the facial nerve, which was likely impinged in the facial canal as a result of the fracture to the temporal bone.

GAS 983, 987; N 20, 63, BP 26, 133; ABR/McM 11

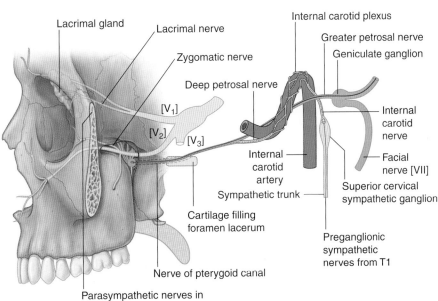

• *GAS* Fig. 8.157A

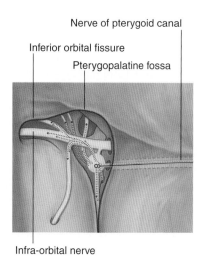

Nerve of pterygoid canal

Inferior orbital fissure

Pterygopalatine fossa

Infra-orbital nerve

Preganglionic parasympathetic nerves	——
Postganglionic parasympathetic nerves	········
Preganglionic sympathetic nerves	——
Postganglionic sympathetic nerves	········

• *GAS* **Fig. 8.157B**

298. D. The fracture to the zygomatic bone, because of proximity, likely distorted the orbit resulting in damage to the structures running within the inferior orbital fissure, where the nerves that transmit secretomotor fibers for the lacrimal gland pass.

A, B. C. E. Damage to the zygomatic nerve would not result in the other symptoms listed.
GAS 927, 986; N 61, 63, 96, BP 26; ABR/McM 11, 52

299. C. The patient suffers from either a damaged nerve or a trapped muscle; the inferior oblique muscle is defective.

A, B. Complete or partial ptosis results from an inability to lift the upper eyelid and will not result from damage to the lower orbit.

D. Inability to depress the adducted eyeball will result from damage to the superior oblique muscle. The nerve to the superior oblique and the muscle itself run superomedially and will therefore not be damaged in this patient.

E. An inability to produce tears will result from parasympathetic damage and will only result from damage to the zygomatic nerve, traveling from the pterygopalatine ganglion, or its zygomaticotemporal branch. (*GAS* Fig. 8.157B).
GAS 927, 929; N BP 26, 96; ABR/McM 52, 53, 54

300. A. The petrous part of the temporal bone houses the middle and inner ear and has the facial canal with the facial nerve passing through it.

B. Damage to the infratemporal fossa will not cause hearing loss or vertigo but will produce additional symptoms.

C, D, E. The middle ear could account for the hearing loss, and the inner ear for hearing loss and vertigo, but not the facial palsy or lack of lacrimation.
GAS 1030; N 110; ABR/McM 57

301. B. The area of damage is in the tympanic membrane, which is supplied by the facial, glossopharyngeal, and vagus nerves.

A. The auriculotemporal and great auricular nerves supply the temporomandibular joint and external ear, respectively.

C. The lesser occipital nerves supply the skin on the posterior aspect of the skull behind the ear.

D. The chorda tympani is responsible for taste to the anterior two-thirds of the tongue and sensation to the middle ear.

E. The lesser petrosal nerve and tympanic plexus carry autonomic innervation to and through the middle ear and are not associated with the external acoustic meatus.
GAS 944, 947; N 107; ABR/McM 57

302. C. The infant's condition is known as *coloboma* and results from failure of the choroid fissure to fuse.

A. Failure of the neuroectoderm to induce the surface ectoderm to differentiate results in failure of the eye to form.

B. Failed obliteration of the intraretinal space results in retinal separation between the pigmented and neural layers.

D. If the optic cup does not overlap the developing lens, the iris will fail to form entirely.

E. If the lens vesicle does not separate from the surface ectoderm, the eye cavities will not form.
N 102; ABR/McM 41

303. B. The ethmoid sinuses are groups of cells located in the ethmoid bone. There are three groups of cells: posterior (drain into the superior nasal meatus), middle (drain into the middle nasal meatus at the ethmoid bulla), and anterior (drain into the middle nasal meatus by way of the ethmoid infundibulum at the semilunar hiatus). This can spread infections from the paranasal sinuses into the nasal cavity, leading to upper respiratory tract infections.

A. The auditory tube runs from the middle ear to the nasopharynx.

C. The nasolacrimal duct indirectly drains the lacrimal gland, which is located on the lateral side of the orbit.

D, E. The sphenoidal sinus drains into the sphenoethmoidal recess.
GAS 1061; N 43–44; ABR/McM 5

304. D. Oblique facial clefts are rare and often bilateral facial anomalies that extend from the upper lip to the medial margin of the orbit. In this condition, the nasolacrimal ducts are open grooves draining the tears from the lacrimal lake that lubricates the conjunctiva. This results from failure of the fusion of the mesenchyme of the maxillary process with the lateral nasal process.

A, B, C. E. Failure of fusion of the medial nasal prominences results in a median cleft lip and palate, while

failure of fusion of the intermaxillary segment with the maxillary processes results in a unilateral cleft lip.
N 31; ABR/McM 16

305. E. Treacher Collins syndrome (craniofacial dysostosis) is an autosomal disorder characterized by malar hypoplasia, underdeveloped mandible, downward slanting palpebral fissures, defects of the lower eyelids and external ears, and abnormalities of the middle and internal ears.

A and B. Failure of the medial nasal prominences to fuse with the medial aspect of the maxillary process produces, or failed fusion of lateral nasal prominences with maxillary processes, will result in a facial cleft, which is not seen in this case.

C. This is a first *arch* syndrome because of failure of neural crest cells to migrate into the first arch during the fourth week of development.

D. Failed migration of neural crest cells to the third and fourth pharyngeal pouches would lead thyroid and parathyroid abnormalities. This is a first arch syndrome due to failure of neural crest cells to migrate during the fourth week of development.
N 63; ABR/McM 16

306. B. The superior cerebellar artery originates immediately before the termination of the basilar artery. It passes lateral below the oculomotor nerve to give blood supply to the anterior and medial parts of the cerebellum. An aneurysm of the superior cerebellar artery would result in oculomotor nerve palsy. This will affect the parasympathetics to the ciliary body and pupillary constrictor resulting in blurry vision, the levator palpebrae superioris resulting in ptosis, and the extrinsic muscles of the eye with the exception of the lateral rectus and superior oblique, resulting in lateral deviation (abduction) of the eye.

A, C, D, E. Damage to oculomotor nerve would cause abduction, not adduction, and complete, not partial, ptosis.
GAS 869–870; N 150, 152, 154; ABR/McM 68

307. C. Hydrocephalus is an abnormal accumulation of CSF in the ventricles of the brain. This can be because of abnormal flow (often blockage in the cerebral aqueduct of Sylvius), impaired reabsorption, or rarely, excessive production of CSF. Communicating hydrocephalus is caused by impaired reabsorption of CSF because of abnormal functioning of the arachnoid granulations, which are responsible for drainage of the CSF into the venous system.

A, B, D, E. In this condition, all the ventricles of the brain become dilated. Incidentally, although the fact that this baby was delivered by cesarean section is in no way responsible for the hydrocephalus, the term "cesarean section" is interesting. Some people think the term is applied because Julius Caesar was delivered through an incision after his mother died during labor. However, that story is probably apocryphal. A more likely explanation is that when Julius Caesar was emperor of the Roman Empire, he issued a series of rules called the Cesarean codes. One of these rules required somebody attending to a woman in labor (probably equivalent to a midwife) to attempt delivery of a viable infant immediately if the mother died during childbirth.
GAS 864; N 111–113; ABR/McM 61, 72

308. C. This patient has gustatory sweating, also called Frey syndrome. When his parotid gland was removed, the postganglionic nerves that innervated the glandular epithelium of his parotid gland were cut, but the nerve cell bodies of those nerves, which are located in the otic ganglion, were undamaged and able to regenerate fibers. These fibers travel with the auriculotemporal nerve, and they "sought out" glandular epithelium. The closest glands are sweat glands in the skin of the face. Under circumstances that normally induce salivation (seeing appetizing food in this case), sweating occurs instead.

A. Ciliary ganglion controls ciliary muscle and sphincter pupillae muscle.

B. Pterygopalatine ganglion controls lacrimation and mucous secretion of nasal cavities and paranasal sinuses.

D. Submandibular ganglion controls salivation from submandibular and sublingual salivary glands.

E. Superior salivatory nucleus contains presynaptic parasympathetic fibers that are carried by facial nerve.

8

Neuroanatomy

Questions

1. A 28-year-old man is brought to the emergency department 40 minutes after he was involved in a motor vehicle collision. He was the unrestrained driver. The patient is alert and oriented to place and person only. Physical examination shows several abrasions on the face and chest. An x-ray of the skull shows minor maxillofacial injuries and a fracture at the foramen ovale. If there is injury to the nerve within the foramen ovale, which of the following clinical findings would most likely be seen?
   A. Loss of jaw jerk reflex
   B. Loss of sensation and taste on the posterior one third of the tongue
   C. Deviation of the tongue toward the side of injury
   D. Loss of sensation to the lower eyelid, cheek and upper lip
   E. Loss of the afferent limb of the corneal reflex

2. A 31-year-old man is brought into the emergency department by his wife after falling 2.13 m (7 ft) from a scaffold inside their house 1 hour ago. He has no history of medical conditions. The patient is awake and oriented to time, place, and person. His pulse is 98/min and blood pressure is 100/85 mm Hg. Physical examination shows a dilated right pupil that deviates downward and to the right. A computed tomography (CT) scan of the head shows a biconvex-shaped collection of blood in the right temporal lobe. Which of the following clinical signs is typical of this patient's condition?
   A. Bitemporal hemianopsia
   B. Left anopsia
   C. Left homonymous hemianopsia with macular sparing
   D. Left upper quadrantanopsia
   E. Left lower quadrantanopsia

3. An 8-year-old boy is brought to the physician because of a 4-month history of persistent headaches. His mother says that most days he wakes up because of a headache and it typically lasts the entire day. He has vomited twice over the past 2 days. His temperature is 37.1°C (98.8°F), pulse is 80/min, respirations are 16/min, and blood pressure is 120/70 mm Hg. The boy appears tired but alert. Physical examination shows that the patient finds it difficult to maintain his balance when asked to walk heel-to-toe in a straight line. He has no vision problems and cranial nerves II–XII are grossly intact. A CT scan of the head shows a tumor located in the posterior cranial fossa. Biopsy confirms the diagnosis of medulloblastoma. Damage to which of the following brain structures is likely responsible for this patient's physical examination findings?
   A. Cerebellar vermis
   B. Medullary pyramids
   C. Medial lemniscus in the midbrain
   D. Medial longitudinal fasciculus in the pons
   E. Cerebral aqueduct

4. A 7-year-old girl is brought to the physician by her parents because of a 2-month history of headaches and vision problems. Her school performance has been declining over the past few months. Her growth and previous well-child checks have been normal. Physical examination shows that the patient is unable to identify the physician's finger in her right and left temporal visual fields. She is able to track the physician's finger using both eyes during the "H test." Which of the following structures is most likely affected in this patient?
   A. Optic radiation in the parietal lobe
   B. Optic radiation in the temporal lobe
   C. Optic nerve
   D. Optic tract
   E. Optic chiasm

5. A 62-year-old man is brought to the emergency department by his wife because of numbness and tingling on the left side of his face and over his right upper and lower extremities. The patient also has been having difficulty swallowing. The patient's wife says his voice has been sounding more hoarse than normal. Physical examination shows a nondistressed man with an ataxic gait, the left pupil is constricted with partial drooping of the eyelid, and there is a loss of the gag reflex. There is decreased sensory and pain sensation on the left side of the face, and right side upper and lower extremities. Which of the following arteries would most likely be occluded?
   A. Anterior spinal artery
   B. Posterior inferior cerebellar artery (PICA)
   C. Anterior inferior cerebellar artery (AICA)
   D. Middle cerebral artery (MCA)
   E. Basilar artery

6. A 65-year-old man comes to the emergency department because of a severe headache that started 2 hours ago. He has a history of tension headaches, but they have never been this intense. His other medical problems include type 2 diabetes and hypertension. He has a 25-pack-year smoking history and drinks 2 to 3 beers a day. His pulse is 110/min and blood pressure is 150/90 mm Hg. He is awake, alert and oriented. Neurologic examination shows his strength 3/5 in his left leg and 5/5 in his right leg. There is a decreased sensation in his entire left lower limb. Motor and sensory sensation in his upper limb and face was 5/5 bilaterally. His vision is not impaired and CNs II–XII are intact. A CT scan of the head shows an area of hypodensity in his right frontal lobe. Injury to which of the following arteries would most likely explain this patient's current condition?
   A. Anterior cerebral artery (ACA)
   B. Middle cerebral artery (MCA)
   C. Posterior cerebral artery (PCA)
   D. Posterior communicating artery
   E. Basilar artery

7. A 68-year-old man comes to the emergency department with a 4-day history of fever and severe right ear pain. His other medical problems include type 2 diabetes, hypertension, and hypercholesterolemia. He smokes a pack of cigarettes a day and drinks 2 to 3 beers on the weekends. His temperature is 39.1°C (102.5°F), pulse is 101/min and blood pressure is 128/80 mm Hg. Physical examination shows swelling and redness of the area behind the ear. Otoscopic examination shows purulent drainage and granulation tissue within the external acoustic meatus. The pathogen causing this clinical picture is likely to gain access to the brain parenchyma using which of the following routes?
   A. External ear → Middle ear → Ethmoid cells → Frontal lobe
   B. External ear → Middle ear → Auditory tube → Cerebellum
   C. External ear → Middle ear → Mastoid cells → Temporal lobe
   D. Middle ear → External ear → Maxillary sinus → Parietal lobe
   E. Middle ear → External ear → Frontal sinus → Frontal lobe

8. A 44-year-old woman comes to the physician because of 4-month history of headaches and vision impairment. She has no other medical problems. Physical examination shows decreased vision in her temporal visual fields bilaterally. A CT scan of the head shows a tumor within the sella turcica with extension into the hypothalamus. A diagnosis of pituitary adenoma is made, and a surgical resection is scheduled. During a follow-up examination, the patient says that she has a significantly increased appetite. She eats multiple times a day and has gained 4.5 kg (10 lb) in the past 2 weeks. The patient's new symptoms can be explained by damage to which of the following structures during the procedure?
   A. Suprachiasmatic nucleus
   B. Posterior hypothalamic nucleus
   C. Anterior hypothalamic nucleus
   D. Ventromedial nucleus
   E. Lateral nucleus

9. A 51-year-old woman comes to the physician because of 6-week history of intermittent pain in the right side of her face. She describes it as a severe, sharp, stabbing pain in her right cheek and jaw that lasts several seconds. The pain occurs at multiple points during the day and is worsened with chewing, brushing her teeth, and smiling. Her other medical problems include hypertension and osteoarthritis. She does not smoke or drink alcohol. Her pulse is 76/min, respirations are 16/min and blood pressure is140/90 mm Hg. Inspection of her face shows no lesions, rashes, or asymmetry. Lightly tapping the face on the right side elicits her symptoms. The affected nerve in this patient provides sensory input into which of the following structures?
   A. Ventral posterolateral nucleus of the thalamus
   B. Ventral posteromedial nucleus of the thalamus
   C. Lateral geniculate nucleus of the thalamus
   D. Medial geniculate nucleus of the thalamus
   E. Ventral lateral nucleus of the thalamus

10. A 56-year-old woman is brought to the emergency department because of a sudden onset of a headache during her breakfast this morning. She is confused and disoriented. Her pulse is 103/min, blood pressure is 156/93 mm Hg, and respirations are 16/min. A CT scan of the head shows evidence of occlusion of the PCA confirming an ischemic stroke. Which of the following symptoms would also present during physical examination?
   A. Contralateral paralysis and loss of sensation of the lower extremities
   B. Broca aphasia with contralateral paralysis and loss of sensation to the face and upper extremities
   C. Contralateral hemianopsia with macular sparing
   D. CN IV palsy
   E. Quadriplegia with loss of facial, tongue, and mouth movements

11. A newborn girl is being evaluated in the neonatal intensive care unit for new-onset seizures. The patient was delivered 2 days ago at 30 weeks' gestation to a 22-year-old primigravida. The delivery was complicated by prolonged labor necessitating forceps-assisted delivery. The patient weighed 2100 g at birth (low birth weight <2500 g). Pulse is 180/min and blood pressure is 60/40 mm Hg. Physical examination shows an irritable infant with bulging fontanelles. Imaging of the brain confirms a germinal matrix hemorrhage. The affected area in this patient can likely be found in which of the following anatomical structures?
   A. Lateral ventricles
   B. Mammillary bodies

C. Pituitary gland

D. Hippocampus

E. Hypothalamus

12. A 63-year-old man is brought to the emergency department because of a right lower extremity weakness, specifically difficulty getting out of bed. He has a history of type 2 diabetes mellitus, and hypertension. His temperature is 37°C (98.6°F), pulse is 112/min and irregular, respirations are 16/min and blood pressure is 145/90 mm Hg. Physical examination of the right lower extremity shows motor power of 1/5, deep tendon reflexes (DTRs) 3+, and a positive Babinski sign. Left lower extremity examination shows motor power of 5/5, DTR 2+ and an absent Babinski sign. An occlusion of which of the following vessels is the most likely cause of these symptoms?

A. Left ACA

B. Left internal carotid artery

C. Right PICA

D. Right PCA

E. Right MCA

13. A 62-year-old man is brought to the emergency department by his wife when she noticed he was having a meaningless conversation with her this morning. She says he was conversing normally the previous night. Physical examination shows fluent speech without comprehension and he is unable to repeat phrases. Which of the following areas correlate with the symptoms presented in this patient?

A. Left inferior frontal gyrus

B. Left superior temporal gyrus

C. Left supramarginal gyrus

D. Superior colliculi

E. Paramedian pontine reticular formation

14. A 35-year-old man is brought to the emergency department because of a sudden onset of a severe headache. The patient says that it is the worst headache of his life. Physical examination shows a tall man that is 1.98 m (6.6 ft), with hypermobile joints and subluxation of the lens superior and temporally. A CT scan of the head shows a ruptured berry aneurysm. Which of the following is the most common site for a berry aneurysm within the circle of Willis?

A. AICA and vertebral artery

B. PCA and posterior communicating artery

C. MCA and posterior communicating artery

D. ACA and MCA

E. ACA and anterior communicating artery

15. A 56-year-old man is brought to the emergency department after he was found lying unconscious in the restroom at work. Prior to going to the restroom, his coworkers say that he had complained of chest pain. His pulse is 48/min, blood pressure is 62/45 mm Hg, and respirations are 8/min. An electrocardiogram (ECG) indicates an acute myocardial infarction. During this time, which of the following regions is the most vulnerable to ischemic damage?

A. Thalamus

B. Spinal cord

C. Pons

D. Medulla

E. Hippocampus

16. A 60-year-old man dies from a progressive neurologic condition. His 25-year-old son is currently presenting with the same symptoms he had at that age. At autopsy, a brain section of the elderly man shows cystic degenerative changes involving a part of the basal ganglia located laterally to the left lateral ventricle. Which of the following structures corresponds with the cystic degeneration?

A. Head of the caudate nucleus

B. Globus pallidus

C. Internal capsule

D. Lentiform nucleus

E. Putamen

17. A 75-year-old woman is brought to the emergency department by her son after a sudden onset of confusion with drooping of the right side of the face this morning. Since this morning, her sense of taste was diminished, and her gait has become unbalanced. Physical examination shows a loss of facial movements and sensation on the right side of the face, ptosis and miosis of the right eye with a diminished corneal reflex, and loss of pain and temperature sensation of the left side upper and lower extremities. The patient's hearing is also decreased on the right side. Which of the following locations is most likely damaged?

A. Medial medulla oblongata

B. Lateral medulla oblongata

C. Lateral pons

D. Medial inferior pons

E. Brainstem

18. A 75-year-old man is brought to the emergency department because of involuntary twitching movements of his right arm that started last night. He was writing when his arm flung the pen across his desk. He has a longstanding history of hypertension and diabetes mellitus. He says he is not taking his medications as prescribed. Physical examination shows wild-swinging repetitive motions of the proximal muscles of his right arm. Which of the following is most likely damaged in this patient?

A. Internal capsule

B. Lentiform nucleus

C. Putamen

D. Substantia nigra

E. Subthalamic nucleus

19. An 8-year-old boy is brought to the emergency department by his parents because of a 3-week history of mild intermittent headaches, vomiting, and fatigue. The headaches and fatigue have progressively worsened over the past week. He appears sluggish and is difficult to arouse. A CT scan of the brain shows the lateral ventricles measure 20 mm in diameter bilaterally (normal range: <10 mm), the third ventricle measures 4 mm (normal range:<5 mm), and the fourth ventricle measures 8 mm (normal range:<9 mm). Which of the following is the most likely source of obstruction in this patient?

A. Arachnoid villi

B. Cerebral aqueduct

C. Interventricular foramen of Monro

D. Foramina of Luschka

E. Foramen of Magendie

20. A 62-year-old woman comes to the emergency department because of a sudden decrease in vision. The patient has a past history of hypertension and type 2 diabetes mellitus. She has no headaches, blurry vision, photophobia, or muscle weakness. Physical examination shows both pupils are 3 mm (normal 2 to 4 mm) and reactive to light. Visual field tests show contralateral superior hemianopsia of the left upper quadrant. Which part of the optic tract has been damaged in this patient?

A. Right optic nerve

B. Optic chiasm

C. Left optic tract

D. Superior optic radiations

E. Inferior optic radiations

21. A 46-year-old man is brought to the emergency department after he was found walking alongside the highway, confused and disoriented. He has a history of alcohol use with numerous hospitalizations for alcoholic intoxication requiring thiamine repletion. Physical examination shows a disheveled man with a stumbling gait and bilateral horizontal nystagmus. A magnetic resonance imaging (MRI) of the head would show pathology involving which of the following structures?

A. Mammillary bodies

B. Basal ganglia

C. Pituitary gland

D. Medial geniculate nucleus

E. Amygdala

22. A 27-year-old man comes to the physician because he has been feeling tired lately. He has been experiencing a "low mood," fatigue, and difficulty concentrating at work over the past 2 months. He also stopped attending his weekly soccer practices because he was no longer interested. The patient does not have any suicidal ideations. The patient is diagnosed with major depressive disorder, and it is decided to start him on a medication which binds to 5HT1 receptors at the raphe nuclei. In what regions of the brain are these structures located?

A. Reticular formation

B. Basal ganglia

C. Basal forebrain

D. Rostral pons

E. Substantia innominata

23. A 63-year-old man comes to the emergency department because of sudden onset of severe headache, neck stiffness, nausea, and vomiting. The patient was watching television at home when he began having a headache. The patient has a 20-year history of hypertension, 20 pack-per-year of cigarette smoking, and polycystic kidney disease. A CT scan of the head shows a ruptured aneurysm arising from the posterior communicating artery. Before rupture, which of the following conditions was the patient at most risk of developing from an aneurysm at this location?

A. Optic atrophy

B. Contralateral superior hemianopsia

C. Ipsilateral oculomotor nerve palsy

D. Bitemporal hemianopsia

E. Horner syndrome

24. A 65-year-old man is brought to the emergency department because of an acute onset of headache and weakness. The patient was resting on his couch when the symptoms started 1 hour ago. He has 20-year history of hypertension, type 2 diabetes mellitus, and hyperlipidemia. His pulse is 90/min, respirations are 17/min, and blood pressure is 155/95 mm Hg. Physical examination shows dysarthria and right-sided facial weakness. Biceps tendon reflex is 3+ and there is 2/5 strength in the right arm. There is also decreased pinprick and temperature sensation over the right side of the body. A CT scan of the head shows an ischemic stroke. What vessel was most likely occluded in this patient?

A. ACA

B. MCA

C. PCA

D. PICA

E. AICA

25. A 42-year-old woman is brought to the emergency department because of an acute onset of left facial weakness. She has a history of hypertension and uncontrolled diabetes. Her pulse is 85/min, blood pressure is 185/110 mm Hg, and respirations are 17/min. A CT scan of the head confirms an ischemic stroke. She is treated with tissue plasminogen activator (tPA) and her blood pressure is managed. Two weeks following the stroke, the patient began to experience difficulty in speech repetition. Her speech is fluent, and comprehension is intact, but she is unable to repeat sentences. The aphasia is thought to be a secondary complication related to the ischemic stroke. Which of the following anatomic structures is most likely damaged?

A. Inferior frontal lobe

B. Superior temporal lobe

C. Arcuate fasciculus

D. Watershed zone of the ACA and MCA

E. Watershed zone of the PCA and MCA

26. A 82-year-old man is brought to the emergency department because of headache, vomiting, and impaired consciousness. The patient has a history of chronic hypertension and has no recent history of falls or trauma. His pulse is 85/min, blood pressure is 155/98 mm Hg, and respirations are 18/min. Physical examination shows neck stiffness, an unsteady gait, and bilateral horizontal nystagmus. There is no hemiparesis. A CT scan of the head shows an intracranial hemorrhage. In which of the following anatomic sites is this hemorrhage most likely present?

A. Thalamus

B. Basal ganglia

C. Pons

D. Cerebellum

E. Cerebral hemisphere

27. A 55-year-old man comes to the emergency department with severe pain around the left eye for the past 5 hours. His symptoms began while watching TV at home. He has a 15-year history of diabetes mellitus and hypertension. On slit lamp examination, there is cupping of the optic disc, and tonometry shows an increase in intraocular pressure. The diagnosis of glaucoma is made. Through which of the following structures does the aqueous humor drain out of the eye?
    A. Trabecular meshwork
    B. Ciliary body
    C. Iris
    D. Choroid
    E. Lens

28. A 82-year-old man is brought to the emergency department because of a sudden onset of left-sided weakness. He has a history of chronic hypertension. A CT scan shows a large hypodensity on the right side of the brain. He is diagnosed with an ischemic stroke and aggressive management is initiated. The patient dies 4 days later. The family has requested an autopsy. At autopsy, which of the following histologic findings would most likely be present?
    A. Red neurons
    B. Neutrophilic infiltration and phagocytosis
    C. Macrophage infiltration and phagocytosis
    D. Reactive gliosis
    E. Glial scarring

29. A 73-year-old man is brought to the physician by his son because of problems with his balance for the past 1 month. The patient's son says that he often misses steps while walking up and down the stairs. His temperature is 36.6°C. (98°F), pulse is 76/min, blood pressure is 116/74 mm Hg, and respirations are 14/min. He had an eye examination 2 weeks ago, which did not show any new problems. Physical examination shows that he can hear and communicate clearly. When asked to close his eyes with his arms raised, he has increased swaying movements, and the examiner had to help him in order to prevent him from falling. Upon placing a vibrating tuning fork on the body prominences of the patient's right or left large toe or fingers, he has a marked decrease in his ability to sense the vibrations. The patient is experiencing a problem in which of the following pathways?
    A. Spinothalamic
    B. Pyramidal
    C. Reticulospinal
    D. Dorsal column
    E. Rubrospinal

30. A 36-year-old woman comes to the physician because of worsening headache and vision problems for the past day. She started taking oral contraceptives 2 weeks ago. She has a BMI of 31 kg/m². Her temperature is 37.2°C (99°F), pulse is 84/min, blood pressure is 130/84 mm Hg, and respirations are 16/min. Physical examination shows mild ptosis, proptosis, periorbital edema, mydriasis, decreased visual acuity, and decreased movements of the extraocular muscles of the left eye. There is diminished pinprick sensation over the left forehead and left mid-third of the face. At the end of the examination, she became lethargic and noncommunicative. Which of the following sites is most likely affected?
    A. Jugular foramen
    B. Cavernous sinus
    C. Optic chiasm
    D. Occipital lobe of the brain
    E. Foramen rotundum

31. A 57-year-old man comes to the emergency department because of persistent left-sided paralysis for the last several hours. He has difficulty moving the left side of his face, left arm, and left leg. He has a history of peptic ulcer disease, hypertension, paroxysmal atrial fibrillation, and ischemic stroke without residual symptoms. His anticoagulation therapy was discontinued last month after he developed a perforated peptic ulcer. Blood pressure is 157/93 mm Hg and pulse is 89/min and irregular. Physical examination shows no sensory deficits. Which of the following structures in the cerebral hemisphere is most likely affected?
    A. Right precentral gyrus
    B. Left precentral gyrus
    C. Right postcentral gyrus
    D. Left postcentral gyrus
    E. Occipital lobe

32. A 19-year-old man is brought to the emergency room after he was punched in his right eye by an unknown person when he was walking back home in the middle of the night. His temperature is 36.6°C (98°F), pulse is 76/min, blood pressure is 116/74 mm Hg, and respirations are 14/min. Physical examinations of the right eye shows eyelid swelling, mild ecchymosis, posteriorly displaced eyeball, comparatively decreased visual acuity, limited superior gaze, and decreased sensation over the mid-third face. An entrapment of which of the following muscles most likely occurred?
    A. Superior oblique
    B. Superior rectus
    C. Inferior oblique
    D. Inferior rectus
    E. Medial rectus

33. A 24-year-old man comes to the physician because of worsening headaches for the past 1 month. He has had episodes of nausea and vomiting for the past 2 days. He has had occasional minor headaches for the past year, which resolve after taking over-the-counter acetaminophen. An MRI of the head shows a cystic enhancing lesion measuring 2.0 × 2.5 cm in the right cerebellar hemisphere. At physical examination, which of the following findings is mostly likely expected to be present in this patient?
    A. Right hemiparesis
    B. Right homonymous hemianopsia
    C. Right tongue deviation

D. Right lower facial droop

E. Right dysdiadochokinesia

34. A 57-year-old man comes to the physician because of fatigue. The patient has a history of well-controlled hypothyroidism. He has no weight gain or cold intolerance. He takes levothyroxine and has no drug allergies. He does not use tobacco or illicit drugs and drinks occasionally. Physical examination shows a shiny tongue and pale palmar creases. His gait is unstable when his eyes are closed, and vibration sense is markedly decreased over the lower extremities. Stool tests are negative for occult blood. Which of the following spinal tracts are damaged in this patient?

    A. Spinoreticular tract

    B. Corticospinal tract

    C. Dorsal column

    D. Spinothalamic tract

    E. Spinocerebellar tract

35. A 62-year-old man comes to the physician because of left shoulder pain that radiates to his back. The patient also has weakness in the left hand. His symptoms started 4 months ago and has been getting progressively worse. The patient has a 30-year smoking history but does not use illicit drugs. He appears awake, alert, oriented, and follows commands. Neurologic examination shows partial left-sided ptosis of the upper eyelid. His pupils are asymmetric in dim light with 2 mm on the left and 4 mm on the right, and both are reactive to light. The pupils become more symmetric in bright light. The left upper extremity has 3/5 strength. This patient has a tumor most likely compressing which of the following structures?

    A. Recurrent laryngeal nerve

    B. Cerebellum

    C. Frontal lobe

    D. Spinal cord

    E. Sympathetic ganglion

36. A 26-year-old woman comes to the physician because of 1-day history of diplopia. She says that the symptoms are aggravated when she is walking downstairs. Her temperature is 36.7°C. (98.2°F), pulse is 76/min, blood pressure is 144/96 mm Hg, and respirations are 18/min. Physical examination shows that when she is asked to move her right eye inward toward her nose and look down, she can look inward but not down. An MRI of the head shows a proximal superior cerebellar artery aneurysm. A loss of function of which muscle is the cause of this patient's symptoms?

    A. Lateral rectus

    B. Medial rectus

    C. Inferior oblique

    D. Levator palpebrae superioris

    E. Superior oblique

37. A 62-year-old man comes to the emergency department because of loss of his right eye vision. He has a history of hypertension, hyperlipidemia, diabetes mellitus type 2, and ischemic heart disease. His temperature is 37.2°C (99°F), pulse is 76/min, blood pressure is 144/96 mm Hg, and respirations are 18/min. Physical examination shows that when light is shone on the right eye, no pupillary constriction is observed in either eye. When the light is shone on the left eye, both pupils constricted. Which of the following nerves is most likely affected?

    A. CN V1

    B. CN III

    C. CN II

    D. CN VII

    E. CN IV

38. A 70-year-old man come to the physician because of headache, difficulties with speech and swallowing, and weight loss. He has a history of prostate cancer which was treated with radical prostatectomy, orchiectomy, and radiotherapy. He has lost 11.3 kg (25 lb) over the last 3 months. His vital signs are within normal limits. Physical examination shows hoarseness, uvular deviation to the left, right soft palate depression, and decreased right-sided gag response. There is atrophy of the right sternocleidomastoid and trapezius muscles. An MRI of the head shows multiple lesions consistent with metastases. Injury to which of the following anatomic structures is most likely responsible for this patient's symptoms?

    A. Foramen ovale

    B. Cavernous sinus

    C. Foramen rotundum

    D. Foramen magnum

    E. Jugular foramen

39. A 76-year-old man is brought to the physician for a routine examination. The man has noted that over the past few years hearing over the phone has become increasingly difficult. He expresses frustration with hearing ongoing conversations at social gatherings when there is excessive background noise. His vital signs are within normal limits. Physical examination shows that air conduction is greater than bone conduction bilaterally. A Weber test is performed. Which of the following describes the best placement of the vibrating tuning fork for this test?

    A. External occipital protuberance

    B. Mastoid process

    C. Vertex of the head

    D. Glabella

    E. Angle of mandible

40. A 54-year-old woman is brought to the emergency department with left-sided body weakness and slurred speech. She has a history of hypertension that is controlled with lifestyle modifications. Her blood pressure is 195/100 mm Hg, temperature is 37.2°C (98.6°F), respirations are 16/min, SpO2% 98 on room air. Physical examination shows significant reduction in motor strength of the left upper and lower extremities. Cranial nerve examination shows a right-sided facial droop, the patient is unable to keep the right eye closed tightly when physician tries to open her eyes; however, she is

able to form furrow lines at the forehead. A CT scan of the head shows a hemorrhagic stroke. At what location of the skull does the cranial nerve involved in the patient's physical examination findings exit the skull?

A. Foramen ovale
B. Foramen cecum
C. Jugular foramen
D. Foramen magnum
E. Stylomastoid foramen

41. A 32-year-old woman comes to the physician because of a 3-day history of fever and pain in her throat. She has no vomiting, abdominal pain, muscle aches, or diarrhea. Her blood pressure is 115/88 mm Hg, temperature is 37.8°C (100.2°F), respirations are 18/min and SpO$_2$% 99 on room air. Physical examination shows normal heart sounds, and the lungs are clear to auscultation. Lymphadenopathy of the cervical lymph nodes is palpated, and the gag reflex is evaluated. The nerve that is responsible for the sensory component of this reflex innervates which of the following muscles?

A. Buccinator
B. Stylohyoid
C. Stylopharyngeus
D. Omohyoid
E. Posterior digastric

42. A 50-year-old woman is brought to the emergency department because of high blood pressure. The patient says that she has lost feelings on the right sight of her face. Her blood pressure is 200/105 mm Hg, temperature is 37.2°C (98.6°F), respirations are 19/min, and SpO$_2$% 96 on room air. Physical examination shows numbness on the right side of her lower face, no weakness in upper or lower extremities, tongue deviation to right side on protrusion, uvula deviated to the left side when asked to say "ah." The lesion causing these symptoms is found in which of the following locations?

A. Central lesion of nerve nuclei
B. Peripheral lesion of nerve nuclei
C. Peripheral nerve lesion
D. Autonomic ganglia lesion
E. Autonomic nerve lesion

43. A 76-year-old man comes to the physician for follow-up examination. The patient has a history of type 2 diabetes mellitus, hypertension, hyperlipidemia, and prostate cancer. He smoked three packs of cigarettes per day since he was 19 years old and he does not drink alcohol. Over the past year the patient has noted that his vision is becoming worse. He says that his vision is blurry, especially at night, which has resulted in him not leaving his home during the night. The patient also adds that he often sees halos around light structures. He has no pain in the eye. His blood pressure is 150/90 mm Hg, temperature is 37.2°C (98.6°F), respirations are 16/min, and SpO$_2$ 99% on room air. Physical examination shows visual acuity of 20/40 in the left eye and 20/80 in the right eye. There is loss of the red-light reflex in the right eye, and the right retina cannot be visualized with

fundoscopy. Which of the following structures is most likely affected?

A. Retina
B. Aqueous humor
C. Ciliary body
D. Canal of Schlemm
E. Lens

44. A 16-year-old girl is brought to the emergency department after being involved in a motor vehicle collision. The girl was unresponsive on the scene. The emergency response team decided to secure the airway by performing a cricothyroidotomy because of extensive facial injuries. Resuscitative efforts are successful, and the girl is later transferred to the intensive care unit. Her family is concerned about her extensive facial injuries and asks if she will have facial deformities from the collision. Reconstructive imaging of the skull is performed and shows damage to the superior orbital fissure. Which of the following functions would be impaired in this patient?

A. Afferent (sensory) limb of corneal reflex
B. Afferent (sensory) limb of pupillary reflex
C. Efferent (motor) limb of pupillary reflex
D. Efferent (motor) limb of corneal reflex
E. A and C
F. B and D

45. A 79-year-old woman is brought to the emergency department because of slurred speech and difficulty walking. She has a 30-year history of hypertension and osteoporosis. Her blood pressure is 160/95 mm Hg, temperature is 37.2°C (98.6°F), respirations are 18/min, and SpO$_2$% 96 on room air. Physical examination shows an elderly lady not in acute distress. Neurologic examination shows flaccid paralysis of the left side of tongue, left-sided hemiparesis, and loss of sensation and proprioception of the trunk and extremities. Which of the following is the location of the nuclei associated with this lesion?

A. Inferior cerebellar peduncle
B. Medial medulla oblongata
C. Medial pons
D. Lateral midbrain
E. Posterior spinal cord

46. A 22-year-old man comes to the physician because he is having difficulty with speech and concentrating on his work assignments. He has a past history of depression. His family history includes a maternal uncle who died at a young age from heart and liver conditions, and a paternal aunt who also died at a young age from a liver condition. He does not use tobacco, stimulants, alcohol, or street drugs. Physical examination shows a yellowish discoloration of the skin. There is also a golden-brown halo surrounding the iris of the eye. Neurologic examination shows cogwheel rigidity of the upper extremities and bradykinesia. A basic metabolic profile shows elevation in liver enzymes. A diagnosis is made that he has an autosomal recessive inheritance pattern involving a mutation on chromosome 13. This

condition results in depositions in which of the following layers of the eye?

A. Pigmented epithelium layer of retina
B. Capsule layer of lens
C. Descemet membrane of cornea
D. Photoreceptor layer of retina
E. Choroid of eye

47. This condition results in depositions in which of the following areas?

A. Basal ganglia
B. Thalamus
C. Mammillary bodies
D. Pineal gland

48. A 15-year-old boy is brought to the emergency department because of fever, nausea, vomiting, and abdominal pain. His parents say that their child has been feeling unwell for the past 2 days and has not been able to attend school. History includes type one diabetes mellitus. His blood pressure is 110/75 mm Hg, temperature is 38.3°C (101°F), respirations are 25/min, and $SpO_2\%$ 97 on room air. Physical examination shows a young man who is somnolent. Respiratory examination shows rapid short breaths. Urine dipstick is positive for ketones. Blood serum studies show hyperglycemia, metabolic acidosis, and severe hyponatremia. The diabetic ketoacidosis protocol is initiated. Two days later the patient develops weakness of the upper and lower extremities, hallucinations, and tremors. The region affected in this condition is supplied by which of the following vessels?

A. PICA
B. PCA
C. Vertebral artery
D. Basilar artery
E. Superior cerebellar artery

49. Which of the following is where the lesion is located?

A. Midbrain
B. Medulla oblongata
C. Thalamus
D. Pons
E. Cerebellum

50. A 58-year-old woman comes to the physician because of fatigue and weight loss for the past year. She has a 50-pack-per-year history of smoking. Physical examination shows drooping of the left eyelid, a constricted left pupil, and loss of sweating on the left side of her face. A CT scan of the chest shows a mass on the upper lobe of the left lung. Loss of function of which of the following muscles is responsible for the drooping of the eyelid in this patient?

A. Orbicularis oculi
B. Pupillary sphincter
C. Levator palpebrae superioris
D. Superior tarsal
E. Superior rectus

51. A 14-year-old boy is brought to the physician because of headaches, fatigue, and loss of vision. He says that the headaches started about a month ago and have been getting worse. Physical examination shows bitemporal hemianopsia. An MRI of the head shows a tumor. A lesion in which of the following will lead to the visual deficits present in this patient?

A. Left optic tract
B. Right optic tract
C. Right Meyer loop
D. Optic chiasm
E. Dorsal optic radiation

52. A 73-year-old man comes to the physician because of a history of multiple falls in the past 6 months and a few episodes of nocturnal urinary incontinence. His sons noticed that their father is exhibiting strange behavior lately and has been experiencing difficulty in remembering past events. His vital signs are within normal limits. Physical examination shows a broad-based clumsy gait. What is the most likely diagnosis?

A. Parkinson disease
B. Syringomyelia
C. Normal pressure hydrocephalus (NPH)
D. Stroke
E. Alzheimer disease

53. A 25-year-old man comes to the physician because of uncontrollable choreiform movements. He has moderate dementia with a severe gait disturbance as well as agitation and problems with his mood. He has a family history of movement disorders. Which of the following findings will most likely be present on MRI in this condition?

A. Cerebellar stroke
B. Atrophy of the head of the caudate nucleus
C. Enhanced ring-like lesions
D. Tumor
E. Subarachnoid hemorrhage

54. A 35-year-old woman comes to the emergency department because of double vision and headache for the past 2 hours. She immigrated from Scandinavia and has a past history of type 1 diabetes that is well controlled with subcutaneous insulin injections. She says that she has experienced weakness and numbness in her arms that worsen with taking a hot shower but resolved spontaneously for the past month. She has no nausea, photophobia, or neck stiffness and her vital signs are within normal limits. Physical examination shows nystagmus. Which of the following is the most likely diagnosis?

A. Meningitis
B. Encephalitis
C. Multiple sclerosis (MS)
D. Rabies
E. Brain tumor

55. A 35-year old woman comes to the emergency department because of increasing weakness of her lower extremities. She was in her usual state of health until approximately 1 week ago when she developed increased difficulty climbing the stairs. She is now unable to stand. Two weeks ago, she had an episode of bloody diarrhea, which she attributes to drinking unpasteurized milk. Physical examination shows

reduced bilateral lower extremity strength with absent patellar reflexes. Which of the following best describes the most likely pathophysiological mechanism behind the patient's condition?

A. Widespread central nervous system (CNS) demyelination secondary to destruction of oligodendrocytes

B. Autoimmune inflammatory demyelination of the CNS due to infection

C. Autoimmune attack of the peripheral Schwann cells due to molecular mimicry

D. Hereditary motor and sensory neuropathy affecting peripheral nerves

E. Loss of corticospinal and cortibulbar tracts due to low serum electrolytes

56. A 22-year-old man comes to the physician because of muscle weakness and frequent falling. He had a recent visit to the emergency department for pneumonia and a bedside ultrasound showed an enlarged heart. He has 8-year history of diabetes. Physical examination shows an abnormal curvature of the upper spine, severe marked muscle weakness (2/5) in all limbs, nystagmus, and loss of DTRs. A genetic condition is suspected and confirmed by genetic studies. Which of the following neurologic symptoms will most likely be found in this patient?

A. Dysarthria

B. Myoclonic seizures

C. Worsening choreiform movements of the limbs

D. Increased proprioception

E. Marked cognitive deficits

Answers

1. **A.** The mandibular division of the trigeminal nerve (V3) exits the skull through the foramen ovale within the sphenoid bone. V3 innervates the lower one third of the face and is responsible for sensation of the cheek, lower lip, anterior part of the pinna, part of the external acoustic meatus, teeth of the mandible, mastoid cells, mucous membranes of cheek, mandible and the anterior two-thirds of the tongue. V3 is also responsible for both the sensory and motor limb of the jaw jerk reflex as it innervates the muscle spindle from the masseter and the masseter muscle itself. Thus, injury to V3 within the foramen ovale will result in loss of the jaw jerk reflex.

   B. Taste and sensation of the tongue is innervated by several cranial nerves. Taste on the anterior two-thirds of the tongue is innervated by the facial nerve (VII) while sensation is innervated by the mandibular branch of trigeminal nerve (V3). Taste and sensation of the posterior one third of the tongue is innervated by the glossopharyngeal nerve (IX). CN IX exits the skull via the jugular foramen.

   C. Motor function of the tongue is controlled by the hypoglossal nerve (XII), which passes through the hypoglossal canal. Injury to XII will result in deviation of the tongue toward the side of the lesion when protruded.

   D. Sensation of the lower eyelid, cheek and upper lip is by the maxillary division of the trigeminal nerve (V2). This nerve exits the skull through the foramen rotundum.

   E. The afferent limb of the corneal reflex is via the ophthalmic branch of the trigeminal nerve (V1). Injury to this nerve within the superior orbital fissure will lead to loss of the ipsilateral corneal reflex. *GAS 887; N 133; ABR/McM 42*

2. **B.** The patient who comes in after a fall with biconvex blood collection on neuroimaging has an epidural hematoma. Epidural hematomas are usually caused by trauma to the head, such as a fall or motor vehicle accident, which results in a skull fracture and rupture of, commonly, the middle meningeal artery. Patients typically present with a lucid interval directly after the injury with rapid deterioration in mental status due to expansion of the hematoma under high arterial pressures that are in a confined space. Uncal herniation is a common complication of supratentorial epidural hematomas. Increased intracranial pressure from the arterial bleed results in transtentorial herniation of the uncus (mesial temporal lobe). Compression of the ipsilateral CN III results in a dilated pupil with the characteristic "down and out" gaze. The ipsilateral PCA can also be affected resulting in contralateral homonymous hemianopsia with macular sparing. As the hematoma occurred on the right side, the patient's left eye would have been affected.

   A. Bitemporal hemianopsia occurs due to compression of the optic chiasm. This is not a common presentation of uncal herniation.

   C. Left anopsia is caused by damage to the left optic nerve, which is spared in uncal herniation.

   D, E. Left lower and upper quadrantanopsia are due to lesions of the right MCA. This artery is not usually affected in uncal herniations. *GAS 879, 1120; N 129; ABR/McM 80*

3. **A.** This young boy is presenting with persistent headaches that are worse in the morning, as well as nausea and vomiting, which are all common symptoms of brain tumors. Medulloblastoma is the second most common childhood brain tumor and typically involves the cerebellum. Damage to the cerebellar vermis is common in medulloblastomas and often results in truncal dystaxia and patients usually present with a wide-based gait. Other symptoms of damage to the cerebellum include nystagmus, vertigo, and dysdiadochokinesia.

   B, C, D. Damage to brainstem structures is not common in medulloblastomas. The medullary pyramids contain fibers primarily from the lateral corticospinal tract and will result in spastic paresis of the limbs.

If the medial lemniscus in the midbrain is affected, the patient will experience decreased touch, vibration and proprioception in the contralateral limbs. Damage to the medial longitudinal fasciculus of the pons results in medial rectus palsy during lateral conjugate gaze and nystagmus when adducting the eye.

E. Compression of the fourth ventricle is a common occurrence in medulloblastoma. However, this results in increased intracranial pressure and symptoms of nausea and vomiting. It does not account for the truncal dystaxia in this patient. *GAS 854–856; N 124; ABR/McM 70–71*

4. **E.** Craniopharyngiomas are common childhood tumors that derive from Rathke pouch remnants and are located near the sella turcica. These tumors compress the **optic chiasm** which results in bitemporal hemianopsia. The nerve fibers from the temporal and nasal retina cross over in the optic chiasm. Compression of the center of the optic chiasm will affect the nerve fibers of the nasal retina of the left and right eye, which would lead to loss of vision in the temporal visual fields of both eyes.

A. Compression of the optic radiations in the parietal lobe, also referred to as the dorsal optic radiation, results in contralateral lower quadrantanopsia.

B. Optic radiations in the temporal lobe, or Meyer loop, contain fibers from the lower retina and damage results in contralateral upper quadrantanopsia.

C. Compression of the optic nerve results in ipsilateral anopsia.

D. Compression of the optic nerve results in contralateral homonymous hemianopsia. *GAS 1064–1065; N 131; ABR/McM 79*

5. **B.** This patient is exhibiting signs and symptoms of lateral medullary (Wallenberg) syndrome, which results from lesions within the PICA. The lateral medulla oblongata is associated with the vestibular nuclei, lateral spinothalamic tract, spinal trigeminal nucleus, nucleus ambiguus, sympathetic fibers and the inferior cerebellar peduncle. A disruption of the vestibular nuclei causes symptoms of vomiting, vertigo, and nystagmus. The loss of the lateral spinothalamic tract will result in loss of pain and temperature of the contralateral upper and lower extremities. A loss of the spinal trigeminal nucleus causes loss of pain and temperature from the ipsilateral side of the face supplied by CN V. A loss of the nucleus ambiguus results in dysphagia and hoarseness and is specific to PICA lesions. The loss of sympathetic fibers causes ipsilateral Horner syndrome. Lastly, the loss of the inferior cerebellar peduncles leads to ataxia and dysmetria. The medulla oblongata contains nuclei related to CNs IX, X, XI, XII. In lateral medullary syndrome, CN X is affected, leading to loss of the gag reflex.

A. A lesion within the anterior spinal artery affects the lateral corticospinal tract, causing contralateral hemiparesis of the upper and lower limbs;

the medial lemniscus, causing loss of contralateral proprioception; and caudal medulla oblongata, particularly the hypoglossal nerve nucleus causing ipsilateral hypoglossal nerve dysfunction, where the tongue deviates ipsilaterally when protruded.

C. A lesion in the AICA leads to the lateral pontine syndrome. Lesions within the lateral pons would disrupt the vestibular nuclei, facial nucleus, spinal trigeminal nucleus, cochlear nuclei, and sympathetic fibers.

D. A MCA lesion would affect the sensory and motor cortex of the contralateral upper limb and face. If the stroke occurs in the dominant hemisphere then aphasia occurs: Broca aphasia if in the frontal lobe and Wernicke aphasia if in the temporal lobe. If the lesion were in the nondominant hemisphere, the patient would experience hemineglect.

E. A basilar artery leads to "locked-in syndrome." The pons, medulla oblongata, lower midbrain, corticospinal tracts, corticobulbar tracts, extraocular cranial nerve nuclei, and paramedian pontine reticular formation are all affected. Only the patient's consciousness is preserved, including blinking. Affected individuals would be quadriplegic, with loss of tongue, mouth, and facial movements. *GAS eFigs. 9.42, 9.43, and 9.52* *GAS 870; N 152; ABR/McM 66*

6. **A.** This patient with the sudden-onset severe headache and cardiovascular risk factors is likely to have a subarachnoid hemorrhage secondary to rupture of an aneurysm. Subarachnoid hemorrhages present acutely as "the worst headache of my life." The junction between the ACA and anterior communicating artery in the circle of Willis is the most common location for saccular aneurysms. Furthermore, this patient experienced hemiparesis and decreased sensation in his left leg, contralateral to the area of hemorrhage noticed on CT scan. The ACA provides blood supply to the anteromedial surface of the brain, which contains the motor and sensory cortices representing the lower limb. A stroke in this region of the brain will result in contralateral paralysis and sensory loss to the lower limb.

B. The MCA supplies the motor and sensory cortices representing the upper limb and face. A stroke in this region would result in contralateral paralysis and loss of sensation. As the MCA also supplies Wernicke area and Broca area, aphasia and hemineglect can occur.

C. The PCA supplies, among other things, the occipital lobe and a stroke would result in vision impairment. Contralateral hemianopsia with macular sparing is a common complication of PCA stroke.

D. Occlusion of the posterior communicating artery can lead to oculomotor nerve palsy.

E. Injury to the basilar artery can result in the "locked-in syndrome": complete paralysis of voluntary muscles of the body except the extraocular muscles. *GAS 870; N 152; ABR/McM 66*

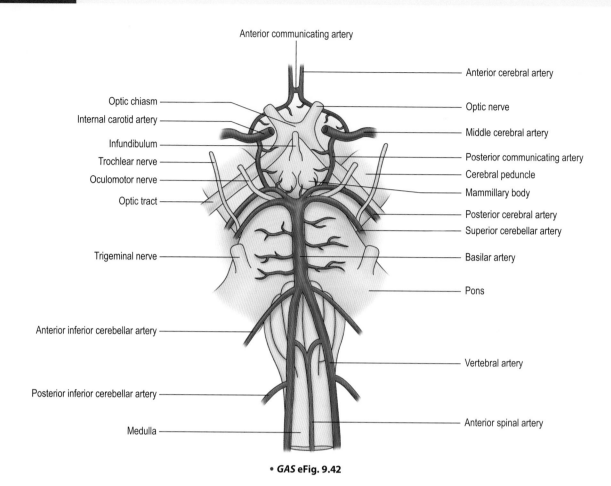

Anterior communicating artery

Optic chiasm

Internal carotid artery

Infundibulum

Trochlear nerve

Oculomotor nerve

Optic tract

Trigeminal nerve

Anterior inferior cerebellar artery

Posterior inferior cerebellar artery

Medulla

Anterior cerebral artery

Optic nerve

Middle cerebral artery

Posterior communicating artery

Cerebral peduncle

Mammillary body

Posterior cerebral artery

Superior cerebellar artery

Basilar artery

Pons

Vertebral artery

Anterior spinal artery

• *GAS* eFig. 9.42

7. C. Malignant otitis externa (MOE) is an infection of the external acoustic meatus. *Pseudomonas* is the most common pathogen and patients with diabetes and immunosuppression are at an increased risk. MOE presents with a fever, severe ear pain, swelling of the mastoid and purulent drainage from the ear. Granulation tissue on the floor of the external acoustic meatus is pathognomonic for the disease. Spread of the infection to the mastoid process or other parts of the skull is common. The bacteria spread from the external ear to the internal ear, pass through the mastoid cells, erode the skull, and enter the brain. Infection of the brain can lead to the formation of brain abscesses.

A. The ethmoid cells are sinuses located between the orbit and the nasal cavity. Bacteria do not typically spread from the internal ear to the sinus.

B. The auditory tube connects the middle ear to the nasopharynx. Travel of bacteria from the auditory tube to the cerebellum is unlikely.

D, E. MOE is an infection of the external ear and does not originate within the internal ear.
GAS 944–947; N 105; ABR/McM 57–58

8. D. Pituitary adenomas are tumors of the anterior pituitary gland. In this patient, the tumor extends past the pituitary stalk and up into the hypothalamus. After surgery involving the hypothalamus, the patient experienced increased appetite and weight gain. This was likely due to damage of the ventromedial nucleus of the hypothalamus. The ventromedial nucleus is considered the "satiety center" of the brain and inhibits the urge to eat when stimulated. Bilateral damage of the nucleus eliminates this inhibition and results in hyperphagia and obesity.

A. The suprachiasmatic nucleus plays a role in regulation of the body's circadian rhythms.

B. The posterior hypothalamic nucleus is responsible for thermoregulation of the body, including heat production and conservation. Damage to this area would result in poikilothermia (inability to thermoregulate).

C. The anterior hypothalamic nucleus also plays a role in thermoregulation by cooling off the body.

E. The lateral nucleus is stimulated by a hormone called ghrelin, which induces hunger and eating. Damage to this nucleus would lead to anorexia, starvation and failure to thrive.
GAS 855; N 158; ABR/McM 79

9. B. The patient with paroxysms of unilateral sharp, stabbing pains in the jaw and cheek has trigeminal neuralgia. Trigeminal neuralgia is a chronic condition that affects the trigeminal nerve and results in electric-like pains in the distribution of the nerve, most commonly V2 and V3. The trigeminal nerve sends sensory

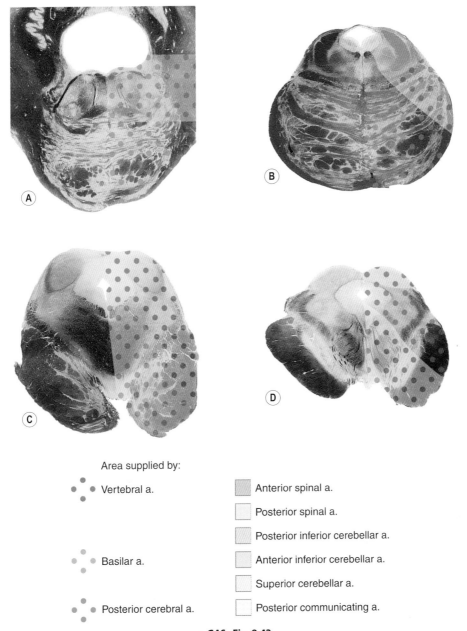

Area supplied by:

⦿ Vertebral a.

⦿ Basilar a.

⦿ Posterior cerebral a.

▨ Anterior spinal a.

☐ Posterior spinal a.

▨ Posterior inferior cerebellar a.

☐ Anterior inferior cerebellar a.

☐ Superior cerebellar a.

☐ Posterior communicating a.

• *GAS* eFig. 9.43

input into the ventral posteromedial nucleus of the thalamus via the trigeminothalamic tract which then projects to the somatosensory cortex.

A. The ventral posterolateral nucleus receives input from the dorsal column/medial lemniscus and spinothalamic tracts.

C. The lateral geniculate nucleus receives visual input from the optic nerve (CN II) and projects to the primary visual cortex in the calcarine sulcus.

D. The medial geniculate nucleus receives auditory input from the superior olivary nucleus and inferior colliculus.

E. The ventral lateral nucleus receives input from the cerebellum and basal ganglia and projects to the motor cortex.

GAS 877; N 121–122; ABR/McM 75

10. C. An infarct in the PCA would affect the occipital lobe, causing visual impairment. The resulting symptom would be contralateral hemianopsia with macular sparing.

A. Contralateral paralysis with loss of sensation of the lower limbs would occur when there is an infarct in the ACA.

B. Contralateral paralysis with contralateral loss of sensation of the upper limb and face occurs with an infarct or lesion within the MCA. If the stoke occurs in the dominant hemisphere then aphasia occurs. If the occlusion was in the temporal lobe then Wernicke aphasia would occur, however, a lesion within the frontal lobe would result in Broca aphasia. If the lesion were in the nondominant hemisphere, the patient would experience hemineglect.

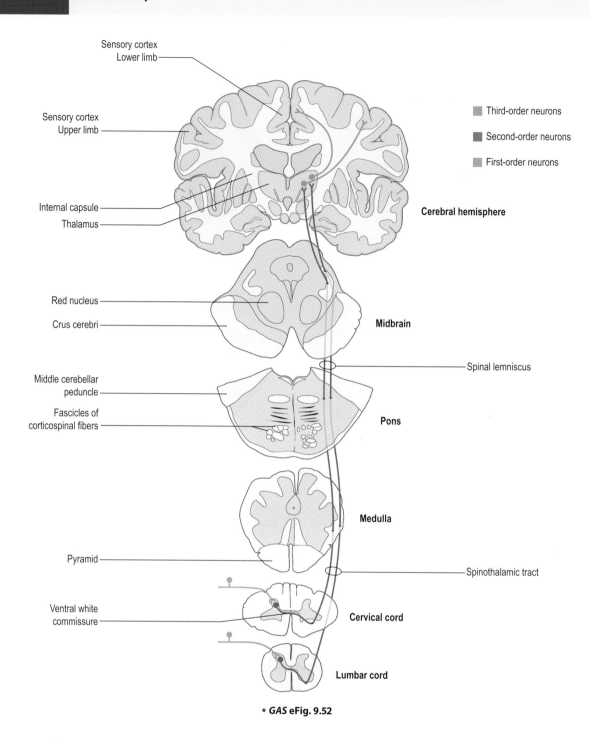

Sensory cortex
Lower limb

Sensory cortex
Upper limb

Third-order neurons

Second-order neurons

First-order neurons

Internal capsule

Thalamus

Cerebral hemisphere

Red nucleus

Crus cerebri

Midbrain

Spinal lemniscus

Middle cerebellar
peduncle

Fascicles of
corticospinal fibers

Pons

Medulla

Pyramid

Spinothalamic tract

Ventral white
commissure

Cervical cord

Lumbar cord

• *GAS eFig. 9.52*

D. An infarct in the PCA would not result in a CN IV palsy.

E. Locked-in syndrome occurs when there is an infarct of the basilar artery causing quadriplegia, and loss of facial and tongue movements. Only consciousness and blinking are preserved.
GAS 870; N 152; ABR/McM 66

11. A. A germinal matrix hemorrhage is a form of intraventricular hemorrhage characterized by bleeding into the subependymal germinal matrix. The germinal matrix is a highly vascularized region, located near the lateral ventricles, from which cells migrate during brain development. Germinal matrix hemorrhage

commonly occurs in premature babies (usually <34 weeks) with perinatal asphyxia. Clinical presentation includes seizures, irritability, bulging fontanelles, and lethargy in neonates.

B, C, D, E. The germinal atrix is located at the head of the caudate nucleus near the lateral ventricles. It is not found near these brain structures.
N 119; ABR/McM 74,

12. A. The ACA supplies the medial surface of the frontal and parietal lobes which are the primary motor and sensory cortices (leg/foot), respectively. Occlusion results in the spastic paresis and anesthesia of the contralateral lower limb.

B. The internal carotid artery's anterior circulation branches are via the anterior and middle cerebral arteries as well as giving rise to the ophthalmic, and anterior and posterior communicating arteries. Occlusion would result in more deficits than spastic paresis of the lower limb.

C. The PICA is a branch of the vertebral artery that supplies the inferior cerebellar peduncle, the lateral medulla oblongata including the lateral spinothalamic tract, nucleus ambiguus and spinal trigeminal nucleus. Occlusion would result in the lateral medullary syndrome or Wallenberg syndrome. Symptoms include decreased pain and temperature sensations of the face and limbs, vertigo, dysmetria, vomiting, decreased gag reflex, nystagmus, dysphagia, hoarseness, and ipsilateral Horner syndrome.

D. The PCA supplies the occipital lobe, lower temporal lobe, midbrain, and thalamus. Occlusion results in contralateral hemianopsia with macular sparing.

E. The MCA gives rise to the lenticulostriate arteries which supply the internal capsule, caudate nucleus, globus pallidus and putamen. Occlusion results in contralateral spastic paralysis and anesthesia of the upper limb/face.

GAS 868–870; N 150–153; ABR/McM 66

13. **B.** This patient is suffering from Wernicke aphasia, as he has fluent aphasia with impaired comprehension and repetition. Wernicke area is located within the superior temporal gyrus.

A. The inferior frontal gyrus is associated with Broca aphasia, which results in nonfluent aphasia with intact comprehension.

C. Damage to the left supramarginal gyrus would result in conduction aphasia, where there is poor repetition but intact comprehension.

D. Damage to the superior colliculi would lead to Parinaud syndrome which, among other things, causes paralysis of upward gaze.

E. Damage to the paramedian pontine reticular formation would cause the eyes to look away from the side of the lesion.

N 116

14. **E.** Berry aneurysms appear at the bifurcations in the circle of Willis. The most common location is the junction of the ACA and the anterior communication artery. A rupture of a berry aneurysm would lead to a subarachnoid hemorrhage or hemorrhagic stroke. The optic chiasm can become compressed, leading to hemianopsia. Berry aneurysms are associated with Ehlers-Danlos syndrome, autosomal dominant polycystic kidney disease, and Marfan syndrome, as seen in this patient with tall stature, hypermobile joints, and subluxation of the lenses.

A, B, C, D. These are not the most common sites for a berry aneurysm.

GAS 873–874; N 150–152; ABR/McM 66–67

15. **E.** Prolonged hypoxia of at least 5 minutes can lead to irreversible damage. Hypoxia may occur due to a stroke or cardiovascular collapse. The regions that are the most vulnerable to ischemic damage include the hippocampus, neocortex, cerebellum, and watershed areas.

A, B, C, D. These areas are less susceptible to ischemic damage compared to the hippocampus.

GAS 871–872

16. **A.** The caudate nucleus is located laterally to the lateral ventricles. It is a C-shaped structure with a head, body, and tail.

B, D, E. The lentiform nucleus is divided into the putamen and globus pallidus nuclei. These lens-shaped nuclei are bounded medially by the caudate nucleus and the thalamus. The lateral boundary is the external capsule.

C. The internal capsule is composed of white-matter axons and is divided into a genu, and anterior and posterior limbs. It runs through the basal ganglia. It separates the lentiform nucleus (globus pallidus and putamen) from the caudate nucleus and thalamus.

N 121; ABR/McM 77

17. **C.** This patient is suffering from a stroke with injury to the AICA, which to leads damage to the lateral pons. This patient would present with damage to the spinocerebellar tracts causing ipsilateral ataxia, spinothalamic tracts causing decreased pain and temperature perception of the contralateral arm and leg, sensory nucleus of the trigeminal nerve causing loss of pain and temperature sensation on the ipsilateral part of the face supplied by CN V, and sympathetic pathways causing an ipsilateral Horner syndrome. With damage to the pons, nuclei related to CNs V, VI, VII, VIII could be involved. The patient exhibits damage to CN VII and CN VIII. Damage to CN VII nuclei results in paralysis of the face, decreased lacrimation, salivation, decreased taste from the anterior two-thirds of the tongue and a diminished corneal reflex. Damage to CN VIII causes ipsilateral hearing loss.

A. Damage to the medial medulla oblongata can occur when there is a lesion of the anterior spinal artery. The resulting symptoms would be due to damage to the lateral corticospinal tract causing hemiparesis of the contralateral upper and lower limbs. There is also damage to the medial lemniscus causing diminished proprioception of the contralateral upper and lower limbs. The medulla oblongata contains nuclei related to CNs IX, X, XI, and XII. The medially located cranial nerve is XII, thus a patient with damage to the medial medulla oblongata would have injury to the hypoglossal nerve causing ipsilateral tongue dysfunction.

B. Damage to the lateral medulla oblongata is seen in Wallenberg syndrome due to an infarct or lesion in the PICA. A patient would present with symptoms of damage to the spinothalamic tract, sensory nucleus of the trigeminal nerve, sympathetic pathway, and the spinocerebellar tract. The medulla oblongata contains nuclei related to CNs IX, X, XI, XII. In Wallenberg syndrome, CN X is affected causing dysphagia, hoarseness, and loss of the gag reflex.

D. Damage to the medial inferior pons would cause contralateral spastic hemiparesis, contralateral loss of light touch/vibratory/kinesthetic sensation, paralysis of gaze on the side of the lesion, and ipsilateral paralysis of the lateral rectus muscle.

E. The hallmark of a brainstem lesion is an alternating syndrome with long tract findings on one side, for example hemiparalysis, and cranial nerve symptoms on the other side.
GAS 869–872; N 128, 151; ABR/McM 67

18. E. This patient has a history of uncontrolled hypertension which is a risk factor for hemorrhagic stroke. Hemorrhagic destruction of the subthalamic nucleus results in the wild, flinging movements of the contralateral limbs.

A. The internal capsule contains the primary motor and sensory white matter tracts in its posterior limb. Damage to the internal capsule would involve both motor and sensory deficits.

B. Lentiform nucleus is the collective name for both the putamen and globus pallidus. Lesions in the lentiform nucleus involve chorea and dystonia and not specifically wild flinging movements.

C. Lesions in the putamen are associated with hepatolenticular degeneration or Wilson disease. Symptoms include "wing beating tremors," asterixis, chorea, neuropsychiatric symptoms, hepatitis, or liver cirrhosis.

D. The loss of pigmented dopaminergic neurons in the substantia nigra results in Parkinson disease. Symptoms include bradykinesia, shuffling gate, cogwheel rigidity, a pill-rolling/resting tremor, masked facies, dementia, and depression.
GAS 871–872

19. C. The ventricular system is comprised of left and right lateral, a third ventricle and a fourth ventricle. The cerebrospinal fluid (CSF) is produced primarily by ependymal cells located at the choroid plexus found within the ventricles. From the lateral ventricles, the CSF flows to the third ventricle via the right and left interventricular foramina of Monro. It then descends to the fourth ventricle via the cerebral aqueduct (of Sylvius) and then into the subarachnoid space via the foramina of Luschka (lateral apertures) and the foramen of Magendie (medial opening). The CSF is then absorbed by arachnoid granulations in the subarachnoid space and drains into the dural venous sinuses.

A, B, D, E Obstruction at any of these structures would lead to enlargement of the third and fourth ventricles.
GAS 865; N 119; ABR/McM 72

20. E. This patient suffered from a temporal lobe lesion affecting the inferior optic radiations. Visual information reaching the retina is inverted and reversed (D). Optic fibers then travel along the optic nerve and meet at the optic chiasm (A&B). At this level, fibers from the left hemi-retina will cross into the left optic tract, and fibers from the right hemi-retina will cross into the left optic tract. The optic tracts then synapse in the thalamus at the lateral geniculate nucleus (C), which then leave as the optic radiations. The inferior optic radiations pass into the temporal lobe and carry information from the upper visual fields; injury at this site will lead to contralateral homonymous superior quadrantanopsia (E). The superior optic radiations pass into the parietal lobe and carry information from the lower visual fields (D). Finally, the upper and lower optic radiations synapse at the primary visual cortex.
N 131; ABR/McM 60

21. A. This patient is suffering from Wernicke-encephalopathy syndrome, which is an acute onset that is potentially reversible and is seen in thiamine deficiency and presents as the triad of encephalopathy, ophthalmoplegia, and ataxia. This syndrome is associated with bilateral necrosis of the mammillary bodies.

B, C, D, E. These structures would not show pathology with Wernicke encephalopathy.
N 118; ABR/McM 66

22. A. The raphe nuclei release serotonin (5HT). They are located in the medial portion of the reticular formation. Dopamine, Gamma-Aminobutyric Acid (GABA), and norepinephrine neurotransmitters are released by neurons from the substantia nigra, nucleus accumbens, locus coeruleus, and the basal nucleus of Meynert, respectively.

B. The substantia nigra is located in the midbrain.

C. The nucleus accumbens is located in the basal forebrain rostral to the preoptic area of the hypothalamus.

D. The locus coeruleus is located in the posterior area of the rostral pons in the upper lateral floor of the fourth ventricle.

E. Finally, the basal nucleus of Meynert is in the substantia innominata.
GAS eFig. 9.99top

23. D. This patient had a ruptured aneurysm arising from the posterior communicating artery. Aneurysms from this location can compress the optic chiasm and disrupts crossing fibers from each contralateral hemi-retina leading to bitemporal hemianopsia.

A. Lesions at the level of the temporal lobe can affect the inferior optic radiations.

B. This patient had a ruptured aneurysm arising from the posterior communicating artery. Aneurysms from this location can compress the optic chiasm and disrupts crossing fibers from each contralateral hemi-retina leading to bitemporal hemianopsia.

C. Aneurysms at the level of the posterior communicating artery can lead to compression of the ipsilateral CN III and cause oculomotor nerve palsy. Chronic compression could also lead to evidence of optic atrophy on fundoscopy (A).

E. Horner syndrome can result from internal carotid artery aneurysms.

GAS 868–871; N 150–152; ABR/McM 66–67

24. **B.** In the parietal lobe, the primary sensory cortex located in the post-central gyrus receives sensory information from the contralateral part of the body, while the primary motor cortex located in the pre-central gyrus controls movement of the contralateral part of the body. Nerve fibers carrying motor and sensory information from different parts of the body terminate in specific areas on the cerebral cortices. These specialized areas are arranged in an orderly fashion. Lesions in certain areas will lead to contralateral spastic paresis and sensory deficits in specific areas of the body.

A. The lower limb is located on the medial side of the brain, which is supplied by the ACA.

C. Going further down the cerebral hemisphere, the arm, hands, and face are located on the lateral side of the cerebral cortices, which is supplied by the MCA.

D. The PCA supplies the occipital lobe, and the PICA is an important artery for supplying the cerebellum and the medulla oblongata.

E. Finally, the AICA supplies the pons so that disruption of this vessel can lead to the lateral pontine syndrome.

GAS 868–871; N 150–152; ABR/McM 65

25. **C.** This patient is suffering from conduction aphasia, which is caused by damage to the arcuate fasciculus, or secondary to any lesion affecting the peri-Sylvian area. This patient's speech will be fluent with intact comprehension and poor repetition.

A. Damage to the inferior frontal lobe would lead to Broca aphasia causing nonfluent aphasia with poor repetition and intact comprehension.

B. Damage to the superior temporal lobe would lead to Wernicke aphasia or receptive aphasia. This patient's speech will be fluent with poor comprehension and repetition.

D. Damage to the watershed zone of the ACA and MCA world lead to transcortical motor aphasia. This patient would have a nonfluent speech with intact comprehension and repetition. E. Damage to the watershed zone of the PCS and MCA would lead to transcortical sensory aphasia, which leads to a fluent speech with good repetition but poor comprehension.

GAS 867; N 116; ABR/McM 65

26. **D.** This patient is experiencing a hemorrhagic stroke in the cerebellum, which leads to ataxia, nystagmus,

occipital headache, neck stiffness, focal weakness, and no hemiparesis.

A. A hemorrhagic stroke in the thalamus would cause contralateral hemiparesis, with the eyes deviated toward hemiparesis with an up-gaze palsy and non-reactive miotic pupil.

B. A hemorrhagic stroke in the basal ganglia would cause contralateral hemiparesis, gaze palsy, and homonymous hemianopsia.

C. A hemorrhagic stroke in the pons would cause a deep coma with paralysis within minutes. The patient's pupils would be pinpoint and reactive.

E. A hemorrhagic stroke in the cerebral lobes would cause contralateral hemiparesis with homonymous hemianopsia and the eyes deviating away from the side of hemiparesis. There is also a high likelihood of seizures.

GAS 871–872

27. **A.** The ciliary body is found between the choroid and the iris (C and D). The ciliary body is made up of the ciliary muscle, which controls the shape of the lens, and the ciliary epithelium, which produces the aqueous humor (B). The aqueous humor continually flows into the posterior chamber and pass through the space between the lens and iris to reach the anterior chamber (C and E). The aqueous humor then drains into the trabecular meshwork to exit the eye via the Schlemm canal.

GAS 936–941; N 100–102; ABR/McM 51

28. **C.** Four days following an ischemic stroke, the most likely histologic finding is macrophage infiltration and phagocytosis which occurs 3 to 5 days post infarction.

A. The first step when neurons undergo the process of ischemia is that the neurons swell and become eosinophilic, which gives them the red color. This red neuron step occurs at 12 to 48 hours following ischemic damage.

B. After the red neuron step, the neurons undergo necrosis and neutrophilic infiltration from 24 to 74 hours.

D. Reactive gliosis occurs 1 to 2 weeks post infarction alongside vascular proliferation.

E. The final step of neuron ischemia is glial scarring, which occurs more than 2 weeks following an infarction.

GAS 871–872

29. **D.** The Romberg test is used to determine if there is any problem with balance with the patient. It tests for a combination of several neurologic systems, namely proprioception, vestibular input, and vision. In this patient, there are no new or existing worsening vision problems. He does not have any vertigo, dizziness, or tinnitus to suggest any problem with vestibular apparatus. But he has a decreased ability to sense vibrations and joint positions, which is proprioception. This function is carried by the dorsal columns of the spinal cord.

A. The spinothalamic tract transmits pain and temperature-related sensation to the cerebrum via the thalamus.

B. The pyramidal tracts are involved in the control of motor functions of the body.

C. The reticulospinal tracts are involved with eye and respiratory muscle movements.

E. Just like pyramidal tracts, the rubrospinal tract governs the flexor and extensor muscles, but more importantly, the muscle tone in the flexor muscle groups of the upper limbs. It plays a crucial role in force, velocity, and direction of movement.

30. B. This patient most likely has cavernous sinus thrombosis. Cavernous sinus houses oculomotor nerve, trochlear nerve, ophthalmic and maxillary branches of the trigeminal nerve, abducens nerve, internal carotid artery. An obese female who recently started taking oral contraceptives is in a prothrombotic state. She presents with progressive headache, diminished visual acuity, proptosis, periorbital edema, decreased mentation, and decreased sensation over the ophthalmic (V1) and maxillary (V2) distributions suggesting increased pressure in the cavernous sinus most likely due to cavernous sinus thrombosis. An increased cavernous sinus pressure decreases the blood flow through the internal carotid artery as it is coursing through it, which is most likely contributing to her worsening mental status.

A. Major neurovascular structures that exit from the jugular foramen include the glossopharyngeal nerve, vagus nerve, accessory nerve, and internal jugular vein. A lesion to the jugular foramen will most likely show physical examination findings of hoarseness, drooping of the soft palate and deviation of the uvula toward the normal side, dysphagia, loss of sensory function from the posterior one-third of the tongue, loss of gag reflex, and sternocleidomastoid and trapezius muscles paresis.

C. A lesion to the optic chiasm will lead to visual field defects.

D. Damage to the occipital lobe will cause visual defects.

E. Foramen rotundum transmits the maxillary nerve (V2). Damage to this nerve will cause a decrease in sensation of the mid-third of the face. It will not cause the other problems that are also seen in the lesions involving the cavernous sinus.

N 116; ABR/McM 65

31. A. This patient has a lesion at the precentral gyrus, which is associated with the primary motor cortex. The precentral gyrus is a prominentgyrus on the surface of the posterior frontal lobe of the brain. The internal pyramidal layer of the precentral cortex contains giant pyramidal neurons called Betz cells, which send long axons to the contralateral motor nuclei of the cranial nerves and to the lower motor neurons in the ventral horn of the spinal cord. These axons form the corticospinal tract. The Betz cells along with their axons are known as upper motor neurons. This patient is predisposed to ischemia to this

region due to his history. Left motor deficits lead us to believe the lesion is on the right side.

B. Left precentral gyrus: The patient is experiencing motor deficits on the left side, which indicates that the lesion would be in the right hemisphere.

C. The postcentral gyrus is the location of the somatosensory cortex. The patient is not experiencing any sensory deficits.

D. The postcentral gyrus is the location of the somatosensory cortex. The patient is not experiencing any sensory deficits.

E. The precentral gyrus is located on the frontal lobe and not in the parietal.

N 116; McM 65

32. D. Trauma to the eye can cause increased pressure in the orbit, creating a fracture. The floor of the orbit is thinner and more likely to crack when exposed to high force like a punch or a baseball hitting the eye. A consequence of the orbital floor fracture is entrapment of the inferior rectus muscle. As a result, the patient will most likely experience a limitation of upward gaze. An eyelid swelling is most likely because of air trapped in the periorbital soft tissue post-trauma. Enophthalmos, or posteriorly displaced eyeball, is commonly encountered. A decrease in visual acuity is expected in traumatic ocular conditions.

A. Superior oblique muscle is innervated by the trochlear nerve (CN IV). The primary function of this muscle is intorsion of the eye in the adducted position; i.e., it is vital when looking toward the nose, as well as when walking down stairs. A loss of function of this muscle can occur due to head trauma, especially if there is damage to the trochlea, which functions as a pulley for the tendon of this muscle.

B. The primary function of the superior rectus muscle is elevation of the eye. It is not close to the orbital floor where a fracture has most likely occurred in this patient.

C. The primary function of the inferior oblique muscle is extorsion of the eye. Also, it is the only muscle that is capable of elevating the eye when it is in a fully adducted position.

E. The medial rectus muscle is responsible for turning the eye medially. It is also not close to the orbital floor where a fracture has most likely occurred in this patient.

GAS 927–933; N 96, 98; ABR/McM 52–54

33. E. The cerebellar hemispheres functions are motor planning and coordination of complex tasks. A lesion to cerebellar hemisphere will show clinical signs in the ipsilateral limbs. Most clinical signs are dysdiadochokinesia, dysmetria, limb ataxia, intention tremor, and scanning speech. Dysdiadochokinesia is incoordination in performing rapidly alternating movements. To test for this, an examiner usually asks the patient to alternately pronate and supinate the hand.

A. Hemiparesis will be a result of insult to the motor pathway of the upper motor neurons. For example, a stroke of the ACA branches supplying the left motor cortex will cause right hemiparesis or paralysis based on the extent of the lesion.

B. A lesion to the left occipital lobe will cause right homonymous hemianopsia.

C. A lesion to left cerebellar hemisphere will cause a left-sided intention tremor. In this patient, there is a cystic lesion in the right cerebellar hemisphere.

D. A lesion in the left cerebral hemisphere or left upper motor neurons will cause right lower facial droop.

GAS 867, 870; N 124–126; ABR/McM 68, 70

34. **C.** This patient has vitamin B12 deficiency due to pernicious anemia. Patients with autoimmune diseases, such as Hashimoto thyroiditis, tend to have other autoimmune comorbidities. A complication of vitamin B12 deficiency is the degeneration of the dorsal columns of the spinal cord (subacute combined degeneration). The onset is gradual and uniform. The pathological findings of subacute combined degeneration consist of patchy losses of myelin in the dorsal and lateral columns. On physical examination, patients can present with glossitis, grey skin, and weakness of legs, arms, and trunk, and tingling and numbness. Romberg test is usually positive in these patients.

A. The spinoreticular tract conveys deep and chronic pain.

B. The corticospinal tract's primary purpose is for voluntary motor control of the body and limbs.

B. The spinothalamic tract is important in the localization of pain and temperature.

E. The spinocerebellar tract conveys proprioceptive information from the body to the cerebellum. It is not affected by vitamin B12 deficiency.

GAS 920, 930; N 172, 213, 230; ABR/McM 194, 195

35. **E.** Pancoast tumor is a tumor of the lung's apex. It is a type of lung cancer defined primarily by its location, situated at the top end of either the right or left lung. It typically spreads to nearby tissues such as the ribs and vertebrae. Most Pancoast tumors are non–small cell cancers. The growing tumor can cause compression of a brachiocephalic vein, subclavian artery, phrenic nerve, recurrent laryngeal nerve, vagus nerve, or, characteristically, compression of asympathetic ganglion, resulting in a range of symptoms known as Horner's syndrome. The classic triad presented in Horner syndrome includes: (1) ptosis, (2) miosis, and (3) anhidrosis.

A. Compression of the recurrent laryngeal nerve would lead to symptoms such as hoarse voice and cough, not Horner's.

B. Compression of the cerebellum would lead to motor-related symptoms, depending on the region being compressed. Miosis would not occur.

C. Damage to the frontal lobe can cause a variety of more noticeable issues such as behavioral changes, and not miosis.

D. Compression of the spinal cord would lead to both sensory and motor deficits. Miosis would not be a symptom.

GAS 920, 930; N 172, 213, 230; McM 194, 195

36. **E.** The superior cerebellar artery is the penultimate branch of the basilar artery. It originates from the basilar artery and runs laterally to supply the superior and medial parts of the cerebellum. In its course, it travels very close to the trochlear nerve. The aneurysm in the superior cerebellar artery in this patient is likely compressing the trochlear nerve. The trochlear nerve innervates the superior oblique muscle, which acts to move the eye downward and laterally. It is the only muscle that can depress the pupil when the eye is adducted. When an individual walks downstairs or reads the newspaper, this eye motion is initiated, and diplopia results if it is not functioning correctly.

A. The abducens nerve innervates the lateral rectus muscle, which abducts the eye.

B. The oculomotor nerve innervates medial rectus muscle, which adducts the eye.

C. The inferior oblique muscle is innervated by the oculomotor nerve. The primary function of the inferior oblique muscle is extorsion of the eye. Also, it is the only muscle that is capable of elevating the eye when it is in a fully adducted position.

D. The levator palpebrae superioris muscle elevates and retracts the upper eyelid. It is innervated by the oculomotor nerve. A loss of function of this muscle will result in complete ptosis.

GAS 870, 889; N 149, 154; ABR/McM 66, 67

37. **C.** The optic nerve carries the sense of vision. A lesion to the optic nerve will lead to blindness on the same side. The optic and oculomotor nerves provide the afferent and efferent limbs, respectively, of the pupillary light reflex. Normally, when light is shone in one eye, both pupils will constrict, that is, there is a direct response and also a consensual response in the other eye. In this patient, his right CN II, that is, the afferent portion of the reflex, is damaged. As such, when the light is shone on the right eye, there is no direct pupillary reaction on the right eye; neither is any signal transmitted for the consensual pupillary light reaction on the left eye. The patient is completely blind on the right side. However, when the light is shone on the left eye of this patient, there is observed ipsilateral and contralateral pupillary light reaction. This suggests that his left CN II, left CN III, and right CN III are intact, but only his right-sided CN II is damaged, likely because of ischemia secondary to his comorbidities of hypertension, hyperlipidemia, and diabetes.

A and D. The ophthalmic division (V1) of the trigeminal nerve provides sensory innervation to the cornea as the afferent portion of the corneal reflex, while the facial nerve (CN VII) innervates the orbicularis oculi, which closes the eyelids as the efferent portion of this reflex. Normally, both eyes will close at the same time. However, these nerves are not part of the pupillary light reflex.

E. The trochlear nerve innervates the superior oblique muscle, which acts to move the eye downward and laterally. It is the only muscle that can depress the pupil when the eye is adducted. When an individual walks downstairs or reads the newspaper, this eye motion is initiated. It plays no role in visual sensation or pupillary light reflex.

GAS 885–886, 889–890; N 143; ABR/McM 78–80

38. E. Metastatic disease is the most common cause of jugular foramen syndrome. This patient with a history of prostate cancer likely has a recurrence of the disease with metastasis. Major neurovascular structures that emit from jugular foramen are glossopharyngeal nerve, vagus nerve, accessory nerve, and internal jugular vein. A lesion to the jugular foramen will most likely show physical examination findings of hoarseness, vocal cord paralysis, drooping of the soft palate and deviation of the uvula toward the normal side, dysphagia, loss of sensory function from the posterior one-third of the tongue, loss of gag reflex, and sternocleidomastoid and trapezius muscle paresis.

A. The foramen ovale transmits the mandibular nerve, accessory meningeal artery, lesser petrosal nerve, and an emissary vein that connects the cavernous sinus with the pterygoid venous plexus. A lesion to this structure does not result in all the symptoms this patient is experiencing.

B. The cavernous sinus houses oculomotor nerve, trochlear nerve, ophthalmic and maxillary divisions of the trigeminal nerve, abducens nerve, and the internal carotid artery. A lesion of this structure does not result in all the symptoms this patient is experiencing.

C. The foramen rotundum transmits maxillary division (V2) of the trigeminal nerve. A lesion to this structure does not result in all the symptoms the patient is experiencing. D. The major structures through foramen magnum are medulla oblongata, the spinal root of cranial nerve XI, vertebral arteries, and anterior and posterior spinal arteries. A lesion of this structure does not result in all the symptoms the patient is experiencing.

GAS 888–891; N 135; ABR/McM 9, 11

39. C. Weber test is a useful screening test for hearing loss. It can indicate unilateral conductive or sensorineural hearing loss, and in tandem with Rinne test can localize and specify the nature of the deficit. The test is performed on the superior aspect of the sagittal suture of the skull, also known as the vertex.

A. The occipital protuberance is a bony elevation near the middle of the occipital bone of the skull. It is not a suitable placement site for the Weber test.

B. The mastoid process is a projection on the temporal bone of the skull. It is not a suitable placement site for the Weber test.

D. The glabella is the region of the face superior to the nose and between the eyebrows. It is not a suitable placement site for the Weber test.

E. The angle of the mandible is the inferoposterior region of the ramus of the mandible. It is not a suitable placement site for the Weber test.

GAS 843–851; N 11, 16, 17, 22; ABR/McM 8, 9, 13

40. E. A hemorrhagic stroke is an interruption of blood flow to the brain due to ruptured blood vessels. Risk factors include hypertension, smoking, and use of oral

contraceptives. Signs and symptoms that present with stroke are dependent on the area affected by the lack of perfusion. A lesion in the CNS of CN VII results in paralysis of muscles of the inferior face on the side contralateral to the lesion. In this lesion, forehead wrinkling is not impaired because it is innervated bilaterally. CN VII travels the posterior cranial fossa, internal acoustic meatus, facial canal, and stylomastoid foramen to emerge from the cranium and give rise to five terminal motor branches (temporal, zygomatic, buccal, marginal mandibular, and cervical).

A. The foramen ovale is behind the foramen rotundum in the greater wing of the sphenoid bone and transmits the maxillary nerve of CN V.

B. The foramen cecum is a depression between the crista galli and the crest of the frontal bone. It may be either blind-ended or carry a vein draining from the nasal mucosa to the superior sagittal sinus.

C. The jugular foramen is a large foramen in the posterior cranial fossa that transmits CN IX, CN X, CN XI, and the internal jugular vein.

D. The foramen magnum is the most prominent feature in the posterior cranial fossa. It transmits the spinal cord, vertebral arteries, and roots of CN XI for part of their course.

GAS 884; N 64; BP 27; ABR/McM 9, 11

41. C. The gag reflex tests CN IX and CN X by stimulation of the back of the throat on each side with a tongue depressor causing muscular contraction of each side of the pharynx. Glossopharyngeal branches provide the afferent limb for this reflex. Stylopharyngeus is the only muscle of those listed that is innervated by CN IX.

A. Buccinator is a muscle of the oral cavity between the maxilla and the mandible. It is innervated by CN V and CN VII.

B. Stylohyoid is a part of the suprahyoid muscles that elevate the hyoid and larynx in relation to swallowing. It is innervated by CN VII.

D. Omohyoid is a part of the infrahyoid muscles that depress the hyoid and larynx during swallowing and speaking. It is innervated by the ansa cervicalis.

E. Posterior digastric is a part of the suprahyoid muscles that elevate the hyoid and larynx in relation to swallowing. It is innervated by CN VII.

GAS 888, 891, 1040–1041; N 70; ABR/McM 45, 47

42. A. A stroke is an interruption of blood flow to the brain. It may be hemorrhagic due to ruptured blood vessels, or ischemic from occlusion of blood vessels. Risk factors include hypertension, smoking, and use of oral contraceptives. Signs and symptoms that present with stroke are dependent on the area affected by the lack of perfusion, but usually include paresis or sensory loss. The signs in this patient include facial numbness and tongue deviation to the right (implicating CN XII) and uvula deviation to the left (implicating CN X) on examination. This suggests a right-sided central lesion, meaning it occurs between the cortex and brainstem nuclei.

B. Lesion of nerve nuclei would occur between the nuclei and the muscles. However, this patient has no weakness in the upper or lower extremities.

C. Nerve lesion would occur outside the CNS and the cranial nerves that would be involved in this clinical presentation.

D. A lesion of autonomic ganglia would present differently than the clinical presentation given. The vagal ganglia are exclusively afferent and would not produce deficient motor activity.

E. This patient has a lesion of CN X and CN XII, not a lesion of autonomic nerves. CN XII carries out only somatic efferent, while CN X carries visceral as well as somatic functions.
GAS 871; N 127–129; ABR/McM 78, 84, 85

43. E. The lens is a transparent biconvex elastic disc that separates the anterior one-fifth of the eyeball from the posterior four-fifths. With increased age, the lenses of the eye become harder and flatter, as well as becoming opaque, thus reducing the focusing power of the lenses. Cataracts are opacities of the lenses visible through the pupil. They are the world's leading cause of blindness. Risk factors include cigarette smoking, diabetes, and advanced age, all of which occur in this patient. On the other hand, glaucoma is increased intraocular pressure leading to progressive vision loss. This is due to a disruption in the normal cycle of production and absorption of aqueous humor. The most common type is primary open-angle glaucoma. This manifests as slow, painless loss of peripheral vision and eventually central vision if left untreated. The vision loss usually presents bilaterally. This patient is less likely to have glaucoma.

A. The retina is a thin sheet of cells that lines the inner posterior surface of the eyeball. Glaucoma is associated with an acquired loss of retinal ganglion cells and axons within the optic nerve.

B. Aqueous humor is the fluid that fills the anterior and posterior chambers of the eye. It supplies nutrients to the avascular cornea and maintains intraocular pressure. If the normal cycle of aqueous humor production and absorption is disrupted, glaucoma can result.

C. The ciliary body serves to anchor the lens via suspensory ligaments. By contraction of its smooth muscle, the ciliary body changes the refractive power of lens (accommodation). Ciliary processes secrete aqueous humor into the posterior chamber which then flows through the pupil into the anterior chamber. Overproduction of aqueous humor relative to absorption can lead to glaucoma.

D. The canal of Schlemm, also called the scleral venous sinus, is a circular venous channel at the junction between the cornea and the iris. It collects aqueous humor from the anterior chamber into episcleral veins. Interference with the drainage into the canal of Schlemm can lead to glaucoma.
GAS 936; N 94, 100–103

44. E. A and C are correct.

A. The corneal reflex is performed by touching the cornea with a wisp of cotton. The afferent (sensory) limb of corneal reflex is performed by CN V, which would not be injured in the patient's lesion.

B. The pupillary reflex involves rapid constriction of the pupil in response to light. The afferent (sensory) limb of pupillary reflex is performed by CN II, which would not be injured in the patient's lesion.

C. This patient has sustained a traumatic physical injury to the superior orbital fissure. The nervous structures passing through the superior orbital fissure include CN III, CN IV, branches of CN V, and CN VI. Of the options given, CN III will be affected as it carries the efferent (motor) limb of the pupillary reflex. The pupillary reflex involves rapid constriction of the pupil in response to light.

D. The corneal reflex is performed by touching the cornea with a wisp of cotton. The efferent (motor) limb of corneal reflex is performed by CN VII, which would not be injured in the patient's lesion.
GAS 885-886, 889-890; N 20, 143; ABR/McM 78-80

45. B. This patient presents with hypoglossal palsy, hemiparesis, and lemniscal sensory loss. This suggests a lesion involving the medial medulla since this would impair CN XII, the medullary pyramids (corticospinal tracts), and medial lemniscus.

A. The inferior cerebellar peduncle contains afferent fibers, including dorsal spinocerebellar tract, cuneocerebellar tract, olivocerebellar tract, and vestibulocerebellar tract. The presentation may present similar to peripheral vestibular disorders.

C. A lesion of the medial pons would affect the corticospinal tract, the medial lemniscus, and CN VI. The presentation would be characterized by spastic hemiparesis, loss of tactile and vibratory sensation, and lateral rectus palsy.

D. A lesion to the lateral midbrain (paramedian midbrain) would affect corticospinal tracts, superior cerebellar peduncle decussation, and CN III. The presentation would be characterized by oculomotor palsy and cerebellar ataxia.

E. A lesion to the posterior spinal cord would affect the dorsal columns and lateral corticospinal tracts. The presentation would be characterized by isolated loss of proprioception and vibratory sensation. GAS eFig. 9.53
GAS 867–870; N 124–125; ABR/McM 66–67

46. C. Wilson disease, also known as hepatolenticular degeneration, is due to a buildup of copper leading to hepatic symptoms such as jaundice, as well as movement dysregulation due to CNS involvement. The golden halo around the iris is a Kayser-Fleischer ring that forms due to deposition of copper in Descemet membrane of the cornea.

A. Pigmented epithelium of the retina is a layer of cuboidal cells extending from the periphery of

Sensory cortex
Lower limb

Sensory cortex
Upper limb

Internal capsule

Thalamus

Cerebral hemisphere

Third-order neurones

Second-order neurones

First-order neurones

Medial lemniscus

Red nucleus

Crus cerebri

Midbrain

Middle cerebellar peduncle

Medial lemniscus

Pons

Nucleus gracilis

Nucleus cuneatus

Internal arcuate fibers

Medulla

Medial lemniscus

Pyramid

Fasciculus gracilis

Fasciculus cuneatus

Cervical cord

Lumbar cord

• *GAS* **eFig. 9.53**

the optic disc to the ora serrata. These cells play a major role in rod and cone component turnover. This layer is not where Kayser-Fleischer rings are formed.

B. The capsule layer of the lens is a basement membrane that covers the surface of the lens. It consists of various classes of collagen fibers, glycosaminoglycans, and glycoproteins. It is not where Kayser-Fleischer rings are formed.

D. Rods and cones are the photoreceptors of the outer retina that respond to light. This layer is not where Kayser-Fleischer rings are formed.

E. The choroid plexus of the eye is in the middle vascular layer of the wall of the eyeball. It is continuous with the ciliary body and iris anteriorly. It is not where Kayser-Fleischer rings are formed.

GAS 939–941; N 101

47. A. Wilson disease, also known as hepatolenticular degeneration, is due to a buildup of copper in different parts of the body. The basal ganglia is made up of nuclei deep to the neocortex that is primarily involved in motor control. As a result, deposition of copper in the basal ganglia leads to motor symptoms such as tremor, dyskinesia, and rigidity.

B. The thalamus is a structure in the diencephalon that is involved in relaying sensory and motor signals, and regulating alertness. The motor symptoms in Wilson disease are not due to a thalamic lesion.

C. Mammillary bodies are brainstem nuclei located inferiorly and posteriorly to the hypothalamus. They are involved with spatial and episodic memory consolidation and storage. Degeneration of the mammillary bodies leads to symptoms such as memory loss and confabulation.

D. The pineal gland is an endocrine gland located in the posterior aspect of the cranial fossa in the brain. It functions primarily in regulating circadian rhythms and wakefulness. The motor symptoms in Wilson disease are not due to a pineal gland lesion.

N 121

48. D. This patient likely had a stroke in the basilar artery secondary to his diabetic ketoacidosis. The basilar artery is formed at the junction of the pons and medulla by the convergence of the vertebral arteries. It supplies blood to the cerebellum, brainstem, thalamus, and occipital and medial temporal lobes of the brain. A lesion to this artery would present with motor symptoms and an altered or decreased level of consciousness.

A. The PICA supplies the posterior inferior cerebellum and the lateral medulla. A lesion to this vessel would likely result in vertigo and truncal ataxia.

B. A lesion of the PCA would present with homonymous hemianopia and sensory loss.

C. A lesion of the vertebral artery could present with vision changes, loss of balance, or bulbar symptoms.

E. A lesion of the superior cerebellar artery would result in vertigo, nystagmus, ataxia, or hemiparesis.

GAS 870; N 150, 154; ABR/McM 66–67

49. D. Osmotic demyelination syndrome (ODS) is a neurologic condition involving severe damage to the myelin sheath of brain stem frequently associated with rapid correction of hyponatremia. Central pontine myelinolysis (CPM) is an acute demyelinating neurologic disorder affecting primarily the central pons. It is characterized by weakness and incoordination of the bulbar muscles, brisk reflexes throughout, including jaw jerk with extensor plantars, dysphagia, dysarthria, and altered mental status. ODS is a well-recognized complication of treatment of patients with severe and prolonged hyponatremia, particularly when corrected too rapidly iatrogenically. This is likely the reason for symptoms in this patient with diabetic ketoacidosis.

C. Extrapontine myelinolysis, with or without pontine involvement, occurs most often in the basal ganglia and thalamus, but much less frequently. Although both conditions share the same pathology, the location of the lesions results in different clinical presentations. The manifestation separation of patients with myelinolysis in central pontine and extrapontine locations is possible on the basis of clinical symptoms. Classically, CPM is associated with dysarthria and dysphagia, due to corticobulbar fiber involvement, as well as an initially flaccid quadriparesis due to lesions in the corticospinal tract. Extrapontine myelinolysis is characterized by tremor and ataxia and may be associated with movement disorders including mutism, parkinsonism, dystonia, and catatonia.

A. Midbrain is not typically the region affected by ODS.

B. Medulla oblongata is not typically the region affected by ODS.

D. Cerebellum is not typically the region affected by ODS.

GAS 870; N 150, 154; ABR/McM 66–67

50. D. The superior tarsal muscle works to keep the upper eyelid raised after the levator palpebrae superioris (Option C)—supplied oculomotor nerve (CN III) has raised the upper eyelid. The superior tarsal muscle is supplied by postganglionic sympathetic fibers originating in the superior cervical ganglion. Damage to some elements of this sympathetic nervous system can inhibit this muscle, causing a drooping eyelid, or partial ptosis. The sympathetic transmission to superior tarsal muscle can be hindered with compression because of Pancoast tumor of the pulmonary apex, owing to the close proximity of the sympathetic trunk, as seen in this case.

A. The facial nerve (CN VII) innervates the orbicularis oculi, which closes the eyelid as the efferent portion of the corneal reflex.

B. The optic nerve (CN II) and oculomotor nerve (CN III) provide the afferent limb and the efferent limb, respectively, of the pupillary light reflex.

E. The primary function of the superior rectus muscle is the elevation of the eye. It is supplied by the oculomotor nerve (CN III).

GAS 918–920, N 94

51. D. A lesion to the optic chiasm will lead to visual field defects bilaterally, and mostly occurs due to the mass effect caused by the pituitary tumor located in the sella turcica. Depending on the extension of compression, it typically presents as bilateral hemianopia causing bilateral loss of outer visual fields.

A. Left optic tract lesions will cause left homonymous hemianopias.

B. Right optic tract lesions will cause right homonymous hemianopias.

C. Right Meyer loop lesions will cause left superior quadrantanopia.

E. Dorsal optic radiation lesions will cause inferior quadrantanopia on the side it carries sensation from.

N 117–118; ABR/McM 59, 66

52. C. NPH presents as a triad of urinary incontinence, gait instability, and dementia ("wet, wobbly, and wacky"). NPH is an abnormal buildup of CSF in the brain's ventricles, or cavities. It occurs if the normal flow of CSF throughout the brain and spinal cord is blocked in some way. This causes the ventricles to enlarge, putting pressure on the brain. NPH can occur in people of any age, but it is most common in the elderly. It may result from a subarachnoid hemorrhage, head trauma, infection, tumor, or complications of surgery. However, many people develop NPH even when none of these factors are present. In these cases the cause of the disorder is unknown.

A. Parkinson disease patients may have a general slowing of movements with correlates to similar symptoms as seen in this case, but this condition does not typically present with the triad as seen in NPH.

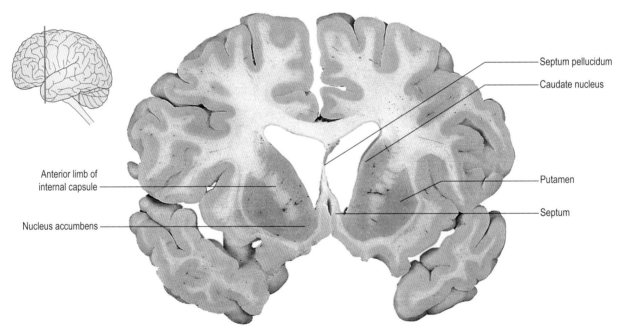

Anterior horn of lateral ventricle

Body of lateral ventricle

Interventricular foramen

Atrium

Third ventricle

Posterior horn of lateral ventricle

Cerebral aqueduct

Fourth ventricle

Inferior horn of lateral ventricle

Lateral recess of fourth ventricle (and foramen of Luschka)

Body of lateral ventricle

Posterior horn of lateral ventricle

Ⓐ Ⓑ

• *GAS* eFig. 9.15

Septum pellucidum

Caudate nucleus

Anterior limb of internal capsule

Nucleus accumbens

Putamen

Septum

• *GAS* eFig. 9.102

B. Syringomyelia results from syrinx expansion from cystic degeneration of the spinal cord resulting in involvement of spinal tract damage involved in pain and temperature, as well as motor functions.

D. A stroke typically results in focal neurologic deficits that can be evident in neurologic exams.

E. Alzheimer disease patients may have a general slowing of movements with correlates with similar symptoms as seen in this case, but this condition does not typically present with the triad as seen in NPH. GAS eFig. 9.15top

GAS 865–866; N 111, 113, 120; ABR/McM 60–62

53. B. Atrophy of the caudate nucleus. Huntington disease is an autosomal dominant disease that results from progressive degeneration of nerve cells in the caudate nucleus of the brain. It limits a person's functional abilities, and causes the individual difficulties with movement, cognition, and psychiatric symptoms. It usually develops early in life after age 20 and there is no cure for this disease.

A. Cerebellar stroke will mostly present with focal neurologic deficits.

C. Enhanced ring-like lesions could be because of infections or malignancy, both of which will likely cause headache, nausea, vomiting, and can be associated with focal neurologic deficits.

D. Tumors can also present with headache due to mass effect, hydrocephalus in case of obstruction of the CSF flow, and nausea and vomiting.

E. Subarachnoid hemorrhage will mostly present with focal neurologic deficits.

N 123; ABR/McM 76

54. C. MS is the most common chronic CNS disease of young adults (20 to 30 years of age), and more common in women. It is commonly seen in regions away from the equator. It also has Uhthoff phenomenon, which is a worsening of neurologic symptoms in MS and other neurologic, demyelinating conditions when the body gets overheated from hot weather, exercise, fever, or saunas and hot tubs. Furthermore, it presents with ocular symptoms, particularly internuclear ophthalmoplegia, which is degeneration of medial longitudinal fasciculus, as well as blurry vision because of demyelination of the optic nerve. Finally, it presents with relapsing neurologic deficits with periods of remission.

A. Meningitis will present with fever, headache, and photophobia. There is typically nuchal rigidity.

B. Encephalitis mostly occurs due to viral etiology, and initially presents with mild flu-like signs and symptoms—such as a fever or headache.

C. Rabies is a viral disease that causes inflammation of the brain; signs can include tingling, prickling, or itching of the affected area from the bites of animals such as bats, raccoons, skunks, and stray dogs that are reservoirs of rabies virus. Flu-like symptoms, such as a fever, headache, muscle aches, loss of appetite, nausea, and tiredness, may also present.

E. Tumor can present with headache due to mass effect, hydrocephalus in case of obstruction of the CSF flow, and nausea and vomiting. This patient does not have these symptoms.

N 11

55. C. Guillain-Barre syndrome (GBS) is a rare disorder in which the body's immune system attacks peripheral Schwann cells due to molecular mimicry, typically after an infection. Consuming raw milk infected with Campylobacter jejuni can lead to diarrheal symptoms. Over time, the body's immune system also attacks healthy nerve cells in the peripheral nervous system in an ascending fashion from lower extremities and up and this leads to weakness, numbness, and tingling, and can eventually cause paralysis.

A. Multiple sclerosis is caused by widespread CNS demyelination secondary to destruction of oligodendrocytes. It does not affect peripheral nerves.

B. In GBS, the nerves affected are peripheral, not central.

D. Charcot-Marie-Tooth disease is one of the hereditary motor and sensory neuropathies of the peripheral nervous system characterized by progressive loss of muscle tissue and touch sensation across various parts of the body.

E. ODS is a well-recognized complication of treatment of patients with severe and prolonged hyponatremia, particularly when corrected too rapidly iatrogenically. *N 12*

56. A. This patient most likely has Becker muscular dystrophy, the milder form of the genetic muscular disorder that primarily affects the skeletal and cardiac muscle. These muscular dystrophies exclusively occur in men. They are caused by different mutations in the same dystrophin gene. The two conditions differ in their severity, age of onset, and rate of progression. Affected children may have delayed motor skills, such as sitting, standing, walking, and speaking. They are usually wheelchair-dependent by adolescence. The signs and symptoms of Becker muscular dystrophy are generally milder and more varied. In most cases, muscle weakness becomes apparent later in childhood or adolescence and worsens at a much slower rate. Respiratory muscles also become weaker over time and there is diminished work of breathing and coughing to clear secretions from the respiratory tract, which makes them susceptible to pneumonia. Patient may also have endocrine conditions, such as diabetes or hypoparathyroidism. Cardiomyopathy typically begins in adolescence; later, heart muscle becomes enlarged, giving rise to dilated cardiomyopathy. There could also be ocular symptoms because of weak muscles, causing nystagmus. A rare but important group of scoliosis is that in which the muscle is abnormal.

Muscular dystrophy is the commonest example. The abnormal muscle does not retain the normal alignment of the vertebral column, and curvature develops as a result. A muscle biopsy is needed to make the diagnosis.

E. Dysarthria is a common neurologic manifestation of these patients and is more likely present than marked cognitive deficits, although mild cognitive deficits are present in many cases.

B. MERRF syndrome, or myoclonic epilepsy with ragged red fibers is a mitochondrial disease. It is extremely rare, and has varying degrees of expressivity due to heteroplasmy. MERRF syndrome affects different parts of the body, particularly the muscles and nervous system. The signs and symptoms of this disorder appear at an early age, generally childhood or adolescence. Patients primarily display myoclonus as their first symptom. There may also be seizures, cerebellar ataxia, myopathy, dementia, optic atrophy, bilateral deafness, peripheral neuropathy, spasticity, or lipomas.

C. Huntington disease presents with worsening choreiform limb movements. Muscular dystrophies characteristically do not have chorea.

D. Muscular dystrophy affects the muscular component of motor skills more than the proprioceptive ability of the patient.

N 8, GAS 74

9

Embryology

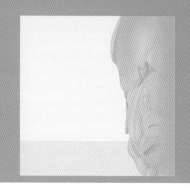

See also other chapters.

Questions

Questions 1–25

1. A 35-year-old pregnant woman comes to the physician for the first time to evaluate her pregnancy. She is in her 30th week of pregnancy and is aware that this is late for an initial evaluation. Ultrasonography examinations shows intrauterine twins, and one twin is surrounded by excessive amniotic fluid, while the other is surrounded by too little. A diagnosis of twin-to-twin transfusion syndrome is made. Which of the following types of pregnancy is most likely the cause of such a condition?
   A. Dichorionic, diamniotic twins
   B. Dichorionic, monoamniotic twins
   C. Monochorionic, monoamniotic twins
   D. Conjoined twins
   E. Monochorionic, diamniotic twins

2. A 35-year-old woman gravida 2, para 0, aborta 1 at 28 weeks' gestation comes to the office for a prenatal visit. Ultrasonography examination shows conjoined twins. This condition is typically caused by incomplete division of embryonic discs. The most common location where conjoined twins connect is which of the following?
   A. Thoracopagus
   B. Dicephalus
   C. Craniopagus
   D. Omphalopagus
   E. Rachipagus

3. A 27-year-old woman gives birth to an infant with severe neurologic symptoms. Physical examination shows cerebral palsy, ataxia, numbness of hand and feet, and weakness of muscles. The woman resides in a fishing town. A diagnosis of Minamata disease is made. Which of the following teratogens consumed by the mother is the most likely cause of this congenital disorder?
   A. Lead
   B. Mercury
   C. Alcohol
   D. Cocaine
   E. Streptomycin

4. A clinical study is designed to evaluate the prevalence of clear cell adenocarcinoma of the vagina between 1966 and 1969. Seven out of eight girls whose mothers had taken a certain agent during pregnancy were diagnosed with this condition. Which of the following teratogens is the most likely agent that pregnant mothers would have consumed to cause this condition in their daughters?
   A. Alcohol
   B. Diethylstilbestrol (DES)
   C. Lithium
   D. Nicotine
   E. Folic acid

5. A 30-year-old pregnant woman, gravida 2, para 0, aborta 1, at 28 weeks' gestation comes to the office for a prenatal visit. As part of prenatal counseling, the woman is informed that during weeks 3–8, the embryo is most susceptible to teratogens because major organs develop. Which of the following exposures during this period would most likely result in congenital deafness, low birth rate, inflammation of the retina, and jaundice?
   A. Toxoplasmosis
   B. Heroin
   C. Mercury poisoning
   D. Alcohol
   E. Tetracycline

6. A 28-year-old woman who became pregnant 10 weeks ago comes to the physician for an evaluation of her pregnancy. She has a house cat, for which she cleans the litterbox and feeds the cat raw meat. The patient appears well, and physical examination shows no abnormalities. Her vital signs are within normal limits for her age of gestation. Laboratory studies shows positive immunoglobulin M (IgM) for a zoonotic parasite. The woman is informed that the fetus has a high risk of developing congenital deafness, having a low birth rate, and developing inflammation of the retina and jaundice. Which of the following teratogens can give rise to these findings?

A. Toxoplasmosis
B. Heroin
C. Mercury poisoning
D. Alcohol
E. Tetracycline

7. A 20-year-old pregnant woman comes to the hospital to give birth. She is sexually active, she has smoked 20 cigarettes daily for the past 5 years, and has no history of recent travel. She delivers a small-for-gestational-age male who is 4 weeks premature. Which of the following teratogens most likely contributed to the low birth rate and premature delivery?
A. Heroin
B. Warfarin
C. Rubella
D. Tetracycline
E. Nicotine

8. A 25-year-old woman comes to the physician for evaluation of her newborn infant. Physical examination of the infant shows a flat philtrum, thin vermilion border, and small palpebral fissures. These craniofacial abnormalities are associated with an agent that can cross the placenta in utero and be secreted by the mammary glands during breastfeeding. Which of the following teratogens is most likely responsible for this condition?
A. Alcohol
B. Warfarin
C. Heroin
D. Rubella
E. Tetracycline

9. A newly married couple comes to a physician for counseling on family planning. The couple hopes to start a family soon. The husband takes medication for hyperlipidemia, and the wife takes medication for epilepsy. The physician explains that with exposure to the current medications taken by the couple, a pregnancy could be complicated by serious birth defects, such as microcephaly, cleft palate, and congenital heart defects. This exposure during pregnancy will most likely cause which of the following?
A. Fetal hydantoin syndrome
B. Fetal alcohol syndrome (FAS)
C. Down syndrome
D. Treacher Collins syndrome
E. DiGeorge syndrome

10. A 6-day-old breast-fed boy is brought to the emergency department by his mother because of poor weight gain and irritability since delivery, and a 2-hour history of vomiting. Imaging studies show a combination of congenital defects including atrial septal defect (ASD), patent ductus arteriosus, hypoplasia of the dorsum of the nose, and pectus carinatum. The mother had not come in for any prenatal visits before parturition. She had heart surgery to repair a mitral valve defect secondary to rheumatic heart disease and continued use of anticoagulant throughout her pregnancy. Which of the following teratogens will most likely explain the baby's congenital defects?

A. Heroin
B. Warfarin
C. Rubella
D. Tetracycline
E. Nicotine

11. A 24-year-old woman comes to the physician because she has not been able to get pregnant for the past 4 years. She is sexually active with her husband and does not use barrier contraception. The patient has been experiencing hot flashes, irregular menses, night sweats, and vaginal dryness. A diagnosis of premature ovarian failure is made, and estrogen replacement therapy is initiated. Which of the following is the organ responsible for secreting estrogen?
A. Anterior pituitary
B. Posterior pituitary
C. Hypothalamus
D. Suprarenal cortex
E. Ovary

12. A 26-year-old overweight woman visits her physician because she has not been able to get pregnant for the past 4 years. She has irregular menstrual periods, decreased breast size, and hair growth on the chest and abdomen. Transvaginal ultrasonography shows a thick band around which of the following reproductive organs?
A. Ovary
B. Posterior wall of the uterus
C. Fimbriae of the uterine (fallopian) tube
D. Isthmus of the uterine (fallopian) tube
E. Ampulla of the uterine (fallopian) tube

13. A 39-year-old woman comes to the physician for in vitro fertilization procedure. Follicle-stimulating hormone (FSH) analogs are injected to stimulate follicles, then human chorionic gonadotropin (hCG) is injected to induce the final oocyte maturation, and lastly the oocyte is retrieved via transvaginal oocyte retrieval. Through which of the following spaces will the needle be inserted through the vaginal wall to reach the ovary?
A. Posterior part of the fornix
B. Lateral part of the fornix
C. Pouch of Morison
D. Retropubic space (of Retzius)
E. Extraperitoneal space

14. A 39-year-old woman comes to the physician for in vitro fertilization procedure. FSH analogs are injected to stimulate follicles, then hCG is injected to induce the final oocyte maturation, and lastly the oocyte is retrieved via transvaginal oocyte retrieval. The retrieved oocyte is arrested at which stage of development?
A. Prophase of meiosis 1
B. Metaphase of meiosis 1
C. Prophase of meiosis 2
D. Metaphase of meiosis 2
E. Telophase of meiosis 2

15. A 35-year-old woman gravida 2, para 0, aborta 1 at 28 weeks' gestation comes to the office for a prenatal visit. She has been experiencing periodic spotting for

the past 2 weeks. Ultrasonography shows implantation of the embryo near the internal os of the uterus. Despite periodic spotting, she experiences no pain during pregnancy. Which of the following best describes this condition?

A. Placenta previa
B. Abruptio placentae
C. Preeclampsia
D. Leiomyoma
E. Pelvic inflammatory disease

16. A 22-year-old pregnant woman comes to the physician because of significant bleeding in her first trimester and pain in the lower back. An ultrasound examination shows an ectopic abdominal pregnancy. Which of the following is the most common place for an ectopic abdominal pregnancy?

A. Rectouterine pouch (of Douglas)
B. Pouch of Morison
C. Retropubic space
D. Extraperitoneal space
E. Retroperitoneal space

17. A 26-year-old man comes to the physician because of 6-month history of a lump in his left testis. A diagnosis of testicular teratocarcinoma is made. This tumor can be loosely referred to as "male pregnancy" because at an early stage the carcinoma contains all three primary germ layers: ectoderm, mesoderm, and endoderm. In normal embryologic development, which of the following processes gives rise to these three primary germ layers?

A. Morulation
B. Gastrulation
C. Craniocaudal folding
D. Cleavage
E. Induction

18. A 20-year-old woman comes to the physician for information regarding trying to become pregnant. A successful pregnancy will lead to the formation of a blastocyst. Which of following best describes the formation of the blastocyst?

A. Blastomere → morula → blastocyst
B. Morula → zygote → blastocyst
C. Blastomere → blastocyst
D. Zygote → blastocyte → blastocyst
E. Morula → blastocyte → blastocyst

19. A 35-year-old woman, gravida 2, para 0, aborta 1, at 28 weeks' gestation comes to the office for a prenatal visit. She has been experiencing periodic spotting for the past 2 weeks. Ultrasonography of the pelvis shows an enlarged uterus and chorionic villi. Laboratory studies show elevated hCG levels for her gestational age. A diagnosis of hydatidiform mole is suspected, a condition characterized by gross edema of the chorionic villi surrounded by trophoblastic cells. The trophoblastic cell normally gives rise to which two cell layers?

A. Ectoderm and endoderm
B. Endoderm and mesoderm
C. Hypoblast and epiblast

D. Neural crest and neural tube
E. Syncytiotrophoblast and cytotrophoblast

20. An obese 40-year-old woman comes to the physician for her third trimester evaluation. Physical examination shows swollen hands. Her blood pressure is 150/85 mm Hg. Blood pressure from prior visits during this pregnancy have been normal. Urine testing shows proteinuria. Ultrasound examination shows a fetus appropriately aged at 33 weeks. An induced labor as treatment for preeclampsia before developing into seizures that may put the mother and infant at risk is initiated. The woman experiences significant pain during the induced labor from the contractions of the uterus. Pain fibers from the uterus travel in which of the following nerves?

A. Sympathetics
B. Parasympathetics
C. Somatic
D. Somatic and sympathetics
E. Sympathetics and parasympathetics

21. A 35-year-old pregnant woman comes to the physician for pregnancy evaluation during her 12th week of pregnancy. She previously had a child with Down syndrome. An ultrasound examination of the nuchal translucency procedure is performed. If the current pregnancy is diagnosed as Down syndrome, which of the following would mostly likely also be seen?

A. Meromelia
B. Hydrocephalus
C. Anencephaly
D. Atrioventricular septal defect
E. Plagiocephaly

22. A 20-year-old man comes to the physician for routine examination. He is 200 cm (6 ft 5 in) tall with unusually long and thin limbs. Physical examination shows a hollowed chest and severe near-sightedness (myopia). Genetic analysis shows a mutation in the fibrillin 1 *(FBN1)* gene, and the patient is diagnosed with Marfan syndrome. A computed tomography (CT) scan of the thorax shows a bulge anterior to the spinal cord and to the left of midline. Which condition is he most likely susceptible to?

A. Ruptured aorta
B. Double inferior vena cava
C. Portal hypertension
D. Hydronephrosis
E. Pyloric stenosis

23. A 3-year-old girl is brought to the emergency department by her mother for the fourth time in a year for a bone fracture. Before social services is called for possible child abuse, a genetic test is performed showing a mutation in the *COL1A1* gene. Physical examination will most likely show which of the following?

A. Pigeon chest
B. Short limbs
C. Yellow sclera
D. Ruptured aorta
E. Stiff joints

24. A 30-year-old pregnant woman gravida 2, para 0, aborta 1 at 30 weeks' gestation comes to the office for a prenatal visit. Her body mass index (BMI) is in the overweight category and she has developed gestational diabetes since her last visit. The physician advises the patient that pregnant women with gestational diabetes are more likely to have babies weighing 4kg (9 lb) or more. During delivery, the physician should be most concerned about which of the following in this expecting mother?
    A. Interspinous distance
    B. Diameter of the pelvic inlet
    C. Anteroposterior (AP) diameter
    D. Placenta previa
    E. Diameter of the pelvic outlet

Questions 26–50

25. A 30-year-old pregnant woman, gravida 2, para 0, aborta 1, at 28 weeks' gestation comes to the office for a follow-up appointment. An ultrasound examination shows a 4-cm mass growing at the base of the infant's spine. Which of the following is the most likely diagnosis?
    A. Incomplete closure of the embryonic neural tube
    B. Remnants of the primitive streak
    C. Swelling or growth of the endothelial cells that line blood vessels
    D. Neuroendocrine tumor arising from neural crest elements of the sympathetic nervous system
    E. Benign nerve sheath tumor of the peripheral nervous system

26. A 9-month-old boy previously diagnosed with Down syndrome is brought to the physician by his parents after they observe a noticeable lump in the back of his neck. He recently had a respiratory infection. An ultrasound examination of the neck shows the presence of fluid. A needle aspiration shows the presence of fluid and white blood cells, an indication of embryonic lymphatic fluid. Magnetic resonance imaging (MRI) of the neck shows failure of the jugular lymph sacs to join the lymphatic system, thereby preventing lymph drainage. Which of the following embryonic conditions could explain this case?
    A. Hemangioma
    B. Thyroglossal cyst
    C. Lingual cyst
    D. Cystic hygroma
    E. Squamous cell carcinoma of the larynx

27. A 30-year-old pregnant woman, gravida 2, para 0, aborta 1, at 28 weeks' gestation comes to the office for a prenatal visit. She is accompanied by her husband, who is short in stature, with short limbs, bowlegs, exaggerated lumbar lordosis, and a large head with frontal bossing. Ultrasonography shows the fetus to have a short humerus. Genetic analysis shows a mutation in the *FGFR3* gene. Which of the following features are most likely to be present in their child?
    A. Pigeon chest (Marfan syndrome)

B. Brittle bones (osteogenesis imperfecta)
C. Trident hand (achondroplasia)
D. Cardiac abnormalities
E. Mental retardation

28. A 25-year-old pregnant woman comes to the emergency department because a heavy vaginal bleeding. A diagnosis of spontaneous abortion is made, likely due to a failure of implantation. Under normal circumstances, at which stage of embryonic development will an embryo most likely implant into the endometrium of the uterus?
    A. Trilaminar embryo
    B. Zygote
    C. Morula
    D. Blastocyst
    E. Bilaminar embryo

29. The following are embryonic changes that occur during development of the upper limbs:
    1. Separate fingers
    2. Limb bud development
    3. Webbed fingers
    4. Digital rays
Which of the following most likely represents the correct order of developmental changes that occur in the upper limbs between weeks 5 and 8?
    A. 2-4-3-1
    B. 3-4-2-1
    C. 2-3-4-1
    D. 4-2-3-1
    E. 1-4-3-2

30. An investigator is studying the incidence of the developmental origins of the arteries that supply blood to the brain. The investigation involves injecting contrast media into the hearts of fetal chicken eggs and studying the arteries that develop in the pharyngeal arches since blood vessels that develop bilaterally in several of these structures supply the cerebral arterial circle (of Willis). Which of the following pairs of pharyngeal arches most likely gives rise to arteries that contribute to the blood vessels in the cerebral arterial circle (of Willis)?
    A. Pharyngeal arches 1 and 2
    B. Pharyngeal arches 2 and 3
    C. Pharyngeal arches 3 and 4
    D. Pharyngeal arches 4 and 5
    E. Pharyngeal arches 4 and 6

31. A 60-year-old man comes to the physician because of a 3-month history of feeling "pins and needles" and sharp pains over his right upper chest and back. Physical examination shows a rash of red, erupted vesicles at the right border of the sternum located a few centimeters above the nipple. Antiviral treatment is initiated for herpes zoster. The patient recovers and is free of pain, and his skin looks free of vesicles. Which of the following structures has the same embryologic origin as the location where the viral particles reside?
    A. Dorsal horn

    B. Ventral horn
    C. Dorsal root ganglion
    D. Conus medullaris
    E. Dura mater

32. A 63-year-old woman is admitted to the emergency department because of 1-day history of severe pleuritic chest pain radiating to the inferior portion of her scapula. The pain is relieved by bending forward and worsened by lying down or during inspiration. Physical examination shows a friction rub sound on auscultation of the lower left sternal border. Which of the following embryonic structures most likely gave rise to the affected structure?
    A. Splanchnopleuric mesoderm
    B. Somatopleuric mesoderm
    C. Septum transversum
    D. Oropharyngeal membrane
    E. Coelomic cleft

33. A 45-year-old man comes to the emergency department because of 2-day history of right leg heaviness, pain swelling and cramping. He also experiences nonspecific back pain and abdominal pain. Physical examination shows scrotal swelling, lower quadrant pain and blood in his urine. A CT scan of his thorax shows the presence of thrombus in a left inferior vena cava. Which of the following structures most likely gave rise to the vein that the thrombus is lodged within?
    A. Right anterior cardinal
    B. Right vitelline
    C. Left vitelline
    D. Left supracardinal
    E. Left anterior cardinal

34. A 9-year-old boy is brought to the emergency department because of a 2-day severe cough and chest pain leading to coughing up blood. The boy appears ill, lethargic, and cyanotic. Physical examination shows a cardiac arrhythmia and a murmur. A diagnosis of Eisenmenger syndrome is made. Which of the following disorders could be the initial congenital defect behind this syndrome?
    A. Ventricular septal defect
    B. Ebstein anomaly
    C. Underdeveloped left ventricle (hypoplastic left heart syndrome)
    D. Common atrioventricular canal
    E. Large foramen secundum

35. A 5-day-old breast-fed boy is brought to the emergency department by his mother because of poor weight gain, irritability, and dyspnea. Physical examination shows marked cyanosis in the lower extremities and harsh cardiac murmurs on auscultation. Echocardiography shows a cardiomegaly and a communication between the left side of the ascending aorta and the right wall of the pulmonary trunk. This condition is due to faulty migration of neural crest cells that led to partial development of which of the following embryologic structures?

    A. Right subclavian artery
    B. Aorticopulmonary septum
    C. Tricuspid valve
    D. Inferior vena cava
    E. Left subclavian artery

36. A 1-year-old girl is brought to the physician because of a 1-month history of a small "strawberry"-like swelling on her scalp that has been growing rapidly. Physical examination confirms a diagnosis of hemangioma. Which of the following embryologic layers gives rise to this vascular tumor?
    A. Mesoderm
    B. Endoderm
    C. Ectoderm
    D. Trophoblast
    E. Syncytiotrophoblast

37. A 55-year-old man comes to the emergency department because of long-standing history of shortness of breath during exertion, coughing, and swelling of the legs and feet. An echocardiography shows severe mitral regurgitation. A minimally invasive mitral valve repair is performed and a percutaneous coronary sinus catheter is placed to deliver retrograde cardioplegia. During the procedure, the catheter stuck in an enlarged valve of the coronary sinus (Thebesian valve). Which of the following embryonic structures gives rise to the structure that the Thebesian valve sits in?
    A. Primitive ventricle
    B. Bulbus cordis
    C. Truncus arteriosus
    D. Left horn of the sinus venosus–left common cardinal vein
    E. Primitive atria

38. A 5-day-old breast-fed boy is brought to the emergency department by his mother because of poor weight gain, irritability, and dyspnea. Oxygenated blood reaches the heart in fetal circulation from the inferior vena cava and passes through a communication between the left and right atria through a portion of the septum secundum. This opening is most likely which of the following?
    A. Foramen ovale
    B. Ductus arteriosus
    C. Foramen primum
    D. Ductus venosus
    E. Truncus arteriosus

39. A 40-year-old woman, gravida 2, para 0, aborta 1, at 28 weeks' gestation comes to the office for a prenatal visit. Ultrasound examination shows abnormal limb development of the fetus with one arm shorter than the other. Which of the following most likely describes this condition?
    A. Meromelia
    B. Central digit ray deformity
    C. Talipes equinovarus
    D. Polydactyly
    E. Syndactyly

40. A 1-day-old breast-fed boy was born with a cleft hand, also known as "lobster-claw hand." This abnormality is caused by the apical ectodermal ridge (AER) failing to properly develop. Which of the following best describes the principal function of the AER?
    A. Establishes the AP axis of the limb bud
    B. Stimulates blood vessel growth into the limb bud
    C. Stimulates cartilage differentiation in the limb bud
    D. Stimulates nerve growth into the limb bud
    E. Stimulates outgrowth of the limb bud

41. A 22-year-old woman gives birth to a 3.6-kg (8 -lb) girl. Physical examination shows two additional toes medial to her left great toe. Which of the following best describes this limb anomaly?
    A. Amelia
    B. Cleft foot
    C. Clubfoot
    D. Polydactyly
    E. Syndactyly

42. A 40-year-old woman comes to the physician because of a 2-week history of progressive headaches, blurred vision, and loss of muscle coordination. Her vital signs are within normal limits. She was diagnosed with a hydatidiform mole 4 years ago when she was pregnant. Laboratory studies show increased levels of hCG. Which of the following is the most likely diagnosis?
    A. Placenta previa
    B. Placenta accreta
    C. Vasa previa
    D. Placenta abruption
    E. Choriocarcinoma

43. A 6-year-old boy brought into the emergency department by his mother because of a 5-day history of vomiting and abdominal pain. His pain is radiating down his back and is worsened when he lays flat on his back. Physical examination shows abdominal tenderness. A CT scan of the abdomen shows a pancreas containing two separate duct systems emptying into the duodenum. One duct is very short and drains only a small portion of the head of the pancreas, while the remainder of the pancreas is drained via the other duct. A diagnosis of pancreas divisum is made. Which of the following most accurately describes this embryologic anomaly?
    A. Formation of a bifid ventral bud
    B. Formation of a bifid dorsal bud
    C. Failure of the dorsal and ventral buds to fuse
    D. Fusion of the dorsal and bifid ventral bud
    E. Nonrotation of the midgut

44. A 4-day-old breast-fed boy is brought to the emergency department by his mother because of poor weight gain and malodorous diarrhea. His mother says that her son cries constantly, especially hours after feeding. The infant has not passed meconium and is small for his age. A CT scan of the abdomen shows obstruction of a small segment of the intestine by a superior mesenteric artery that is wrapping itself around the segment. The condition is diagnosed as a type IIIb intestinal atresia (also known as Christmas tree or apple peel deformity). Which of the following arteries is mostly likely also affected?
    A. Middle colic/right colic/ileocolic artery
    B. Splenic artery
    C. Inferior mesenteric artery
    D. Left renal artery
    E. Left gastric artery

45. A 32-year-old man comes to the emergency department because of a 2-day history of severe abdominal pain. Physical examination shows rebound tenderness localizing below the edge of the liver. Laboratory studies show a leucocyte count of 18,000/mm³. A CT scan of the abdomen shows an abnormal mass anterior to the right kidney. A diagnosis of appendicitis because of an inflamed subhepatic appendix is suspected. Which of the following would have most likely caused the appendix to develop in this position?
    A. Rubella infection
    B. Malrotation of the midgut
    C. Failure of migration of the neural crest cells
    D. Meckel diverticulum
    E. Failure of lateral folds to close

46. A 6-hour-old girl is examined in the neonatal intensive care unit. During delivery, the newborn was cyanotic with an Apgar score of 0. A CT scan shows right ventricular hypertrophy, ventricular septal defect, overriding of the aorta, and pulmonary valve stenosis. Which of the following conditions is most likely associated with this clinical picture?
    A. Pulmonary atresia
    B. Hepatosplenomegaly
    C. Cardiomegaly
    D. Anal atresia
    E. Meckel diverticulum

47. A 4-hour-old boy with respiratory distress is examined in the neonatal intensive care unit. During physical examination, his symptoms are alleviated when placed in the prone position. Which of the following most likely explains his symptoms?
    A. Down syndrome
    B. Treacher Collins syndrome
    C. Pierre Robin sequence
    D. Patent ductus arteriosus
    E. Bronchopulmonary dysplasia

48. A 5-year-old boy is brought the physician by his parents for a follow-up examination. The parents say that sometimes he does not respond when they talk to him. Physical examination shows a small jaw, large mouth, flat cheekbones, and malformed pinna. The patient had one surgery to correct a congenital cleft palate. Which of the following most likely describes this boy's embryologic defect?
    A. Trisomy 13
    B. Defect in *FBN1* gene
    C. Failure of fusion of medial nasal prominences

D. Failure of rostral neuropore to close

E. Failure of neural crest migration into the first pharyngeal arch

49. A 37-year-old man comes to the emergency department because of a 6-hour history of severe headache initially started as toothache. He has a large facial swelling that had previously been painless until this admission. A CT scan of the head shows a tumor in the posterior part of the mandible. A biopsy shows a benign type of ameloblastoma. During normal development, which of the following develops from the cells responsible for the development of this tumor?

A. Enamel

B. Alveolar bone

C. Cementum

D. Periodontal ligaments

E. Pulp

50. A 6-year-old boy is brought to the physician by his parents for a routine physical examination. During eye examination, a wormlike structure is projecting from the optic disc. This finding is diagnosed as persistence of the distal portion of the hyaloid artery. Which of the following does the proximal portion of the hyaloid vessels eventually become?

A. Optic artery and vein of the retina

B. Optic artery and vein of the lens

C. Central artery and vein of the retina

D. Central artery and vein of the lens

E. Supraorbital vessels

Questions 51–56

51. A 14-month-old boy is brought to the physician for evaluation of his eyes. His parents noticed that when photos of their child were taken, his eyes appeared white instead of red from the camera flash. Physical examination of the eye shows poor vision in the right eye. A CT scan of the head shows calcifications within the right intraorbital mass. The patient is diagnosed with retinoblastoma. Which of the following structures share the same embryologic origin as the structure that this tumor develops from?

A. The optic nerve

B. Lens

C. Sclera

D. Sphincter pupillae muscle of the iris

E. Vitreous body

52. A 3-year-old girl is brought to the physician by his parents because of developmental delay. A CT scan of the head shows partial atresia of the cerebellum. Which of the following is the embryologic origin of the atretic organ?

A. Telencephalon

B. Diencephalon

C. Mesencephalon

D. Metencephalon

E. Myelencephalon

53. A 55-year-old man comes to the physician because he can no longer go bike riding without getting breathless. He also says these occurrences are associated with chest pain. Auscultation of the heart shows a cardiac murmur. Echocardiography shows aortic stenosis. Which of the following is the embryologic origin of the aorta?

A. Bulbus cordis

B. Truncus arteriosus

C. Sinus venosus

D. Ductus arteriosus

E. Ductus venosus

54. A 45-year-old pregnant woman, gravida 2, para 0, aborta 1, at 28 weeks' gestation comes to the office for a prenatal visit. An ultrasound examination shows decreased amniotic fluid surrounding the fetus. Which of the following medications is responsible for this condition?

A. Angiotensin-converting enzyme (ACE) inhibitors

B. Aminoglycosides

C. Tetracyclines

D. Lithium

E. Folate antagonists

55. A 2-week-old boy is brought to the emergency department by his parents because of poor feeding, wheezing, coughing, and a hoarse cry. Imaging shows a double-arched aorta resulting in a ring around the trachea and esophagus. Which of the following is the most likely embryologic origin of this condition?

A. Failure of the distal part of the right aorta to disappear

B. Failure of the fifth aortic arch to disappear

C. Failure of the first aortic arch to disappear

D. Failure of the second aortic arch to disappear

E. Failure of the sixth aortic arch to disappear

56. A 25-year-old pregnant woman, gravida 2, para 0, aborta 1, at 28 weeks' gestation comes to the office for a prenatal visit. An ultrasound examination shows increased amniotic fluid surrounding the fetus. Which of the following is most likely to increase amniotic pressure?

A. Renal hypoplasia

B. Esophageal atresia

C. Ureter obstruction

D. Potter syndrome

E. Down syndrome

Answers

Answers 1–25

1. E. In monochorionic diamniotic twins, the single placenta (due to as yet unknown factors) develops blood vessel connections between the umbilical vessels of the twins. These connections result in an unbalanced blood supply known as twin–twin transfusion syndrome (TTTS). In TTTS, the donor twin does not get enough blood and the recipient twin becomes volume overloaded. In an attempt to reduce its blood volume, the recipient twin increases urine production, eventually resulting in polyhydramnios. At the same time, the donor twin produces less than the usual amount of urine leading to oligohydramnios. As the disease progresses, the donor produces so little urine that its bladder may not be seen on ultrasound. The twin becomes wrapped up by its amniotic membrane (known as a "stuck" twin). Often the polyhydramnios of the recipient twin is the first thing noticed by the patient due to a sudden increase in the size of the uterus. *This condition is only possible when twins share a single chorion but have separate amniotic sacs.*
   See Moore KL, Persaud TVN, Torchia MG: Before We Are Born, ed 8, 2013, pp. 85–88

2. A. Failure of complete division or fusion of adjacent embryonic discs leads to conjoined twins. These are always monozygotic and share a single chorion, placenta, and amniotic sac. The most common site of attachment is an anterior union of the thoracic regions called thoracopagus where the twins are joined at the anterior chest wall. The original "Siamese twins" were of this latter type. The second most common site of attachment is omphalopagus.
   85–88

3. B. Minamata disease is a severe neurologic syndrome caused by methyl mercury poisoning. It can be acquired or congenital, following maternal mercury ingestion as in this case. Accumulation of methyl mercury from maternal ingestion of fish and shellfish or pork (due to certain pesticide contamination) is the primary cause.
   A. Lead poisoning can cause permanent learning and behavioral disorders
   C. Alcohol exposure can result in FAS, which has a wide spectrum including mental and growth retardation plus morphogenetic disturbances.
   D. Cocaine exposure can cause microcephaly, neurobehavioral disturbances, spontaneous abortion, and urogenital disturbances.
   E. Streptomycin exposure can result in vestibulocochlear (cranial nerve [CN] VIII) nerve defects.
   317

4. B. DES is a synthetic nonsteroidal estrogen once commonly used in pregnant women to prevent breast engorgement, among many other uses. Prenatal exposure increases risk of multiple conditions including vaginal clear cell adenocarcinoma and reproductive tract malformations. It has since been proven to be toxic and teratogenic.
   A. FAS from maternal alcoholism has a wide spectrum of congenital defects including mental and growth retardation plus morphogenetic disturbances.
   C. Lithium causes heart and great vessel abnormalities in utero.
   D. Nicotine causes premature delivery, conotruncal defects, and urinary tract abnormalities (Table 9.1).
   E. Folic acid is not a teratogen.
   312–319

5. A. Toxoplasmosis is an infectious teratogen that causes jaundice, intracranial calcifications and chorioretinitis, microcephaly, microphthalmia, and hydrocephalus.
   B. Heroin is a behavioral teratogen that causes small birth weight, central nervous system dysfunction, and small head circumference.
   C. Mercury can lead to cerebral atrophy, spasticity, seizures, and mental deficiency
   D. Alcohol exposure can result in FAS, which has a wide spectrum of congenital defects including mental and growth retardation plus morphogenetic disturbances.
   E. Tetracycline causes tooth and bone defects including yellow discoloration and hypoplasia.
   312–319

6. A. Infectious teratogens include toxoplasmosis, which causes jaundice, intracranial calcifications and chorioretinitis, microcephaly, microphthalmia, and hydrocephalus.
   B. Methadone and heroin are behavioral teratogens that result in small birth weight, central nervous system dysfunction, and small head circumference.
   C. Mercury can lead to cerebral atrophy, spasticity, seizures, and mental deficiency.
   D. Alcohol exposure can result in FAS, which has a wide spectrum of congenital defects including mental and growth retardation plus morphogenetic disturbances.
   E. Tetracycline causes tooth and bone defects including yellow discoloration and hypoplasia.
   312–319

7. E. Nicotine can cause premature delivery, low birth weight, and poor physical growth due to its constrictive effect on uterine blood vessels. It also causes conotruncal defects and urinary tract abnormalities.
   A. Heroin is a behavioral teratogen and presents with small birth weight, central nervous system dysfunction, and small head circumference.
   B. Warfarin can be associated with nasal hypoplasia, stippled epiphyses, hypoplastic phalanges, eye anomalies, and mental deficiency.
   C. Congenital rubella syndrome presents with cataracts, cardiac defects, and deafness among other defects.
   D. Tetracycline exposure can cause tooth and bone defects, including yellow discoloration and hypoplasia.
   312–319

---

*Subsequent cross-references to *Before We Are Born* list page numbers only.

TABLE 9.1	Some Teratogens Known to Cause Human Birth Defects
Agents	**Most Common Congenital Anomalies**
Drugs	
Alcohol	Fetal alcohol syndrome (FAS); intrauterine growth restriction (IUGR); mental deficiency; microcephaly; ocular anomalies; joint abnormalities; short palpebral fissures; fetal alcohol spectrum disorders (FASDs); cognitive and neurobehavioral disturbances
Androgens and high doses of progestogens	Varying degree of masculinization of female fetuses; ambiguous external genitalia (labial fusion and clitoral hypertrophy)
Methotrexate	IUGR; skeletal and renal defects
Cocaine	IUGR; prematurity; microcephaly; cerebral infarction; urogenital anomalies; neurobehavioral disturbances
Diethylstilbestrol	Abnormalities of uterus and vagina; cervical erosion and ridges
Isotretinoin (12-cis-retionic acid)	Craniofacial abnormalities; neural tube defects such as spina bifida cystica; cardiovascular defects; cleft palate; thymus aplasia
Lithium carbonate	Various anomalies, usually involving the heart and great vessels
Methotrexate	Multiple anomalies, especially skeletal, involving the face, cranium, limbs, and vertebral column
Misoprostol	Abnormal development of the limbs, ocular defects, cranial nerve defects, and autism spectrum disorders
Phenytoin (Dilantin)	Fetal hydantoin syndrome; IntraUterine Growth Restriction (IUGRI) microcephaly; mental retardation; ridged metopic suture; inner epicanthal folds; eyelid ptosis; broad, depressed, nasal bridge; phalangeal hypoplasia
Tetracycline	Stained teeth; hypoplasia of enamel
Thalidomide	Abnormal development of the limbs; meromelia (partial absence of limb) and amelia (complete absence of the limb); facial anomalies; systemic anomalies (e.g., cardiac and kidney defects and ocular anomalies)
Trimethadione	Abnormal development of the limbs; V-shaped eyebrows; low-set ears; cleft lip and/or palate
Valproic acid	Craniofacial anomalies; neural tube defects; often hydrocephalus; heart and skeletal defects; poor postnatal cognitive development
Warfarin	Nasal hypoplasia; stippled epiphyses; hypoplastic phalanges; eye anomalies; mental deficiency
Chemicals	
Methylmercury	Cerebral atrophy; spasticity; seizures; mental deficiency
Polychlorinated biphenyls	IUGR; skin discoloration
Infections	
Cytomegalovirus	Microcephaly; chorioretinitis; sensorineural loss; delayed psychomotor and mental development; hepatosplenomegaly; hydrocephaly; cerebral palsy; brain (periventricular) calcification
Herpes simplex virus	Skin vesicles and scarring; chorioretinitis; hepatomegaly; thrombocytopenia; petechiae; hemolytic anemia; hydranencephaly
Human parvovirus B19	Fetal anemia; nonimmune hydrops fetalis; fetal death
Rubella virus	IUGR; postnatal growth retardation; cardiac and great vessel abnormalities; microcephaly; sensorineural deafness; cataract; microphthalmos; glaucoma; pigmented retinopathy; mental deficiency; neonatal bleeding; hepatosplenomegaly; osteopathy; tooth defects
Toxoplasma gondii	Microcephaly; mental deficiency; microphthalmia; hydrocephaly; chorioretinitis; cerebral calcifications; hearing loss; neurologic disturbances
Treponema pallidum	Hydrocephalus; congenital deafness; mental deficiency; abnormal teeth and bones
Varicella virus	Cutaneous scars (dermatome distribution); neurologic anomalies (e.g., limb paresis, hydrocephaly, seizures); cataracts; microphthalmia; Horner syndrome; optic atrophy; nystagmus; chorioretinitis; microcephaly; mental deficiency; skeletal anomalies (e.g., hypoplasia of limbs, fingers, and toes); urogenital anomalies
High levels of ionizing radiation	Microcephaly; mental deficiency; skeletal anomalies; growth retardation; cataracts

From Moore KL, Persaud TVN, Torchia MG: *Before We Are Born*, ed 8, Philadelphia: Elsevier, 2013, p. 303.

8. **A.** Fetal alcohol syndrome (FAS) is associated with intrauterine growth restriction (IUGR), mental deficiency, microcephaly, ocular anomalies, joint abnormalities, and small palpebral fissures.

   B. Warfarin can be associated with nasal hypoplasia, stippled epiphyses, hypoplastic phalanges, eye anomalies, and mental deficiency.

   C. Women who use heroin during pregnancy greatly increase their risk of serious pregnancy complications. These risks include poor fetal growth, premature rupture of membranes, premature birth, and stillbirth.

   D. Rubella virus is associated with various anomalies such as IUGR, postnatal growth retardation, cardiac and great vessel abnormalities, microcephaly, sensorineural deafness, cataract, microphthalmos (also referred to as microphthalmia), glaucoma, pigmented retinopathy, mental deficiency, neonate bleeding, hepatosplenomegaly, osteopathy, and tooth defects.

   E. Tetracycline exposure can be associated with stained teeth and hypoplasia of enamel.
   312–319

9. **A.** Fetal hydantoin syndrome occurs in 5%–10% of children born to mothers treated with phenytoin or hydantoin anticonvulsants. The usual pattern of defects consists of IUGR, microcephaly, mental deficiency, ridged frontal suture, inner epicanthal folds, eyelid ptosis, broad depressed nasal bridge, nail and/or distal phalangeal hypoplasia, and hernias.

   B. FAS: IUGR, mental deficiency, microcephaly, ocular anomalies, joint abnormalities, and short palpebral fissures.

   C. Trisomy 21 (Down syndrome), the most common chromosomal numerical abnormality resulting in birth defects (intellectual disability, abnormal facies, heart malformations), is usually caused by nondisjunction. The risk of meiotic nondisjunction increases with increasing maternal age.

   D. Treacher Collins syndrome is characterized by craniofacial deformities, such as absent cheekbones.

   E. Infants with DiGeorge syndrome are born without a thymus and parathyroid glands and have defects in their cardiac outflow tracts.
   306–316

10. **B.** Warfarin is associated with nasal hypoplasia, stippled epiphyses, hypoplastic phalanges, eye anomalies, and mental deficiency.

    A. Women who use heroin during pregnancy greatly increase their risk of serious pregnancy complications. These risks include poor fetal growth, premature rupture of the membranes, premature birth, and stillbirth.

    C. Rubella virus is associated with various anomalies such as IUGR, postnatal growth retardation, cardiac and great vessel abnormalities, microcephaly, sensorineural deafness, cataract, microphthalmos, glaucoma, pigmented retinopathy, mental deficiency, neonate bleeding, hepatosplenomegaly, osteopathy, and tooth defects.

    D. Tetracycline is associated with stained teeth and hypoplasia of enamel.

    E. Nicotine can cause premature delivery, low birth weight, and poor physical growth due to its constrictive effect on uterine blood vessels. It also causes conotruncal defects and urinary tract abnormalities.
    312–317

11. **E.** The ovaries are almond-shaped reproductive glands that produce oocytes. They are located close to the lateral pelvic walls on each side of the uterus. The ovaries also produce estrogen and progesterone, the hormones responsible for the development of secondary sex characteristics and regulation of pregnancy.

    A. FSH is produced by the anterior pituitary gland, which stimulates the development of ovarian follicles and the production of estrogen by the follicular cells. Luteinizing hormone (LH) serves as the "trigger" for ovulation (release of secondary oocyte) and stimulates the follicular cells and corpus luteum to produce progesterone.

    B. The posterior pituitary contains oxytocin and vasopressin and does not produce estrogen.

    C. Gonadotropin-releasing hormone (GnRH) is secreted from the hypothalamus and stimulates the production and secretion of FSH and LH from the anterior pituitary.

    D. The suprarenal cortex produces mineralocorticoids, glucocorticoids, and androgens, not estrogen
    10, 14–17

12. **A.** Polycystic ovary syndrome (PCOS) is a syndrome of ovarian dysfunction along with the cardinal features of hyperandrogenism and polycystic ovary morphology. Its clinical manifestations include menstrual irregularities, signs of androgen excess (e.g., hirsutism), and obesity. The ultrasound criteria for the diagnosis of a polycystic ovary are eight or more subcapsular follicular cysts less than 10 mm in diameter and increased ovarian stroma.

    B. The posterior wall of the uterus is not assessed as part of the ultrasound criteria for the diagnosis of polycystic ovaries.

    C. Fimbriae of the uterine (fallopian) tube are not assessed as part of the ultrasound criteria for the diagnosis of polycystic ovaries.

    D. Isthmus of the uterine (fallopian) tube is not assessed as part of the ultrasound criteria for the diagnosis of polycystic ovaries.

    E. Ampulla of the uterine (fallopian) tube is not assessed as part of the ultrasound criteria for the diagnosis of polycystic ovaries.
    14–19

13. **A.** Each ovary is attached to the back of the broad ligament by the mesovarium. The posterior wall of the vagina is longer than the anterior wall and the posterior part of the fornix is deeper than the other parts of the fornix.

    B. The posterior location and proximity of the ovary to the posterior fornix allows for easiest and least invasive access through the posterior, not lateral, part of the fornix.

C. The posterior part of the fornix is covered by peritoneum in the front of the rectouterine pouch (of Douglas) so ideal insertion would not take this path.

D. The retropubic space of Retzius lies between the bladder and the pubic symphysis. The need would not take this path.

E. The extraperitoneal space, or space in the abdomen and pelvis that lies outside the peritoneum, would not be encountered in an ideal path starting from the vaginal wall.

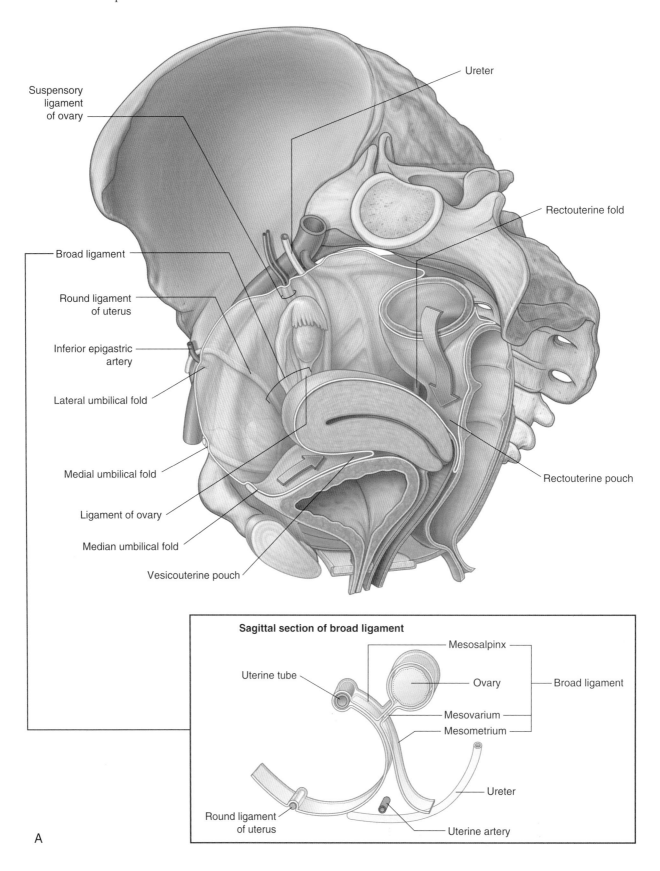

Suspensory ligament of ovary

Broad ligament

Round ligament of uterus

Inferior epigastric artery

Lateral umbilical fold

Medial umbilical fold

Ligament of ovary

Median umbilical fold

Vesicouterine pouch

Ureter

Rectouterine fold

Rectouterine pouch

Sagittal section of broad ligament

Uterine tube

Mesosalpinx

Ovary

Broad ligament

Mesovarium

Mesometrium

Ureter

Round ligament of uterus

Uterine artery

A

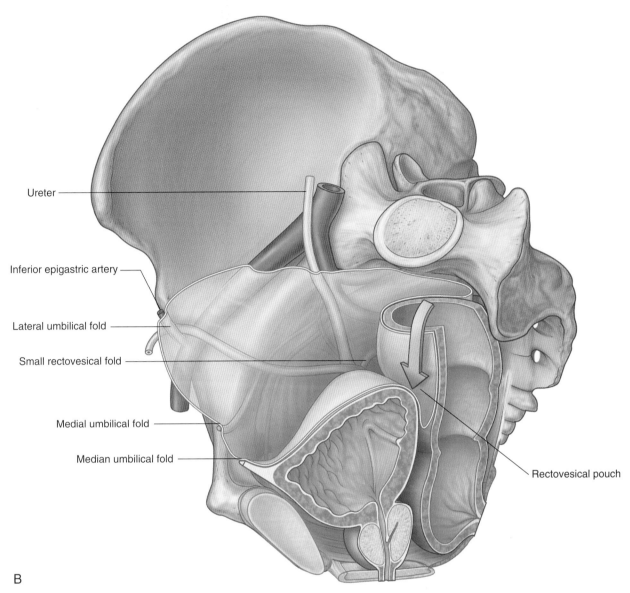

Ureter

Inferior epigastric artery

Lateral umbilical fold

Small rectovesical fold

Medial umbilical fold

Median umbilical fold

Rectovesical pouch

B

• *GAS* **Fig. 5.59**

14–18

14. A. Primary oocytes begin the first meiotic divisions before birth, but completion of prophase in meiosis 1 does not occur until adolescence. The follicular cells surrounding the primary oocytes secrete a substance, oocyte maturation inhibitor, which arrests the meiotic process of the oocyte.
B. The only phase that is completed in primary oocytes is interphase of meiosis 1, not metaphase 1.
C, D, E. At the onset of puberty, primary oocytes resume meiosis and transition to secondary oocytes arrested at metaphase of meiosis 2. Meiosis 2 is then completed during ovulation of the menstruation cycle.
14–19

15. A. Placenta previa is defined as a placenta that has implanted into the lower segment of the uterus. It is now classified as either major, in which the placenta is covering the internal os of the uterus, or minor, when the placenta is sited within the lower segment of the uterus, but does not cover the internal os of the uterus.

The mother will present with painless bleeding, often recurrent in the third trimester, and ultrasound scans will demonstrate the abnormal location of the placenta. The bleeding occurs due to separation of the placenta as the lower segment develops in the third trimester.
B. A placental abruption is separation of a normally positioned placenta from the uterine wall.
C. Preeclampsia is a serious disorder that occurs during pregnancy, usually after the 20th week of gestation. Maternal hypertension, proteinuria, and edema are essential features of this condition.
D. Leiomyoma is a benign tumor of smooth muscle (fibroid).
E. Pelvic inflammatory disease is characterized by inflammation and infection arising from the endocervix leading to endometritis, salpingitis, oophoritis, pelvic peritonitis, and, subsequently, formation of tubo-ovarian and pelvic abscesses.
80–82

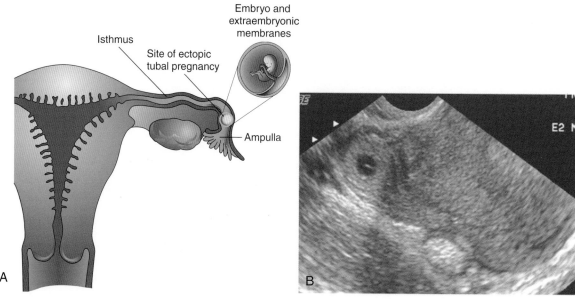

Isthmus

Site of ectopic
tubal pregnancy

Embryo and
extraembryonic
membranes

Ampulla

A

B

• **Fig. 9.1**

16. A. Ectopic pregnancy is the existence of a pregnancy outside the normal confines of the uterus or abnormally in the uterus. Although the uterine (fallopian) tube is the most common site of an ectopic pregnancy, it can also occur in the abdominal cavity, and when that is the case, the rectouterine pouch (of Douglas) is the most common site.

   B. The pouch of Morison or hepatorenal recess is the space between the liver and the right kidney and is not usually a site for ectopic pregnancy.

   C. The retropubic space is an extraperitoneal space between the pubic symphysis and the urinary bladder. It is a very unlikely site for ectopic pregnancy.

   D. Ectopic pregnancies rarely exist at the extraperitoneal space.

   E. Ectopic pregnancies rarely exist at the retroperitoneal space (Fig. 9.1).
   32–34

17. B. Gastrulation occurs in early embryogenesis and is the process by which the blastula is reorganized into a three-layered structure (i.e., ectoderm, mesoderm, and endoderm).

   A. Morulation involves the cleavage or division of the fertilized ovum usually into a 16-cell structure that resembles a ball.

   C. Craniocaudal folding is a process that occurs with lateral folding of the embryo that transforms it from a flat disc into a three-dimensional tube within the body.

   D. Cleavage is the process of division of the fertilized ovum.

   E. Induction is the physiologic and chemical signal to stimulate cells to differentiate.
   35–38

18. A. After fertilization of the ovum, cleavage commences with the formation of blastomere and then a 16-cell morula. Fluid would then enter the cavity of the morula with the formation of a blastocyst. The blastocyst will then invade the endometrial wall.

   B. Before the blastomere can become the blastocyte, it must undergo mitotic divisions to yield the morula.

   C. The fertilization of an ovum immediately results into a one-celled diploid zygote. The zygote undergoes 4 rounds of mitosis to yield the morula.

   D. The zygote stage is followed by the development of a morula.

   E. Upon the completion of the morula, fluid enters the morula to form a cavitation resulting in the formation of the blastocyst.
   21–24

19. E. Upon trophoblastic invasion of the endometrium, the trophoblastic cells produce two cell layers: the syncytiotrophoblast is the outer layer that is related to the endometrial wall while the cytotrophoblast is the inner layer, which usually gives rise to the chorionic villi.

   A, B. The ectoderm, endoderm, and mesoderm are body germ layers produced during gastrulation.

   C. Hypoblast and epiblast cells are derived from the inner cell mass of the blastocyst, and the epiblast will ultimately, under gastrulation, form the germ layers.

   D. Neural crest cells do not give rise to the syncytiotrophoblast and cytotrophoblast; the neural tube forms the central nervous system.
   21–24

20. A. Pain fibers from organs and structures above the pelvic pain line will follow the sympathetic nerve fibers. Recall that the uterine fundus and body are located above the most inferior part of the pelvic peritoneal reflection, which is known as the pelvic pain line.

   B. Pain fibers from structures below the pelvic pain line will follow the parasympathetic nerves: the uterus is above the pelvic pain line.

C, D. The uterus is a visceral organ and as such will not have somatic innervations.

E. Pain fibers from the uterus are visceral afferent fibers and will run primarily with sympathetic fibers.
7–10

21. D. Down syndrome is a congenital abnormality involving triplication of chromosome 21. It is more common in children of women who become pregnant at 35 years or older (advanced maternal age is a risk factor).

A. Meromelia is the partial absence of one or more extremities. Meromelia has been associated with several etiologies including, but not limited to, chromosomal abnormalities, genetic disorders, environmental exposures in utero (namely, thalidomide) or as a complication of chorionic villus sampling.

B. Hydrocephalus is the enlargement of the cerebral ventricles because of excess cerebrospinal fluid (CSF). Fetal hydrocephalus is most commonly due to obstruction of the cerebral aqueduct that may result from the faulty circulation of CSF through the cerebral ventricles. Hydrocephalus is most seen in etiologies such as a tumor, hemorrhage, or an arachnoid cyst.

C. Anencephaly is due to the failure of rostral neuropore closure at day 25 of neurulation. On ultrasonography, anencephaly would present with a missing brain and polyhydramnios.

E. Plagiocephaly, colloquially known as Flat Head Syndrome, is a post-natal condition in which there is asymmetric flattening of the neonate's skull due to an imbalanced positioning when supine.
45, 235–236, 247–248, 271, 306–307

22. A. Marfan syndrome affects the connective tissue supporting the body's joints and organs (e.g., heart, aorta, and eyes). Abnormalities in the connective tissue are due to mutations in a single protein building block (amino acid) in the fibrillin-1 protein. This leads to a severe reduction in the amount of fibrillin-1 available to form microfibrils, and elasticity in many tissues is decreased. In Marfan syndrome elastic fibers are significantly reduced, eventually leading to aortic aneurysm and rupture. The thoracic aorta is contained in the posterior mediastinum. It begins at the lower border of the fourth thoracic vertebra, where it is continuous with the aortic arch, and ends in front of the lower border of the 12th thoracic vertebra at the aortic hiatus, where it becomes the abdominal aorta.

B. Double inferior vena cava is not typically seen in Marfan Syndrome.

C. Portal hypertension is more commonly present in patients with a long history of liver disease, typically presents in patients with cirrhotic livers. It is not associated with Marfan Syndromes.

D. Hydronephrosis occurs due to impaired urine flow distal to the renal pelvis. The most common cause of hydronephrosis is renal calculi.

E. Pyloric stenosis is a congenital hypertrophy of the pyloric sphincter that typically presents in neonates as projectile, non-bilious vomiting.

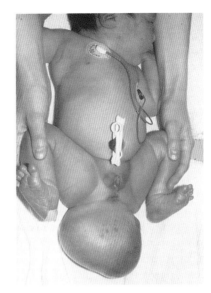

• Fig. 9.2

225–229

23. B. The *COL1A1* gene produces a component of type I collagen called the pro-α1(I) chain. Mutation of the gene leads to reduced production of pro-α1(I) chains and future reduced type I collagen. A shortage of this critical protein underlies the bone fragility and other characteristic features of osteogenesis imperfecta. Osteogenesis imperfecta has four types (I, II, III, and IV). In addition to more severe bone problems (fractures), features of these conditions can include blue sclerae, hearing loss, short stature, respiratory problems, and a disorder of tooth development. Discoloration of the sclera gives the appearance of a blue or blue gray color. This is due to the thinning of the sclera caused by a defective type I collagen; as a result, the choroidal veins are evident, giving the appearance of a blue color.

A. Pectus excavatum, colloquially known as pigeon chest, is one of the common features in Marfan Syndrome. On physical examination, Marfan Syndrome presents with skeletal abnormalities such as long extremities, arachnodactyly, scoliosis, and hypermobile joints. It is due to a mutation of FBN1 gene and results in a faulty fibrillin-1 glycoprotein.

C. Yellow sclera is a common presentation of jaundice and results from hyperbilirubinemia (conjugated or unconjugated). It does not present with fragile bone.

D. Marfan syndrome can present with the spontaneous rupture of aorta but is not associated with brittle bones presenting with frequent fractures.

E. Stiff joints are a common presentation of patients with arthritis. Arthritis typically presents in patients in their fourth decade of age and older.
225–229

24. A. During embryogenesis, poorly controlled diabetes mellitus in the mother is associated with a twofold to threefold increase in the incidence of birth defects such as macrosomia, which is diagnosed as birth weight greater than 8 pounds 13 ounces (4000 g), regardless of gestational age. Fetal macrosomia makes vaginal delivery difficult and puts the baby at risk of injury during birth. Therefore, cesarean section is recommended, during which epidural anesthesia is given. Hence the interspinous distance is of concern. Other common anomalies with maternal diabetes mellitus include holoprosencephaly (failure of the forebrain to divide into hemispheres), meroencephaly (partial absence of the brain), sacral agenesis, congenital heart defects, and limb anomalies.

B, C, E. Fetuses noted to have macrosomia must be delivered via C-section as vaginal birth predisposes them to a higher probability of injury during birth. Diameters of the pelvic inlet, pelvic outlet, or anteroposterior are considerations for vaginal delivery, not epidural anesthesia.

D. Placenta previa involves placement of the placenta over the cervix. This can complicate vaginal deliveries, but is not related to gestational diabetes.
318–319

25. B. Remnants of the primitive streak (a thick linear band of epiblast at the beginning of week 3) may persist and give rise to a large tumor known as a sacrococcygeal teratoma. Because it is derived from pluripotent primitive streak cells, the tumor contains tissues derived from all three germ layers in incomplete stages of differentiation. Sacrococcygeal teratomas are the most common tumors in newborn infants and have an incidence of approximately 1 in 27,000. These tumors are usually surgically excised promptly and the prognosis is good (Fig. 9.2).

A. A growing mass would not be present in myelomeningocele

C. Hemangioma is not usually found in this region

D. Neuroblastoma more commonly develops from a suprarenal gland

E. Neurofibromas incorporate additional cellular structures and are often cutaneous
38–29, 45

Answers 26–50

26. D. Cystic hygromas are large swellings that usually appear in the inferolateral part of the neck and consist of large, single or multilocular, fluid-filled cavities. Hygromas may be present at birth, but they often enlarge and become evident during later infancy. Hygromas are believed to arise from parts of a jugular lymph sac that are pinched off, or from lymphatic spaces that do not establish connections with the main lymphatic channels, whereas a thyroglossal cyst is a fibrous cyst that forms from a persistent thyroglossal duct. Lingual cysts in the tongue may be derived from remnants of the thyroglossal duct. They may enlarge and produce pharyngeal pain, dysphagia (difficulty in swallowing), or both.

A. Hemangiomas, also known as strawberry hemangiomas, are benign vascular tumors that present as bright red plaques on the skin. They typically regress spontaneously.

B. Thyroglossal duct cyst is the remnant of the pathway of the thyroid from the base of the tongue. It commonly presents in the midline of the neck and moves with the protrusion of the tongue and swallowing.

C. Lingual cyst are rare congenital tumors of the oropharynx and presents with an enlarged tongue.

E. Squamous cell carcinoma of the larynx is a malignant tumor that commonly presents in older patients with a history of consuming alcohol and smoking.
222

27. C. The *FGFR3* gene provides instructions for making a protein called fibroblast growth factor receptor 3. These proteins play a role in several important cellular processes, including regulation of cell growth and division, determination of cell type, formation of blood vessels, wound healing, and embryo development. Mutations in the *FGFR3* gene cause more than 99% of cases of achondroplasia. In achondroplasia (autosomal dominant disorder) the problem is not in forming cartilage but in converting it to bone (endochondral ossification at the epiphysial cartilage plates), particularly in the long bones of the limbs. Other features include an average-size trunk, short arms and legs with particularly short upper arms and thighs, and limited range of motion at the elbows. The head is enlarged (macrocephaly) with a prominent forehead and a "scooped out" nose (flat nasal bone). Fingers are typically short and the ring finger and middle fingers may diverge, giving the hand a three-pronged (trident) appearance. In addition, lordosis and kyphosis of the vertebral column may be present.

A. Pigeon chest is more likely to be seen with Marfan syndrome than achondroplasia

B. Brittle bones are associated with osteogenesis imperfecta, rather than achondroplasia

D. Cardiac abnormalities are not more likely to be present than a "trident hand" in this case

E. Mental retardation is not more likely to be present than a "trident hand" in this case
236–238, 310

28. D. Implantation of the blastocyst begins at the end of the first embryonic week and normally occurs in the endometrium of the uterus, usually superiorly in the body of the uterus and slightly more often on the posterior than on the anterior wall. The blastocyst begins to implant on approximately the sixth day of the luteal phase.

A. The trilaminar embryo develops at 3 weeks, after implantation into the endometrium of the uterus

B. The fertilization of an ovum immediately results in a one-celled diploid zygote. Implantation does not occur at this stage.

C. A zygote undergoes four round of mitosis to yield a morula. Implantation does not occur at this stage.

E. The bilaminar embryo develops at 2 weeks, after implantation into thc endometrium of the uterus.
33

29. A. Development of the upper limb begins at 26–27 days after fertilization with the appearance of the upper limb

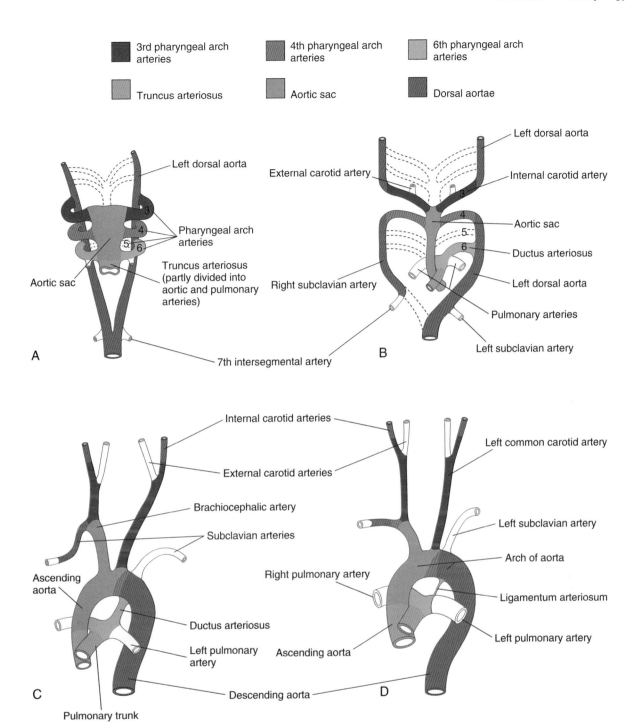

• **Fig. 9.3**

buds; at 33–36 days the hand plates are formed and the digital rays are present; at 44–46 days notches form between digital rays, and at 49–51 days webbed fingers are distinct. Separate fingers appear at 52–53 days.

B, C. Webbed fingers do not develop before digital rays.

D. Digital rays do not develop before limb buds.

E. Separate fingers do not develop before limb buds.
58–60

30. C. Pharyngeal arches 3 and 4 give rise to the common carotid artery, internal carotid artery, the aortic arch, and subclavian artery. The cerebral arterial circle (of Willis) is formed by arteries that take their origin from these structures.

A. Arches 1 and 2 give rise to the maxillary artery, external carotid artery, stapedial artery, and hyoid artery, which do not contribute to the cerebral arterial circle (of Willis).

B. Although arch 3 participates in the formation of the cerebral arterial circle (of Willis), second arch structures do not.

D. Arch 5 is rudimentary (if present) and has no derivatives.

E. Arch 6 gives rise to the aortic arches, pulmonary artery, and ductus arteriosus but does not contribute to the cerebral arterial circle (of Willis) (Fig. 9.3).

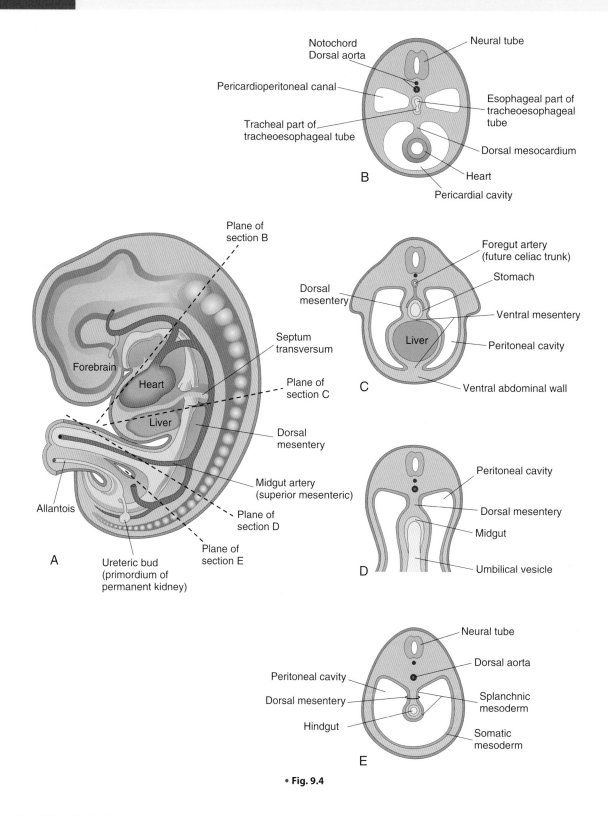

• **Fig. 9.4**

101–102, 214–215

31. C. After initial infection, the herpes zoster virus can remain latent in the dorsal root ganglion until the body becomes immunocompromised or stressed and then reappears as a vesicular rash along one of the dermatomes, in the condition called shingles. The dorsal root ganglion sensory neurons are derivatives of neural crest cells. Other neural crest cell derivatives include the pia mater, chromaffin cells of the suprarenal medulla, thyroid parafollicular cells, Schwann cells, melanocytes, cranial nerves, connective tissue, and some bones of the skull and face. There are usually 21 pairs of denticulations on the paired denticulate ligaments, which take their origin from the pia mater and attach to the dura mater.

A. The dorsal horn is part of the spinal cord and therefore derived from neural tube

B. The ventral horn is part of the spinal cord and therefore derived from neural tube
D. The conus medullaris is part of the spinal cord and therefore derived from neural tube
E. The dura mater is of mesenchymal origin.
254–258

32. B. The structure involved is likely the parietal pleura, a derivative of the somatopleuric mesoderm. The lateral plate mesoderm gives rise to somatopleuric mesoderm and splanchnopleuric mesoderm. The somatopleuric mesoderm is the dorsal layer that is associated with ectoderm, which forms the body wall lining and dermis.

A. The splanchnopleuric mesoderm, the ventral layer of the lateral mesoderm, is associated with endoderm; this forms the viscera and heart.
C. The septum transversum forms the central tendon of the diaphragm.
D. The oropharyngeal membrane forms a septum between the primitive mouth and pharynx.
E. The coelomic cleft is formed during the division of the coelomic cavity and does not relate to the development of the pleura (Fig. 9.4).
40, 53

33. D. The left inferior vena cava results from regression of the right supracardinal vein while the left supracardinal vein persists.

A, E. The right anterior cardinal vein and left cardinal veins contribute to the formation of the internal jugular veins and superior vena cava (with the common cardinal veins).

B, C. The vitelline veins, during development, drain the yolk sac; they contribute to the formation of the hepatic veins, hepatic portal vein, and distal part of the inferior vena cava.
190–193

34. A. Eisenmenger syndrome or tardive cyanosis is the process in which a left-to-right shunt caused by a congenital heart defect causes increased flow through the pulmonary vasculature, causing pulmonary hypertension. This in turn causes increased pressure in the right side of the heart and reversal of the shunt into a right-to-left shunt. Eisenmenger syndrome is a cyanotic heart defect characterized by a long-standing intracardiac shunt caused commonly by ventricular septal defects.

B. In Ebstein anomaly, the septal leaflet of the tricuspid valve is displaced toward the apex of the right ventricle of the heart. There is subsequent atrialization of part of the right ventricle (which is now contiguous with the right atrium). This causes the right atrium to enlarge and the anatomic right ventricle to be small. Here there is an initial right-to-left shunt that results in a cyanotic baby.
C. With the underdeveloped left ventricle, both the aorta and left ventricle are underdeveloped before birth, and the aortic and mitral valves are each too small to allow sufficient blood flow. As blood returns from the lungs to the left atrium, it must pass through an ASD to the right side of the heart. In this defect babies appear cyanotic.

D. In the common atrioventricular canal defect the heart has one common chamber due to defects in the formation of its septae. Patients develop pulmonary hypertension by the second year of life.
E. In a large foramen secundum (foramen ovale), the ASD does lead to pulmonary hypertension but has a much slower progression. Symptoms usually appear after the third decade of life.
204–212

35. B. Aorticopulmonary septum is the correct answer. The cardiac neural crest cells are involved in the development of the muscle and connective tissue walls of large arteries, parts of the cardiac septum, and parts of the thyroid and parathyroid glands and thymus. The aorticopulmonary septum is derived specifically from the cardiac neural crest cells; once formed it separates the aorta and pulmonary trunk and fuses with the interventricular septum within the heart during development.

A. The right subclavian artery takes its origin from the fourth pharyngeal arch.
C. The tricuspid valve is formed from proliferation of tissue around the atrioventricular canal.
D. The inferior vena cava takes its origin from the vitelline veins.
E. The left subclavian artery takes its origin from the left seventh intersegmental artery
204–212

36. A. A hemangioma is a benign endothelial cell tumor. It is characterized by an increased number of normal or abnormal vessels filled with blood. Hemangiomas usually appear in the first weeks of life and grow most rapidly over the first 6 months. A hemangioblast is the common precursor for blood vessels and blood formation induced by vascular endothelial growth factor secreted by surrounding mesoderm.

B. The endoderm forms the epithelial lining of the primitive gut, respiratory tract, tympanic cavity and auditory tube, and the allantois and vitelline duct.
C. The ectoderm gives rise to the central nervous system, the peripheral nervous system, the sensory epithelium of the ear, nose, and eye, the epidermis, hair, and nails, the sebaceous, mammary, and pituitary glands, and the enamel of the teeth.
D. Trophoblast become cells that form the outer layer of a blastocyst and that provide nutrients to the embryo and later develop into a large part of the placenta. They are the first cells to differentiate from the fertilized egg.
E. A syncytiotrophoblast is the epithelial lining of the placental villi, which will penetrate the walls of the uterus to establish maternofetal circulation.
293

37. D. The left horn of the sinus venosus gives rise to the coronary sinus.

A, E. The primitive atria and ventricles will give rise to the atria and ventricles, respectively.

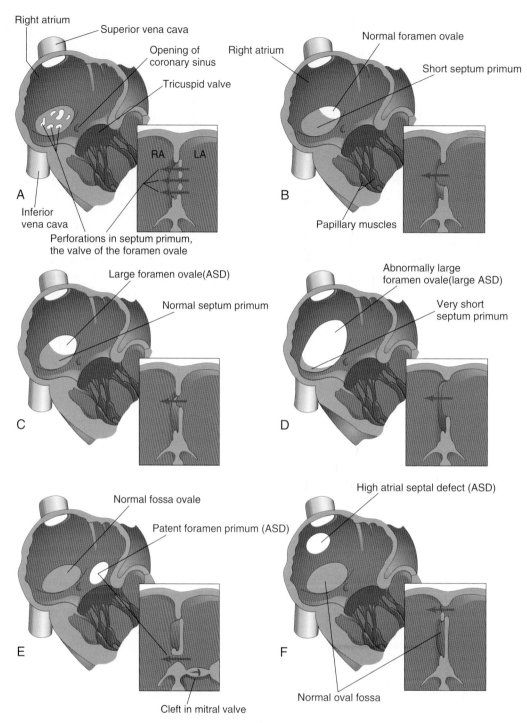

A. Right atrium · Superior vena cava · Opening of coronary sinus · Tricuspid valve · Inferior vena cava · Perforations in septum primum, the valve of the foramen ovale · RA · LA

B. Right atrium · Normal foramen ovale · Short septum primum · Papillary muscles

C. Large foramen ovale(ASD) · Normal septum primum

D. Abnormally large foramen ovale(large ASD) · Very short septum primum

E. Normal fossa ovale · Patent foramen primum (ASD) · Cleft in mitral valve

F. High atrial septal defect (ASD) · Normal oval fossa

• **Fig. 9.5**

B, C. The bulbus cordis and truncus arteriosus gives rise to the smooth parts of the right and left ventricles and their corresponding arteries.

  190–196

38. A. In the fetal heart, the left and right atria communicate with each other by an opening in the septum secundum referred to as the foramen ovale.

  B. The ductus arteriosus is a vessel that connects the left pulmonary artery and the aortic arch in the fetus.

  C. The foramen primum is the perforation in the inferior septum primum, which is closed off as it fuses to the endocardial cushion.

  D. The ductus venosus is the vessel that connects the left umbilical vein to the inferior vena cava.

  E. The truncus arteriosus will give rise to the aorta and pulmonary trunk (Fig. 9.5).

  197–201

39. A. Meromelia is the partial absence of a limb (amelia is total absence).

B, E. Syndactyly refers to fused digits, and polydactyly is an excess in the number of digits. Central digit ray formation is the underlying mechanism for syndactyly

    C. Talipes equinovarus is a malrotation of the foot, more commonly referred to as clubfoot.

    D. Polydactyly refers to supernumerary digits of the hands or feet

    241, 249

40. E. The AER secretes growth factor, which initiates outgrowth of the limb mesenchyme that initiates formation of the limb bud.

    241–243

41. D. Polydactyly describes the presence of supernumerary digits of the hands and feet.

    A. Amelia is complete absence of a limb.

    B. Cleft foot occurs when one or more digital rays fail to develop, causing absence of the central digits.

    C. Clubfoot is a malrotation of the foot around the limb axis

    E. Syndactyly is absence of digits either due to failure of digital rays to form or incomplete apoptosis.

    241, 249

42. E. Typically after the diagnosis of hydatidiform mole, all the invasive trophoblastic tissue is carefully removed. Once invasive trophoblastic tissue remains, hCG levels rise above normal levels, eventually developing into a choriocarcinoma, a malignancy that can spread to the brain. Once this occurs, the patient experiences headaches, blurred vision, and motor dysfunctions. Such tissue produces this hormone. In this case the trophoblastic tissue has developed into a malignant choriocarcinoma and metastasized to the brain, causing her symptoms such as blurred vision.

    A. Placenta previa is a condition in which the placenta, due to its low position, separates from the uterine wall during dilation of the cervix during labor

    B. Placenta accreta is the condition that the placenta rapidly grows into the uterine wall and remains attached during labor causing significant bleeding

    C. Vasa previa is the condition in which the fetal vessels run near the opening of the uterus placing them at risk or rupture during labor

    D. Placenta abruption is early separation of the placenta from the uterus.

    144–147

43. C. The dorsal and ventral pancreatic buds normally fuse to form the adult pancreas. The ventral duct, although smaller, becomes the terminal portion of the main pancreatic duct.

    A, B, D. A bifid ventral bud, when fusing to the dorsal bud, typically leads to the formation of an annular pancreas, which is a band of pancreatic tissue that wraps around the duodenum.

    E. Nonrotation of the midgut would result in displacement of the entire pancreas.

    144–147

44. A. The superior mesenteric artery is closely related to the duodenum and gives rise to the middle colic, right colic, and ileocolic arteries. Therefore any of these vessels may be affected.

    B, E. The splenic and left gastric arteries are branches of the celiac trunk and lie superior to the intestines.

    C. The inferior mesenteric artery branches of the abdominal aorta are located too inferiorly.

    D. The left and right renal arteries branch from the aorta retroperitoneally and are not related to the intestinal tract.

    144–145

45. B. Misplacement of a normally formed appendix is due to malrotation of the midgut.

    A. Rubella infection leads to a myriad of birth defects including cataracts and cardiac problems but not gastrointestinal problems.

    C. Neural crest cells do not directly contribute to the formation of the gastrointestinal tract

    D. Meckel diverticulum is an outpouching of the ileum and may become infected, mimicking the symptoms of appendicitis, but would not be found subhepatically.

    E. Failure of the lateral folds to close will form neural tube defects.

    144–150

46. D. VACTERL syndrome is a cooccurrence of birth defects. It commonly occurs in mothers who are 13–19 years of age who have taken progesterone-estrogen birth control pills during the critical stage of development. The acronym stands for Vertebral, Anal, Cardiac, Tracheal, Esophageal, Renal, and Limb anomalies. Tetralogy of Fallot is a common heart defect seen with VACTERL syndrome.

    A. Pulmonary atresia is a heart disease in which the pulmonary valve leaflets are fused resulting in the blockage of blood circulation to the lungs. Pulmonary atresia commonly presents with cyanosis, dyspnea, easy fatigue and feeding problems in a newborn. It does not present with the mentioned CT findings.

    B. Hepatosplenomegaly may be one of the presenting signs in a patient with Gaucher disease; a lysosomal storage disease that leads to an accumulation of sphingolipids in the liver, spleen, and bone marrow. It does not present with the mentioned CT findings

    C. Cardiomegaly is a presenting sign of a long history of heart disease. It would be uncommon to see cardiomegaly in a young patient with Tetralogy of Fallot.

    E. Meckel diverticulum is an embryological remnant of the vitelline duct that results in a congenital outpouching of the small intestine. It is commonly diagnosed using Meckel scintigraphy and is commonly 2 inches long and 2 feet from the ileocecal valve.

    315

47. C. Pierre Robin sequence (also called Robin sequence) is usually not inherited, but when it is, it is autosomal dominant. It is due to the failure of neural crest cells to migrate to the first pharyngeal arch. This results in a hypoplastic mandible (micrognathia), which results in

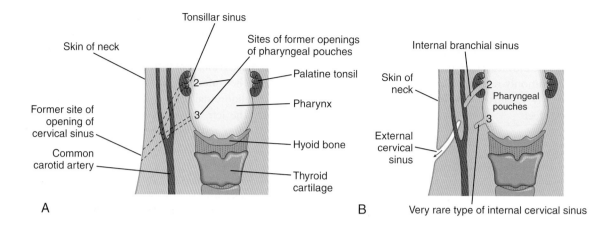

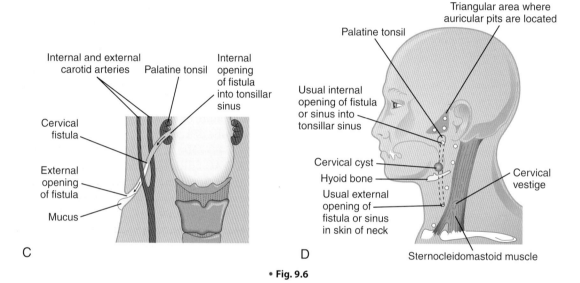

• **Fig. 9.6**

posterior displacement of the tongue and obstruction of the elevation and fusion of the palatine shelves leading to a cleft palate. Respiratory symptoms are common in patients with Pierre Robin sequence particularly when the baby is placed on his/her back (supine).
A. Down syndrome is a result of trisomy 21; patients present with slanted palpebral fissures, cardiac anomalies, and impaired cognitive function.
B. Treacher Collins is a first arch syndrome, but it also includes other craniofacial anomalies such as disfigured external ears and impaired hearing.
D. Patent ductus arteriosus is a cardiac anomaly due to failure of closure of the ductus arteriosus at birth that usually presents with a holosystolic murmur.
E. Bronchopulmonary dysplasia is a respiratory syndrome seen in newborns and characterized by lung inflammation and scarring. Patients will have respiratory distress when lying in any position (Fig. 9.6).
109

48. E. Treacher Collins syndrome (craniofacial dysostosis) is an autosomal disorder characterized by malar hypoplasia, downward-slanting palpebral fissures, defects of the lower eyelids and external ears, and sometimes abnormalities of the middle and internal ear. This is a first arch syndrome

due to failure of neural crest cells to migrate into the first arch during the fourth week of development.
A. Trisomy 13, also called Patau syndrome, is a chromosomal condition associated with severe intellectual disability and physical abnormalities in many parts of the body including microphthalmia, cleft lip and palate, and brain and spinal cord anomalies.
B. Defect in the *FBN1* gene leads to Marfan syndrome.
C. Failure of fusion of the medial nasal prominences leads only to cleft lip and palate
D. Failure of closure of the rostral neuropore leads to meroencephaly or anencephaly.
109

49. A. Tooth development (odontogenesis) usually begins in the sixth to eighth weeks. This development occurs from ectodermal tissue in three stages: bud stage, cap stage, and bell stage. The enamel usually develops in the advanced bell stage when cells of the inner enamel epithelium develop into ameloblasts, which produce and deposit enamel in the form of rods over the dentine.
B, C, D, E. Alveolar bone, cementum, periodontal ligaments, and pulp all develop from mesenchymal tissue, not ectoderm.
296–298

50. C. In the area of the embryo that becomes the eyes, the optic cup (an invagination of the neuroectoderm) is formed. This is connected to the developing brain by the optic stalk. Linear grooves called retinal fissures develop in the optic cups and along the optic stalks. These fissures contain vascular mesenchyme, which develop into the hyaloid artery and vein. The hyaloid vessels supply the optic cup and lens. As the retinal fissures fuse, these vessels are enclosed within the primordial optic nerve. The distal portion usually degenerates, but the proximal portion becomes the central artery and vein of the retina.
277–284

Answers 51–56

51. D. Retinoblastoma is a malignant carcinoma of the retina. The retina develops from the inner and outer layers of the optic cup, which is an invagination of the neuroectoderm. The outer thin layer becomes the inner pigment epithelium of the retina, while the inner layer becomes the light sensitive neural retina. The sphincter pupillae muscle of the iris develops from the neuroectoderm of the optic cup.
- **A.** The optic nerve develops from the optic stalk.
- **B.** The lens develops from surface ectoderm.
- **C.** The sclera develops from the mesoderm.
- **E.** The vitreous body develops from the mesoderm
279–282

52. D. The brain develops from the neural tube. By the 28th day, the caudal and rostral neuropores close, leading to the development of three primary brain vesicles: prosencephalon (forebrain), mesencephalon (midbrain), and rhombencephalon (hindbrain). By the fifth week, the forebrain subdivides into the telencephalon and diencephalon, while the mesencephalon remains undivided; the hindbrain subdivides into the metencephalon and myelencephalon. The metencephalon gives rise to the pons and cerebellum.
- **A.** The telencephalon gives rise to the cerebral hemispheres
- **B.** The diencephalon gives rise to the thalamus, hypothalamus, and epithalamus
- **C.** The mesencephalon becomes midbrain structures
- **E.** The myelencephalon becomes the medulla oblongata
259–268

53. B. The arch of the aorta develops from the truncus arteriosus, which is the cranial part of the primitive heart tube. It also gives rise to the pulmonary trunk.
- **A.** The bulbus cordis develops into the conus arteriosus of the right ventricle.

- **C.** The sinus venosus has two horns: a right horn that develops into the smooth sinus venarum of the right atrium and a left horn that develops into the coronary sinus.
- **D.** The ductus arteriosus connects the fetal pulmonary trunk to the aorta allowing for blood to bypass the pulmonary circulation.
- **E.** The ductus venosus connects the umbilical vein to the inferior vena cava allowing blood to bypass the hepatic circulation in the fetus.
190–196

54. A. The condition described in the vignette is oligohydramnios (reduced amniotic fluid). Some medications, such as ACE inhibitors, may cause polyhydramnios when administered during pregnancy.
- **B.** Aminoglycosides may cause ototoxicity.
- **C.** Tetracyclines may lead to discolored teeth and inhibited bone growth.
- **D.** Lithium is implicated in Ebstein's anomaly.
- **E.** Folate antagonists are responsible for neural tube defects.
130–135

55. A. A double arch of the aorta is a rare cardiac anomaly. There is the formation of a right and left arch of the aorta, which occurs due to a persistence of the distal part of the right dorsal aorta. This creates a vascular ring around the trachea and esophagus with resulting compression of these structures. Babies present with wheezing aggravated by crying, feeding, and flexion of the neck.
- **B.** Pharyngeal arch 5 is rudimentary (if present) and has no derivatives.
- **C, D.** Pharyngeal arches 1 and 2 give rise to the maxillary artery, external carotid artery, stapedial artery, and hyoid artery
- **E.** Pharyngeal arch 6 gives rise to the pulmonary artery and ductus arteriosus
214

56. B. Increase in amniotic fluid volume and pressure is called polyhydramnios. Esophageal atresia prevents the passage of excessive amniotic fluid into the stomach and intestines where it is absorbed. Fluid is eventually passed through the umbilical arteries into the placenta for removal into the maternal bloodstream. This leads to a buildup of amniotic fluid and polyhydramnios.
- **A.** Renal hypoplasia leads to a decrease in the amniotic fluid (oligohydramnios).
- **C.** Ureteric obstruction leads to a decrease in the amniotic fluid (oligohydramnios).
- **D, E.** Potter and Down syndromes have other associated anomalies.
84, 130, 138

Credits

Chapter 1

- **Fig. 1.1** From Bogart, B.I., Ort, V.H., 2007. Elsevier's Integrated Anatomy and Embryology. Elsevier, Philadelphia, p. 260, Fig. 9-18.
- **Fig. 1.4** Courtesy of A.E. Chudley, MD, Children's Hospital and University of Manitoba, Winnipeg, Manitoba, Canada. From Moore, K.L., Persaud, T.V.N., Torchia, M.G., 2013. Before We Are Born, eighth ed. Elsevier, Philadelphia, p. 253, Fig. 16-10.
- **Fig. 1.5** From Manaster, B.J., May, D.A., Disler, D.G., 2013. Musculoskeletal Imaging: The Requisites, fourth ed. Elsevier, Philadelphia, p. 146, Fig. 9-9.

***GAS* Fig. 2.20, *GAS* Fig. 2.21, *GAS* Fig. 2.31, *GAS* Fig. 2.34, *GAS* Fig. 2.46, *GAS* Fig. 2.49** From Drake, R.L., Vogl, A.W., Mitchell, A.W.M., 2015. Gray's Anatomy for Students, third ed. Elsevier, Philadelphia.

Chapter 2

- **Figs. 2.10 to 2.12** From Moore, K.L., Persaud, T.V.N., Torchia, M.G., 2013. Before We Are Born, eighth ed. Elsevier, Philadelphia, p. 199, Fig. 14-10.

***GAS* Fig. 3.9, *GAS* Fig. 3.16, *GAS* Fig. 3.34, *GAS* Fig. 3.46, *GAS* Fig. 3.71, *GAS* Fig. 3.75, GAS Fig. 3.77, *GAS* Fig. 3.88, *GAS* Fig. 3.102, *GAS* Fig. 3.108** From Drake, R.L., Vogl, A.W.., Mitchell, A.W.M., 2015. Gray's Anatomy for Students, third ed. Elsevier, Philadelphia.

Chapter 3

- **Fig. 3.9** From Jazayeri, S.B., Shahlaee, A., 2013. A 2.5-month-old infant with refractory vomiting and failure to thrive. Gastroenterology 144, e3–e4.

***GAS* Fig. 4.22, *GAS* Fig. 4.27, *GAS* Fig. 4.29, *GAS* Fig. 4.38, *GAS* Fig. 4.41, *GAS* Figs. 4.47 to 4.50, *GAS* Fig. 4.57, *GAS* Fig. 4.63, *GAS* Fig. 4.64, *GAS* Fig. 4.66, *GAS* Fig. 4.79, *GAS* Fig. 4.80, *GAS* Fig. 4.83, *GAS* Fig. 4.86, *GAS* Fig. 4.93, *GAS* Fig. 4.97, *GAS* Fig. 4.100, *GAS* Fig. 4.102, *GAS* Fig. 4.104, *GAS* Fig. 4.106, *GAS* Fig. 4.107, *GAS* Fig. 4.121, *GAS* Fig. 4.122, *GAS* Fig. 4.126, *GAS* Fig. 4.127, *GAS* Fig. 4.132, *GAS* Fig. 4.139, *GAS* Fig. 4.140, *GAS* Fig. 4.155, *GAS* Fig. 4.157** From Drake, R.L., Vogl, A.W., Mitchell, A.W.M., 2015. Gray's Anatomy for Students, third ed. Elsevier, Philadelphia.

Chapter 4

***GAS* Fig. 5.7, *GAS* Fig. 5.12, *GAS* Figs. 5.15 to 5.17, *GAS* Fig. 5.34, *GAS* Fig. 5.46, *GAS* Fig. 5.54, *GAS* Fig. 5.57, *GAS* Fig. 5.58, *GAS* Fig. 5.65, *GAS* Fig. 5.69, *GAS* Fig. 5.75, *GAS* Fig. 5.78** From Drake, R.L., Vogl, A.W., Mitchell, A.W.M., 2015. Gray's Anatomy for Students, third ed. Elsevier, Philadelphia.

Chapter 5

- **Fig. 5.3** From Weir, J., Abrahams, P., 2003. Imaging Atlas of Human Anatomy, third ed. Elsevier, Philadelphia.

***GAS* Fig. 6.16, *GAS* Fig. 6.30, *GAS* Fig. 6.38, *GAS* Fig. 6.41, *GAS* Fig. 6.50, *GAS* Fig. 6.98, *GAS* Fig. 6.99, *GAS* Fig. 6.105, *GAS* Fig. 6.110, *GAS* Fig. 6.119** From Drake, R.L., Vogl, A.W., Mitchell, A.W.M., 2015. Gray's Anatomy for Students, third ed. Elsevier, Philadelphia.

Chapter 6

- **Fig. 6.10** From Neligan, P.C., Chang, J., 2013. Plastic Surgery, third ed., vol 6. In: Upper Extremity, Elsevier, Philadelphia, p. 761, Fig. 34.23.
- **Fig. 6.14** From Preston, D.C., Shapiro, B.E., 1998. Median neuropathy. In: Electromyography and Neuromuscular Disorders: Clinical- Electrophysiologic Correlations. Butterworth-Heinemann, Boston.

***GAS* Fig. 7.22, *GAS* Fig. 7.24, *GAS* Fig. 7.39, *GAS* Fig. 7.50, *GAS* Fig. 7.52, *GAS* Fig. 7.57, *GAS* Fig. 7.69, *GAS* Fig. 7.72, *GAS* Fig. 7.73, *GAS* Fig. 7.83, *GAS* Fig. 7.86, *GAS* Fig. 7.87, *GAS* Fig. 7.90, *GAS* Fig. 7.103, *GAS* Fig. 7.109** From Drake, R.L., Vogl, A.W., Mitchell, A.W.M., 2015. Gray's Anatomy for Students, third ed. Elsevier, Philadelphia.

Chapter 7

- **Fig. 7.23** From Netter, F., 2014. Atlas of Human Anatomy, sixth ed. Elsevier, Philadelphia. All rights reserved. www.netter images.com.

***GAS* Fig. 8.33, *GAS* Fig. 8.35, *GAS* Fig. 8.38, *GAS* Figs. 8.44 to 8.46, *GAS* Fig. 8.65, *GAS* Fig. 8.66, *GAS* Fig. 8.72, *GAS* Fig. 8.84, *GAS* Fig. 8.103, *GAS* Fig. 8.116, *GAS* Fig. 8.120, *GAS* Fig. 8.121, *GAS* Fig. 8.146, *GAS* Fig. 8.153, *GAS* Fig. 8.159, *GAS* Fig. 8.169, *GAS* Fig. 8.176, *GAS* Fig. 8.190, *GAS* Fig. 8.192, *GAS* Fig. 8.193, *GAS* Fig. 8.217, *GAS* Fig. 8.235, *GAS* Fig. 8.239, *GAS* Fig. 8.257** From Drake, R.L., Vogl, A.W., Mitchell, A.W.M., 2015. Gray's Anatomy for Students, third ed. Elsevier, Philadelphia.

Chapter 8

***GAS* Figs. e9.15, e9.42, e9.43, e9.52, e9.53, e9.99** From Drake, R.L., Vogl, A.W., Mitchell, A.W.M., 2020. Gray's Anatomy for Students, fourth ed. Elsevier, Philadelphia.

Chapter 9

- **Figs. 9.1 to 9.7** From Moore, K.L., Persaud, T.V.N., Torchia, M.G., 2013. Before We Are Born, eighth ed. Elsevier, Philadelphia, p. 32.

***GAS* Fig. 5.58** From Drake, R.L., Vogl, A.W., Mitchell, A.W.M., 2015. Gray's Anatomy for Students, third ed. Elsevier, Philadelphia.

Index

Page numbers followed by *f* and *t* indicate figures and tables respectively.